ANOPHELES MOSQUITOES - NEW INSIGHTS INTO MALARIA VECTORS

Edited by **Sylvie Manguin**

In memory of my mother who showed me the way.

Anopheles mosquitoes - New insights into malaria vectors

http://dx.doi.org/10.5772/3392
Edited by Sylvie Manguin

Contributors

Indra Vythilingam, Jeffery Hii, Vas Dev, Vinod P. Sharma, Jan Conn, Martha Quinones, Marinete Povoa, Wej Choochote, Atiporn Saeung, Donald R. Roberts, Richard Tren, Kimberly Hess, Papa Makhtar Drame, Anne Poinsignon, Alexandra Marie, Souleymane Doucoure, Herbert Noukpo, Sylvie Cornélie, Franck Remoué, Ralph E. Harbach, Claire Garros, Jean- Pierre Dujardin, Claudio R. Lazzari, Chloé Lahondère, Pierre Carnevale, Richard Allan, Claire Duchet, Wannapa Suwonkerd, Michael J. Bangs, Wanapa Ritthison, Christophe Boëte, Uli Beisel, Gregory C. Lanzaro, Yoosook Lee, Nigel Beebe, Tanya L. Russell, Thomas R. Burkot, Neil F. Lobo, Robert D. Cooper, Eliska Rejmankova, Nicole Achee, John Grieco, Vincent Corbel, Raphael N'Guessan, Valérie Obsomer, Steve J Connor, Nicolas Titeux, Pietro Ceccato, Christelle Vancutsem, Gregory Duveiller, Marc Coosemans, Jean-Francois Pekel, Lies Durnez, Marianne Sinka, Sylvie Manguin, Chung Thuy Ngo, Krajana Tainchum, Waraporn Juntarajumnong, Theeraphap Chareonviriyaphap, Estelle Jumas-Bilak, Anne-Laure Michon, Christophe Antonio Nkondjio, Frédéric Simard, George K Christophides, Mathilde Gendrin, Catherine Walton, Katy Morgan, Pradya Somboon, Diego Ayala, Ibrahima Dia, Moussa Wamdaogo Guelbeogo

Published by InTech

Janeza Trdine 9, 51000 Rijeka, Croatia

Publishing Process Manager Dragana Manestar
Typesetting InTech DTP Team
Cover InTech Design Team

Additional hard copies can be obtained from orders@intechopen.com

Anopheles mosquitoes - New insights into malaria vectors, Edited by Sylvie Manguin
p. cm.
ISBN 978-953-51-1188-7

For EU product safety concerns:
IN TECH d.o.o., Prolaz Marije Krucifikse Kozulić 3, 51000 Rijeka, Croatia,
info@intechopen.com or visit our website at intechopen.com.

Meet the editor

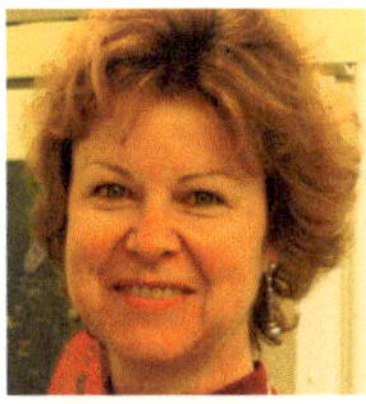

Sylvie Manguin is a full-time Research Professor at the Institute of Research for Development (IRD), based at University of Montpellier. She is a leading medical entomologist and academician researcher whose main interest concerns mosquitoes involved in the transmission of pathogenic agents, especially Anopheles vectors of malaria agents. She has developed studies on these mosquitoes from three continents (Asia, Africa, Americas) including species identification, population genetics, phylogenetic, vectorial capacities, spatial surveillance, midgut microbiota, immunological markers and vector control. She is the author of 75 indexed publications, four book chapters, and three books including "Biodiversity of malaria in the World" (John Libbey Ed.) that won the award of the International Festival of Medical Education Book (EDIMED). She is a member of the Editorial Boards of the Malaria Journal and Acta Tropica and serves as reviewer in several international institutions and more than 20 scientific journals.

Contents

Preface

First of all I would like to thank Sylvie Manguin, Editor of this book, who compiled 24 chapters that present current knowledge on malaria vector taxa. By asking me to preface this book, Sylvie got me out of my "bubble of Auvergne Region" and reconnected me with a scientific community that I had indeed never abandoned. It is with great pleasure that I found in this book the contributions of my former students and friends.

At the end of the second millennium, I had more or less put my pen down while the threat of global warming posed a major concern for the development and extension of vector-borne diseases. Particularly pessimistic forecasts predicted an extension of malaria up to the Polar Circle. However, no geographic expansion of malaria has been noticed in the last 20 years [1]. At most, the disease has reappeared on the Korean Peninsula where it was eradicated in the 1950s [2, 3]. Also, no particular invasion of *Anopheles* species has been observed as opposed to the global invasion of *Aedes albopictus* [4].

After the failure of the World Programme of Malaria Eradication (1950), WHO (World Health Organization) proposed at the Conference of Amsterdam (1992) a new strategy based on the treatment of all clinical cases using all chemo-therapeutic compounds, in particular the artemisinin-based combination therapy (ACT). Vector control was a principal component of prevention. The use of insecticide-treated nets (ITN) has been shown to be effective in all epidemiological situations, and the pyrethroids used to impregnate the nets (permethrin, deltamethrin, lambdacyhalothrin, etc), besides protecting sleepers, has a beneficial impact on all members of communities where these nets are used [5, 6].

In last 20 years, manufacturers produced long-lasting insecticidal nets (LLIN) using fabrics that retain insecticide activity from three to five years (even after more than 15 washes). These LLINs are well accepted by users, and more than 24 million nets have been distributed in the Afrotropical Region alone. In 1992, it was expected that implementation of this new strategy would initially reduce malaria mortality by 50% [6]. However, accurate data on malaria deaths is very difficult to obtain; this mainly rural disease often eludes official statistics and the results of different studies vary widely depending on the sources. The most recent estimates provided by Murray et al. in 2012 [7] give a more nuanced trend with the malaria mortality burden being larger than previously estimated, especially in adults. This study estimated that in 2010 malaria was the cause of 1.24 million deaths compared to 655,000 deaths reported by WHO, and in the Afrotropical Region infant mortality (children < 5 years old) due to malaria was estimated to be 24% *versus* 16% based on the WHO malaria report estimates [8]. These figures, although imprecise, provide a current estimate of the impact of malaria worldwide, which falls far short of the expected results despite the enormous financial expenditures of the WHO, charitable organizations, foundations and national initiatives.

Currently, the spectrum of resistance to many, if not the majority, of insecticides continues to pose a serious threat to all control programs, and alternate methods of control are of very limited efficacy [9]. Larval control by insecticides or insect growth regulators (IGR) is limited to specific habitats, such as the oases of Oman. Hopes are now based on genetic control by transgenic mosquitoes. Research underway for more than 20 years has not produced a means of controlling malaria on a continental scale such as Africa where it endures without a solution for sustained control. We are still left with expectation.

Finally, one cannot ignore the considerable work on the systematics of *Anopheles* mosquitoes. In addition to the creation of the subgenus *Baimaia* by Harbach, Rattanarithikul & Harrison, many new species have been described or are waiting to be described [10, 11], especially in Asia where the majority of the vectors belong to species complexes [4]. Southeast Asia with the *Anopheles dirus* complex and New Guinea with the *Anopheles farauti* complex, both comprised of eight species, represent 'hot spots' of *Anopheles* biodiversity. Species complexes include vectors and non-vectors and the identification of the vector species poses a real problem that can be solved by the new techniques apparent in the book.

This book, describing new insights and innovative approaches to the study of malaria vectors, contributes to a passionate aim of society – the eradication of malaria as a cause of morbidity and mortality in the poorest populations of the world.

Prof. Jean Mouchet
Emeritus Research Professor at IRD
Langeac, France

References

[1] Reiter P. Global warming and malaria: knowing the horse before hitching the cart. Malaria Journal 2008;7 Suppl 1:S3.

[2] Manguin S, Carnevale P, Mouchet J, Coosemans M, Julvez J, Richard-Lenoble D, et al. Biodiversity of malaria in the world. Paris, France: John Libbey Eurotext; 2008.

[3] Mouchet J, Carnevale P, Coosemans M, Julvez J, Manguin S, Richard-Lenoble D, et al. Biodiversité du paludisme dans le monde. Paris, France: John Libbey Eurotext; 2004.

[4] Manguin S, Boëte C. Global impact of mosquito biodiversity, human vector-borne diseases and environmental change: InTech; 2011.

[5] Carnevale P, Robert V, Boudin C, Halna JM, Pazart L, Gazin P, et al. La lutte contre le paludisme par des moustiquaires imprégnées au Burkina Faso. Bull Soc Pathol Exot Filiales 1988;81:832-846.

[6] Lengeler C, Cattani JA, De Savigny D. Net Gain. A new method for the preventing malaria deaths. Geneva: WHO; 1996.

[7] Murray CJ, Rosenfeld LC, Lim SS, Andrews KG, Foreman KJ, Haring D, et al. Global malaria mortality between 1980 and 2010: a systematic analysis. Lancet 2012;379:413-431.

[8] WHO. World malaria report. In: WHO, editor. WHO global malaria program. Geneva: WHO; 2011. p. 278.

[9] malERA Consultative Group. A research agenda for malaria eradication: vector control. PLoS Med 2011;8:e1000401.

[10] Harbach RE. The classification of genus *Anopheles* (Diptera: Culicidae): a working hypothesis of phylogenetic relationships. Bull Entomol Res 2004;94:537-553.

[11] Harbach RE, Rattanarithikul R, Harrison BA. *Baimaia,* a new subgenus for *Anopheles kyondawensis* Abraham, a unique crabhole-breeding anopheline in Southeast Asia. The Proceedings of the Entomological Society of Washington 2005;107.

Preface from the Editor

In a global public health context, the genus *Anopheles* is by far the most important group of pathogen-carrying mosquitoes due to their exclusive involvement in the transmission of human malaria parasites. To properly control malaria, an entirely preventable and treatable disease, the current recommended interventions advocated by WHO [1] include vector control through the use of insecticide-treated nets (ITNs), periodic indoor residual spraying (IRS) and, in some specific settings, larval control. During the past decade, coverage with vector control interventions have increased substantially in sub-Saharan Africa; for example, reaching 53% of households with at least one ITN in 2012. However, WHO has also observed that *"due to fewer deliveries of ITNs and increasing mosquito resistance to insecticides, recent successes in malaria vector control may be jeopardized."* [1]. As vector control is a very effective means of malaria control, a better understanding of *Anopheles* populations is a key element for reaching the goal of malaria elimination in the future [2].

A large amount of scientific knowledge and technical advances concerning these mosquitoes has accumulated over the past century, and in recent decades the advent of novel technologies have accelerated the acquisition of new information. In fact, the current trend of research and new findings as a consequence of the renewed emphasis for controlling malaria using vector control is rapidly expanding our understanding of *Anopheles* mosquitoes. The 24 chapters of this book present some of the latest research on important malaria vectors using innovative approaches supported by state-of-the-art methodologies covering a wide array of study disciplines on the biology, genetics, distribution, pathogen transmission, and the application of these findings in the improvement of current vector control strategies.

This book is divided into five sections. Section 1: Focuses on the reliable identification and classification of certain species, an area that has been fraught with past difficulties for accurately differentiating the individual sibling species placed within taxonomic complexes. The precise identification of a species must be linked to their specific role and importance in the transmission of malaria agents that can dramatically differ from their morphologically indistinguishable sibling species. Section 2: Provides up-to-date information on the genetic diversity, bionomics and distribution of the dominant vector species of Latin America, Africa, Asia, and Southwest Pacific as presented in nine chapters. Section 3: Presents a better understanding of environmental aspects linked to larval habitat ecology and spatial surveillance of *Anopheles* vectors having found increasing utility in the last decade. Section 4: Pathogen transmission is presented with a focus on *Plasmodium knowlesi,* an emerging public health problem in Southeast Asia, along with transmission influencing factors such as thermoregulation during blood feeding and the role of mosquito midgut microbiota as possible means to control disease by transmission blocking approach. Section 5: Reviews the current status on insecticide resistance, innovative approaches to vector control, and new tools to evaluate control efficacy based on *Anopheles* saliva biomarkers and perspectives for using transgenic mosquitoes.

A total of 71 authors, from 20 countries on five continents (Africa, Asia, Australia, America, and Europe), with internationally recognized expertise, have generously participated in this book and I am extremely grateful to all for their time and energy to contribute to new and innovative topics on *Anopheles*. The originality of this book, published as 'open access' by InTech, is to offer a detailed description and analysis of new concepts, paradigms and innovative approaches on the understanding of *Anopheles* mosquitoes and the development of better weapons to control the vector.

I am also profoundly grateful to Professor Jean Mouchet, my mentor and the one of generations of medical entomologists, who kindly accepted to write a preface for this book. I also thank Ms. Dragana Manestar for her valuable support and assistance in publishing this book. This publication should benefit not only medical entomologists, but also students, scientists, public health managers, and decision makers interested in malaria and its vectors.

Sylvie Manguin, PhD
Institute of Research for Development (IRD)
Montpellier, France

References

[1] WHO. WHO malaria report. In: WHO, editor. WHO global malaria program. Geneva: WHO; 2012. p. 260.

[2] malERA Consultative Group. A research agenda for malaria eradication: vector control. PLoS Med 2011;8:e1000401.

Section 1

Species Identification and Phylogeny of *Anopheles*

Chapter 1

The Phylogeny and Classification of *Anopheles*

Ralph E. Harbach

Additional information is available at the end of the chapter

http://dx.doi.org/10.5772/54695

1. Introduction

Anopheles was introduced as a genus of mosquitoes in 1818 by Johann Wilhelm Meigen [1], a German entomologist famous for his revolutionary studies of Diptera. Little was done on the taxonomy of *Anopheles* until the discovery during the last two decades of the 19th century that mosquitoes transmit microfilariae and malarial protozoa, which initiated a drive to collect, name and classify these insects. In 1898, the Royal Society and the Rt. Hon. Joseph Chamberlain, Secretary of State for the Colonies of Britain, appointed a Committee to supervise the investigation of malaria. On 6 December 1898, Mr. Chamberlain directed the Colonies to collect and send mosquitoes to the British Museum (Natural History) (Figure 1), and in 1899 the Committee appointed Frederick V. Theobald to prepare a monograph on the mosquitoes of the world, which was published in five volumes between 1901 and 1910 [2–6]. As a consequence, many new generic names were introduced in an effort to classify numerous new mosquito species into seemingly natural groups. Theobald proposed 18 genera for species of *Anopheles* based on the distribution and shape of scales on the thorax and abdomen. Four of these proposed genera, *Cellia, Kerteszia, Nyssorhynchus* and *Stethomyia*, are currently recognized as subgenera of *Anopheles* and the other 14 are regarded as synonyms of one or other of subgenera *Anopheles, Cellia* or *Nyssorhynchus*. Theobald, however, was not the only person to propose generic names for species of *Anopheles*. During the first three decades of the 20th century, 37 genera (including the 18 recognized by Theobald) were established for species of *Anopheles* [7].

As additional new species were discovered, it became increasingly apparent that Theobald's system of classification was neither practical nor natural. Frederick Knab in North America, one of the early critics of Theobald's classification, stated that "the subject was made needlessly difficult by hasty work and by the sub-division of the old genus *Anopheles* into numerous ill-defined and fancifully differentiated genera. The intricacies of this 'system,' unwarranted from both a scientific and practical standpoint, even the trained entomologist could not tread with safety, and to others it could be no less than hopeless or disastrous" [8]. Consequently, during the two decades following the completion of Theobald's monograph in 1910, significant changes were made toward a much more conservative system of classification, culminating in the reduction of 38 genus-group names (including *Anopheles*) to the recognition of the single genus *Anopheles*.

The current subgeneric classification of *Anopheles* is based primarily on the number and positions of specialized setae on the gonocoxites of the male genitalia (Figure 2), and this basis of classification has been accepted since it was introduced by Sir (Samuel) Rickard Christophers in 1915 [9]. Christophers proposed three generic subdivisions, which F.M. Edwards [10] and Francis Metcalf Root [11] formally recognized as subgenera *Anopheles*, *Myzomyia* (=*Cellia*) and *Nyssorhynchus*. Edwards adopted this system and added subgenus *Stethomyia* in his classical treatise on family Culicidae published in 1932 [12]. This system recognized *Kerteszia* as an informal group within subgenus *Nyssorhynchus*. *Kerteszia* was elevated to subgeneric status by W.H.W. Komp [13]. Subgenus *Lophopodomyia* was proposed by P.C.A. Antunes in 1937 [14] and subgenus *Baimaia* was introduced by Ralph E. Harbach and his colleagues in 2005 [15].

Genus *Anopheles* currently includes 465 formally named species that are disproportionately divided between seven subgenera: *Anopheles* (cosmopolitan, 182 species), *Baimaia* (Oriental, one species), *Cellia* (Old World, 220 species), *Kerteszia* (Neotropical, 12 species), *Lophopodomyia* (Neotropical, six species), *Nyssorhynchus* (Neotropical, 39 species) and *Stethomyia* (Neotropical, five species) [16]. Four of the subgenera, *Anopheles*, *Cellia*, *Kerteszia* and *Nyssorhynchus*, include the species that transmit human malarial parasites. Most vector species of *Anopheles* have been found to comprise complexes of sibling species.

2. Classification of genus *Anopheles*

The aim of classification is to group and categorize biological entities that share some unifying characteristics. Classification has been defined by Ernst Mayr & W.J. Bock [17] as "The arrangement of similar entities (objects) in a hierarchical series of nested classes, in which each more inclusive higher-level class is subdivided comprehensively into less inclusive classes at the next lower level." These classes (groups) are known as **taxa** (singular: **taxon**). The level of a taxon in a hierarchical classification is referred to as a **taxonomic rank** or **category**. Ideally, taxonomic categories should denote equivalent phylogenetic rank; however, in practice they are basically subjective groupings of subordinate taxa that are presumed to represent monophyletic groups of species that are assigned to taxonomic ranks based on shared morphological and biological characteristics that are not a measure of phylogenetic equivalence. For this reason, the taxonomic categories of genus *Anopheles*, including the formal rank of subgenus, should not be considered to represent equivalent phylogenetic ranks.

http://dx.doi.org/10.5772/54695

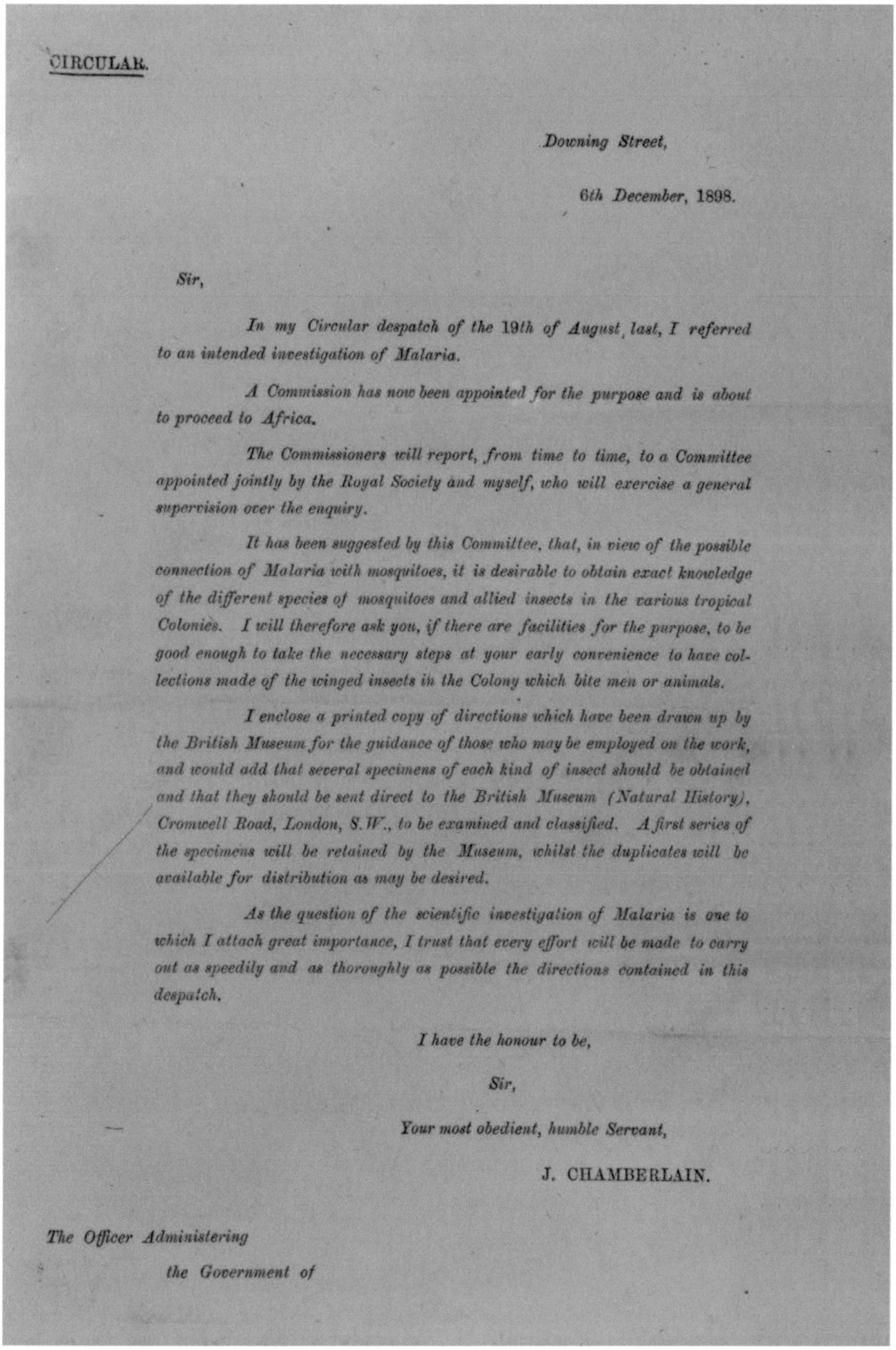

CIRCULAR.

Downing Street,

6th December, 1898.

Sir,

In my Circular despatch of the 19*th of August last, I referred to an intended investigation of Malaria.*

A Commission has now been appointed for the purpose and is about to proceed to Africa.

The Commissioners will report, from time to time, to a Committee appointed jointly by the Royal Society and myself, who will exercise a general supervision over the enquiry.

It has been suggested by this Committee, that, in view of the possible connection of Malaria with mosquitoes, it is desirable to obtain exact knowledge of the different species of mosquitoes and allied insects in the various tropical Colonies. I will therefore ask you, if there are facilities for the purpose, to be good enough to take the necessary steps at your early convenience to have collections made of the winged insects in the Colony which bite men or animals.

I enclose a printed copy of directions which have been drawn up by the British Museum for the guidance of those who may be employed on the work, and would add that several specimens of each kind of insect should be obtained and that they should be sent direct to the British Museum (Natural History), Cromwell Road, London, S.W., to be examined and classified. A first series of the specimens will be retained by the Museum, whilst the duplicates will be available for distribution as may be desired.

As the question of the scientific investigation of Malaria is one to which I attach great importance, I trust that every effort will be made to carry out as speedily and as thoroughly as possible the directions contained in this despatch.

I have the honour to be,

Sir,

Your most obedient, humble Servant,

J. CHAMBERLAIN.

The Officer Administering
the Government of

Figure 1. Letter issued from Downing Street on 6 December 1898 directing the British Colonies to collect and send mosquitoes to the British Museum (Natural History).

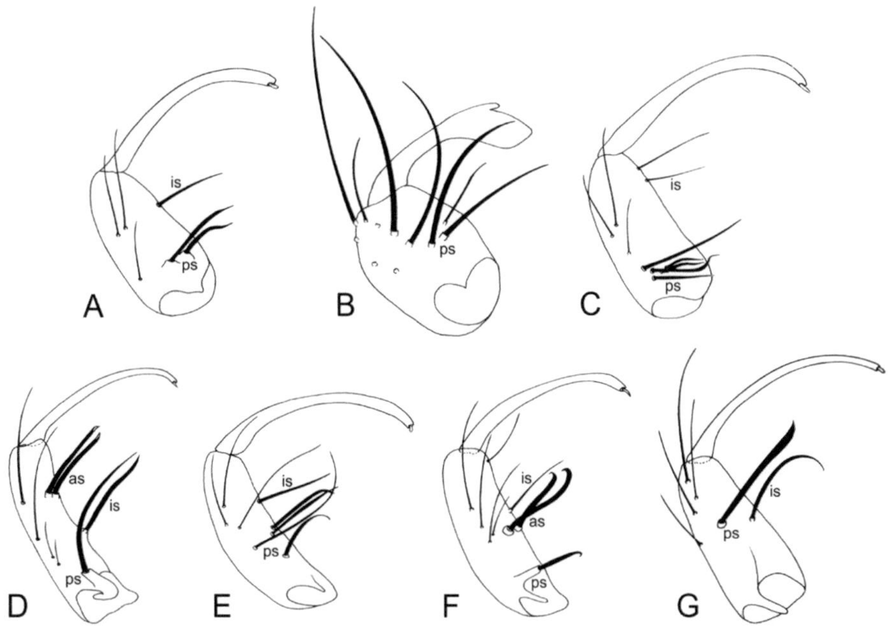

Figure 2. Subgenera of *Anopheles* – specialized setae on the gonocoxites of the male genitalia (after Harbach & Kitching [18]): A, *Anopheles*; B. *Baimaia*; C, *Cellia*; D, *Kerteszia*; E, *Lophopodomyia*; F, *Nyssorhynchus*; G, *Stethomyia*. as, accessory setae; is, inner seta; ps, parabasal seta(e).

Infrasubgeneric categories (taxonomic ranks below subgenus) have no formal status under the *International Code of Zoological Nomenclature* [19]. They are convenience categories only, often based on superficial similarities that may not indicate natural relationships. The informal categories used in the classification of *Anopheles* include Sections, Series, Groups, Subgroups and Complexes (see Appendix 1).

Unlike formal taxonomic categories, which precede the name of the taxonomic unit, for instance family Culicidae, genus *Anopheles* and species *gambiae*, the names of informal taxonomic categories follow the name of the taxonomic unit, for example the Pyretophorus Series, Hyrcanus Group or Gambiae Complex, which are written in Roman (i.e. non-italic) script with the first letter capitalized. It should be stressed that both formal and informal taxonomic entities are conceptual constructs invented by taxonomists for the purpose of creating some order in the diversity of species. For example, the species *gambiae* and the Hyrcanus Group, which are human-conceived taxonomic concepts, cannot be observed as entities or visualized under a microscope.

The internal classification of genus *Anopheles* (between genus and species levels) is based primarily on the schemes proposed by Edwards [12], John A. Reid & Kenneth L. Knight [20], Alexis Grjebine [21], M.T. Gillies & Botha de Meillon [22], Reid [23], Michael E. Faran [24] and Kenneth J. Linthicum [25]. These schemes were reviewed, amalgamated and updated in 1994 [26] and updated again in 2004 and 2012 [27,16 respectively]. The three largest subgenera, i.e. *Anopheles*, *Cellia* and *Nyssorhynchus*, are divided into hierarchical systems of informal taxonomic categories (Appendix 1; examples shown in Figure 3). Subgenus *Anopheles* is divided into two Sections based on the shape of the pupal trumpet. The Laticorn Section was created for species with a wide funnel-shaped trumpet having the longest axis transverse to the stem, and the Angusticorn Section for species with a semi-tubular trumpet having the longest axis vertical more or less in line with the stem [20]. Subgenus *Nyssorhynchus* is divided into three Sections based on unique combinations of larval, pupal and adult characters [28]. Subgenus *Cellia* and the Sections of subgenera *Anopheles* and *Nyssorhynchus* are divided into Series, the larger Series are divided into species Groups, and some Groups are further divided into Subgroups and species Complexes. Most of the groupings at each level of classification are presumed to represent natural groups of species, thus implying phylogenetic relationships, but much additional basic taxonomic research is needed before the formal and informal taxa can be firmly established as monophyletic entities. The internal classification of the genus (subgenera and infrasubgeneric groups) is detailed in Appendix 1. An alphabetical list of all formally named, currently recognized species and their position in the classification is provided in Appendix 2. Similarly, all currently known sibling species complexes are listed in Appendix 3, and the unnamed and provisionally designated species of the complexes and their position in the classification are listed in Appendix 4.

3. Phylogeny of *Anopheles*

Anopheles is undoubtedly the most studied and best known genus of mosquitoes, largely because of their great impact on human health. As vectors of causative agents of malaria and filariasis, *Anopheles* mosquitoes have affected the lives of more humans than any other insects. As a matter of fact, *Anopheles* is one of few groups of eukaryote organisms that have had an impact on human evolution – the emergence of sickle cell anemia as a mode of resistance to malarial protozoa. As a result of more than a century of studies by medical entomologists, taxonomists and geneticists, 537 species of *Anopheles* are currently known and most have been formally named (87%) (Appendix 2), but until recently little work has been done to understand the evolution and phylogenetic relationships of these mosquitoes.

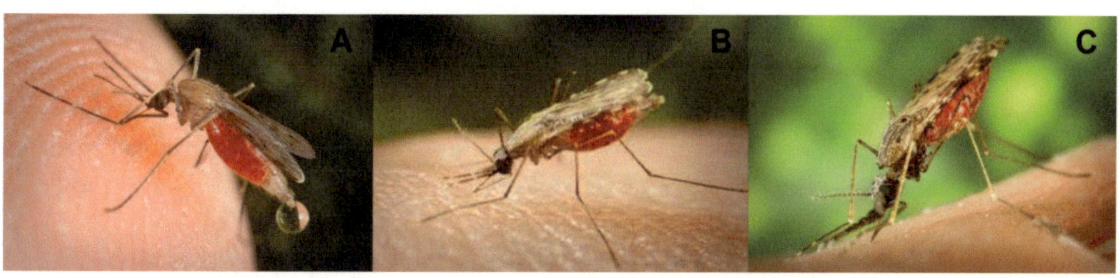

Figure 3. Hierarchical classification (from specific to general) of A. *Anopheles freeborni*, Freeborni Subgroup, Maculipennis Group, Anopheles Series, Angusticorn Section, Subgenus *Anopheles*; B. *Anopheles minimus*, Minimus Complex, Minimus Subgroup, Funestus Group, Myzomyia Series, Subgenus *Cellia*; C. *Anopheles albimanus*, Albimanus Series, Albimanus Section, Subgenus *Nyssorhynchus*.

The phylogenetic studies of anopheline mosquitoes conducted to date are summarized in Appendix 5. In view of the impact of malaria on human health, it is not surprising that most of these studies have dealt with species Groups, Subgroups and Complexes that include vectors of human malarial protozoa. It is obvious that the evolutionary relationships of malaria vectors and their closest allies have received more attention than other groups. However, none of these studies can be regarded as complete in terms of taxonomic coverage of any group, and the field of disease vector systematics presents many opportunities for further research. Phylogenetic patterns are used to interpret bionomic features such as differences in the nature of blood-feeding by adult females, feeding behavior and the occurrence of immature stages in aquatic habitats.

Mosquitoes probably evolved in the Jurassic [12,29,30] (146–200 Mya)[1], along with the early mammals, first birds and first flowering plants. Unfortunately, due to the paucity of mosquito fossils, there is no direct indication of the evolutionary history of anopheline mosquitoes. The second oldest fossil mosquito, *Paleoculicis minutus* [31] from the Late Cretaceous (66.0–100.5 Mya), has morphological features that indicate a closer affinity with culicine than anopheline mosquitoes, which suggests that this ancestral lineage is younger than the lineage that gave rise to subfamily Anophelinae. *Anopheles* (*Nyssorhynchus*?) *dominicanus* [32] and *An.* (?) *rottensis* [33] are the only fossil anopheline mosquitoes. The former is from the mid-Tertiary (about 15–45 Mya) and the latter is from the Late Oligocene of Germany (approximately 25 Mya). If the anopheline mosquitoes are indeed ancestral to all other Culicidae [18,34], it would appear from available fossil evidence that extant groups may have evolved in the Cenozoic Era (<66.0 Mya). From divergence times based on sequence data for nuclear protein-coding genes and fossil calibration points, it appears that major mosquito lineages date to the Early Cretaceous (100.5–145.0 Mya), and the ancestral lineage of anophelines may have appeared as early as the Jurassic (~145 Mya) [34].

Anopheles is the nominotypical genus of subfamily Anophelinae. In addition to *Anopheles* (cosmopolitan), the subfamily includes two other genera: *Bironella* (Australasian) and *Chagasia* (Neotropical). Cladistic analyses of morphological data and DNA sequences of various ribosomal, mitochondrial and nuclear genes strongly support the placement of *Chagasia* in an ancestral relationship to all other anophelines [18,34–41].

In 2000, Sallum et al. [40] performed the first phylogenetic analysis of subfamily Anophelinae, based on morphological characters. The results indicated that genus *Anopheles* is paraphyletic because it included genus *Bironella*. Subgenera *Kerteszia*, *Nyssorhynchus*, *Cellia*, *Lophopodomyia* and *Stethomyia*, along with genus *Bironella*, were found to be monophyletic taxa dispersed among various Series and species Groups of subgenus *Anopheles*. The Christya Series of subgenus *Anopheles* was placed with *Kerteszia* + *Nyssorhynchus* and this clade was sister to *Cellia* + all other anophelines except *Chagasia*.

Two years later, Sallum et al. [41] conducted a molecular analysis of anopheline relationships based on ribosomal (18S, 28S) and mitochondrial (COI, COII) DNA sequences. The results of

1 Geological ages of eras and periods follow the geological timescale determined by the International Commission on Stratigraphy (http://www.stratigraphy.org).

that study cannot be compared directly with the results of their earlier study [40] because significantly fewer taxa were included in the analyses. Nevertheless, the molecular data corroborated the paraphyly of genus *Anopheles* relative to *Bironella* and the sister-group relationship of *Kerteszia* and *Nyssorhynchus,* and supported the monophyly of the other subgenera and genus *Bironella,* which was reconstructed as the sister to *Lophopodomyia* rather than *Stethomyia.*

In 2005, Harbach & Kitching [36] revised and expanded the phylogenetic analysis of Sallum et al. [40], with special consideration of the specialized setae of the male gonocoxites (Figure 2) that diagnose the subgenera. Parsimony analysis of the data set under implied weighting supported the monophyly of subgenera *Cellia, Kerteszia* and *Nyssorhynchus,* and the sister relationship of *Kerteszia* + *Nyssorhynchus.* Subgenus *Anopheles* was recovered as a polyphyletic lineage basal to a monophyletic clade consisting of *Kerteszia* + *Nyssorhynchus* and *Cellia* in a sister-group relationship. *Bironella, Lophopodomyia* and *Stethomyia* were firmly nested within subgenus *Anopheles,* which would be paraphyletic even if these taxa were subsumed within it. Subgenus *Baimaia,* represented by *An. kyondawensis,* was supported as the sister of *Bironella* + all other *Anopheles. Bironella* and *Stethomyia,* contrary to the earlier study of Sallum et al. [40], were also supported as monophyletic clades separate from subgenus *Anopheles.* The preferred cladogram of Harbach & Kitching (Figures 4 and 5) is taken here to represent the best available estimate of anopheline phylogeny and evolutionary relationships because it is based on a greater number of taxonomic groups and homologous characters than all other hypotheses published to date.

A later analysis of subgenus *Anopheles* by Collucci & Sallum [42] included 38 species representing the same Series (6) and species Groups (15) of the subgenus that were included in the study of Sallum et al. [40]. The data were analyzed using successive approximations character weighting (SACW) and implied weighting (IW). Most of the relationships between members of the subgenus were either moderately or poorly supported. The Laticorn Section was recovered as a monophyletic clade in the IW analysis, suggesting that the laticorn development of the pupal trumpet is a derived condition for subgenus *Anopheles.* In the SACW analyses, members of the group comprised a paraphyletic lineage relative to the Cycloleppteron Series. The Angusticorn Section was recovered as a polyphyletic assemblage in both analyses. These results are contradicted by those of Sallum et al. [40] and Harbach & Kitching [36] who found that neither section is monophyletic. Below the section level of classification, only the Lophoscelomyia and Arribalzagia Series were recovered as monophyletic assemblages. The Myzorhynchus Series was paraphyletic relative to the Cycloleppteron, Christya and Arribalzagia Series, and the Anopheles Series was polyphyletic. Surprisingly, the two species of the Cycloleppteron Series included in the analyses were not grouped together, suggesting that the series is not monophyletic. In contrast, the Arribalzagia, Christya, Cycloleppteron, Lophoscelomyia and Myzorhynchus Series were recovered as monophyletic assemblages in the IW analysis of Harbach & Kitching (Figure 4). Furthermore, with the removal of subgenus *Baimaia,* the remaining species of the Anopheles Series included in their analysis also formed a monophyletic group. With the exception of the Pseudopunctipennis Group, all the species groups represented in the analysis of Collucci & Sallum (Aitkenii, Albotaeniatus, Culiciformis,

Hyrcanus, Plumbeus, Umbrosus Groups) were recovered as monophyletic assemblages with moderate to strong support [the Pseudopunctipennis Group was also found to be polyphyletic in the study of Harbach & Kitching (Figure 4)]. The Hyrcanus Group was paired with *An. coustani*, which corroborates previous hypotheses of a close relationship between the Hyrcanus and Coustani Groups [20,36,40,43]. Unfortunately, the analyses of Collucci & Sallum are biased by the selection of outgroup taxa whose interrelationships with the ingroup taxa were unresolved in previous studies. Thus, the results of their study cast doubt on their assertion that subgenus *Anopheles* is monophyletic. Based on the relationships recovered by Harbach & Kitching, subgenus *Anopheles* would be monophyletic if subgenus *Lophopodomyia* were to be reduced to the status of a species Group of the Anopheles Series (Figure 4). The Anopheles Series is a morphologically diverse assemblage of species and informal taxonomic groups, a number of which at one time or another were deemed to merit recognition as subgenera [20]. Sallum et al. [40] also found the Anopheles Series to be polyphyletic, but with its members interspersed in a complexity of inter-group relationships rather than arrayed in a pectinate sequence (Figure 4).

All phylogenetic studies conducted to date have demonstrated the monophyly of subgenera *Cellia* [36,38–41], *Kerteszia* [36,38–41,44] and *Nyssorhynchus* [36,38–41], and the sister pairing of *Kerteszia* and *Nyssorhynchus* [36,40,41]. The sister relationship of *Cellia* and the two New World subgenera is not inconsistent with the molecular analyses of Sallum et al. [41] if *Lophopodomyia* + *Bironella* is excluded from the clade that contains *Kerteszia* + *Nyssorhynchus*, but it differs markedly from the results of their earlier study based on morphology and a larger number of taxa [40], which placed *Kerteszia* + *Nyssorhynchus*, along with *An. implexus* (Christya Series), in a sister-group relationship with *Cellia* + a clade comprised of *Bironella*, *Lophopodomyia*, *Kerteszia* and *Nyssorhynchus*. *Anopheles implexus* (Christya Series) is sister to the terminal clade formed by *Kerteszia*, *Nyssorhynchus* and *Cellia* in Figure 4.

4. Distribution and phylogeography of *Anopheles*

Interpreting the current distributions of anophelines in an evolutionary context is problematic. The supercontinent of Pangaea existed in the Late Paleozoic and Early Mesozoic Eras from about 300–200 Mya and gradually separated 200–145 Mya into the two supercontinents of Laurasia and Gondwana [45]. As noted above, evidence from DNA sequence data and fossil calibration points [34] indicates that ancestral anophelines diverged from ancestral culicines about 217 Mya (230–192 Mya), before the complete splitting of Pangaea. If this was the case, then the separation of *Anopheles* and *Bironella* about 54 Mya (75.8–37.1 Mya, end of the Cretaceous to near the end of the Eocene Epoch of the Cenozoic) [34] must have occurred after the separation of Gondwana into multiple continents, i.e. Africa, South America, India, Antarctica and Australia, in the Cretaceous. Atlantica (the land mass that comprised present-day South America and Africa) separated from eastern Gondwana (the land mass that comprised Antarctica, India and Australia) 150–140 Mya. South America started to separate from Africa in a south-to-north direction during the Middle Cretaceous (about 125–115 Mya) [46]. At the same time, Madagascar and India began to separate from Antarctica, and separated from each other 100–90 Mya during the Cenomanian and Turonian Stages of the Late Cretaceous. India continued to move northward and collided with Eurasia about 35 Mya. Laurasia split to give rise to North America/Greenland and Eurasia about 60–55 Mya. Africa began to move northeastward toward Europe and South America moved northward to separate from Antarctica. North and South America were joined by the Isthmus of Panama during the Pliocene, approximately 3.7–3.0 Mya.

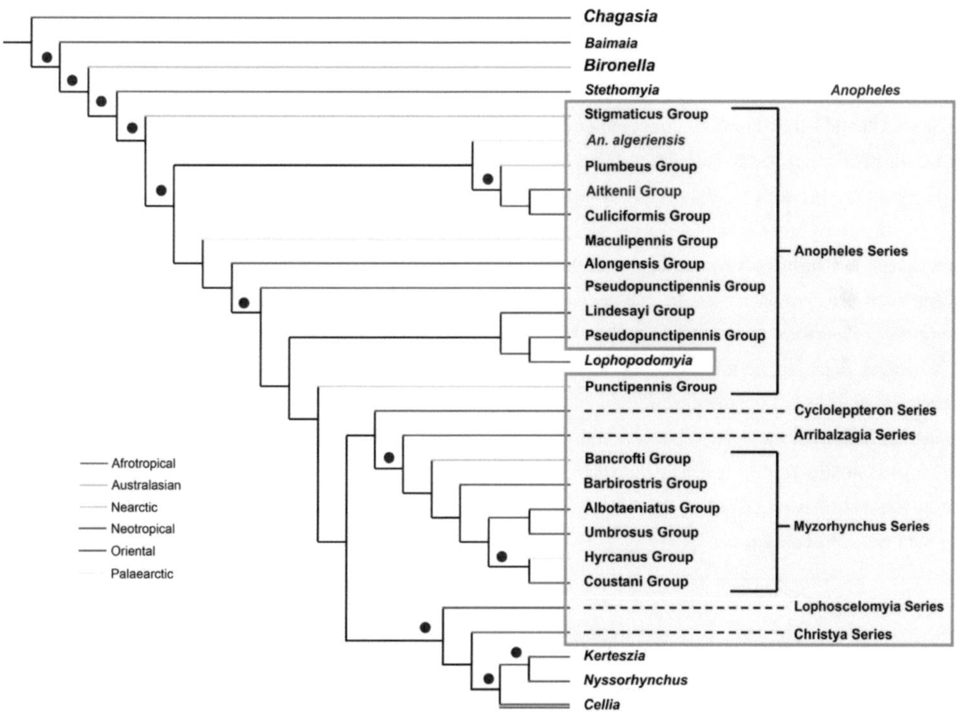

Figure 4. Phylogeny of subfamily Anophelinae, modified from Harbach & Kitching [36], indicating relationships within subgenus *Anopheles*. Filled circles indicate Bremer support values greater than 0.8.

Belkin [47] hypothesized that anophelines initially differentiated in the American Mediterranean Region. In concert with this postulate, Harbach & Kitching [36] suggested a possible New World origin of subfamily Anophelinae based on the basal placement of *Chagasia* relative to *Anopheles* + *Bironella* in their phylogeny of mosquito genera. Based on a phylogeny of 16 anopheline species inferred from sequences of two protein-coding nuclear genes and the Neotropical distribution of *Chagasia* and four of the seven subgenera of *Anopheles*, Krzywinski et al. [39] agreed with the hypothesis that South America was the center of origin of Anophelinae. However, as will be seen below, more recent studies suggest a different scenario for the evolution of the extant groups of the subfamily. This scenario closely reflects Christophers [48] insightful observations:

Subgenus *Anopheles* appears to be the oldest of the predominant subgenera, not only on [morphological grounds], but by reason of its worldwide distribution and the greater diversity and distinctness of its forms; almost every species of the subgenus appears to be as distinctive as are the species groups of subgenus *Myzomyia* [=*Cellia*], if not more so.

Nyssorhynchus appears to be a Neotropical development from some pre-*Anopheles* form, whilst the group *Arribalzagia* appears to be a highly specialized development of subgenus *Anopheles*.

Myzomyia shows every evidence of being a new and actively disseminating branch, as is suggested by its complete absence from the New World. Had it been once disseminated throughout North America it is unlikely that it would have been eliminated from the whole continent so completely as to leave not a single species in this area, though there is no actual proof that this did not occur. The apparent affinity between the group *Neomyzomyia* and subgenus *Nyssorhynchus* suggests an intermediate ancestor, though not necessarily one in the south, *i. e.*, such affinity does not prove or suggest a land-connection between Australia and South America, as the common ancestor may have been derived from the north and later eliminated. [next paragraph omitted]

The date of isolation of South America, judging by the history of mammals, would be from the middle of the Eocene, when connections between North and South America were severed, until the end of the Pliocene (*Zittel*). The anopheline fauna, therefore, arose from elements which pre-dated this period, and there were already subgenus *Anopheles*-like forms, as well as some earlier type from which *Nyssorhynchus* arose.

At some unknown period a similar special development took place, resulting in an early form (*Neomyzomyia*) of subgenus *Myzomyia*. This form appears to have once been distributed throughout the Oriental, Ethiopian [i.e. Afrotropical], and Australian Regions, and to have later undergone some regression, eventually remaining in greatest strength in the Australian Region.

Edwards, in reviewing the fossil remains of mosquitoes, notes that probably all the main divisions of the family [Culicidae] existed in Mid-Tertiary much as they do today, and with almost identical characters, and considers that, though no fossil *Anopheles* have been found, there can be no doubt from its morphology that this is also an old genus, probably older than any culicine form.

Based on the relationships shown in Figure 4, distributions of the principal group taxa (Appendix 6) and the geological dates listed above, it would appear that the ancestral lineage of *Anopheles* existed before the breakup of Pangaea and subsequently diversified into the modern subgenera and species after the separation of the continents. This would explain the cosmopolitan distribution and greater diversity of subgenus *Anopheles*, but not the earlier divergence of genus *Chagasia* and subgenus *Stethomyia*, which are confined to the Neotropical Region, the Oriental subgenus *Baimaia* and the Australasian genus *Bironella* (Figure 4). *Chagasia* possess several features that characterize species of subfamily Culicinae, including the strongly arched mesonotum, trilobed scutellum (Figure 6) and setae on the postpronotum. Based on these shared features, *Chagasia* has been considered an ancient group showing affinities with non-anophelines and phylogenetic analyses of morphological data and DNA sequences of various ribosomal, mitochondrial and nuclear genes strongly support its placement in an ancestral relationship to all other anophelines [33,35–41]. From the foregoing, however, it is inferred here that *Chagasia*, with only seven species, is a relic of a once more widely distributed taxon that is now confined to residual areas of South and Central America. It is also possible, although less likely, that *Chagasia*, as suggested by the late John N. Belkin for other mosquitoes [47], may have originated through hybridization between early anopheline and culicine forms.

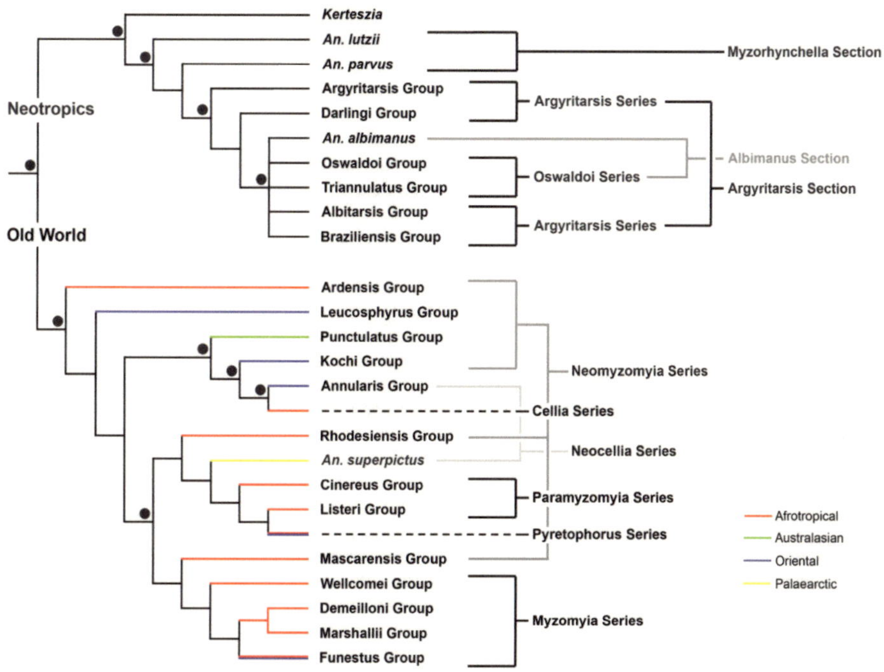

Figure 5. Phylogeny of subgenera *Cellia*, *Kerteszia* and *Nyssorhynchus*, modified from Harbach & Kitching [36], indicating relationships within subgenera *Cellia* and *Nyssorhynchus*. Filled circles indicate Bremer support values greater than 0.8.

Similarly, *Bironella* (as suggested by Christophers [48]), *Baimaia* and *Stethomyia*, with few species and restricted distributions, are also the remnants of once much more widely distributed forms. The isolation of ancestral members of subgenus *Anopheles* in South America also explains the uniqueness of the extant Neotropical fauna of the subgenus, especially the well-differentiated Arribalzagia Series. In accordance with this hypothesis, the following groups are also probably residual elements of once more widely distributed ancestral forms of subgenus *Anopheles*: the Afrotropical Christya Series (two species), the Australasian Atratipes (two species) and Stigmaticus (six species) Groups, the Oriental Alongensis (two species) and Culiciformis (three species) Groups, the Oriental Lophoscelomyia Series (five species) and the Neotropical Cycloleppteron Series (two species). It is noteworthy that the extant members of the relict groups are not vectors of human malarial parasites.

As noted previously, subgenus *Anopheles* has an almost world-wide distribution. Species are found at elevations from coastal areas to mountainous terrain in temperate, subtropical and tropical areas, but are absent from the majority of the Pacific Islands, including the large ones of New Zealand, Fiji and New Caledonia. The sole species of subgenus *Baimaia* has been found only in forested hilly and mountainous areas between 14° and 17° north on either side of the

Thai-Myanmar border and at a location near the Thai-Laos border in Thailand, and is probably also a relict taxon that has retained generalized ancestral features of the male genitalia [36]. Most species of subgenus *Cellia* have distributions in the Afrotropical, Australasian and Oriental Regions, but some species occur in southern areas of the Palaearctic. Species of *Cellia* are conspicuously absent from the majority of the islands of the Pacific, including New Zealand, Fiji and New Caledonia. Species of subgenus *Kerteszia* are found in the Neotropical Region, from Veracruz State in Mexico through Central America and Atlantic South America, along the Andes and along the coast, to the States of Misiones in Argentina and Rio Grande do Sul in Brazil, and also occur south along the Pacific Coast of South America to the State of El Oro, Ecuador. The subgenus is absent from all islands of the West Indies except Trinidad, and from most of the vast expanse of the Amazon basin in South America [49]. Species of subgenus *Lophopodomyia* are known to occur in areas of Panama and northern South America (Brazil, Colombia, Ecuador, French Guiana and Venezuela). Species of subgenus *Nyssorhynchus* are restricted to the Neotropical Region, except for *An. albimanus*, which extends into the Nearctic Region (northern Mexico and along the Rio Grande River in Texas). Finally, species of subgenus *Stethomyia* principally occur in southern Central America (Costa Rica and Panama) and northern South America (Brazil, Colombia, French Guiana, Guyana, Suriname and Venezuela), but one or two species are known to occur on the islands of Trinidad and Tobago and as far south as Peru and Bolivia.

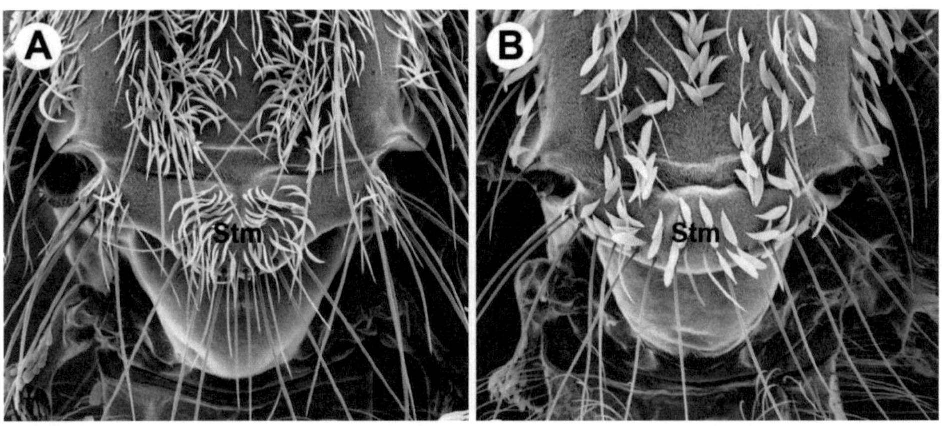

Figure 6. Two forms of the mosquito scutellum (Stm): A, trilobed scutellum of *Chagasia* and species of subfamily Culicinae; B, evenly rounded scutellum of *Anopheles*, with few exceptions. Original images from Harbach & Kitching [18].

Subgenera *Kerteszia, Lophopodomyia, Nyssorhynchus* and *Stethomyia*, and the Arribalzagia and Cycloleppteron Series of subgenus *Anopheles* are special to the Neotropical Region, where they probably originated following the separation of South America and Africa. The derived position of subgenera *Cellia* and *Kerteszia* + *Nyssorhynchus* relative to subgenus *Anopheles* (Figure 4) supports the hypothesis that the stem lineage of these subgenera originated in Gondwana and diverged following the separation of Atlantica to give rise to *Cellia* in Africa and *Kerteszia* and *Nyssorhynchus* in South America. It is interesting to note that *Lophopodo-*

myia and the Pseudopunctipennis Group are sister taxa in Figure 4, which is plausible in view of the hypothesized evolution of these groups from Neotropical ancestors. The Pseudopunctipennis Group is nearly restricted to the Neotropics, except for *An. franciscanus* and a minor extension of *An. pseudopunctipennis* into the Nearctic Region, which undoubtedly occurred relatively recently, after the land bridge formed to connect North and South America 3.7–3.0 Mya. Except for these two species, all *Anopheles* species in the Nearctic Region are members of the Anopheles Series of subgenus *Anopheles*. Half of the species of the Holarctic Maculipennis Group (24 species) occur in the Nearctic Region and the other half occur in the Palaearctic. This indicates that the Maculipennis Group must have evolved in the Northern Hemisphere prior to the separation of North America and Eurasia during the Paleocene and Eocene Epochs (60–55 Mya). The Plumbeus Group includes species in the Nearctic (2), Neotropical (4) and Palaearctic (3) Regions. Its position in the cladogram shown in Figure 4 is based on *An. judithae*, a Nearctic species. This group may be what paleontologists call a "stem group" [50], a paraphyletic or polyphyletic assemblage of species that share features of extinct taxa. The spotted distribution of these "living fossil" species suggests that their extinct relatives, ancestral forms of the Anopheles Series, existed before the separation of Pangaea. This bodes well with Christophers & Barraud's 1931 hypothesis [51] that the eggs of species of the Plumbeus Group are primitive compared to other species of subgenus *Anopheles*.

Species in subgenus *Cellia* are confined to the Eastern Hemisphere, with members in the Afrotropical, Australasian, Oriental and Palaearctic regions (Figure 5, Appendix 6). The Afrotropical Region is characterized by a large number of species of subgenus *Cellia* and relatively few species of subgenus *Anopheles*. The Myzomyia Series is especially dominant, but species of the Neocellia, Neomyzomyia and Pyretophorus Series also occur in the region. The Myzomyia, Neocellia and Pyretophorus Series are represented in the Afrotropical and Oriental Regions, but no species, species groups or subgroups of these series (with the exception of the Minimus Subgroup) are common to both regions (see Appendix 6). The Myzomyia Series is a dominant group in Africa, where *An. funestus* is a principal malaria vector [52,53]. Related species of the Funestus Group, including *An. minimus* and other members of the Minimus Subgroup, are major vectors of malarial parasites in southern Asia [52,54]. Evidence from phylogenetic analyses of mitochondrial DNA (ITS2 and D3 sequences) indicates that the Funestus Group originated in the Afrotropical Region [55]. The Neocellia Series also includes several important malaria vectors in southern Asia, notably *An. stephensi* and members of the Maculatus Group [52,54]. The Pyretophorus Series includes the formidable malaria vectors of the Gambiae Complex in Africa and important vectors of the Sundaicus and Subpictus Complexes in Southeast Asia [53,54]. The morphology-based phylogeny of Anthony et al. [56] indicates that the Pyretophorus Series originated in Africa and suggests that the capacity to vector malarial parasites is an ancestral condition subsequently lost independently in several lineages.

The anopheline fauna of the Australasian Region also shows evidence of isolation, but not to the degree indicated by the Neotropical fauna. The isolation appears to be more recent, corresponding to the separation of Australia from Antarctica between 37.0–33.5 Mya. The region includes a preponderance of species of the Neomyzomyia Series of subgenus *Cellia*, which may signal a relatively recent arrival from the Oriental Region, with some diversification. Members of the Neomyzomyia Series are the only *Anopheles* in the South Pacific [47]. Species groups of the series are confined to the Afrotropical (Ardensis, Mascarensis, Pauliani, Ranci, Rhodesiensis and Smithii Groups), Australasian (Punctulatus Group, Lungae Complex and unassigned species) or Oriental Region (Kochi, Leucosphyrus and Tessellatus Groups) (Appendix 6). The Neomyzomyia Series has been regarded as the most primitive series of subgenus *Cellia* based on egg morphology and the reduced or non-existent cibarial armature of females [57–59], and is thought to have originated in Africa and subsequently disperse eastward to the Oriental and Australasian Regions [52,59]. None of the African species of the Neomyzomyia Series, except for *An. nili*, are major vectors of malaria. In comparison, most species of the Oriental Leucosphyrus and Australasian Punctulatus Groups of the Neomyzomyia Series are important vectors of both primate and human malarial parasites. The Cellia and Paramyzomyia Series of subgenus *Cellia* are restricted to the Afrotropical Region, except for *An. pharoensis* (Cellia Series) and *An. multicolor* (Paramyzomyia Series) which occur in adjacent arid areas of the Palaearctic (Sahara and Middle East). It seems reasonable to hypothesize that those series that are presently represented by groups in the Afrotropical, Australasian and Oriental Regions arose before eastern Gondwana (Antarctica, India and Australia) fragmented. The Mascarensis, Pauliani and Ranci Groups are confined to Madagascar, which supports the hypothesis that the ancestral forms of at least these groups of the Neomyzomyia Series existed before Madagascar separated from India 100–90 Mya.

Human malaria probably evolved in Africa along with its mosquito hosts and other primates. Modern humans arose in Africa about 200,000 years ago and dispersed into Eurasia [60], reaching Australia about 40,000 years ago. Migration into the New World occurred about 15–20 millennia ago, and most of the Pacific Islands were colonized by four thousand years ago. The point here is that the rise and dispersal of modern humans occurred long after the formation of the continents and the evolution of the major groups of *Anopheles*. Consequently, it seems reasonable to assume that human malarial parasites accompanied humans during their migration out of Africa and were passed on to species of *Anopheles* in other regions that had the ecological, physiological and behavioural attributes required to propagate infections and maintain transmission. These taxa were surely already adapted to feeding on primates, including the ancestors of *Homo sapiens*, and were capable of developing and transmitting the *Plasmodium* species specific to those hosts.

Comprehensive information on the dominant malaria vectors of the world, most of which are presumably recently evolved members of sibling species complexes (Appendix 3), is summarized in a series of publications (and a chapter of this book) by M. Sinka and a team of regional experts and technical advisors – the Americas [61], Africa, Europe and the Middle East [53], the Asia-Pacific Region [54] – that culminated in a thorough review of the principal malaria vector taxa of the world [62]. At present, 96 formally named species of *Anopheles* are members of 26 sibling species complexes (Appendix 4). Twenty of these nominal species actually consist of more than one species, which all together comprise a total of 67 species. Excluding the name-bearing type species, the 58 species, plus five other unnamed species that are not members of species complexes, a total of 72 species, have yet to be given formal Latin names (Appendix 4).

5. Conclusion

A more robust phylogeny of *Anopheles* mosquitoes than is currently available may be of use in the fight against malaria. Foley et al. [37] suggested that it may help "by elucidating descent relationships of genes for refractoriness, insecticide resistance, and genetically determined ecological and behavioral traits important to malaria transmission." Interrupting the life cycle of malarial parasites by genetically manipulating vector receptiveness to infection is a potential approach to malaria control. A natural classification of *Anopheles* predictive of biological and ecological traits could facilitate the manipulation of vector genomes by informing the dynamics of introduced genes. Obviously, co-evolutionary studies of parasites and vectors require phylogenies for the mosquitoes. This must far exceed the taxon-limited (exemplar-based) studies conducted to date as they do not provide a basis for gaining insights into interspecific and co-evolutionary relationships of vectors and parasites.

It seems fitting to end here with a comment concerning interspecific hybridization, which was mentioned above in relation to genus *Chagasia* in the Neotropical Region. Although anopheline species occur in sympatry in most ecosystems, hybridization has only been detected at very low levels between certain members of species complexes in subgenus *Cellia*, e.g. *An. gambiae* with both *An. arabiensis* and *An. bwambae* in Africa [63,64], *An. dirus* and *An. baimaii* in Thailand [65] and *An. minimus* and *An. harrisoni* in Vietnam [66]. However, as advocated by Belkin [47], hybridization could provide sufficient genetic variation to permit adaptation to new habitats. Hybridization may occur regularly between some species, particularly widely distributed species that are morphologically similar. It could have played a role in the speciation and evolution of *Anopheles* mosquitoes and the pathogens they transmit.

Appendix 1 — The internal classification of genus *Anopheles*

Subgenus	Section	Series	Group	Subgroup	Complex	Author
Anopheles						[1]
	Angusticorn					[20]
		Anopheles				[12]
					Claviger	[67]
			Alongensis			[68]
			Aitkenii			[10]
			Atratipes			[69]

Subgenus	Section	Series	Group	Subgroup	Complex	Author
			Culiciformis			[20]
			Lindesayi			[20]
					Gigas	[70]
					Lindesayi	[70]
			Maculipennis			[20]
				Maculipennis		[71]
				Quadrimaculatus		[71]
				Freeborni		[71]
			Plumbeus			[20]
			Pseudopunctipen-nis			[20]
			Punctipennis			[20]
					Crucians	[72]
			Stigmaticus			[20]
		Cycloleppteron				[12]
		Lophoscelomyia				[12]
			Asiaticus			[23]
				Asiaticus		[73]
				Interruptus		[73]
	Laticorn					[20]
		Arribalzagia				[74]
		Christya				[75]
		Myzorhynchus				[12]
			Albotaeniatus			[20]
			Bancroftii			[20]
			Barbirostris			[20]
				Barbirostris		[23]
					Barbirostris	[76]
				Vanus		[23]
			Coustani			[20]
			Hyrcanus			[77]
				Lesteri		[78]
				Nigerrimus		[78]

Subgenus	Section	Series	Group	Subgroup	Complex	Author
			Umbrosus			[79]
				Baezai		[73]
				Letifer		[23]
				Separatus		[73]
				Umbrosus		[73]
Baimaia						[15]
Cellia						[80]
		Cellia				[75]
			Squamosus			[21]
		Myzomyia				[75]
			Demeilloni			[22]
			Funestus			[81]
				Aconitus		[82]
				Culicifacies		[81]
				Funestus		[81]
				Minimus		[82]
					Fluviatilis	[83]
					Minimus	[84]
				Rivulorum		[81]
			Marshallii			[22]
					Marshallii	[85]
			Wellcomei			[22]
		Neocellia				[75]
			Annularis			[23]
					Annularis	[86]
					Nivipes	[87]
			Jamesii			[73]
			Maculatus			[88]
				Maculatus		[73]
				Sawadwongporni		[73]
		Neomyzomyia				[75]
					Annulipes	[89]

Subgenus	Section	Series	Group	Subgroup	Complex	Author
					Longirostris	[90]
					Lungae	[47]
			Ardensis			[22]
					Nili	[22]
			Kochi			[73]
			Leucosphyrus			[91]
				Hackeri		[92]
				Leucosphyrus		[93]
					Dirus	[94]
					Leucosphyrus	[92]
				Riparis		[93]
			Mascarensis			[26]
			Pauliani			[21]
			Punctulatus			[95]
					Farauti	[96]
			Ranci			[21]
				Ranci		[21]
				Roubaudi		[21]
			Rhodesiensis			[22]
			Smithii			[22]
			Tessellatus			[73]
		Paramyzomyia				[51]
			Cinereus			[22]
			Listeri			[22]
		Pyretophorus				[12]
					Gambiae	[97]
			Ludlowae			[73]
					Sundaicus	[98]
			Subpictus			[73]
					Subpictus	[99]
Kerteszia						[100]
					Cruzii	[101]

Subgenus	Section	Series	Group	Subgroup	Complex	Author
Lophopodomyia						[14]
Nyssorhynchus						[102]
	Albimanus					[103]
		Albimanus				[24]
		Oswaldoi				[24]
			Oswaldoi			[24]
				Oswaldoi		[24]
					Nuneztovari	[104]
				Strodei		[24]
					Benarrochi	[105]
			Triannulatus		Triannulatus	[24]
	Argyritarsis					[103]
		Albitarsis				[25]
			Albitarsis			[25]
					Albitarsis	[106]
			Braziliensis			[25]
		Argyritarsis				[25]
			Argyritarsis			[25]
			Darlingi			[25]
			Lanei			[25]
			Pictipennis			[25]
	Myzorhynchella					[107]
Stethomyia						[80]

Appendix 2

Alphabetical list of formally named species of *Anopheles* and their position in the classification of the genus. For species Complexes, see Appendices 3 and 4; for authorship of species, visit http://mosquito-taxonomic-inventory.info/valid-species-list.

Species	Subgenus	Section	Series	Group	Subgroup
aberrans	*Anopheles*	Angusticorn	Anopheles	Aitkenii	

Species	Subgenus	Section	Series	Group	Subgroup
acaci	*Anopheles*	Angusticorn	Anopheles	Aitkenii	
acanthotorynus	*Stethomyia*				
aconitus	*Cellia*		Myzomyia	Funestus	Aconitus
ahomi	*Anopheles*	Laticorn	Myzorhynchus	Barbirostris	Vanus
ainshamsi	*Cellia*		Neocellia		
aitkenii	*Anopheles*	Angusticorn	Anopheles	Aitkenii	
albertoi	*Nyssorhynchus*	Albimanus	Oswaldoi	Oswaldoi	Strodei
albimanus	*Nyssorhynchus*	Albimanus	Albimanus		
albitarsis	*Nyssorhynchus*	Argyritarsis	Albitarsis	Albitarsis	
albotaeniatus	*Anopheles*	Laticorn	Myzorhynchus	Albotaeniatus	
algeriensis	*Anopheles*	Angusticorn	Anopheles		
alongensis	*Anopheles*	Angusticorn	Anopheles	Alongensis	
amictus	*Cellia*		Neomyzomyia		
anchietai	*Anopheles*	Laticorn	Arribalzagia		
annandalei	*Anopheles*	Angusticorn	Lophoscelomyia	Asiaticus	
annularis	*Cellia*		Neocellia	Annularis	
annulatus	*Cellia*		Neomyzomyia		
annulipalpis	*Anopheles*	Angusticorn	Cycloleppteron		
annulipes	*Cellia*		Neomyzomyia		
anomalophyllus	*Nyssorhynchus*	Albimanus	Oswaldoi	Oswaldoi	Oswaldoi
antunesi	*Nyssorhynchus*	Myzorhynchella			
apicimacula	*Anopheles*	Laticorn	Arribalzagia		
apoci	*Cellia*		Myzomyia		
aquasalis	*Nyssorhynchus*	Albimanus	Oswaldoi	Oswaldoi	Oswaldoi
arabiensis	*Cellia*		Pyretophorus		
arboricola	*Anopheles*	Angusticorn	Anopheles	Plumbeus	
ardensis	*Cellia*		Neomyzomyia	Ardensis	
argenteolobatus	*Cellia*		Cellia		
argyritarsis	*Nyssorhynchus*	Argyritarsis	Argyritarsis	Argyritarsis	
argyropus	*Anopheles*	Laticorn	Myzorhynchus	Hyrcanus	
artemievi	*Anopheles*	Angusticorn	Anopheles	Maculipennis	Maculipennis

http://dx.doi.org/10.5772/54695

Species	Subgenus	Section	Series	Group	Subgroup
arthuri	*Nyssorhynchus*	Albimanus	Oswaldoi	Oswaldoi	Strodei
aruni	*Cellia*		Myzomyia	Funestus	Funestus
asiaticus	*Anopheles*	Angusticorn	Lophoscelomyia	Asiaticus	Asiaticus
atacamensis	*Nyssorhynchus*	Argyritarsis	Argyritarsis	Pictipennis	
atratipes	*Anopheles*	Angusticorn	Anopheles	Atratipes	
atroparvus	*Anopheles*	Angusticorn	Anopheles	Maculipennis	Maculipennis
atropos	*Anopheles*	Angusticorn	Anopheles	Maculipennis	
aurirostris	*Cellia*		Neomyzomyia		
austenii	*Cellia*		Myzomyia	Marshallii	
auyantepuiensis	*Kerteszia*				
azaniae	*Cellia*		Myzomyia		
azevedoi	*Cellia*		Paramyzomyia	Cinereus	
aztecus	*Anopheles*	Angusticorn	Anopheles	Maculipennis	
baezai	*Anopheles*	Laticorn	Myzorhynchus	Umbrosus	Baezai
baileyi	*Anopheles*	Angusticorn	Anopheles	Lindesayi	
baimaii	*Cellia*		Neomyzomyia	Leucosphyrus	Leucosphyrus
baisasi	*Cellia*		Neomyzomyia	Leucosphyrus	Leucosphyrus
balabacensis	*Cellia*		Neomyzomyia	Leucosphyrus	Leucosphyrus
balerensis	*Anopheles*	Laticorn	Myzorhynchus	Albotaeniatus	
bambusicolus	*Kerteszia*				
bancroftii	*Anopheles*	Laticorn	Myzorhynchus	Bancroftii	
barberellus	*Cellia*		Myzomyia		
barberi	*Anopheles*	Angusticorn	Anopheles	Plumbeus	
barbirostris	*Anopheles*	Laticorn	Myzorhynchus	Barbirostris	Barbirostris
barbumbrosus	*Anopheles*	Laticorn	Myzorhynchus	Barbirostris	Vanus
barianensis	*Anopheles*	Angusticorn	Anopheles	Plumbeus	
beklemishevi	*Anopheles*	Angusticorn	Anopheles	Maculipennis	Quadrimaculatus
belenrae	*Anopheles*	Laticorn	Myzorhynchus	Hyrcanus	
bellator	*Kerteszia*				
benarrochi	*Nyssorhynchus*	Albimanus	Oswaldoi	Oswaldoi	Strodei
bengalensis	*Anopheles*	Angusticorn	Anopheles	Aitkenii	

Species	Subgenus	Section	Series	Group	Subgroup
berghei	*Cellia*		Myzomyia	Marshallii	
bervoetsi	*Cellia*		Myzomyia		
boliviensis	*Kerteszia*				
borneensis	*Anopheles*	Angusticorn	Anopheles	Aitkenii	
bradleyi	*Anopheles*	Angusticorn	Anopheles	Punctipennis	
braziliensis	*Nyssorhynchus*	Argyritarsis	Albitarsis	Braziliensis	
brevipalpis	*Anopheles*	Laticorn	Myzorhynchus	Umbrosus	
brevirostris	*Anopheles*	Laticorn	Myzorhynchus	Umbrosus	
brohieri	*Cellia*		Myzomyia	Marshallii	
brucei	*Cellia*		Myzomyia	Funestus	Rivulorum
brumpti	*Cellia*		Cellia		
brunnipes	*Cellia*		Myzomyia		
bulkleyi	*Anopheles*	Angusticorn	Lophoscelomyia		
bustamentei	*Anopheles*	Laticorn	Arribalzagia		
buxtoni	*Cellia*		Neomyzomyia	Ardensis	
bwambae	*Cellia*		Pyretophorus		
calderoni	*Anopheles*	Laticorn	Arribalzagia		
caliginosus	*Anopheles*	Laticorn	Myzorhynchus	Coustani	
cameroni	*Cellia*		Neomyzomyia	Rhodesiensis	
campestris	*Anopheles*	Laticorn	Myzorhynchus	Barbirostris	Barbirostris
canorii	*Stethomyia*		Neomyzomyia	Smithii	
carnevalei	*Cellia*		Neomyzomyia	Ardensis	
caroni	*Cellia*				
carteri	*Cellia*		Myzomyia	Demeilloni	
chiriquiensis	*Anopheles*	Angusticorn	Anopheles	Pseudopunctipennis	
chodukini	*Anopheles*	Laticorn	Myzorhynchus	Hyrcanus	
christyi	*Cellia*		Pyretophorus		
cinctus	*Cellia*		Neomyzomyia	Ardensis	
cinereus	*Cellia*		Paramyzomyia	Cinereus	
claviger	*Anopheles*	Angusticorn	Anopheles		
clowi	*Cellia*		Neomyzomyia	Punctulatus	

Species	Subgenus	Section	Series	Group	Subgroup
colledgei	*Anopheles*	Angusticorn	Anopheles	Stigmaticus	
collessi	*Anopheles*	Laticorn	Myzorhynchus	Umbrosus	Letifer
comorensis	*Cellia*		Pyretophorus		
concolor	*Anopheles*	Angusticorn	Anopheles		
confusus	*Cellia*		Myzomyia	Funestus	Funestus
corethroides	*Anopheles*	Angusticorn	Anopheles	Stigmaticus	
costai	*Anopheles*	Laticorn	Arribalzagia		
coustani	*Anopheles*	Laticorn	Myzorhynchus	Coustani	
cracens	*Cellia*		Neomyzomyia	Leucosphyrus	Leucosphyrus
crawfordi	*Anopheles*	Laticorn	Myzorhynchus	Hyrcanus	Lesteri
cristatus	*Cellia*		Neomyzomyia	Leucosphyrus	Riparis
cristipalpis	*Cellia*		Cellia		
crucians	*Anopheles*	Angusticorn	Anopheles	Punctipennis	
cruzii	*Kerteszia*				
crypticus	*Anopheles*	Laticorn	Myzorhynchus	Coustani	
cucphuongensis	*Anopheles*	Angusticorn	Anopheles	Alongensis	
culicifacies	*Cellia*		Myzomyia	Funestus	Culicifacies
culiciformis	*Anopheles*	Angusticorn	Anopheles	Culiciformis	
cydippis	*Cellia*		Cellia	Squamosus	
daciae	*Anopheles*	Angusticorn	Anopheles	Maculipennis	Maculipennis
dancalicus	*Cellia*		Neocellia		
darlingi	*Nyssorhynchus*	Argyritarsis	Argyritarsis	Darlingi	
daudi	*Cellia*		Pyretophorus		
deaneorum	*Nyssorhynchus*	Argyritarsis	Albitarsis	Albitarsis	
deemingi	*Cellia*		Neomyzomyia	Ardensis	
demeilloni	*Cellia*		Myzomyia	Demeilloni	
diluvialis	*Anopheles*	Angusticorn	Anopheles	Maculipennis	Quadrimaculatus
dirus	*Cellia*		Neomyzomyia	Leucosphyrus	Leucosphyrus
dispar	*Cellia*		Neocellia	Maculatus	
distinctus	*Cellia*		Myzomyia	Wellcomei	
domicola	*Cellia*		Myzomyia		

Species	Subgenus	Section	Series	Group	Subgroup
donaldi	*Anopheles*	Laticorn	Myzorhynchus	Barbirostris	Barbirostris
dravidicus	*Cellia*		Neocellia	Maculatus	Maculatus
dthali	*Cellia*		Myzomyia		
dualaensis	*Cellia*		Neomyzomyia		
dunhami	*Nyssorhynchus*	Albimanus	Oswaldoi	Oswaldoi	Oswaldoi
dureni	*Cellia*		Neomyzomyia	Ardensis	
earlei	*Anopheles*	Angusticorn	Anopheles	Maculipennis	Freeborni
eiseni	*Anopheles*	Angusticorn	Anopheles	Pseudopunctipennis	
ejercitoi	*Anopheles*	Laticorn	Myzorhynchus	Albotaeniatus	
elegans	*Cellia*		Neomyzomyia	Leucosphyrus	Leucosphyrus
engarensis	*Anopheles*	Laticorn	Myzorhynchus	Hyrcanus	
eouzani	*Cellia*		Neomyzomyia	Ardensis	
epiroticus	*Cellia*		Pyretophorus		
erepens	*Cellia*		Myzomyia	Wellcomei	
erythraeus	*Cellia*		Myzomyia		
ethiopicus	*Cellia*		Myzomyia		
evandroi	*Anopheles*	Laticorn	Arribalzagia		
evansae	*Nyssorhynchus*	Albimanus	Oswaldoi	Oswaldoi	Oswaldoi
faini	*Cellia*		Neomyzomyia	Smithii	
farauti	*Cellia*		Neomyzomyia	Punctulatus	
fausti	*Anopheles*	Angusticorn	Anopheles	Plumbeus	
filipinae	*Cellia*		Myzomyia	Funestus	Aconitus
flavicosta	*Cellia*		Myzomyia		
flavirostris	*Cellia*		Myzomyia	Funestus	Minimus
fluminensis	*Anopheles*	Laticorn	Arribalzagia		
fluviatilis	*Cellia*		Myzomyia	Funestus	Minimus
fontinalis	*Cellia*		Myzomyia		
forattinii	*Anopheles*	Laticorn	Arribalzagia		
fragilis	*Anopheles*	Angusticorn	Anopheles	Aitkenii	
franciscanus	*Anopheles*	Angusticorn	Anopheles	Pseudopunctipennis	
franciscoi	*Anopheles*	Laticorn	Myzorhynchus	Barbirostris	Barbirostris

Species	Subgenus	Section	Series	Group	Subgroup
freeborni	*Anopheles*	Angusticorn	Anopheles	Maculipennis	Freeborni
freetownensis	*Cellia*		Myzomyia	Demeilloni	
freyi	*Anopheles*	Laticorn	Myzorhynchus	Barbirostris	
funestus	*Cellia*		Myzomyia	Funestus	Funestus
fuscicolor	*Anopheles*	Laticorn	Myzorhynchus	Coustani	
fuscivenosus	*Cellia*		Myzomyia	Funestus	Rivulorum
gabaldoni	*Anopheles*	Laticorn	Arribalzagia		
galvaoi	*Nyssorhynchus*	Albimanus	Oswaldoi	Oswaldoi	Oswaldoi
gambiae	*Cellia*		Pyretophorus		
garnhami	*Cellia*		Myzomyia	Demeilloni	
georgianus	*Anopheles*	Angusticorn	Anopheles	Punctipennis	
gibbinsi	*Cellia*		Myzomyia	Marshallii	
gigas	*Anopheles*	Angusticorn	Anopheles	Lindesayi	
gilesi	*Lophopodomyia*				
goeldii	*Nyssorhynchus*	Albimanus	Oswaldoi	Oswaldoi	Oswaldoi
gomezdelatorrei	*Lophopodomyia*				
gonzalezrinconesi	*Kerteszia*				
grabhamii	*Anopheles*	Angusticorn	Cycloleppteron		
grassei	*Cellia*		Neomyzomyia	Pauliani	
greeni	*Cellia*		Neocellia	Maculatus	
grenieri	*Cellia*		Neomyzomyia	Pauliani	
griveaudi	*Cellia*		Neomyzomyia	Ranci	
guarani	*Nyssorhynchus*	Myzorhynchella			
guarao	*Anopheles*	Laticorn	Arribalzagia		
hackeri	*Cellia*		Neomyzomyia	Leucosphyrus	Hackeri
hailarensis	*Anopheles*	Laticorn	Myzorhynchus	Hyrcanus	
halophylus	*Nyssorhynchus*	Albimanus	Oswaldoi	Triannulatus	
hamoni	*Cellia*		Neomyzomyia	Smithii	
hancocki	*Cellia*		Myzomyia	Marshallii	
hargreavesi	*Cellia*		Myzomyia	Marshallii	
harperi	*Cellia*		Myzomyia	Marshallii	

Species	Subgenus	Section	Series	Group	Subgroup
harrisoni	*Cellia*		Myzomyia	Funestus	Minimus
hectoris	*Anopheles*	Angusticorn	Anopheles	Pseudopunctipennis	
heiheensis	*Anopheles*	Laticorn	Myzorhynchus	Hyrcanus	
hermsi	*Anopheles*	Angusticorn	Anopheles	Maculipennis	Freeborni
hervyi	*Cellia*		Neocellia		
hilli	*Cellia*		Neomyzomyia		
hinesorum	*Cellia*		Neomyzomyia	Punctulatus	
hodgkini	*Anopheles*	Laticorn	Myzorhynchus	Barbirostris	Barbirostris
homunculus	*Kerteszia*				
hughi	*Cellia*		Myzomyia	Marshallii	
hunteri	*Anopheles*	Laticorn	Myzorhynchus	Umbrosus	
hyrcanus	*Anopheles*	Laticorn	Myzorhynchus	Hyrcanus	
implexus	*Anopheles*	Laticorn	Christya		
incognitus	*Cellia*		Neomyzomyia		
indefinitus	*Cellia*		Pyretophorus	Subpictus	
ininii	*Nyssorhynchus*	Albimanus	Oswaldoi	Oswaldoi	Oswaldoi
insulaeflorum	*Anopheles*	Angusticorn	Anopheles	Aitkenii	
intermedius	*Anopheles*	Laticorn	Arribalzagia		
interruptus	*Anopheles*	Angusticorn	Lophoscelomyia	Asiaticus	Interruptus
introlatus	*Cellia*		Neomyzomyia	Leucosphyrus	Leucosphyrus
inundatus	*Anopheles*	Angusticorn	Anopheles	Maculipennis	Quadrimaculatus
irenicus	*Cellia*		Neomyzomyia	Punctulatus	
jamesii	*Cellia*		Neocellia	Jamesii	
janconnae	*Nyssorhynchus*	Argyritarsis	Albitarsis	Albitarsis	
jebudensis	*Cellia*		Neomyzomyia	Smithii	
jeyporiensis	*Cellia*		Myzomyia	Funestus	
judithae	*Anopheles*	Angusticorn	Anopheles	Plumbeus	
karwari	*Cellia*		Neocellia		
keniensis	*Cellia*		Myzomyia	Demeilloni	
kingi	*Cellia*		Neomyzomyia	Ardensis	
kleini	*Anopheles*	Laticorn	Myzorhynchus	Hyrcanus	

http://dx.doi.org/10.5772/54695

Species	**Subgenus**	**Section**	**Series**	**Group**	**Subgroup**
kochi	*Cellia*		Neomyzomyia	Kochi	
kokhani	*Cellia*		Neomyzomyia		
kolambuganensis	*Cellia*		Neomyzomyia		
koliensis	*Cellia*		Neomyzomyia	Punctulatus	
kompi	*Stethomyia*				
konderi	*Nyssorhynchus*	Albimanus	Oswaldoi	Oswaldoi	Oswaldoi
koreicus	*Anopheles*	Laticorn	Myzorhynchus	Barbirostris	
kosiensis	*Cellia*		Myzomyia	Marshallii	
kweiyangensis	*Anopheles*	Laticorn	Myzorhynchus	Hyrcanus	
kyondawensis	*Baimaia*				
labranchiae	*Anopheles*	Angusticorn	Anopheles	Maculipennis	Maculipennis
lacani	*Cellia*		Neomyzomyia	Ranci	Roubaudi
laneanus	*Kerteszia*				
lanei	*Nyssorhynchus*	Argyritarsis	Argyritarsis	Lanei	
latens	*Cellia*		Neomyzomyia	Leucosphyrus	Leucosphyrus
leesoni	*Cellia*		Myzomyia	Funestus	Minimus
lepidotus	*Kerteszia*				
lesteri	*Anopheles*	Laticorn	Myzorhynchus	Hyrcanus	Lesteri
letabensis	*Cellia*		Myzomyia	Marshallii	
letifer	*Anopheles*	Laticorn	Myzorhynchus	Umbrosus	Letifer
leucosphyrus	*Cellia*		Neomyzomyia	Leucosphyrus	Leucosphyrus
lewisi	*Anopheles*	Angusticorn	Anopheles	Maculipennis	
liangshanensis	*Anopheles*	Laticorn	Myzorhynchus	Hyrcanus	
limosus	*Cellia*		Pyretophorus		
lindesayi	*Anopheles*	Angusticorn	Anopheles	Lindesayi	
listeri	*Cellia*		Paramyzomyia	Listeri	
litoralis	*Cellia*		Pyretophorus		
lloreti	*Cellia*		Myzomyia	Demeilloni	
longipalpis	*Cellia*		Myzomyia	Funestus	Funestus
longirostris	*Cellia*		Neomyzomyia		
lounibosi	*Cellia*		Neomyzomyia	Rhodesiensis	

Species	Subgenus	Section	Series	Group	Subgroup
lovettae	*Cellia*		Neomyzomyia	Smithii	
ludlowae	*Cellia*		Pyretophorus	Ludlowae	
lungae	*Cellia*		Neomyzomyia		
lutzii	*Nyssorhynchus*	Myzorhynchella			
macarthuri	*Cellia*		Neomyzomyia	Leucosphyrus	Riparis
machardyi	*Cellia*		Neomyzomyia	Ardensis	
maculatus	*Cellia*		Neocellia	Maculatus	Maculatus
maculipalpis	*Cellia*		Neocellia		
maculipennis	*Anopheles*	Angusticorn	Anopheles	Maculipennis	Maculipennis
maculipes	*Anopheles*	Laticorn	Arribalzagia		
majidi	*Cellia*		Myzomyia		
malefactor	*Anopheles*	Laticorn	Arribalzagia		
maliensis	*Cellia*		Neomyzomyia	Ardensis	
manalangi	*Anopheles*	Laticorn	Myzorhynchus	Barbirostris	Vanus
mangyanus	*Cellia*		Myzomyia	Funestus	Aconitus
marajoara	*Nyssorhynchus*	Argyritarsis	Albitarsis	Albitarsis	
marshallii	*Cellia*		Myzomyia	Marshallii	
marteri	*Anopheles*	Angusticorn	Anopheles		
martinius	*Anopheles*	Angusticorn	Anopheles	Maculipennis	Maculipennis
mascarensis	*Cellia*		Neomyzomyia	Mascarensis	
mattogrossensis	*Anopheles*	Laticorn	Arribalzagia		
maverlius	*Anopheles*	Angusticorn	Anopheles	Maculipennis	Quadrimaculatus
mediopunctatus	*Anopheles*	Laticorn	Arribalzagia		
melanoon	*Anopheles*	Angusticorn	Anopheles	Maculipennis	Maculipennis
melas	*Cellia*		Pyretophorus		
mengalangensis	*Anopheles*	Angusticorn	Anopheles	Lindesayi	
meraukensis	*Cellia*		Neomyzomyia		
merus	*Cellia*		Pyretophorus		
messeae	*Anopheles*	Angusticorn	Anopheles	Maculipennis	Maculipennis
millecampsi	*Cellia*		Neomyzomyia	Ardensis	
milloti	*Cellia*		Neomyzomyia	Pauliani	

http://dx.doi.org/10.5772/54695

Species	Subgenus	Section	Series	Group	Subgroup
minimus	*Cellia*		Myzomyia	Funestus	Minimus
minor	*Anopheles*	Laticorn	Arribalzagia		
mirans	*Cellia*		Neomyzomyia	Leucosphyrus	Hackeri
moghulensis	*Cellia*		Neocellia		
montanus	*Anopheles*	Laticorn	Myzorhynchus	Albotaeniatus	
mortiauxi	*Cellia*		Myzomyia	Marshallii	
moucheti	*Cellia*		Myzomyia		
mousinhoi	*Cellia*		Myzomyia	Marshallii	
multicinctus	*Cellia*		Neomyzomyia	Ardensis	
multicolor	*Cellia*		Paramyzomyia	Listeri	
murphyi	*Cellia*		Cellia		
namibiensis	*Anopheles*	Laticorn	Myzorhynchus	Coustani	
natalensis	*Cellia*		Neomyzomyia	Ardensis	
nataliae	*Cellia*		Neomyzomyia		
neivai	*Kerteszia*				
nemophilous	*Cellia*		Neomyzomyia	Leucosphyrus	Leucosphyrus
neomaculipalpus	*Anopheles*	Laticorn	Arribalzagia		
nigerrimus	*Anopheles*	Laticorn	Myzorhynchus	Hyrcanus	Nigerrimus
nigritarsis	*Nyssorhynchus*	Myzorhynchella			
nilgiricus	*Anopheles*	Angusticorn	Anopheles	Lindesayi	
nili	*Cellia*		Neomyzomyia	Ardensis	
nimbus	*Stethomyia*				
nimpe	*Anopheles*	Laticorn	Myzorhynchus	Hyrcanus	
nitidus	*Anopheles*	Laticorn	Myzorhynchus	Hyrcanus	Nigerrimus
nivipes	*Cellia*		Neocellia	Annularis	
njombiensis	*Cellia*		Myzomyia	Marshallii	
noniae	*Anopheles*	Angusticorn	Lophoscelomyia	Asiaticus	
notanandai	*Cellia*		Neocellia	Maculatus	Sawadwongporni
notleyi	*Cellia*		Neomyzomyia	Ranci	Roubaudi
novaguinensis	*Cellia*		Neomyzomyia		
nuneztovari	*Nyssorhynchus*	Albimanus	Oswaldoi	Oswaldoi	Oswaldoi

Species	Subgenus	Section	Series	Group	Subgroup
obscurus	*Anopheles*	Laticorn	Myzorhynchus		
occidentalis	*Anopheles*	Angusticorn	Anopheles	Maculipennis	Freeborni
oiketorakras	*Lophopodomyia*				
okuensis	*Anopheles*	Laticorn	Christya		
omorii	*Anopheles*	Angusticorn	Anopheles	Plumbeus	
oryzalimnetes	*Nyssorhynchus*	Argyritarsis	Albitarsis	Albitarsis	
oswaldoi	*Nyssorhynchus*	Albimanus	Oswaldoi	Oswaldoi	Oswaldoi
ovengensis	*Cellia*		Neomyzomyia	Ardensis	
pallidus	*Cellia*		Neocellia	Annularis	
palmatus	*Anopheles*	Angusticorn	Anopheles	Aitkenii	
paltrinierii	*Cellia*		Neocellia		
paludis	*Anopheles*	Laticorn	Myzorhynchus	Coustani	
pampanai	*Cellia*		Myzomyia	Funestus	Aconitus
papuensis	*Anopheles*	Angusticorn	Anopheles	Stigmaticus	
paraliae	*Anopheles*	Laticorn	Myzorhynchus	Hyrcanus	Lesteri
parangensis	*Cellia*		Pyretophorus		
parapunctipennis	*Anopheles*	Angusticorn	Anopheles	Pseudopunctipennis	
parensis	*Cellia*		Myzomyia	Funestus	Funestus
parvus	*Nyssorhynchus*	Myzorhynchella			
pattoni	*Cellia*		Neocellia		
pauliani	*Cellia*		Neomyzomyia	Pauliani	
peditaeniatus	*Anopheles*	Laticorn	Myzorhynchus	Hyrcanus	Lesteri
perplexens	*Anopheles*	Angusticorn	Anopheles	Punctipennis	
persiensis	*Anopheles*	Angusticorn	Anopheles	Maculipennis	Maculipennis
peryassui	*Anopheles*	Laticorn	Arribalzagia		
petragnani	*Anopheles*	Angusticorn	Anopheles		
peytoni	*Anopheles*	Angusticorn	Anopheles	Aitkenii	
pharoensis	*Cellia*		Cellia		
philippinensis	*Cellia*		Neocellia	Annularis	
pholidotus	*Kerteszia*				
pictipennis	*Nyssorhynchus*	Argyritarsis	Argyritarsis	Pictipennis	

Species	Subgenus	Section	Series	Group	Subgroup
pilinotum	*Anopheles*	Angusticorn	Anopheles	Aitkenii	
pinjaurensis	*Anopheles*	Angusticorn	Anopheles	Aitkenii	
plumbeus	*Anopheles*	Angusticorn	Anopheles	Plumbeus	
pollicaris	*Anopheles*	Laticorn	Myzorhynchus	Barbirostris	Barbirostris
powderi	*Anopheles*	Angusticorn	Anopheles	Plumbeus	
powelli	*Anopheles*	Angusticorn	Anopheles	Stigmaticus	
pretoriensis	*Cellia*		Neocellia		
pristinus	*Nyssorhynchus*	Myzorhynchella			
pseudobarbirostris	*Anopheles*	Laticorn	Myzorhynchus	Bancroftii	
pseudojamesi	*Cellia*		Neocellia	Jamesii	
pseudomaculipes	*Anopheles*	Laticorn	Arribalzagia		
pseudopictus	*Anopheles*	Laticorn	Myzorhynchus	Hyrcanus	
pseudopunctipennis	*Anopheles*	Angusticorn	Anopheles	Pseudopunctipennis	
pseudosinensis	*Anopheles*	Laticorn	Myzorhynchus	Hyrcanus	Nigerrimus
pseudostigmaticus	*Anopheles*	Angusticorn	Anopheles	Stigmaticus	
pseudosundaicus	*Cellia*		Pyretophorus		
pseudotibiamaculatus	*Lophopodomyia*				
pseudowillmori	*Cellia*		Neocellia	Maculatus	
pujutensis	*Cellia*		Neomyzomyia	Leucosphyrus	Hackeri
pulcherrimus	*Cellia*		Neocellia		
pullus	*Anopheles*	Laticorn	Myzorhynchus	Hyrcanus	
punctimacula	*Anopheles*	Laticorn	Arribalzagia		
punctipennis	*Anopheles*	Angusticorn	Anopheles	Punctipennis	
punctulatus	*Cellia*		Neomyzomyia	Punctulatus	
pursati	*Anopheles*	Laticorn	Myzorhynchus	Hyrcanus	Nigerrimus
quadriannulatus	*Cellia*		Pyretophorus		
quadrimaculatus	*Anopheles*	Angusticorn	Anopheles	Maculipennis	Quadrimaculatus
rachoui	*Anopheles*	Laticorn	Arribalzagia		
radama	*Cellia*		Neomyzomyia	Pauliani	
rageaui	*Cellia*		Neomyzomyia	Smithii	
rampae	*Cellia*		Neocellia	Maculatus	Sawadwongporni

Species	Subgenus	Section	Series	Group	Subgroup
ranci	*Cellia*		Neomyzomyia	Ranci	Ranci
rangeli	*Nyssorhynchus*	Albimanus	Oswaldoi	Oswaldoi	Oswaldoi
recens	*Cellia*		Neomyzomyia	Leucosphyrus	Hackeri
reidi	*Anopheles*	Laticorn	Myzorhynchus	Barbirostris	Vanus
rennellensis	*Cellia*		Neomyzomyia	Punctulatus	
rhodesiensis	*Cellia*		Neomyzomyia	Rhodesiensis	
riparis	*Cellia*		Neomyzomyia	Leucosphyrus	Riparis
rivulorum	*Cellia*		Myzomyia	Funestus	Rivulorum
rodhaini	*Cellia*				
rollai	*Kerteszia*				
rondoni	*Nyssorhynchus*	Albimanus	Oswaldoi	Oswaldoi	Strodei
roperi	*Anopheles*	Laticorn	Myzorhynchus	Umbrosus	Letifer
roubaudi	*Cellia*		Neomyzomyia	Ranci	Roubaudi
ruarinus	*Cellia*		Neomyzomyia	Rhodesiensis	
rufipes	*Cellia*		Neocellia		
sacharovi	*Anopheles*	Angusticorn	Anopheles	Maculipennis	Maculipennis
salbaii	*Cellia*		Neocellia		
samarensis	*Anopheles*	Laticorn	Myzorhynchus	Umbrosus	
sanctielii	*Nyssorhynchus*	Albimanus	Oswaldoi	Oswaldoi	Oswaldoi
saperoi	*Anopheles*	Laticorn	Myzorhynchus	Albotaeniatus	
saungi	*Cellia*		Neomyzomyia		
sawadwongporni	*Cellia*		Neocellia	Maculatus	Sawadwongporni
sawyeri	*Nyssorhynchus*	Argyritarsis	Argyritarsis	Argyritarsis	
scanloni	*Cellia*		Neomyzomyia	Leucosphyrus	Leucosphyrus
schueffneri	*Cellia*		Neocellia	Annularis	
schwetzi	*Cellia*		Myzomyia		
separatus	*Anopheles*	Laticorn	Myzorhynchus	Umbrosus	Separatus
seretsei	*Cellia*		Paramyzomyia	Listeri	
sergentii	*Cellia*		Myzomyia	Demeilloni	
seydeli	*Cellia*		Myzomyia	Marshallii	
shannoni	*Anopheles*	Laticorn	Arribalzagia		

http://dx.doi.org/10.5772/54695

Species	Subgenus	Section	Series	Group	Subgroup
similissimus	*Anopheles*	Laticorn	Myzorhynchus	Umbrosus	
sinensis	*Anopheles*	Laticorn	Myzorhynchus	Hyrcanus	
sineroides	*Anopheles*	Laticorn	Myzorhynchus	Hyrcanus	
sintoni	*Anopheles*	Angusticorn	Anopheles	Culiciformis	
sintonoides	*Anopheles*	Angusticorn	Anopheles	Culiciformis	
smaragdinus	*Anopheles*	Angusticorn	Anopheles	Maculipennis	Quadrimaculatus
smithii	*Cellia*		Neomyzomyia	Smithii	
solomonis	*Cellia*		Neomyzomyia		
somalicus	*Cellia*		Neomyzomyia	Ardensis	
splendidus	*Cellia*		Neocellia	Jamesii	
squamifemur	*Lophopodomyia*				
squamosus	*Cellia*		Cellia	Squamosus	
stephensi	*Cellia*		Neocellia		
stigmaticus	*Anopheles*	Angusticorn	Anopheles	Stigmaticus	
stookesi	*Cellia*		Neomyzomyia		
stricklandi	*Anopheles*	Angusticorn	Anopheles	Aitkenii	
strodei	*Nyssorhynchus*	Albimanus	Oswaldoi	Oswaldoi	Strodei
subpictus	*Cellia*		Pyretophorus	Subpictus	
sulawesi	*Cellia*		Neomyzomyia	Leucosphyrus	Hackeri
sundaicus	*Cellia*		Pyretophorus	Ludlowae	
superpictus	*Cellia*		Neocellia		
swahilicus	*Cellia*		Cellia		
symesi	*Anopheles*	Laticorn	Myzorhynchus	Coustani	
takasagoensis	*Cellia*		Neomyzomyia	Leucosphyrus	Leucosphyrus
tasmaniensis	*Anopheles*	Angusticorn	Anopheles	Atratipes	
tchekedii	*Cellia*		Myzomyia		
tenebrosus	*Anopheles*	Laticorn	Myzorhynchus	Coustani	
tessellatus	*Cellia*		Neomyzomyia	Tessellatus	
theileri	*Cellia*		Myzomyia	Wellcomei	
theobaldi	*Cellia*		Neocellia		
thomasi	*Stethomyia*				

Species	Subgenus	Section	Series	Group	Subgroup
tibiamaculatus	*Anopheles*	Angusticorn	Anopheles	Pseudopunctipennis	
tigertti	*Anopheles*	Angusticorn	Anopheles	Aitkenii	
torresiensis	*Cellia*		Neomyzomyia	Punctulatus	
triannulatus	*Nyssorhynchus*	Albimanus	Oswaldoi	Triannulatus	
trinkae	*Nyssorhynchus*	Albimanus	Oswaldoi	Oswaldoi	Oswaldoi
turkhudi	*Cellia*		Paramyzomyia	Cinereus	
umbrosus	*Anopheles*	Laticorn	Myzorhynchus	Umbrosus	Umbrosus
vagus	*Cellia*		Pyretophorus	Subpictus	
vaneedeni	*Cellia*		Myzomyia	Funestus	Funestus
vanhoofi	*Cellia*		Neomyzomyia	Smithii	
vanus	*Anopheles*	Laticorn	Myzorhynchus	Barbirostris	Vanus
vargasi	*Lophopodomyia*				
varuna	*Cellia*		Myzomyia	Funestus	Aconitus
vernus	*Cellia*		Neomyzomyia	Ardensis	
veruslanei	*Anopheles*	Laticorn	Arribalzagia		
vestitipennis	*Anopheles*	Laticorn	Arribalzagia		
vietnamensis	*Anopheles*	Laticorn	Myzorhynchus	Hyrcanus	Lesteri
vinckei	*Cellia*		Neomyzomyia	Ardensis	
walkeri	*Anopheles*	Angusticorn	Anopheles	Maculipennis	
walravensi	*Cellia*		Myzomyia		
watsonii	*Cellia*		Neomyzomyia		
wellcomei	*Cellia*		Myzomyia	Wellcomei	
wellingtonianus	*Anopheles*	Angusticorn	Anopheles	Lindesayi	
whartoni	*Anopheles*	Laticorn	Myzorhynchus	Umbrosus	Letifer
willmori	*Cellia*		Neocellia	Maculatus	
wilsoni	*Cellia*		Neomyzomyia	Smithii	
xelajuensis	*Anopheles*	Angusticorn	Anopheles	Plumbeus	
xui	*Anopheles*	Laticorn	Myzorhynchus	Hyrcanus	
yaeyamaensis	*Cellia*		Myzomyia	Funestus	Minimus
ziemanni	*Anopheles*	Laticorn	Myzorhynchus	Coustani	

Appendix 3

Sibling species complexes of *Anopheles* – formally named and unnamed species. The Maculatus, Maculipennis and Punctulatus Complexes are now considered to be super-complexes referred to as "Groups" with subordinate complexes. Likewise, the Culicifacies Complex is considered to be a Subgroup.

Subgenus *Anopheles*

Barbirostris Complex [76]
barbirostris
Claviger Complex [67]
claviger
petragnani
Crucians Complex [72]
bradleyi
crucians A
crucians B
crucians C
crucians D
crucians E
georgianus
Gigas Complex [70]
baileyi
gigas
gigas s.l.
Lindesayi Complex [70]
lindesayi
mengalangensis
nilgiricus
wellingtonianus
Maculipennis Group [20]
atropos
aztecus
lewisi
walkeri
Maculipennis Subgroup [71]
artemievi
atroparvus
daciae
labranchiae
maculipennis
martinius
melanoon
messeae
persiensis
sacharovi
Quadrimaculatus Subgroup [21]
beklemishevi
diluvialis
inundatus
maverlius
quadrimaculatus
smaragdinus
Freeborni Subgroup [71]
earlei
freeborni
hermsi
occidentalis

Subgenus *Cellia*

Annularis Complex [86]
annularis A
annularis B
pallidus
philippinensis
schueffneri
Annulipes Complex [89]
annulipes A
annulipes B
annulipes C
annulipes D
annulipes F
annulipes G
annulipes H
annulipes I
annulipes J
annulipes K
annulipes L
annulipes M
annulipes N
annulipes O
annulipes P
annulipes Q
Culicifacies Subgroup [108]
culicifacies A
culicifacies B
culicifacies C
culicifacies D
culicifacies E
Dirus Complex [93]
aff. *takasagoensis*
baimaii
cracens
dirus
elegans
nemophilous
scanloni
takasagoensis
Fluviatilis Complex [83]
fluviatilis S
fluviatilis T
fluviatilis U
Gambiae Complex [96]
arabiensis
bwambae
comorensis
gambiae
melas
merus
quadriannulatus
quadriannulatus B
Leucosphyrus Complex [91]
baisasi
balabacensis
introlatus
latens
leucosphyrus
Longirostris Complex [90]
Genotype A
Genotype B
Genotype C1
Genotype C2
Genotype D
Genotype E
Genotype F
Genotype G
Genotype H
Lungae Complex [47]
lungae
nataliae
solomonis
Maculatus Group [88]
dispar
greeni
pseudowillmori
willmori
Maculatus Subgroup [73]
dravidicus
maculatus
Sawadwongporni Subgroup [73]
notanandai
rampae
sawadwongporni
Marshallii Complex [85]
hughi
kosiensis
letabensis
marshallii
Minimus Complex [84]
harrisoni
minimus
yaeyamaensis
Nivipes Complex [70,87]
nivipes cytotype 1
nivipes cytotype 2
Nili Complex [22]
carnevalei
nili
ovengensis
somalicus
Punctulatus Group [94]
clowi
koliensis
punctulatus
rennellensis
sp. nr *punctulatus*
Farauti Complex [94,109]
farauti
farauti 4
farauti 5
farauti 6
farauti 8
hinesorum
irenicus
torresiensis
Subpictus Complex [95]
subpictus A
subpictus B
subpictus C
subpictus D
Sundaicus Complex [97]
epiroticus
sundaicus
sundaicus B
sundaicus C
sundaicus D
sundaicus E
Superpictus Complex [110]
superpictus A
superpictus B

Subgenus *Kerteszia*

Cruzii Complex [101]
cruzii A
cruzii B
cruzii C

Subgenus *Nyssorhynchus*

Albitarsis Complex [106]
albitarsis
albitarsis F
albitarsis G
albitarsis H
albitarsis I
deaneorum
janconnae
lineage nr *janconnae*
marajoara
oryzalimnetes
Benarrochi Complex [105]
benarrochi
benarrochi B
Nuneztovari Complex [104,111]
goeldii
nuneztovari B/C
nuneztovari A
Triannulatus Complex [112,113]
halophylus
triannulatus
triannulatus C

Appendix 4

Unnamed and provisionally designated members of species complexes and their position in the classification of genus *Anopheles* (Sections of subgenera *Anopheles* and *Nyssorhynchus* are omitted). Excluding nominotypical members, the list includes 72 species that require formal Latin names.

Species	Authors	Subgenus	Series	Group	Subgroup	Complex
albitarsis sp. F,G,H,I	[114,115]	*Nyssorhynchus*	Albitarsis	Albitarsis		Albitarsis
annularis sp. A,B	[86]	*Cellia*	Neocellia	Annularis		Annularis
annulipes sp. A–Q	[89]	*Cellia*	Neomyzomyia			Annulipes
Anopheles CP Form	[116]	*Nyssorhynchus*	Oswaldoi	Oswaldoi	Strodei	
barbirostris clades I–IV	[117]	*Anopheles*	Barbirostris	Barbirostris	Barbirostris	Barbirostris
benarrochi sp. B	[105]	*Nyssorhynchus*	Oswaldoi	Oswaldoi	Strodei	Benarrochi
crucians sp. A–E	[72]	*Anopheles*	Anopheles	Punctipennis		Crucians
cruzii sp. A,B,C	[118]	*Kerteszia*				
culicifacies sp. A–E	[108]	*Cellia*	Myzomyia	Funestus	Culicifacies	Culicifacies
farauti sp. 4,5,6	[109,119]	*Cellia*	Neomyzomyia	Punctulatus		Farauti
fluviatilis sp. S,T,U	[83]	*Cellia*	Myzomyia	Funestus	Minimus	Fluviatilis
funestus-like sp.	[120]	*Cellia*	Myzomyia	Funestus	Funestus	
gigas s.l. (Thailand)	[70]	*Anopheles*	Anopheles	Lindesayi		Gigas
hyrcanus sp_{IR}	[121]	*Anopheles*		Hyrcanus		
janconnae, lineage nr	[122]	*Nyssorhynchus*	Albitarsis	Albitarsis		Albitarsis
longipalpis Type A	[123]	*Cellia*	Myzomyia	Funestus	Minimus	
longipalpis Type C	[123]	*Cellia*	Myzomyia	Funestus	Funestus	
longirostris Genotypes A,B,C1,C2,D,E,F,G,H	[90]	Cellia	Neomyzomyia			Longirostris
marajoara lineages 1,2	[124]	*Nyssorhynchus*	Albitarsis	Albitarsis		Albitarsis
nivipes (2 cytotypes)	[87]	*Cellia*	Neocellia	Annularis		Nivipes
nuneztovari sp. A	[125]	*Nyssorhynchus*	Oswaldoi	Oswaldoi	Oswaldoi	Nuneztovari
nuneztovari B/C	[104]	*Nyssorhynchus*	Oswaldoi	Oswaldoi	Oswaldoi	Nuneztovari
punctulatus, sp. nr	[126]	*Cellia*	Neomyzomyia	Punctulatus		

Species	Authors	Subgenus	Series	Group	Subgroup	Complex
quadriannulatus sp. B	[127]	*Cellia*	Pyretophorus			Gambiae
subpictus sp. A-D	[99]	*Cellia*	Pyretophorus	Subpictus		Subpictus
sundaicus sp. B-E	[98,128]	*Cellia*	Pyretophorus	Ludlowae		Sundaicus
superpictus sp. A,B	[110,129]	*Cellia*	Neocellia			Superpictus
takasagoensis, aff.	[130]	*Cellia*	Neomyzomyia	Leucosphyrus	Leucosphyrus	Dirus
triannulatus sp. C	[113]	*Nyssorhynchus*	Oswaldoi	Triannulatus		Triannulatus

Appendix 5

Phylogenetic studies of *Anopheles* mosquitoes. Groups included in the table are those recognized herein. None of the studies included all taxa that comprise the group investigated, but those marked with an asterisk (*) included the majority of species. Nucleotide sequences include *COI, COII, cyt b, ND4, ND5* and *ND6* from mitochondrial DNA (mtDNA); *D2, D3, 18S, ITS1* and *ITS2* from ribosomal DNA (rDNA); *EF-1α*, G_6pd and *white* from nuclear DNA.

Group	Data set	Authors
Genus *Anopheles*	Morphology	[40]
		[36]
	cyt b, ND5, D2	[38]
	ND5, D2, G_6pd*, white*	[39]
	COI, COII, D2	[41]
	18S	[131]
Subgenus *Anopheles*	Morphology	[42]
	COII	[37]
Anopheles Series		
Maculipennis Group	Chromosomes	[132]
	ITS2	[71]* [133,134]
Maculipennis Subgroup	*ITS2*	[135]
Freeborni and Quadrimaculatus Subgroups	*D2*	[136]
Myzorhynchus Series	*ITS2, COI, COII*	[137,139]
Barbirostris Complex	*ITS2, COI*	[117]
Hyrcanus Grou	*ITS2*	[139,140] [141]*

Group	Data set	Authors
	ITS2, COI	[142]
Subgenus *Cellia*	Chromosomes	[143,144]
	COII	[37]
Myzomyia Series	Chromosomes	[143,144]
	COII, D3	[82]
Funestus Group	*ITS2, COII, D3*	[55]*
	COII, D3	[81]*
Minimus Subgroup	*COII, D3*	[145]
Minimus Complex	*D3, ITS2*	[146]*
Neocellia Series	Chromosomes	[87]
Annularis Group	*ITS2, COII, D3, ND5*	[147]
	D3, ITS2	[148]
Maculatus Group	*ITS2, COII, D3*	[149–151]
Neomyzomyia Series	*ITS2, COI, COII, EF-1α*	[89]
Annulipes Complex	*COI, ND6*	[152]
Leucosphyrus Group		
Punctulatus Group	*ITS2*	[153]
	18S	[154]
Farauti Complex	*ITS1*	[109]
Pyretophorus Series	Morphology	[56]*
	Chromosomes	[144]
	COII	[37]
Gambiae Complex	Chromosomes	[155]
	rDNA, mtDNA	[156]
Sundaicus Complex	mtDNA	[157]
	ITS2, D2, COI, ND4	[158]
	white	[114]
	cyt b, ITS2, COI	[128]
Subgenus *Kerteszia*	Morphology	[44]
Subgenus *Nyssorhynchus*	*ITS2*	[159]
Albimanus Section	Morphology	[24]
Argyritarsis Section	Morphology	[25]
Myzorhynchella Section	*ITS2, COI, white*	[160]

Appendix 6

Summary of the formal and informal group taxa (species complexes omitted) of genus *Anopheles*. The zoogeographic distribution and the number of formally named and informally designated species (in parentheses) are given for each taxon. Minor extensions of one or more species of a group into an adjacent zoogeographic region are disregarded. C = cosmopolitan; NW = New World; OW = Old World; Af = Afrotropical; Au = Australasian; Ne = Nearctic; Nt = Neotropical; Or = Oriental; Pa = Palaearctic.

Subgenus *Anopheles* – C (191)
Angusticorn Section – OW, NW (95)
Anopheles Series – OW and NW (88)
Alongensis Group – Or (2)
Aitkenii Group – Or (13)
Atratipes Group – Au (2)
Culiciformis Group – Or (3)
Lindesayi Group – Or (7)
Maculipennis Group – Ne, Pa (20)
Maculipennis Subgroup – Pa (10)
Quadrimaculatus Subgroup – Ne (5), Pa (1)
Freeborni Subgroup – Ne (4)
Plumbeus Group – Ne (2), Nt (4), Pac (3)
Pseudopunctipennis Group – Ne (7)
Punctipennis Group – Ne (9)
Stigmaticus Group – Au (6)
Cycloleppteron Series – Ne (2)
Lophoscelomyia Series – Or (4)
Unassigned – (1)
Asiaticus Group – (4)
Unassigned – (2)
Asiaticus Subgroup – (1)
Interruptus Subgroup – (1)
Laticorn Section – Af, Au, Nt, Or, Pa (96)
Arribalzagia Series – Ne (24)
Christya Series – Af (2)
Myzorhynchus Series – Af, Au, Or, Pa (70)
Albotaeniatus Group – Or (4), Pa (1)
Bancroftii Group – Au/Or (2)
Barbirostris Group – Or (16)
Unassigned – (2)
Barbirostris Subgroup – (9)
Vanus Subgroup – (5)
Coustani Group – Af (9)
Hyrcanus Group – Pa (26)
Unassigned – (17)
Lesteri Subgroup – (5)
Nigerrimus Subgroup – (4)
Umbrosus Group – Or (12)
Unassigned – (5)
Baezai Subgroup – (1)
Letifer Subgroup – (4)
Separatus Subgroup – (1)
Umbrosus Subgroup – (1)

Subgenus *Baimaia* – Or (1)

Subgenus *Cellia* – OW (233)
Cellia Series – Af (8)
Unassigned – (6)
Squamosus Group – (2)
Myzomyia Series – Af, Or (71)
Unassigned – Af (16)
Demeilloni Group – Af (7)
Funestus Group – Af, Or (29)
Unassigned – (1)
Aconitus Subgroup – Or (5)
Culicifacies Subgroup – Or (5)
Funestus Subgroup – Af (7)
Minimus Subgroup – Af (1), Or (6)
Rivulorum Subgroup – Af (4)
Marshallii Group – Af (15)
Wellcomei Group – Af (4)
Neocellia Series – Af, Or, Pal (24)
Unassigned – Af, Or, Pa (14)
Annularis Group – Or (7)
Jamesii Group – Or (3)
Maculatus Group – Or (9)
Unassigned – (4)
Maculatus Subgroup – (2)
Sawadwongporni Subgroup – (3)
Neomyzomyia Series – Af, Au, Or (121)
Unassigned – Af, Au, Or (42)
Ardensis Group – Af (18)
Kochi Group – Or (1)
Leucosphyrus Group – O (21)
Hackeri Subgroup – (5)
Leucosphyrus Subgroup – (13)
Riparis Subgroup – (3)
Mascarensis Group – Af (1)
Pauliani Group – Af (5)
Punctulatus Group – Au (13)
Ranci Group – Af (5)
Unassigned – (1)
Ranci Subgroup – (1)
Roubaudi Subgroup – (3)
Rhodesiensis Group – Af (5)
Smithii Group – Af (9)
Tessellatus Group – Or (1)
Paramyzomyia Series – Af, Pa (6)
Cinereus Group – Af (2), Pa (1)
Listeri Group – Af (2), Pa (1
Pyretophorus Series – Af (10), Or (12)

Subgenus *Kerteszia* – Nt (14)

Subgenus *Lophopodomyia* – Nt (6)

Subgenus *Nyssorhynchus* – Nt (38)
Albimanus Section – (24)
Albimanus Series – (1)
Oswaldoi Series – (23)
Oswaldoi Group – (21)
Oswaldoi Subgroup – (14)
Strodei Subgroup – (7)
Triannulatus Group – (3)
Argyritarsis Section – (14)
Albitarsis Series – (8)
Albitarsis Group – (7)
Braziliensis Group – (1)
Argyritarsis Series – (6)
Argyritarsis Group – (2)
Darlingi Group – (1)
Lanei Group – (1)
Pictipennis Group – (2)
Myzorhynchella Section – (6)

Subgenus *Stethomyia* – Ne (5)

Author details

Ralph E. Harbach*

Address all correspondence to: r.harbach@nhm.ac.uk

Department of Life Sciences, Natural History Museum, London, UK

Three new species of *Anopheles* were formally described and named while the book was in press: *An.* (*Anopheles*) *vanderwulpi* (= *An. barbirostris* clade II) [161]; *An.* (*Cellia*) *amharicus* (= *An. quadriannulatus* sp. B) and *An.* (*Cellia*) *coluzzii* (= molecular M form of *An. gambiae*) [162]. *Anopheles* (*Anopheles*) *kunmingensis* (Laticorn Section, Myzorhynchus Series, Hyrcanus Group) was inadvertently omitted from Appendix 2 during preparation of the chapter. Thus, the genus now includes 469 formally named species and 70 species that require formal Latin names.

References

[1] Meigen JW. Systematische Beschreibung der bekannten europäischen zweiflügeligen Insekten. Volume 1. Aachen; 1818.

[2] Theobald FV. A Monograph of the Culicidae or Mosquitoes. Volume 1. London: British Museum (Natural History); 1901.

[3] Theobald FV. A Monograph of the Culicidae or Mosquitoes. Volume 2. London: British Museum (Natural History); 1901.

[4] Theobald FV. A Monograph of the Culicidae or Mosquitoes. Volume 3. London: British Museum (Natural History); 1903.

[5] Theobald FV. A Monograph of the Culicidae or Mosquitoes. Volume 4. London: British Museum (Natural History); 1907.

[6] Theobald FV. A Monograph of the Culicidae or Mosquitoes. Volume 5. London: British Museum (Natural History); 1910.

[7] Knight KL, Stone A. A catalog of the mosquitoes of the world (Diptera: Culicidae). Second edition. Thomas Say Foundation 1977;6 1–611.

[8] Knab F. The species *of Anopheles* that transmit human malaria. American Journal of Tropical Diseases and Preventive Medicine 1913;1 33–43.

[9] Christophers SR. The male genitalia of *Anopheles*. Indian Journal of Medical Research 1915;3 371–394.

[10] Edwards FW. A revision of the mosquitos [*sic*] of the Palaearctic Region. Bulletin of Entomological Research 1921;12 263–351.

[11] Root FM. The male genitalia of some American *Anopheles* mosquitoes. American Journal of Hygiene 1923;31 264–279.

[12] Edwards FW. Genera Insectortum. Diptera, Fam. Culicidae. Fascicle 194. Bruxelles: Desmet-Verteneuil; 1932.

[13] Komp WHW. The species of the subgenus *Kerteszia* of *Anopheles* (Diptera, Culicidae). Annals of the Entomological Society of America 1937;30 492–529.

[14] Antunes PCA. A new *Anopheles* and a new *Goeldia* from Colombia (Dipt. Culic.). Bulletin of Entomological Research 1937;28 69–73.

[15] Harbach RE, Rattanarithikul R, Harrison BA. *Baimaia*, a new subgenus for *Anopheles kyondawensis* Abraham, a unique crabhole-breeding anopheline in southeastern Asia. Proceedings of the Entomological Society of Washington 2005;107 750–761.

[16] Harbach RE. Mosquito Taxonomic Inventory. http://mosquito-taxonomic-inventory.info/ (accessed on 1 April 2013).

[17] Mayr E, Bock WJ. Classifications and other ordering systems. Journal of Zoological Systematics and Evolutionary Research 2002;40 169–194.

[18] Harbach RE, Kitching IJ. Phylogeny and classification of the Culicidae (Diptera). Systematic Entomology 1998;23 327–370.

[19] International Commission on Zoological Nomenclature. International Code of Zoological Nomenclature. Fourth Edition. London: International Trust for Zoological Nomenclature; 1999.

[20] Reid JA, Knight KL. Classification within the subgenus *Anopheles* (Diptera, Culicidae). Annals of Tropical Medicine and Parasitology 1961;55 474–488.

[21] Grjebine A. Faune de Madagascar. XXII. Insecies Diptéres Culicidae Anophelinae. Paris: Centre National de la Recherche Scientifique, Office de la Recherche Scientifique et Technique Outre-Mer; 1966.

[22] Gillies MT, de Meillon B. The Anophelinae of Africa South of the Sahara (Ethiopian Zoogeographical Region). Publications of the South African Institute for Medical Research 1968;54 1–343.

[23] Reid JA. Anopheline mosquitoes of Malaya and Borneo. Studies from the Institute for Medical Research Malaya 1968;31 1–520.

[24] Faran ME. Mosquito studies (Diptera, Culicidae) XXXIV. A revision of the Albimanus Section of the subgenus *Nyssorhynchus* of *Anopheles*. Contributions of the American Entomological Institute 1980;15(7) 1–215.

[25] Linthicum KJ. A revision of the Argyritarsis Section of the subgenus *Nyssorhynchus* of *Anopheles* (Diptera: Culicidae). Mosquito Systematics 1988;20 98–271.

[26] Harbach RE. Review of the internal classification of the genus *Anopheles* (Diptera: Culicidae): the foundation for comparative systematics and phylogenetic research. Bulletin of Entomological Research 1994;84 331–342.

[27] Harbach RE. The classification of genus *Anopheles* (Diptera: Culicidae): a working hypothesis of phylogenetic relationships. Bulletin of Entomological Research 2004;94 537–553.

[28] Peyton EL, Wilkerson RC, Harbach RE. Comparative analysis of the subgenera *Kerteszia* and *Nyssorhynchus* of *Anopheles* (Diptera: Culicidae). Mosquito Systematics 1992;24 51–69.

[29] Borkent A, Grimaldi DA. The earliest fossil mosquito (Diptera: Culicidae), in mid-Cretaceous amber. Annals of the Entomological Society of America 2004;97 882–888.

[30] Bertone MA, Courtney GW, Wiegmann BM. Phylogenetics and temporal diversification of the earliest true flies (Insecta: Diptera) based on multiple nuclear genes. Systematic Entomology 2008;33 668–687.

[31] Poinar Jr JO, Zavortink TJ, Pike T, Johnston PA. *Paleoculicis minutus* (Diptera: Culicidae) n. gen., n. sp., from Cretaceous Canadian amber, with a summary of described fossil mosquitoes. Acta Geologica Hispanica 2000;35 119–128.

[32] Zavortink TJ, Poinar Jr GO. *Anopheles* (*Nyssorhynchus*) *dominicanus* sp. n. (Diptera: Culicidae) from Dominican amber. Annals of the Entomological Society of America 2000;93 1230–1235.

[33] Statz G. Neue Dipteren (Nematocera) aus dem Oberoligocän von Rott. II. Teil. V. Familie Culicidae (Stechmücken). Palaeontographica 1944;95(A) 108–120, 6 pls.

[34] Reidenbach KR, Cook S, Bertone MA, Harbach RE, Wiegmann BM, Besansky NJ. Phylogenetic analysis and temporal diversification of mosquitoes (Diptera: Culicidae) based on nuclear genes and morphology. BMC Evolutionary Biology 2009;9 298.

[35] Besansky NJ, Fahey GT. Utility of the *white* gene in estimating phylogenetic relationships among mosquitoes (Diptera: Culicidae). Molecular Biology and Evolution 1997;14 442–454.

[36] Harbach RE, Kitching IJ. Reconsideration of anopheline phylogeny (Diptera: Culicidae: Anophelinae) based on morphological data. Systematics and Biodiversity 2005;3 345–374.

[37] Foley DH, Bryan JH, Yeates D, Saul A. Evolution and systematics of *Anopheles*: insights from a molecular phylogeny of Australasian mosquitoes. Molecular Phylogenetics and Evolution 1998;9 262–275.

[38] Krzywinski J, Wilkerson RC, Besansky N. Evolution of mitochondrial and ribosomal gene sequences in Anophelinae (Diptera: Culicidae): implications for phylogeny reconstruction. Molecular Phylogenetics and Evolution 2001;18 479–487.

[39] Krzywinski J, Wilkerson RC, Besansky N. Toward understanding Anophelinae (Diptera, Culicidae) phylogeny: insights from nuclear single copy genes and the weight of evidence. Systematic Biology 2001;50 540–556.

[40] Sallum MAM, Schultz TR, Wilkerson RC. Phylogeny of Anophelinae (Diptera Culicidae) based on morphological characters. Annals of the Entomological Society of America 2000;93 745–775.

[41] Sallum MAM, Schultz TR, Foster PG, Aronstein K, Wirtz RA, Wilkerson RC. Phylogeny of Anophelinae (Diptera: Culicidae) based on nuclear ribosomal and mitochondrial DNA sequences. Systematic Entomology 2002;27 361–382.

[42] Collucci E, Sallum MAM. Cladistic analysis of the subgenus *Anopheles* (*Anopheles*) Meigen (Diptera: Culicidae) based on morphological characters. Memórias do Instituto Oswaldo Cruz 2007;102 277–291.

[43] Harrison BA, Scanlon JE. Medical entomology studies – II. The subgenus *Anopheles* in Thailand (Diptera: Culicidae). Contributions of the American Entomological Institute 1975;12(1) iv + 1–307.

[44] Collucci E, Sallum MAM. Phylogenetic analysis of the subgenus *Kerteszia* of *Anopheles* (Diptera: Culicidae: Anophelinae) based on morphological characters. Insect Systematics and Evolution 2003;34 361–372.

[45] Merali Z, Skinner BJ. Visualizing Earth Science. John Wiley: Hoboken, New Jersey; 2009.

[46] Valencio D, Vilas JF. Age of the separation of South America and Africa. Nature 1969;223 1353–1354.

[47] Belkin JN. The Mosquitoes of the South Pacific *(Diptera, Culicidae)* [*sic*]. Volumes I and II. Berkeley & Los Angeles: University of California Press; 1962.

[48] Christophers SR. The fauna of British India, Including Ceylon and Burma. Diptera. Vol. IV. Family Culicidae. Tribe Anophelini. London, Taylor and Francis; 1933.

[49] Zavortink TJ. Mosquito studies (Diptera, Culicidae) XXIX. A review of the subgenus *Kerteszia* of *Anopheles*. Contributions of the American Entomological Institute 1973;9(3) 1–54.

[50] Smith AB. Systematics and the Fossil Record: Documenting Evolutionary Patterns. Oxford: Blackwell Scientific Publications; 1994.

[51] Christophers SR, Barraud PJ. The eggs of Indian *Anopheles* with descriptions of the hitherto undescribed eggs of a number of species. Records of the Malaria Survey of India 1931;2 161–192.

[52] Mattingly PF. The Biology of Mosquito-Borne Disease. The Science of Biology Series 1. London: George Allen & Unwin Ltd; 1969.

[53] Sinka ME, Bangs MJ, Manguin S, Coetzee M, Mbogo CM, Hemingway J, Patil AP, Temperley WH, Gething PW, Kabaria CW, Okara RM, Van Boeckel T, Godfray HCJ, Harbach RE, Hay SI. The dominant *Anopheles* vectors of human malaria in Africa, Europe and the Middle East: occurrence data, distribution maps and bionomic précis. Parasites & Vectors 2010;3 117.

[54] Sinka ME, Bangs MJ, Manguin S, Chareonviriyaphap T, Patil AP, Temperley WH, Gething PW, Elyazar IRF, Kabaria CW, Harbach RE, Hay SI. The dominant *Anopheles* vectors of human malaria in the Asia-Pacific region: occurrence data, distribution maps and bionomic précis. Parasites & Vectors 2011;4 89.

[55] Garros C, Harbach RE, Manguin S. Systematics and biogeographical implications of the phylogenetic relationships between members of the Funestus and Minimus Groups of *Anopheles* (Diptera: Culicidae). Journal of Medical Entomology 2005;42 7–18.

[56] Anthony TG, Harbach RE, Kitching IJ. Phylogeny of the Pyretophorus Series of *Anopheles* subgenus *Cellia* (Diptera: Culicidae). Systematic Entomology 1999;24 193–205.

[57] Evans AM. Mosquitoes of the Ethiopian Region. II.–Anophelini adults and early stages. London: British Museum (Natural History); 1938.

[58] Gillies MT. Notes on the eggs of some East African *Anopheles*. Annals of Tropical Medicine and Parasitology 1955;49 158–160.

[59] Mattingly PF. Mosquito eggs III. Mosquito Systematics Newsletter 1969;1 41–50.

[60] Stringer C. The Origin of our Species. London: Penguin Books Ltd; 2011.

[61] Sinka ME, Rubio-Palis Y, Manguin S, Patil AP, Temperley WH, Gething PW, Van Boeckel T, Kabaria CW, Harbach R.E, Hay SI. The dominant *Anopheles* vectors of human malaria in the Americas: occurrence data, distribution maps and bionomic précis. Parasites & Vectors 2010;3 72.

[62] Sinka ME, Bangs MJ, Manguin S, Rubio-Palis Y, Chareonviriyaphap T, Coetzee M, Mbogo CM, Hemingway J, Patilm AP, Temperley WH, Gething PW, Kabaria CW, Okara RM, Burkot TR, Harbach RE, Hay SI. A global map of dominant malaria vectors. Parasites & Vectors 2012;5 69.

[63] Besansky NJ, Lehmann T, Fahey GT, Fontenille D, Braack LEO, Hawley WA, Collins FH. Patterns of mitochondrial variation within and between African malaria vectors, *Anopheles gambiae* and *An. arabiensis*, suggest extensive gene flow. Genetics 1997;147 1817–1828.

[64] Thelwell NJ, Huisman RA, Harbach RE, Butlin RK. Evidence for mitochondrial introgression between *Anopheles bwambae* and *Anopheles gambiae*. Insect Molecular Biology 2000;9 203–210.

[65] Walton C, Handley JM, Collins FH, Baimai V, Harbach RE, Deesin V, Butlin RK. Genetic population structure and introgression in *Anopheles dirus* mosquitoes in Southeast Asia. Molecular Ecology 2001;10 569–580.

[66] Van Bortel W, Trung HD, Manh ND, Roelants P, Verlé P, Coosemans M. Identification of two species within the *Anopheles minimus* complex in northern Vietnam and their behavioural divergences. Tropical Medicine and International Health 1999;4 257–265.

[67] Coluzzi M, Sacca G, Feliciangeli D. Il complesso *A. claviger* nella sottoregione mediterranea. Cahiers ORSTROM, série Entomologie médicale et Parasitologie 1965; 97–102.

[68] Vu TP, Nguyen DM,Tran DH, Nguyen NV. *Anopheles* (*Anopheles*) *cucphuongensis*: a new species from Vietnam (Diptera: Culicidae). *Mosquito Systematics* 1990;22 145–148.

[69] Lee DJ, Hicks MM, Griffiths M, Debenham ML, Bryan JH, Russell RC, Geary M, Marks EN. The Culicidae of the Australasian Region. Volume 5. Nomenclature, synonymy, literature, distribution, biology and relation to disease. Genus *Anopheles*. Subgenera *Anopheles, Cellia*. Monograph Series, Entomology Monograph No. 2. Canberra: Australian Government Publishing Service; 1987.

[70] Harrison BA, Rattanarithikul R, Peyton EL, Mongkolpanya K. Taxonomic changes, revised occurrence records and notes on the Culicidae of Thailand and neighboring countries. Mosquito Systematics 1991;22 196–227.

[71] Linton Y. Systematics of the Holarctic *maculipennis* complex. Systematics Symposium: 70th Annual Meeting of the American Mosquito Control Association, February 22–26, 2004, Savannah, Georgia.

[72] Wilkerson RC, Reinert JF, Li C. Ribosomal DNA ITS2 sequences differentiate six species in the *Anopheles crucians* complex (Diptera: Culicidae). Journal of Medical Entomology 2004;41 392–401.

[73] Rattanarithikul R, Harrison BA, Harbach RE, Panthusiri P, Coleman RE. Illustrated Keys to the mosquitoes of Thailand. IV. *Anopheles*. Southeast Asian Journal of Tropical Medicine and Public Health 2006;37(suppl. 2) 1–128.

[74] Root FM. The classification of American *Anopheles* mosquitoes. American Journal of Hygiene 1922;2 321–322.

[75] Christophers SR. Provisional list and reference catalogue of the Anophelini. Indian Medical Research Memoirs 1924;3 1–105.

[76] Satoto TBT. Cryptic species within *Anopheles barbirostris* van der Wulp, 1884, inferred from nuclear and mitochondrial gene sequence variation. PhD Thesis. University of Liverpool; 2001.

[77] Reid JA. The *Anopheles hyrcanus* group in south–east Asia (Diptera: Culicidae). Bulletin of Entomological Research 1953;44 5–76.

[78] Harrison BA. A new interpretation of affinities within the *Anopheles hyrcanus* complex of Southeast Asia. Mosquito Systematics 1972;4 73–83.

[79] Reid JA. The *Anopheles umbrosus* group (Diptera: Culicidae). Part 1: systematics, with descriptions of two new species. Transactions of the Royal Entomological Society of London 1950;101 281–318.

[80] Theobald FV. The classification of the Anophelina. Journal of Tropical Medicine 1902;5 181–183.

[81] Garros C, Harbach RE, Manguin S. Morphological assessment and molecular phylogenetics of the Funestus and Minimus Groups of *Anopheles* (*Cellia*). Journal of Medical Entomology 2005;42 522–536.

[82] Chen B, Butlin RK, Harbach RE. Molecular phylogenetics of the Oriental members of the Myzomyia Series of *Anopheles* subgenus *Cellia* (Diptera: Culicidae) inferred from nuclear and mitochondrial DNA sequences. Systematic Entomology 2003;28 57–69.

[83] Sarala KS, Nutan N, Vasantha K, Dua VK, Malhotra MS, Yadav RS, Sharma VP. Cytogenetic evidence for three sibling species in *Anopheles fluviatilis* (Diptera: Culicidae). Annals of the Entomological Society of America 1994;87 116–121.

[84] Green CA, Gass RF, Munstermann LE, Baimai V. Population-genetic evidence for two species in *Anopheles minimus* in Thailand. Medical and Veterinary Entomology 1990;4 25–34.

[85] Gillies MT, Coetzee M. A supplement to the Anophelinae of Africa south of the Sahara (Afrotropical Region). Publications of the South African Institute for Medical Research 1987;55 1–143.

[86] Atrie B, Subbarao SK, Pillai MKK, Rao SRV, Sharma VP. Population cytogenetic evidence for sibling species in *Anopheles annularis* (Diptera: Culicidae). Annals of the Entomological Society of America 1999;92 243–249.

[87] Green CA, Harrison BA, Klein TA, Baimai V. Cladistic analysis of polytene chromosome rearrangements in anopheline mosquitoes, subgenus *Cellia*, series *Neocellia*. Canadian Journal of Genetics and Cytology 1985;27 123–133.

[88] Rattanarithikul R, Green CA. Formal recognition of the species of the *Anopheles maculatus* group (Diptera: Culicidae) occurring in Thailand, including the descriptions of two new species and a preliminary key to females. Mosquito Systematics 1987;18 246–278.

[89] Foley DH, Wilkerson RC, Cooper RD, Volovsek ME, Bryan JH. A molecular phylogeny of *Anopheles annulipes* (Diptera: Culicidae) sensu lato: The most species-rich anopheline complex. Molecular Phylogenetics and Evolution 2007;43 283–297.

[90] Alquezaar DE, Hemmerter S, Cooper RD, Beebe NW. Incomplete concerted evolution and reproductive isolation at the rDNA locus uncovers nine cryptic species within *Anopheles longirostris* from Papua New Guinea. BMC Evolutionary Biology 2010;10 392.

[91] Reid JA. A preliminary account of the forms of *Anopheles leucosphyrus* Dönitz (Diptera: Culicidae). Proceedings of the Royal Entomological Society of London Series B Taxonomy 1949;18 42–53.

[92] Sallum MAM, Peyton EL, Wilkerson RC. Six new species of the *Anopheles leucosphyrus* group, reinterpretation of *An. elegans* and vector implications. Medical and Veterinary Entomology 2005;19 158–199.

[93] Peyton EL. A new classification for the Leucosphyrus Group of *Anopheles* (*Cellia*). Mosquito Systematics 1990;21 197–205.

[94] Sallum MAM, Peyton EL, Harrison BA, Wilkerson RC. Revision of the Leucosphyrus group of *Anopheles* (*Cellia*) (Diptera, Culicidae). Revista Brasileira de Entomologia 2005;49(Supl. 1) 1–152.

[95] Schmidt ER, Foley DH, Hartel GF, Williams GM, Bryan JH. Descriptions of the *Anopheles* (*Cellia*) *farauti* complex of sibling species (Diptera: Culicidae) in Australia. Bulletin of Entomological Research 2001;91 389–410.

[96] Schmidt ER, Foley DH, Bugoro H, Bryan JH. A morphological study of the *Anopheles punctulatus* group (Diptera: Culicidae) in the Solomon Islands, with a description of *Anopheles* (*Cellia*) *irenicus* Schmidt, sp.n. Bulletin of Entomological Research 2003;93 515–526.

[97] White GB. *Anopheles bwambae* sp.n., a malaria vector in the Semliki Valley, Uganda, and its relationships with other sibling species of the *An. gambiae* complex (Diptera: Culicidae). Systematic Entomology 1985;10 501–522.

[98] Sukowati S, Baimai V, Harun S, Dasuki Y, Andris H, Efriwati M. Isozyme evidence for three sibling species in the *Anopheles sundaicus* complex from Indonesia. Medical and Veterinary Entomology 1999;13 408–414.

[99] Suguna SG, Rathinam KG, Rajavel AR, Dhanda V. Morphological and chromosomal descriptions of new species in the *Anopheles subpictus* complex. Medical and Veterinary Entomology 1994;9 88–94.

[100] Theobald FV. A catalogue of the Culicidae in the Hungarian National Museum, with descriptions of new genera and species. Annales Musei Nationalis Hungarici 1905;3 61–119, figures legends + 4 pls.

[101] Ramirez CC, Dessen EM. Chromosomal evidence for sibling species of the malaria vector *Anopheles cruzii*. Genome 2000;43 143–151.

[102] Blanchard R. Nouvelle note sur les moustiques. Comptes Rendus Hebdomadaires des Séances et Mémoires de la Société de Biologie 1902;54 793–795.

[103] Levi Castillo R. Atlas de los Anofelinos Sudamericanos. Quayaquil, Ecuador: Sociedad Filantrópica de Guayas; 1949.

[104] Sierra DM, Velez ID, Linton Y-M. Malaria vector *Anopheles* (*Nyssorhynchus*) *nuneztovari* comprises one genetic species in Colombia based on homogeneity of nuclear ITS2 rDNA. Journal of Medical Entomology 2004;41 302–307.

[105] Ruiz F, Quiñones ML, Erazo HF, Calle DA, Alzate JF, Linton Y-M. Molecular differentiation of *Anopheles* (*Nyssorhynchus*) *benarrochi* and *An.* (*N.*) *oswaldoi* from Southern Colombia. Memorias do Instituto Oswaldo Cruz 2005;100 155–160.

[106] Wilkerson RC, Parsons TJ, Klein TA, Gaffigan TV, Bergo E, Consolim J. Diagnosis by random amplified polymorphic DNA polymerase chain reaction for four cryptic species related to *Anopheles* (*Nyssorhynchus*) *albitarsis* (Diptera: Culicidae) from Paraguay, Argentina, and Brazil. Journal of Medical Entomology 1995;32 697–704.

[107] Peyton EL, Wilkerson RC, Harbach RE. Comparative analysis of the subgenera *Kerteszia* and *Nyssorhynchus* of *Anopheles* (Diptera: Culicidae). Mosquito Systematics 1992;24 51–69.

[108] Kar I, Subbarao SK, Eapen A, Ravendaran J, Satyanarayana TS, Raghavendra K, Nanda N, Sharma VP. Evidence for a new malaria vector species, species E, within the *Anopheles culicifacies* complex (Diptera: Culicidae). Journal of Medical Entomology 1999;36 595–600.

[109] Bower JE, Dowton M, Cooper RD, Beebe NW. Intraspecific concerted evolution of the rDNA ITS1 in *Anopheles farauti* sensu stricto (Diptera: Culicidae) reveals recent patterns of population structure. Journal of Molecular Evolution 2008;67 397–411.

[110] Oshaghi MA, Yaghobi-Ershadi MR, Shemshad Kh, Pedram M, Amani H. The *Anopheles superpictus* complex: introduction of a new malaria vector complex in Iran. Bulletin de la Société de Pathologie exotique 2008;101 429–434.

[111] Conn J, Puertas YR, Seawright JA. A new cytotype *of Anopheles nuneztovari* from western Venezuela and Colombia. Journal of the American Mosquito Control Association 1993;9 294–301.

[112] Rosa-Freitas MG, Lourenço-de-Oliveira R, de Carvalho-Pinto CJ, Flores-Mendoza F, Silva-do-Nascimento TF. Anopheline species complexes in Brazil. Current knowledge of those related to malaria transmission. Memorias do Instituto Oswaldo Cruz 1998;93 651–655.

[113] Silva-do-Nascimento TR, Lourenço-de-Oliveira R. Diverse population dynamics of three *Anopheles* species belonging to the Triannulatus Complex (Diptera: Culicidae). Memorias do Instituto Oswaldo Cruz 2007;102 975–982.

[114] Brochero HHL, Li C, Wilkerson RC. A newly recognized species in the *Anopheles* (*Nyssorhynchus*) *albitarsis* complex (Diptera: Culicidae) from Puerto Carreño, Colombia. American Journal of Tropical Medicine and Hygiene 2007;76 1113–1117.

[115] Ruiz-Lopez F, Wilkerson RC, Conn JE, McKeon SN, Levin DM, Quiñones ML, Póvoa MM, Linton Y-M. DNA barcoding reveals both known and novel taxa in the Albitarsis Group (*Anopheles*: *Nyssorhynchus*) of Neotropical malaria vectors. Parasites & Vectors 2012;5 44.

[116] Sallum MAM, Foster PG, dos Santos CLS, Flores DC, Motoki MT, Bergo ES. Resurrection of two species from synonymy of *Anopheles* (*Nyssorhynchus*) *strodei* Root, and characterization of a distinct morphological form from the Strodei Complex (Diptera: Culicidae). Journal of Medical Entomology 2010;47 504–526.

[117] Paredes-Esquivel C, Donnelly MJ, Harbach RE, Townson H. A molecular phylogeny of mosquitoes in the *Anopheles barbirostris* subgroup reveals cryptic species: implications for identification of disease vectors. Molecular Phylogenetics and Evolution 2009;50 141–151.

[118] Ramirez CC, Dessen EM. Chromosome differentiated populations of *Anopheles cruzii*: evidence for a third sibling species. Genetica 2000;108 73–80.

[119] Foley DH, Paru R, Dagoro H, Bryan JH. Allozyme analysis reveals six species within the *Anopheles punctulatus* complex of mosquitoes in Papua New Guinea. Medical and Veterinary Entomology 1993;7 37–48.

[120] Spillings BL, Brooke BD, Koekemoer LL, Chiphwanya J, Coetzee M, Hunt RH. A new species concealed by *Anopheles funestus* Giles, a major malaria vector in Africa. American Journal of Tropical Medicine and Hygiene 2009;81 510–515.

[121] Djadid ND, Jazayeri H, Gholizadeh S, Pashaeirad S, Zakeri S. First record of a new member of *Anopheles* Hyrcanus Group from Iran: molecular identification, diagnosis, phylogeny, status of kdr resistance and *Plasmodium* infection. Journal of Medical Entomology 2009;46 1084–1093.

[122] Gutiérrez LA, Orrego LM, Gómez GF, López A, Luckhart S, Conn JE, Correa MM. A new mtDNA COI gene lineage closely related to *Anopheles janconnae* of the Albitarsis complex in the Caribbean region of Colombia. Memorias do Instituto Oswaldo Cruz 2010;105 1019–1025.

[123] Koekemoer LL, Misiani EA, Hunt RH, Kent RJ, Norris DE, Coetzee M. Cryptic species within *Anopheles longipalpis* from southern Africa and phylogenetic comparison with members of the *An. funestus* group. Bulletin of Entomological Research 2009;99 41–49.

[124] McKeon SN, Lehr MA, Wilkerson RC, Ruiz JF, Sallum MA, Povoa MM., Conn JE, Lima JBP. Lineage divergence detected in the malaria vector *Anopheles marajoara* (Diptera: Culicidae) in Amazonian Brazil. Malaria Journal 2010;9 271.

[125] Conn J. A genetic study of the malaria vector *Anopheles nuneztovari* from western Venezuela. Journal of the American Mosquito Control Association 1990;6 400–405.

[126] Foley DH, Cooper RD, Bryan JH. A new species within the *Anopheles punctulatus* complex in Western Province, Papua New Guinea. Journal of the American Mosquito Control Association 1995;11 122–127.

[127] Hunt RH, Coetzee M, Fettene M. The *Anopheles gambiae* complex: a new species from Ethiopia. Transactions of the Royal Society of Tropical Medicine and Hygiene 1998;92 231–235.

[128] Dusfour I, Michaux JR, Harbach RE, Manguin S. Speciation and phylogeography of the Southeast Asian *Anopheles sundaicus* complex. Infection, Genetics and Evolution 2007;7 484–493.

[129] Oshaghi MA, Shemshad Kh, Yaghobi-Ershadi MR, Pedram M, Vatandoost H, Abaie MR, Akbarzadeh K, Mohtarami F. Genetic structure of the malaria vector *Anopheles superpictus* in Iran using mitochondrial cytochrome oxidase (COI and COII) and morphologic markers: A new species complex? Acta Tropica 2007;101 241–248.

[130] Takano KT, Nguyen NTH, Nguyen BTH, Sunahara T, Yasunami, M, Nguyen MD, Takagi M. Partial mitochondrial DNA sequences suggest the existence of a cryptic species within the Leucosphyrus group [*sic*] of the genus *Anopheles* (Diptera: Culicidae), forest malaria vectors, in northern Vietnam. Parasites & Vectors 2010;3 41.

[131] Bargues MD, Latorre JM, Morchon R, Simon F, Escosa R, Aranda C, Sainz S, Fuentes MV, Mas-Coma S. rDNA sequences of *Anopheles* species from the Iberian Peninsula and an evaluation of the 18S rRNA gene as phylogenetic marker in Anophelinae. Journal of Medical Entomology 2006;43 508–517.

[132] White GB. Systematic reappraisal of the *Anopheles maculipennis* complex. Mosquito Systematics 1978;10 13–44.

[133] Gordeev M, Goriacheva I, Shaikevitch E, Ejov M. Variability of the second internal transcribed spacer of the ribosomal DNA among five Palaearctic species of anopheline mosquitoes. European Mosquito Bulletin 2004;17 14–19.

[134] Djadid ND, Gholizadeh S, Tafsiri E, Romi R, Gordeev M, Zakeri S. Molecular identification of Palearctic [*sic*] members of *Anopheles maculipennis* in northern Iran. Malaria Journal 2007;6-6 (10 pp.).

[135] Marinucci M, Romi R, Mancini M, Di Luca M, Severini C. Phylogenetic relationships of seven palearctic [*sic*] members of the *maculipennis* complex inferred from ITS2 sequence analysis. Insect Molecular Biology 1999;8 469480.

[136] Porter CH, Collins FH. Phylogeny of Nearctic members of the *Anopheles maculipennis* species group derived from the D2 variable region of 28S ribosomal RNA. Molecular Phylogenetics and Evolution 1996;6 178–188.

[137] Saeung A, Otsuka Y, Baimai V, Somboon P, Pitasawat B, Tuetan B, Junkum A, Takaoka H, Choochote W. Cytogenetic and molecular evidence for two species in the *Anopheles barbirostris* complex (Diptera: Culicidae) in Thailand. Parasitology Research 2007;101 1337–1344.

[138] Saeung A, Baimai V, Otsuka Y, Rattanarithikul R, Somboon P, Junkum A, Tuetun B, Takaoka H, Choochote W. Molecular and cytogenetic evidence of three sibling species of the *Anopheles barbirostris* form A (Diptera: Culicidae) in Thailand. Parasitology Research 2008;102 499–507.

[139] Ma Y-J, Qu F-Y. *Anopheles hyrcanus* complex from China: sequence differences of ribosomal DNA second internal transcribed spacer and phylogenetic analyses. Entomological Knowledge 2002;39 209–214 (in Chinese).

[140] Ma Y, Xu J. The Hyrcanus Group of *Anopheles* (*Anopheles*) in China (Diptera: Culicidae): species discrimination and phylogenetic relationships inferred by ribosomal DNA internal transcribed spacer 2 sequences. Journal of Medical Entomology 2005;42 610–619.

[141] Hwang UW. Revisited ITS2 phylogeny of *Anopheles* (*Anopheles*) Hyrcanus [*sic*] group mosquitoes: reexamination of unidentified and misidentified ITS2 sequences. *Parasitology Research*, 2007;101 885–894.

[142] Paredes-Esquivel C, Harbach RE, Townson H. Molecular taxonomy of members of the *Anopheles hyrcanus* group from Thailand and Indonesia. Medical and Veterinary Entomology 2011;25 348–352.

[143] Green CA. Cladistic analysis of mosquito chromosome data (*Anopheles* (*Cellia*) Myzomyia). Journal of Heredity 1982;73 2–11.

[144] Pape T. Cladistic analyses of mosquito chromosome data in *Anopheles* subgenus *Cellia* (Diptera: Culicidae). Mosquito Systematics 1992;24 1–11.

[145] Sharpe RG, Harbach RE, Butlin RK. Molecular variation and phylogeny of the Minimus Group of *Anopheles* subgenus *Cellia* (Diptera: Culicidae). Systematic Entomology 2000;25 265–272.

[146] Sawabe K, Takagi M, Tsuda Y, Tuno N. Molecular variation and phylogeny of the *Anopheles minimus* complex (Diptera: Culicidae) inhabiting Southeast Asian countries, based on ribosomal DNA internal transcribed spaces, ITS1 and 2, and the 28S D3 sequences. Southeast Asian Journal of Tropical Medicine and Public Health 2003;34 771–780.

[147] Morgan K, O'Loughlin M, Mun-Yik F, Linton Y-M, Somboon P, Min S, Htun PT, Nambanya S, Weerasinghe I, Sochantha T, Prakash A, Walton C. Molecular phyloge-

netics and biogeography of the Neocellia Series of *Anopheles* mosquitoes in the Oriental Region. Molecular Phylogenetics and Evolution 2009;52 588–601.

[148] Alam MT, Das MK, Dev V, Ansari MA, Sharma YD. PCR-RFLP method for the identification of four members of the *Anopheles annularis* group of mosquitoes (Diptera: Culicidae). Transactions of the Royal Society of Tropical Medicine and Hygiene 2007;101 239–244.

[149] Ma Y, Qu F, Dong X, Zhou H. Molecular identification of *Anopheles maculatus* complex from China. Chinese Journal of Parasitology and Parasitic Diseases 2002;20 321–324 (in Chinese).

[150] Ma Y, Shizhu L, Jiannong X. Molecular identification and phylogeny of the Maculatus Group of *Anopheles* mosquitoes (Diptera: Culicidae) based on nuclear and mitochondrial DNA sequences. Acta Tropica 2006;99 272–280.

[151] Walton C, Somboon P, Harbach RE, Zhang S, Weerasinghe I, O'Loughlin SM, Phompida S, Sochantha T, Tun-Lin W, Chen B, Butlin RK. Molecular identification of mosquito species in the *Anopheles annularis* group in southern Asia. Medical and Veterinary Entomology 2007;21 30–35.

[152] Sallum MAM, Foster PG, Li C, Sithiprasasna R, Wilkerson RC. Phylogeny of the Leucosphyrus Group of *Anopheles* (*Cellia*) Diptera: Culicidae) based on mitochondrial gene sequences. Annals of the Entomological Society of America 2007;100 27–35.

[153] Beebe NW, Ellis JT, Cooper RD, Saul A. DNA sequence analysis of the ribosomal DNA ITS2 region for the *Anopheles punctulatus* group of mosquitoes. Insect Molecular Biology 1999;8 381–390.

[154] Beebe NW, Cooper RE. Distribution and evolution of the *Anopheles punctulatus* group (Diptera: Culicidae) in Australia and Papua New Guinea. International Journal of Parasitology 2002;32 563–574.

[155] Coluzzi M, Sabatini A, Petrarca V, Di Deco MA. Chromosomal differentiation and adaptation to human environments in the *Anopheles gambiae* complex. Transactions of the Royal Society of Tropical Medicine and Hygiene 1979;73 483–497.

[156] Besansky NJ, Powell JR, Caccone A, Hamm DM, Scott JA, Collins FH. Molecular phylogeny of the *Anopheles gambiae* complex suggests genetic introgression between principal malaria vectors. Proceedings of the National Academy of Science, USA 1994;91 6885–6888.

[157] Caccone A, Garcia BA, Powell JR. Evolution of the mitochondrial DNA control region in the *Anopheles gambiae* complex. Insect Molecular Biology 1996;6 51–59.

[158] Wilkerson RC, Foster PG, Li C, Sallum MAM. Molecular phylogeny of Neotropical *Anopheles* (*Nyssorhynchus*) *albitarsis* species complex (Diptera: Culicidae). Annals of the Entomological Society of America 2005;98 918–925.

[159] Marrelli MT, Floeter-Winter LM, Malafronte RS, Tadei WP, Lourenço-de-Oliveira R, Flores-Mendoza C, Marinotti O. Amazonian malaria vector anopheline relationships interpreted from ITS2 rDNA sequences. Medical and Veterinary Entomology 2005;19 208–218.

[160] Bourke BP, Nagaki SS, Bergo ES, da Cruz Cardoso J, Sallum MAM. Molecular phylogeny of the Myzorhynchella Section of *Anopheles* (*Nyssorhynchus*) (Diptera: Culicidae): genetic support for recently described and resurrected species. Memórias do Instituto Oswaldo Cruz 2011;106 705–715.

[161] Townson H, Dyer N, McAlister E, Satoto TBT, Boewono DT, Bangs MJ & Harbach RE Systematics of *Anopheles barbirostris* van der Wulp and a sibling species of the Barbirostris Complex (Diptera: Culicidae) in eastern Java, Indonesia. Systematic Entomology 2013;38: 180–191.

[162] Coetzee M, Hunt RH, Wilkerson R, della Torre A, Coulibaly MB & Besansky NJ *Anopheles coluzzii* and *Anopheles amharicus*, new members of the *Anopheles gambiae* complex. Zootaxa 2013;3619: 246–274.

Chapter 2

Systematic Techniques for the Recognition of *Anopheles* Species Complexes

Wej Choochote and Atiporn Saeung

Additional information is available at the end of the chapter

http://dx.doi.org/10.5772/54853

1. Introduction

Throughout the world, 528 species of *Anopheles* mosquitoes have been discovered, and approximately 80 of them play an important role as vectors of malaria, filarial nematode and encephalitis virus. Among these, at least 20 taxa represent species complexes, which comprise about 115 sibling species members. The existence of species complexes in *Anopheles* vectors leads to difficulty in precisely identifying sibling species (isomorphic species) and/or subspecies (morphologically/cytologically polymorphic races) members that possess identical morphology or minimal morphological distinction. In addition, those members may differ in biological characteristics (e.g., microhabitats, resting and biting behavior, sensitivity or resistance to insecticides, susceptible or refractory to malaria parasites, etc.), which can be used to determine their potential for transmitting disease agents. Incorrect identification of individual members in *Anopheles* species complexes may result in failure to distinguish between a vector and non-vector, and lead to complications and/or unsuccessful vector control [1-5].

So far, at least 1 and 2 traditional techniques have been used widely for the recognition of sibling species and/or subspecies members at post- and pre-mating barriers. For post-mating barriers; the hybridization or crossing experiment, using the artificial mating technique to determine hybrid non-viability, sterility or breakdown, is still a useful tool for recognizing *Anopheles* species complexes. Detailed genetic incompatibility, including lack of insemination, embryonation, hatchability, larval survival, pupation, emergence, adult sex distortion, abnormal reproductive system and complete or incomplete (some cases only at the inversion heterozygote regions) asynaptic salivary gland polytene chromosomes are useful criteria for elucidating sibling species and subspecies status. However, a point worth noting is that an isofemale line (isoline) colony established from the combinative characters of morphological and/or cytological markers has to be considered seriously. A laboratory raised colony established from a naturally mixed population should be omitted, since it may be a mixture of cryptic species [6-10]. In addition, many *Anopheles* species do not reproduce in captivity. As for pre-mating barriers; examination of the polytene chromosomes in wild-caught adult females, and/or progenies of iso-female lines, provides clear evidence that different specific mate recognition systems (SMRS) exist. The total absence or significantly deficient number of heterozygotes for an inversion in a sympatric population entirely indicates the presence of reproductive isolation within a taxon [10-12]. Nonetheless, at least 4 problems have been raised regarding this matter, i.e., (1) a skilled person is needed to prepare a perfect chromosome and make an identification, (2) homosequential banding species cannot be employed, e.g., *An. maculipennis* complex [13] and *An. barbirostris* complex [14-17], (3) a relatively large amount of sample materials are required to perform the Hardy-Weinberg equilibrium, which cannot be applied to small numbers of rare species specimens that are caught during specific seasons, and (4) it cannot be performed in allopatric anopheline populations. Electrophoretic variations at enzyme loci are not only useful for identification of sibling species, but also for the correct identification of morphologically cryptic *Anopheles* species. Variations at a locus thus enable detection of reproductive isolation within populations, resulting from positive assortative (preferential) mating [10-11, 18]. Nevertheless, at least 2 problems have been raised regarding this technique, i.e., (1) specimens must be fresh or frozen until analysis, and (2) its use must be similar to that of the polytene chromosome, as it requires a relatively large amount of sample materials to perform the Hardy-Weinberg equilibrium and cannot be performed in allopatric anopheline populations, as previously described.

Regarding the modernized technique; molecular investigation of some specific genomic markers, e.g., ribosomal DNA (ITS2, D2, D3, IGS) and mitochondrial DNA (COI, COII, Cyt b, ND5), has been used extensively as a tool to characterize and/or diagnose cryptic members in the intra-taxa of *Anopheles* mosquitoes, and the advantage of this PCR-based technique is that few nanograms of DNA are required from preserved specimens [19]. Nonetheless, controversy arose when only comparative DNA sequence analyses of some specific genomic regions were used as first hand criteria to differentiate between the status of specific species, sibling species and subspecies within the taxon *Anopheles*. For example, based on a comparison of the D3 domain of 28S (28S-D3), *An. fluviatilis* S has been considered as synonymous to the *An. minimus* species C [20-22]. However, subsequent investigation of the conspecificity of these two species, based on ITS2 and D2-D3 domains of 28S rDNA regions, suggests that *An. fluviatilis* S and *An. minimus* C, do not deserve to be synonymous [23]. Similar results were also obtained in the determining on specific species status between *An. lesteri* and *An. paraliae* [unpublished data]. The comparative DNA sequence analyses between *An. lesteri* strain from Korea and *An. paraliae* strain from Thailand revealed low pairwise genetic distance for COI (0.007-0.017) and COII (0.008-0.011) regions with 4-9 and 5-7 base substitutions, respectively, whereas a considerable genetic distance (0.040) was obtained in ITS2 region with 16 base substitutions. Supportively, the phylogenetic trees demonstrated that these two species were separated from each other with a 74-100% bootstrap value for 3 regions. It was interesting to note that *An. lesteri* and *An. paraliae* were distinguished appreciably by DNA sequence data, however, were confirmed to be genetically compatible by the crossing experiments. Remarkably, prior to reaching a definite conclusion of specific species, sibling species and subspecies status within the taxon *Anopheles*, crossing experiments need to be carried out intensively using iso-female lines established from sympatric and/or allopatric populations, which relate to morphological variants, cytogenetic forms and/or comparative DNA sequence analyses of some specific regions.

2. Formation of robust systematic procedures

In light of the advantages and disadvantages of the techniques mentioned above, 3 techniques, i.e., the crossing experiment, molecular investigation and cytogenetic markers (characteristics of metaphase karyotypes) were selected, and they formed the robust systematic procedures for the recognition of *Anopheles* species complexes [24] (Figure 1).

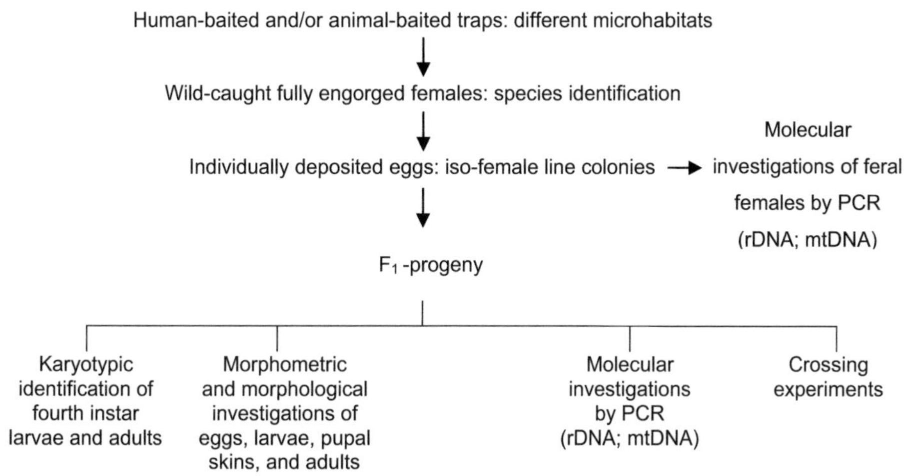

Figure 1. Summarized flow chart for robust systematic procedures

By following the flow chart: (1) try to collect anopheline mosquitoes that are distinct in their behavior (e.g., biting humans or animals with relation to different microhabitats and/or locations), (2) try to record morphological variation(s) as far as possible during the species identification process of wild-caught females, (3) establish an iso-female line colony by allowing gravid females to lay eggs individually, (4) conduct molecular investigation of laid-egg feral females to obtained a robust DNA marker, with this step usually taking about 1 week. Since development of the F_1-progeny usually takes about 2 weeks from first instar larvae to adults, the metaphase karyotype investigation of fourth instar larvae, newly emerged adult females and males is performed in order to (5) obtain a cytogenetic marker (karyotypic form), (6) if molecular investigation fails in the step of laid-egg feral female it will be performed in F_1-progeny, (7) carry out morphometric and morphological investigations of eggs, larvae, pupal skins and adults to confirm precise species identification, and (8) perform the important step of crossing experiments among iso-female line colonies by using a karyotypic marker (or form) related to a DNA marker (large sequence divergence or very low intraspecific sequence variation) of each iso-female line colony.

Regarding techniques necessary for success in operating robust systematic procedure: 3 important techniques were developed by the authors, and they have been proven as efficient and necessary for the robust systematic recognition of sibling species and/or subspecies members within the taxon *Anopheles* species complex. They are: (1) the establishment of a healthy iso-female line colony that is the backbone of population-genetic study on *Anopheles* vectors, since it provides healthy larval and adult progenies for preparation of attractive metaphase and salivary gland polytene chromosomes, and potent adults for crossing experiments. The inability to establish a healthy iso-female line colony that can be colonized for many consecutive generations is the principle cause of failure in a population-genetic study of *Anopheles* vectors, (2) the technique for metaphase chromosome preparations in adult females and males by intrathoracic inoculation [25] and that for fourth instar larval brains [14] using extracted solution derived from dried seeds and rhizomes of a decoration plant (*Gloriosa superba* L.), instead of synthetic colchicine solution, and (3) modified technique for salivary gland polytene chromosome preparations in fourth instar larvae [26]. Detailed and important procedures regarding the 3 techniques are as follows:

3. Techniques for establishment of a healthy iso-female line colony of difficult-to-rear anophelines

An iso-female line colony of *An. campestris*-like Form E, Thai strain [14] was established from 1 wild-caught fully engorged adult female collected from a human-baited trap reared successfully under laboratory conditions for 98 consecutive generations and used as a role model for other fresh-water breeding anopheline species.

4. Procedures

4.1. Transportation of wild-caught anophelines

Wild-caught fully engorged adult females collected from human- and/or animal-baited traps in the field were kept in a plastic cup (8.5 cm in diameter and 11 cm in depth, lined inside with filter paper), with a pad of cotton wool soaked with 10% sucrose solution placed on top of the covering screen. It was covered with a translucent plastic bag in order to keep humid conditions in the cup and delay rapid drying of the soaked cotton wool (Figure 2a). It was stored in a humid chamber using a picnic foam-box (18 x 26 x 39 cm) to maintain humidity and temperature (Figure 2b). Then it was transported to the insectarium for colonization and biological studies. All of the experiments were performed in the insectarium at 27±2 ºC, 70-80% relative humidity, and illumination from a combination of natural daylight from a glass-window and fluorescent lighting was provided for approximately 12 hours a day.

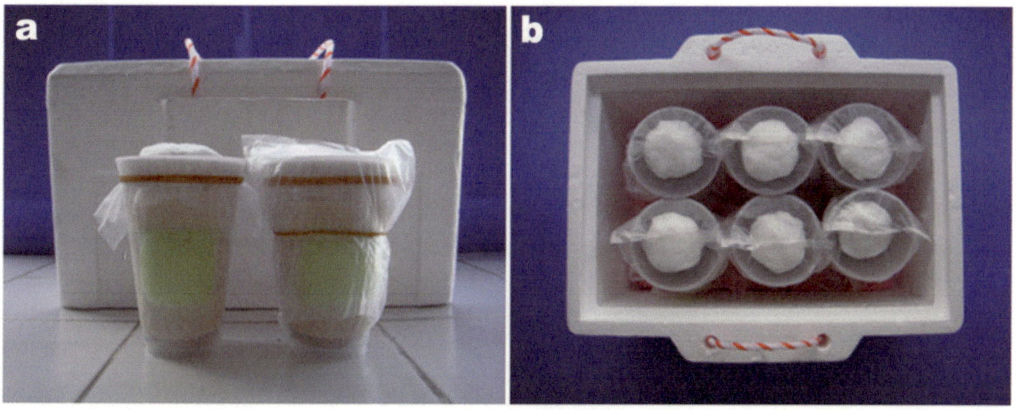

Figure 2. (a) A screen-topped plastic cup with a pad of soaked cotton wool placed on top of the covering screen (left), covered with a translucent plastic bag (right), and a humid chamber derived from a picnic foam-box (background). (b) Top view of the humid chamber showing 6 plastic cups placed on a wet towel lined the bottom (pink colour) and 10-15 ice cubes

4.2. Egg laying

After the engorged adult female was maintained for 4-5 days and/or until gravid in the insectarium, it was placed in a screen-topped oviposition plastic-cup (6 cm in diameter and 7 cm in depth) containing 25 ml of natural water (brought from a basin that was used for tap-water production). Wet filter paper lined the inside of the screen-topped was covered with a black plastic sheet (Figure 3a-c). The eggs attached to the moist side of the filter paper and/or floating on the water surface were rinsed and transferred to white plastic tray (25 x 36 x 6 cm) containing 1,500 ml rearing water (equal part of natural water and distilled water) with wet filter paper lining the inside. During the embryonation period, the eggs were exposed to a 40-watt light instead of sunlight, for warming the eggs until hatching (Figure 3d).

4.3. Rearing of larvae, pupae and adults

After egg hatching, first instar larvae were transferred daily from an ovipot to a white plastic tray (25 x 36 x 6 cm) containing 2,000 ml rearing water and approximately 15 stems of garden grass (*Axonopus compressus*), and 80 first instar larvae were reared in each tray. The rearing tray was covered with a transparent plastic sheet for reducing the need to change and/or re-fill the tray with rearing water during the larval development process (Figure 4a-b). An extra and/or a standard formula of fish food consisting approximately of protein 47.5%, oil 6.5%, fibre 2.0%, ash 10.5%, moister 6.0% and additives of vitamins A (29,770 IU/kg), D3 (1,860 IU/kg), E (200 mg/kg), L-ascorbyl-2-polyphosphate (138 mg/kg), lecithin, l-lysine monochlorhydrate, and citric acid was used as larval nutrient. Fine fish food was placed in a vial covered with a nylon screen (34 x 43 threads per cm^2) and sprinkled on the water until the food particles stopped spreading across the water's surface. First and second instar larvae were fed twice daily, and this schedule was increased to 3-5 times daily after most of the larvae reached third and fourth instars, respectively. Before each feeding, floating clumps of excess food were

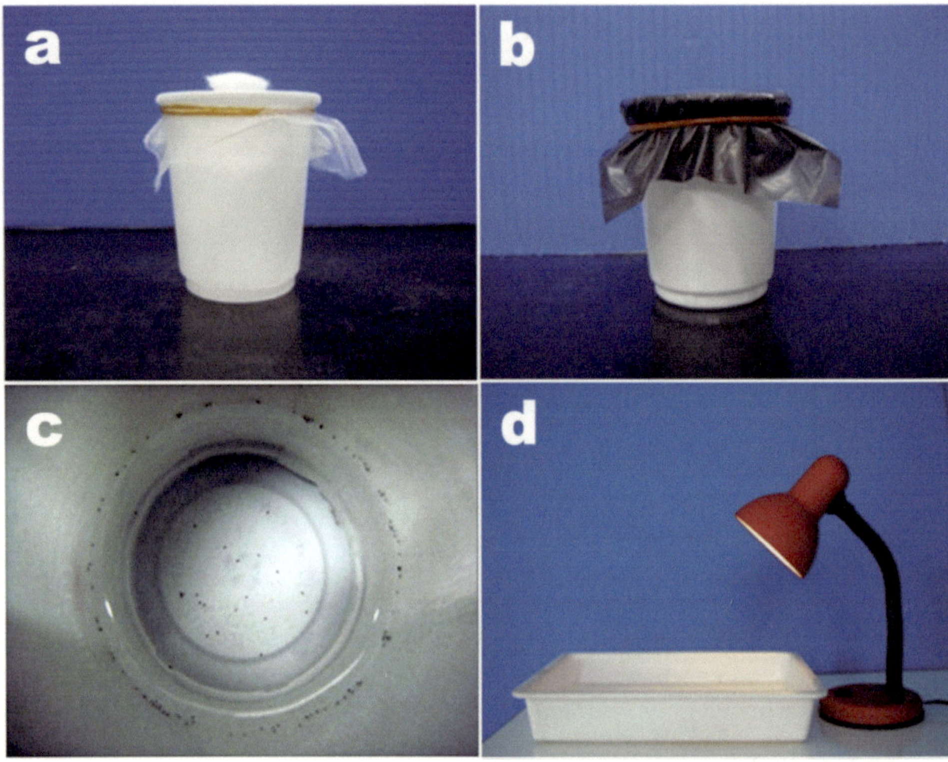

Figure 3. (a) A screen-topped oviposition plastic-cup, (b) covered with a black plastic sheet, and (c) top view of the plastic cup showing egg-batch after 12-hours-oviposition of a gravid adult female. (d) Eggs placed in a white plastic tray and exposed to a 40-watt light

removed by dragging a sheet of typing-paper across the water's surface. Any larvae trapped on the paper during the cleaning process were dislodged by rinsing the paper in a tray of rearing water and returning it to the rearing tray. After pupation, approximately 100 pupae placed in a plastic cup (14.5 cm in diameter and 6 cm in depth) containing 150 ml of distilled water were kept in a 30 x 30 x 30 cm cage, and the emerged adults were provided with both 10% sucrose solution and 5% multivitamin syrup solution (consisting approximately of vitamins A: 2,000 I.U., D: 200 I.U., E: 1.50 I.U., B1: 0.70 mg, B2: 0.85 mg, B6: 0.35 mg and C: 17.50 mg, nicotinamide: 9.00 mg, orange juice: 0.50 g and cod liver: 0.10 g per 100 ml solution) saturated in cotton wool coiled around a small piece of wood and placed in a small bottle. Increased humidity to promote adult survival was provided by covering the cage with a wet towel overlaid with a black plastic sheet (Figure 4c). One-day-old males were removed daily from the cage and kept in a screen-topped plastic cup (lined inside with filter paper), where they were provided with a 5% multivitamin syrup solution through a pad of soaked cotton wool, which was placed on top of the screen and changed daily. In order to keep humid conditions in the cup and delay rapid drying of the cotton wool soaked in 5% multivitamin syrup solution, the screen-top was covered with a translucent plastic bag (Figure 4d).

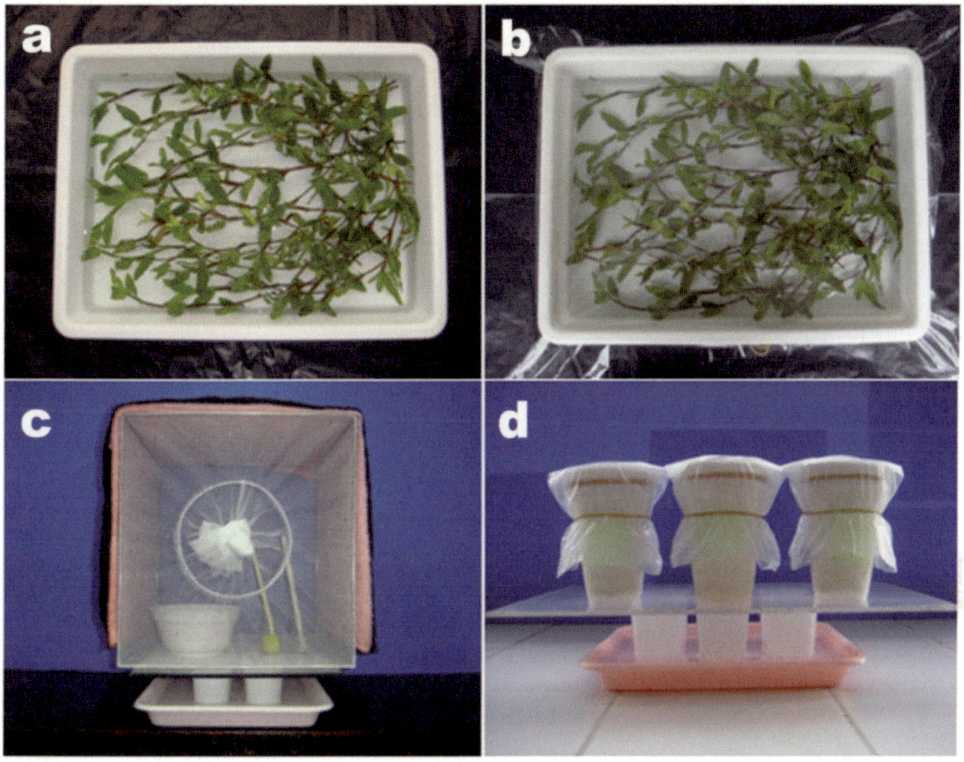

Figure 4. (a) Top view of a white plastic tray placed with 15 stems of garden grass, and (b) covered with a transparent plastic sheet. (c) Adult rearing cage partially covered with a wet towel (pink colour) and a black plastic-sheet with plastic container for holding pupae, and two bottles with cotton wicks, one containing 10% sucrose solution and another 5% multivitamin syrup solution. (d) Adult males being kept in a screen-topped plastic cup (lined inside with filter paper) with a pad of cotton wool soaked in 5% multivitamin syrup solution and the top covered with a translucent plastic bag to maintain humidity.

4.4. Suitable blood-feeding condition

Comparative direct feeding ability on white rat in a 30 x 30 x 30 cm cage, and artificial feeding ability on human heparinized-blood (obtained from human volunteers whom sign the consent form) in a plastic cup (8.5 cm in diameter and 11 cm in depth, lined inside with filter paper) (Figure 5), of female *An. campestris*-like Form E at different ages ranging from 1 to 10 days, demonstrated that in the cage, adult females aged of 3, 4, 5 and 6 days were successful in feeding on the blood of white rats, with feeding rates of 30%, 39%, 62% and 43%, respectively. Interestingly, the adult females aged 3, 4, 5, and 6 days succeeded in artificial feeding on human heparinized-blood in the plastic cup at higher rates than direct feeding on white rat in the cage in all experiments by yielding feeding rates of 62%, 68%, 78% and 61%, respectively. Nevertheless, the engorged females that derived from 2 feeding methods were used satisfactorily for the maintenance of an iso-female line laboratory-raised colony of *An. campestris*-like Form E. One difficulty and/or failure in rearing mosquitoes in the laboratory was the subsequent generation's refusal to feed on blood, particularly from small laboratory animals such as guinea pig, white rat, golden hamster, etc. This leads to direct feeding from human volunteers, especially at the beginning of the first to fifth generations of the colony. However, to solve this problem, forced artificial feeding on human heparinized-blood by *An. campestris*-like Form E was successful in this study and has been used routinely up to this time. Nonetheless, a point to be kept in mind is that only the healthy progenies of laboratory-raised colonies could be used successfully. Additionally, the use of direct blood feeding of subsequent mosquito progenies from human volunteers is a potentially dangerous method and should be given up entirely, since at least 4 reports have declared that *An. peditaeniatus* [27], *An. subpictus* [28-29] and *An. barbirostris* [30] have been incriminated as secondary vectors of Japanese encephalitis virus, which is possibly transmitted vertically.

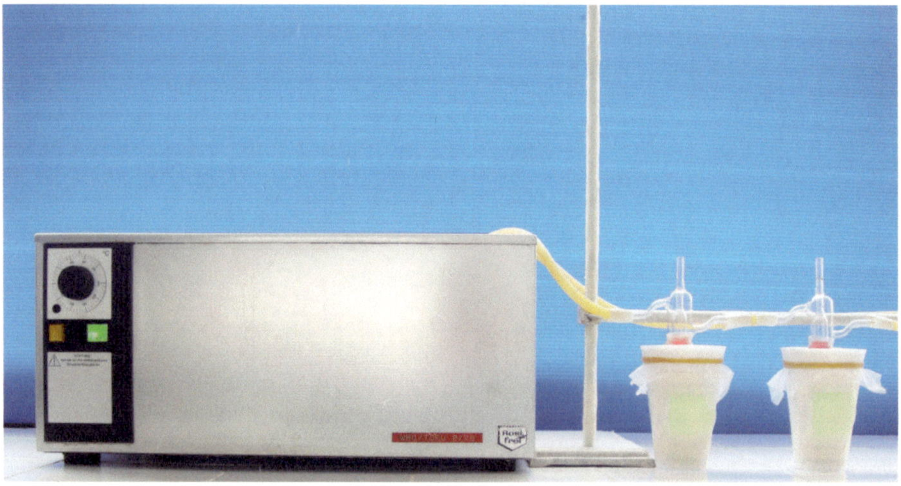

Figure 5. Artificial feeding system. A warm water-bath at 40°C, with a water pump placed inside, is connected to glass inlet and outlet feeding-chambers by rubber tubes. Thin paraffin-membrane covers the bottom tip of the feeding chambers, which are filled with human heparinized-blood, and the bottom tip is in close contact with 50 fasted adult female *An. campestris*-like Form E that are inside a screen-topped paper cup.

4.5. Ability of free mating in a 30 cm cubed cage and male ability to mate artificially

One of the difficulties in the colonization of anopheline mosquitoes in the laboratory might be due to adults not being capable of copulation in a small and/or standard cage (30 x 30 x 30 cm). Thus, in order to determine the adaptive stenogamy of *An. campestris*-like Form E, the newly emerged females and males co-habitated at a ratio of 200/300, in a 30 x 30 x 30 cm cage for one week [31-32]. The results indicated that *An. campestris*-like Form E failed to mate freely in the cage at a 0% insemination rate (from experiments repeated 3 times), indicating strong eurygamy. Thus, the artificial mating methods as described by [33-34] were used. The best age for artificial mating in male *An. campestris*-like Form E was 5-days-old (100% mating rate, 86.67% insemination rate). Nonetheless, males aged 4 and 8 days old could be used satisfactorily (93.33-100% mating rates, 80-82.14% insemination rates) (Table 1).

Day after emergence*	No. successfully mated females (%)	No. insemination (%)
1	11 (36.67)	0 (0)
2	23 (76.67)	18 (78.26)
3	23 (76.67)	18 (78.26)
4	30 (100)	24 (80.00)
5	30 (100)	26 (86.67)
6	28 (93.33)	23 (82.14)
7	28 (93.33)	24 (85.71)
8	28 (93.33)	23 (82.14)
9	26 (86.67)	16 (61.54)
10	23 (76.67)	11 (47.83)

*Thirty males for each experiment.

Table 1. Artificial mating ability of *An. campestris*-like Form E males

4.6. Searching for a suitable oviposition-condition

Many anopheline colonies have been reported to adapt easily to oviposit eggs in the cage on various types of simple ovipots, e.g., petridish, crystallizing dish, terra-cotta bowl, white plastic cup, black cup, etc. [35-39]. In the case of using 20 gravid adult females of *An. campestris*-like Form E put in a 30 x 30 x 30 cm cage for 12 hours (starting from 18.00-06.00 hours), the results revealed that 0, 0, 279, 0 and 0 eggs per an oviposited-plastic cup (9 cm in diameter and 10.5 cm in depth, containing 80 ml of natural water) were found in experiments 1, 2, 3, 4 and 5, respectively; whereas the forced laying of eggs by placing 20 gravid adult females in an oviposited-plastic cup (details mentioned above in paragraph 2 "Egg laying") in the same size and conditions as used in the cage, a massive number of eggs, i.e., 1,273, 1,318, 1,705, 2,180 and 1,501 eggs per cup, were recovered for experiments 1, 2, 3, 4 and 5, respectively (Figure 6). The high yield of eggs recovered from the latter experiment appears to result in the fact that the close-system of an oviposited-plastic cup provided significantly higher relative humidity than a cage or open-system. The air-rich water molecules in high relative humidity are the important attractants to gravid female alfactometer, which indicates suitable or acceptable oviposition sites [40]. Thus, in oviposition of *An. campestris*-like Form E and other anopheline species in our laboratory, this method has been used routinely up until now.

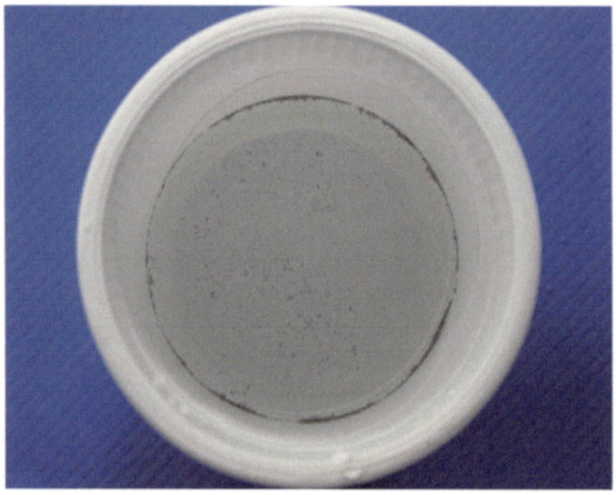

Figure 6. Top view of ovipot derived from a plastic cup showing massive egg-batches after 12-hours-oviposition of the 20 gravid adult females

4.7. Other important factors

Throughout the larval rearing period, the number of larvae, rearing conditions in the tray, and food were the most important factors, not only for routine rearing, but also special rearing in order to obtain a high yield of metaphase and polytene chromosomes, which were necessary for population-genetic study of anophelines. Stressful rearing-conditions, e.g., the overcrowding of larvae in a rearing tray (in this study, 80 larvae per 25 x 36 x 6 cm tray was an appropriate number for *An. campestris*-like Form E), and the use of inappropriate water medium and food would lead to a rapid drop in and/or loss of a colony. Also, this would result in low larval and pupal survival rates, adult F_1-progenies refusing to take blood meal, difficulty in artificial mating of adult females and males and/or failure to inseminate sperm into mated-female spermathecae, short life span of adult females and males, mated gravid adult females laying fewer numbers of eggs and/or failure to lay eggs, and low egg-hatchability. Thus, any rearing system, which is an important first step that leads to obtaining healthy larvae, would be a promising method for successfully establishing a colony, particularly an iso-female line colony, which is more difficult and complicated to establish than a mixed colony. As mentioned previously, food was one of the most important factors for obtaining healthy larvae, thus, several kinds of larval food were tested for use and comparison, e.g., mouse pellets, cat and dog biscuits and various formulas of fish food. The results indicated that the standard formula of fish food as mentioned in paragraph 3 ("Rearing of larvae, pupae and adults"), proved to be an excellent larval food for *An. campestris*-like Form E. It is expected that this fish food formula was also ideal for other anopheline species with rearing difficulties. The use of equal part of natural water and distilled water as the larval rearing medium also proved to be promising. Trials using boiled tap-water, filtered tap-water, polarized water and deionized water yielded unsatisfactory outcomes by providing low larval survival, particularly through subsequent progenies. The addition of garden grass to the larval rearing tray, as stated by [31], resulted in high larval survival for *An. campestris*-like Form E. Using few stems of garden grass, or withdrawing it, would lead to low larval survival and/or weak larvae for rearing subsequent generations. Using slightly more or less than 15 stems of garden grass, depending upon the size of the stems, and size and number of leaves, proved to improve conditions to a suitable level for larval rearing, since the grass provided a resting place for larvae, rendered shade as in natural breeding sites (rice paddy, ponds and swamps associated with water plants) [41-42], and aerated the medium. Its roots were also very important for maintaining clear and clean rearing medium by using larval waste products and unconsumed food as fertilizer, which determined the obvious active growth of grass in the rearing tray. Finally, we hope that the detailed information concerning rearing aspects of *An. campestris*-like Form E will prove to be important for the establishment of other anopheline species that have been previously difficult to rear.

Notes: By following the systematic rearing procedures as detail-mentioned above, at least 23 *Anopheles* species were successful reared in our insectarium, i.e., subgenus *Anopheles* [*An. argyropus* (F_{23}), *An. barbirostris* species A1 (F_{86}), *An. belenrae* (F_{26}), *An. campestris*-like Form E (F_{98}), *An. crawfordi* (F_{23}), *An. lesteri* (F_{60}), *An. nigerrimus* (F_{23}), *An. nitidus* (F_{28}), *An. paraliae* (F_{24}), *An. peditaeniatus* (F_{23}), *An. pullus* (F_{24}), *An. pursati* (F_{24}) and *An. sinensis* (F_{28})]; and *Cellia* [*An. harrisoni* (F_{51}), *An. jamesii* (F_{10}), *An. jeyporiensis* (F_5), *An. karwari* (F_{13}), *An. kochi* (F_{25}), *An. nivipes* (F_{12}), *An. pampanai* (F_{11}), *An. philippinensis* (F_{12}), *An. splendidus* (F_{10}) and *An. tessellatus* (F_{27})].

5. Techniques for metaphase and polytene chromosome preparations

5.1. Rearing condition of mosquitoes for chromosome preparations

The methods for rearing conditions were generally routine as mentioned in paragraph 3, except, 10 first instar larvae per tray were used to obtain a high yield of metaphase chromosomes from larval brains, ovaries and testes, and polytene chromosomes from larval salivary glands. Comparative outcome rates of metaphase chromosomes from larval brains and polytene chromosomes from larval salivary glands between routine (80 larvae) and special (10 larvae) rearing revealed as follows: (1) metaphase chromosomes: experiment 1 [10 larvae (87.50%) vs. 80 larvae (33.33%)], 2 [10 larvae (75.00%) vs. 80 larvae (30.00%)] and 3 [10 larvae (77.78%) vs. 80 larvae (30.00%)]; and (2) salivary gland polytene chromosomes: experiment 1 [10 larvae (80.00%) vs. 80 larvae (50.00%)], 2 [10 larvae (66.67%) vs. 80 larvae (50.00%)] and 3 [10 larvae (100.00%) vs. 80 larvae (66.67%)]. Thus, a special rearing with 10 larvae was used routinely for chromosome preparation.

5.2. Preparation of metaphase chromosomes from adult females and males and fourth instar larvae

5.2.1. Preparation of 0.5% and 1% solutions of dried Gloriosa superba *seed and rhizome powders*

Summarized flow chart for normal saline-extracted *Gl. superba* seed and rhizome powders, as follows:

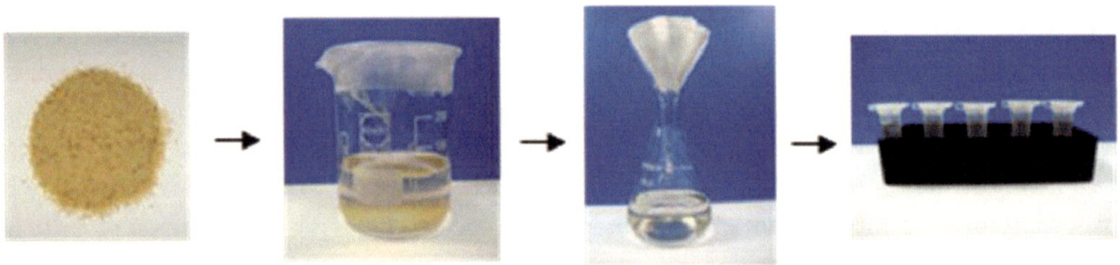

0.5 g of dried seed powder or 1 g of dried rhizome powder → Macerated in 100 ml of 0.85% sodium chloride solution for 6 hours at 27±2 °C, and kept at 4 °C for 14-16 hours (or in a refrigerator) → Filtrated → 1 ml of filtrate filled in a 1.5-ml microcentrifuge tube, and kept at -20 °C*

*By keeping at this condition, the colchicine-like activity in the filtrate stays stable for at least 2 years.

Notes: colchicine solution has been used widely at a concentration of 0.05-1% for metaphase chromosome preparation in the cytogenetic study of eukaryotic organisms, e.g., protozoans [43], helminthes [44-45], snails [46], insects [8, 47-50], and plants [51-52]. Spindle formation or microtubule polymerization inhibits arresting mitosis at the metaphase [53-54]. The alkaloid colchicine was isolated from a plant named autumn crocus or meadow saffron (*Colchicum autumnale* L., Family Liliaceae) in 1820 by Pelletier and Caventou [53]. At present, the commercial products derived from this plant are merchandised extensively and used worldwide. Recently, systematic and continuous studies evaluated the colchicine-like activity of a common decorative plant found widely in tropical countries, Dong Deung (*Gl. superba*, Family Liliaceae) [55], which highlighted the benefits of this plant used for metaphase chromosome preparation in mosquitoes [14, 24, 56-58]. Various concentrations and/or extracted-fractions of dried *Gl. superba* seed and rhizome powders yielded similar metaphase rates and an average number of metaphase chromosomes per positive mosquito to synthetic colchicine solution, indicating that these extracts could be used to replace colchicine. In addition, the authors also mentioned that considerable budget savings could be realized by using their techniques.

Other benefits include a decorative plant that can be bought at many shops in Thailand's flower-markets, and it is hoped elsewhere in tropical countries. It can be grown easily in small-spaced land and outdoors with general fertilizers (e.g., simple formula chemical fertilizer, organic fertilizer and animal manure), which are necessary to promote its growth. It takes about 5-7 months to grow from small budding-rhizomes into mature tree with flowers and green pods (Figure 7a-d).

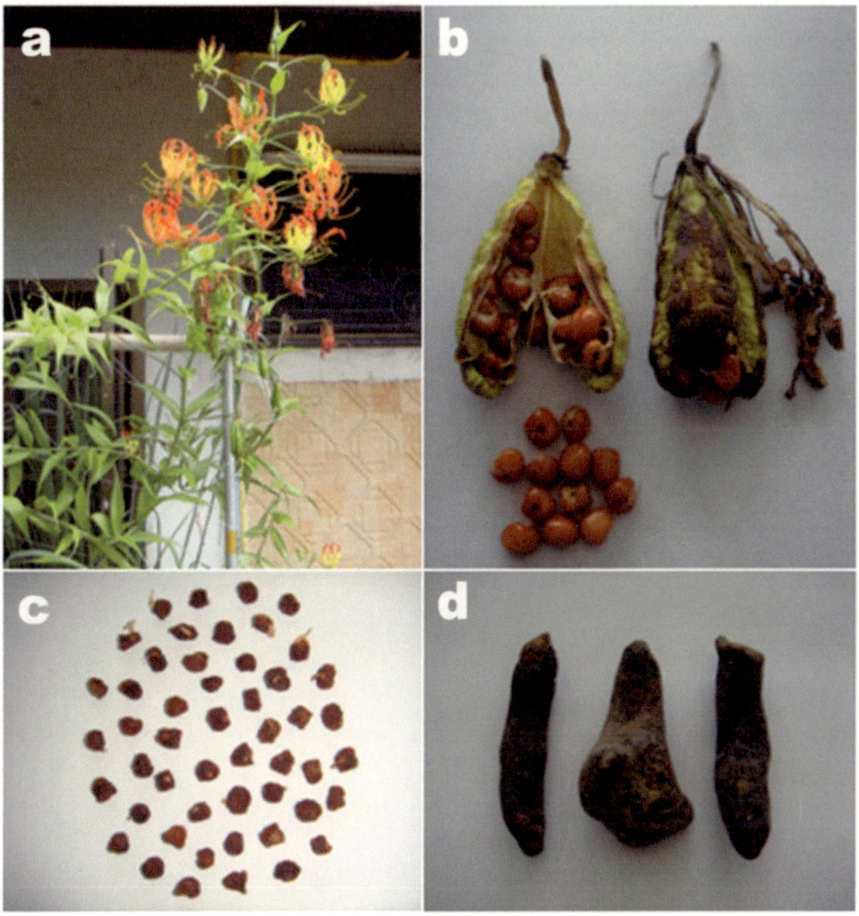

Figure 7. Showing a common decorative plant, Dong Deung (*Gl. superba*). (a) Dong Deung trees with beautiful flowers and green pods, (b) Ripe and broken Dong Deung pods with reddish-orange seeds, (c) Dried Dong Deung seeds and (d) Dried Dong Deung rhizomes

5.2.2. Preparation of the metaphase chromosomes from adult females and males and fourth instar larvae

5.2.2.1. Procedures

Metaphase chromosomes for adult females and males were prepared using the modified techniques described by [25]. The newly emerged adult females and males aged up to about 6-12 hours were starved, anaesthetized with ether and placed on their side on a slide under a binocular microscope. A needle was made by drawing out a glass capillary tube in a flame until the pointed end was approximately 80-100 µm in diameter; the shorter the needle the easier it was to handle. An inoculation was made into the post-spiracular area of the mesothorax, and a filtrate of 0.5% solution of dried *Gl. superba* seed powder was introduced into each mosquito by gently blowing down the attached rubber tube. The volume of inoculums could be controlled by observing the extension of abdomen until it was similar in size to the fully-engorged mosquitoes post fed on 10% sucrose solution. A few minutes after inoculation, most of the mosquitoes had recovered completely. Five inoculated mosquitoes were then kept in a 10-ml test tube (1.5 cm in diameter and 10 cm in length), with cotton wool soaked by 3 drops of distilled water closing the opened-side in order to provide adequate moisture. Then, the cotton wool was sealed with paraffin and the test tube held in an insectarium at 27±2 °C and 70-80% relative humidity for 3 hours (Figure 8a-c).

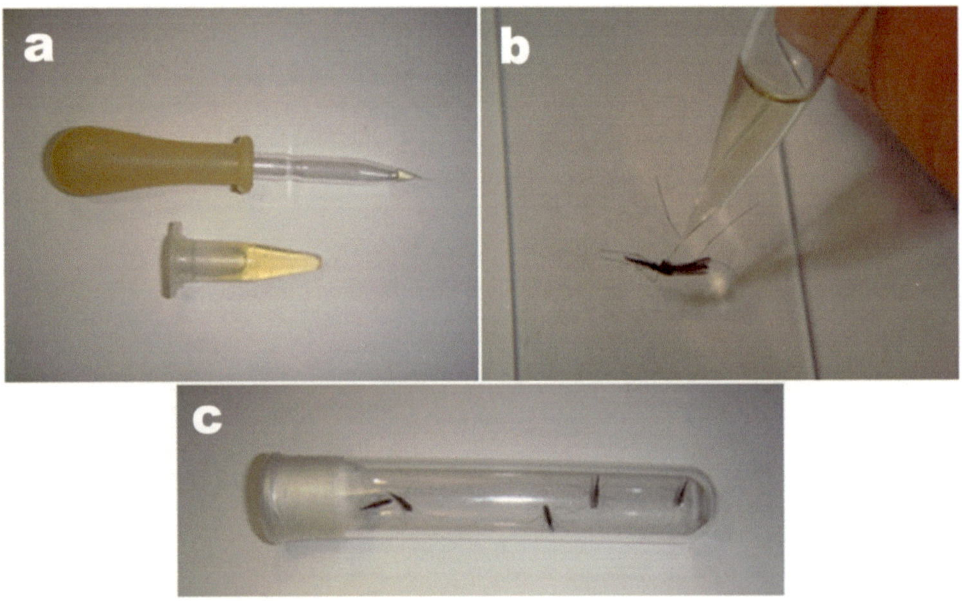

Figure 8. (a) Lower row: 1 ml filtrate of 0.5% solution of dried *Gl. superba* seed powder filled in a 1.5-ml microcentrifuge tube, and upper row: an inoculation glass-needle filled with a filtrate. (b) Intra-thoracic inoculation of a filtrate into the post-spiracular area of the mesothorax. (c) Five inoculated mosquitoes kept in a 10-ml test tube

The inoculated mosquitoes were dissected in a small drop of 1% hypotonic sodium citrate solution on a siliconized slide by pulling out the last abdominal segment to obtain the ovaries or testes under a binocular microscope. The organs obtained were left in 1% hypotonic sodium citrate solution for 10 minutes, and then transferred to a small drop of Carnoy's fixative on a siliconized slide for at least 2 minutes. Then, a drop of 60% acetic acid was added, and the organs were torn and mixed well with dissecting needles. A drop of cell suspension was placed on a clean microscopic slide on a warming plate at about 45–50°C. Droplets of cells were released slowly from a Pasteur pipette to form a circular trail of monolayer cells. The dried slides were stained with 20% Giemsa in phosphate buffer pH 7.2 for 1 hour, rinsed with deionized water, air-dried at room temperature, mounted in Permount® (Fisher, Fairlawn, NJ, USA) and examined under a green filter compound microscope. Metaphase karyotypes were identified by following the standard descriptions (Figure 9) [59-60].

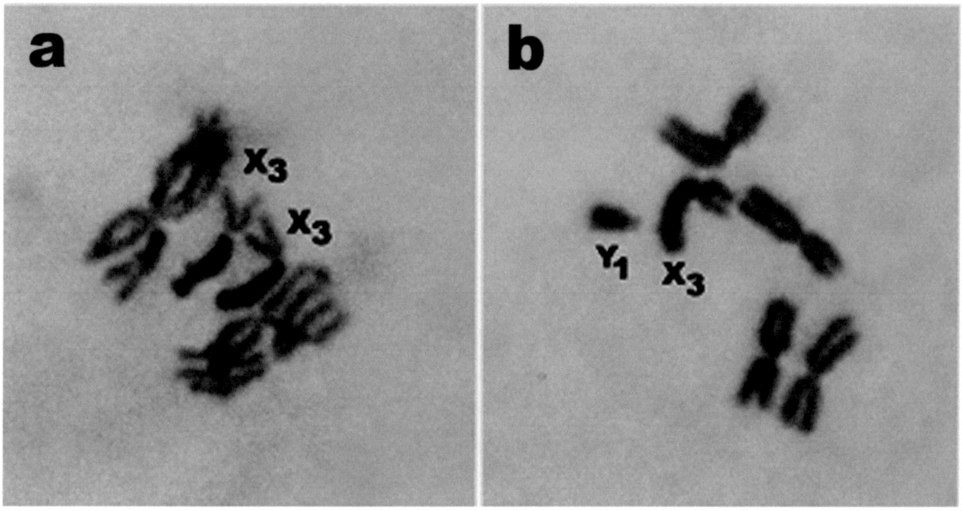

Figure 9. Metaphase chromosomes of *An. paraliae* Form A. (a) Ovary chromosomes, showing homozygous large submetacentric X_3 chromosomes. (b) Testis chromosomes, showing large submetacentric X_3 and small telocentric Y_1 chromosomes

The techniques for metaphase chromosome preparations in fourth instar larvae mainly followed those described above, except for the 5 fourth instar larvae that were incubated with a 1 ml filtrate of 0.5% dried *Gl. superba* seed powder solution in a 10-ml test tube for two hours. Then, the larval brains were excised, fixed, smeared, stained with Giemsa, mounted and examined under a green filter compound microscope (Figure 10).

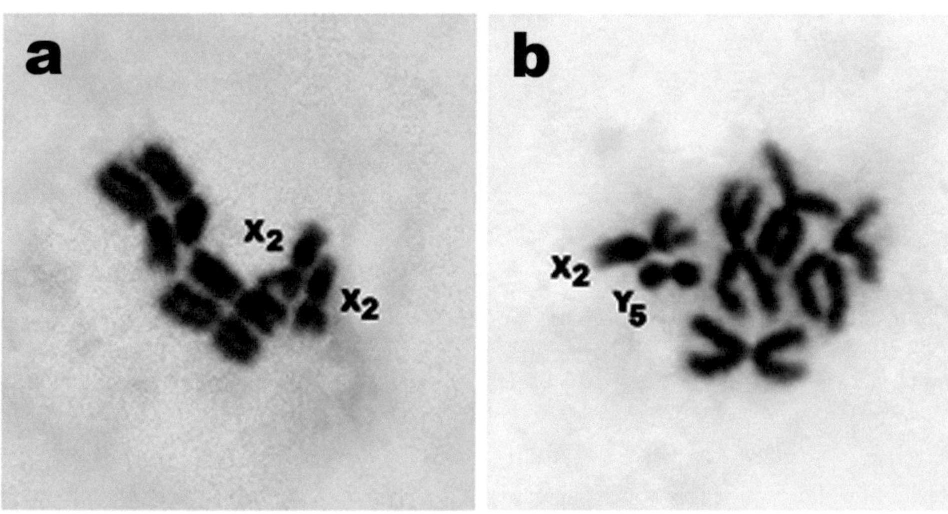

Figure 10. Metaphase chromosomes from brains of *An. campestris*-like Form E. (a) Showing homozygous submetacentric X_2 chromosomes. (b) Showing submetacentric X_2 and small metacentric Y_5 chromosomes

5.3. Preparation of the polytene chromosome from larval salivary glands

5.3.1. Procedures

Salivary gland polytene chromosomes were prepared using the slightly modified published techniques [26, 61]. The early fourth instar larvae were removed from the rearing tray by a dropper and rinsed in clean distilled water. A healthy larva with flared-thorax in appearance was picked up with forceps, attached to filter paper to remove excess water, placed on a siliconized slide filled with a drop of 1% hypotonic sodium citrate solution, and then dissected under a binocular microscope. The head was cut off, and one dissecting needle was inserted through the anterior end of thorax to posterior end. Then, another dissecting needle was scratched along the line of the inserted needle to tear the thorax integument, open the thorax and take out the internal organs before the thorax and abdomen were transferred into a drop of 15% acetic acid on a siliconized slide. The bilobed salivary glands were removed from the thorax using dissecting needles, and only the whitish anterior lobe of each salivary gland was transferred into a small drop of 45% acetic acid on a siliconized slide and left for 1 minute. After that, one drop of 2% aceto-lactic orcein stain was added. After 15 minutes of staining, a grease-free 22 mm^2 coverslip was placed on the stained salivary glands. The preparation was wrapped firmly in filter paper and gently pressed with a thumb to squash and spread the chromosomes. Then, the coverslip edges were sealed with transparent nail varnish. The prepared chromosomes were scrutinized under a green filter compound microscope. The arm of the polytene chromosomes was identified by following the standard map (Figure 11) [61].

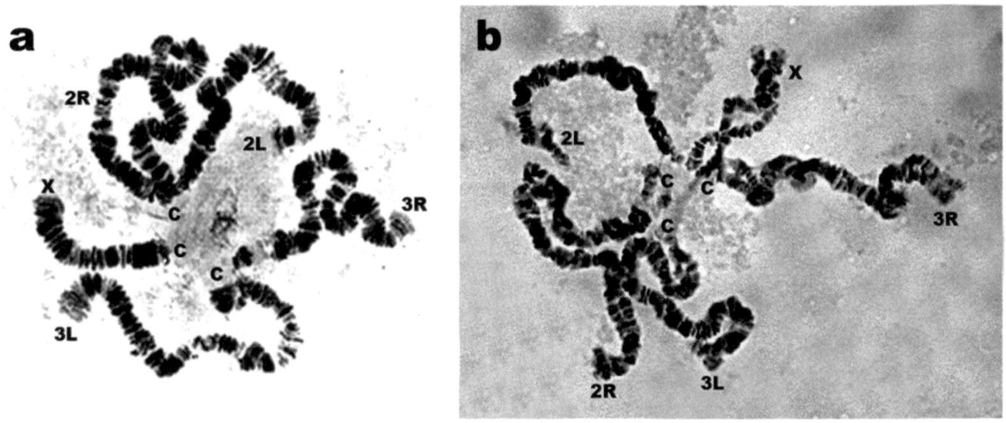

Figure 11. (a) Complete synaptic salivary gland polytene chromosome of *An.campestris*-like Form E. (b) Homosequential asynapsis in all autosomes and the X chromosome from crosses between *An.campestris*-like Form E and *An. barbirostris* species A1

Notes: by application of this robust systematic procedure, 5 sibling species members have recently been recognized in the taxon *An. barbirostris* complex within 2 years [14-16]. In addition, 8 species comprising a total of 26 subspecies (cytological forms) have been recognized during the past decade, i.e., *An. vagus* Forms A and B [62], *An. pullus* Forms A and B (= *An.*

yatsushiroensis) [62], *An. sinensis* Forms A and B [64-66], *An. aconitus* Forms B and C [67], *An. barbirostris* species A1 (Forms A, B, C and D) and A2 (Forms A and B) [14-16], *An. campestris*-like Forms B, E, and F [68], *An. peditaeniatus* Forms B, C, D, E [69], and *An. paraliae* Forms A, B, C, D and E [unpublished data].

6. Conclusion

The formation of robust systematic procedures is highly anticipated, based on the crossing experiments between iso-female lines using cytological markers (characteristics of metaphase chromosomes/karyotypic forms). Together with this information, the data on comparative sequence analyses of some specific genomic regions (rDNA and mtDNA) would bring success in recognizing and reliably identifying sibling species and/or subspecies members within the taxon of other *Anopheles* species complexes. In addition, the detailed techniques necessary for the establishment of difficult-to-rear anopheline species, which yield high rates of attractive metaphase and polytene chromosomes and potent adults for crossing experiments, would be main keys leading to successful study on the population-genetic structure of *Anopheles* vectors. These factors are important for studying the biology, behavior of *Anopheles* species, as well as for an epidemiology and a control approach of the targeted vector species.

Acknowledgements

Sincere thanks are extended to the Thailand Research Fund (TRF Advanced Research Scholar: BRG/14/2545 and BRG5380021, and TRF Senior Research Scholar: RTA5480006), the Thailand Research Fund through the Royal Golden Jubilee Ph.D. Program (Grant No. PHD/0044/2546, PHD/0052/2548, PHD/0082/2549, PHD/0031/2550, PHD/0297/2551 and PHD/0356/2552), Biodiversity Research and Training Program (Grant No. BRT R_249004, 250009 and 252005: 2006-2009), and Faculty of Medicine Research Fund, Chiang Mai University, Chiang Mai, Thailand, for their continuous financial support in the population-genetic study of *Anopheles* vectors in Thailand.

Author details

Wej Choochote* and Atiporn Saeung

*Address all correspondence to: wchoocho@mail.med.cmu.ac.th

Department of Parasitology, Faculty of Medicine, Chiang Mai University, Chiang Mai, Thailand

References

[1] Foley DH, Beebe N, Torres E, Saul A (1996) Misidentification of a Philippine malaria vector revealed by allozyme and ribosomal DNA markers Am. J. Trop. Med. Hyg. 54: 46-48.

[2] Van Bortel W, Harbach RE, Trung HD, Roelants P, Backeljau T, Coosemans M (2001) Confirmation of *Anopheles varuna* in vietnam, previously misidentified and mistargeted as the malaria vector *Anopheles minimus*. Am. J. Trop. Med. Hyg. 65: 729-732.

[3] World Health Organization (2007) Anopheline species complexes in South and South-East Asia. SEARO Technical Publication No. 57. WHO Regional Office for South-East Asia, New Delhi. 102 p.

[4] Singh OP, Nanda N, Dev V, Bali P, Sohail M, Mehrunnisa A, Adak T, Dash AP (2010) Molecular evidence of misidentification of *Anopheles minimus* as *Anopheles fluviatilis* in Assam (India). Acta Trop. 113: 241-244.

[5] Harbach RE (2012) Genus *Anopheles* Meigen, 1818. Available: http://mosquito-taxonomic-inventory.info/genus-anopheles-meigen-1818. Accessed 2012 May 14.

[6] Kanda T, Takai K, Chiang GL, Cheong WH, Sucharit S (1981) Hybridization and some biological facts of seven strains of the *Anopheles leucosphyrus* group (Reid, 1968). Jap. J. Sanit. Zool. 32: 321-329.

[7] Baimai V, Andre RG, Harrison BA, Kijchalao U, Panthusiri L (1987) Crossing and chromosomal evidence for two additional sibling species within the taxon *Anopheles dirus* Peyton and Harrison (Diptera: Culicidae) in Thailand. Proc. Entomol. Soc. Wash. 89: 157-166.

[8] Baimai V, Poopittayasataporn A, Kijchalao U (1988) Cytological differences and chromosomal rearrangements in four members of the *Anopheles dirus* complex (Diptera: Culicidae) in Thailand. Genome 30: 372–379.

[9] Sawadipanich Y, Baimai V, Harrison BA (1990) *Anopheles dirus* species E: Chromosomal and crossing evidence for another member of the Dirus complex. J. Am. Mosq. Control Assoc. 6: 477-481.

[10] Subbarao SK (1998) Anopheline species complexes in South-East Asia. WHO. Tech. Publ. SEARO. 18: 1-82.

[11] Peterson HE (1980) A comment on "mate recognition systems". Evolution 34: 330-331.

[12] Green CA, Rattanarithikul R, Charoensub A (1992) Population genetic confirmation of species status of the malaria vectors *Anopheles willmori* and *An. pseudowillmori* in Thailand and chromosome phylogeny of the Maculatus group of mosquitoes. Med. Vet. Entomol. 6: 335-341.

[13] Coluzzi M (1970) Sibling species in *Anopheles* and their importance to malariology. Misc. Publ. Ent. Soc. Am. 7: 63-77.

[14] Saeung A, Otsuka Y, Baimai V, Somboon P, Pitasawat B, Tuetun B, Junkum A, Takaoka H, Choochote W (2007) Cytogenetic and molecular evidence for two species in the *Anopheles barbirostris* complex (Diptera: Culicidae) in Thailand. Parasitol. Res. 101: 1337-1344.

[15] Saeung A, Baimai V, Otsuka Y, Rattanarithikul R, Somboon P, Junkum A, Tuetun B, Takaoka H, Choochote W (2008) Molecular and cytogenetic evidence of three sibling species of the *Anopheles barbirostris* Form A (Diptera: Culicidae) in Thailand. Parasitol. Res. 102: 499-507.

[16] Suwannamit S, Baimai V, Otsuka Y, Saeung A, Thongsahuan S, Tuetun B, Apiwathnasorn C, Jariyapan N, Somboon P, Takaoka H, Choochote W (2009) Cytogenetic and molecular evidence for an additional new species within the taxon *Anopheles barbirostris* (Diptera: Culicidae) in Thailand. Parasitol. Res. 104: 905-918.

[17] Saeung A (2012) *Anopheles* (Diptera: Culicidae) species complex in Thailand: Identification, distribution, bionomics and malaria-vector importance. Int. J. Parasitol. Res. 4: 75-82.

[18] Green, CA, Gass RF, Munstermann LE, Baimai V (1990) Population-genetic evidence for two species in *Anopheles minimus* in Thailand. Med. Vet. Entomol. 4: 25-34.

[19] Collins FH, Paskewitz SM (1996) A review of the use of ribosomal DNA (rDNA) to differentiate among cryptic *Anopheles* species. Insect Mol. Biol. 5: 1-9.

[20] Harbach RE (2004) The classification of genus *Anopheles* (Diptera: Culicidae): a working hypothesis of phylogenetic relationships. Bull. Entomol. Res. 94: 537-553.

[21] Garros C, Harbach RE, Manguin S (2005) Morphological assessment and molecular phylogenetics of the Funestus and Minimus Groups of *Anopheles* (*Cellia*). J. Med. Entomol. 42: 522–536.

[22] Chen B, Butlin RK, Pedro PM, Wang XZ, Harbach RE (2006) Molecular variation, systematics and distribution of the *Anopheles fluviatilis* complex in southern Asia. Med. Vet. Entomol. 20: 33–43.

[23] Singh OP, Chandra D, Nanda N, Sharma SK, Htun PT, Adak T, Subbarao SK, Dash AP (2006) On the conspecificity of *Anopheles fluviatilis* species S with *Anopheles minimus* species C. J. Biosci. 31: 671-677.

[24] Saeung A (2010) Genetic study of *Anopheles barbirostris*. Ph.D. Thesis, Chiang Mai University. 110 p.

[25] Choochote W, Rongsriyam Y, Tookyang B, Pakdicharoen A, Likitvong K (1992) A technique for chromosome preparation in adult mosquitoes. Mosq-Borne Dis. Bull. 9: 20-22.

[26] Kanda T (1979) Improved techniques for the preparation of polytene chromosomes for some *Anopheles* mosquitoes. Mosq. News 39: 568-574.

[27] Mourya DT, Ilkal MA, Mishra AC, Jacob PG, Pant U, Ramanujam S, Mavale MS, Bhat HR, Dhanda V (1989) Isolation of Japanese encephalitis virus from mosquitoes collected in Karnataka state, India during 1985 to 1987.Trans. R. Soc. Trop. Med. Hyg. 83: 550-552.

[28] George S, George JP, Rao JA (1987) Isolation of Japanese encephalitis and West Nile viruses from mosquitoes collected in Kolar district of Karnataka state during 1977-79. Indian J. Med. Res. 85: 235-238.

[29] Thenmozhi V, Rajendran R, Ayanar K, Manavalan R, Tyagi BK (2006) Long-term study of Japanese encephalitis virus infection in *Anopheles subpictus* in Cuddalore district, Tamil Nadu, South India. Trop. Med. Int. Hlth. 11: 288-293.

[30] Chakravarty SK, Sarkar JK, Chakravarty MS, Mukherjee MK, Mukherjee KK, Das BC, Hati AK (1975) The first epidemic of Japanese encephalitis studied in India-virological studies. Indian J. Med. Res. 63: 77-82.

[31] Choochote W, Sucharit S, Abeyewickreme W (1983) A note on adaptation of *Anopheles annularis* Van Der Wulp, Kanchanaburi, Thailand to free mating in a 30 x 30 x 30 cm cage. Southeast Asian J. Trop. Med. Public Health, 14: 559-560.

[32] Choochote W, Sucharit S, Khamboonruang C, Somboon P, Maleewong W, Suwapanit P (1985) Adaptation of various species and strains of *Anopheles* mosquitoes to natural copulation in a 30 cm cube cage. J. Parasit. Trop. Med. Ass. Thailand 8: 44-47.

[33] Baker RH, French WL, Kitzmiller JB (1962) Induced copulation in *Anopheles* mosquitoes. Mosq. News 22: 16-17.

[34] Ow Yang CK, Sta Maria FL, Wharton RH (1963) Maintenance of a laboratory colony of *Anopheles maculatus* by artificial mating. Mosq. News 23: 34-35.

[35] Chomcharn Y (1979) The study of *Plasmodium falciparum* in Thailand with respect to the mosquito vector, *Anopheles balabacensis* baisas and the effect of primaquine on the gametocytes and sporogony. Ph.D. Thesis, Mahidol University. pp. 46-48.

[36] Gerberg EJ, Barnard DR, Ward RA (1994) Procedures for laboratory rearing of specific mosquitoes, In: Manual for mosquito rearing and experimental techniques. Louisiana: Allen Press. pp. 41-45.

[37] Bangs MJ, Soelarto T, Barodji, Wicaksana BP, Boewono DT (2002) Colonization of *Anopheles maculatus* from Central Java, Indonesia. J. Am. Mosq. Control Assoc. 18: 359-363.

[38] Kim SJ, Choochote W, Jitpakdi A, Junkum A, Park SJ, Min GS (2003) Establishment of a self-mating mosquito colony of *Anopheles sinensis* from Korea. Korean J. Entomol. 33: 267-271.

[39] Da Silva AN, Dos Santos CC, Lacerda RN, Santa Rosa EP, De Souza RT, Galiza D, Sucupira I, Conn JE, Póvoa MM (2006) Laboratory colonization of *Anopheles aquasalis* (Diptera: Culicidae) in Belém, Pará, Brazil. J. Med. Entomol. 43: 107-119.

[40] Clements AN (1999) The biology of mosquitoes. Vol. 2. Sensory reception and behavior. Oxon, UK: CABI Publishing.

[41] Reid JA (1968) Anopheline mosquitoes of Malaya and Borneo. Stud. Inst. Med. Res. Malaya 31: 1-520.

[42] Harrison BA, Scanlon JE (1975) Medical entomology studies-II. The subgenus *Anopheles* in Thailand (Diptera: Culicidae). Contrib. Am. Entomol. Inst. 12: 1-307.

[43] Yuh YS, Liu JY, Shaio MF (1997) Chromosome number of *Trichomonas vaginalis*. J. Parasitol. 83: 551-553.

[44] Petkeviciute RA (1996) Chromosome study in the progenetic cestode *Cyathocephalus truncatus* (Cestoda: Spathebothriidea). Int. J. Parasitol. 26: 1211-1216.

[45] Hirai H, Toguchi I, Saitoh Y, Kawanaka M, Sugiyama H, Habe S, Okamoto M, Hirata M, Shimada M, Tiu WU, Lai K, Upatham ES, Agatsuma T (2000) Chromosomal differentiation of the *Schistosoma japonicum*. Int. J. Parasitol. 30: 441-452.

[46] Petkeviciute R, Staneviciute G, Kiseliene V (1995) Mitotic chromosomes of *Sphaerostomum bramae* (Muller, 1776) Szidat, 1944. J. Helminthol. 69: 347-349.

[47] Baker RH, Aslamkhan M (1969) Karyotypes of some Asian mosquitoes of the subfamily culicinae (Diptera: Culicidae). J. Med. Entomol. 6: 44-52.

[48] Baimai V (1977) Chromosomal polymorphisms of constitutive heterochromatin and inversions in *Drosophila*. Genetics 85: 85-93.

[49] Bermard J, Max K (1977) Heterochromatin variation in *Cryptobothrus chrysophorus*. Chromosoma 65: 59-79.

[50] Nunamarker RA, Brown SE, Knudson DL (1996) Metaphase chromosomes of *Culicoides variipennis* (Diptera: Ceratopogonidae). J. Med. Entomol. 35: 871-873.

[51] Vosa CG (1973) Heterochromatin recognition and analysis of chromosome variation in *Scilla sibirica*. Chromosoma 43: 269-278.

[52] Marks GE (1976) Variation of Giemsa banding patterns in the chromosomes of *Anemone blanda*. Chromosoma 5: 179-184.

[53] Insel PA (1996) Analgesic-antipyretic and anti-inflammatory agents and drugs employed in the treatment of gout. In: Hardman JG, Limbird LE, editors. The pharmacological basis of therapeutic, 9th ed. McGraw-Hill, New York. pp. 647-649.

[54] Haraguchi T, Kaneda T, Hiraoka Y (1997) Dynamics of chromosomes and microtubules visualized by multiple wavelength fluorescence imaging in living mammalian cells: effects of mitotic inhibitors on cell cycle progression. Genes. Cells 2: 369-380.

[55] Smitinand T (1980) Thai plant names: Botanical names-ver-nacular names. Royal Forest Department, Bangkok.

[56] Jitpakdi A, Choochote W, Insun D, Tippawangkosol P, Keha P, Pitasawat B (1999) Screening of ten plant species for metaphase chromosome preparation in adult mosquitos (Diptera: Culicidae) using an inoculation technique. J. Med. Entomol. 36: 892-895.

[57] Choochote W, Pitasawat B, Jitpakdi A, Rattanachanpichai E, Riyong D, Leemingsawat S, Wongkamchai S (2001) The application of ethanol-extracted *Gloriosa superba* for metaphase chromosome preparation in mosquitoes. Southeast Asian J.Trop. Med. Public Health, 32: 76-82.

[58] Choochote W, Rongsriyam K, Pitasawat B, Jitpakdi A, Rattanachanpichai E, Junkum A, Tuetun B, Chaiwong P (2004) Evaluation of the colchicine-like activity of *Gloriosa superba*-extracted fractions for mosquito (Diptera: Culicidae) cytogenetic study. J. Med. Entomol. 41: 672-676.

[59] Baimai V, Rattanarithikul R, Kijchalao U (1993) Metaphase karyotypes of *Anopheles* of Thailand and Southeast Asia: I. The Hyrcanus group. J. Am. Mosq. Control Assoc. 9: 59-67.

[60] Baimai V, Rattanarithikul R, Kijchalao U (1995) Metaphase karyotypes of *Anopheles* of Thailand and Southeast Asia: IV, The Barbirostris and Umbrosus species groups, subgenus *Anopheles* (Diptera: Culicidae). J. Am. Mosq. Control Assoc. 11: 323-328.

[61] White GB, Coluzzi M, Zahar AR (1975) Review of cytogenetic studies on anopheline vectors of malaria. WHO/MAL/75, 489. 35 p.

[62] Choochote W, Jitpakdi A, Sukontason K, Chaithong U, Wongkamchai S, Pitasawat B, Jariyapan N, Suntaravitun T, Rattanachanpichai E, Sukontason K, Leemingsawat S, Rongsriyam Y (2002) Intraspecific hybridization of two karyotypic forms of *Anopheles vagus* (Diptera: Culicidae) and the related egg surface topography. Southeast Asian J. Trop. Med. Public Health, 33 (suppl 3): 29-35.

[63] Park SJ, Choochote W, Jitpakdi A, Junkum A, Kim SJ, Jariyapan N (2003) Evidence for a conspecific relationship between two morphologically and cytologically different forms of Korean *Anopheles pullus* mosquito. Mol. Cells 16: 354-360.

[64] Choochote W, Jitpakdi A, Rongsriyam Y, Komalamisra N, Pitasawat B, Palakul K (1998) Isoenzyme study and hybridization of two forms of *Anopheles sinensis* (Diptera: Culicidae) in Northern Thailand. Southeast Asian J. Trop. Med. Public Health, 29: 841-848.

[65] Min GS, Choochote W, Jitpakdi A, Kim SJ, Kim W, Jung J, Junkum A (2002) Intraspecific hybridization of *Anopheles sinensis* (Diptera: Culicidae) strains from Thailand and Korea. Mol. Cells 14: 198-204.

[66] Park MH, Choochote W, Kim SJ, Somboon P, Saeung A, Tuetan B, Tsuda Y, Takagi M, Joshi D, Ma Y, Min GS (2008) Non-reproductive isolation among four allopatric strains of *Anopheles sinensis* in Asia. J. Am. Mosq. Control Assoc. 24: 489-495.

[67] Junkum A, Jitpakdi A, Jariyapan N, Komalamisra N, Somboon P, Suwonkerd W, Saejeng A, Bates PA, Choochote W 2005. Evidence to support two conspecific cytological races on *Anopheles aconitus* in Thailand. J. Vector Ecol. 30: 213-224.

[68] Thongsahuan S, Baimai V, Otsuka Y, Saeung A, Tuetun B, Jariyapan N, Suwannamit S, Somboon P, Jitpakdi A, Takaoka H, Choochote W (2009) Karyotypic variation and geographic distribution of *Anopheles campestris*-like (Diptera: Culicidae) in Thailand. Mem. Inst. Oswaldo Cruz 104: 558-566.

[69] Choochote W (2011) Evidence to support karyotypic variation of the mosquito, *Anopheles peditaeniatus* in Thailand. J. Insect Sci. 11: 10.

Chapter 3

Genetic and Phenetic Approaches to *Anopheles* Systematics

Claire Garros and Jean-Pierre Dujardin

Additional information is available at the end of the chapter

http://dx.doi.org/10.5772/56090

1. Introduction

The *Anopheles* genus is probably one of the best studied genera among insects of medical importance. Of more than 500 species currently listed in the world about sixty species are vectors of malaria agents and about thirty species are responsible for most of the transmission [1-3]. The important epidemiological role of anopheline species has motivated many studies of taxonomy and systematics with traditional tools. With the advent of molecular tools, the development of informatics databases and new mathematical concepts on shape, characterizing insects has become more and more accurate. Molecular tools based on the nucleotide polymorphism of DNA have allowed the identification of cryptic diversity, confirming and refining previous findings suggesting the existence of many species groups or complexes of sibling species. The development of international genetic sequence database collaborationshttp://www.insdc.org, http://www.barcodinglife.com/ allowed the use of reference sequences for species identification. Although not well developed, the same need for informatic databases arose for traditional taxonomy.

Despite the general acknowledge that traditional taxonomy is important, the decline in taxonomy and skills basis for identifying and describing biodiversity is a striking reality. Retiring taxonomists are leaving orphan reference collections - most often not digitalized - and associated catalogues or literature. Taxonomy being not considered as "big science", few students are entering the field. This has particularly negative effects when dealing with arthropod pests, nuisances or vector species because the corollary is that taxonomic expertise is lost and would drastically be missing if the sanitary situation requires it. Meanwhile the development of molecular identification tools, recent mathematical developments motivated by the need for quantifying morphological characters [4], a new field has progressively emerged, called "modern" or "geometric" morphometrics, allowing to quantify and to visualize morphological differences between taxa.

Both these new tools reinforcing the taxonomic research are not only welcome, they are also highly needed. Entomological investigations for surveillance activities or research purposes collect usually large numbers of individuals (sometimes in bad shape) which means time-consuming identification process. The problem may become intractable when species diversity is high and, as in the *Anopheles* genus, when cryptic diversity occurs (sibling species, isomorphic species, cryptic species, etc.). In case of emerging vector-borne diseases or newly invasive species, the first question asked by health managers, scientists and public authorities to evaluate the risk for animal and public health, and to implement vector control measures, is: "what is this species?". To answer such question implies quick and rapid identification of the species responsible for the nuisance or the pathogen transmission. Therefore, under these circumstances, it does not come as a surprise if entomologists and epidemiologists have looked for new techniques that can speed up the process of reliably identifying specimens and sometimes of delimiting taxa. In the present chapter, we describe two independent approaches which can be used alternatively or in complement to each other: the molecular and the morphometric approaches.

2. Molecular identification of Anopheline species

Before the development and use of molecular assays for the identification of individual specimens, cytogenetics technique was widely used for Anopheline species. This method has proved to be extremely informative, not only for species identification but also in the analysis of population structure and determining the existence of sibling species. However, the required expertise for cytogenetics has limited its large scale application. Allozymes have also widely been used but the need for individuals to be stored in liquid nitrogen constrained the collection. Since the 1990s, the development of techniques for DNA amplification primarily by Polymerase Chain Reaction (PCR) in research laboratories together with the analysis of DNA polymorphism has taken precedence over all other techniques of identification to the species level. The huge expansion of molecular identification assays is related to their sensitivity, reliability and speed to generate high number of identifications. Moreover, these assays can be applied to all stages of development, sex, and on whole specimen or parts (e.g. legs). The first complex for which biologists have designed and validate species specific probes is for the *An. gambiae* Complex[1], because of its obvious epidemiological importance in the Afrotropical region. Over time, a host of techniques have been developed with as common a species-specific amplification for determining an individual's membership in a taxon (Table 1). We do not intend to make an exhaustive presentation of all the molecular identification assays developed to date for *Anopheles* species and complexes, but rather to provide guidance on those most employed, with their advantages and disadvantages, as well as detail and review the relative merits of three different tools for species identification.

---

1 We follow the recommendations as stated in references (1, 2) for the naming of sibling species complex and species group.

Biogeographic region	Complex or Group	Assays	References
Afrotropical	*An. gambiae, An. arabiensis, An. quadriannulatus, An. melas*	multiplex AS PCR	[5]
	An. bwambae, An. gambiae	multiplex AS PCR	[6]
	An. gambiae, An. arabiensis	RFLP PCR	[7]
	An. funestus, An. vaneedeni	RFLP PCR	[8]
	An. funestus, An. vaneedeni, An. rivulorum, An. leesoni	SSCP PCR	[9]
	An. funestus, An. leesoni, An. parensis, An. vaneedeni, An. rivulorum	multiplex AS PCR	[10]
	An. gambiae Complex	RFLP PCR	[11]
	An. quadriannulatus sp. B, *An. gambiae Complex*	multiplex AS PCR	[12, 13]
	An. funestus, An. leesoni, An. parensis, An. vaneedeni, An. rivulorum-like, *An. rivulorum*	multiplex AS PCR	[14]
	An. nili typical form, An. ovengensis, An. carnevalei	multiplex AS PCR	[15]
	An. nili, An. carnevalei, An. somalicus, An. ovengensis	multiplex AS PCR	[15]
	An. bwambae	AS PCR	[16]
	An. gambiae /An. arabiensis as one group *and An. quadriannulatus/An. melas/An. merus* as a second group	quantitative	[17]
	An. moucheti Complex *(An. bervoetsi, An. moucheti, An. nigeriensis)*	AS PCR	[18]
	An. gambiae, An. arabiensis	quantitative	[19]
	An. gambiae, An. arabiensis, An. quadriannulatus/An. melas/An. merus as one group	quantitative	[20]
	An. funestus, An. funestus-like, *An. parensis, An. rivulorum, An. vaneedeni, An. leesoni, An. longipalpis*	multiplexe AS PCR	[21]
	An. parensis, An. leesoni, An. vaneedeni, An. rivulorum, An. funestus	quantitative	[22]
	An. gambiae, An. arabiensis	LAMP	[23]
	An. funestus, An funestus-like, *An. parensis, An. rivulorum, An. vaneedeni, An. leesoni*	RFLP PCR	[24]

Biogeographic region	Complex or Group	Assays	References
Palearctic	*An. atroparvus, An. sacharovi, An. melanoon, An. messeae, An. labranchiae, An. maculipennis s.s.*	multiplex AS PCR	[25]
	An. atroparvus, An. labranchiae, An. maculipennis, An. martinius, An melanoon, An. messeae, An. sacharovi	heteroduplex PCR	[26]
	An. claviger, An. petragnani	multiplex AS PCR	[27]
	An. maculipennis Group (*An. maculipennis, An. labranchiae, An. atroparvus, An. sacharovi, An. melanoon, An. messeae, An. beklemishevi*)	multiplex AS PCR	[28, 29]
Oriental	*An. lesteri* (Syn. *An. anthropophagus*), *An. sinensis*	RFLP PCR	[30]
	An. dirus Complex *(An. dirus s.s, An. cracens, An. scanloni, An. baimaii)*	multiplex AS PCR	[31]
	An. aconitus, An. varuna, An. minimus, An. harrisoni, An. jeyporiensis	RFLP PCR	[32]
	An. dispar, An. greeni	RFLP PCR	[33]
	An. minimus and An. harrisoni, hybrids AC, *An. aconitus, An. pampanai, An. varuna*	multiplex AS PCR	[34]
	An. minimus and *An. harrisoni,* hybrids AC, *An. aconitus, An. pampanai, An. varuna*	Multiplex AS and SSCP PCR	[35]
	An. dirus Complex (former species A, B, C and D)	multiplex AS PCR	[36]
	An. dirus Complex (former species A, B, C/D)	multiplex AS PCR	[37]
	An. aconitus, An. varuna, An. minimus, An. harrisoni, An. jeyporiensis	multiplex AS PCR	[38]
	An. culicifacies Complex (*An. culicifacies* species A and D/species B, C and E)	multiplex AS PCR	[39, 40]
	An. culicifacies Complex *(An. culicifacies* species A, B, C, D, E*)*	RFLP PCR	[41, 42]
	An. maculatus, An. dravidicus, An. pseudowillmori, An. sawadwongporni, An. rampae	multiplex AS PCR	[43]
	An. sundaicus Complex (*An. sundaicus, An. epiroticus, An. sundaicus* E)	AS PCR	[44]
	An. annularis Complex (*An. annularis, An. nivipes, An. philippinensis, An. pallidus, An. schueffneri*)	multiplex AS PCR	[45]

Biogeographic region	Complex or Group	Assays	References
	An. annularis Complex (species A and B) and *An. annularis* Group (*An. nivipes, An. philippinensis, An. annularis and An. pallidus*)	RFLP PCR	[46, 47]
	An. annularis Group (*An. annularis, An. nivipes, An. pallidus, An. philippinensis, An. schueffneri*)	AS PCR	[48]
	An. fluviatilis, An. culicifacies, An. varuna and *An. aconitus, An. annularis, An. pallidus, An. philippinensis*	multiplex AS PCR	[49]
Afrotropical and Oriental	*An. funestus, An. parensis, An. rivulorum, An. vaneedeni, An. leesoni, An. aconitus, An. minimus, An. harrisoni, An. pampanai, An. varuna*	multiplex AS PCR	[50]
	An. funestus, An. parensis, An. rivulorum, An. vaneedeni, An. leesoni, An. aconitus, An. minimus, An. harrisoni, An. pampanai, An. varuna	RFLP PCR	[51]
Neotropical	*An. benarrochi, An. oswaldoi*	RFLP PCR	[52]
	An. fluminensis	multiplex AS PCR	[53]
	An. albitarsis, An. nuneztovari, An. rangeli, An. albimanus, An. triannulatus, An. punctimacula, An. darlingi	RFLP PCR	[54]
	An. benarrochi, An. darlingi, An. nuneztovari, An. konderi, An. rangeli, An. triannulatus sensu lato, An. forattinii, An. mattogrossensis, An. peryassui	RFLP PCR	[55]
Australasian	*Punctulatus* Group (*An. farauti* no. 1-7, *An. punctulatus, An. sp. near punctulatus, An. koliensis*)	RFLP PCR	[56]
	Punctulatus Group (*An. punctulatus s.s., Anopheles koliensis,* and *An. farauti* species complex [eight cryptic species])	multiplex AS PCR	[57, 58]

Table 1. List of references of developed molecular identification assays for different anopheline species.

2.1. RFLP-PCR assays

RFLP-PCR (Restriction Fragment Length Polymorphism) assay is based on the amplification of a known locus of the genome and its subsequent digestion by a restriction enzyme (Fig. 1A).

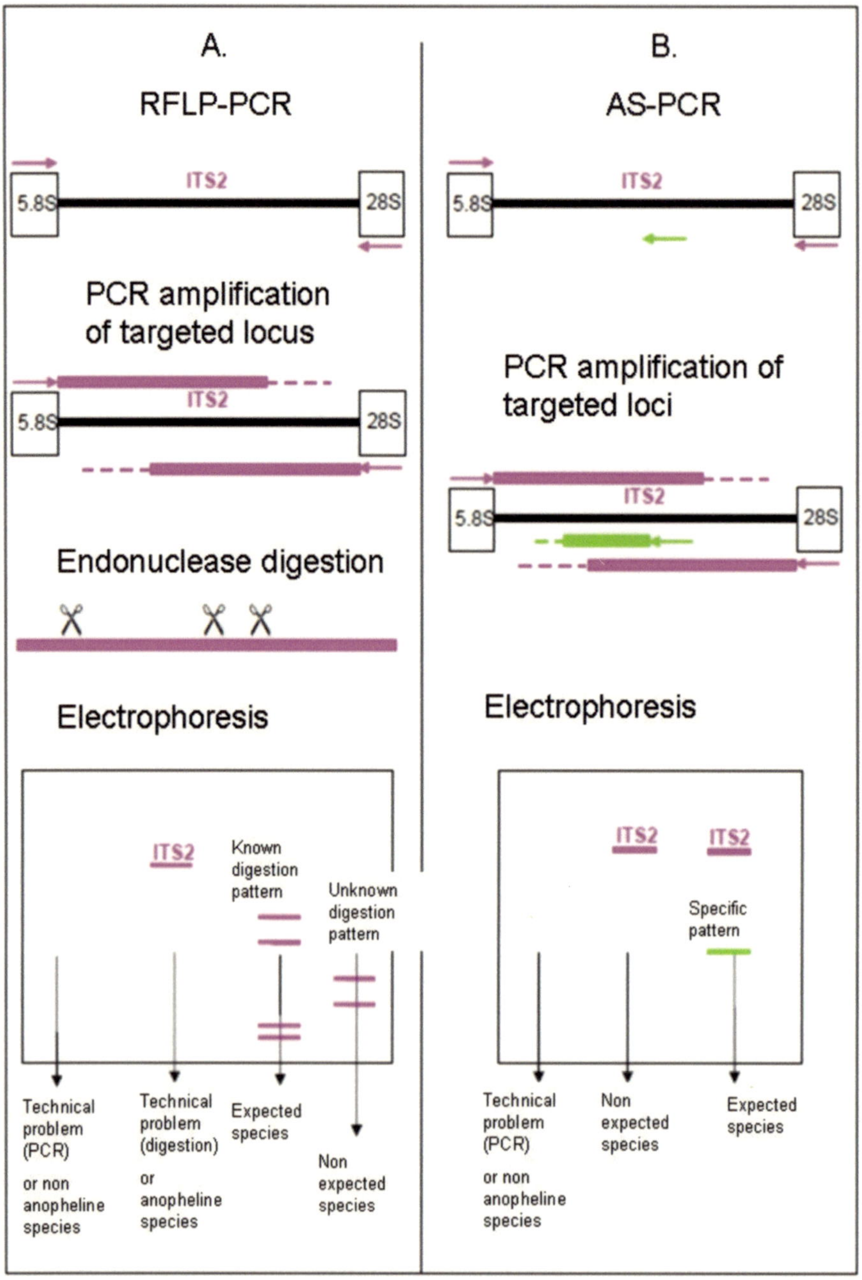

Figure 1. Comparison of RFLP PCR (A) and AS PCR (B) methods and outputs.

The identification of different taxa is made through the polymorphism of the region targeted DNA, revealed by the endonuclease, and resulting in different digestion profiles. Each species is characterized by a digestion profile with bands of different sizes. The need for two steps (amplification and digestion) is time-consuming (digestion can take between 1-3 hours) and expensive. However, an identification assay based on this method is particularly appropriate in the case of entomological survey where anopheline fauna of a region is not known. Indeed, such assay is a priori non-selective and all species encountered give a digestion profile. Examples of RFLP-PCR assays include work on the M and S molecular forms of *An. gambiae*, *An. funestus* Group, *An. punctulatus* Group, *An. minimus* Complex, *An. oswaldoi* Group and Arribalzagia Series (Table 1).

2.2. SSCP-PCR assays

PCR (SSCP PCR) is based on the nucleotide mutations in PCR products [59]. The SSCP-PCR (Single Strand Conformation Polymorphism) requires after the PCR amplification a step of heat denaturation of the PCR products, which are cooled very quickly to generate the formation of secondary structures of single stranded DNA. These formations migrate differentially based on their size and conformation, linked to polymorphism of the targeted region. Migration profile is species-specific and thus allows species identification. However, this method is also time-consuming (in particular with electrophoresis of several hours), and can pose problems of reproducibility. It requires special equipment and the use of polyacrylamide gel, more expensive than agarose gels. This kind of assay is not recommended for the identification of a large number of specimens. Some examples of SSCP-PCR tests include work on the *An. funestus* Group, including Asian species of the *An. minimus* and *An. aconitus* Subgroups (Table 1).

2.3. AS-PCR or PASA assays

The generalization of partial or complete sequencing of many genomes allowed the development of identification assays based on a single step easier to implement and above all faster. These assays have been named allele-specific (AS-PCR) or PCR amplification of specific alleles (PASA) (Fig. 1B). This kind of assay is very specific and robust. It allows to quickly screen a large number of specimens, it is the most common technique currently being developed (Table 1). The basis of these assays is the identification of target amplification of a region of size known and specific to the different taxa studied. This assay therefore requires prior development of primers specific to each taxa and appropriate evaluation of the intraspecific variation of the targeted DNA region. Most recently developed identification tests are AS-PCR based focusing on the ITS2 differences [10, 15, 18, 25, 27-29, 31, 34, 38-40, 53, 58, 60, 61]; older assays targeted the IGS region (*An. gambiae* Complex) [5, 6, 12, 13].

Usually assays are developed to identify several species in a single PCR. When the primers are combined in a single amplification reaction, it is called "multiplex PCR". When developing a molecular identification assay, primers must first be checked for specificity. Moreover, an internal positive control is highly recommended; outcomes must be "amplification" rather than "no-amplification". Indeed, non-amplifications are indistinguishable from a technical problem such as false negative.

The choice of the locus of hybridization primers can be done either from a systematic sequencing of the regions of interest in the species studied, or from a random screening of regions not localized on the genome. In the first case, a prior sequencing of DNA regions studied is necessary. The choice of primers is then made on the basis of nucleotide differences observed between taxa on the target area in order to obtain fragments of specific sizes of each species (more than 25 bp difference). Thus, the identification is based on the length polymorphism amplified DNA fragments. In the second case, the selection of specific primers is made from screening random non-localized regions of the genome. Screening can highlight size of the amplified fragments specific taxa, and in this case be used for identification. Once bands of specific species are being recognized, they are cloned and sequenced. The fragment generated is called SCAR (Sequence Characterized Amplified Region). Of these nucleotide sequences are defined pairs of primers specific for the species to be identified. The combination of different primers may vary: 1) two pairs of primers for two different amplifications [62], 2) a pair of universal external primers and internal specific primers [63], 3) an universal primer and several species specific primers [10, 13, 15, 31], or 4) several amplifications with species specific pair of primers [37] (Fig. 2).

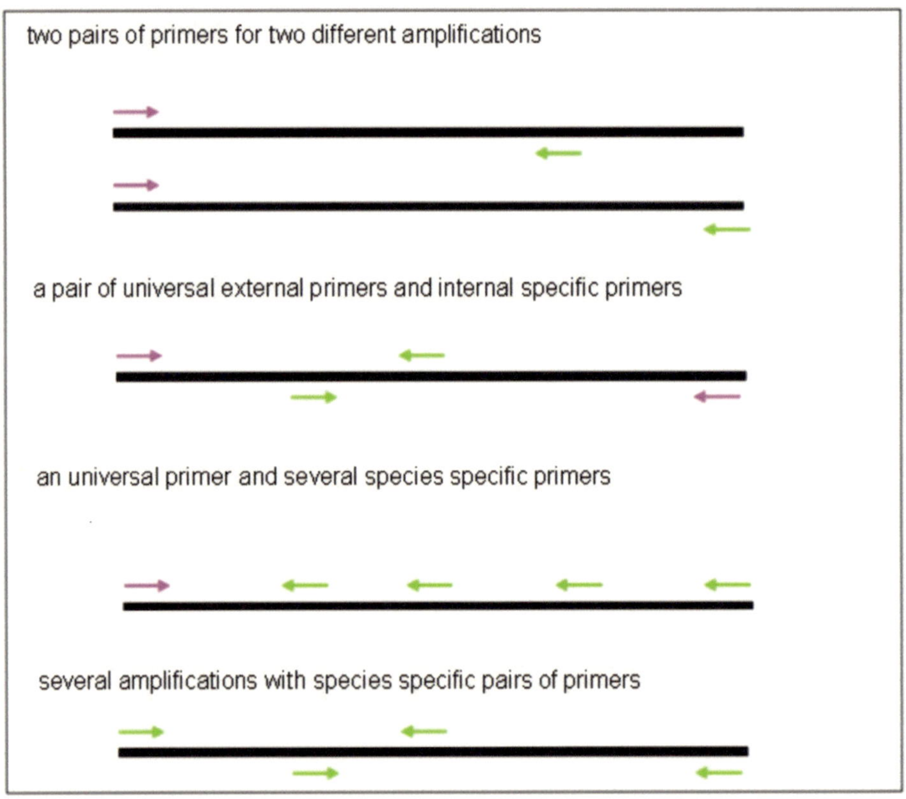

Figure 2. Different types of AS PCR.

2.4. Molecular identification using quantitative assays

The methods described above are qualitative and determine to which species a given individual belongs. However, despite their usefulness for species identification, they are not suitable for quantifying samples with large numbers of mixed species. Moreover, disadvantages of the conventional PCR approaches include the requirement for post-PCR processing (gel electrophoresis of PCR products) and manual scoring of test samples which can be prone to error due to the similar amplicon sizes generated by certain species. For *Anopheles* species, different high-throughput methods based on real-time PCR have been described. These recent assays are based on TaqMan single nucleotide polymorphism (SNP) genotyping and are "closed tube" approaches that require only a single step to characterize a mosquito DNA sample. Unlike conventional AS-PCR, these assays do not require processing of samples by agarose gel electrophoresis, which is time consuming, restricts throughput and requires the use of the safety hazard ethidium bromide (Table 1, *An. funestus* Group and *An. gambiae* Complex). One should expect the development of such assays in the future.

2.5. Species identification and barcode database

The initiative to barcode living forms was set out by [64] and since then the debate on "DNA taxonomy" has not ended with serious concerns about empirical approaches associated with DNA barcode data and their potential to impede rather than enhance the practice of taxonomy and the dissemination of reliable taxonomic information [65]. DNA barcoding is a new technique that uses the variations in short, standardized gene regions (Folmer region of the Cytochrome oxidase I, COI) can be used to identify known species and to discover new ones. This is possible because the variation within each species is low relative to the differences among species. Since its development in 2003, the application of this technology has grown from straightforward taxonomic identification to such fields as biodiversity monitoring and ecosystem reconstruction, with new uses emerging in public health, agriculture, economics and trade, and law enforcement. If a specimen is damaged or fragmented, at an immature stage of development, or part of an undiscovered cryptic species, even specialists may be unable to make identification. Barcoding solves these problems because non-specialists can obtain barcodes from tiny amounts of tissue, in many cases even when it has been digested. The principle relies on specimen identification using a partial sequence for COI. Investigators will identify specimen by first extracting its DNA, then amplifying and sequencing COI before comparing the sequence from the query with COI sequences for all known species. The use of DNA sequences in Diptera predates the formal proposal of DNA barcoding. Particularly extensive is the use of DNA sequences for *Anopheles* genus DNA barcoding aims at providing a new identification tool for unidentified specimens or cryptic diversity (see also http://www.barcodinglife.com/index.php/Taxbrowser_Taxonpage?taxid=7809). DNA barcoding is now pursued today by the Consortium for the Barcode of Life (CBOL) (see also http://www.barcodeoflife.org/). To maximize adherence of barcoding projects to the global barcoding landscape, guideline for DNA extraction, amplification and sequencing (for high through put studies especially) have been released on the CBOL website. Moreover, the consortium created a reserved keyword namely BARCODE when new sequences submissions into International Nucleotide Sequence Database meet the standards established by the consortium.

3. Modern morphometrics applied to mosquitoes with emphasis on the *Anopheles* genus

In modern morphometrics, size and shape are derived from a configuration of landmarks collected on a non-articulated part, often a single organ. Mosquito species diagnostic using geometric morphometrics generally makes use of the wings because these structures are almost bidimensional and relatively rigid, reducing digitizing error. The most common technique is the landmark-based approach. A few anatomical landmarks available on a wing (or any measurable part of the body) are submitted to specialized analyses to provide size and shape information, with the further possibility to visualize shape changes. A few landmarks do not completely describe the wing, nor do they describe the complete body. However, provided there is anatomical correspondence among individual landmarks, only a partial capture of shape is needed to allow valid comparisons among populations and species. There are also other technical approaches, in particular for those cases where landmarks are not conspicuous. The reader should refer to the following references for detailed information on morphometrics such as mathematical approaches and statistical procedures [4, 66-75].

3.1. Why morphometrics?

Various arguments, not only related to cost/effectiveness, should convince most laboratories to apply modern morphometrics. The method is inexpensive. Modern morphometric techniques (at least 2D techniques) do not require more equipment than the one already present in any laboratory of entomology: optical devices (binocular microscope), computers and internet connection. They do not require from entomologists any new practice other than the usual dissecting and mounting, thus new personal is not necessary. The method is fast. While the dissection and sample preparation step might be time consuming, something which itself depends on the group of insects or the organ under study, the morphometric analysis is fast. Various hundreds of specimens can be measured (digitized) in one week, and the analytical steps can be performed in a few days or less. In spite of being fast, the method cannot pretend to quickly identify thousands of specimens. This could be improved with the progress of some specialized software aiming at the automatic digitization of mosquito wings [76]. Although some entomological knowledge is required, there is no need to be an expert in the insect group under study, a skill which is disappearing anyway since a few decades as stated above [77, 78]. The required skill in morphometrics is the same whatever the taxonomic group under study: it is mainly the ability to use specialized software. Morphometric study is a non-traumatic approach, in the sense that it does not impede the application on the same specimens of most other characterizing techniques, including molecular techniques. Actually, the technique could be applied in complement to almost any other kind of study. There are indeed many circumstances in which morphologically distinct species cannot be identified anymore because diagnostic characters were destroyed by the technique of capture or lost in the transport from field to laboratory. Some diagnostic morphologic characters are just a few scales on a given place of the body, and these precious scales are not visible any more on damaged specimens. As an example, the Asian anopheline species *An. dirus* and *An. cracens*, or the

Neotropical *An. marajoara* (*An. marajoensis*) and *An. braziliensis*, are distinguished on the basis of a labile tuft of scales [79-82].

In our experience, obstacles to adopt the strategy to use modern morphometrics in complement of other identification techniques - or as a main approach - are relatively easy to overcome. Modern morphometrics relies on sophisticated mathematical developments. They only require an intuitive understanding to allow a biological interpretation of the data. In the same way as molecular biologists have learned to use different specialized software, morphometricians have to assimilate the use of one or more dedicated software.

Unexpectedly, the picture step may be a problematic one. It is often the only financial investment needed in some laboratories to start applying modern morphometrics. No need however for a sophisticated optico-informatic device to capture the images. Current digital cameras applied to the binocular provide enough resolution and simpler use, even a simple scanner can provide reliable pictures [83]. The resolution, or size, of the picture, must be identical for each image. It should be as high as possible, but there is no rigid rule: the picture has to be taken with the idea to see the anatomical landmarks of interest. An important point is to keep an accurate information of size: size scale should be associated with the pictures. Unless a clear scale could be associated with each picture (Fig. 3), optical zooms should be avoided. And finally, there is no need for a complex imaging software: specialized and free software exists which only need the picture file as input.

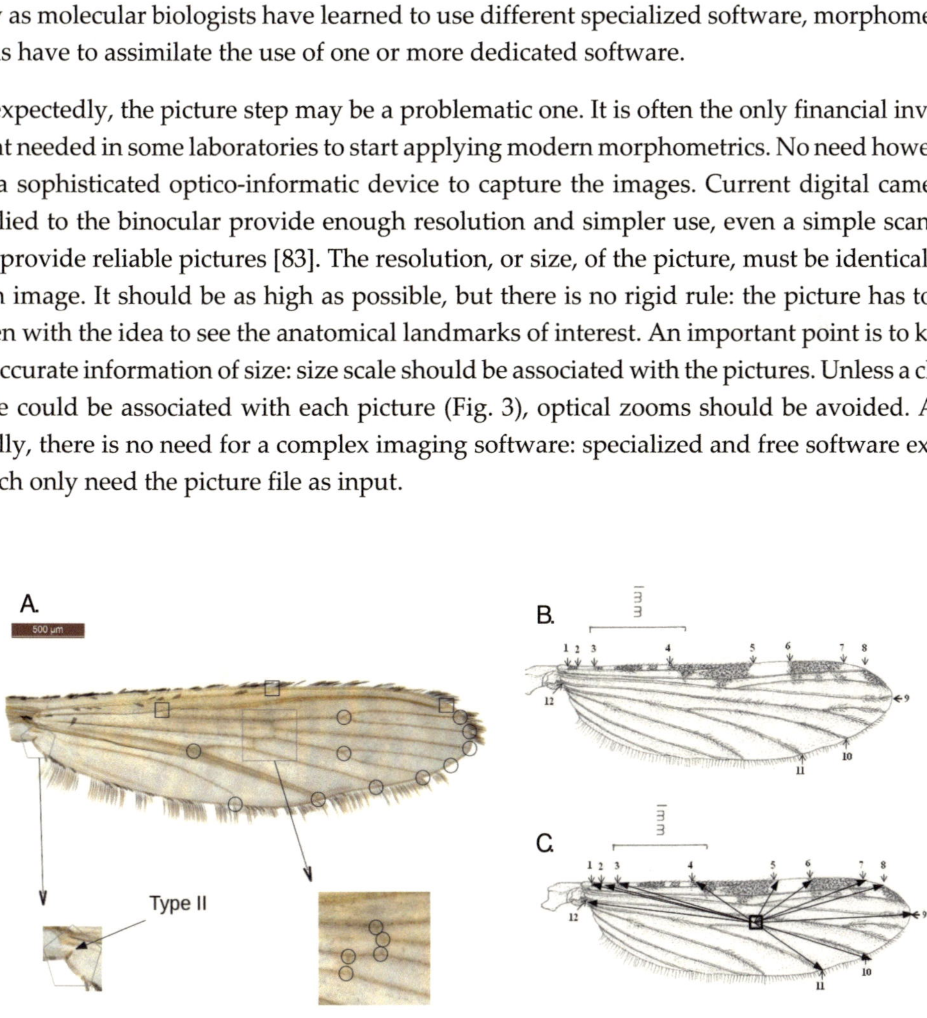

Figure 3. A. Landmarks (LM) type I are the centers of the circles or squares. Circles indicate easily recognized LM, squares may be difficult to localize from one individual to another and are not often used. Landmark type II is the top of the curve making the transition between alula and posterior margin of the wing. The scales of the wing have been removed. B. Figure presented in [84]. Landmarks 8, 9, 10, 11 and 12 are homologous landmarks. The remaining landmarks (from 1 to 7) are defined by the transition between black and white scales. Courtesy of Nicolas Jaramillo (University of Antioquia, Medellin, Colombia). C. The centroid size is computed from the distances (in pixels) between the centroid of the configuration (black square) and each one of the landmarks. The coordinates (x,y) of the centroid position are the arithmetic average of all the x and y coordinates. Modified from [84].

3.2. Shape and size in modern morphometrics

Numerical data of shape are x,y coordinates of anatomical landmarks. Depending on the kind of landmarks, homologous landmarks or pseudo-landmarks, shape is the relative position of anatomical points (Fig. 3) or it is a sequence of points describing the contour of an organ (Fig. 4). Accordingly, different statistics apply, involving the Procrustes superimposition to the consensus configuration [72], or the elliptic Fourier analysis [85], respectively. In both approaches, shape changes can be visualized (Fig. 4).

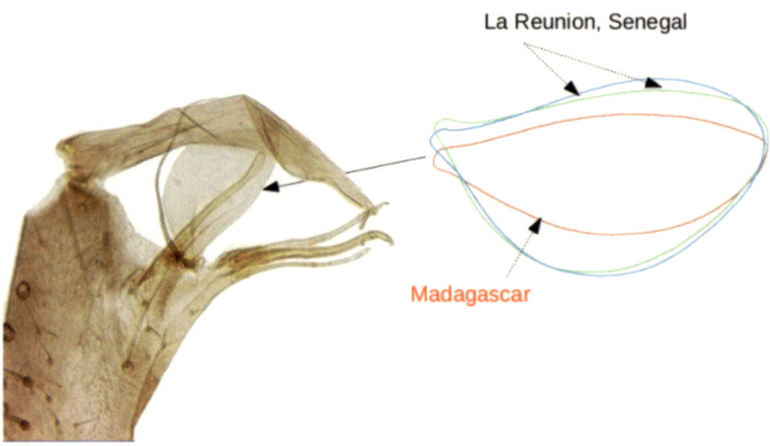

Figure 4. Estimated contours of the male genital leaflet of *Culex* from the Univittatus Subgroup (Pipiens Group) in Madagascar, Senegal and La Reunion. Inverse elliptic Fourier analysis disclosed two shapes allowing non-overlapping separation between Madagascar and other countries. The shape difference, corresponded to genetically differentiated populations, commensurate with speciation (Boussés et al., unpublished data)

Size estimator in modern morphometrics is a single variable which is separate from the set of shape variables. It is thus possible to test for statistical relationship between size and shape (allometry). The landmark-based approach provides a global estimator of size using the totality of wing landmarks, which is called "centroid size" (Fig. 3). It provides information about size changes in as many directions as from the centroid to each landmarks. The centroid size of the wing is highly correlated to the traditional length and width of the wing [86], but not well correlated to smaller inter-landmark distances of the wing [66]. The size of an outline can be estimated in various ways, as for instance the perimeter of the outline or, better, the square root of its area.

In spite of providing many Type I landmarks, the mosquito wing is not easy to digitize because of the presence of scales on the veins. Scales can hide the area where two veins are crossing, so that the user has to guess the likely anatomical point of interest. One strategy is to make an estimation of the digitizing error and consider that with good scores the results can be submitted for publication. The digitizing error can be reduced by using the mean value of repeated measurements [87]; this can be performed also by taking the mean of left and right wings [88]. Phase contrast microscope can improve the relative transparency of the scales helping to localize the junction of two veins [89, 90]. Scales can be tentatively removed before digitizing the wings. Different techniques are used, from mechanical (Fig. 5) to chemical treatment [87, 91-93].

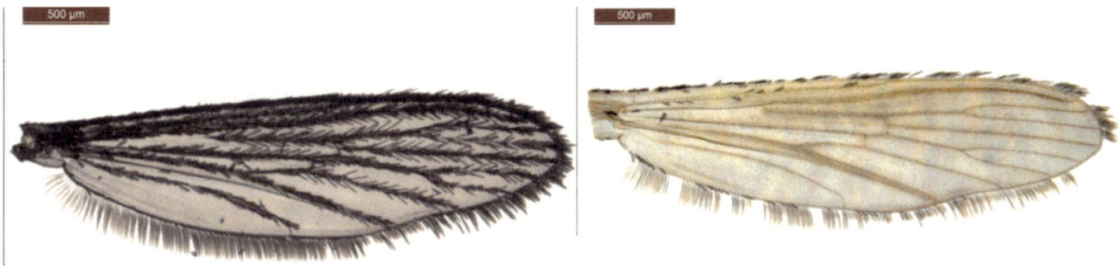

Figure 5. Mechanical scales removal on a *Culex* wing, as processed at the ©EID Méditerranée, Montpellier, France. Courtesy of Guillaume Lacour and Lucie Marquereau.

There is maybe a fourth response to that problem, which is to consider that the scale color could define landmarks. Indeed, especially in some groups of the *Anopheles* genus, scales have marked different colors at specific locations, producing a black and white pattern having an upmost importance as taxonomic characters. As long as the transition between black and white scales could be considered as the junction of different tissues, these landmarks could be assimilated to Type I landmarks. Calle et al [84] obtained remarquable results making use of these scale-defined landmarks together with the more classical landmarks (see landmarks 1 to 7 of Fig. 3B).

3.3. Distinguishing groups: size or shape?

Taxonomists know of many species being consistently larger or smaller than others, giving size character an undisputed importance for species recognition. Moreover, the size of the wing acquired a renewed importance because of its likely association with wing beat frequencies mediating assortative matings [94, 95]: Stanford et al [96] found an agreement between size differences between incipient species of *An. gambiae* and their known level of assortative mating. In species recognition or distinction, a good discrimination between groups means not only to reveal statistically significant differences, but also to allow little overlapping between them, and this is generally best achieved through the comparison of shapes (instead of sizes). In addition to be more discriminant, shape is generally a more stable feature than size with regards to environmental variation. For these reasons, less overlapping and more stability, interspecific differences revealed by shape are generally of more taxonomic utility than size differences between species. As long as shape variation is not the passive consequence of size variation, i.e. an allometric effect of size differences, shape should be the main source of taxonomic information. However, the observed shape differences between groups after Procrustes analysis are not exchangeable to other groups [73], making it difficult to export the results. Even if not independent, size and shape can also be combined to improve species delimitation [97]

3.4. The need for morphometrics database

For taxonomic use, it is not only necessary to adopt powerful tools exploring morphological similarities, it is also important to share the results. Whenever a piece of DNA is distinguishing two taxa, it can be published, stored as a sequence in the Gene Bank and shared with other biologists or taxonomists. When a morphological, qualitative character is discovered allowing to distinguish two taxa, it can be published and shared with other people. Unfortunately, shape variables are sample dependent and cannot be shared in the same way as genetic or morphologic characters [73]. As shape variables are derived from raw coordinates of landmarks, the temptation would be to use the raw coordinates as reference data. However, when the objective is to distinguish very similar or cryptic species, the measurement error (ME) may represent a significant obstacle. ME is always higher between two users than between two measurements from the same user, so that in any circumstance a one-user data set is the most reliable set of data [73]. Two solutions are presently developed to adapt modern morphometrics to a more acceptable taxonomic use: (i) to share machine-computed coordinates [76], or (ii) to share images instead of coordinates. The latter initiative is already running for bees (http://apiclass.mnhn.fr). It is in development for mosquitoes as a bank of reference images at http://mom-clic.com/clic-bank under the name CLIC (Collection of Landmarks for Identification and Characterization). The need for such a database is underestimated because, as it can be deduced from the low number of works on *Anopheles*, the power of morphometrics to identify taxa is itself probably underestimated. The chances of successful identification would then depend on the relevance of reference images, on their level of shape divergence and on the classification techniques.

3.5. Applications to *Anopheles* sp.

While there have been sporadically traditional morphometric studies to help species diagnostic in the *Anopheles* genus [98-104], there have been very few studies adopting the modern approach.

Apparently, mosquito wings show very similar venation patterns among different species and higher taxa, including different tribes. However, Dujardin [66] showed that *Anopheles* sp. could be distinguished from other genera of mosquitoes, based on their venation pattern using 13 landmarks. Regarding species complex, some attempts were made to separate the species of the *An. dirus* Complex (former *An. dirus* species A from Thailand, *An. dirus* species B from Malaysia) using traditional morphometric techniques applied to pupae and larvae [100]. However it may become impossible to identify slightly damaged specimens. In spite of similar size, the separation based on the wing venation pattern was satisfactory in both sexes, even when using rough mounting of wings on scotch tape. Latter study used old laboratory strains, so that an additional effect of morphological divergence could have enhanced the results. Similar studies are required on field specimens.

Vincente et al [87] studied the intraspecific variation of *An. atroparvus* in various countries of Europe at 21 landmarks, adding one Portuguese population of *An. maculipennis*. Authors showed an overlapping on the first principal component of shape between allopatric *An. maculipennis* and *An. atroparvus*. The objective of the study was not to examine the discriminating power of landmark-based morphometrics to separate both species, a task for which the discriminant analysis was more indicated. Notably, size could show drastic differences among populations, interfering with interspecific shape variation.

Five members of the *Nyssorhynchus* Subgenus were compared for wing and leg dimensions with promising results [98]. A few years later, Calle et al [84] used the landmark-based approach to compare 11 members of the same subgenus, some of them were cryptic species living in sympatry. A notable specificity of this study was the combined use of standard wing landmarks with some landmarks at the transition between black and white scales. The technique was able to correctly assign 97% of individuals to their respective species in the Argyritarsis Section (*An. braziliensis*, *An. darlingi* and *An. marajoara*) and 86% of individuals in the Albimanus Section (*An. albimanus*, *An. aquasalis*, *An. benarrochi*, *An. nuneztovari*, *An. oswaldoi*, *An. rangeli*, *An. strodei*, and *An. triannulatus*). These results are noticeable since some of these species are cryptic species, or species with overlapping variability of diagnostic characters, a few of them living in sympatry. In the Argyritarsis Section, shape-based reclassification scores were very high (97% for *An. darlingi* and *An. braziliensis*, and 100% for *An. marajoara*). *An. braziliensis* and *An. marajoara* differ by the presence or absence of tuft of scales in the abdominal segment II as well as by the color of scales of the abdominal segment VIII, with some other characters presenting overlapping variation. As for many morphologically close species of mosquitoes, the identification can be made very difficult on damaged specimens. The three species were collected from different geographic areas, which could also explain their significant size differences. In the Albimanus Section, *An. triannulatus* and *An. rangeli* did not show any overlapping in the morphospace described by shape, but they also strongly differed by size, with *An. triannulatus* being the smallest species and *An. rangeli* the largest one. To distinguish *An. rangeli* from *An. nuneztovari* may be much more difficult and need the examination of immature stages. The wing venation pattern could recognize 84% of *An. rangeli* and 90% of *An. nuneztovari*. High reclassification scores were also obtained when comparing *An. aquasalis* and *An. nuneztovari*. *An. aquasalis* is an important vector in Venezuela, while not in Colombia, and, without a very detailed morphological examination, it could be morphologically confounded with the Venezuelian vector *An. nuneztovari*. The wing venation pattern could distinguish these two species with scores as high as 90% [84]. In some parts of its distribution in Brazil, *An.* (*Kerteszia*) *cruzii* are sympatric with secondary vectors like *An. homunculus* and *An. bellator*. Identification of these species based on female specimens is often jeopardised by polymorphisms, overlapping morphological characteristics and damage caused to specimens during collection. Pairwise cross-validated reclassification showed that geometric morphometrics could distinguish between the three species with a reliability rate varying from 78 to 88% [105].

4. Conclusions

The taxonomy of the *Anopheles* greatly benefits from the powerful information provided by DNA sequences. The identification and detection of *Anopheles* species, especially cryptic and sibling species, are readily achieved using molecular identification assays. The DNA sequences are an invaluable source of phylogenetic information, which is not to say that for species recognition, DNA sequences should be the only alternative to traditional morphological approaches.

We presented here the interest to take into account the modern morphometric alternative for its ability to separate morphologically indistinguishable species, as well as for its unbeatable speed and low cost. Despite promising outcomes, the recent morphometric techniques were not often applied to distinguish anopheline species, and other possibilities, for instance the ones making use of artificial intelligence, were even not considered.

As long as a phenetic approach provides satisfactory scores of species classification, and when the objective is to identify species, its combination with molecular methods could help reducing costs. An integrative approach would not only be less expensive, it would preserve the interest of biologists for the morphological interaction with environmental changes and speciation events.

Acknowledgements

To Nicolas Jaramillo (Antioqui University, Medellin, Colombia), Lincoln Suesdek (Sao Paulo University, Brazil), and Sylvie Manguin (IRD, Montpellier, France) for critical reading.

Author details

Claire Garros[1*] and Jean-Pierre Dujardin[2]

*Address all correspondence to: claire.garros@cirad.fr

1 Cirad, UMR 15 Contrôle des Maladies Animales Exotiques et Emergentes, Montpellier, France

2 MIVEGEC, UMR 224 IRD, UMR 5290 CNRS-IRD-UMI-UMII, IRD, Montpellier, France

References

[1] Harbach RE. Review of the internal classification of the genus *Anopheles* (Diptera: Culicidae): the foundation for comparative systematics and phylogenetic research. Bulletin of Entomological Research. 1994;84:331-42.

[2] Harbach RE. The classification of genus *Anopheles* (Diptera: Culicidae): a working hypothesis of phylogenetic relationships. Bulletin of Entomological Research. 2004;94:537-53.

[3] Harbach RE. Mosquito Taxonomic Inventory http://mosquito-taxonomic-inventoryinfo/. 2012.

[4] Sneath P, Sokal R. The principles of numerical taxonomy W.H Freeman; 1963. Available from: http://books.google.fr/books?id=HP-6AAAAIAAJ&dq=numerical%20taxonomy&hl=fr&source=gbs_book_other_versions.

[5] Scott JA, Brogdon WG, Collins FH. Identification of single specimens of the *Anopheles gambiae* complex by the polymerase chain reaction. American Journal of Tropical Medicine and Hygiene. 1993 Oct;49(4):520-9.

[6] Townson H, Onapa AW. Identification by rDNA-PCR of *Anopheles bwambae*, a geothermal spring species of the *An. gambiae* complex. Insect Molecular Biology. 1994 Nov;3(4):279-82.

[7] Favia G, della Torre A, Bagayoko M, Lanfrancotti A, Sagnon N, Toure YT, et al. Molecular identification of sympatric chromosomal forms of *Anopheles gambiae* and further evidence of their reproductive isolation. Insect Molecular Biology. 1997 Nov; 6(4):377-83.

[8] Koekemoer LL, Coetzee M, Hunt RH. Hpall endonuclease distinguishes between two species in the *Anopheles funestus* group. Insect Molecular Biology. 1998 Aug;7(3): 273-7.

[9] Koekemoer LL, Lochouarn L, Hunt RH, Coetzee M. Single-strand conformation polymorphism analysis for identification of four members of the *Anopheles funestus* (Diptera: Culicidae) group. Journal of Medical Entomology. 1999 Mar;36(2):125-30.

[10] Koekemoer LL, Kamau L, Hunt RH, Coetzee M. A cocktail polymerase chain reaction assay to identify members of the *Anopheles funestus* (Diptera: Culicidae) group. American Journal of Tropical Medicine and Hygiene. 2002 Jun;66(6):804-11.

[11] Fanello C, Santolamazza F, della Torre A. Simultaneous identification of species and molecular forms of the *Anopheles gambiae* complex by PCR-RFLP. Medical Veterinary Entomology. 2002 Dec;16(4):461-4.

[12] Fettene M, Koekemoer LL, Hunt RH, Coetzee M. PCR assay for identification of *Anopheles quadriannulatus* species B from Ethiopia and other sibling species of the *Anopheles gambiae* complex. Medical Veterinary Entomology. 2002 Jun;16(2):214-7.

[13] Fettene M, Temu EA. Species-specific primer for identification of *Anopheles quadriannulatus* sp. B (Diptera: Culicidae) from Ethiopia using a multiplex polymerase chain reaction assay. Journal of Medical Entomology. 2003;40(1):112-5.

[14] Cohuet A, Simard F, Toto JC, Kengne P, Coetzee M, Fontenille D. Species identification within the *Anopheles funestus* group of malaria vectors in Cameroon and evidence for a new species. American Journal of Tropical Medicine and Hygiene. 2003 Aug;69(2):200-5.

[15] Kengne P, Awono-Ambene P, Antonio-Nkondjio C, Simard F, Fontenille D. Molecular identification of the *Anopheles nili* group of African malaria vectors. Medical Veterinary Entomology. 2003;17:67-74.

[16] Besansky NJ, Collins FH, Townson H. A species-specific PCR for the identification of the malaria vector *Anopheles bwambae*. Annals of Tropical Medicine and Parasitology. 2006 Apr;100(3):277-80.

[17] Bass C, Williamson MS, Wilding CS, Donnelly MJ, Field LM. Identification of the main malaria vectors in the *Anopheles gambiae* species complex using a TaqMan real-time PCR assay. Malaria Journal. 2007;6:155.

[18] Kengne P, Antonio-Nkondjio C, Awono-Ambene HP, Simard F, Awolola TS, Fontenille D. Molecular differentiation of three closely related members of the mosquito species complex, *Anopheles moucheti*, by mitochondrial and ribosomal DNA polymorphism. Medical Veterinary Entomology. 2007 Jun;21(2):177-82.

[19] Walker ED, Thibault AR, Thelen AP, Bullard BA, Huang J, Odiere MR, et al. Identification of field caught *Anopheles gambiae s.s.* and *Anopheles arabiensis* by TaqMan single nucleotide polymorphism genotyping. Malaria Journal. 2007;6:23.

[20] Bass C, Williamson MS, Field LM. Development of a multiplex real-time PCR assay for identification of members of the *Anopheles gambiae* species complex. Acta Tropica. 2008 Jul;107(1):50-3.

[21] Koekemoer LL, Misiani EA, Hunt RH, Kent RJ, Norris DE, Coetzee M. Cryptic species within *Anopheles longipalpis* from southern Africa and phylogenetic comparison with members of the *An. funestus* group. Bulletin of Entomological Research. 2009 Feb;99(1):41-9.

[22] Vezenegho SB, Bass C, Puinean M, Williamson MS, Field LM, Coetzee M, et al. Development of multiplex real-time PCR assays for identification of members of the *Anopheles funestus* species group. Malaria Journal. 2009;8:282.

[23] Bonizzoni M, Afrane Y, Yan G. Loop-mediated isothermal amplification (LAMP) for rapid identification of *Anopheles gambiae* and *Anopheles arabiensis* mosquitoes. American Journal of Tropical Medicine and Hygiene. 2009 Dec;81(6):1030-4.

[24] Choi KS, Coetzee M, Koekemoer LL. Simultaneous identification of the *Anopheles funestus* group and *Anopheles longipalpis* type C by PCR-RFLP. Malaria Journal. 2010;9:316.

[25] Proft J, Maier WA, Kampen H. Identification of six sibling species of the *Anopheles maculipennis* complex (Diptera: Culicidae) by a polymerase chain reaction assay. Parasitology Research. 1999 Oct;85(10):837-43.

[26] Romi R, Boccolini D, Di Luca M, La Rosa G, Marinucci M. Identification of the sibling species of the *Anopheles maculipennis* complex by heteroduplex analysis. Insect Molecular Biology. 2000 Oct;9(5):509-13.

[27] Kampen H, Sternberg A, Proft J, Bastian S, Schaffner F, Maier WA, et al. Polymerase chain reaction-based differentiation of the mosquito sibling species *Anopheles claviger s.s.* and *Anopheles petragnani* (Diptera: Culicidae). American Journal of Tropical Medicine and Hygiene. 2003 Aug;69(2):195-9.

[28] Kampen H. Integration of *Anopheles beklemishevi* (Diptera: Culicidae) in a PCR assay diagnostic for palaearctic *Anopheles maculipennis* sibling species. Parasitology Research. 2005 Sep;97(2):113-7.

[29] Kampen H. The ITS2 ribosomal DNA of *Anopheles beklemishevi* and further remarks on the phylogenetic relationships within the *Anopheles maculipennis* group of species (Diptera: Culicidae). Parasitology Research. 2005 Sep;97(2):118-28.

[30] Gao Q, Beebe NW, Cooper RD. Molecular identification of the malaria vectors *Anopheles anthropophagus* and *Anopheles sinensis* (Diptera: Culicidae) in central China using polymerase chain reaction and appraisal of their position within the Hyrcanus group. Journal of Medical Entomology. 2004 Jan;41(1):5-11.

[31] Walton C, Handley JM, Kuvangkadilok C, Collins FH, Harbach RE, Baimai V, et al. Identification of five species of the *Anopheles dirus* complex from Thailand, using allele-specific polymerase chain reaction. Medical Veterinary Entomology. 1999 Feb; 13(1):24-32.

[32] Van Bortel W, Trung HD, Roelants P, Harbach RE, Backeljau T, Coosemans M. Molecular identification of *Anopheles minimus s.l.* beyond distinguishing the members of the species complex. Insect Molecular Biology. 2000 Jun;9(3):335-40.

[33] Torres EP, Foley DH, Saul A. Ribosomal DNA sequence markers differentiate two species of the *Anopheles maculatus* (Diptera: Culicidae) complex in the Philippines. Journal of Medical Entomology. 2000 Nov;37(6):933-7.

[34] Kengne P, Trung HD, Baimai V, Coosemans M, Manguin S. A multiplex PCR-based method derived from random amplified polymorphic DNA (RAPD) markers for the identification of species of the *Anopheles minimus* group in Southeast Asia. Insect Molecular Biology. 2001 Oct;10(5):427-35.

[35] Sharpe RG, Hims MM, Harbach RE, Butlin RK. PCR-based methods for identification of species of the *Anopheles minimus* group: allele-specific amplification and single-strand conformation polymorphism. Med Vet Entomol. 1999 Jul;13(3):265-73.

[36] Huong NT, Sonthayanon P, Ketterman AJ, Panyim S. A rapid polymerase chain reaction based method for identification of the *Anopheles dirus* sibling species. Southeast Asian Journal of Tropical Medicine and Public Health. 2001 Sep;32(3):615-20.

[37] Manguin S, Kengne P, Sonnier L, Harbach RE, Baimai V, Trung HD, et al. SCAR markers and multiplex PCR-based identification of isomorphic species in the *Anopheles dirus* complex in Southeast Asia. Medical Veterinary Entomology. 2002 Mar;16(1): 46-54.

[38] Phuc HK, Ball AJ, Son L, Hanh NV, Tu ND, Lien NG, et al. Multiplex PCR assay for malaria vector *Anopheles minimus* and four related species in the Myzomyia Series from Southeast Asia. Medical Veterinary Entomology. 2003 Dec;17(4):423-8.

[39] Singh OP, Dinesh Chandra, Nutan Nanda, Raghavendra K, Sujatha Sunil, Sharma SK, et al. Differentiation of members of the *Anopheles fluviatilis* species complex by an allele-specific polymerase chain reaction based on 28S ribosomal DNA sequences. American Journal of Tropical Medicine and Hygiene. 2004;70(1):27-32.

[40] Singh OP, Goswami G, Nanda N, Raghavendra K, Chandra D, Subbarao SK. An allele-specific polymerase chain reaction assay for the differentiation of members of *Anopheles culicifacies* complex. Journal of Biosciences. 2004;29(3):101-6.

[41] Goswami G, Singh OP, Nanda N, Raghavendra K, Gakhar SK, Subbarao SK. Identification of all members of the *Anopheles culicifacies* complex using allele-specific polymerase chain reaction assays. American Journal of Tropical Medicine and Hygiene. 2006 Sep;75(3):454-60.

[42] Goswami G, Raghavendra K, Nanda N, Gakhar SK, Subbarao SK. PCR-RFLP of mitochondrial cytochrome oxidase subunit II and ITS2 of ribosomal DNA: markers for the identificationof members of the *Anopheles culicifacies* complex (Diptera: Culicidae). Acta Tropica. 2005;95:92-9.

[43] Walton C, Somboon P, O'Loughlin SM, Zhang S, Harbach RE, Linton YM, et al. Genetic diversity and molecular identification of mosquito species in the *Anopheles maculatus* group using the ITS2 region of rDNA. Infection, Genetics and Evolution. 2007 Jan;7(1):93-102.

[44] Dusfour I, Blondeau J, Harbach RE, Vythilingham I, Baimai V, Trung HD, et al. Polymerase chain reaction identification of three members of the *Anopheles sundaicus* (Diptera: Culicidae) complex, malaria vectors in Southeast Asia. Journal of Medical Entomology. 2007 Sep;44(5):723-31.

[45] Walton C, Somboon P, Harbach RE, Zhang S, Weerasinghe I, O'Loughlin SM, et al. Molecular identification of mosquito species in the *Anopheles annularis* group in southern Asia. Medical Veterinary Entomology. 2007 Mar;21(1):30-5.

[46] Alam MT, Das MK, Dev V, Ansari MA, Sharma YD. Identification of two cryptic species in the *Anopheles* (*Cellia*) *annularis* complex using ribosomal DNA PCR-RFLP. Parasitology Research. 2007 Apr;100(5):943-8.

[47] Alam MT, Das MK, Dev V, Ansari MA, Sharma YD. PCR-RFLP method for the identification of four members of the *Anopheles annularis* group of mosquitoes (Diptera: Culicidae). Transactions of the Royal Society of Tropical Medicine and Hygiene. 2007 Mar;101(3):239-44.

[48] Swain S, Mohanty A, Mahapatra N, Parida SK, Marai NS, Tripathy HK, et al. The development and evaluation of a single step multiplex PCR for simultaneous detection of *Anopheles annularis* group mosquitoes, human host preference and *Plasmodium fal-*

ciparum sporozoite presence. Transactions of the Royal Society of Tropical Medicine and Hygiene. 2009 Nov;103(11):1146-52.

[49] Swain S, Mohanty A, Tripathy HK, Mahapatra N, Kar SK, Hazra RK. Molecular identification and phylogeny of Myzomyia and Neocellia series of *Anopheles* subgenus *Cellia* (Diptera: Culicidae). Infection, Genetics and Evolution. 2010 Oct;10(7):931-9.

[50] Garros C, Koekemoer LL, Coetzee M, Coosemans M, Manguin S. A single multiplex assay to identify major malaria vectors within the African *Anopheles funestus* and the Oriental *An. minimus* Groups. American Journal of Tropical Medicine and Hygiene. 2004;70(6):583-90.

[51] Garros C, Koekemoer LL, Kamau L, Awolola TS, Van Bortel W, Coetzee M, et al. Restriction fragment length polymorphism method for the identification of major African and Asian malaria vectors within the *Anopheles funestus* and *An. minimus* groups. American Journal of Tropical Medicine and Hygiene. 2004 Mar;70(3):260-5.

[52] Ruiz F, Quinones ML, Erazo HF, Calle DA, Alzate JF, Linton YM. Molecular differentiation of *Anopheles* (*Nyssorhynchus*) *benarrochi* and *An.* (*N.*) *oswaldoi* from southern Colombia. Memorias do Instituto Oswaldo Cruz. 2005 Apr;100(2):155-60.

[53] Brelsfoard CL, Fritz GN, Rodriguez R. Sequence analysis of the rDNA internal transcribed spacer 2 and polymerase chain reaction identification of *Anopheles fluminensis* (Diptera: Culicidae: Anopheles) in Bolivia. Journal of Medical Entomology. 2006 May;43(3):460-6.

[54] Zapata MA, Cienfuegos AV, Quiros OI, Quinones ML, Luckhart S, Correa MM. Discrimination of seven *Anopheles* species from San Pedro de Uraba, Antioquia, Colombia, by polymerase chain reaction-restriction fragment length polymorphism analysis of its sequences. American Journal of Tropical Medicine and Hygiene. 2007 Jul;77(1): 67-72.

[55] Matson R, Rios CT, Chavez CB, Gilman RH, Florin D, Sifuentes VL, et al. Improved molecular technique for the differentiation of neotropical anopheline species. American Journal of Tropical Medicine and Hygiene. 2008 Mar;78(3):492-8.

[56] Beebe NW, Saul A. Discrimination of all members of the *Anopheles punctulatus* complex by polymerase chain reaction--restriction fragment length polymorphism analysis. American Journal of Tropical Medicine and Hygiene. 1995 Nov;53(5):478-81.

[57] Henry-Halldin CN, Nadesakumaran K, Keven JB, Zimmerman AM, Siba P, Mueller I, et al. Multiplex assay for species identification and monitoring of insecticide resistance in *Anopheles punctulatus* group populations of Papua New Guinea. American Journal of Tropical Medicine and Hygiene. 2012 Jan;86(1):140-51.

[58] Henry-Halldin CN, Reimer L, Thomsen E, Koimbu G, Zimmerman A, Keven JB, et al. High throughput multiplex assay for species identification of Papua New Guinea

malaria vectors: members of the *Anopheles punctulatus* (Diptera: Culicidae) species group. American Journal of Tropical Medicine and Hygiene. 2011 Jan;84(1):166-73.

[59] Orita M, Suzuki Y, Sekiya T, Hayashi K. A rapid and sensitive detection of point mutations and genetic polymorphisms using polymeras chain reaction. Genomics. 1989;5:874-9.

[60] Koekemoer LL, Hargreaves K, Hunt RH, Coetzee M. Identification of *Anopheles parensis* (Diptera: Culicidae) using ribosomal DNA internal transcribed spacer (ITS2) sequence variation. African Entomology. 2002;10:235-9.

[61] Thanaphum S, Green CA, Baimai V, Gass RF, Gingrich JB. Genetic linkage relationships of eight enzyme/electromorph loci in *Anopheles minimus.* Genetica. 1990;82:63-72.

[62] Paskewitz SM, Collins FH. Use of the polymerase chain reaction to identify mosquito species of the *Anopheles gambiae* complex. Medical Veterinary Entomology. 1990 Oct; 4(4):367-73.

[63] Porter CH, Collins FH. Species-diagnostic differences in a ribosomal DNA internal transcribed spacer from the sibling species *Anopheles freeborni* and *Anopheles hermsi* (Diptera : Culicidae). American Journal of Tropical Medicine and Hygiene. 1991 Aug; 45(2):271-9.

[64] Hebert PD, Ratnasingham S, deWaard JR. Barcoding animal life: cytochrome c oxidase subunit 1 divergences among closely related species. Proceedings of the Biological Sciences. 2003 Aug 7;270 Suppl 1:S96-9.

[65] Meier R. DNA sequences in taxonomy : opportunities and challenges. In: Wheele QD, editor. The new taxonomy. Tempe, USA: Arizona State University; 2008.

[66] Dujardin JP. Modern morphometrics of medically important insects. In: M. Tibayrenc E, editor. Genetics and evolution of infectious diseases. 2011. p. 473-501.

[67] Kendall D. Shape-manifolds, procrustean metrics and complex projective spaces. Bulletin of the London Mathematical Society. 1984;16:81-121.

[68] Kendall D. A survey of the statistical theory of shape. Statistical Science. 1989;4:87-120.

[69] Adams DC. Methods for shape analysis of landmark data from articulated structures. Evolutionary Ecology Research. 1999;1(8):959-70.

[70] Rohlf FJ, Archie J. A comparison of Fournier methods for the description of wing shape in mosquitoes (Diptera : Culicidae). Systematic Zoology. 1984;33:302-17.

[71] Rohlf FJ, Marcus LF. A revolution in morphometrics. TREE. 1993;8(4):129-32.

[72] Bookstein FL. Morphometric tools for landmark data. Geometry and Biology. New York: Cambridge University Press; 1991.

[73] Dujardin JP, Kaba D, Henry A. The exchangeability of shape. BMC Research Notes. 2010;3:266.

[74] Dujardin JP, Slice DE. Contributions of morphometrics to medical entomology: John Wiley and sons Inc.; 2006.

[75] Lestrel PE. Morphometrics for life science: World Scientific Publishing; 2000.

[76] Houle D, Mezey J, Galpern P, Carter A. Automated measurement of *Drosophila* wings. BMC Evolutionary Biology. 2003;3:25.

[77] Reeves WC. Concerns about the future of medical entomology in tropical medicine research. American Journal of Tropical Medicine and Hygiene. 1989 Jun;40(6):569-70.

[78] Scoble MJ, Clark BR, Godfray HCJ, Kitching IJ, Mayo SJ. Revisionary taxonomy in a changing e-landscape. Tijdschrif voor Entomologie. 2007;150:305-17.

[79] Sallum MAM, Peyton EL, Harrison BA, Wilkerson RC. Revision of the Leucosphyrus group of *Anopheles* (*Cellia*) (Diptera, Culicidae). Revista Brasileira de Entomologia. 2005;49:1-152.

[80] Sallum MAM, Peyton EL, Wilkerson RC. Six new species of the *Anopheles leucosphyrus* Group, with reinterpretation of *An. elegans* and vector implications. Medical Veterinary Entomology. 2005;19(158-199).

[81] Rattanarithikul R, Harrison BA, Harbach RE, Panthusiri P, Coleman R. Illustrated keys to the mosquitoes of Thailand iv. *Anopheles*. Southeast Asian J Trop Med Public Health. 2006;37(2):1-128.

[82] Gonzales R, Carrejo N. Introduccion al estudio taxonomico de *Anopheles* de Colombia. Calves y notas de distribucion: Cali : Editorial Litocencoa; 2007.

[83] Kaba D, Ravel S, Acapovi-Yao G, Solano P, Allou K, Bosson-Vanga H, et al. Phenetic and genetic structure of tsetse fly populations (*Glossina palpalis palpalis*) in southern Ivory Coast. Parasit Vectors. 2012 5:153.

[84] Calle DA, Quinones ML, Erazo HF, Jaramillo N. Differentiation by geometric morphometrics among 11 *Anopheles* (*Nyssorhynchus*) in Colombia. Biomedica. 2008;28:371-85.

[85] Kuhl FP, Giardinia C. Elliptic Fournier features of a closed contour. Computer Graphics and Image Processing. 1982;18(236-258).

[86] Morales Vargas ER, Ya-umphan P, Phumala-Morales N, Komalamisra N, Dujardin JP. Climate associated size and shape changes in *Aedes aegypti* populations from Thailand. Infection, Genetics and Evolution. 2010;10(4):580-5.

[87] Vicente JL, Sousa CA, Alten B, Caglar SS, Falcuta E, Latorre JM, et al. Genetic and phenotypic variation of the malaria vector *Anopheles atroparvus* in southern Europe. Malaria Journal. 2011;10:5.

[88] Henry A, Thongsripong P, Fonseca-Gonzelez I, Jamarillo-Ocampo N, Dujardin JP. Wing shape of dengue vectors from around the world. Infection, Genetics and Evolution. 2010; 10(2):207-14.

[89] Jirakanjanakit N, Leemingsawat S, Thongrungkiat S, Apiwathnasorn C, Singhaniyom S, Bellec C, et al. Influence of larval density or food variation on the geometry of the wing of *Aedes* (*Stegomyia*) *aegypti*. Tropical Medicine and International Health. 2007 Nov;12(11):1354-60.

[90] Jirakanjanakit N, Leemingsawat S, Dujardin JP. The geometry of the wing of *Aedes* (*Stegomyia*) *aegypti* in isofemale lines through successive generations. Infection, Genetics and Evolution. 2008 Jul;8(4):414-21.

[91] Aytekin AM, Alten B, Caglar SS, Ozbel Y, Kaynas S, Simsek FM, et al. Phenotypic variation among local populations of phlebotomine sand flies in southern Turkey. Journal of Vector Ecology. 2007;32(2):226-34.

[92] Prudhomme J, Gunay F, Rahola N, Ouanaimi F, Guernaoui S, Boumezzough A, et al. Wing size and shape variation of *Phlebotomus papatasi* (Diptera : Psychosidae) populations from the south and north slopes of the Atlas Mountains in Morroco. Journal of Vector Ecology. 2012;37(1):137-47.

[93] Motoki MT, Suesdek L, Sallum MAM. Wing geometry of *Anopheles darlingi* Root (Diptera : Culicidae) in five major Brazilian ecoregions. Infection, Genetics and Evolution. 2012;12(6):1246-52.

[94] Cator LJ, Arthur BJ, Harrington LC, Hoy RR. Harmonic convergence in the love songs of the dengue vector mosquito. Science. 2009;323(5917):1077-9.

[95] Cator LJ, Ng'habi K, Hoy RR, Harrington LC. Sizing up a mate : variation in production and response to acoustic signals in *Anopheles gambiae*. Behavioural Ecology. 2010;21:1033-9.

[96] Sanford MR, Demirci B, Marsden CD, Lee Y, Cornel AJ, Lanzaro GC. Morphological differentiation may mediate mate-choice between incipient species of *Anopheles gambiae s.s.* PLoS One. 2011;6(11): e27920.

[97] Mutanen M, Pretorius E. Subjective visual evaluation versus traditional and geometric morphometrics in species delimitation : a comparison of moth genitalia. Systematic Entomology. 2007;32:371-86.

[98] Calle DA, Quinones ML, Erazo HF, Jaramillo N. Morphometric discrimination of females of five species of *Anopheles* of the subgenus *Nyssorhynchus* from Southern and northwest Colombia. Memorias do Instituto Oswaldo Cruz. 2002;97(8):1191-5.

[99] Petrarca V, Sabatinelli G, Touré Y, Di Deco MA. Morphometrics multivariate analysis of field samples of adult *Anopheles arabiensis* and *An. gambiae s.s.* (Diptera : Culicidae). Journal of Medical Entomology. 1998;35:16-25.

[100] Hii JL. Multivariate morphometrics for the immature stages of the *Anopheles balabacensis* complex (Diptera : Culicidae). Mosquito Systematics. 1986;18(2):125-33.

[101] Linley JR, Lounibos LP, Conn J. A description and morphometrics analysis of the egg of four south American populations of *Anopheles* (*Nyssorhynchus*) *aquasalis* (Diptera : Culicidae). Mosquito Systematics. 1993;25(3):198-214.

[102] Linley JR, Kaiser PE. The egg of *Anopheles punctipennis* and *Anopheles perplexens* (Diptera : Culicidae). Mosquito Systematics. 1994;26(2):43-56.

[103] Rodriguez MH, Chavez B, Hernandez-Avila JE, Orozco A, Arredondo-Jimenez JI. Description and morphometric analysis of the eggs of *Anopheles vestitipennis* (Diptera : Culicidae) from southern Mexico. Journal of Medical Entomology. 1999;36(1): 78-87.

[104] Lounibos LP, Coetzee L, Duzak D, Nishimura N, Linley JR, Service MW, et al. A description and morphometric analysis of eggs of species of the *Anopheles gambiae* complex. Journal of the American Mosquito Control Association. 1999;15(2):157-85.

[105] Lorenz C, Suesdek L, editors. Rapid microevolution and altitudinal preference in populations of *Anopheles cruzii* in the Atlantic forest of Sao Paulo/Brazil. eSOVE meeting; 2012; Montpellier.

Section 2

Genetic Diversity and Distribution of Dominant Vector Species

Chapter 4

Global Distribution of the Dominant Vector Species of Malaria

Marianne E. Sinka

Additional information is available at the end of the chapter

http://dx.doi.org/10.5772/54163

1. Introduction

Human malarial protozoa are transmitted by mosquitoes of the genus *Anopheles*. There are 465 formally recognised species and more than 50 unnamed members of species complexes [1]. Approximately 70 of these species have the capacity to transmit human malaria parasites [2] and 41 are considered here to be dominant vector species/species complexes (DVS), capable of transmitting malaria at a level of major concern to public health [3, 4] (Tables 1-3).

The aim of this chapter is to document the distribution of these DVS using global and regional maps. In addition, behavioural summaries are provided for the most important species, i.e. those on each continent that are considered the most dangerous and responsible for most malaria transmission, and hence have the greatest impact on human health. Only the primary vectors in those regions with current and problematic malaria transmission are discussed further here (i.e. the vectors of Europe and the Middle-East are not included – but more details can be found in Sinka *et al.* [5]) The regions covered include the Americas, Africa and the Asian-Pacific.

The maps presented (e.g. Figure 1) provide species location information and highlight the existence of a greater number of vector species than is often considered, many in sympatry, across the malarial zones. Amongst these DVS, there are often important behavioural characteristics that must be considered if successful vector control is to be applied. For example, some species do not always enter houses to bite, are most active in the early evening, and prefer to rest outdoors after feeding, such as many of the species common in South America (e.g. *An. albopictus, An. marajoara, An. nuneztovari*), *An. dirus* in South-East Asia and *An. farauti* in the Australian-Pacific region. Others are highly opportunistic in their feeding habits (including *An. darlingi*, the most 'dominant' south American species amongst the South American DVS); biting readily indoors or out. As such, a large investment in insecticide treated bednets (ITNs) or insecticide residual spraying (IRS) will not reduce malaria transmission where such species occur. Thus, to appreciate where different malaria control methods are best applied, one must know what *Anopheles* species exists in an area *and* understand their behaviour. A map clearly and simply addresses the first of these needs, and if accompanied by a behavioural summary, than informed decisions about how to combat malaria transmission can be made.

Maps clearly illustrate the spatial extent of a species' distribution. Often, even within a single *Anopheles* species range, behaviour can vary depending on location. The best known example is the *An. gambiae* complex. The *An. gambiae* complex was initially considered as a single species. Clear differences in behaviour reported across its distribution caused it to be examined more closely and now this complex is considered to include eight species [1, 6] including the DVS: *An. arabiensis, An. gambiae, An melas* and *An. merus. Anopheles arabiensis,* is considered mostly zoophilic, when compared to the highly anthropophilic *An. gambiae,* but still plays a very important role in malaria transmission – indeed, its presence and propensity to rest outdoors is attributed (amongst other factors) to the 'failure' of the mass indoor residual spraying program intended to control malaria in Nigeria during the Garki project [7]. Variability in behaviour within the *An. gambiae* species (rather than the complex) is also commonly reported [5]. Such spatially dependant variability amongst the DVS will be discussed further within this chapter.

The maps presented in this chapter are not a comprehensive analysis of all anophelines. They show only those species designated as DVS; a categorisation initially based on information taken from a number of authoritative reviews [8-12] ([10] translated and updated:[13]) and with additional guidance from a technical advisory group of vector experts [3, 5, 14, 15]. This chapter will also briefly touch upon the methodology behind creating the distribution maps for these DVS including what information is needed to ensure increasingly accurate maps can be produced in future.

2. Global

The global DVS map (Figure 1) gives a clear overview of the variability in vector complexity across the world. Africa appears to show a relatively simple picture of a small number of highly dominant species covering large areas of the continent and although the 'secondary DVS' are not shown (see Figure 4), even with their influence, the comparative complexity between African and Asia is very different. The Asian-Pacific region has 19 DVS [14] (16 of which are shown on the multi-species maps presented here (Figures 1 & 5) – see below) whereas Africa has only seven DVS [5], with the three 'primary' DVS shown on the global map (Figure 1 - see below). Of the 19 species in the Asian-Pacific, nine are now considered species complexes, whereas of the seven African DVS, only *An. nili* is a confirmed species complex (the *An. gambiae* complex is not included here, as specific individual members of the complex are categorised within these seven African DVS) [1, 6, 16]. It is unclear what is the cause of the high diversity of vectors found in the Asian-Pacific region, but it may be simply a factor of the large number of islands, and hence a consequence of limitations in dispersal and specialisation within a restricted environment. Whatever the reason, the Asian-Pacific region maintains a high number of vectors and species complexes and even within individual species, behaviours can vary hugely depending on location (e.g. *An. annularis* – see below).

http://dx.doi.org/10.5772/54163

North America (excluding Mexico) shows a simple vector profile (Figure 2). There are only two species considered here as DVS: *An. freeborni* found in northwestern USA and the *An. quadrimaculatus* complex, found in the southern regions of the country. In Latin America, however, the situation is a little more complex. Despite a number of sympatric species on the continent, *An. darlingi* is considered the most important vector in the neotropical region [13] and hence is shown dominating all localities where it occurs. In Central America this species does not have such a great influence and both *An. albimanus* and *An. pseudopunctipennis* are considered of greater importance.

The individual regions (Americas, Africa, and Asia-Pacific) are discussed in more detail in the following sections.

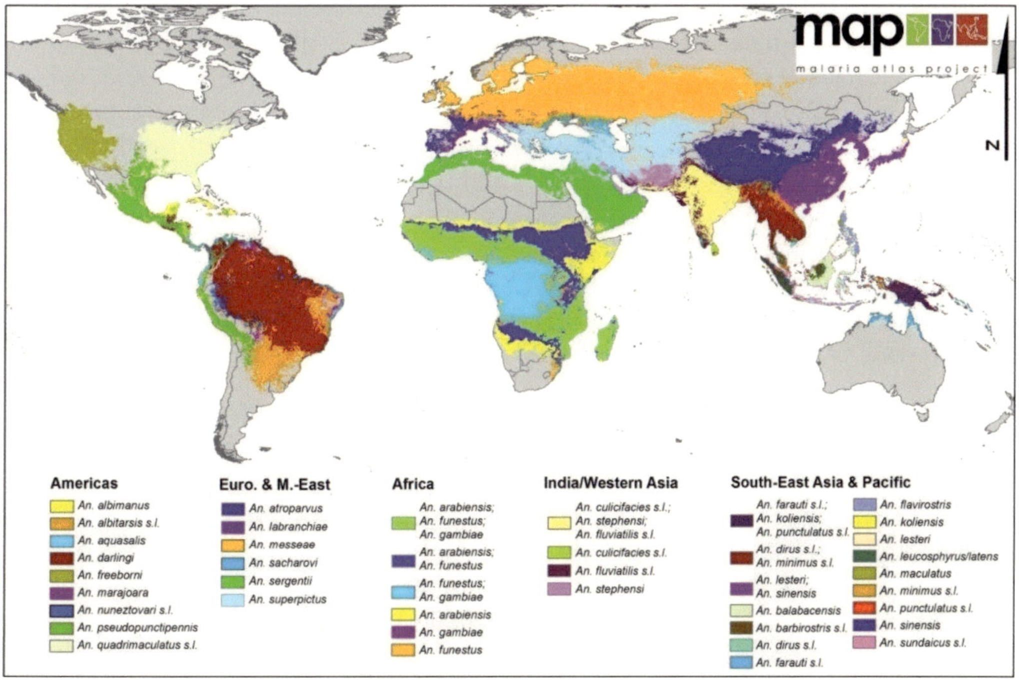

Figure 1. The global distribution of 34 DVS. (Map reproduced from Sinka *et al.* [4]); s.l.: *sensu lato*, meaning 'in the broad sense' referring to species complex

3. The Americas

On a global scale, the nations of the Americas benefit from having the lowest *P. falciparum* morbidity, with stable risk areas typically having low levels of endemicity ($PfPR_{2\text{-}10} \leq 5\%$) [17]. Such reduced levels of malaria transmission coupled with continuing reports of decreasing mortality and morbidity for all major *Plasmodium* species across the region (e.g. between 2000 and 2007) [18] have been credited to an increasing use of integrated vector control [19].

Integrated vector control/management relies on a number of factors, but foremost (as given in the World Health Organisation (WHO), strategic framework for integrated vector management [20]) is the 'selection of proven vector control methods based on knowledge of local vector biology and ecology, disease transmission and morbidity'; essentially, knowing which vector species is present and understanding how it behaves.

There are nine DVS in the Americas (Figure 2, Table 1) [15], with two species having their distributions contained entirely within North America (*An. freeborni* and *An. quadrimaculatus*), and the remaining six species encompassing areas from southern North America, through Central America and into South America, incorporating the northern reaches of Argentina. As stated above, in South America, *An. darlingi* is considered to be the most important of the DVS where it is found [13]. However there is increasing evidence of the importance of other species, including members of the *An. albitarsis* complex (e.g. *An. marajoara*), that may have a higher influence in malaria transmission than previously thought [21]. As such, and due to the dominance across the continent indicated by the *An. darlingi* distribution in Figure 2, single species maps are also shown for *An. albitarsis, An. marajoara, An. nuneztovari* and *An. pseudopunctipennis* (Figure 3).

Many of the American species show great variability in their adult behaviour, with most showing little preference for biting either humans or animals [15] (Table 1), tending to feed on whichever host they first encounter. This variability is also reflected in their propensity to bite both indoors and out. Overall, the majority of DVS in the Americas will rest outside after biting (Table 1, [15]).

Despite similar adult behaviour amongst many of the South American DVS, there are a number of behavioural characteristics found in the larval stages that do differentiate the species (Table 1). For example *An. aquasalis,* whose name means salt (salis) water (aqua), is a vector found in coastal environments. Its larvae prefer clear, non-polluted water bodies such as mangrove swamps, lagoons and ditches [22, 23]. They can develop in fresh water sites, but it is considered a poor competitor in such habitats, especially against *An. albimanus* [15], which may be causal in tending to restrict the range of *An. aquasalis* to brackish locations.

Anopheles darlingi larvae are characteristically associated with patches of floating debris found along river margins in rural and lowland forested areas [24]. *Anopheles marajoara* is also found in lowland areas but is more common in secondary forests and is able to adapt to environments that have undergone some human intervention [21, 25] which may be a causal factor in its increasing dominance over *An. darlingi* in some localities. Forest clearance and pollution will decrease sites suitable for *An. darlingi* but increase the availability of sunlit marshy areas and ponds more suitable for *An. marajoara* [21, 26].

The *An. pseudopunctipennis* complex is known to be able to survive and transmit malaria at altitudes higher than many other DVS, up to 3000 m [27, 28]. Its larvae also have a defining characteristic; an apparent obligate association with filamentous *Spirogyra*-type green algae [23, 27, 29-31] (Table 1). Indeed, the removal of such algae has been shown to be a viable method of control for this species [31].

http://dx.doi.org/10.5772/54163

Species	Larval site characteristics	Host		Biting		Resting		Other
		Anthropo-philic	Zoophilic	Endophagic	Exophagic	Endophilic	Exophilic	
An. albimanus	Sunlit, brackish or fresh, clear, still or flowing water, containing higher plants or algae	•	•		•		•	Bites at dusk/night
An. albitarsis complex	Sunlit, fresh, clear or turbid, still water with some higher plants or algae	•	•	•	•	○	•	Bites at dusk/night
An. aquasalis	Sunlit, brackish or fresh, clear or turbid, still or flowing water with some higher plants or algae	•	•	•	•	-	•	An ability to utilise brackish coastal larval habitats raises this species from a relatively poor vector to a DVS. Has been found biting in the day but mostly bites at dusk/night
An. darlingi	Shaded (occasionally sunlit), fresh (occasionally brackish), clear or turbid, still or flowing water with higher plants or algae	•	○	•	•	-	•	Bites at dusk, night and dawn
An. freeborni	Sunlit, fresh, clear, still water with higher plants or algae	•	•	•	•	-	•	Bites at dusk, night and dawn
An. marajoara	Sunlit (occasionally shaded), fresh, clear or turbid, still or flowing water with higher plants or algae	•	•	•	•	-	•	Bites at dusk/night
An. nuneztovari complex	Sunlit or shaded, fresh, clear or turbid, still or flowing water with higher plants or algae		•		•	-	•	Bites at dusk, night and dawn
An. pseudopunctipennis	Sunlit, brackish or fresh, clear or turbid, still or flowing water with higher plants or algae	•	•	•	•	•	•	Larval habitats are strongly associated with filamentous algae, and species can exist at high altitudes (up to 3000 m). Bites at night
An. quadrimaculatus complex	Sunlit, fresh, clear or turbid, still water with higher plants or algae. Occasionally no vegetation		•	-	•	-	•	Bites at dusk, night and dawn and occasionally in the day

Table 1. Summary of bionomics of the DVS of the Americas (created by cross referencing TAG and literature searches). Filled dot (•) indicates typical behaviour, open dot (○) indicates non-typical behaviour but examples exist, and dashes (-) indicate no data.

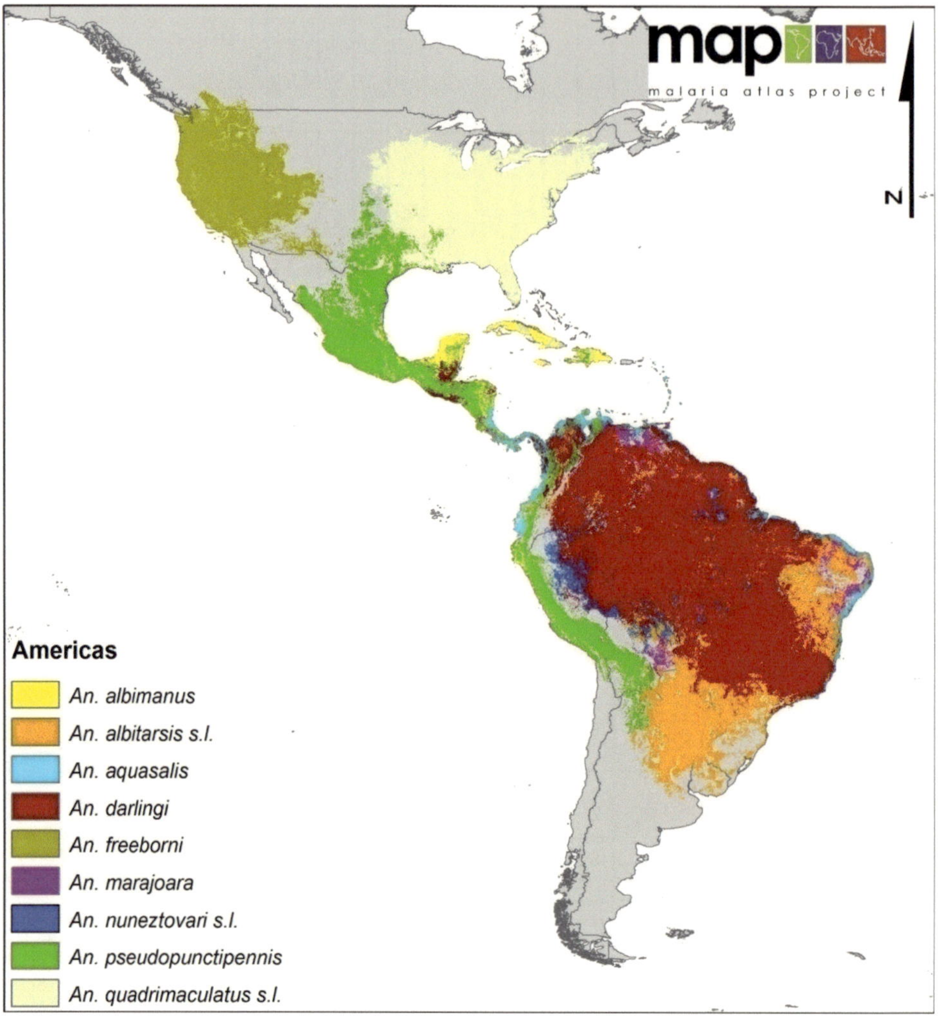

Figure 2. Multi-species map of the nine DVS of the Americas (map reproduced from Sinka *et al.* [4])

4. Africa

Across the huge and variable landscape of the African continent, there is a corresponding variability in the intensity of malaria transmission [32, 33]. Sub-saharan Africa is, however, home to localities suffering from the highest global malaria transmission levels, and hence, morbidity and mortality of malaria [17, 32, 34-36]; a consequence of the wide spread presence of the most effective and efficient vector currently known, *An. gambiae* [37, 38]. *Anopheles gambiae* is a member of the *An. gambiae* complex, which also contains other DVS including *An. arabiensis, An. merus* and *An. melas* [6, 39-42]. Also found in Africa is the widespread *An.*

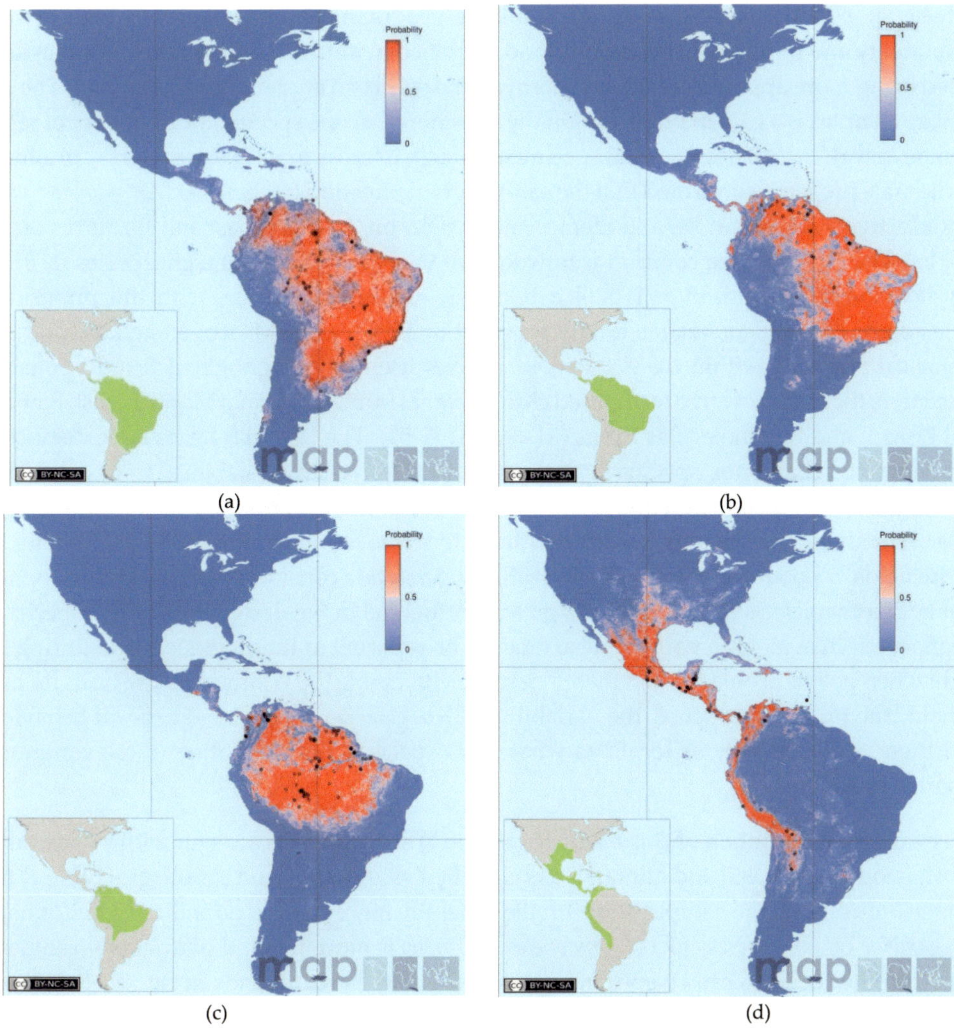

Figure 3. Predicted distribution maps for a) *An. albitarsis* s.l. (n = 138); b) *An. marajoara* (n = 56); c) *An. nuneztovari* (n = 171); d) *An. pseudopunctipennis* (n = 156). The insert map in each shows the expert opinion distribution for that species (Maps reproduced from Sinka et al, [15]).

funestus subgroup of which *An. funestus* is another highly effective vector, and possibly the first species to adapt to make use of humans as a food/blood source [43]. The more restricted, but still highly anthropophilic *An. moucheti* and the more widespread *An. nili* complex add to a suite of vectors within Africa that have proved highly efficient in malaria transmission and equally difficult to control [5].

Figure 1 shows those vector species that can be considered the 'primary' DVS of Africa: *An. gambiae, An. arabiensis* and *An. funestus*. Figure 4 indicates the more 'secondary' DVS, including *An. moucheti, An. nili, An. melas* and *An. merus*. Examining only the 'primary' species (Figure 1), the vector situation in Africa appears relatively simple. However for each of these species to have an extensive spread across such a large geographical area suggests a high level of adaptability and plasticity in behaviours and tolerances within all of these DVS. This plasticity is becoming more apparent as the taxonomy of the species complexes are untangled. The *An. gambiae* complex is a case in point. Originally considered as one species, the discovery of saline tolerant larval '*An. gambiae*' coastal specimens which, in cross mating experiments, produced sterile male progeny, confirmed that the salt-water tolerant and fresh-water '*An. gambiae*' were reproductively incompatible, and identified *An. melas* on the west coast and *An. merus* on the east [44-47]. The Gambiae complex is now known to consist of at least eight species [1, 6] yet this taxonomic categorisation is still a relatively recent occurrence, with the provisional inclusion of *An. quadriannulatus* B only reported in 1998 [6, 48]. Moreover, behavioural and ecological plasticity within the *An. gambiae* species itself have highlighted further potential speciation; there are now five recognised chromosomal forms (Savanna, Mopti, Forest, Bamako and Bissau) and two molecular forms (M and S) [49-51]. The M and S forms have distinctive and separate behaviours, specifically in terms of preferred larval habitats, with the S form utilising larval sites considered typical for *An. gambiae* (i.e. temporary pools or puddles that only occur after rain) whereas larvae from the M form are found in more permanent sites such as rice fields or flooded areas [52-57]. Overall, *An. gambiae* is considered highly anthropophilic (Table 2), a characteristic that is held as greatly influential in the designation of this species as the most effective malaria vector. It also tends to be reported as biting indoors and during the night when people are asleep and therefore more vulnerable [5]. Although these traits do tend to hold true in a general sense, the variability of *An. gambiae* does extend to adult behaviour and there are a number of localities where this species does not follow these commonly reported behaviours [5].

The extensive distribution of *An. arabiensis* (Figure 1) also indicates a vector with a wide range of behaviours [40, 58, 59] and although it is classified as zoophilic and exophagic (Table 2) this is often only reported in comparison with the generally highly anthropophilic and endophagic *An. gambiae* or *An. funestus* [5, 60]. *Anopheles arabiensis* is more tolerant of drier environments than the other DVS, as can be seen in Figure 1 where its range extends north (the Sahel) and south (desert and steppe of Namibia and Botswana) beyond those of either *An. gambiae* or *An. funestus.* It is noticeably absent from the humid, forested areas of western Africa (Figure 1).

Despite the zoophilic label, the feeding behaviour of *An. arabiensis* varies greatly depending upon location, host availability and the local genotype [40, 58, 59, 61] and there is some suggestion that *An. arabiensis* populations are more anthropophilic, endophilic and endophagic in western Africa whereas those in the east are more zoophilic and exophilic [62].

Beside the apparent inability to exist in the forested west of Africa, *An. arabiensis* appears to tolerate a much greater range of larval sites than *An. gambiae*. Similar to its sibling, it makes use of sunlit, temporary, shallow fresh-water habitats and the larger more permanent sites as characterised by *An. gambiae* M form, but it is also able to survive in flowing water, turbid or polluted sites and even, on occasion, brackish habitats [5, 63-66]. It readily makes use of rice fields, although its propensity for sunlit water means it is primarily found when the rice plants are small and larval numbers reduce substantially as the plants mature [67-70]. The adapta-

http://dx.doi.org/10.5772/54163

Species	Larval site characteristics	Host		Biting		Resting		Other
		Anthropo-philic	Zoophilic	Endophagic	Exophagic	Endophilic	Exophilic	
An. arabiensis	Sunlit (occasionally shaded), fresh (occasionally brackish), clear or turbid, still or flowing water with higher plants or algae (occasionally without vegetation)	•	•	○	•	○	•	Bites at dusk/night and occasionally at dawn. Species shows high behavioural plasticity and readily adapts in response to control
An. funestus	Sunlit or shaded, fresh (occasionally brackish), clear, still or flowing water with higher plants or algae (occasionally without vegetation)	•	○	•	•	•	○	Bites at dusk, but mainly during the night and to a lesser extent at dawn
An. gambiae	Sunlit (occasionally shaded), fresh (occasionally brackish), clear or turbid, still or flowing water with or without higher plants or algae	•	○	•	•	•	•	Larval site characteristics are influenced by molecular and/or chromosomal form
An. melas	Sunlit or shaded, fresh or brackish, clear or turbid, still water with higher plants or algae	•	•	•	•	○	•	Unlike other DVS, *An melas* densities tend to link to tides rather than rainfall
An. merus	Sunlit or shaded, fresh or brackish, clear or turbid, still water with higher plants or algae	•	•	○	•	○	•	Despite also being a coastal vector, *An. merus* is not influenced by tides like *An. melas*, nor can it tolerate the same levels of salinity.
An. moucheti	Sunlit (occasionally shaded), fresh, clear (occasionally turbid), still or flowing water with higher plants or algae	•	○	•	○	•	○	Range entirely restricted to equatorial forests. This vector is highly anthropophilic and endophilic.
An. nili complex	Sunlit or shaded, fresh, clear, still or flowing water with higher plants or algae	•	○	•	•	•	•	Behaviour depends on sibling, with *An. nili* being highly anthropophilic and the most important vector of the complex

Table 2. Summary of bionomics of the DVS of Africa (created by cross referencing TAG and literature searches) Filled dot (•) indicates typical behaviour, open dot (○) indicates non-typical behaviour but examples exist, and dashes (-) indicate no data.

bility, plasticity and general tendencies for *An. arabiensis* to feed outdoors on animals (Table 2) means that this species does not readily succumb to traditional methods of control such as IRS or ITNs [59, 71, 72].

Anopheles funestus, is a highly adaptable species with a large distribution across sub-saharan Africa (Figure 1). It is also a highly effective vector, and in some cases, due to a relatively high longevity plus a preference for human blood and late night biting (Table 2), is even more efficient at transmitting malaria than *An. gambiae* [38, 40, 73]. *Anopheles funestus* is the only member within the Funestus Subgroup regarded as an important vector [73], and can only be morphologically distinguished from other members at certain stages in their development, again highlighting the importance of correct species identification [38, 40, 73, 74]. Indeed, for this subgroup, such identification is rarely reported, and hence the distributions illustrated here (Figure 1) cannot distinguish the true range of this specific vector. For example in Ethiopia, only one known study has performed PCR identifications of the Funestus Group [75], indicating that only *An. parensis* (a non-vector member of the Funestus Subgroup) is present.

Anopheles funestus is a highly anthropophilic mosquito [5, 38, 76, 77] and its endophilic behaviour adds to a suite of behaviours that enhance its ability to effectively transmit malaria [5]. It is comparably consistent in its behaviour and has been subject to successful control via both IRS and ITNs, but some populations have shown a rapid development of insecticide resistance to pyrethroids which was considered the primary cause of epidemic malaria reported in South Africa in the late 1990s [73, 78].

The larvae of *An. funestus* are found in large permanent or semi-permanent bodies of fresh-water such as swamps, large ponds or lake edges [5]. They are also associated with rice cultivation in some localities, favouring older fields with mature rice plants [79-81].

5. Asia

The region of Central, South and East Asia is home to 46% of the global populations at risk (PAR) of stable falciparum malaria [82] and suffers a particularly high impact of vivax malaria, with an estimated 82% of the world's PAR of *P. vivax* transmission [83]. Indeed within the 'top 10' of countries with the highest global *P. vivax* PAR estimates, seven are from Asia (China, Indonesia, Pakistan, Vietnam, the Philippines, Myanmar and Thailand) [84]. The complexity of the vector situation in the Asian-Pacific region increases the problems associated with understanding the vector/transmission environment. This region has a greater number of DVS than any other and amongst these, there are a greater number of species complexes and taxonomic complexities than anywhere else [1, 6, 16].

With at least nine out of 19 DVS found in the Asian-Pacific now considered as a species complex [1, 6], the impetus to correctly identify both the vectors and their behaviours at a specific location is even greater in this region than elsewhere. Indeed, even within those species not currently considered as part of a complex, behavioural variability is common, depending upon location, and in some cases to such an extent that a species considered a vector in one location

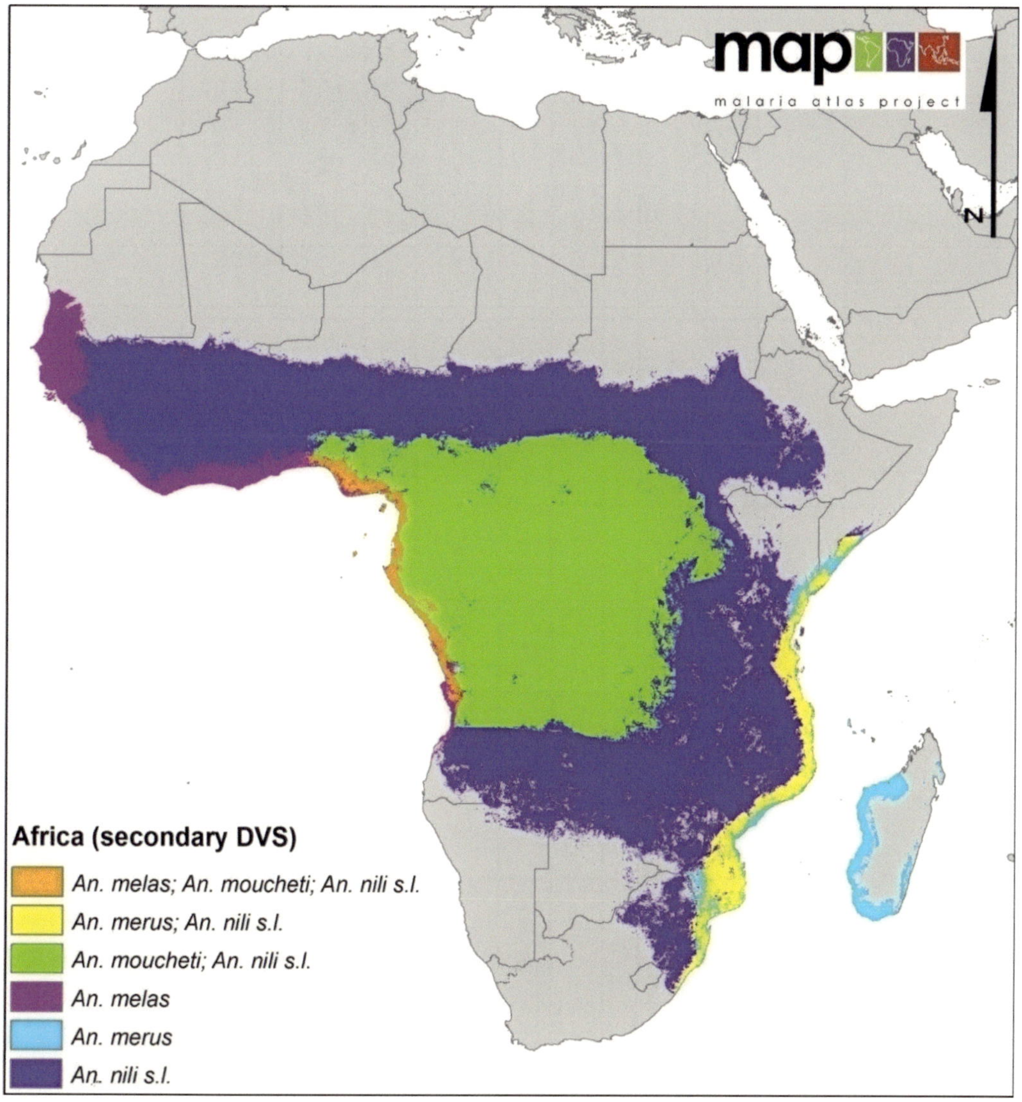

Figure 4. Multi-species map of Africa indicating the distributions of the four 'secondary' but still important, DVS. (map reproduced from Sinka et al. [4]).

may be only of secondary importance, or even a non vector in another [14]. For example, *An. annularis* has a range extending across India, down through South-East Asia, across many of the Indonesian islands down to and including Timor Island [14]. However, it only has a focal role in malaria transmission in selected areas of India. Elsewhere it is considered of little importance [85-91] (hence, *An. annularis,* along with *An. aconitus* and *An. subpictus*; all listed in Table 3 as DVS, are not included in the multi-species maps shown here in Figure 1 and Figure 5, as overall, they do not have as great an impact in malaria transmission as other species in the region).

Species	Larval site characteristics	Host		Biting		Resting		Other
		Anthropo-philic	Zoophilic	Endophagic	Exophagic	Endophilic	Exophilic	
An. aconitus	Sunlit, fresh, clear (occasionally turbid), still or flowing water with higher plants and algae (occasionally without vegetation)	○	•	•	•	○	•	Particularly favours both coast plain and upland rice fields as larval sites
An. annularis	Sunlit, fresh, clear (occasionally turbid), still or flowing water with higher plants and algae (occasionally without vegetation)	○	•	•	•	•	○	Vector role depends on location. Possible complex of two (species A and B) siblings, but these do not appear to be linked to variable vector capacity
An. balabacensis	Shaded (occasionally sunlit), fresh, still water with or without higher plants or algae	•	-	•	•	•	○	Primarily found in forested environments
An. barbirostris complex	Sunlit or shaded, clear or turbid, still or flowing water with higher plants or algae (occasionally without vegetation)	○	•	○	•	○	•	The siblings within the complex are yet to be fully resolved and their distributions are unclear.
An. culicifacies complex	Sunlit, fresh (occasionally brackish) clear (occasionally turbid), still or flowing water with or without higher plants or algae	•	•	•	•	•	○	Bionomics dependent on sibling: Sp E = Anthropophilic; Sp A, B, C , D = Zoophilic)
An. dirus complex	Shaded, fresh, clear or turbid, still water without vegetation	•	○	•	•	-	•	Bionomics dependent on sibling but the two main vectors are *An. dirus* and *An. baimaii*. *Anopheles scanloni* is also anthropophilic but plays more focal role in transmission in Thailand
An. farauti complex	Sunlit or shaded, fresh or brackish, clear or turbid, stagnant (occasionally flowing) water with higher plants or algae (occasionally without vegetation)	•	○	•	•	○	•	*Anopheles farauti*, *An. hinesorum* and *An. farauti* No. 4 are the only siblings considered to be important malaria vectors
An. flavirostris	Shaded, fresh, clear, flowing (occasionally still) water with higher plants or algae (occasionally without vegetation)	○	•	•	•	○	•	Historically confused/misidentified as *An. minimus*. All records of *An. minimus* from the Philippines, Sabah (Malaysia) and Indonesia are now considered to be *An. flavirostris*
An. fluviatilis complex	Sunlit, fresh, flowing (occasionally still), water with higher plants or algae (occasionally without vegetation)	•	•	•	•	•	•	Bionomics dependent on sibling. Species S is the most anthropophilic and endophilic and is the main vector of the complex. Species T and U are primarily zoophilic, exophagic and exophilic and non or poor vectors in India.

Table 3a. Summary of bionomics of the DVS of the Asian-Pacific (created by cross referencing TAG and literature searches) Filled dot (•) indicates typical behaviour, open dot (○) indicates non-typical behaviour but examples exist, and dashes (-) indicate no data.

http://dx.doi.org/10.5772/54163

Species	Larval site characteristics	Host		Biting		Resting		Other
		Anthropophilic	Zoophilic	Endophagic	Exophagic	Endophilic	Exophilic	
An. koliensis	Sunlit (occasionally shaded), fresh, clear, still water with higher plants or algae (occasionally without vegetation)	•	○	•	•	○	•	Currently considered a single species but new evidence suggests it may be a complex of two or more species
An lesteri	Shaded, fresh water with higher plants or algae	•	•	?	?	•	-	*Anopheles lesteri* is synonymous with *An. anthropophagus.*
An. leucospyrus/latens	Shaded, fresh, clear or turbid, still water	•	-	•	•	-	•	Most reported information for *An. leucosphyrus* probably actually refers to *An. latens*
An. maculatus (group)	Sunlit (occasionally shaded), fresh, clear (occasionally turbid), still or flowing water with higher plants or algae (occasionally without vegetation)	○	•	•	•	○	•	Vector role of individual species is unclear due to previous misidentifications based solely on overlapping morphological characteristics and due to apparent variability within species depending on location
An. minimus complex	Shaded (occasionally sunlit), fresh, clear, still or flowing water with higher plants or algae (occasionally without vegetation)	•	•	•	•	•	•	Within the complex, only *An. minimus* and *An. harrisoni* are current vectors of malaria
An. punctulatus complex	Sunlit (occasionally shaded), fresh, clear or turbid, still water without vegetation (occasionally with higher plants or algae)	•	○	•	•	○	•	Within the complex, only *An. punctulatus* is a known vector of malaria
An. sinensis complex	Fresh, clear, still (occasionally flowing) water with higher plants or algae (occasionally without vegetation)	○	•	-	•	-	•	Possibly refractory to *P. falciparum* but an important vector of *P. vivax*
An. stephensi	Sunlit or shaded, fresh (occasionally brackish), clear or turbid still (occasionally flowing) water with higher plants or algae (occasionally without vegetation)	○	•	•	○	•	-	One of the few anophelines able to flourish in urban areas
An. subpictus complex	Sunlit, brackish or fresh, clear or turbid, still (occasionally flowing) water with higher plants or algae (occasionally without vegetation)	○	•	•	•	•	○	The complex is currently considered to consist of four siblings: Species A, B, C and D although there is some confusion in the identification of Sp. B in some localities (may be a member of *An. sundaicus* complex)
An. sundaicus complex	Sunlit (occasionally shaded, brackish (occasionally fresh), clear or turbid, still (occasionally flowing) water with higher plants or algae (occasionally without vegetation)	•	○	•	•	•	•	The complex is currently considered to consist of four allopatric siblings:

Table 3b. Summary of bionomics of the DVS of the Asian-Pacific (created by cross referencing TAG and literature searches) Filled dot (•) indicates typical behaviour, open dot (○) indicates non-typical behaviour but examples exist, and dashes (-) indicate no data.

Unfortunately the high number of vectors in this region, and their complexity, have not equated to a higher level of knowledge, despite considerable effort from local scientists as well as from US military entomologists during WWII and the Vietnam War. Indeed, amongst all 41 DVS mapped [5, 14, 15], the two species with the lowest number of occurrence points, were both from the Asian-Pacific region (*An. leucosphyrus*/*An. latens* (12 points) and *An. balabacensis* (14 points)). There are also limitations when attempting to categorise vector behaviour as again, some species are very poorly studied, or those data that do exist are compromised by unreliable identifications due to the lack of robust techniques that are now available. Hence the summaries given here should be considered as potentially transient and may be updated as more data is collected and systematic PCR-based assays for species identification are applied [92-94]. Accepting these caveats, it must also be noted that the behavioural information presented is the culmination of a comprehensive review of the published literature combined with the 'on the ground' knowledge of highly competent and experienced experts and as such, do represent the best currently available species distribution maps and bionomics knowledge. Here focus is on the species and species complexes designated as the most influential across the region, including *An. culicifacies, An. fluviatilis* and *An. stephensi* across the Indian subcontinent; *An. dirus* and *An. minimus* within south-east Asia and the DVS members of the Punctulatus Group in the Pacific region. More detailed bionomics information and single species distribution maps for all 19 Asian-Pacific DVS are given in Sinka *et al.* [14].

5.1. Indian subcontinent (Bangladesh, Bhutan, India, Nepal, Pakistan, Sri Lanka)

The Indian subcontinent is densely populated giving rise to very high figures for the population at risk from malaria, however, the levels of risk are typically lower than those found in sub-saharan Africa. The majority of people at risk are living in areas of low endemicity (<5% prevalence) or areas of unstable malaria transmission where the disease is not endemic. This is true for both falciparum and vivax malaria. A smaller number of people living in India itself are at risk of much higher levels of falciparum malaria (>40% prevalence), possibly equalling the levels of risk found in sub-saharan Africa although there is a need for more data to support these figures [82].

The range of the *An. culicifacies* complex extends far beyond the Indian subcontinent; it also encompasses large areas of Southeast Asia including Vietnam, Cambodia, Lao PDR and southern China and reaches as far as Yemen in the Middle East with a small distribution in Eritrea as well as Nepal, India, Pakistan and Sri Lanka [14] (Figure 1). Despite this extensive distribution, the complex has only been studied in any detail in India and Sri Lanka [95-100]. Of the five species (A, B, C, D, E) of the complex, four are considered vectors in India (A, C, D and E) [101]. Of these four, species E is a particularly efficient vector due to its highly anthropophilic and endophilic behaviour and is considered the most important vector of both *P. falciparum* and *P. vivax* in southern India and Sri Lanka [102, 103]. The remaining three species (A, C and D) are primarily zoophilic and tend to be considered as playing more minor roles in malaria transmission [97]. Indeed, the highly zoophilic behaviour of Species B means it is often considered a non-vector [99, 104].

Members of the complex are found at a wide range of altitudes, from plains to hilly and mountainous areas [100]. The habitats they utilise are also varied and include forested and deforested ecotypes and irrigated areas. Consequentially, the larval sites they inhabit are also wide-ranging and include man-made habitats such as irrigation canals, borrow pits, domestic wells, tanks and gutters as well as natural sites such as stream margins and rock pools [96, 100, 101, 104-107]. A tolerance to brackish water has also been reported [96, 108], although fresh-water sites appear to be preferred. With many aspects of behaviour dependent on sibling, further investigations, coupled with confirmed identifications of each species, are needed before targeted vector control can be applied.

Again, despite a large distribution (Figure 1) [14], the behaviour and ecology of the *An. fluviatilis* complex has only been studied in any detail in two countries: India and Iran. The complex consists of three species, currently and informally designated species S, T and U [109] and an as yet unconfirmed form V [110]. The complex is distributed widely across the forested hills and mountains of southwestern Asia (Iran, Pakistan, Afghanistan, India, Nepal, Bangladesh and Myanmar) [104, 111-114]. Members of the complex also exhibit behavioural differences, with the anthropophilic and endophilic *An. fluviatilis* S categorised as a highly efficient vector in India [112], whereas both the zoophilic Species T and U, which also tend to feed and rest outdoors, are considered poor or non-vectors [115, 116]. However, species T is considered an important vector in Pakistan, Nepal and Iran [117, 118]. The larvae of this complex are associated with slow-flowing water in streams or river margins [119-124] (Table 3a).

The ability of the larval stages of *An. stephensi* (Table 3b) to develop in urban areas, making use of artificial containers such as domestic wells, overhead water tanks, room coolers, cisterns and roof gutters and in water bodies in construction sites and other industrial localities, brings malaria transmission into densely populated areas including the major cities of India such as Delhi [125, 126]. In general, malaria is considered to be a disease confined to rural environments, as a simple consequence of the tendency of anophelines to search for clean and unpolluted larval habitats and thus the existence of *An. stephensi* in such areas is a defining characteristic of the species.

Anopheles stephensi is found across the Indian subcontinent [14], extending from the Arabian Peninsula, through Iran and Iraq, across to Bangladesh, southern China, Myanmar and Thailand (Figure 1) [127-129]. It is typically described as an endophilic and endophagic species despite a tendency to bite outdoors during warmer months when people are more active outdoors [130, 131]. Host availability seems to be a driver to a variable anthropophily for this species, and therefore in urban areas, there appears to be a greater tendency for biting humans [132, 133], and therefore an increased risk of malaria transmission.

5.2. Southeast Asia (Cambodia, Laos, Myanmar, Thailand, Vietnam)

Human populations in Southeast Asia, with the exception of Myanmar, are typically exposed to low levels of falciparum and vivax malaria endemicity, unstable malaria transmission or are living in malaria-free areas. The majority of the population in Myanmar live in areas with low malaria endemicity but significant numbers live in areas of moderate (5-40% prevalence) and high (>40% falciparum prevalence or >7% vivax prevalence) risk. There is increasing evidence that knowlesi malaria is transmitted from monkeys to humans in this region, particularly in the South, but the level of risk is currently unmeasured [82, 83, 134, 135].

The Dirus and Minimus complexes both contain species considered particularly efficient in transmitting malaria. Indeed, the *An. dirus* complex, due to its longevity and the highly anthropophilic behaviour of its members (Table 3a), is considered to be the dominant vector group in any area where its species exist [136]. However, due to its close relationship with members of the Leucosphyrus Complex, there has been considerable confusion in its identity in the published literature [137]. Species of the *An. dirus* complex are forest dwellers, existing in mountains and foothills, cultivated forests and forest fringes. There are eight members, *An. dirus* (formerly *An. dirus* species A), *An. cracens* (formerly sp. B), *An. scanloni* (formerly sp. C), *An. baimaii* (formerly sp. D), *An. elegans* (formerly sp. E), *An. nemophilous* (formerly sp. F), *An. takasagoensis* and the recently added species informally named *An.* Aff. *Takasagoensis* [138-142]. Of these species, *An. dirus* and *An. baimaii* are vectors of particular note [143-146]. As mentioned above, they are both highly anthropophilic, but their efficiency in transmitting both vivax and falciparum malaria is enhanced through biting humans both in and outdoors and of avoiding most conventional control methods by resting mainly outdoors (Table 3a) [111, 143, 145, 147-150].

Larvae are typically found in small, temporary, shallow and shaded pools of fresh water within the forest environment, such as puddles, pits, animal footprints, wheel ruts, hollow logs and slow flowing streams (Table 3a) [151-154].

Species of the *An. minimus* complex are also found in the hilly forested regions, but unlike the Dirus Complex, are restricted to mainland Southeast Asia (Figure 1) [14]. The complex contains three sibling species, *An. minimus* (formerly species A), *An. harrisoni* (formerly sp. C) and *An. yaeyamaensis* (formerly sp. E) [155-157]. This latter species has a very restricted distribution, only being found in the Ryukyu Archipelago in southern Japan, where it was considered a major malaria vector before the successful eradication of the disease in 1962 [158, 159]. Both *An. minimus* and *An. harrisoni* are, however, still considered primary vectors across their range, which encompasses much of Southeast Asia [14], although all historical records of *An. minimus* in Indonesia are now considered to actually be *An. flavirostris. Anopheles minimus* has a more adaptable nature than *An. harrisoni* allowing it to occupy a large variety of habitats, including dense canopy forests to open rice fields [14] and therefore has a greater distribution. *Anopheles harrisoni* tends to be restricted to deforested agricultural sites [160, 161]. *Anopheles minimus* is also highly variable in its behaviour (Table 3b), being an opportunistic mosquito, although in some reports this may be a consequence of the species complex not being fully identified [160]. Larvae of the *An. minimus* complex are found in small or moderate streams with slow-running, clear water. Females lay their eggs in the partially shaded grassy margins (Table 3b)[162-165]. Larvae have also been found in water containers in Hanoi [166].

Anopheles minimus is considered primarily anthropophilic, but its choice of blood meal can also be influenced by the availability of alternative animal hosts such as domestic cattle [148, 167, 168]. Biting habit is also variable (Table 3b), and dependent on location, with reports of endophagic behaviour in India, Thailand and central Vietnam, but exophagic behaviour in Cambodia and northern Vietnam [148, 165, 169]. The same is found for resting behaviour, although there appears to be a large influence of the use of IRS on resting location and population densities for this species [170, 171]. Overall, *An. harrisoni* appears more consistent in behaviour, generally reported as exophagic, exophilic and zoophilic and thus potentially the less dominant vector [172, 173].

5.3. Asia-Pacific (Indonesia, Papua New Guinea, Philippines, Solomon Islands, Vanuatu, Timor Leste)

Human populations in the Asia-Pacific, with the exception of Papua New Guinea and Indonesian Papua, typically live in areas with low levels of falciparum and vivax malaria endemicity (<5% prevalence), or unstable malaria transmission or that are malaria-free. The majority of the population in Papua New Guinea live in areas with low malaria endemicity (<5% prevalence) but significant numbers live in areas of moderate (5-40% prevalence) risk. [82, 83].

The DVS in the Asia-Pacific region (as categorised here) are dominated by three of the 12 members of the Punctulatus Group, namely *An. farauti* complex, *An. koliensis* and *An. punctulatus* complex (Figure 5). *Anopheles farauti* complex has the widest distribution of these vectors (and of the Punctulatus Group as a whole), extending from the Maluku island group (Indonesia) in the west to Vanuatu in the east, including northern Australia in between. Of the eight species within the *An. farauti* complex, only three are considered to be main vectors, *An. farauti* s.s., *An. hinesorum* (formerly *An. farauti* No. 2) and *An. farauti* No. 4, although there is some, albeit limited and circumstantial, evidence of *An. farauti* No. 6 as a primary vector in the highlands, river valleys and intramontane plains of New Guinea [174, 175].

Despite being the most studied member of the Punctulatus Group, there are still many unknowns regarding the ecology and behaviour of the species of the *An. farauti* complex, with added uncertainty due to apparent variability in behaviour depending on location (based on reports of undifferentiated members of the complex). However, there are some trends that appear relatively consistent, for example, members seem to be mainly anthropophilic, although they will feed on domestic livestock, birds and other animals where available (Table 3a) [14]. Both endo- and exophagic feeding on humans has been reported, and some, albeit limited, endophilic behaviour. On the whole, females tend to be early biters (18.00 – 20.00), biting and resting outdoors [14, 176].

The larvae of *An. farauti* complex are able to make use of a large variety of water sources, both sunlit and shaded, but tend to be found in natural, rain-fed temporary pools through to semi-permanent/permanent bodies of ground water, often with floating or emergent vegetation. Within the complex, a defining trait of *An. farauti* s.s. is its ability to tolerate brackish larval sites, and hence this species is found mainly on the coast in pools within mangroves containing high organic debris and subject to tidal fluctuations. They are also found in natural swamps, oxbows, fish ponds, ditches, borrow pits and pools along stream or river margins [14]. Other members of the complex may have greater or lesser salinity tolerance, but this is one uncertainty that still needs to be confirmed, along with many other aspects of behaviour within the complex.

Anopheles koliensis plays an important role in transmitting malaria wherever it is found, possibly due to its strong anthropophily (Table 3b). Its range is essentially limited to New Guinea Island (Figure 5) with only a patchy distribution in the Solomon Islands, where it is absent in some areas despite a presence of apparently suitable environments [177-179]. Where it is found, it will bite in or outdoors, but is rarely found resting indoors [180]. The larvae of this species are found in more permanent habitats than those of either the *An. farauti* or *An. punctulatus* complexes [180, 181]. Typical larval sites include sunlit irrigation ditches, and ponds containing floating and/or emergent vegetation, often in close association with humans. They are never found in brackish water [14].

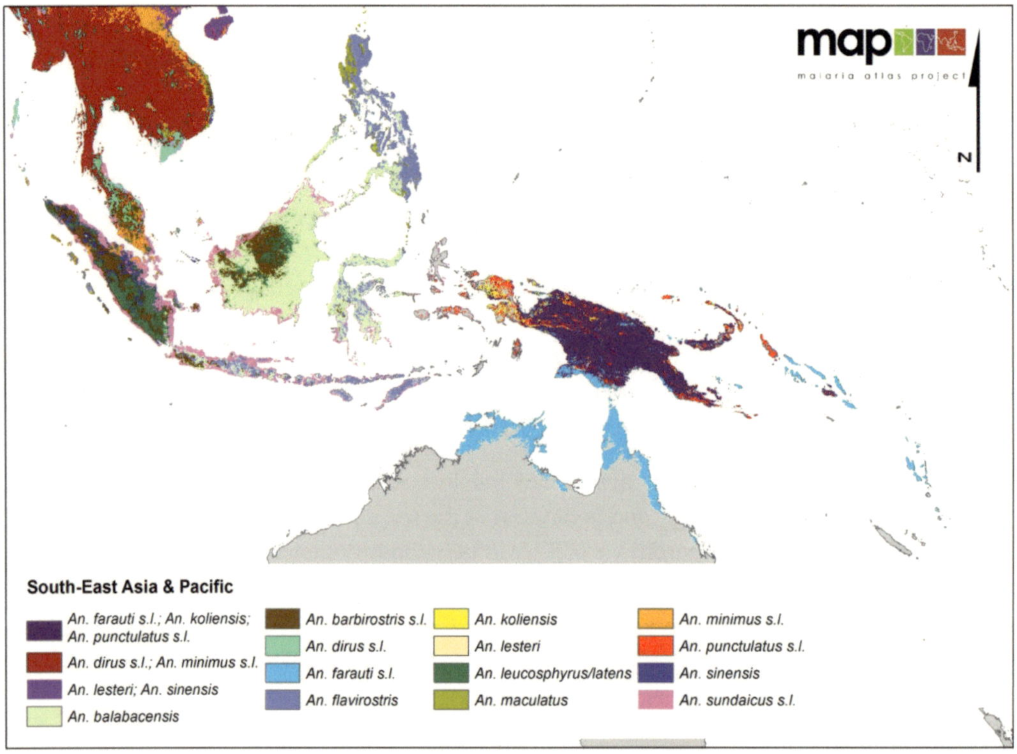

Figure 5. Multi-species map of South-East Asia and the Asia-Pacific region indicating the distribution of 13 DVS of particular importance. (map reproduced from Sinka et al. [4]).

The last DVS in this region is a member of the *An. punctulatus* complex. The complex contains two species, *An. punctulatus* and *An.* sp. near *punctulatus* [182] of which the latter is relatively uncommon and restricted to a few remote highland localities on New Guinea Island where little is known of its ability to transmit malaria. On the other hand, *Anopheles punctulatus* is a highly efficient malaria vector across much of its range, which extends within lowland valleys and plains, and up to altitudes of 2000m across New Guinea Island and the Solomon Islands [174], although its impact and importance as a vector appears reduced in this eastward end of its range [14, 178, 179]. As with other vectors within the Punctulatus Group, *An. punctulatus* feeds readily on humans both in and outdoors and is mainly found resting outdoors (Table 3b) [181, 183, 184]. This species is particularly adept at exploiting disturbed environments, such as those caused by land clearance or areas subject to drought conditions, where receding rivers result in small temporary pools rapidly colonised by larvae. Such colonisations can result in explosive adult populations and subsequent severe and unpredictable outbreaks of malaria [185, 186]. The typical larval sites utilised by this species reflect the conditions found in such disturbed ecologies, i.e. scattered temporary pools of fresh water, generally sunlit and shallow, containing either clear or turbid water with little or no vegetation [14]. Eggs can cope with some level of desiccation and larvae can survive in damp mud for several days during drought conditions [183]. They are also able to withstand high water temperatures (over 40°C) where they grow rapidly with particularly short development time (5-9 days to adults), occasionally resorting to cannibalism to survive, (Bangs, pers com; [14]).

6. Map methodology

A full description of the methodology used to create the individual and multi-species maps is given in Sinka *et al* [15] and Sinka *et al* [4].

The maps presented here were created using the Boosted Regression Tree (BRT) environmental niche modelling method [187, 188]. This method uses spatially defined presence data and environmental and climatic variables to identify the conditions that typify a species' habitat. The model then identifies all locations where such conditions exist and therefore other localities where the species could potentially occur (i.e. its fundamental niche). It also provides an estimate of the probability of occurrence, i.e. applying a numerical value to indicate the conditions within the acceptable range of a species. The multi-species maps show only presence pixels with a probability value greater than 0.5 for each species.

To create the multi-species maps, the individual species distributions were overlaid ensuring the most dominant species (established through consultation with a technical advisory group of vector experts) was uppermost. Where more than one species was considered dominant in an area the species distributions were merged.

7. Conclusions

The maps given in this chapter are presented with the caveat that they represent only the beginning of a process to establish the distribution of these vectors. As with all species distribution modelling, the accuracy of the output is limited by the amount and quality of the data that is available to the model. The data must be accurately geo-referenced and reflect the true and full identity of the species to be modelled. Our maps were created using the most comprehensive database of species occurrence currently available, yet still, for many of the DVS, the quality of the data is ambiguous and the quantity is poor. However, as more reliable and repeatable methods of species identification are developed, species occurrence data and the corresponding bionomics will be better understood as the taxonomy of many of these species are resolved. Moreover, a greater commitment for data sharing between research groups, public health officials, modellers and map makers is beginning to increase the quantity and quality of data available and subsequently, increasingly accurate maps and a greater understanding of transmission dynamics, combined with the benefits of targeted vector control, is making the prospect of the global elimination of malaria a much more realistic goal.

Acknowledgements

The information detailed in this chapter is based on a study originally conceived by Simon Hay and completed in collaboration with an esteemed group of vector experts, who were generous with both their time and expertise, and without whom, the bionomics sections would be a great deal shorter and the maps a great deal poorer. I would therefore like to thank Michael J. Bangs, Theeraphap Chareonviriyaphap, Maureen Coetzee, Ralph E. Harbach, Janet Hemingway, Sylvie Manguin, Charles M. Mbogo and Yasmin Rubio-Palis. Thanks also to Catherine Moyes for providing malaria parasite backgound information and for proof reading this work.

Author details

Marianne E. Sinka*

Address all correspondence to: marianne.sinka@zoo.ox.ac.uk

Spatial Ecology and Epidemiology Group, Tinbergen Building, Department of Zoology, University of Oxford, South Parks Road, Oxford, UK

References

[1] Genus *Anopheles* Meigen, 1818. *Mosquito Taxonomic Inventory* [database on the Internet]2011 [cited 2 December 2011]. Available from: http://mosquito-taxonomic-inventory.info.

[2] Service MW, Townson H. The *Anopheles* vector. In: Gilles HM, Warrell DA, editors. Essential Malariology. Fourth edition ed. London: Arnold; 2002. p. 59-84.

[3] Hay SI, Sinka ME, Okara RM, Kabaria CW, Mbithi PM, Tago CC, Benz D, Gething PW, Howes RE, Patil AP, Temperley WH, Bangs MJ, Chareonviriyaphap T, Elyazar IR, Harbach RE, Hemingway J, Manguin S, Mbogo CM, Rubio-Palis Y, Godfray HC. Developing global maps of the dominant *Anopheles* vectors of human malaria. PLoS Med. 2010;7(2):e1000209.

[4] Sinka ME, Bangs MJ, Manguin S, Rubio-Palis Y, Chareonviriyaphap T, Coetzee M, Mbogo CM, Hemingway J, Patil AP, Temperley WH, Gething PW, Kabaria CW, Burkot TR, Harbach RE, Hay SI. A global map of dominant malaria vectors. Parasit Vectors. 2012;5(69).

[5] Sinka ME, Bangs MJ, Manguin S, Coetzee M, Mbogo CM, Hemingway J, Patil AP, Temperley WH, Gething PW, Kabaria CW, Okara RM, Van Boeckel T, Godfray HCJ, Harbach RE, Hay SI. The dominant *Anopheles* vectors of human malaria in Africa, Europe and the Middle East: occurrence data, distribution maps and bionomic précis. Parasit Vectors. 2010;3(1):117.

[6] Harbach RE. The classification of genus *Anopheles* (Diptera: Culicidae): a working hypothesis of phylogenetic relationships. Bull Entomol Res. 2004;94(6):537-53.

[7] Collins FH, Paskewitz SM. Malaria: current and future prospects for control. Annu Rev Entomol. 1995;40:195-219.

[8] Service MW. Appendix II. Characteristics of some major *Anopheles* vectors of human malaria. In: Gilles HM, Warrell DA, editors. Bruce-Chwatt's Essential Malariology. Third ed. London: Edward Arnold; 1993. p. 305-10.

[9] Service MW. The *Anopheles* vector. In: Gilles HM, Warrell DA, editors. Bruce-Chwatt's Essential Malariology. Third ed. London: Edward Arnold; 1993. p. 96-123.

[10] Mouchet J, Carnevale P, Coosemans M, Julvez J, Manguin S, Richard-Lenoble D, Sircoulon J. Biodiversité du paludisme dans le monde. Montrouge, France: John Libbey Eurotext; 2004.

[11] Kiszewski A, Mellinger A, Spielman A, Malaney P, Sachs SE, Sachs J. A global index representing the stability of malaria transmission. Am J Trop Med Hyg. 2004;70(5): 486-98.

[12] White GB. Malaria. Geographical distribution of arthropod-borne diseases and their principal vectors Geneva: World Health Organization, Division of Vector Biology and Control1989 Contract No.: WHO/VBC/89967.

[13] Manguin S, Carnevale P, Mouchet J, Coosemans M, Julvez J, Richard-Lenoble D, Sircoulon J. Biodiversity of malaria in the world. Montrouge, France: John Libbey Eurotext; 2008.

[14] Sinka ME, Bangs MJ, Manguin S, Chareonviriyaphap T, Patil AP, Temperley WH, Gething PW, Elyazar IR, Kabaria CW, Harbach RE, Hay SI. The dominant *Anopheles* vectors of human malaria in the Asia-Pacific region: occurrence data, distribution maps and bionomic précis. Parasit Vectors. 2011;4:89.

[15] Sinka ME, Rubio-Palis Y, Manguin S, Patil AP, Temperley WH, Gething PW, Van Boeckel T, Kabaria CW, Harbach RE, Hay SI. The dominant *Anopheles* vectors of human malaria in the Americas: occurrence data, distribution maps and bionomic précis. Parasit Vectors. 2010 Aug 16;3(1):72.

[16] Manguin S, Boëte C. Global impact of mosquito biodiversity, human vector-borne diseases and environmental change. In: Lopez-Pujol J, (ed.). The importance of biological interactions in the study of biodiversity. Rijeka, Croatia: InTech open access Publisher; 2011. p. 390.

[17] Hay SI, Guerra CA, Gething PW, Patil AP, Tatem AJ, Noor AM, Kabaria CW, Manh BH, Elyazar IR, Brooker S, Smith DL, Moyeed RA, Snow RW. A world malaria map: *Plasmodium falciparum* endemicity in 2007. PLoS Med. 2009 Mar 24;6(3):e1000048.

[18] WHO/PAHO (World Health Organization/Pan American Health Organization). Malaria in the Americas: time series epidemiological data from 2000 to 2007. Washington DC: Pan American Health Organization, Regional Office for the Americas 2008.

[19] WHO/PAHO (World Health Organization/Pan American Health Organization). Regional strategic plan for malaria in the Americas 2006-2010. Washington, DC: Pan American Health Organization, Regional Office for the Americas 2006.

[20] WHO (World Health Organization). Global strategic framework for integrated vector management. Geneva: World Health Organization 2004.

[21] Conn JE, Wilkerson RC, Segura MN, de Souza RT, Schlichting CD, Wirtz RA, Povoa MM. Emergence of a new neotropical malaria vector facilitated by human migration and changes in land use. Am J Trop Med Hyg. 2002;66(1):18-22.

[22] Grillet ME, Montañez H, Berti J. Estudio biosistemático y ecológico de *Anopheles aquasalis* y sus implicaciones para el control de la malaria en el estado Sucre: II. Ecología de sus criaderos. Bol Dir Malariol San Amb 1998;38(1):38-46.

[23] Manguin S, Peyton EL, James AC, Roberts DR. Apparent changes in the abundance and distribution of *Anopheles* species on Grenada Island. J Am Mosq Control Assoc. 1993;9(4):403-7.

[24] Brochero HL, Rey G, Buitrago LS, Olano VA. Biting activity and breeding sites of *Anopheles* species in the municipality Villavicencio, Meta, Colombia. J Am Mosq Control Assoc. 2005;21(2):182-6.

[25] Moreno JE, Rubio-Palis Y, Acevedo P. Identificación de criaderos de anofelinos en un área endémica del estado Bolívar, Venezuela. Bol Malariol San Amb 2000;40:21-30.

[26] Moreno JE, Rubio-Palis Y, Paez E, Perez E, Sanchez V. Abundance, biting behaviour and parous rate of anopheline mosquito species in relation to malaria incidence in gold-mining areas of southern Venezuela. Med Vet Entomol. 2007 Dec;21(4):339-49.

[27] Manguin S, Roberts DR, Peyton EL, Rejmankova E, Pecor J. Characterization of *Anopheles pseudopunctipennis* larval habitats. J Am Mosq Control Assoc. 1996;12(4): 619-26.

[28] Rubio-Palis Y, Zimmerman RH. Ecoregional classification of malaria vectors in the neotropics. J Med Entomol. 1997 Sep;34(5):499-510.

[29] Bond JG, Novelo-Gutierrez R, Ulloa A, Rojas JC, Quiroz-Martinez H, Williams T. Diversity, abundance, and disturbance response of Odonata associated with breeding sites of *Anopheles pseudopunctipennis* (Diptera: Culicidae) in southern Mexico. Environ Entomol. 2006 Dec;35(6):1561-8.

[30] Bond JG, Quiroz-Martinez H, Rojas JC, Valle J, Ulloa A, Williams T. Impact of environmental manipulation for *Anopheles pseudopunctipennis* Theobald control on aquatic insect communities in southern Mexico. J Vector Ecol. 2007 Jun;32(1):41-53.

[31] Bond JG, Rojas JC, Arredondo-Jimenez JI, Quiroz-Martinez H, Valle J, Williams T. Population control of the malaria vector *Anopheles pseudopunctipennis* by habitat manipulation. Proc Biol Sci. 2004 Oct 22;271(1553):2161-9.

[32] Hay SI, Guerra CA, Tatem AJ, Atkinson PM, Snow RW. Urbanization, malaria transmission and disease burden in Africa. Nat Rev Microbiol. 2005 Jan;3(1):81-90.

[33] Hay SI, Rogers DJ, Toomer JF, Snow RW. Annual *Plasmodium falciparum* entomological inoculation rates (EIR) across Africa: literature survey, internet access and review. Trans R Soc Trop Med Hyg. 2000;94(2):113-27.

[34] Fontenille D, Simard F. Unravelling complexities in human malaria transmission dynamics in Africa through a comprehensive knowledge of vector populations. Comp Immunol Microbiol Infect Dis. 2004 Sep;27(5):357-75.

[35] Guerra CA, Gikandi PW, Tatem AJ, Noor AM, Smith DL, Hay SI, Snow RW. The limits and intensity of *Plasmodium falciparum* transmission: implications for malaria control and elimination worldwide. PLoS Med. 2008 Feb;5(2):e38.

[36] Hay SI, Okiro EA, Gething PW, Patil AP, Tatem AJ, Guerra CA, Snow RW. Estimating the global clinical burden of *Plasmodium falciparum* malaria in 2007. PLoS Med. 2010;7(6):e100029.

[37] Coluzzi M. The clay feet of the malaria giant and its African roots: hypotheses and inferences about origin, spread and control of *Plasmodium falciparum*. Parassitologia. 1999 Sep;41(1-3):277-83.

[38] Gillies MT, de Meillon B. The Anophelinae of Africa South of the Sahara (Ethiopian zoogeographical region). 2nd ed. Johannesburg: The South African Institute for Medical Research; 1968.

[39] Temu EA, Minjas JN, Coetzee M, Hunt RH, Shift CJ. The role of four anopheline species (Diptera: Culicidae) in malaria transmission in coastal Tanzania. Trans R Soc Trop Med Hyg. 1998 Mar-Apr;92(2):152-8.

[40] Gillies MT, Coetzee M. A supplement to the Anophelinae of Africa south of the Sahara (Afrotropical region). Johannesburg: The South African Institute for Medical Research; 1987.

[41] Cuamba N, Mendis C. The role of *Anopheles merus* in malaria transmission in an area of southern Mozambique. J Vector Borne Dis. 2009 Jun;46(2):157-9.

[42] Bryan JH. *Anopheles gambiae* and *A. melas* at Brefet, The Gambia, and their role in malaria transmission. Ann Trop Med Parasitol. 1983 Feb;77(1):1-12.

[43] Charlwood JD, Smith T, Kihonda J, Heiz B, Billingsley PF, Takken W. Density-independent feeding success of malaria vectors (Diptera: Culicidae) in Tanzania. Bull Entomol Res. 1995 Mar;85(1):29-35.

[44] Gelfand HM. *Anopheles gambiae* Giles and *Anopheles melas* Theobald in a coastal area of Liberia, West Africa. Trans R Soc Trop Med Hyg. 1955 Nov;49(6):508-27.

[45] Muirhead-Thomson RC. Studies on salt-water and fresh-water *Anopheles gambiae* on the East African coast. Bull Entomol Res. 1951;41:487-502.

[46] Muirhead-Thomson RC. Studies on *Anopheles gambiae* and *A. melas* in and around Lagos. Bull Entomol Res. 1948;38:527-58.

[47] Muirhead-Thomson RC. Studies on the breeding places and control of *Anopheles gambiae* and *A. gambiae* var. *melas* in coastal districts of Sierra Leone. Bull Entomol Res. 1946;36:185-252.

[48] Hunt RH, Coetzee M, Fettene M. The *Anopheles gambiae* complex: a new species from Ethiopia. Trans R Soc Trop Med Hyg. 1998 Mar-Apr;92(2):231-5.

[49] Coluzzi M, Petrarca V, Dideco MA. Chromosomal inversion intergradation and incipient speciation in *Anopheles gambiae*. B Zool. 1985;52(1-2):45-63.

[50] Della Torre A, Fanello C, Akogbeto M, Dossou-yovo J, Favia G, Petrarca V, Coluzzi M. Molecular evidence of incipient speciation within *Anopheles gambiae* s.s. in West Africa. Insect Mol Biol. 2001;10(1):9-18.

[51] Fanello C, Petrarca V, della Torre A, Santolamazza F, Dolo G, Coulibaly M, Alloueche A, Curtis CF, Toure YT, Coluzzi M. The pyrethroid knock-down resistance gene in the *Anopheles gambiae* complex in Mali and further indication of incipient speciation within *An. gambiae* s.s. Insect Mol Biol. 2003;12(3):241-5.

[52] Caputo B, Nwakanma D, Jawara M, Adiamoh M, Dia I, Konate L, Petrarca V, Conway DJ, Della Torre A. *Anopheles gambiae* complex along The Gambia river, with particular reference to the molecular forms of *An. gambiae* s.s. Malar J. 2008 Sep 22;7(1):182.

[53] Costantini C, Ayala D, Guelbeogo WM, Pombi M, Some CY, Bassole IH, Ose K, Fotsing JM, Sagnon N, Fontenille D, Besansky NJ, Simard F. Living at the edge: biogeographic patterns of habitat segregation conform to speciation by niche expansion in *Anopheles gambiae*. BMC Ecol. 2009 May 21;9(1):16.

[54] Della Torre A, Costantini C, Besansky NJ, Caccone A, Petrarca V, Powell JR, Coluzzi M. Speciation within *Anopheles gambiae*-the glass is half full. Science. 2002 Oct 4;298(5591):115-7.

[55] Della Torre A, Tu ZJ, Petrarca V. On the distribution and genetic differentiation of *Anopheles gambiae* s.s. molecular forms. Insect Biochem Molec. 2005 Jul;35(7):755-69.

[56] Diabate A, Dabire RK, Heidenberger K, Crawford J, Lamp WO, Culler LE, Lehmann T. Evidence for divergent selection between the molecular forms of *Anopheles gambiae*: role of predation. BMC Evol Biol. 2008 Jan 11;8(1):5.

[57] Diabate A, Dabire RK, Kim EH, Dalton R, Millogo N, Baldet T, Simard F, Gimnig JE, Hawley WA, Lehmann T. Larval development of the molecular forms of *Anopheles gambiae* (Diptera: Culicidae) in different habitats: a transplantation experiment. J Med Entomol. 2005;42(4):548-53.

[58] Sharp BL, Lesueur D. Behavioral variation of *Anopheles arabiensis* (Diptera: Culicidae) populations in Natal, South Africa. Bull Entomol Res. 1991 Mar;81(1):107-10.

[59] White GB. *Anopheles gambiae* complex and disease transmission in Africa. Trans R Soc Trop Med Hyg. 1974;68(4):278-301.

[60] White GB. The *Anopheles gambiae* complex and malaria transmission around Kisumu, Kenya. Trans R Soc Trop Med Hyg. 1972;66(4):572-81.

[61] White GB, Rosen P. Comparative studies on sibling species of *Anopheles gambiae* Giles complex (Dipt: Culicidae). II. Ecology of Species A and B in savanna around Kaduna, Nigeria, during transition from wet to dry season. Bull Entomol Res. 1973;62(4):613-25.

[62] Tirados I, Costantini C, Gibson G, Torr SJ. Blood-feeding behaviour of the malarial mosquito *Anopheles arabiensis*: implications for vector control. Med Vet Entomol. 2006;20(4):425-37.

[63] Shililu J, Mbogo C, Ghebremeskel T, Githure J, Novak R. Mosquito larval habitats in a semi-arid ecosystem in Eritrea: impact of larval habitat management on *Anopheles arabiensis* populations. Am J Trop Med Hyg. 2007 Jan;76(1):103-10.

[64] Shililu J, Ghebremeskel T, Seulu F, Mengistu S, Fekadu H, Zerom M, Ghebregziabiher A, Sintasath D, Bretas G, Mbogo C, Githure J, Brantly E, Novak R, Beier JC. Larval habitat diversity and ecology of anopheline larvae in Eritrea. J Med Entomol. 2003;40(6): 921-9.

[65] Kamau L, Munyekenye GO, Vulule JM, Lehmann T. Evaluating genetic differentiation of *Anopheles arabiensis* in relation to larval habitats in Kenya. Infect Genet Evol. 2007 Mar;7(2):293-7.

[66] Abdullah MA, Merdan AI. Distribution and ecology of the mosquito fauna in the southwestern Saudi Arabia. J Egypt Soc Parasitol. 1995 Dec;25(3):815-37.

[67] Mwangangi JM, Muturi EJ, Shililu JI, Muriu S, Jacob B, Kabiru EW, Mbogo CM, Githure JI, Novak RJ. Environmental covariates of *Anopheles arabiensis* in a rice agroecosystem in Mwea, Central Kenya. J Am Mosq Control Assoc. 2007 Dec;23(4):371-7.

[68] Mwangangi JM, Muturi EJ, Shililu J, Muriu SM, Jacob B, Kabiru EW, Mbogo CM, Githure J, Novak R. Survival of immature *Anopheles arabiensis* (Diptera: Culicidae) in aquatic habitats in Mwea rice irrigation scheme, central Kenya. Malar J. 2006;5:114.

[69] Mwangangi J, Shililu J, Muturi E, Gu WD, Mbogo C, Kabiru E, Jacob B, Githure J, Novak R. Dynamics of immature stages of *Anopheles arabiensis* and other mosquito species (Diptera: Culicidae) in relation to rice cropping in a rice agro-ecosystem in Kenya. J Vector Ecol. 2006 Dec;31(2):245-51.

[70] Mutero CM, Blank H, Konradsen F, van der Hoek W. Water management for controlling the breeding of *Anopheles* mosquitoes in rice irrigation schemes in Kenya. Acta Trop. 2000;76(3):253-63.

[71] Ameneshewa B, Service MW. Resting habits of *Anopheles arabiensis* in the Awash River valley of Ethiopia. Ann Trop Med Parasitol. 1996;90(5):515-21.

[72] Coluzzi M, Sabatini A, Petrarca V, Di Deco MA. Chromosomal differentiation and adaptation to human environments in the *Anopheles gambiae* complex. Trans R Soc Trop Med Hyg. 1979;73(5):483-97.

[73] Coetzee M, Fontenille D. Advances in the study of *Anopheles funestus*, a major vector of malaria in Africa. Insect Biochem Mol Biol. 2004 Jul;34(7):599-605.

[74] Cohuet A, Simard F, Toto JC, Kengne P, Coetzee M, Fontenille D. Species identification within the *Anopheles funestus* group of malaria vectors in Cameroon and evidence for a new species. Am J Trop Med Hyg. 2003;69(2):200-5.

[75] Weeto MM, Koekemoer LL, Kamau L, Hunt RH, Coetzee M. Evaluation of a species-specific PCR assay for the *Anopheles funestus* group from eleven African countries and Madagascar. Trans R Soc Trop Med Hyg. 2004 Mar;98(3):142-7.

[76] Antonio-Nkondjio C, Kerah CH, Simard F, Awono-Ambene P, Chouaibou M, Tchuinkam T, Fontenille D. Complexity of the malaria vectorial system in Cameroon: contribution of secondary vectors to malaria transmission. J Med Entomol. 2006;43(6): 1215-21.

[77] Awolola TS, Oyewole IO, Koekemoer LL, Coetzee M. Identification of three members of the *Anopheles funestus* (Diptera: Culicidae) group and their role in malaria transmission in two ecological zones in Nigeria. Trans R Soc Trop Med Hyg. 2005;99(7):525-31.

[78] Hargreaves K, Koekemoer LL, Brooke BD, Hunt RH, Mthembu J, Coetzee M. *Anopheles funestus* resistant to pyrethroid insecticides in South Africa. Med Vet Entomol. [Article]. 2000 Jun;14(2):181-9.

[79] Carnevale P, Guillet P, Robert V, Fontenille D, Doannio J, Coosemans M, Mouchet J. Diversity of malaria in rice growing areas of the Afrotropical region. Parassitologia. 1999;41(1-3):273-6.

[80] Chandler JA, Highton RB, Hill MN. Mosquitoes of the Kano Plain, Kenya. I. Results of indoor collections in irrigated and nonirrigated areas using human bait and light traps. J Med Entomol. 1975 Dec 30;12(5):504-10.

[81] Sogoba N, Doumbia S, Vounatsou P, Bagayoko MM, Dolo G, Traore SF, Maiga HM, Toure YT, Smith T. Malaria transmission dynamics in Niono, Mali: the effect of the irrigation systems. Acta Trop. 2007 Mar;101(3):232-40.

[82] Gething PW, Patil AP, Smith DL, Guerra CA, Elyazar IR, Johnston GL, Tatem AJ, Hay SI. A new world malaria map: *Plasmodium falciparum* endemicity in 2010. Malar J. 2011;10:378.

[83] Gething PW, Elyazar IRF, Moyes CM, Smith DL, Battle KE, Guerra CA, Patil AP, Tatem AJ, Howes RE, Myers MF, George DB, Horby P, Wertheim HF, Price R, Müller I, Baird JK, Hay SI. A long neglected world malaria map: *Plasmodium vivax* endemicity in 2010. PLoS Negl Trop Dis. 2012;6(9):e1814.

[84] Guerra CA, Howes RE, Patil AP, Gething PW, Van Boeckel TP, Temperley WH, Kabaria CW, Tatem AJ, Manh BH, Elyazar IRF, Baird KJ, Snow RW, Hay SI. The international limits and population at risk of *Plasmodium vivax* transmission in 2009. PLoS Negl Trop Dis. 2010;4(8):e774.

[85] Dash AP, Bendley MS, Das AK, Das M, Dwivedi SR. Role of *An. annularis* as a vector of malaria in inland of Orissa. J Commun Dis. 1982;14:224.

[86] Ghosh KK, Chakraborty S, Bhattacharya S, Palit A, Tandon N, Hati AK. *Anopheles annularis* as a vector of malaria in rural West Bengal. Indian J Malariol. 1985;22(2):65-9.

[87] Gunasekaran K, Sahu SS, Parida SK, Sadanandane C, Jambulingam P, Das PK. Anopheline fauna of Koraput District, Orissa state, with particular reference to transmission of malaria. Indian J Med Res. 1989;89:340-3.

[88] Mahapatra N, Marai NS, Ranjit MR, Parida SK, Hansdah DP, Hazra RK, Kar SK. Detection of *Plasmodium falciparum* infection in *Anopheles* mosquitoes from Keonjhar District, Orissa, India. J Vector Borne Dis. 2006;43(4):191-4.

[89] Prakash A, Bhattacharyya DR, Mohapatra PK, Mahanta J. Role of the prevalent *Anopheles* species in the transmission of *Plasmodium falciparum* and *P. vivax* in Assam state, north-eastern India. Ann Trop Med Parasitol. 2004;98(6):559-68.

[90] Ramasamy R, De Alwis R, Wijesundere A, Ramasamy MS. Malaria transmission at a new irrigation project in Sri Lanka: the emergence of *Anopheles annularis* as a major vector. Am J Trop Med Hyg. 1992;47(5):547-53.

[91] Rao TR. The anophelines of India, 2nd edition. New Delhi: Malaria Research Centre, Indian Council of Medical Research 1984.

[92] Garros C, Koekemoer LL, Coetzee M, Coosemans M, Manguin S. A single multiplex assay to identify major malaria vectors within the African *Anopheles funestus* and the Oriental *An. minimus* groups. Am J Trop Med Hyg. 2004 Jun;70(6):583-90.

[93] Walton C, Somboon P, O'Loughlin SM, Zhang S, Harbach RE, Linton YM, Chen B, Nolan K, Duong S, Fong MY, Vythilingum I, Mohammed ZD, Trung HD, Butlin RK.

Genetic diversity and molecular identification of mosquito species in the *Anopheles maculatus* group using the ITS2 region of rDNA. Infect Genet Evol. 2007 Jan;7(1):93-102.

[94] Walton C, Handley JM, Kuvangkadilok C, Collins FH, Harbach RE, Baimai V, Butlin RK. Identification of five species of the *Anopheles dirus* complex from Thailand, using allele-specific polymerase chain reaction. Med Vet Entomol. 1999 Feb;13(1):24-32.

[95] Surendran SN, Abhayawardana TA, De Silva BG, Ramasamy R, Ramasamy MS. *Anopheles culicifacies* Y-chromosome dimorphism indicates sibling species (B and E) with different malaria vector potential in Sri Lanka. Med Vet Entomol. 2000;14(4): 437-40.

[96] Jude PJ, Dharshini S, Vinobaba M, Surendran SN, Ramasamy R. *Anopheles culicifacies* breeding in brackish waters in Sri Lanka and implications for malaria control. Malar J. 2010 Apr 21;9(1):106.

[97] Subbarao SK, Sharma VP. Anopheline species complexes and malaria control. Indian J Med Res. 1997;106:164-73.

[98] Amerasinghe PH, Amerasinghe FP, Konradsen F, Fonseka KT, Wirtz RA. Malaria vectors in a traditional dry zone village in Sri Lanka. Am J Trop Med Hyg. 1999;60(3): 421-9.

[99] Subbarao SK. The *Anopheles culicifacies* complex and control of malaria. Parasitol Today. 1988;4(3):72-5.

[100] Barik TK, Sahu B, Swain V. A review on *Anopheles culicifacies*: from bionomics to control with special reference to Indian subcontinent. Acta Trop. 2009 Feb;109(2):87-97.

[101] Sharma VP. Fighting malaria in India. Curr Sci. 1998;75:1127-40.

[102] Surendran SN, De Silva BG, Srikrishnaraj KA, Ramasamy MS, Ramasamy R. Establishment of species E, not B as the major vector of malaria in the *Anopheles culicifacies* complex in the country. Proc Sri Lanka Assoc Advmt Sci. 2003;59:18.

[103] Subbarao SK, Vasantha K, Raghavendra K, Sharma VP, Sharma GK. *Anopheles culicifacies*: siblings species composition and its relationship to malaria incidence. J Am Mosq Control Assoc. 1988;4(1):29-33.

[104] Vatandoost H, Shahi H, Abai MR, Hanafi-Bojd AA, Oshaghi MA, Zamani G. Larval habitats of main malaria vectors in Hormozgan Province and their susceptibility to different larvicides. Southeast Asian J Trop Med Public Health. 2004;35 Suppl 2:22-5.

[105] Surendran SN, Ramasamy R. Some characteristics of the larval breeding sites of *Anopheles culicifacies* species B and E in Sri Lanka. J Vector Borne Dis. 2005;42(2):39-44.

[106] Sabesan S, Krishnamoorthy K, Jambulingam P, Rajendran G, Kumar NP, Rajagopalan PK. Breeding habitats of *Anopheles culicifacies* in Rameswaram Island. Indian J Med Res. 1986;84:44-52.

[107] Amerasinghe FP, Ariyasena TG. Larval survey of surface water-breeding mosquitoes during irrigation development in the Mahaweli Project, Sri Lanka. J Med Entomol. 1990;27(5):789-802.

[108] Roberts D. Mosquitoes (Diptera: Culicidae) breeding in brackish water: female ovipositional preferences or larval survival? J Med Entomol. 1996 Jul;33(4):525-30.

[109] Subbarao SK, Nanda N, Vasantha K, Dua VK, Malhotra MS, Yadav RS, Sharma VP. Cytogenetic evidence for three sibling species in *Anopheles fluviatilis*. Ann Entomol Soc Am. 1994;87:116-21.

[110] Chen B, Butlin RK, Pedro PM, Wang XZ, Harbach RE. Molecular variation, systematics and distribution of the *Anopheles fluviatilis* complex in southern Asia. Med Vet Entomol. 2006;20(1):33-43.

[111] Nandi J, Kaul SM, Sharma SN, Lal S. Anthropophily of anophelines in Duars of West Bengal and other regions of India. J Commun Dis. 2000;32(2):95-9.

[112] Nanda N, Yadav RS, Subbarao SK, Joshi H, Sharma VP. Studies on *Anopheles fluviatilis* and *Anopheles culicifacies* sibling species in relation to malaria in forested hilly and deforested riverine ecosystems in northern Orissa, India. J Am Mosq Control Assoc. 2000;16(3):199-205.

[113] Bhatt RM, Kohli VK. Biting rhythms of some anophelines in central Gujarat. Indian J Malariol. 1996;33(4):180-90.

[114] Malakar P, Das S, Saha GK, Dasgupta B, Hati AK. Indoor resting anophelines of north Bengal. Indian J Malariol. 1995;32(1):24-31.

[115] Nanda N, Joshi H, Subbarao SK, Yadav RS, Shukla RP, Dua VK, Sharma VP. *Anopheles fluviatilis* complex: host feeding patterns of species S, T, and U. J Am Mosq Control Assoc. 1996;12(1):147-9.

[116] Sharma SK, Nanda N, Dutta VK. Studies on the bionomics of *Anopheles fluviatilis* s.l. and the sibling species composition in the foothills of Shiwalik Range, India. Southeast Asian J Trop Med Public Health. 1995;26(3):566-72.

[117] Eshghi N, Motabar M, Javadian E, Manoutcheri AV. Biological features of *Anopheles fluviatilis* and its role in the transmission of malaria in Iran. Trop Geogr Med. 1976 Mar; 28(1):41-4.

[118] Naddaf SR, Oshaghi MA, Vatandoost H, Assmar M. Molecular characterization of *Anopheles fluviatilis* species complex in the Islamic Republic of Iran. East Mediterr Health J. 2003;9(3):257-65.

[119] Shukla RP, Pandey AC, Kohli VK, Ojha VP, Sharma VP. Bionomics of vector anophelines in District Naini Tal, Uttar Pradesh. Indian J Malariol. 1995;32(4):153-63.

[120] Shukla RP, Nanda N, Pandey AC, Kohli VK, Joshi H, Subbarao SK. Studies on bionomics of *Anopheles fluviatilis* and its sibling species in Nainital District, U.P. Indian J Malariol. 1998;35(2):41-7.

[121] Reisen WK, Pradhan SP, Shrestha JP, Shrestha SL, Vaidya RG, Shrestha JD. Anopheline mosquito (Diptera: Culicidae) ecology in relation to malaria transmission in the inner and outer terai of Nepal, 1987-1989. J Med Entomol. 1993;30(4):664-82.

[122] Hanafi-Bojd AA, Vatandoost H, Jafari R. Susceptibility status of *Anopheles dthali* and *An. fluviatilis* to commonly used larvicides in an endemic focus of malaria, southern Iran. J Vector Borne Dis. 2006;43(1):34-8.

[123] Gunasekaran K. Age composition, natural survival and population growth of *Anopheles fluviatilis* James, 1902, the major malaria vector in the endemic belt of Koraput District, Orissa, India. Southeast Asian J Trop Med Public Health. 1994;25(1):196-200.

[124] Bhatt RM, Srivastava HC, Pujara PK. Biology of malaria vectors in central Gujarat. Indian J Malariol. 1994;31(2):65-76.

[125] Batra CP, Reuben R. Breeding of *Anopheles stephensi* (Liston) in wells and cisterns in Salem, Tamil Nadu. Indian J Med Res. 1979 Dec;70 Suppl:114-22.

[126] Batra CP, Mittal PK, Adak T, Subbarao SK. Efficacy of Agnique MMF monomolecular surface film against *Anopheles stephensi* breeding in urban habitats in India. J Am Mosq Control Assoc. 2006;22(3):426-32.

[127] Vatandoost H, Oshaghi MA, Abaie MR, Shahi M, Yaaghoobi F, Baghaii M, Hanafi-Bojd AA, Zamani G, Townson H. Bionomics of *Anopheles stephensi* Liston in the malarious area of Hormozgan Province, southern Iran, 2002. Acta Trop. 2006;97(2):196-203.

[128] Manouchehri AV, Javadian E, Eshighy N, Motabar M. Ecology of *Anopheles stephensi* Liston in southern Iran. Trop Geogr Med. 1976 Sep;28(3):228-32.

[129] Krishnan KS. *A. stephensi* Liston, 1901. Vectors of Malaria in India. 2nd ed. Delhi: National Society of India for Malaria and Other Mosquito-born Disease; 1961. p. 39-58.

[130] Zaim M, Ershadi MR, Manouchehri AV, Hamdi MR. The use of CDC light traps and other procedures for sampling malaria vectors in southern Iran. J Am Mosq Control Assoc. 1986;2(4):511-5.

[131] Reisen WK. Population dynamics of some Pakistan mosquitoes: the impact of residual organophosphate insecticide spray on anopheline relative abundance. Ann Trop Med Parasitol. 1986;80(1):69-75.

[132] Sweet WC, Rao B. Races of *Anopheles stephensi* Liston, 1901. Ind Med Gaz. 1937;72:665-74.

[133] Singh OP. Bionomics of malaria vectors in India: Malaria Research Centre 2002.

[134] Cox-Singh J, Singh B. Knowlesi malaria: newly emergent and of public health importance? Trends Parasitol. 2008 Sep;24(9):406-10.

[135] Vythilingam I. *Plasmodium knowlesi* and *Wuchereria bancrofti*: their vectors and challenges for the future. Front Syst Biol. 2012;3(115).

[136] Rosenberg R, Andre RG, Somchit L. Highly efficient dry season transmission of malaria in Thailand. Trans R Soc Trop Med Hyg. 1990;84(1):22-8.

[137] Manguin S, Garros C, Dusfour I, Harbach RE, Coosemans M. Bionomics, taxonomy, and distribution of the major malaria vector taxa of *Anopheles* subgenus *Cellia* in Southeast Asia: An updated review. Infect Genet Evol. 2008 Nov 29;8:489-503.

[138] Peyton EL, Harrison BA. *Anopheles* (*Cellia*) *dirus*, a new species of the Leucosphyrus Group from Thailand (Diptera: Culicidae). Mosq Syst. 1979;11(1):40-52.

[139] Peyton EL, Harrison BA. *Anopheles* (*Cellia*) *takasagoensis* Morishita 1946, an additional species in the Balabacensis Complex of Southeast Asia (Diptera: Culicidae). Mosq Syst. 1980;12(3):335-47.

[140] Peyton EL, Ramalingam S. *Anopheles* (*Cellia*) *nemophilous*, a new species of the Leucosphyrus Group from peninsular Malaysia and Thailand (Diptera: Culicidae). Mosq Syst. 1988;20:272-99.

[141] Sallum MA, Peyton EL, Wilkerson RC. Six new species of the *Anopheles leucosphyrus* group, reinterpretation of *An. elegans* and vector implications. Med Vet Entomol. 2005;19(2):158-99.

[142] Takano KT, Nguyen NT, Nguyen BT, Sunahara T, Yasunami M, Nguyen MD, Takagi M. Partial mitochondrial DNA sequences suggest the existence of a cryptic species within the Leucosphyrus group of the genus *Anopheles* (Diptera: Culicidae), forest malaria vectors, in northern Vietnam. Parasit Vectors. 2010;3:41.

[143] Dutta P, Bhattacharyya DR, Khan SA, Sharma CK, Mahanta J. Feeding patterns of *Anopheles dirus*, the major vector of forest malaria in north east India. Southeast Asian J Trop Med Public Health. 1996;27(2):378-81.

[144] Manguin S, Bangs MJ, Pothikasikorn J, Chareonviriyaphap T. Review on global co-transmission of human *Plasmodium* species and *Wuchereria bancrofti* by *Anopheles* mosquitoes. Infect Genet Evol. 2010 Mar;10(2):159-77.

[145] Prakash A, Bhattacharyya DR, Mohapatra PK, Mahanta J. Malaria transmission risk by the mosquito *Anopheles baimaii* (formerly known as *An. dirus* species D) at different hours of the night in North-east India. Med Vet Entomol. 2005;19(4):423-7.

[146] Rattanarithikul R, Konishi E, Linthicum KJ. Detection of *Plasmodium vivax* and *Plasmodium falciparum* circumsporozoite antigen in anopheline mosquitoes collected in southern Thailand. Am J Trop Med Hyg. 1996;54(2):114-21.

[147] Vythilingam I, Phetsouvanh R, Keokenchanh K, Yengmala V, Vanisaveth V, Phompida S, Hakim SL. The prevalence of *Anopheles* (Diptera: Culicidae) mosquitoes in Sekong Province, Lao PDR in relation to malaria transmission. Trop Med Int Health. 2003;8(6): 525-35.

[148] Trung HD, Bortel WV, Sochantha T, Keokenchanh K, Briet OJ, Coosemans M. Behavioural heterogeneity of *Anopheles* species in ecologically different localities in Southeast Asia: a challenge for vector control. Trop Med Int Health. 2005;10(3):251-62.

[149] Misra SP, Nandi J, Narasimham MV, Rajagopal R. Malaria transmission in Nagaland, India. Part I. Anophelines and their seasonality. J Commun Dis. 1993;25(2):62-6.

[150] Baimai V. Population cytogenetics of the malaria vector *Anopheles leucosphyrus* group. Southeast Asian J Trop Med Public Health. 1988;19(4):667-80.

[151] Prakash A, Bhattacharyya DR, Mohapatra PK, Mahanta J. Physico-chemical characteristics of breeding habitats of *Anopheles dirus* (Diptera: Culicidae) in Assam, India. J Environ Biol. 2002 Jan;23(1):95-100.

[152] Prakash A, Bhattacharyya DR, Mohapatra PK, Mahanta J. Breeding and day resting habitats of *Anopheles dirus* in Assam, India. Southeast Asian J Trop Med Public Health. 1997;28(3):610-4.

[153] Oo TT, Storch V, Becker N. Studies on the bionomics of *Anopheles dirus* (Culicidae: Diptera) in Mudon, Mon State, Myanmar. J Vector Ecol. 2002;27(1):44-54.

[154] Htay A, Minn S, Thaung S, Mya MM, Than SM, Hlaing T, Soe S, Druilhe P, Queuche F. Well-breeding *Anopheles dirus* and their role in malaria transmission in Myanmar. Southeast Asian J Trop Med Public Health. 1999;30(3):447-53.

[155] Harbach RE, Garros C, Manh ND, Manguin S. Formal taxonomy of species C of the *Anopheles minimus* sibling species complex (Diptera: Culicidae). Zootaxa. 2007;1654:41-54.

[156] Harbach RE, Parkin E, Chen B, Butlin RK. *Anopheles* (*Cellia*) *minimus* Theobald (Diptera: Culicidae): neotype designation, characterization, and systematics. Proc Entomol Soc Wash. 2006;108(1):198-209.

[157] Somboon P, Rory A, Tsuda Y, Takagi M, Harbach RE. Systematics of *Anopheles* (*Cellia*) *yaeyamaensis* sp. n., alias species E of the *An. minimus* complex of southeastern Asia (Diptera: Culicidae). Zootaxa. 2010;2651:43-51.

[158] Farid MA, Chen CT, Hsu TC, Liu SY. Report of WHO evaluation team on malaria eradication in the Ryukyu Islands, 1965. Geneva1966.

[159] Miyagi I, Toma T, Malenganisho WL, Uza M. Historical review of mosquito control as a component of malaria eradication program in the Ryukyu Archipelago. Southeast Asian J Trop Med Public Health. 1996;27(3):498-511.

[160] Garros C, Van Bortel W, Trung HD, Coosemans M, Manguin S. Review of the Minimus Complex of *Anopheles*, main malaria vector in Southeast Asia: from taxonomic issues to vector control strategies. Trop Med Int Health. 2006 Jan;11(1):102-14.

[161] Rongnoparut P, Ugsang DM, Baimai V, Honda K, Sithiprasasna R. Use of a remote sensing-based geographic information system in the characterizing spatial patterns for

Anopheles minimus A and C breeding habitats in western Thailand. Southeast Asian J Trop Med Public Health. 2005 Sep;36(5):1145-52.

[162] Rattanarithikul R, Green CA, Panyim S, Noigamol C, Chanaimongkol S, Mahapibul P. Larval habitats of malaria vectors and other *Anopheles* mosquitoes around a transmission focus in northwestern Thailand. J Am Mosq Control Assoc. 1995;11(4):428-33.

[163] Khan SA, Handique R, Tewari SC, Dutta P, Narain K, Mahanta J. Larval ecology and mosquito fauna of upper Brahmaputra valley, northeast India. Indian J Malariol. 1998;35(3):131-45.

[164] Harrison BA. Medical entomology studies - XIII. The Myzomyia Series of *Anopheles* (*Cellia*) in Thailand, with emphasis on intra-interspecific variations (Diptera: Culicidae). Contrib Am Entomol Inst (Ann Arbor). 1980;17:1-195.

[165] Dev V. *Anopheles minimus*: its bionomics and role in the transmission of malaria in Assam, India. Bull World Health Organ. 1996;74(1):61-6.

[166] Van Bortel W, Trung HD, Manh ND, Roelants P, Verle P, Coosemans M. Identification of two species within the *Anopheles minimus* complex in northern Vietnam and their behavioural divergences. Trop Med Int Health. 1999;4(4):257-65.

[167] Dev V, Bhattacharyya PC, Talukdar Rupjyoti. Transmission of malaria and its control in the northeastern region of India. J Assoc Physicians India. 2003;51:1073-6.

[168] Chareonviriyaphap T, Prabaripai A, Bangs MJ, Aum-Aung B. Seasonal abundance and blood feeding activity of *Anopheles minimus* Theobald (Diptera: Culicidae) in Thailand. J Med Entomol. 2003;40(6):876-81.

[169] Suthas N, Phorn S, Udom C, Cullen JE. The behaviour of *Anopheles minimus* Theobald (Diptera: Culicidae) subjected to different levels of DDT selection pressure in northern Thailand. Bull Entomol Res. 1986;76:303-12.

[170] Ismail IA, Notananda V, Schepens J. Studies on malaria and responses of *Anopheles balabacensis balabacensis* and *Anopheles minimus* to DDT residual spraying in Thailand. I. Pre-spraying observations. Acta Trop. 1974;31(2):129-64.

[171] Garros C, Marchand RP, Quang NT, Hai NS, Manguin S. First record of *Anopheles minimus* C and significant decrease of *An. minimus* A in central Vietnam. J Am Mosq Control Assoc. 2005 Jun;21(2):139-43.

[172] Van Bortel W, Trung HD, Sochantha T, Keokenchan K, Roelants P, Backeljau T, Coosemans M. Eco-ethological heterogeneity of the members of the *Anopheles minimus* complex (Diptera: Culicidae) in Southeast Asia and its consequences for vector control. J Med Entomol. 2004 May;41(3):366-74.

[173] Sungvornyothin S, Muenvorn V, Garros C, Manguin S, Prabaripai A, Bangs MJ, Chareonvirlyaphap T. Trophic behavior and biting activity of the two sibling species of the *Anopheles minimus* complex in western Thailand. J Vector Ecol. 2006 Dec;31(2): 252-61.

[174] Cooper RD, Waterson DG, Frances SP, Beebe NW, Sweeney AW. Speciation and distribution of the members of the *Anopheles punctulatus* (Diptera: Culicidae) group in Papua New Guinea. J Med Entomol. 2002;39(1):16-27.

[175] Cooper RD, Waterson DG, Frances SP, Beebe NW, Pluess B, Sweeney AW. Malaria vectors of Papua New Guinea. Int J Parasitol. 2009 Jun 5;39(13):1495-501.

[176] Bugoro H, Cooper RD, Butafa C, Iro'ofa C, Mackenzie DO, Chen CC, Russell TL. Bionomics of the malaria vector *Anopheles farauti* in Temotu Province, Solomon Islands: issues for malaria elimination. Malar J. 2011;10:133.

[177] Ebsworth P, Bryan JH, Foley DH. Ecological distribution of mosquito larvae of the *Anopheles punctulatus* group on Niolam (Lihir) Island, Papua New Guinea. J Am Mosq Control Assoc. 2001;17(3):181-5.

[178] Cooper RD, Frances SP. Malaria vectors on Buka and Bougainville Islands, Papua New Guinea. J Am Mosq Control Assoc. 2002;18(2):100-6.

[179] Beebe NW, Bakote'e B, Ellis JT, Cooper RD. Differential ecology of *Anopheles punctulatus* and three members of the *Anopheles farauti* complex of mosquitoes on Guadalcanal, Solomon Islands, identified by PCR-RFLP analysis. Med Vet Entomol. 2000;14(3): 308-12.

[180] Charlwood JD, Graves PM, Alpers MP. The ecology of the *Anopheles punctulatus* group of mosquitoes from Papua New Guinea: a review of recent work. P N G Med J. 1986;29(1):19-26.

[181] Charlwood JD. The influence of larval habitat on the ecology and behavior of females of the Punctulatus Group of *Anopheles* mosquitoes from Papua New Guinea. In: Lounibos LP, Rey JR, Frank JH, editors. Ecology of mosquitoes: Proceedings of a workshop. Vero Beach: Florida Medical Entomology Laboratory; 1985. p. 399-406.

[182] Beebe NW, Cooper RD, Morrison DA, Ellis JT. A phylogenetic study of the *Anopheles punctulatus* group of malaria vectors comparing rDNA sequence alignments derived from the mitochondrial and nuclear small ribosomal subunits. Mol Phylogenet Evol. 2000 Dec;17(3):430-6.

[183] Lee DJ, Hicks MM, Griffiths M, Debenham ML, Bryan JH, Russell RC, Geary M, Marks EN. The Culicidae of the Australasian Region. Volume 5. Nomenclature, synonymy, literature, distribution, biology and relation to disease. Genus *Anopheles*. Subgenera *Anopheles, Cellia*. Canberra: Australian Government Publishing Service; 1987.

[184] Charlwood JD. A differential response to mosquito nets by *Anopheles* and *Culex* mosquitoes from Papua New Guinea. Trans R Soc Trop Med Hyg. 1986;80(6):958-60.

[185] Spenser T, Spenser M, Venters D. Malaria vectors of Papua New Guinea. P N G Med J. 1974;17(1):22-30.

[186] Bangs MJ, Subianto DB. El Nińo and associated outbreaks of severe malaria in highland populations in Irian Jaya, Indonesia: a review and epidemiological perspective. Southeast Asian J Trop Med Public Health. 1999 Dec;30(4):608-19.

[187] De'ath G. Boosted trees for ecological modeling and prediction. Ecology. 2007 Jan;88(1): 243-51.

[188] Elith J, Leathwick JR, Hastie T. A working guide to boosted regression trees. J Anim Ecol. 2008 Jul;77(4):802-13.

Chapter 5

Phylogeography, Vectors and Transmission in Latin America

Jan E. Conn, Martha L. Quiñones and
Marinete M. Póvoa

Additional information is available at the end of the chapter

http://dx.doi.org/10.5772/55217

1. Introduction

The overall focus of this chapter is the impact of phylogeographic studies on information pertinent to vector control, and an update on the relative importance and taxonomic status of five malaria vectors, some of which are species complexes, in the subgenus *Nyssorhynchus*: *Anopheles albimanus* Wiedmann, Albitarsis Complex, *Anopheles aquasalis* Curry, *Anopheles darlingi* Root, and *Anopheles nuneztovari* s.l. Gabaldón, considering literature predominantly since 2000. This cut-off date is to avoid repetition or overlap with some of the same subjects that have been covered in other places [1-4].

It is also of interest to vector control and elimination programs that, since 2000 and a more recent compilation that included a list of confirmed or potential Latin American malaria vectors [5], some vector species have been implicated in additional regions or countries by enzyme-linked immunosorbent assay [ELISA; 6], PCR techniques [7], VecTest [8] or more definitive biological and epidemiological evidence has been provided. Examples of these include *An. rangeli* Gabaldón, Cova Garcia and Lopez, initially implicated in Amapá state, Brazil [9] and subsequently in Putumayo, southern Colombia [10]; and *An. triannulatus*, (Neiva and Pinto) incriminated more broadly from Amazonian Brazil [11], then locally from Amapá, Brazil [12]. Furthermore, based on high frequency, biting behavior, seasonality, ELISA and nested-PCR, for the first time, *An. rondoni* (Neiva and Pinto) has been implicated in Matapá, Pará state, Brazil [13]. This is an understudied species, and its potential as a vector in other localities and regions in its distribution (Argentina, Bolivia, Brazil) is worth investigating.

A relatively early summary of information on the five most important malaria vectors in Latin America was published in 1986 [14]. This publication focused on four species in the *Nysso-*

rhynchus subgenus: *Anopheles albimanus, Anopheles aquasalis, Anopheles darlingi, Anopheles nuneztovari* and one in the *Anopheles* subgenus, *Anopheles pseudopunctipennis* Theobald. Naturally, more than 20 years later, this list of five is debatable, although most researchers would still consider *An. darlingi* to be the primary vector overall, and *An. albimanus* to be one of the most important. Nevertheless, some aspects of this publication are still relevant, and it serves as a useful historical introduction.

A review published in 2012 [15] summarized the overall findings of much of the available literature on genetic diversity of malaria vectors, including those in Latin America, and concluded that Pleistocene (0.01-2.6 mya; 16) environmental changes have been the primary drivers of divergence, at least at the species and population levels. These changes and earlier ones during the Miocene (2.6-5.3 mya)/Pliocene (5.3-23.0 mya) were hypothesized to have influenced the phylogeography of some co-distributed neotropical vector species, including *Anopheles darlingi* and selected Albitarsis Complex members [17].

2. Biology and vector status

2.1. *An. albimanus*

Throughout its broad, mostly coastal distribution (Figure 1), *Anopheles albimanus* is an important local vector and is considered to be ecologically adaptable (18). In general this species is crepuscular, zoophilic, exophagic, exophilic and seasonally abundant (19-20). Despite heteogeneity of several attributes, such as host-feeding behaviour, longevity, insecticide resistance and susceptibility to Plasmodium species, thoughout its distribution, it has maintained single species status (20).

2.1.1. Colombia

An. albimanus is distributed in Colombia along the Atlantic and Pacific coasts (Figure 1). It is the main malaria vector on the Pacific coast, but its presence is considered a risk factor in other regions, even where malaria transmission is low [22]. Adult abundance of *An. albimanus* is associated with malaria transmission. The El Niño-Southern Oscillation Event (ENSO), that affects global climatic conditions every 2 to 7 years, has been strongly associated with increases in malaria cases, particularly in areas where *An. albimanus* is the main malaria vector, such as the Pacific coast [23]. *An. albimanus* breeding sites are very diverse, ranging from temporary small ponds to lagoons, and even include artificial containers. Its human biting rates can range between a few specimens per night night up to thousands, depending on the availablity of breeding sites in and around villages. Despite its considerable distribution on both coasts, *An. albimanus* has been found naturally infected with *P. vivax* only along the Pacific [24] (Table 1). In this region, its biting activity shows at least two peaks, one around midnight and a second one of less intensity before dawn, both indoors and outdoors [4]. Consistent use of insecticide-treated nets (ITNs) in this region could potentially reduce malaria transmission risk. In the Buenaventura peri-urban area, around 20% of the bites occur indoors and the main biting activity is outside houses between 18-21h. Then, at midnight, there is a second peak inside houses. Finally, between 05-06h, activity increases again outdoors [4].

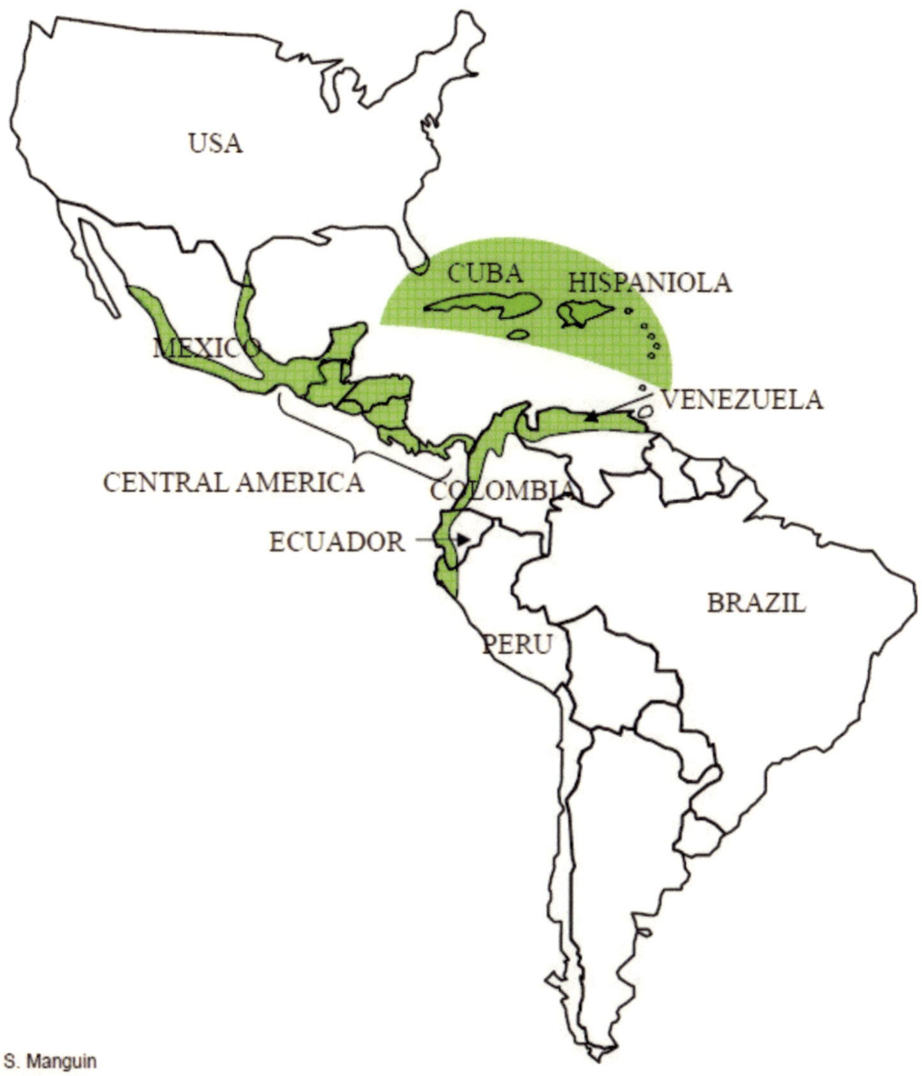

Figure 1. Distribution of *Anopheles albimanus* highlighted in green [21].

Taxon	Country	Local transmission	Regional transmission	Evidence	Reference
An. albimanus	Colombia		Pacific region	ELISA, PCR	24
Albitarsis Complex*	Brazil	Marabá, Pará; Matapi River, Amapá; Amazon region; Macapá, Amapá; N. Amazon region, Roraima; Boa Vista, Roraima; Serra do Navio, Amapá	Amazon region	ELISA, PCR, VecTest	9; 11-13; 25-28; Póvoa 2010 (unpub. data)
	Colombia	Puerto Carreño, Vichada		ELISA	29
	Venezuela	Sifontes, Bolivar		ELISA	30-31
An. aquasalis	Brazil	São Luis, Maranhão; Belém, Pará		ELISA	32-33
	Guyana	Mahdia		VecTest	34
	Suriname	Brokobondo; Galibi; Paramaribo		ELISA	35
	Venezuela	coastal areas			1
An. darlingi	Brazil	Marabá, Pará; Belém, Pará; Matapi River, Amapa; Macapá, Amapá; Boa Vista, Roraima; Serra do Navio, Amapá; Pará, N. Brazil; Anajás, Pará; Goianesia do Para, Pará	Amazon region	ELISA, PCR	9; 11-13; 25; 27-28; 33; 36-37; Póvoa 2012 (unpub. data)
	Colombia	Puerto Carreño, Vichada; Quibdó, Chocó; Dibulla, Guajira	Córdoba; Villavicencio, Meta; Putumayo	ELISA	4; 10; 29; 38-41
	French Guiana	Camopi; Saint Georges de l'Oyapock; Maroni River; Upper Maroni Amazonian forest; Village of Loca; Village of Twenke		ELISA	42-45
	Peru		eastern region	ELISA	46
	Suriname	Maroni River		ELISA	43; 47

Taxon	Country	Local transmission	Regional transmission	Evidence	Reference
	Venezuela	Sifontes, Bolivar; Upper Orinoco River (southern)		ELISA	30-31; 48
An. nuneztovari s.l.	Brazil	Matapi River, Amapa; Serra do Navio, Amapá; Anajás, Pará	Amazon region	ELISA	9; 11-12; 37
	Colombia	Tierralta, Córdoba		ELISA	38
	French Guiana	Saint Georges de l'Oyapock		ELISA	42
	Venezuela	Ocidente de Venezuela		ELISA	49

*, Reference 27 refers to *Anopheles albitarsis* E (now *An. janconnae*) and Póvoa 2010 (unpublished data) refers to the first evidence of *An. oryzalimnetes* as a potential vector. References 12 and 25 refer to *An. marajoara* as a vector, while the remaining references refer to *An. albitarsis* s.l. as vectors.

Table 1. Regional South American vectors subgenus *Nyssorhynchus*: evidence for malaria vector status.

2.1.2. Peru

An. albimanus in Peru is considered the main malaria vector along the Pacific coast, particularly in the north, where it is seasonal, and linked to agriculture [50]. Due to high insecticide application, mainly in rice fields, *An. albimanus* is resistant to all insecticides used in public health in this area [51]. Flooded rice fields provide ideal mosquito breeding habitat and *An. albimanus* density is associated with rice crops. Since 2005, the Peruvian Minister of Health, together with the Agricultural sector, implemented a modified irrigation system, so that the fields are dry for a week, and then intermittently irrigated, resulting in a decrease in mosquito larvae by 87% [52]. An important follow-up question would be whether this *An. albimanus* larval control has actually resulted in a decrease in malaria incidence rate (MIR), or in local *An. albimanus* adult female abundance, as measured by human biting rate (HBR) and entomological inoculation rate (EIR).

In several other South American countries (Ecuador, Panama, Venezuela) where *An. albimanus* is a malaria vector, as determined by sporozoite detection or other comparable information in earlier studies, data based on newer techniques are not available. However, some recent investigations have drawn attention to new distributions or larval habitat characterizations that pinpoint areas of fruitful potential research and possible targets for control measures [53-56].

2.2. Albitarsis Complex

Presently, there are eight recognized species (*An. albitarsis* s.s., *An. albitarsis* F, *An. albitarsis* G, *An. albitarsis* I, *An. deaneorum*, *An. janconnae*, *An. marajoara*, *An. oryzalimnetes)* and one lineage (*An. albitarsis* H) in the Albitarsis Complex [57]. The species described as near *An. janconnae* from Colombia [58] is now considered to be *An. albitarsis* I [57]. The overall distribution of members of this complex is wide-ranging, including both Central and South America, as well as some Caribbean Islands [59] (Figure 2).

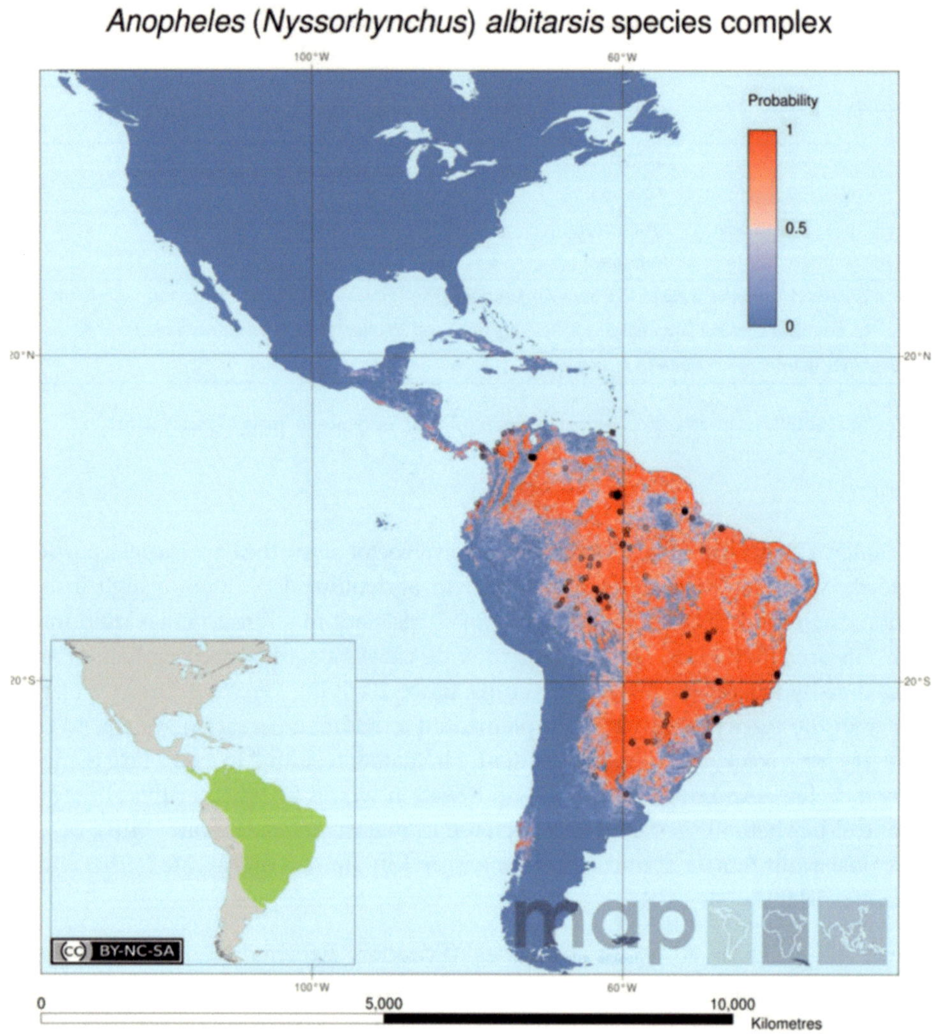

Figure 2. This map shows the predicted probability of occurrence of *An. albitarsis* in the Americas [2]

2.2.1. Brazil

Six species of the Albitarsis Complex are known from Brazil to date: *An. albitarsis* s.s., *An. albitarsis* G, *An. deaneorum*, *An. janconnae*, *An. marajoara*, and *An. oryzalimnetes*, [57,60] (Figure 3). The most broadly distributed member of this complex is *An. marajoara* Galvão and Damasceno [57,59]. It can be very abundant locally [12], and its breeding site types vary from swampy shores of lakes and ponds to small road puddles; it is generally associated with sunlight and often with aquatic or semi-aquatic vegetation [59]. It has been found infected by *Plasmodium falciparum* (Welsh), *Plasmodium vivax* (Grassi & Feletti) 210 and *P. vivax* 247, and *Plasmodium malariae* (Grassi & Feletti), and is a peri-urban as well as a rural vector, depending on locality, availability of breeding sites and hosts [12, 25]. It is also associated with deforested areas of the Vale do Ribeira in the southeastern Atlantic Forest of Brazil [61]. Although the EIR in Amapá state, Brazil was found to be lower than that of *An. darlingi*, it is an important local vector, at least in lowland rainforest in parts of the eastern Amazon [12, 62].

The distribution of *An. janconnae* Wilkerson and Sallum [classified previously as *An. albitarsis* E; [27, 60] appears to be limited to northern Amazonian Brazil, including along the Amazon River [57, 60]. Larval habitat types in several localities in Roraima state ranged from marsh to seepages to stream margins, and, based on analyses of several environmental variables, *An. janconnae* could be classified as a habitat specialist [McKeon, Conn & Povoa, unpublished data, 2012]. *An. janconnae* was incriminated as a local malaria vector around Boa Vista, the capital of Roraima state [27]. It is likely that the infected specimens identified as *An. albitarsis* s.l. from this region [26, 28] (Table 1), are *An. janconnae*, at least according to the geographic distribution [57].

An.oryzalimnetes (Wilkerson and Motoki), previously *An. albitarsis* B [60] has a broad distribution in Brazil that includes the Amazon region and southern Brazil [57]. It is frequently associated with rice fields, and is anthropophilic [60]. It was determined to be positive by ELISA for *Plasmodium* in Pará state [M.M. Povoa 2010, unpublished data], and may play a role in local transmission.

2.2.2. Colombia

At least three members of *An. albitarsis* s.l. are present in Colombia. *Anopheles marajoara* (some collections of which, according to the map [57], may be *An. albitarsis* I) is widely distributed [22], and its biology is similar to that described above under *An. marajoara* in Brazil. It is conisidered to be a regional vector in Colombia [22, 39, 63]. In the municipality of Puerto Carreno in eastern Colombia near the Venezuelan border, it was detected infected with *P. falciparum* [29] at a surprisingly high rate (1.92%; 3/152 specimens infected). Here, its peak biting time was 18-19h, with a minor peak from 20-21h, and it was collected both indoors and outdoors. It is suggested that together with *An. darlingi*, the dominant vector in the area, it is responsible for maintaining local malaria transmission in this municipality [29].

The second member of the complex is sympatric with *An. darlingi* in the east, and probably involved in malaria transmission. This species has been identified by various names, including *An. allopha, An. marajoara*, near *An. janconnae* [58], and most recently as *An. albitarsis* I [57]. Its known distribution thus far is restricted to Colombia. Relatively little is known about its biology, because of species identification issues, and there is no direct evidence yet for its involvement in malaria transmission. It appears that the specimens from Vichada, Colombia, identified as *An. marajoara* [64], are *An. albitarsis* I [57], so the distribution of *An. marajoara* in Colombia, and its involvement in malaria transmission, need re-evaluation.

The third species, *An. albitarsis* F, was first described from Puerto Carreño, near the Venezuelan border, [65]. In this locality it was found in sympatry with *An. darlingi* and a species in the Albitaris Complex now defined as *An. albitarsis* I. Its distribution is hypothesized to include Colombia, Venezuela and Trinidad [57]. Because it can easily be confused morphologically with *An. marajoara*, and it is found in regions of malaria endemnicity, this species is of some epidemiological importance.

2.2.3. *Venezuela*

It now appears that at least *An. albitarsis* I and possibly also *An. albitarsis* F are present is Venezuela [57]. Furthermore, *An. albitarsis* I could be sympatric in some regions with *An. marajoara* (the identification of which needs to be confirmed in Venezuela using molecular techniques), a local vector of *P. vivax* in western Venezuela [66]. *An. marajoara* also plays a significant role, together with *An. darlingi*, in malaria transmission in five localities in southern Venezuela [30-31]. In this gold mining region, where transmission is yearlong, the peak biting time, (19-21h, mostly before midnight), was comparable with most other reports of *An. marajoara*. Although *An. marajoara* was feeding both indoors and outdoors, it was significantly exophagic.

2.3. *Anopheles aquasalis*

This brackish-water breeder is found along the Pacific as far south as Ecuador and along the Atlantic to southern Brazil [1,14] (Figures 3,4). It is rarely found far from the ocean, but it can tolerate quite low salt ion concentrations, and has been detected in freshwater springs. It can be present in enormous numbers in marshy coastal areas, so that even if it is not extremely susceptible to *Plasmodium*, it can maintain malaria transmission when its abundance is high, especially during the rainy season [67]. It persists as an important local vector in Sucre state, eastern Venezuela, where a series of pioneering studies have identified hotspots of local transmission that are very useful for prevention and control efforts [68-69]. It has also been incriminated as a vector of *P. falciparum* and [or] *P. vivax* in Maranhão [32] and Pará states in Brazil [33, 70]. In Linden and Madia, Guyana [34], *An. aquasalis* was detected infected with *P. vivax* using VecTest, but the total sample size of anophelines collected was very small (n=45). In three towns in Suriname, Paramaribo, Brokopondo and Galibi, *An. aquasalis* was also detected infected with *Plasmodium* by ELISA [35], and is likely responsible for local, coastal transmission in this region.

2.4. *Anopheles darlingi*

The species considered to be the most important vector in the Amazon basin is *Anopheles darlingi* [2,3] (Figure 5). It is anthropophilic, adaptive and it has been incriminated in many localities in many countries, where it is often labeled a national vector (Table 1). As such, it has been the focus of a very wide range of research, monitoring and control efforts, and the publication for the first time of its complete genome is an exciting new development (GenBank accession number ADMH00000000).

2.4.1. Bolivia

An. darlingi is distributed in the northeastern Bolivian Amazon, in the departments of Pando, Beni and Santacruz de la Sierra, along the border with Brazil [71]. It shows a biting peak between 19-21h, with 83% of the bites occurring before 22h, when most local people go to bed. After this time, numbers decline, with little or no activity between 02:30-05h [72]. There have been relatively few studies on this species in Bolivia, and data are very scarce.

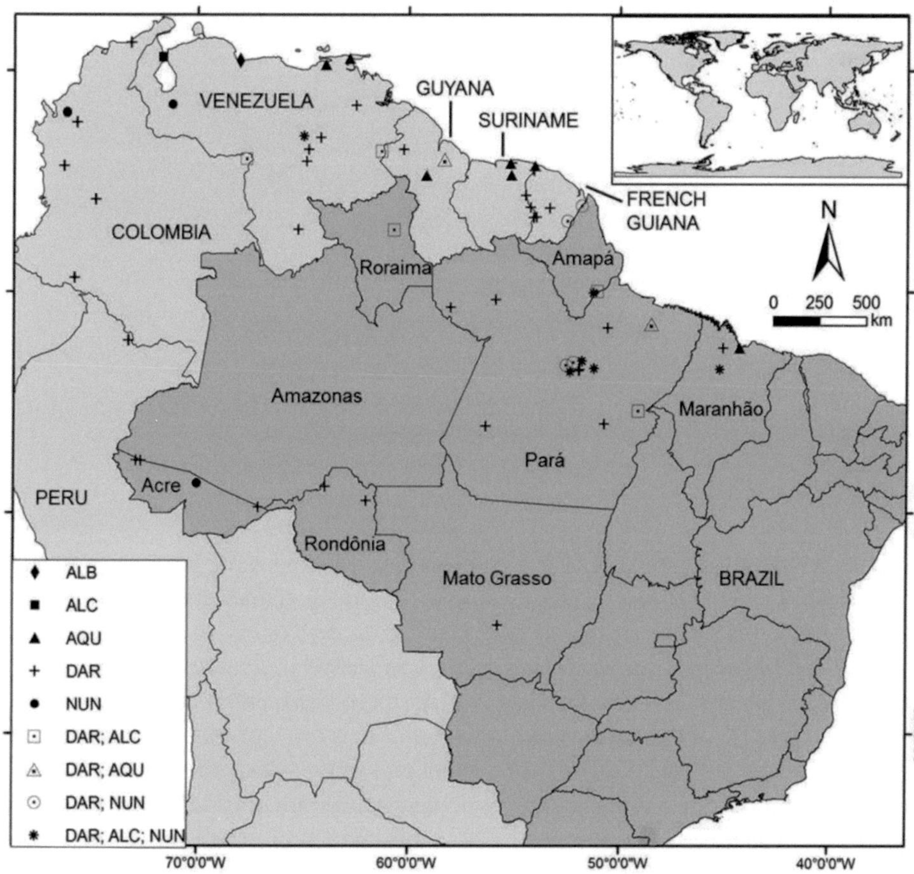

Figure 3. South American localities where malaria vectors have been incriminated by various methods since the year 2000. Species codes: ALB, *Anopheles albimanus*; ALC, Albitarsis Complex; AQU, *An. aquasalis*; DAR, *An. darlingi*; NUN, *An. nuneztovari*. The darker grey area is Brazil.

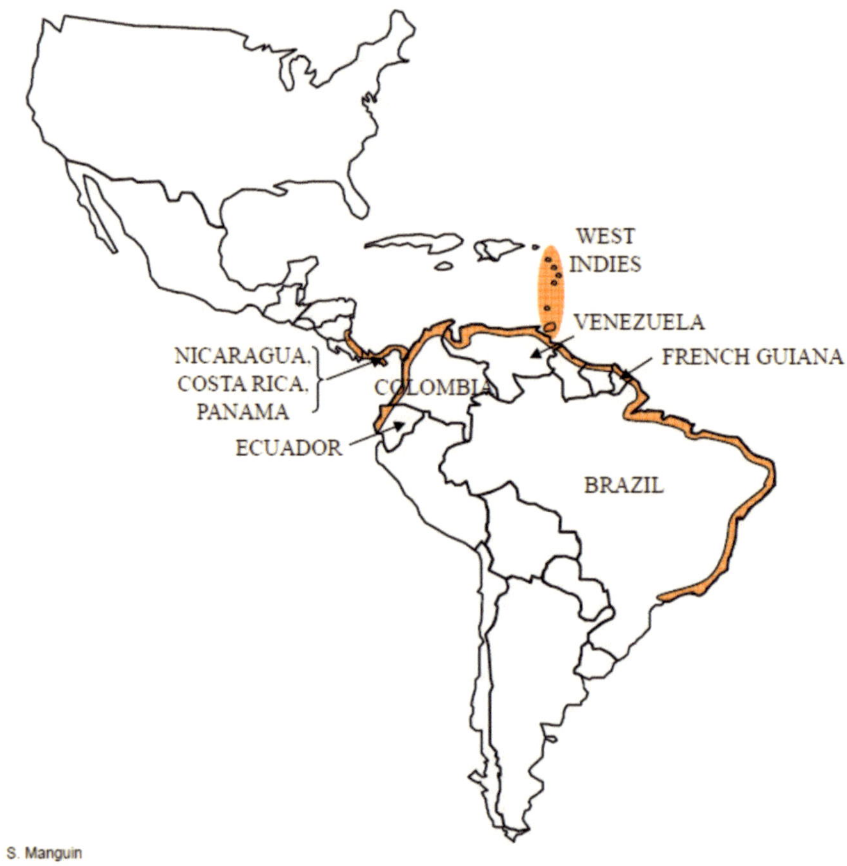

Figure 4. Distribution of *Anopheles aquasalis* highlighted in orange [21]

2.4.2. Brazil

Most of the newest incriminations of the continued involvement of *An. darlingi* in malaria transmission originate in Amazonian Brazil (Table 1, Figure 3). Rather than summarizing each new investigation, this section focuses on the findings on *An. darlingi* in a longitudinal study that investigated bloodmeal hosts, transmission, and seasonal abundance in three riverine villages along the Matapí River in Amapa state, northern Amazonian Brazil [12, 62, 73]. An ELISA analysis for IgG of common vertebrates found that the highest human blood indices (HBI) were in *An. darlingi* and *An. marajoara*. What was unexpected was that the HBIs of *An. darlingi* varied significantly among the three villages, which are only 1.5-7.0 km apart, likely because of host availability. It was found to be important to conduct a census of animals in each locality to be able to interpret the HBI results correctly. Even though *An. darlingi* was the most abundant species collected at human landing catches in each village, the HBI of *An. darlingi* resting collections, from under houses or in vegetation, ranged from 0.017-0.405, demonstrating how opportunistic this species can be, despite its anthropophily [12]. From the same study sites 113,117 mosquitoes collected from 2003-2005 were analyzed by ELISA. For this part of the study, *An. darlingi* and *An. marajoara* had the highest proportion of positives and also the highest EIRs, and thus the highest human-vector contact. Nevertheless, *An. darlingi* is still considered to be more important in this study area than *An. marajoara* because of its higher EIR [12]. Seasonal abundance was measured for 32 consecutive months of collection and showed that *An. darlingi* was most abundant during the wet-dry transition period between June and August, and that a strong positive correlation of *An. darlingi* abundance with rainfall lagged by several months. The latter finding may indicate that rainfall could be an important factor in predicting vector abundance, at least locally.

2.4.3. Colombia

The distribution of *An. darlingi* in Colombia is widespread but heterogeneous, and hypothesized to be interrupted by the Andes. It is found mainly south and east of the Andes, including the Amazon region, bordering Brazil and Peru, but also north and west of the Andes, along

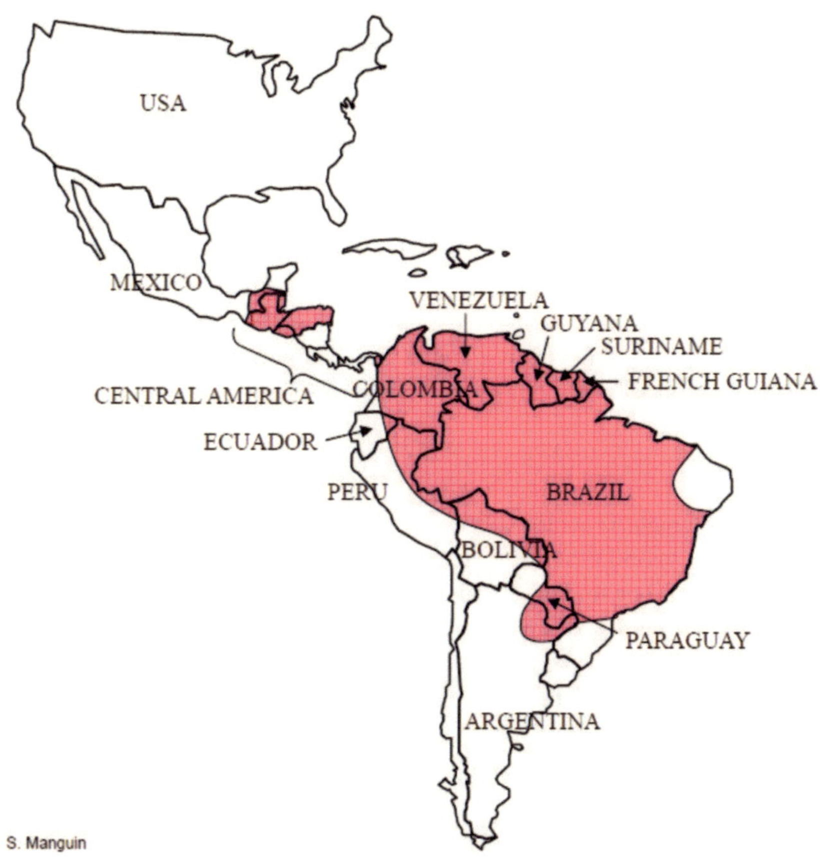

Figure 5. Distribution of *Anopheles darlingi* highlighted in pink [21].

the main Colombian rivers (such as Magdalena, Cauca and Atrato) [22, 74]. *An. darlingi* is the main malaria vector throughout its distribution. Although associated with forest environments, it was also detected in the peri-urban area of the cities of Quibdó (Chocó) and Villavicencio (Meta), where malaria transmission occurs [40]. Breeding sites are the typical streams with slow water movement, but stationary water bodies such as natural and constructed fish ponds also provide good habitats. Similar to Peru (see below), the biting behaviour in Colombia is mostly before midnight, from 18-24h, with a smaller peak at sunrise (05-06h), but there is also persistant biting activity throughout the night [39].

2.4.4. French Guiana

In French Guiana, there has been renewed activity on malaria vectors, with most findings incriminating *An. darlingi* as the primary vector (Table 1). Between 2000-2002 in three Amerindian villages in the Upper-Maroni region of the Amazon forest, *An. darlingi* bit throughout the night, with peaks at 21:30-03:30h and again after 05:30h [44]. The biting rate was very high (255.5 bites/person/night) and specimens were infected with *P. falciparum, P. vivax* and *P. malariae*. Behavior was characterized as endo-exophagic and exophilic. The malaria transmission risk exists all year but probably it is greater during the rainy season when vectorial capacity was estimated to be higher [44]. A combination of ITNs and repellent is recommended; IRS is not efficient because of the housing materials and relative inaccessibility of this region. A second study in the Maroni area compared villages of Amerindian Wayanas and the Aloukous [45]. Significant findings include: the peak local malaria case reporting is the same timeframe (August to October) as the highest IMT (numbers of infected mosquitoes surviving long enough to transmit) of *An. darlingi*; the possibility that the persistent yearlong transmission is focused or perhaps limited to the Amerindian villages; and different bionomics of *An. darlingi* in the two villages which lead investigators to conclude that in this region there may exist two distinctive subspecies of *An. darlingi*. An analysis of collections from 2006-2011, in several regions of French Guiana, detected *An. darlingi* infected by *P. vivax* from Camopi and Saint Georges de l'Oyapock, both near the Oyapock River along the eastern border with Brazil [42].

2.4.5. Peru

An. darlingi is the main malaria vector species in eastern Amazonian Peru, the area with the highest malaria transmission in the country. It invaded this region in the 1990s [75], and its distribution now includes peri-urban settlements around the city of Iquitos, Loreto province. This change has been attributed to logging, agriculture and urban expansion, associated with deforestation [76-77]. To date, its greatest abundance is associated with areas of at least partial deforestation [78]. The main breeding sites in the Peruvian Amazon are streams and river margins in forested areas [77], however, the density of fish ponds has shown a positive association with malaria cases along roads in Loreto, suggesting that such ponds could be important local sources of this species [79]. *An. darlingi* was found naturally infected with *P. vivax* and *P. falciparum* in Loreto [46]. The human biting activity, which is similar indoors and outdoors, peaks two hours after sunset [77]. Because of the early evening biting peak, personal protection may be necessary to supplement bed-net use.

2.4.6. *Panama*

An. darlingi was recently detected in Panamá for the first time, in the eastern Darien region, near the border with Colombia, associated with the highest prevalence of drug-resistant *P. falciparum* [80]. This species was only collected by human landing catch, and not recorded in light traps, confirming its high anthropophily. Despite the extension and increased frequency of deforestation in Panama, *An. darlingi* has been detected only in the east. Its discovery suggests that unplanned deforestation should be avoided to prevent further expansion of this very anthropophilic species, and hence potential *P. falciparum* transmission, to other regions in the country.

2.4.7. *Suriname*

A timely and important new development in Suriname is the apparent collapse of populations of *An. darlingi* in the sparsely inhabited interior, in and around three study communities, correlated with two main factors: the introduction of ITNs and climatic events, *i.e.*, unusual flooding which coincided with the beginning of the control activities in 2006 [47]. However, it should be noted that indoor residual spraying (IRS), active case detection (ACD), and a public awareness campaign also were implemented throughout the interior in 2006. As the authors point out, for Suriname, the next challenge is to try to find ways to use these methods to reduce or eliminate transmission among the gold-mining communities, where people are very mobile, and often active (not using ITNs) during potential biting times of *An. darlingi*. The latter are notoriously plastic, and vary locally and regionally. An important determination will be whether these results [47] can serve as a model for some communities where *An. darlingi* and malaria transmission are endemic in other countries.

2.4.8. *Venezuela*

Investigations along the Upper Orinoco River, southern Venezuela from 1994-1995 confirmed that *An. darlingi* was responsible for most, if not all of the local transmission of *P. falciparum*, *P. vivax* and *P. malariae* [48], that children under the age of 10 were at greatest risk, and that the EIR of *An. darlingi* was 129 positive bites/person/year. In a gold-mining region in southern Venezuela, studies from 1999-2000 [30-31] also determined that *An. darlingi* was one of two main vectors (the other was *An. marajoara* but see above under Albitarsis Complex). Surprisingly, many of the bionomic aspects of the two species in the five localities studied were quite similar (both more abundant during the rainy season, both biting indoors and outdoors with pronounced endophagic behavior), although *An. marajoara* was more abundant overall. The most striking bionomics difference between the two species was the peak biting time: *An. darlingi* bit throughout the night with two minor peaks (23-0h and 03-04h), whereas *An. marajoara* had a peak from 19-21h [30-31].

2.5. *Anopheles nuneztovari* s.l.

Anopheles nuneztovari s.l. is restricted to northern and Amazonian South America (Figure 6) and has been considered to be two genetically, ecologically and epidemiologically distinctive geographic populations, with the perception that the Colombian/western Venezuelan population was a regional vector (anthrophophilic and endo-exophagic) and the Amazonian population, mostly zoophilic and exophagic, was not [1, 5, 11]. Initially, evidence for malaria transmission by *An. nuneztovari* s.l. was found predominantly in Colombia and western Venezuela [22, 49]. However, a series of positive ELISA results and incriminations of malaria transmission involvement from localities in the Brazilian Amazon (Table 1; Figure 3) since 2000 soon undermined this relatively simple view. *An. goeldii*, which had been synonymized with *An. nuneztovari*, was resurrected as a valid species [81]. This work proposed different geographical distributions for each species, with *An. goeldii* in the Amazon region and *An. nuneztovari* more restricted to Colombia and Venezuela. The report of the discovery of *An. nuneztovari* infected with *Plasmodium* from Saint Georges de l'Oyapock, French Guiana, using results from a longitudinal study (2006-2011) is of at least local relevance, but it will be taxonomically important to determine whether this species is actually *An. nuneztovari*, or might possibly be *An. goeldii*, since susceptibility of *An. goeldii* to *Plasmodium* has not yet been tested [42].

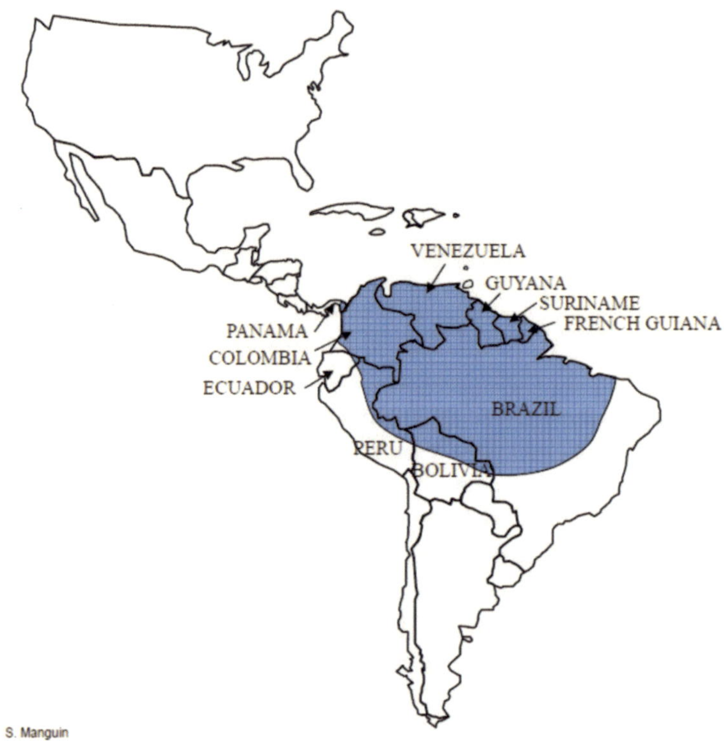

Figure 6. Distribution of *Anopheles nuneztovari* s.l. highlighted in blue [21].

An. nuneztovari s.l. is widely distributed in Colombia [22], particularly in the east, along the Venezuelan frontier, in the northwest region (Departments of Córdoba and Antioquia), where approximately 50% of the malaria cases occur, and in some areas along the Pacific

Coast in the west, notably along the San Juan river (Chocó), and in the Buenaventura area (Valle). Specimens from Tierralta, Córdoba, a region of crop and livestock production, where *An. nuneztovari* s.l. was the most abundant species collected by human landing catches, were infected by *P. vivax* [38]. The breeding sites include small, permanent ponds, sunlit flooded pastures, and it has been determined that aquaculture ponds are one of this species' most frequent breeding places. In the west, in Cimitarra (Santander), such ponds, characterized as permanent, completely exposed to sun and containing emerging vegetation, particularly grasses, represent approximately 81% of the breeding sites [63]. In Colombia, *An. nuneztovari* s.l. shows differing biting behavior by region. An exophagic tendency has been described in the northwest (Córdoba) [82], whereas in the east (Santander), a more endophagic behavior has been described [63]. The endophagic-exophilic variability makes control by residual insecticides very difficult.

3. Phylogeography

3.1. *Anopheles albimanus*

An exemplary study, based on large sample sizes using microsatellite markers and a mtDNA *ND5* gene fragment, laid the groundwork for several *Anopheles albimanus* phylogeographic ideas [83]. These researchers detected restricted gene flow that they hypothesized to be the result of the physical barrier of the Central American Cordillera. Recent work, more geographically focused on one country or a region, with additional local sampling, provides additional insights into phylogeography in Central America [20, 85] and Colombia [84].

A mitochondrial DNA *COI* gene fragment and microsatellites were used to test for congruence with biogeographical provinces [86] in Colombia. In this case [84], one population, Turbo, was from Magdalena (Caribbean), three were from Maracaibo (Caribbean), and the four were from Choco (Pacific). The eight populations tested were clearly differentiated into two coastal regions, Caribbean and Pacific, with evidence for a late Pleistocene expansion (estimated to 21,994 years ago) or a selective sweep. Even though there was evidence for historical restrictions to gene flow (*COI* data), the microsatellites detected contemporary gene flow between the regions. Interestingly, a SAMOVA analysis found an unusual division. Only the three most easterly populations along the Caribbean coast grouped together. The fourth and most western Caribbean population, Turbo, was consistently more closely related to the four Pacific populations. Taken together, these data suggest possible semi-permeable boundaries among the three biogeographical provinces tested. Most relevant to malaria is the fact that the evidence for contemporary gene flow indicates that insecticide resistance genes, for example, could spread readily in these Colombian regions [84].

An. albimanus from Central America was examined using a fragment of the mtDNA *COI* gene to test the original hypothesis [83]. Physical barriers to gene flow were not detected (i.e., the Central America Cordillera was porous for *An. albimanus*) and contemporary isolation by distance was not supported [20]. Three divergent, co-occuring haplotype groups were detected using a statistical parsimony network, and these were not evenly distributed across Costa Rica and Panama. A new hypothesis suggested that they could be the result of multiple introductions into the region, probably caused by historical fragmentation and subsequent secondary contact. A more wide-ranging study incorporated the samples from Colombia [84], Ecuador, and Nicaragua with those from Costa Rica and Panama [20] and added two molecular fragments: the nuclear *white* gene and the ITS2. A SAMOVA analysis defined three large population demes, one from Nicaragua, Costa Rica and the Atlantic coast of western Panama; a second one incorporating the Pacific coast of western Panama, central-eastern Panama and the Caribbean Colombian coast; and a third one restricted to the Pacific coast of Colombia and Ecuador [85]. There were also four haplogroups, based on the *COI* fragment, which differed little from those found in the earlier Panamanian study [20] except for the addition of a fourth, restricted to the Pacific coast of Colombia and Ecuador, and separated by 18 mutation steps from its nearest haplogroup. Interestingly, because it tracks an earlier history, the *white* gene network showed much less divergence, supporting the overall conclusion that the primary time-frame for anopheline divergence at the species level is Pleistocene [15]. In summary, the combined *An. albimanus* data set strongly supported the presence of a single species in this region, which was expected, but also found very robust evidence for Pleistocene geographic fragmentation followed by range expansion across southern Central America [85].

3.2. The Albitarsis Complex

Following the newest revelations about the number of species (eight) plus a novel lineage (*An. albitarsis* H) in *An. albitarsis* s.l. [57], parts of an earlier study on the biogeography and population genetics of this complex [17] need to be reconsidered and modified. This is particularly the case for *An. janconnae*, which is more restricted than thought (under the taxonomic name of *An. albitarsis* E), the expanded distribution of *An. albitarsis* F (which now includes Venezuela and Trinidad as well as Colombia), the complexities of the distribution of *An. marajoara*, which really may have a very broad range, newly described *An. albitarsis* G, distributed along the Brazilian Amazon, and *An. albitarsis* I, restricted to northwestern Colombia [57]. Despite these problems, one recent study can be used to illustrate the phylogeography of at least *An. albitarsis* G [as far as it is known; 57] and part of the range of *An. marajoara* [87]. *An. albitarsis* G [lineage 2 in reference 87] may be restricted to localities near the Amazon River or its tributaries. It has little population structure and the small subdivisions that were detected in haplotype networks were unrelated to geographic locality. The evidence from the mtDNA *COI* fragment used in this study indicates that this lineage is older than *An. marajoara* [lineage 1 in reference 87]. On the other hand, the *white* gene and ITS2 data detected a single network between *An. albitarsis* G and *An. marajoara*, indicating that the divergence is recent. The most compelling result in this study concerning *An. marajoara* is that SAMOVA defined two population demes along the Amazon River, splitting this species into western and eastern entities with differing genetic characteristics. The boundary is located near Rio Jari in Amapá state, not far from one detected in *An. darlingi* [88] and an earlier one seen in a study of *An. nuneztovari* s.l. using restriction fragment length analysis of the mtDNA genome [89]. For *An. marajoara*, this boundary is permeable, since there were shared haplotypes on either side [87]. A denser sampling of all three species could more rigorously test whether this is the result of underlying geological boundaries or perhaps more recent climatic events.

3.3. *An. darlingi*

Several studies on the phylogeography of *An. darlingi* have been undertaken. The earliest one [90] used the mtDNA *COI* fragment and detected a significant genetic division between Central America/northwestern Colombia, and the rest of South America. According to the statistical parsimony network, the more widespread and ancestral haplotypes were in Amazonian and southern South America, suggesting that the Central American/Colombian haplotypes may have originated there. This division was also supported by sequences of the *white* gene, which found two genotypes, genotype I, restricted to the Amazon, and genotype II, in northwestern Colombia and Venezuela, and Central America [91]. A microsatellite analysis of 1,376 samples also strongly supported the initial *COI* genetic division, and found substantial structure within the Amazon Basin [91]. The conclusion was that there were two main drivers for this division: differences in effective population size among the divisions, and physical distances between the populations. A more sophisticated analysis of the mtDNA *COI* fragment included additional Brazilian samples and excluded the Central American samples [88]. These researchers detected six main population groups in South America, and found ancestral distribution to be central Amazonia. They proposed that populations became isolated by three barriers: the Amazon River, the Andes and the southeastern Brazilian coastal ranges. They also found that limited dispersal across some landscape types has promoted differentiation between other proximate populations. A local study of *An. darlingi* in Córdoba and Antioquia, Colombia, using mtDNA *COI*, microsatellites and the *white* gene [74] supported the earlier geographic hypothesis [90], discovering that the five populations tested were more closely related to the Central American populations of *An. darlngi* that they were to South American *An. darlingi*. Because of local high gene flow among the five populations, similar control strategies could be implemented in these two contiguous Colombian states. Similarly, newly detected *An. darlingi* from Panama were most closely related to Colombian and Central American *An. darlingi* [80]. Concordant phylogeographies were determined for the two neotropical vectors *An. darlingi* and *An. triannulatus* [92]. With the mtDNA *COI* fragment, SAMOVA detected four similar population subdivisions: one in southern coastal Brazil, two in central Brazil and one northeast of the Amazon. Both species originated south of the Amazon River and seem to have followed a similar expansion pathway to their present-day distributions. Other neotropical anophelines with similar distributions may share a common spatial and demographic history with these species, and remain to be evaluated.

3.4. *An. aquasalis*

The only study that attempted to analyse *An. aquasalis* within a phylogeographic framework was conducted using a fragment of the mtDNA *COI* gene with specimens from five localities on either side of the Amazon, in Amapá and Pará states, Brazil [93]. The most important findings from this study inferred that despite the width of the mouth of the Amazon, this freshwater delta was not a barrier for the salt-water tolerant *An. aquasalis*, likely because of so much tidal mixing, and the numerous islands and channels in the region. However, gene flow was restricted, based on isolation by distance that was detected using a Nested Clade Analysis [94]. The relative regional importance of *An. aquasalis* as a malaria vector has waned since the earlier publications [1, 14], so there may be fewer opportunities to pursue phylogeographic questions, especially because the distribution is relatively limited. However, no one has compared specimens from the Atlantic and Pacific coasts, and it is possible that population structure similar to that found for *An. albimanus* [85], could be detected in *An. aquasalis,* considering that both species share a relatively narrow coastal distribution in South America, and were subjected to the same kinds of Pleistocene environmental changes.

3.5. *An. nuneztovari* s.l.

The revision of the taxonomic status of *An. nuneztovari* s.l., that now includes *An. nuneztovari* s.s. and *An. goeldii* [81] has implications for the interpretation of the first study of *An. nuneztovari* phylogeography, which focused on the nuclear *white* gene [95]. Five lineages were detected [95], 2 and 3 in Colombia/Venezuela and 1, 4 and 5 in Amazonian Brazil. The earliest divergence, during the Pliocene (5.3-23.0 mya), is between Colombia and Venezuela west of the Andes (lineage 3) and Amazonian lineage 4. The most likely hypothesis to explain this divergence is an early uplift of the East Andean Cordillera [96]. Curiously, the levels of genetic divergences among the five lineages were high, although the minimum spanning network of the haplotypes connected all of them. There were five localities where two lineages were sympatric: in Brazil - Boa Vista, Roraima state; Altamira, Pará state and near Pôrto Velho, Rondonia state; Guayaramerín, Beni, Bolivia; and Rio Socuavó, Zulia, Venezuela. These localities are of special interest, since they may be admixture zones or hotspots of divergence. The simplest hypothesis to explain the five lineages taxonomically is that the two in Colombia/ Venezuela are *An. nuneztovari* s.s. and the three in Brazil are *An. goeldii*. The sharing of haplotypes across the Andes, between eastern and western Venezuela [95], is congruent with and supports findings for *An. albimanus* [83], The Albitarsis Complex [57] and *An. darlingi* (Conn, unpublished data) that have hypothesized that the eastern Andean Cordillera is only a partial barrier for anopheline mosquitoes.

A second phylogeographic study was undertaken with some of the same samples, plus new ones from Amazonian Brazil, using a mtDNA *COI* fragment [97], which charts a more recent history of divergence, all within the Pleistocene, compared with the *white* gene fragment. In this work, there were two major monophyletic clades, I and II. Specimens from Bolivia/ Colombia/Venezuela represent the most basal subclade, IIC; whereas the Amazonian specimens were found in clades I and II-A and II-B. There were also several localities of sympatry among the clades: five in Amapá, Amazonas and Pará states, Amazonian Brazil, and one in Suriname. None of these are the same as the ones detected by the *white* gene study, perhaps suggesting that these were later areas of sympatry. There was an intriguing connection detected between the specimens from Colombia/Venezuela and those from Amazonian Bolivia, which had previously been seen when sequences of the rDNA ITS2 were used [98]. This may be the signature of the marine incursion hypothesis [95]. One of clades I, II-A or II-B likely represents *An. goeldii*, but additional analyses are needed to determine which one, and also to test the hypothesis of multiple species in the Amazon.

http://dx.doi.org/10.5772/55217

4. Conclusions

There have been many changes in the incrimination, identification and several new insights into the phylogeography of the species discussed in this chapter. The most important taxonomic changes are those in the Albitarsis Complex, with the discovery of two new species, *An. albitarsis* G and I, and a new lineage, *An. albitarsis* H. Nothing is known about their involvement in malaria transmission, although their ranges all include malaria endemic areas, or their local contribution to diversity or to a better understanding of the complex patterns of Amazonian biogeography and phylogeography. The relative paucity of new work on *An. aquasalis* is a reminder that its relative importance appears to be lessening, although it is still likely to be important locally, particularly when in high abundance. Obviously, the importance of *An. darlingi* in still on the rise in several localities in many countries, attributable mainly to its remarkable adaptability and association with landscape changes. The resurrection of *An. goeldii* from synonymy is also a milestone, because it provides a first step toward resolving a longstanding discussion about the possible importance of *An. nuneztovari* s.l. in local transmission in Amazonian Brazil. It may also clarify some aspects of the recent phylogeographic inferences based on *white* and the mtDNA *COI* genes. Lastly, the detection of concordant phylogeographies, one of which is *An. darlingi* in Brazil, depict a clear path towards future research which will have important epidemiological consequences.

Acknowledgements

We thank Ricardo Guimarães (LabGeo/IEC/SVS) for creating the map in Figure 3. We thank Sara Bickersmith for tireless work on the table, editorial suggestions, and slight modifications to the map. Some of the unpublished work cited here was funded by a grant from the National Institutes of Health (USA) to JEC (AI R01 54139-02) and a grant from CNPq (Brazil) to MMP.

Author details

Jan E. Conn[1*], Martha L. Quiñones[2] and Marinete M. Póvoa[3]

*Address all correspondence to: jconn@wadsworth.org

1 Department of Biomedical Sciences, School of Public Health, State University of New York-Albany and Griffin Laboratory, Wadsworth Center, New York State Department of Health, Albany, New York, USA

2 Martha L. Quiñones, Faculty of Medicine, National University of Colombia, Bogotá D.C., Colombia

3 Section of Parasitology, Instituto Evandro Chagas, Secretariat of Health Surveillance, Ministry of Health, Belém, Pará, Brazil

References

[1] Lounibos LP, Conn JE. Malaria vector heterogeneity in South America. American Entomologist 2000;46 238-249.

[2] Sinka ME, Rubio-Palis Y, Manguin S, Patil AP, Temperley WH, Gething PW, Van Boeckel T, Kabaria CW, Harbach RE, Hay SI. The dominant *Anopheles* vectors of human malaria in the Americas: occurrence data, distribution maps and bionomic précis. Parasites & Vectors 2010;3 72.

[3] Hiwat H, Bretas G. Ecology of *Anopheles darlingi* Root with respect to vector importance: a review. Parasites & Vectors 2011;4 177.

[4] Montoya-Lerma J, Solarte YA, Giraldo-Calderón GI, Quiñones ML, Ruiz-López F, Wilkerson RC, González R. Malaria vector species in Colombia: a review. Memórias do Instituto Oswaldo Cruz 2011;106: 223-238.

[5] Marrelli MT, Sallum MAM, Marinotti O. The second internal transcribed spacer of nuclear ribosomal DNA as a tool for Latin American anopheline taxonomy – a critical review. Memórias do Instituto Oswaldo Cruz 2006;101(8) 817-832.

[6] Wirtz RA, Burkot TR, Graves PM, Andre RG. Field evaluation of enzyme-linked immunosorbent assays for *Plasmodium falciparum* and *Plasmodium vivax* sporozoites in mosquitoes (Diptera: Culicidae) from Papua New Guinea. Journal of Medical Entomology 1987;24(4) 433-437.

[7] Snounou G, Viriyakosol S, Jarra W, Thaithong S, Brown KN. Identification of the four human malaria parasite species in field samples by the polymerase chain reaction and detection of a high prevalence of mixed infections. Molecular and Biochemical Parasitology 1993;58(2) 283-292.

[8] Ryan JR, Davé K, Collins KM, Hochberg L, Sattabongkot J, Coleman RE, Dunton RF, Bangs MJ, Mbogo CM, Cooper RD, Schoeler GB, Rubio-Palis Y, Magris M, Romer LI, Padilla N, Quakyi IA, Bigoga J, Leke RG, Akinpelu O, Evans B, Walsey M, Patterson P, Wirtz RA, Chan AS. Extensive multiple test center evaluation of the VecTest malaria antigen panel assay. Medical and Veterinary Entomology 2002;17 321-332.

[9] Póvoa MM, Wirtz RA, Lacerda RN, Miles MA, Warhurst D. Malaria vectors in the municipality of Serra do Navio, State of Amapá, Amazon Region, Brazil. Memorias do Instituto Oswaldo Cruz 2001;96(2) 179-184

[10] Quiñones ML, Ruiz F, Calle DA, Harbach RE, Erazo HF, Linton YM. 2006. Incrimination of *Anopheles (Nyssorhynchus) rangeli* and *An. (Nys.) oswaldoi* as natural vectors of *Plasmodium vivax* in Southern Colombia. Memórias do Instituto Oswaldo Cruz 2006;101 617-623.

[11] Tadei WP, Dutary Thatcher B. Malaria vectors in the Brazilian amazon: *Anopheles* of the subgenus *Nyssorhynchus*. Revista do Instituto de Medicina Tropical de São Paulo 2000;42(2) 87-94.

[12] Galardo AK, Arruda M, D'Almeida Couto AA, Wirtz R, Lounibos LP, Zimmerman RH. Malaria vector incrimination in three rural riverine villages in the Brazilian Amazon. American Journal of Tropical Medicine and Hygiene 2007;76(3) 461-469.

[13] da Rocha JAM, de Oliveira SB, Póvoa MM, Moreira LA, Krettli AU. Malaria vectors in areas of *Plasmodium falciparum* epidemic transmission in the Amazon region, Brazil. American Journal of Tropical Medicine and Hygiene 2008;78(6) 872-877.

[14] Fleming G. Biologia y ecologia de los vectores de la malaria en las Americas. PAHO/WHO, 1986; PNSP-86-72, Washington, 54 pp.

[15] Loaiza JR, Bermingham E, Sanjur OI, Scott ME, Bickersmith SA, Conn JE. Review of genetic diversity in malaria vectors (Culicidae: Anophelinae). Infection, Genetics, and Evolution 2012;12(1) 1-12.

[16] Gibbard PL, Head MJ. IUGS ratification of the Quaternary System/Period and the Pleistocene Series/Epoch with a base at 2.58 Ma. Quaternaire 2009; 20 271-272.

[17] Conn JE, Mirabello LM. The biogeography and population genetics of neotropical vector species. Heredity 2007;99 245-256.

[18] Faran ME. Mosquito studies (Diptera: Culicidae) XXXIV. A revision of the *Albimanus* section of the subgenus *Nyssorhynchus* of *Anopheles*. Contributions of the Annals of the Entomological Institute 1980;15 1-215.

[19] Breeland SG. Studies on the ecology of *Anopheles albimanus*. American Journal of Tropical Medicine and Hygiene 1972;21 751-754.

[20] Loaiza JR, Scott ME, Bermingham E, Rovira J, Conn JE. Evidence for Pleistocene population divergence and expansion of *Anopheles albimanus* in Southern Central America. American Journal of Tropical Medicine and Hygiene 2010;82(1) 156-164.

[21] Manguin S, Carnevale P, Mouchet J, Coosemans M, Julvez J, Richard-Lenoble D, Sircoulon J. Biodiversity of malaria in the world. France: John Libbey Eurotext Ed.; 2008.

[22] Olano VA, Brochero H, Saenz R, Quinones M. Molina J. Mapas preliminares de la distribucion de especies de *Anopheles* vectores de malaria en Colombia. Biomedica 2001; 21 402–408.

[23] Poveda G, Rojas W, Quiñones ML, Velez IV, Mantilla RI, Ruiz D, Zuluaga JS, Rua GL. Coupling between Annual and ENSO Timescales in the Malaria - Climate Association in Colombia. Environmental Health Perspectives 2001;109(5) 489-493.

[24] Gutiérrez LA, Naranjo N, Jaramillo LM, Muskus C, Luckart S, Conn JE, Correa MM. Natural infectivity of *Anopheles* species from the Pacific and Atlantic regions of Colombia. Acta Tropica 2008;107(2) 99-105.

[25] Conn JE, Wilkerson RC, Segura MN, de Souza RT, Schlichting CD, Wirtz RA, Póvoa MM. Emergence of a new neotropical malaria vector facilitated by human migration and changes in land use. American Journal of Tropical Medicine and Hygiene 2002;66(1) 18-22.

[26] de Barros FS, Honório NA, Arruda ME. Mosquito anthropophily: implications on malaria transmission in the Northern Brazilian Amazon. Neotropical Entomology 2010;39(6) 1039-1043.

[27] Póvoa MM, de Souza RT, Lacerda RN, Rosa ES, Galiza D, de Souza JR, Wirtz RA, Schlichting CD, Conn JE. The importance of *Anopheles albitarsis* E and *An. darlingi* in human malaria transmission in Boa Vista, state of Roraima, Brazil. Memórias do Instituto Oswaldo Cruz 2006;101(2) 163-168.

[28] da Silva-Vasconcelos A, Kató MY, Mourão EN, de Souza RT, Lacerda RN, Sibajev A, Tsouris P, Póvoa MM, Momen H, Rosa-Freitas MG. Biting indices, host-seeking activity and natural infection rates of anopheline species in Boa Vista, Roraima, Brazil from 1996 to 1998. Memórias do Instituto Oswaldo Cruz 2002;97(2) 151-161.

[29] Jiménez P, Conn JE, Wirtz R, Brochero H. *Anopheles* (Diptera: Culicidae) vectores de malaria en el municipio de Puerto Carreño, Vichada, Colombia. Biomedica 2012;32 13-21.

[30] Moreno JE, Rubio-Palis Y, Páez E, Pérez E, Sánchez V, Vaccari E. Malaria entomological inoculation rates in gold mining areas of Southern Venezuela. Memorias do Instituto Oswaldo Cruz 2009;104(5) 764-768.

[31] Moreno JE, Rubio-Palis Y, Páez E, Pérez E, Sánchez V. Abundance, biting behavior and parous rate of anopheline mosquito species in relation to malaria incidence in gold-mining areas of southern Venezuela. Medical and Veterinary Entomology 2007;21(4) 339-349.

[32] Ribeiro MCT, Goncalves EDD, Tauil PL, da Silva AR. Epidemiological aspects of a malaria focus in the districts of São Luis, MA. Revista da Sociedade Brasileira de Medicina Tropical 2005;38(3) 272-274.

[33] Póvoa MM, Conn JE, Schlichting CD, Amaral JC, Segura MN, da Silva AN, dos Santos CC, Lacerda RN, de Souza RT, Galiza D, Santa Rosa EP, Wirtz RA. Malaria vectors, epidemiology, and the re-emergence of *Anopheles darlingi* in Belém, Pará, Brazil. Journal of Medical Entomology 2003;40(4) 379-386.

[34] Laubach HE, Validum L, Bonilla JA, Agar A, Cummings R, Mitchell C, Cuadrado RR, Palmer CJ. Identification of *Anopheles aquasalis* as a possible vector of malaria in Guyana, South America. West Indian Medical Journal 2001;50(4) 319-21.

[35] Póvoa MM. 2002. Report on Malaria transmission in Suriname. 5p

http://dx.doi.org/10.5772/55217

[36] dos Santos RL, Padilha A, Costa MD, Costa EM, Dantas-Filho Hde C, Póvoa MM. Malaria vectors in two indigenous reserves of the Brazilian Amazon. Revista de Saúde Pública 2009;43(5) 859-868.

[37] dos Santos RL, Sucupira IM, Lacerda RN, Fayal A da S, Póvoa MM. Entomological survey and infectivity during malaria outbreak in the Anajás municipality, Pará State. Revista da Sociedade Brasileira de Medicina Tropical 2005;38(2) 202-204.

[38] Gutiérrez LA, González JJ, Gómez GF, Castro MI, Rosero DA, Luckart S, Conn JE, Correa MM. Species composition and natural infectivity of anthropophilic *Anopheles* (Diptera: Culicidae) in the states of Córdoba and Antioquia, Northwestern Colombia. Memórias do Instituto Oswaldo Cruz 2009;104(8) 1117-1124.

[39] Brochero HL, Rey G, Buitrago LS, Olano VA. Biting activity and breeding sites of *Anopheles* species in the municipality Villavicencio, Meta, Colombia. Journal of the American Mosquito Control Association 2005;21(2) 182-186.

[40] Ochoa J, Osorio L. Epidemiologia de malaria urbana en Quibdó, Chocó. Biomedica 2006;26 278-285.

[41] Herrera M, Orjuela LI, Peñalver C, Quiñones ML. Characterization of the *Anopheles* species present in two ecologically different regions in La Guajira, northern Colombia. In Clark G & Rubio-Palis. Mosquito Vector Biology and Control in Latin America - a 19th Symposium. Journal of the American Mosquito Control Association 2009;25(4):486-499.

[42] Dusfour I, Issaly J, Carinci R, Gaborit P, Girod R. Incrimination of *Anopheles (Anopheles) intermedius* Peryassú, *An. (Nyssorhynchus) nuneztovari* Gabaldón, *An. (Nys.) oswaldoi* Peryassú as natural vectors of *Plasmodium falciparum* in French Guiana. Memórias do Instituto Oswaldo Cruz 2012;107(3) 429-432.

[43] Hiwat H, Issaly J, Gaborit P, Somai A, Samjhawan A, Sardjoe P, Soekhoe T, Girod R. Behavioral heterogeneity of *Anopheles darlingi* (Diptera: Culicidae) and malaria transmission dynamics along the Maroni River, Suriname, French Guiana. Transactions of the Royal Society of Tropical Medicine and Hygiene 2010;104(3) 207-213.

[44] Girod R, Gaborit P, Carinci R, Issaly J, Fouque F. *Anopheles darlingi* bionomics and transmission of *Plasmodium falciparum, Plasmodium vivax*, and *Plasmodium malariae* in American villages of the Upper-Maroni Amazonian forest, French Guiana. Memórias do Instituto Oswaldo Cruz 2008;103(7) 702-710.

[45] Fouque F, Gaborit P, Carinci R, Issaly J, Girod R. 2010. Annual variations in the number of malaria cases related to two different patterns of *Anopheles darlingi* transmission potential in the Maroni area of French Guiana. Malaria Journal 2010;9 80.

[46] Flores-Mendoza C, Fernández R, Escobedo-Vargas KS, Vela-Perez Q, Schoeler GB. Natural *Plasmodium* infections in *Anopheles darlingi* and *Anopheles benarrochi* (Diptera: Culicidae) from Eastern Peru. Journal of Medical Entomology 2004; 41(3) 489-494.

[47] Hiwat H, Mitro S, Samjhawan A, Sardjoe P, Soekhoe T, Takken W. Collapse of *Anopheles darlingi* populations in Suriname after introduction of insecticide-treated nets (ITNs); malaria down to near elimination level. American Journal of Tropical Medicine and Hygiene 2012;86(4) 649-655.

[48] Magris M, Rubio-Palis Y, Menares C, Villegas L. Vector bionomics and malaria transmission in the Upper Orinoco River, Southern Venezuela. Mem Inst Oswaldo Cruz 2007;102(3) 303-311.

[49] Rubio-Palis Y. 2000. *Anopheles* (*Nyssorhynchus*) de Venezuela: taxonomia, bionomía, ecología e importancia médica. Escuela de Malariología y Saneamiento Ambiental "Dr. Arnoldo Gabaldon" y Proyecto Control de Enfermedades Endémicas, Maracay, Venezuela.

[50] Guthmann JP, Hall AJ, Jaffar S, Palacios A, Lines J, Llanos-Cuentas A. Environmental risk factors for clinical malaria: a case-control study in the Grau region of Peru. Transactions of the Royal Society of Tropical Medicine and Hygiene 2001;95(6) 577-583.

[51] Vargas F, Córdova O, Alvardo A. Determinación de la Resistencia a insecticidas en *Aedes aegypti, Anopheles albimanus* y *Lutzomyia peruensis* procedentes del Norte Peruano. Revista Peruana de Medicina Experimental y Salud Publica 2006;23(4) 259-264.

[52] DIGESA-Direccion General de Salud Ambiental, Ministerio de Salud de Perú. Plan de Implementación de la Estrategia de Riego con Secas Intermitentes en el Cultivo de Arroz para el Control Vectorial de la Malaria en Regiones Priorizadas del Perú. Lima, Perú, 2011. 33p.

[53] Loaiza JR, Bermingham E, Scott ME, Rovira JR, Conn JE. Species composition and distribution of adult *Anopheles* (Diptera: Culicidae) in Panama. Journal of Medical Entomology 2008;45(5) 841-851.

[54] Pinault LL, Hunter FF. New highland distribution records of multiple *Anopheles* species in the Ecuadorian Andes. Malaria Journal 2011;11(10) 236.

[55] Pinault LL, Hunter FF. Larval habitat associations with human land uses, roads, rivers, and land cover for *Anopheles albimanus, A. pseudopunctipennis,* and *A. punctimacula* (Diptera: Culicidae) in coastal and highland Ecuador. Frontiers in Physiology 2012;3 59.

[56] Pinault LL, Hunter FF. Characterization of larval habitats of *Anopheles albimanus, Anopheles pseudopunctipennis, Anopheles punctimacula,* and *Anopheles oswaldoi* s.l. populations in lowland and highland Ecuador. Journal of Vector Ecology 2012;37(1) 124-136.

[57] Ruiz-Lopez F, Wilkerson RC, Conn JE, McKeon SN, Levin DM, Quiñones ML, Póvoa MM, Linton YM. DNA barcoding reveals both known and novel taxa in the Albitar-

sis Group (*Anopheles: Nyssorhynchus*) of Neotropical malaria vectors. Parasites & Vectors 2012;5:44.

[58] Gutiérrez LA, Orrego LM, Gómez GF, López A, Luckart S, Conn JE, Correa MM. A new mtDNA COI gene lineage closely related to *Anopheles janconnae* of the Albitarsis complex in the Caribbean region of Colombia. Memórias do Instituto Oswaldo Cruz 2010;105 1019-1025.

[59] Linthicum KJ. A revision of the Argyritarsis Section of the subgenus *Nyssorhynchus* of *Anopheles* (Diptera: Culicidae). Mosquito Systematics 1988;20(2) 98-271.

[60] Motoki MT, Wilkerson RC, Sallum MAM. The *Anopheles albitarsis* complex with the recognition of *Anopheles oryzalimnetes* Wilkerson and Motoki, n. sp. and *Anopheles janconnae* Wilkerson and Sallum, n. sp. (Diptera: Culicidae). Memórias do Instituto Oswaldo Cruz 2009;104(6) 823-850.

[61] Laporta GZ, Ramos DG, Ribeiro MC, Sallum MA. Habitat suitability of *Anopheles* vector species and association with human malaria in the Atlantic Forest in southeastern Brazil. Memórias do Instituto Oswaldo Cruz 2011;106 Suppl 1:239-45.

[62] Galardo AK, Zimmerman RH, Lounibos LP, Young LJ, Galardo CD, Arruda M, D'Almeida Couto AA. Seasonal abundance of anopheline mosquitoes and their association with rainfall and malaria along the Matapí River, Amapí, Brazil. Medical and Veterinary Entomology 2009;23 335-349.

[63] Brochero H, Pareja PX, Ortiz G, Olano VA. Sitios de cría y actividad de picadura de especies de *Anopheles* en el municipio de Cimitarra, Santander, Colombia. Biomedica 2006;26(2) 269-277.

[64] Brochero H, Li C, Wilkerson RC, Conn JE, Ruiz-García. Genetic structure of *Anopheles (Nyssorhynchus) marajoara* (Diptera: Culicidae) in Colombia. American Journal of Tropical Medicine and Hygiene 2010;83(3) 585-595.

[65] Brochero HL, Li C, Wilkerson RC. A newly recognized species in the *Anopheles (Nyssorhynchus) albitarsis* complex (Diptera: Culicidae) from Puerto Carreño, Colombia. American Journal of Tropical Medicine and Hygiene 2007;76(6) 1113-1117.

[66] Rubio-Palis Y, Wilkerson R, Guzman H. Morphological characters of adult *Anopheles (Nyssorhynchus) marajoara* in Venezuela. Journal of the American Mosquito Control Association 2003;19(2)107-114.

[67] Forattini OP. Culicidologia médica: identificação, biologia, epidemiologia, Vol. II., Edusp, São Paulo, 2002. 864 pp.

[68] Grillet ME, Eudes Martínez JE, Barrera R. Malaria hot spot areas: implications for effective and targeted interventions in Venezuela. Boletin de Malariología y Salud Ambiental 2009;49(2) 193-208.

[69] Grillet ME, Barrera R, Martínez JE, Berti J, Fortin MJ. Disentangling the effect of local and global spatial variation on a mosquito-borne infection in a neotropical heteroge-

neous environment. American Journal of Tropical Medicine and Hygiene 2010;82(2) 194-201.

[70] da Silva Ade N, Fraiha-Neto H, dos Santos CC, Segura Mde N, Amaral JC, Gorayeb Ide S, Lacerda RN, Sucupira IM, Pimentel LN, Conn JE, Póvoa MM. Anophelines in Belém, Pará, Brazil: current and retrospective data. Cadernos de Saude Publica 2006;22(8) 1575-1585.

[71] Lardeux F, Chávez T, Rodríguez R, Torrez L. *Anopheles* of Bolivia: new records with an updated and annotated checklist. Comptes Rendus Biologies 2009;332(5) 489-499.

[72] Harris AF, Matias-Arnéz A, Hill N. Biting time of *Anopheles darlingi* in the Bolivian Amazon and implications for control of malaria. Transactions of the Royal Society of Tropical Medicine and Hygiene 2006;100(1) 45-47.

[73] Zimmerman RH, Galardo AK, Lounibos LP, Arruda M, Wirtz R. Bloodmeal hosts of *Anopheles* species (Diptera: Culicidae) in a malaria-endemic area of the Brazilian Amazon. Journal of Medical Entomology 2006;43(5) 947-956.

[74] Gutiérrez LA, Gómez GF, González JJ, Castro MI, Luckart S, Conn JE, Correa MM. Microgeographic genetic variation of the malaria vector *Anopheles darlingi* Root (Diptera: Culicidae) from Córdoba and Antioquia, Colombia. American Journal of Tropical Medicine and Hygiene 2010;83(1) 38-47.

[75] Aramburu Guarda J, Ramal Asayag C, Witzig R. Malaria reemergence in the Peruvian Amazon region. Emerging Infectious Diseases 1999;5 209-215.

[76] Turell MJ, Sardelis MR, Jones JW, Watts DM, Fernandez R, Carbajal F, Pecor JE, Klein TA. Seasonal distribution, biology, and human attraction patterns of mosquitoes (Diptera: Culicidae) in a rural village and adjacent forested site near Iquitos, Peru. Journal of Medical Entomology 2008;45(6) 1165-1172.

[77] Reinbold-Wasson DD, Sardelis MR, Jones JW, Watts DM, Fernandez R, Carbajal F, Pecor JE, Calampa C, Klein TA, Turell MJ. Determinants of *Anopheles* seasonal distribution patterns across a forest to periurban gradient near Iquitos, Peru. American Journal of Tropical Medicine and Hygiene 2012;86(3) 459-463.

[78] Vittor AY, Gilman RH, Tielsch J, Glass G, Shields T, Lozano WS, Pinedo-Cancino V, Patz JA. The effect of deforestation on the human-biting rate of *Anopheles darlingi*, the primary vector of Falciparum malaria in the Peruvian Amazon. American Journal of Tropical Medicine and Hygiene 2006:74(1) 3-11.

[79] Maheu-Giroux M, Casapía M, Soto-Calle VE, Ford LB, Buckeridge DL, Coomes OT, Gyorkos TW. Risk of malaria transmission from fish ponds in the Peruvian Amazon. Acta Tropica. 2010 115(1-2);112-118.

[80] Loaiza J, Scott M, Bermingham E, Rovira J, Sanjur O, Conn JE. *Anopheles darlingi* (Diptera: Culicidae) in Panama. American Journal of Tropical Medicine and Hygiene 2009;81(1) 23-26.

[81] Calado DC, Foster PG, Bergo ES, dos Santos CLS, Galardo AKR, Sallum MAM. Resurrection of *Anopheles goeldii* from synonymy with *Anopheles nuneztovari* (Diptera, Culicidae) and a new record for *Anopheles dunhami* in the Brazilian Amazon. Memórias do Instituto Oswaldo Cruz 2008;103(8) 791-799.

[82] Parra-Henao G, Alarcón-Pineda EP. Observaciones sobre la bionomía de *Anopheles* spp. (Diptera: Culicidae) en el municipio Valencia, departamento Córdoba, Colombia. Boletín de Malariologia y Saneamiento Ambiental 2008;48 95-98.

[83] Molina-Cruz A, de Mérida AM, Mills K, Rodríguez F, Schoua C, Yurrita MM, Molina E, Palmieri M, Black WC 4th. Gene flow among *Anopheles albimanus* populations in Central America, South America, and the Caribbean assessed by microsatellites and mitochondrial DNA. American Journal of Tropical Medicine and Hygiene 2004;71(3) 350-359.

[84] Gutiérrez LA, Naranjo NJ, Cienfuegos AV, Muskus CE, Luckhart S, Conn JE, Correa MM. Population structure analyses and demographic history of the malaria vector *Anopheles albimanus* from the Caribbean and the Pacific regions of Colombia. Malaria Journal 2009;8 259.

[85] Loaiza JR, Scott ME, Bermingham E, Sajur OI, Wilkerson R, Rovira J, Gutiérrez LA, Correa MM, Gríjalva MJ, Birnberg L, Bickersmith S, Conn JE. Late Pleistocene environmental changes lead to unstable demography and population divergence of *Anopheles albimanus* in the northern Neotropics. Molecular Phylogenetics and Evolution 2010b;57(3) 1341-1346.

[86] Morrone JJ. Biogeographic areas and transition zones of Latin America and the Caribbean Islands based on panbiogeographic and cladistic analyses of the entomofauna. Annual Review of Entomology 2006;51 467-494.

[87] McKeon SN, Lehr MA, Wilkerson RC, Ruiz JF, Sallum MA, Lima JBP, Póvoa MM, Conn JE. Lineage divergence detected in the malaria vector *Anopheles marajoara* (Diptera: Culicidae) in Amazonian Brazil. Malaria Journal 2010;9 271.

[88] Pedro PM, Sallum MAM. Spatial expansion and population structure of the neotropical malaria vector, *Anopheles darlingi* (Diptera: Culicidae). Biological Journal of the Linnean Society 2009;97 854-866.

[89] Conn JE, Mitchell SE, Cockburn AF. Mitochondrial DNA analysis of the neotropical malaria vector *Anopheles nuneztovari*. Genome 1998;41(3) 313-327.

[90] Mirabello LM, Conn JE. Molecular population genetics of the malaria vector *Anopheles darlingi* in Central and South America. Heredity 2006;96 311-321.

[91] Mirabello L, Vineis JH, Yanoviak SP, Scarpassa VM, Póvoa MM, Padilla N, Achee NL, Conn JE. Microsatellite data suggest significant population structure and differentiation within the malaria vector *Anopheles darlingi* in Central and South America. BMC Ecology 2008;8 3.

[92] Pedro PM, Uezu A, Sallum MAM. Concordant phylogeographies of 2 malaria vectors attest to common spatial and demographic histories. Journal of Heredity 2010;101(5) 618-627.

[93] Fairley TL, Póvoa MM, Conn JE. Evaluation of the Amazon River delta as a barrier to gene flow for the regional malaria vector, *Anopheles aquasalis* (Diptera: Culicidae) in northeastern Brazil. Journal of Medical Entomology 2002;39(6) 861-869.

[94] Templeton AR, Routman E, Phillips CA. Separating population structure from population history: a cladistics analysis of the geographical distribution of mitochondrial DNA haplotypes in the tiger salamander, *Ambystoma tigrinum*. Genetics 1995;140(2) 767-782.

[95] Mirabello LM, Conn JE. Population analysis using the nuclear *white* gene detects Pliocene/Pleistocene lineage divergence within *Anopheles nuneztovari* in South America. Medical and Veterinary Entomology 2008;22 109-119.

[96] de Fátima Rossetti D, Mann de Toledo P, Góes AM. New geological framework for Western Amazonia (Brazil) and implications for biogeography and evolution. Quaternary Research 2005; 63 78-89.

[97] Scarpassa VM, Conn JE. Mitochondrial DNA detects a complex evolutionary history with Pleistocene epoch divergence for the neotropical malaria vector *Anopheles nuneztovari* s.l. American Journal of Tropical Medicine and Hygiene 2011;85(5) 857-867.

[98] Fritz GN, Conn J, Cockburn AF, Seawright JA. Sequence analysis of the ribosomal DNA internal transcribed spacer 2 from populations of *Anopheles nuneztovari* (Diptera: Culicidae). Molecular Biology and Evolution 1994; 11 406-416.

Chapter 6

Speciation in *Anopheles gambiae* — The Distribution of Genetic Polymorphism and Patterns of Reproductive Isolation Among Natural Populations

Gregory C. Lanzaro and Yoosook Lee

Additional information is available at the end of the chapter

http://dx.doi.org/10.5772/56232

1. Introduction

The African malaria vector, *Anopheles gambiae,* is characterized by multiple polymorphic chromosomal inversions and has become widely studied as a system for exploring models of ecological speciation. An attempt to develop a molecular diagnostic for the chromosomal forms of *A. gambiae* s.s. led to the development of a PCR-based diagnostic to differentiate M and S molecular forms based on a marker located on the X chromosome. Near complete reproductive isolation between M and S molecular forms has led to the suggestion that *A. gambiae* is in early stages of speciation. Comparative genomic studies have been applied to gain an understanding of the evolutionary process resulting in these forms, but models based on these studies currently lack consensus. Furthermore, various studies suggest further subdivisions within each molecular form. These topics are discussed and suggestions for further research needed to elucidate the population structure of *A. gambiae* are presented.

2. *Anopheles gambiae* species complex

Among the global vectors of human malaria arguably the most important species belong to the *Anopheles gambiae* complex, which include the most widespread and potent vectors of malaria in sub-Saharan Africa. The *Anopheles gambiae* species complex includes eight sibling species: *A. gambiae* s.s. Giles, *A. arabiensis* Patton, *A. bwambae* White, *A. melas* Theobald, *A. merus* Dönitz, *A. quadriannulatus* Theobald, *A. amharicus* Hunt, Coetzee and Fettene and *A. comorensis* Brunhes, le Goff and Geoffroy [1-4]. The status of these species was established via the demonstration of F_1 hybrid sterility among crosses between populations [4-8], morphological features [9] and fixed differences in chromosomal inversions [5, 10]. Although the species cannot be reliably distinguished morphologically they do differ in terms of their ecology and geographic distributions (Figure 1). Two species, *A. merus* and *A. melas,* are associated with saltwater larval habitats and so are restricted in distribution to brackish water breeding sites along the east and west coasts respectively. A third saltwater species, *A. bwambae,* is only known to occur in association with hot springs in Semliki Forest National Park in eastern Uganda. The species, *A. quadriannulatus* and *A. amharicus* are primarily zoophilic and are not considered to be involved in the transmission of malaria. *A. quadriannulatus* occurs in southeastern Africa and *A. amharicus* in Ethiopia [2, 4]. A population on the island of Grande Comore in the Indian Ocean was described as a distinct species, *A. comorensis,* on the basis of morphological characters [9]. Little is known about the biology of *A. comorensis*. The two remaining freshwater species, *A. gambiae sensu stricto* (hereafter referred to as *A. gambiae)* and *A. arabiensis,* have the broadest geographic distribution and are the most important vectors of human malaria (Figure 1) [11, 12]. *A. gambiae* has been the most studied with respect to molecular and population genetics, and its whole genome sequence was published in 2002 [13].

Natural populations of *A. gambiae* have an extremely complex genetic structure that has been the subject of a great deal of research, a summary of which will be the focus of this chapter. Populations of *A. gambiae* are thought to be undergoing speciation and have been the focus of numerous studies aimed at evaluating speciation models [14-16]. Discrete subpopulations of *A. gambiae* have been defined in two ways: *chromosomal form* and *molecular form*. Recently the M molecular form of *A. gambiae* was elevated to species status and designated *Anopheles coluzzii* Coetzee *et al.* [4]. We retain the designation M and S forms to facilitate discussion of the recent literature.

3. Chromosomal forms of *Anopheles gambiae*

Chromosomal forms. The *A. gambiae* genome is organized on three chromosomes: two submetacentric autosomes and X/Y sex chromosomes, with males being the heterogametic sex. For descriptive purposes the autosomes are divided into two "arms" at the centromere. The longer arm is referred to as the right arm and the shorter the left arm. A high degree of chromosomal polymorphism, in the form of paracentric inversions, has been described in populations of *A. gambiae.* In a recent study Pombi *et al.* [18] describe 82 rare and 7 common inversions observed in natural populations. Inversions are not randomly distributed among chromosomes, but occur most often on the right arm of chromosome 2 (2R). Cytogenetic analysis is facilitated by the presence of giant polytene chromosomes in the cells of certain tissues. In early studies, the salivary glands of larvae were the source of material, but more recently ovarian nurse cells are used (the latter are easier to obtain and make better preparations for microscopic examination). Polytene chromosomes contain light and dark banding patterns that serve as critical landmarks for the determination of karyotypes (Figure 2). Protocols for the preparation of polytene chromosomes for karyotyping are available on-line at [19].

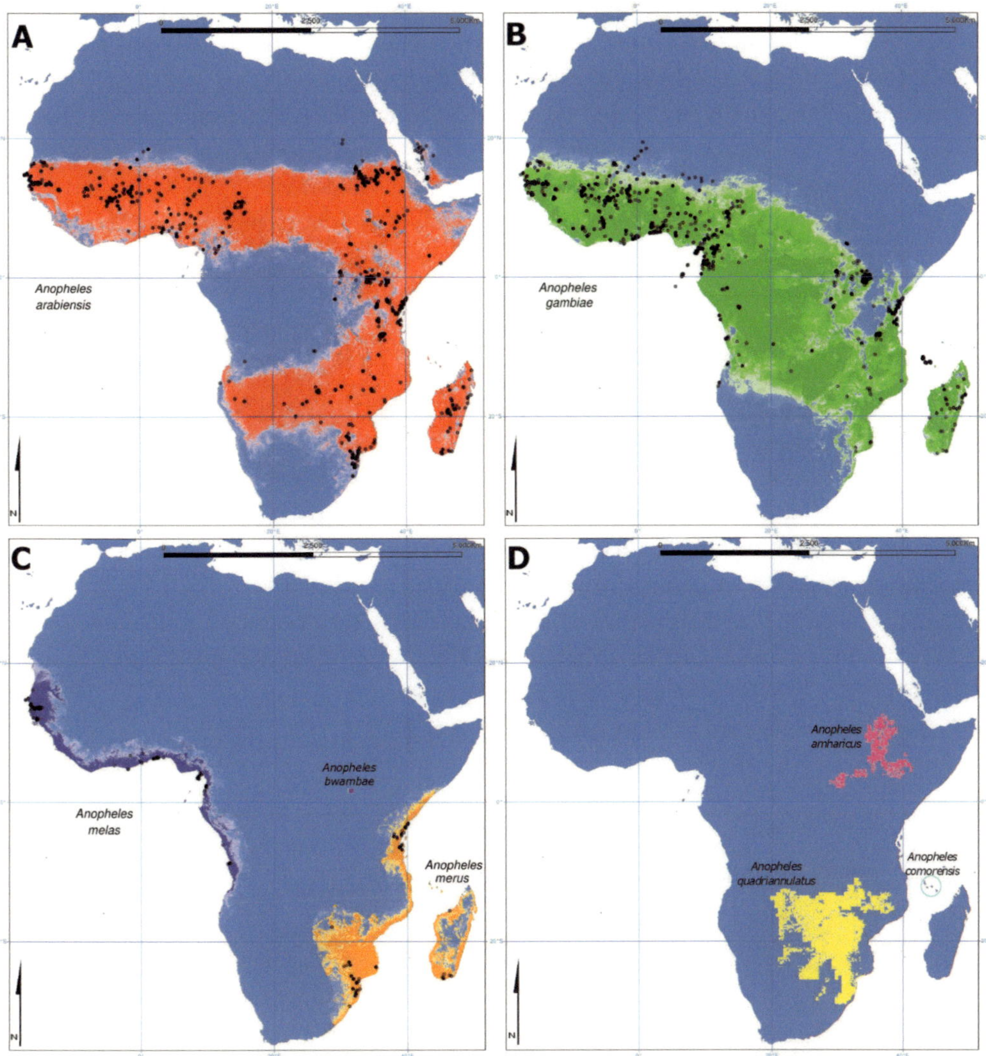

Figure 1. Geographic distribution of members of the *A. gambiae* complex. A: *A. arabiensis* (red); B: *A. gambiae s.s.* (green); C: *A. melas* (Blue), *A. merus* (orange), and *A. bwambae* (cyan); D: *A. quadriannulatus* (former species A) (yellow), *A. amharicus* (former *A. quadriannulatus* B) (magenta) and *A. comorensis* (cyan circle). Data and maps adapted from [17] and [14].

There is general agreement that inversions represent coadapted gene complexes that may enable individuals carrying them to occupy different ecological niches. The nonrandom distribution of inversion breakpoints along the chromosomes [18] and the distribution of inversion frequencies throughout the geographical ranges of the species strongly suggest that at least some of the inversions are maintained by selection that allows different species and, in the case of *A. gambiae*, populations, to survive and exploit a wide variety of habitats [21-23]. The best example is the strong association of inversions 2La and 2Rb with aridity, with the frequency of these inversions being highest in drier areas and even increasing in frequency during the dry season at single sites that experience distinct wet and dry seasons [21, 23, 24]. Specific inversion configurations are associated with specific habitats, leading to the term "ecophenotype" frequently applied to describe individuals carrying certain combinations of inversions [25]. Chromosomal forms have been defined based on the configuration of five paracentric chromosome inversions on the right arm of chromosome 2 (2Rj, b, c, d and u) and one on the left arm of chromosome 2 (2La). Based on this, five chromosomal forms of *A. gambiae* have been described and named *Mopti, Bamako, Bissau, Forest* and *Savanna* according to the geographic regions from which they were first collected and indicating an association of each with a particular type of habitat, as illustrated in Figure 3 [10]. Chromosomal forms are defined as follows: [1] the *Forest* form characterized by the typical non-inverted arrangement 2R+/+, 2L+/+, or by a single inversion polymorphism due to inversion 2Rb, 2Rd or 2La; [2] *Bissau* characterized by high frequencies of the 2Rd inversion and standard 2L+ arrangement; [3] *Savanna* exhibiting high frequencies of 2Rb and 2La inversions as well as polymorphism involving the 2Rcu arrangements and polymorphism in the j, d and the rare k inversion; [4] *Bamako* characterized by the fixed 2Rjcu arrangement and polymorphism in the 2Rb inversion; [5] *Mopti* showing high frequencies of 2Rbc, 2Ru and nearly fixed for 2La (Figure 2). The *Savanna* form has the broadest distribution occurring throughout sub-Saharan Africa, the *Mopti* form predominates in drier habitats in West Africa, the *Forest* form occurs in wetter habitats in Africa, the *Bamako* form occurs in habitats along the Niger River in West Africa and the *Bissau* form is restricted to West Africa (Figure 3) [26, 27].

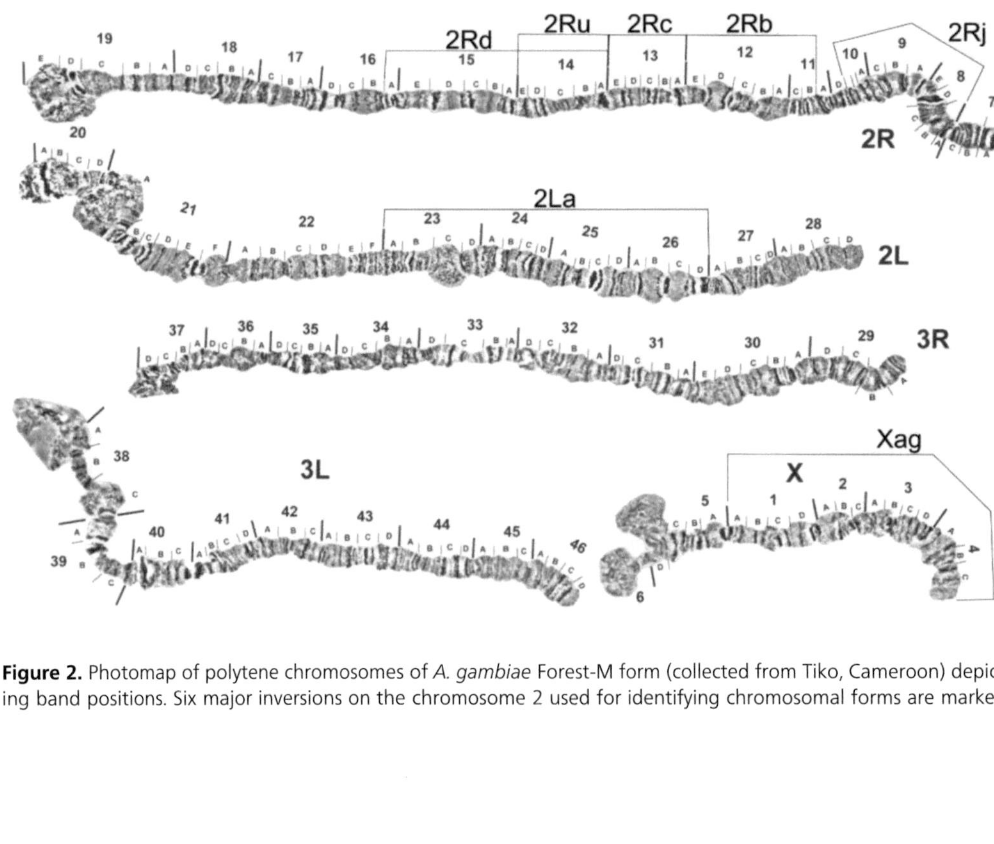

Figure 2. Photomap of polytene chromosomes of *A. gambiae* Forest-M form (collected from Tiko, Cameroon) depicting band positions. Six major inversions on the chromosome 2 used for identifying chromosomal forms are marked.

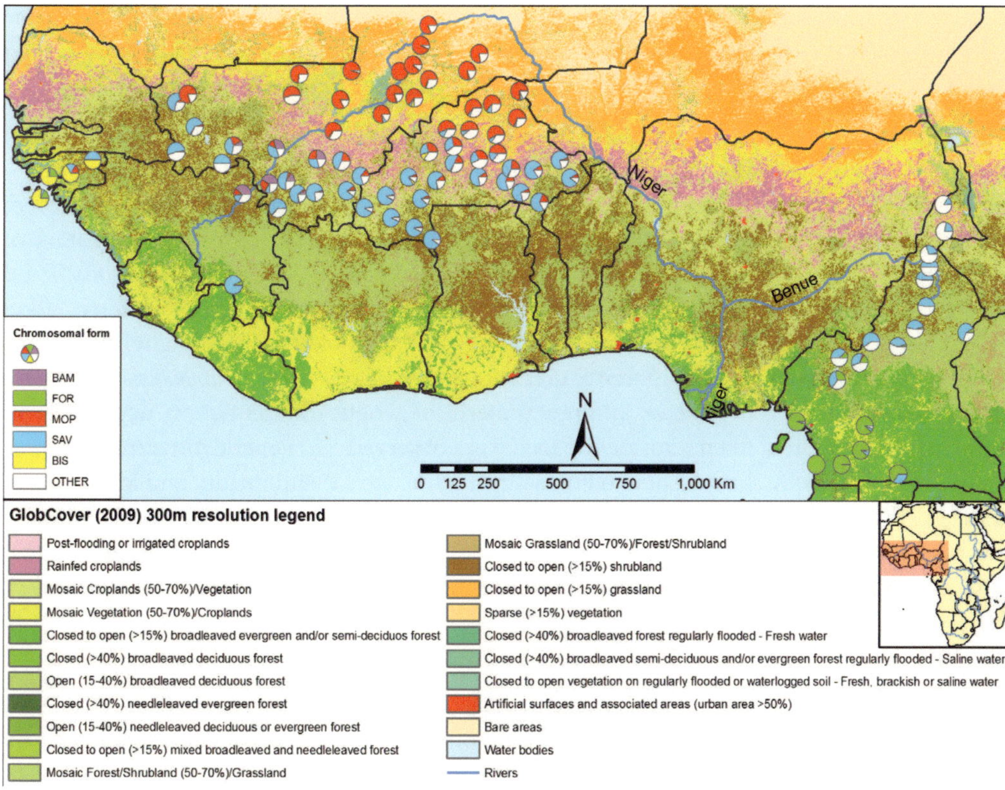

Figure 3. Distribution of chromosomal forms in West and Central Africa. Data from *PopI* [27]. BAM stands for *Bamako* chromosomal form, FOR for *Forest*, MOP for *Mopti*, SAV for *Savanna* and BIS for *Bissau*. OTHER refers to samples with karyotypes that do not fit any described chromosomal form designation.

The Xag inversions is fixed and used as a diagnostic marker to distinguish *A. gambiae* from other species in the complex. Chromosome photomap adapted from: [20]

It has furthermore been suggested that the chromosomal forms are to some extent reproductively isolated and represent distinct species or incipient species that have evolved or are evolving via a process described as "ecotypic speciation" [15, 25]. Studies of karyotype frequencies at sites where the *Bamako*, *Mopti* and *Savanna* forms occur in sympatry have revealed significant departures from the Hardy-Weinberg equilibrium (H-W) [10, 28-30]. Specifically, heterokaryotypes representing hybrids between the *Savanna* form and the other two were under-represented and *Bamako*/*Mopti* hybrids were never encountered. This observation led to the suggestion that there is partial reproductive isolation between *Savanna* and the other forms, nearly complete isolation between the *Bamako* and *Mopti* forms and that these forms represent incipient species. However, hybridization experiments involving crosses between the *Bamako* and *Mopti* forms resulted in viable offspring, demonstrating a lack of post-mating reproductive barriers between them [29, 31]. An estimate of genetic distance (based on allozyme frequencies) [32] between the *Bamako* and *Mopti* forms was reported as 0.015 [33], a value not higher than that typically found between local populations of a single mosquito species. We found that genotypic frequencies in a population composed of three chromosomal forms in Mali did not depart from Hardy-Weinberg expectations, suggesting that this population represents a single gene pool (Lanzaro, unpublished).

It should be emphasized that although these studies do not support reproductive isolation among chromosomal forms, they do not disprove it. Pre-mating isolating mechanisms may act as a barrier between subpopulations, even if post-mating mechanisms have not evolved, and isolation may be recent, so that not enough time has passed for the accumulation of substantial allozyme divergence between the forms. Lanzaro *et al.* [34] conducted a study based on 21 microsatellite loci distributed over the genome, examining genetic differentiation between the *Bamako* and *Mopti* forms in the villages of Banambani and Selinkenyi, Mali. This study revealed strong genetic differentiation between *A. gambiae* and *A. arabiensis,* used here as an outgroup. Within *A. gambiae,* different patterns of genetic differentiation, depending on the genomic location of the microsatellite loci, were observed. No genetic differentiation was found on the 3rd and X-chromosome whereas strong linkage disequilibrium and low levels of genetic differentiation were found for loci located on the 2nd chromosome in association with the inversions that occur there [34]. Similar results were obtained in a study also using microsatellites distributed on all three chromosomes for samples collected in the villages of Selinkenyi, Soulouba, and Kokouna, Mali [35].

Gene flow, like other forces, may be higher in some parts of the genome and lower in others. For example, favorable genes can still be exchanged successfully even when barriers to gene flow are strong. Such genes could be at loci that confer local adaptations and at any linked loci. The significance of this is that gene flow, even if estimated accurately, may still fail to account for variation among different parts of the genome. This effect may be particularly strong for genes contained within inversions, both because of potentially strong selection and because of linkage imposed by the reduced recombination associated with inversions. This effect was explored by Tripet et al. [36] in a study in which they examined divergence for microsatellite loci contained within the *j* and *b* inversions compared with loci outside of inversions. Indeed they did find elevated divergence estimated from loci contained within the inversions relative to those outside. This pattern of divergence, with a strongly non-random distribution over the genome, was later described as a 'mosaic genome architecture' in a paper by Wang-Sattler et al. [37]. As we shall see, this concept was later refined based on high resolution genome-wide analysis, ultimately leading to the recognition of 'islands of speciation' in the *A. gambiae* genome.

Using the chromosomal form concept to define genetically discrete populations is problematic because there is substantial overlap in inversions that define them, probably due to some level of contemporary gene flow. This creates ambiguities in assigning individuals to form, diminishing the utility of the chromosomal form concept for defining reproductive boundaries among populations. For example, in a recent survey of populations in Mali, we found that 26% of 2,459 individuals could not be assigned to a chromosomal form and in Cameroon 39% of 632 individuals could likewise not be assigned (Figure 3, data available at *PopI* [27]).

The role of chromosome inversions in A. gambiae evolution: Ecotypic Speciation. The chromosomal or ecotypic model of speciation was first described for anopheline mosquitoes by Coluzzi [38] and is the prevailing model applied to the chromosomal forms of *A. gambiae* [14, 15]. This model is founded on the observation that certain paracentric inversions that are polymorphic in *A. gambiae* are non-randomly distributed in nature. These are thought to contain multi-locus genotypes that are adaptive to specific aquatic habitats occupied by the immature stages of the mosquito. Under this model, populations carrying alternate gene arrangements would inhabit different, spatially isolated habitats. Genetic divergence, enhanced by reduced recombination associated with the inversions, would then evolve. Ultimately divergence would include genes resulting in reproductive isolation (reduced fitness in hybrids or behavioral differences preventing between form mating), explaining the observed deficiency of inversion heterozygotes. This model was initially adopted to describe the evolution of chromosomal forms of *A. gambiae* [15, 21, 28], but now has become the model for explaining the evolution of the molecular forms as described below [16, 39-42].

The most thorough evaluation of the ecotypic speciation model has been its application to the *Bamako* and *Savanna* forms in Mali [15]. Central to this evaluation is the observation of niche partitioning with respect to larval habitat. This observation was based on a PCR identification method developed for detecting the 2R*j* inversion [43] among larval samples collected in rock pools vs. more typical larval sites (puddles/ponds) in the village of Banambani, Mali. We evaluated this PCR method on a set of 85 field-collected adults previously scored for the 2R*j* genotype cytogenetically. In total, we selected 25 2R*j* homozygotes (*j*/*j*), 40 2R*j* heterozygotes ($+_j/j$) and 20 2R*j* standard ($+_j/+_j$) from the villages of Banambani, Selinkenyi, Tinko and Seroume, Mali. The 2R*j* PCR was accurate in calling 2R*j* homozygotes (*j*/*j*) (100%) in all villages regardless of the presence of the 2R*c* and *u* inversions (Table 1). However, the PCR was much less accurate for the standard arrangement for 2R*j* ($+_j/+_j$), resulting in consistent false identification as 2R*j* heterozygotes ($+_j/j$) in 11 cases and 2Rj (*j*/*j*) homozygotes in 5 cases. Moreover, all true heterozytoes ($+_j/j$) were misidentified as either *j*/*j* (N=13) or $+_j/+_j$ (N=7). The low accuracy rate (=48.2%) of the 2R*j* diagnostic PCR casts doubt on this sole example of niche partitioning (rock pool vs. other) in larval habitat distinguishing the two forms.

The 2R*j* inversion polymorphism in Mali shows two mating patterns in different parts of the species range in this country. At sites along the Senegal River (e.g. villages of Sebetou, Seroume, Bantinngoungou, and Tinko), 2R*j* inversion heterozygotes are commonly found and 2R*j* karyotypes are in Hardy-Weinberg expectation (HWE). On the other hand, at sites along the Niger River and its tributaries (e.g. villages of Banambani, Doneguebougou, Senou, Kela, Selinkenyi, Soulouba, Yorobougoula, Kokouna), a severe deficiency of 2R*j* heterozygotes are observed and 2R*j* genotypes are not in HWE (Figure 4).

In the literature the *Bamako* form includes three genotypes, *jcu*/*jcu*, *jcu*/*jbcu*, and *jbcu*/*jbcu*, all homozygous for *j* [21]. Other individuals carrying 2R*j* inversion but not *c* and *u* inversions such as *jbd*/*jbd*, and *jb*/*b*, commonly found along the Senegal River, cannot be classified under the current definitions for chromosomal forms. 94% of the 2R*j* homozygotes along the Niger River are *Bamako* forms, while no *Bamako* forms are found along the Senegal River.

Overall these results weaken the argument that paracentric inversions play a role in the evolution of reproductive isolation via divergent selection (ecotypic speciation), both because

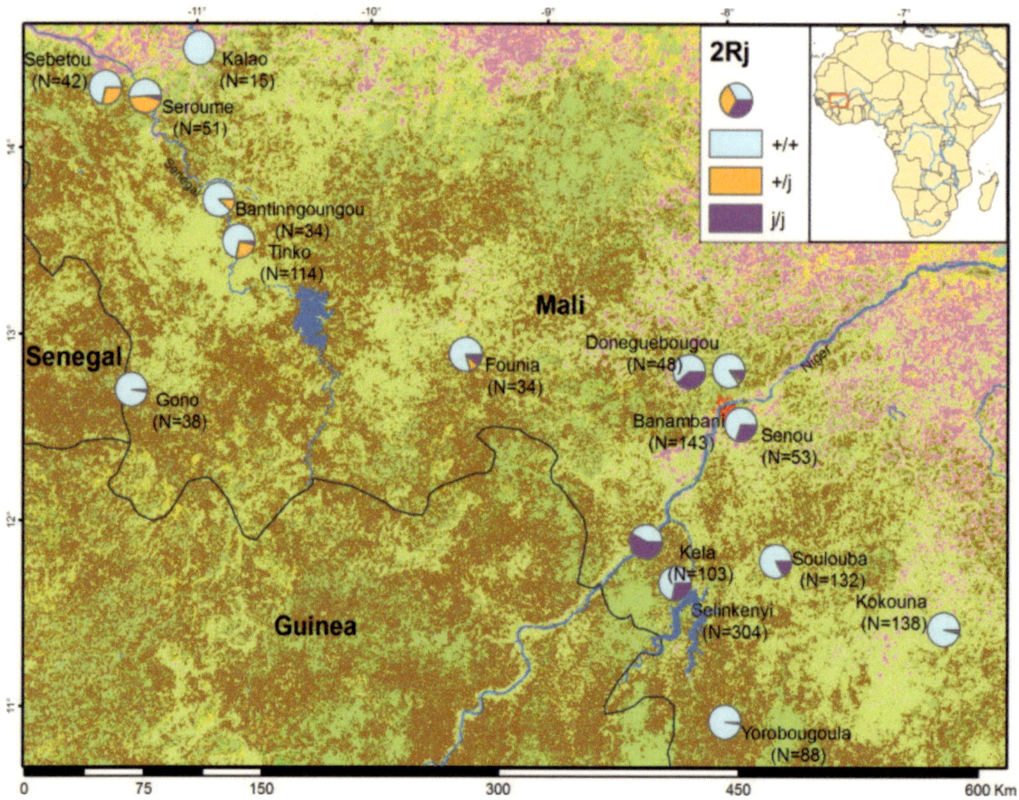

Figure 4. 2R*j* inversion distribution in Mali. For legend of the GlobCover 2009 land cover type used as background, see Figure 2.

		Run 1			Run 2		
2Rj	N	match	mismatch	NA*	match	mismatch	NA*
j/j	25	24	0	1	24	0	1
$+_j$/j	20	0	**20**	0	0	**19**	1
$+_j/+_j$	40	17	**14**	9	16	**16**	8

Table 1. Evaluation of 2R*j* genotyping via a PCR identification method. Samples were karyotyped microscopically prior to being assayed using the PCR protocol of Coulibaly *et al.* [43] * NA stands for 'no amplification'

they cast doubt on the association of inversions with distinct larval habitats and on evidence for reproductive isolation between individuals that differ with respect to the inversions they carry (e.g. a lack of *j* inversion heterozygotes). Genome-wide comparisons of individuals with and without inversions have been conducted and these cast doubt on the role of inversions as forming "coadapted gene complexes". These results are described in detail below.

The role of chromosome inversions in A. gambiae evolution: Comparative Genomics. Central to the "ecotypic speciation" model as applied to *A. gambiae* is the notion that inversions contain multi-locus genotypes that are adaptive to different environments. These "coadapted gene complexes" arise and are maintained as the consequence of reduced recombination within and around the inversion. Ultimately these become, either directly or indirectly, associated with reproductive isolation. One expectation arising from this phenomenon, assuming that reproductive isolation is incomplete or has evolved recently, is higher levels of genetic divergence in regions of the genome contained within the inversion relative to elsewhere in the genome. Indeed, in a genome-wide scan comparing individuals with and without the 2L*a* inversion, significantly higher divergence was observed in a 3 Mb region of the genome within and proximal to the inversion [44]. However, in a subsequent study that included a comparison of inverted and uninverted genomes for the four common 2R inversions (*j*, *b*, *c* and *u*), a region of the genome spanning ~26 Mb, divergence was limited to just one small region (~100 kb) in the 2R*u* inversion [45]. In both studies the Affymetrix *Plasmodium/Anopheles* Genome Microarray (*P/A* array), which contains 142,065 25bp probes, representing roughly 13,000 predicted genes, was used. Lack of divergence associated with the inversions hypothesized to be driving the "ecotypic speciation" process was unexpected. Several explanations were provided including that divergence between the inversion arrangements escaped detection due to shared ancestral polymorphism, extensive recombination within the inversions (gene flux) and limits to the resolution of the microarray they used [45].

In a more recent study [46] the genomes of individuals homozygous for the *jbcu* arrangement (*Bamako* form) were compared with individuals homozygous for the standard arrangement, $+_j+_b+_c+_u$ (*Savanna* form). In this case all individuals were of the S molecular form (unlike the comparisons made in the White et al. [45] study, which were a mixture of M and S form individuals). In addition, Lee et al. [46] utilized an *A. gambiae* whole genome tiling microarray (WGTM) which provides a far higher resolution of the genome than the *P/A* array (probe density = 1 probe per 100,000bp for the *P/A* array; 1 probe per 17bp for the WGTM). As in the White et al. [45] study, this new study revealed very little divergence associated with the chromosome 2R inversions. However, a 3Mb region of the genome on the X chromosome, proximal to the centromere was observed. This is the same region of the genome that contains the sequence divergence used to define the M and S molecular forms (discussed in detail in the following sections). X chromosome divergence is associated with reproductive isolation observed between both the M and S molecular forms and between the *Bamako* and *Savanna* chromosomal forms. These results suggest that the 2R inversions may not be involved in either the evolution or maintenance of reproductive isolation among *A. gambiae* populations.

4. Molecular forms of *Anopheles gambiae*

Defining Molecular Forms. An attempt to develop a molecular diagnostic for the chromosomal forms of *A. gambiae* identified 10 nucleotide residues that differ between the *Mopti* and the *Savanna* or *Bamako* chromosomal forms in a 2.3 kb fragment at the 5′ end of the rDNA IGS region located on the X chromosome [47]. These findings led to the development of a PCR-based diagnostic to differentiate *Mopti* chromosomal forms from *Bamako* and *Savanna* forms based on a single base pair substitution at the 540th nucleotide position in a 28S rDNA amplimer sequence. *Mopti* form individuals carry a C/C genotype and both *Bamako* and *Savanna* individuals a T/T genotype (Genbank accession number AF470112-6) [48]. Individuals carrying C/C are referred to as M molecular form and those carrying the T/T genotype are known as S molecular form. There is good correspondence between the M molecular form and the *Mopti* chromosomal form in Burkina Faso and Mali, however, the *Bamako* and *Savanna* chromosomal forms cannot be distinguished (both are of the S molecular form). The association of M and S molecular forms and chromosomal forms breaks down at other locations in West Africa. For example, in western Senegal and Gambia the association between the *Savanna* chromosomal form and S molecular form does not hold [49] and the *Forest* form contains both M and S individuals. The M and S molecular forms, therefore, largely fail as a diagnostic for chromosomal form. However, the significance of the M and S forms of *A. gambiae* goes well beyond their utility as proxies for identifying chromosomal forms. The molecular form concept has now largely replaced chromosomal form for defining discrete sub-populations of *A. gambiae*, that are to some extent reproductively isolated.

M and S forms occur in sympatry at many sites in West and Central Africa, and typically there is a high degree of reproductive isolation between the two forms. M/S hybrids (C/T genotype) produced in the laboratory did yield clearly distinguishable hybrid patterns in females. Surprisingly, however, field collected individuals carrying "hybrid" karyotypes (putative hybrids between different chromosomal forms) did not produce results consistent with their being hybrid, but rather produced either M or S patterns [48]. This observation supports the notion that certain karyotypes, thought to be fixed in one chromosomal form or another, are in fact shared, occurring commonly in one form and rarely in another, due to ancestral polymorphism and/or ongoing gene flow [40, 50]. This diagnostic now forms the basis of recognizing two distinct subpopulations of *A. gambiae*, known as *molecular forms* (M and S).

Alternate methods for distinguishing M and S forms. The original PCR-based diagnostic used to distinguish the M and S forms [48] was further developed into a method using a restriction digestion of PCR amplimers that allowed distinguishing *A. gambiae* from one of its sibling species *A. arabiensis* while simultaneously distinguishing M from S [51]. This was useful in the field since *A. arabiensis* and both the M and S forms are morphologically indistinguishable and commonly occur in sympatry at study sites throughout West and Central Africa. In 2008, a new method for distinguishing the M and S forms was discovered which takes advantage of polymorphism in insertion sites for a group of retrotransposons known as short interspersed elements (SINEs). One of the SINE insertion sites, located on the X chromosome and referred to as SINE X6.1, was found to be fixed in the M form and absent in the S form. In subsequent studies, in which multiple M/S diagnostic methods were employed, some discrepancies in results were observed [52]. These were most common in populations where M/S hybridization is common, for example in Guinea-Bissau.

Relationships between the M and S forms. Understanding the relationship between the two molecular forms has been the focus of an intense and ongoing research effort. The S form has the broadest distribution occurring throughout sub-Saharan Africa, whereas the M form occurs throughout West and parts of Central Africa. With the exception of a single site in northern Zimbabwe [53], M is absent from eastern Africa (Figure 5) [49].

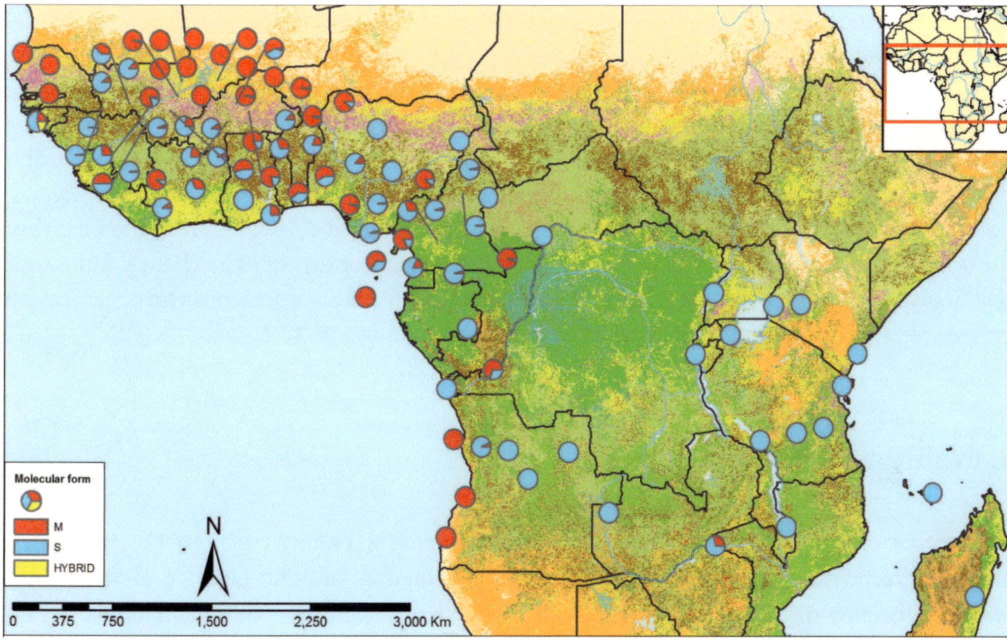

Figure 5. Distribution of molecular forms in Sub-Saharan Africa. For legend of the GlobCover 2009 land cover type used as background, see Figure 2. Data from [27, 40, 49, 50, 54]

Although the M and S forms are largely reproductively isolated in most places where they occur together, this is not true everywhere. Hybridization between forms occurs rarely (~1%) in Mali [55] and reproductive isolation between M and S appears to be complete in Cameroon [56]. In The Gambia, M/S hybrids were identified from a number of sites at frequencies as high as 16.7% of the *A. gambiae* individuals sampled [57] and in Guinea-Bissau hybrids were recovered in over 20% of the individuals assayed [58, 59]. A cryptic subgroup of *A. gambiae* known as the "Goundry" population collected in Burkina Faso was recently found to be composed of 36% M/S hybrids [60]. The Goundry population discovered in the Sudan Savanna zone of Burkina Faso in larval collections but absent in indoor adult collection of the same locality, suggesting that adult stage of Goundry populations mostly rest outdoors [60, 61]. These results suggest that linkage between the M and S alleles and those genes that directly affect reproductive isolation has broken down in a much broader geographic area than previously suggested. Therefore, the notion of an M form and an S form that are largely reproductively isolated (incipient species) and that hybridization only occurs in the "Far-West" region of Africa [62] is an oversimplification.

In the laboratory, chromosomal and molecular forms, including the *Bamako* and *Savanna* forms, appear to display no post-zygotic isolation [31, 63, 64]. Analysis of sperm recovered from inseminated females [55] and the composition of mating swarms [65] support the existence of strong, but not complete, pre-mating reproductive isolation between the M and S molecular forms in nature.

The two molecular forms display phenotypic divergence in different locations within their geographic range [66]. Most notable among these phenotypic differences include differential insecticide resistance [67], desiccation resistance [68], larval habitat segregation [69], and wing morphological differentiation [70]. It has been proposed that the mechanism responsible for promoting divergence is pre-zygotic [63] and associated with mate selection either during swarm formation [71, 72] or within a swarm [65]. Diabate et al. found evidence of clustering of swarms composed of individuals of a single molecular form within the village of Donéguébougou, Mali [71]. Mixed swarms of M and S forms were found elsewhere (Burkina Faso) but the occurrence of mixed swarms was lower than the frequency expected by chance. Manoukis *et al.* analyzed the shape of male swarms and suggested that a difference in swarm organization between M and S forms may enhance the behavioral isolation of the two forms [72].

5. Evolution of the M and S forms

Comparative genomics. Early studies aimed at describing patterns of genetic divergence among chromosomal forms revealed what was termed a "mosaic genome architecture", with divergence distributed non-randomly over the genome (as described above, [29]). Comparisons of the M and S forms revealed a similar pattern. Initial work examined the distribution of microsatellite DNA polymorphism showing exceptionally high divergence in a region of the genome proximal to the centromere on the X chromosome, near the rDNA locus used to define the two forms [35, 73]. High levels of M/S form divergence on the X chromosome was substantiated through detailed examination of the centromeric region using DNA sequencing [74, 75].

The first high density genome-wide comparison of M and S was conducted by Turner et al. [76] using samples collected in Cameroon. They utilized an Affymetrix *Plasmodium/Anopheles* Genome Microarray which contains 142,065 25bp probes representing roughly 13,000 predicted genes. Divergence between the M and S genomes was very low and restricted to three discrete regions, one on the X chromosome (corresponding with the location identified in the microsatellite studies) and two on chromosome 2, one on 2L and one very small (37kb) region on 2R. In total, these diverged regions cover less than 2.8Mb, roughly 1% of the genome. In a subsequent study, utilizing the same microarray, but with samples collected in Mali, the small 2R region of divergence was not observed, and so this small region was considered not to contribute to reproductive isolation between the two forms [77]. Later a third diverged region was observed on the left arm of chromosome 3L and this region, like the X and chromosome 2L regions, was proximal to the centromere [16]. Taken together these studies revealed that the M and S genomes are diverged over only about 3% of their genomes and that this divergence is organized into 3 small regions located near the centromere on the X, 2L and 3L chromosomes, with the remainder of their genomes essentially undifferentiated. These regions of divergence have been considered to represent *islands of speciation* because it is thought that they contain genes that are directly involved in reproductive isolation.

Islands of speciation model. The widely held interpretation of this work is that *A. gambiae* forms represent incipient species, but with enough gene flow to prevent their genomes from diverging in all but a few, relatively small regions [34, 35, 37, 76, 77]. This interpretation is consistent with recent genic models of speciation that predict the existence of small regions of divergence between incipient species in the presence of some degree of gene flow (Figure 6) [78, 79]. The observation that putative "*islands of speciation*" in *A. gambiae* are located proximal to centromeres, where levels of recombination are known to be low, is likewise consistent with models that consider speciation to be driven by genes located in regions of the genome with reduced crossing-over [80, 81].

Incidental islands model. White et al. [16] developed PCR-RFLP assays to detect SNPs that occurred in each of the three islands of speciation and that were diagnostic for the M and S forms. They genotyped a total of 517 individuals including both M and S forms from Mali, Burkina Faso, Cameroon and Kenya. They found complete association among the three unlinked islands in 512 of the 517 individuals genotyped (275 M form and 237 S). Of the five exceptional genotypes, three were heterozygous at all three loci, suggesting these represented F_1 hybrids. To account for the nearly complete linkage between the three diverged islands they suggest that gene flow between M and S must be nearly zero. The presence of F_1 hybrids suggests that they have such low fitness that they contribute little to gene flow between the forms. As mentioned above F_1 hybrids generated in the laboratory show no evidence of intrinsically low fitness, so it is assumed that these are maladapted to conditions in nature. Additional support for very low levels of between form gene flow come from comparisons of M and S based on high-density, genome-wide SNP genotyping [41] and whole genome sequences [42] which revealed widespread divergence between the M and S genomes. Collectively these studies propose an alternative model referred to as the "incidental islands" model [82, 83], which states that reproductive isolation between M and S is complete and that the observed islands of divergence may be incidental, meaning that the divergence observed in areas proximal to centromeres do not necessarily represent the location of genes underlying reproductive isolation but the divergence is due to segregating ancestral variation and not due to contemporary gene flow.

In summary, two opposing models exist that describe the relationship between the M and S forms. The "genomic islands of speciation" model suggests that divergence between the M and S genomes is restricted to small regions (~3% of the genome) that may contain the genes responsible for reproductive isolation between forms and that ongoing gene flow is responsible for very low levels of divergence over the remaining 97% of the genome. The second model, the "incidental islands of divergence" model, suggests that divergence between the two forms is far more extensive and widely distributed over the genome, that gene flow between the two forms is nearly zero and that the M and S forms therefore represent distinct species (Figure 6D).

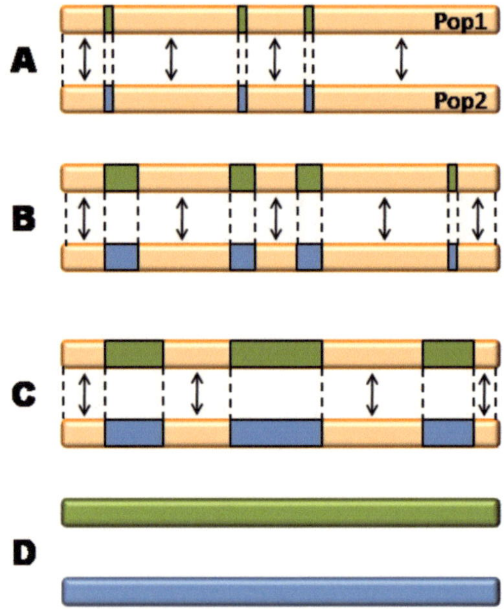

Figure 6. A: Stage 1 - Population/races with differential adaptation; reproductive isolation (RI) not apparent. Green box represents diverged loci specific to Population 1 (Pop1) and Blue represents diverged loci specific to Pop2. Arrows indicate regions of gene flow. B: Stage 2 - Transition between races and species with some degree of RI; population may fuse or diverge. C: Stage 3 - Divergent populations beyond the point of fusion but still share a portion of their genome via gene flow; good species. D: Stage 4 - Species with complete RI. Adapted from [79].

6. Further sub-divisions within molecular forms

Although most discussions consider M and S as the major and biologically relevant subdivisions of *A. gambiae* there is evidence that the two can be further subdivided into population groups that are significantly diverged.

Subdivision within the S form. In a continent-wide survey Lehmann et al. [73] found that S form populations fall into two well defined clades, based on analysis of microsatellite DNA. They refer to these clades as the Northwest (Nigeria, Gabon, Democratic Republic of Congo, NW Kenya) and Southeast (SW Kenya, Tanzania, Malawi) divisions. Wang-Sattler et al. [37] also conducted an analysis based on microsatellite DNA and likewise report that the S form in eastern Africa (Kenya) are distinct from S form populations in the west (Mali). In addition to the East vs. West division between allopatric S form populations is the division of sympatric S form populations in Mali. These are described in detail above (Section 2). In brief, the S form in Mali is divided into the *Bamako* and *Savanna* chromosomal forms which display strong asssortative mating where they occur in sympatry at sites along the Niger River ([21], also see Figure 4). These two populations can be distinguished by the *j* inversion, which is fixed in the *Bamako* form and absent in the *Savanna*. Interestingly, although the two share the X-linked allele that defines them as S molecular form, a detailed analysis revealed that they are strongly diverged at a 3Mb region of the X chromosome, proximal to the centromere [46].

Subdivision within the M form. A comparison of the M form in Mali and the M form in Cameroon has revealed that the two are very different genetically, in fact, divergence between these two is higher than the level of divergence between the M and S forms [23]. This observation has led to a recognition of two, distinct M form groups, the Mopti-M form, which is polymorphic with respect to the 2R *b*, *c*, and u chromosome inversions and the Forest-M form which lacks inversions on chromosome 2L and 2R [23, 84]. In addition to genetic divergence the Forest-M and Mopti-M forms differ in their ecology. The Mopti-M in Mali is most common in the dry northern part of the country whereas Forest-M is absent in the dry northern part of Cameroon and is restricted to the wet southern part of the country [23]. This observation lends support the notion that chromosome inversions are involved in adaptation to arid environments.

The Goundry form. Genetic analysis of *A. gambiae* larvae from roadside pools in Burkina Faso and adults collected from inside nearby houses revealed the occurrence of a genetically distinct population present in the larval sample, but absent from adult collections [60]. The larval population differed from the adult population with respect to the distribution of microsatellite alleles (F_{ST}=0.15), the presence of M/S hybrids (35% in the larval population, <1% in adults) and in the frequency of the 2L*a* inversion (2L*a* = 58% in larval population, 96% in adults). This distinct larval population is called the Goundry form, after one of the village collection sites. Based on these results it is supposed that the Goundry form is a unique form in which the adults rest nearly exclusively outdoors (exophilic) and which, although they carry the X-linked genetic markers that distinguish the M and S forms, the assortative mating associated with these markers is absent. Adults of the Goundry form have never been collected. Adults reared from larvae of the Goundry form were found to have increased susceptibility to infection with *P. falciparum* in laboratory experiments. [60]

7. Future directions

Reconciliation of the opposing speciation models and clarification of new "forms" await the resolution of a number of outstanding questions concerning interactions between the M and S forms. It is clear that the determination of the frequency of hybrid individuals requires that individuals be identified using multi-locus genotypes at unlinked loci, such as those employed by White et al. [16], as opposed to the widely used single locus X-linked markers. This would allow not only the recognition of F_1 hybrids but backcross individuals as well. Determination of the frequencies of both F_1 and backcross genotypes would provide information on the level of introgression. Moreover, multi-locus approach will allow identification of hybrid males. The application of this method to populations throughout the sympatric range of M and S would allow a description of spatial heterogeneity in levels of introgression that could be related to key environmental parameters that include mating cues that sustain assortative mating within forms as well as conditions that favor the survival of hybrid genotypes.

Author details

Gregory C. Lanzaro* and Yoosook Lee

*Address all correspondence to: gclanzaro@ucdavis.edu

Department of Pathology, Microbiology and Immunology School of Veterinary Medicine University of California Davis, CA, USA

References

[1] White GB. *Anopheles bwambae* sp.n, a Malaria Vector in the Semliki Valley, Uganda, and Its Relationships with Other Sibling Species of the *An. gambiae* Complex (Diptera, Culicidae). Syst Entomol. 1985;10(4):501-22.

[2] Hunt RH, Coetzee M, Fettene M. The *Anopheles gambiae* complex: a new species from Ethiopia. Trans R Soc Trop Med Hyg. 1998 Mar-Apr;92(2):231-5. PubMed PMID: 9764342. Epub 1998/10/09. eng.

[3] Harbach R. Mosquito Taxonomic Inventory http://mosquito-taxonomic-inventory.info/2012 [cited 2013]. Available from: http://mosquito-taxonomic-inventory.info/sites/mosquito-taxonomic-inventory.info/files/Anopheles%20classification_25.pdf.

[4] Coetzee M, Hunt RH, Wilkerson R, della Torre A, Coulibaly MB, Besansky N. *Anopheles coluzzii* and *Anopheles amharicus*, new members of the *Anopheles gambiae* complex. Zootaxa. 2013;3619(2):246-74.

[5] Davidson G, Hunt RH. The crossing and chromosome characteristics of a new, sixth species in the *Anopheles gambiae* complex. Parassitologia. 1973 Apr-Aug;15(1):121-8. PubMed PMID: 4788353. Epub 1973/04/01. eng.

[6] Davidson G. Insecticide resistance in *Anopheles gambiae* Giles: a case of simple mendelian inheritance. Nature. 1956 Oct 20;178(4538):863-4. PubMed PMID: 13369563. Epub 1956/10/20. eng.

[7] Davidson G. The Five Mating-Types in the *Anopheles gambiae* Complex. Riv Malariol. 1964 Dec;43:167-83. PubMed PMID: 14318975. Epub 1964/12/01. eng.

[8] Davidson G. *Anopheles gambiae,* a Complex of Species. Bull World Health Organ. 1964;31:625-34. PubMed PMID: 14278001. Pubmed Central PMCID: PMC2555133. Epub 1964/01/01. eng.

[9] Brunhes J, LeGoff G, Geoffroy B. Afrotropical *Anopheles*.1. Description of new species and modifications of taxonomical status (Diptera:Culicidae). Ann Soc Entomol Fr. 1997 Jun;33(2):173-83. PubMed PMID: WOS:A1997XM01900005. French.

[10] Coluzzi M, Sabatini A, Petrarca V, Di Deco MA. Chromosomal differentiation and adaptation to human environments in the *Anopheles gambiae* complex. Trans R Soc Trop Med Hyg. 1979;73(5):483-97. PubMed PMID: 394408. Epub 1979/01/01. eng.

[11] Gillies M, De Meillon B. The Anophelinae of Africa south of Sahara. Johannesburg: The South African Institute for Medical Research, 1968 Contract No.: 54.

[12] Coetzee M, Craig M, le Sueur D. Distribution of African malaria mosquitoes belonging to the *Anopheles gambiae* complex. Parasitol Today. 2000 Feb;16(2):74-7. PubMed PMID: 10652493. Epub 2000/02/01. eng.

[13] Holt RA, Subramanian GM, Halpern A, Sutton GG, Charlab R, Nusskern DR, et al. The genome sequence of the malaria mosquito *Anopheles gambiae*. Science. 2002 Oct 4;298(5591):129-49. PubMed PMID: 12364791. Epub 2002/10/05. eng.

[14] Ayala FJ, Coluzzi M. Chromosome speciation: humans, Drosophila, and mosquitoes. Proc Natl Acad Sci U S A. 2005 May 3;102 Suppl 1:6535-42. PubMed PMID: 15851677. Pubmed Central PMCID: PMC1131864. Epub 2005/04/27. eng.

[15] Manoukis NC, Powell JR, Toure MB, Sacko A, Edillo FE, Coulibaly MB, et al. A test of the chromosomal theory of ecotypic speciation in *Anopheles gambiae*. Proc Natl Acad Sci U S A. 2008 Feb 26;105(8):2940-5. PubMed PMID: 18287019. Pubmed Central PMCID: PMC2268564. Epub 2008/02/22. eng.

[16] White BJ, Cheng C, Simard F, Costantini C, Besansky NJ. Genetic association of physically unlinked islands of genomic divergence in incipient species of *Anopheles gambiae*. Mol Ecol. 2010 Mar;19(5):925-39. PubMed PMID: 20149091. Epub 2010/02/13. eng.

[17] Sinka ME, Bangs MJ, Manguin S, Coetzee M, Mbogo CM, Hemingway J, et al. The dominant *Anopheles* vectors of human malaria in Africa, Europe and the Middle East: occurrence data, distribution maps and bionomic precis. Parasit Vectors. 2010;3:117. PubMed PMID: 21129198. Pubmed Central PMCID: PMC3016360. Epub 2010/12/07. eng.

[18] Pombi M, Caputo B, Simard F, Di Deco MA, Coluzzi M, della Torre A, et al. Chromosomal plasticity and evolutionary potential in the malaria vector *Anopheles gambiae* sensu stricto: insights from three decades of rare paracentric inversions. BMC Evol Biol. 2008;8:309. PubMed PMID: 19000304. Pubmed Central PMCID: PMC2654565. Epub 2008/11/13. eng.

[19] Cornel A. *A. gambiae* s.l. Ovarian Polytene Chromosome Preparation. 2010. In: Methods in *Anopheles* Research [Internet]. CDC/ATCC/NIH/NIAID. 2nd. [242-7]. Available from: http://www.mr4.org/Portals/3/MR4_Publications/Anopheles%20Protocol%20Manual%20Second%20Ed%20v2011/2011%20Complete%20Manual%20PDF%20TOC.pdf.

[20] Dorn P, Noireau F, Krafsur ES, Lanzaro GC, Cornel AJ. Genetics of major insect vectors. In: Tibayrenc M, editor. Genetics and evolution of infectious diseases. Boston: Elsevier; 2011. p. 411-72.

[21] Touré YT, Petrarca V, Traoré SF, Coulibaly A, Maiga HM, Sankare O, et al. The distribution and inversion polymorphism of chromosomally recognized taxa of the *Anopheles gambiae* complex in Mali, West Africa. Parassitologia. 1998 Dec;40(4):477-511. PubMed PMID: 10645562. Epub 2000/01/25. eng.

[22] Coluzzi M, Sabatini A, della Torre A, Di Deco MA, Petrarca V. A polytene chromosome analysis of the *Anopheles gambiae* species complex. Science. 2002 Nov 15;298(5597):1415-8. PubMed PMID: 12364623. Epub 2002/10/05. eng.

[23] Lee Y, Cornel AJ, Meneses CR, Fofana A, Andrianarivo AG, McAbee RD, et al. Ecological and genetic relationships of the Forest-M form among chromosomal and molecular forms of the malaria vector *Anopheles gambiae* sensu stricto. Malar J. 2009;8:75. PubMed PMID: 19383163. Pubmed Central PMCID: PMC2680901. Epub 2009/04/23. eng.

[24] Cheng C, White BJ, Kamdem C, Mockaitis K, Costantini C, Hahn MW, et al. Ecological genomics of *Anopheles gambiae* along a latitudinal cline: a population-resequencing approach. Genetics. 2012 Apr;190(4):1417-32. PubMed PMID: 22209907. Pubmed Central PMCID: PMC3316653. Epub 2012/01/03. eng.

[25] Coluzzi M, Sabatini A, Petrarca V, Di Deco MA. Behavioural divergences between mosquitoes with different inversion karyotypes in polymorphic populations of the *Anopheles gambiae* complex. Nature. 1977 Apr 28;266(5605):832-3. PubMed PMID: 865604. Epub 1977/04/28. eng.

[26] della Torre A, Costantini C, Besansky NJ, Caccone A, Petrarca V, Powell JR, et al. Speciation within *Anopheles gambiae*--the glass is half full. Science. 2002 Oct 4;298(5591):115-7. PubMed PMID: 12364784. Epub 2002/10/05. eng.

[27] Lee Y, Collier TC, Manoukis NC, Lozano-Fuentes S, Vallejo EE, Yan W, et al. An Individual-level Population Genomics Database for Arthropod Disease Vectors (PopI). Davis, CA2004 [updated 2012; cited 2012]. Available from: https://grassi2.ucdavis.edu/.

[28] Bryan JH, Di Deco MA, Petrarca V, Coluzzi M. Inversion polymorphism and incipient speciation in *Anopheles gambiae* s.str. in The Gambia, West Africa. Genetica. 1982;59:167-76.

[29] Coluzzi M, Petrarca V, Di Deco MA. Chromosomal inversion intergradation and incipient speciation in *Anopheles gambiae*. Bollettino di Zoologia. 1985;52(1-2):45-63.

[30] Taylor C, Touré YT, Carnahan J, Norris DE, Dolo G, Traoré SF, Edillo FE, Lanzaro GC. Gene flow among populations of the malaria vector, *Anopheles gambiae*, in Mali, West Africa. Genetics. 2001;157(2):743-50.

[31] Persiani A, Di Deco MA, Petrangeli G. [Laboratory observation of inversion polymorphisms originating from the crossing of various populations of *Anopheles gambiae* s.s]. Ann Ist Super Sanita. 1986;22(1):221-3. PubMed PMID: 3752798. Epub 1986/01/01. Osservazioni di laboratorio su polimorfismi da inversione originati da incrocitra popolazioni diverse di *Anopheles gambiae* s.s. ita.

[32] Nei M. Genetic Distance between Populations. Am Nat. 1972;106(949):283-&. PubMed PMID: WOS:A1972M475000002. English.

[33] Cianchi R, Villani F, Touré YT, Petrarca V, Bullini L. Electrophoretic study of different chromosomal forms of *Anopheles gambiae* s.s. Parassitologia. 1983;25:239-41.

[34] Lanzaro GC, Toure YT, Carnahan J, Zheng L, Dolo G, Traore S, et al. Complexities in the genetic structure of *Anopheles gambiae* populations in west Africa as revealed by microsatellite DNA analysis. Proc Natl Acad Sci U S A. 1998 Nov 24;95(24):14260-5. PubMed PMID: 9826688. Pubmed Central PMCID: PMC24361. Epub 1998/11/25. eng.

[35] Wang R, Zheng L, Toure YT, Dandekar T, Kafatos FC. When genetic distance matters: measuring genetic differentiation at microsatellite loci in whole-genome scans of recent and incipient mosquito species. Proc Natl Acad Sci U S A. 2001 Sep 11;98(19): 10769-74. PubMed PMID: 11553812. Pubmed Central PMCID: PMC58550. Epub 2001/09/13. eng.

[36] Tripet F, Dolo G, Lanzaro GC. Multilevel analyses of genetic differentiation in *Anopheles gambiae* s.s. reveal patterns of gene flow important for malaria-fighting mosquito projects. Genetics. 2005 Jan;169(1):313-24. PubMed PMID: 15677750. Pubmed Central PMCID: PMC1448890. Epub 2005/01/29. eng.

[37] Wang-Sattler R, Blandin S, Ning Y, Blass C, Dolo G, Touré YT, della Torre A, Lanzaro GC, Steinmetz LM, Kafatos FC, Zheng L. Mosaic genome architecture of the *Anopheles gambiae* species complex. PLoS One. 2007 2007 Nov 28;2(11):e1249.

[38] Coluzzi M. Spatial distribution of chromosomal inversions and speciation in Anopheline mosquitoes. Prog Clin Biol Res. 1982;96:143-53. PubMed PMID: 7178155. Epub 1982/01/01. eng.

[39] Nosil P, Funk DJ, Ortiz-Barrientos D. Divergent selection and heterogeneous genomic divergence. Mol Ecol. 2009 Feb;18(3):375-402. PubMed PMID: 19143936. Epub 2009/01/16. eng.

[40] Simard F, Ayala D, Kamdem GC, Pombi M, Etouna J, Ose K, et al. Ecological niche partitioning between *Anopheles gambiae* molecular forms in Cameroon: the ecological side of speciation. BMC Ecol. 2009;9:17. PubMed PMID: 19460146. Pubmed Central PMCID: PMC2698860. Epub 2009/05/23. eng.

[41] Neafsey DE, Lawniczak MK, Park DJ, Redmond SN, Coulibaly MB, Traore SF, et al. SNP genotyping defines complex gene-flow boundaries among African malaria vec-

tor mosquitoes. Science. 2010 Oct 22;330(6003):514-7. PubMed PMID: 20966254. Epub 2010/10/23. eng.

[42] Lawniczak MK, Emrich SJ, Holloway AK, Regier AP, Olson M, White B, et al. Widespread divergence between incipient *Anopheles gambiae* species revealed by whole genome sequences. Science. 2010 Oct 22;330(6003):512-4. PubMed PMID: 20966253. Epub 2010/10/23. eng.

[43] Coulibaly MB, Pombi M, Caputo B, Nwakanma D, Jawara M, Konate L, et al. PCR-based karyotyping of *Anopheles gambiae* inversion 2Rj identifies the BAMAKO chromosomal form. Malar J. 2007;6:133. PubMed PMID: 17908310. Pubmed Central PMCID: PMC2134931. Epub 2007/10/03. eng.

[44] White BJ, Santolamazza F, Kamau L, Pombi M, Grushko O, Mouline K, et al. Molecular karyotyping of the 2La inversion in *Anopheles gambiae*. Am J Trop Med Hyg. 2007 Feb;76(2):334-9. PubMed PMID: 17297045. Epub 2007/02/14. eng.

[45] White BJ, Cheng C, Sangare D, Lobo NF, Collins FH, Besansky NJ. The population genomics of trans-specific inversion polymorphisms in *Anopheles gambiae*. Genetics. 2009 Sep;183(1):275-88. PubMed PMID: 19581444. Pubmed Central PMCID: PMC2746151. Epub 2009/07/08. eng.

[46] Lee Y, Collier TC, Sanford MR, Marsden CD, Fofana A, Cornel AJ, et al. Chromosome Inversions, Genomic Differentiation and Speciation in the African Malaria Mosquito *Anopheles gambiae*. PLoS One. 2013.

[47] Favia G, Lanfrancotti A, Spanos L, Siden-Kiamos I, Louis C. Molecular characterization of ribosomal DNA polymorphisms discriminating among chromosomal forms of *Anopheles gambiae* s.s. Insect Mol Biol. 2001 Feb;10(1):19-23. PubMed PMID: 11240633. Epub 2001/03/10. eng.

[48] Favia G, della Torre A, Bagayoko M, Lanfrancotti A, Sagnon N, Toure YT, et al. Molecular identification of sympatric chromosomal forms of *Anopheles gambiae* and further evidence of their reproductive isolation. Insect Mol Biol. 1997 Nov;6(4):377-83. PubMed PMID: 9359579. Epub 1997/11/14. eng.

[49] della Torre A, Tu Z, Petrarca V. On the distribution and genetic differentiation of *Anopheles gambiae* s.s. molecular forms. Insect Biochem Mol Biol. 2005 Jul;35(7): 755-69. PubMed PMID: 15894192. Epub 2005/05/17. eng.

[50] Costantini C, Ayala D, Guelbeogo WM, Pombi M, Some CY, Bassole IH, et al. Living at the edge: biogeographic patterns of habitat segregation conform to speciation by niche expansion in *Anopheles gambiae*. BMC Ecol. 2009;9:16. PubMed PMID: 19460144. Pubmed Central PMCID: PMC2702294. Epub 2009/05/23. eng.

[51] Fanello C, Santolamazza F, della Torre A. Simultaneous identification of species and molecular forms of the *Anopheles gambiae* complex by PCR-RFLP. Med Vet Entomol. 2002 Dec;16(4):461-4. PubMed PMID: 12510902. Epub 2003/01/04. eng.

[52] Santolamazza F, Caputo B, Calzetta M, Vicente JL, Mancini E, Petrarca V, et al. Comparative analyses reveal discrepancies among results of commonly used methods for *Anopheles gambiae* molecular form identification. Malar J. 2011;10:215. PubMed PMID: 21810255. Pubmed Central PMCID: PMC3170251. Epub 2011/08/04. eng.

[53] Masendu HT, Hunt RH, Govere J, Brooke BD, Awolola TS, Coetzee M. The sympatric occurrence of two molecular forms of the malaria vector *Anopheles gambiae* Giles sensu stricto in Kanyemba, in the Zambezi Valley, Zimbabwe. Trans R Soc Trop Med Hyg. 2004 Jul;98(7):393-6. PubMed PMID: 15138074. Epub 2004/05/13. eng.

[54] della Torre A, Fanello C, Akogbeto M, Dossou-yovo J, Favia G, Petrarca V, et al. Molecular evidence of incipient speciation within *Anopheles gambiae* s.s. in West Africa. Insect Mol Biol. 2001 Feb;10(1):9-18. PubMed PMID: 11240632. Epub 2001/03/10. eng.

[55] Tripet F, Toure YT, Taylor CE, Norris DE, Dolo G, Lanzaro GC. DNA analysis of transferred sperm reveals significant levels of gene flow between molecular forms of *Anopheles gambiae*. Mol Ecol. 2001 Jul;10(7):1725-32. PubMed PMID: 11472539. Epub 2001/07/27. eng.

[56] Wondji C, Frederic S, Petrarca V, Etang J, Santolamazza F, Della Torre A, et al. Species and populations of the *Anopheles gambiae* complex in Cameroon with special emphasis on chromosomal and molecular forms of Anopheles gambiae s.s. J Med Entomol. 2005 Nov;42(6):998-1005. PubMed PMID: 16465741. Epub 2006/02/10. eng.

[57] Caputo B, Nwakanma D, Jawara M, Adiamoh M, Dia I, Konate L, et al. *Anopheles gambiae* complex along The Gambia river, with particular reference to the molecular forms of *An. gambiae* s.s. Malar J. 2008;7:182. PubMed PMID: 18803885. Pubmed Central PMCID: PMC2569043. Epub 2008/09/23. eng.

[58] Oliveira E, Salgueiro P, Palsson K, Vicente JL, Arez AP, Jaenson TG, et al. High levels of hybridization between molecular forms of *Anopheles gambiae* from Guinea Bissau. J Med Entomol. 2008 Nov;45(6):1057-63. PubMed PMID: 19058629. Epub 2008/12/09. eng.

[59] Marsden CD, Lee Y, Nieman CC, Sanford MR, Dinis J, Martins C, et al. Asymmetric introgression between the M and S forms of the malaria vector, *Anopheles gambiae*, maintains divergence despite extensive hybridization. Mol Ecol. 2011 Dec;20(23): 4983-94. PubMed PMID: 22059383. Pubmed Central PMCID: PMC3222736. Epub 2011/11/09. eng.

[60] Riehle MM, Guelbeogo WM, Gneme A, Eiglmeier K, Holm I, Bischoff E, et al. A cryptic subgroup of *Anopheles gambiae* is highly susceptible to human malaria parasites. Science. 2011 Feb 4;331(6017):596-8. PubMed PMID: 21292978. Pubmed Central PMCID: PMC3065189. Epub 2011/02/05. eng.

[61] Crawford JE, Bischoff E, Garnier T, Gneme A, Eiglmeier K, Holm I, et al. Evidence for Population-Specific Positive Selection on Immune Genes of *Anopheles gambiae*. G3

(Bethesda). 2012 Dec;2(12):1505-19. PubMed PMID: 23275874. Pubmed Central PMCID: PMC3516473. Epub 2013/01/01. eng.

[62] Caputo B, Santolamazza F, Vicente JL, Nwakanma DC, Jawara M, Palsson K, et al. The "far-west" of *Anopheles gambiae* molecular forms. PLoS One. 2011;6(2):e16415. PubMed PMID: 21347223. Pubmed Central PMCID: PMC3039643. Epub 2011/02/25. eng.

[63] Diabate A, Dabire RK, Millogo N, Lehmann T. Evaluating the effect of postmating isolation between molecular forms of *Anopheles gambiae* (Diptera: Culicidae). J Med Entomol. 2007 Jan;44(1):60-4. PubMed PMID: 17294921. Epub 2007/02/14. eng.

[64] Di Deco MA, Petrarca V, Villani F, Coluzzi M. Polimorfismo cromosomico d inversioni paracentriche ed eccesso degli eterocariotipi in ceppi di *Anopheles allevati* in laboratorio. Parassitologia. 1980;22:304-7.

[65] Diabate A, Dabire RK, Kengne P, Brengues C, Baldet T, Ouari A, et al. Mixed swarms of the molecular M and S forms of *Anopheles gambiae* (Diptera: Culicidae) in sympatric area from Burkina Faso. J Med Entomol. 2006 May;43(3):480-3. PubMed PMID: 16739404. Epub 2006/06/03. eng.

[66] Lehmann T, Diabate A. The molecular forms of *Anopheles gambiae*: a phenotypic perspective. Infect Genet Evol. 2008 Sep;8(5):737-46. PubMed PMID: 18640289. Pubmed Central PMCID: PMC2731232. Epub 2008/07/22. eng.

[67] Tripet F, Wright J, Cornel A, Fofana A, McAbee R, Meneses C, et al. Longitudinal survey of knockdown resistance to pyrethroid (kdr) in Mali, West Africa, and evidence of its emergence in the Bamako form of *Anopheles gambiae* s.s. Am J Trop Med Hyg. 2007 Jan;76(1):81-7. PubMed PMID: 17255234. Epub 2007/01/27. eng.

[68] Lee Y, Meneses CR, Fofana A, Lanzaro GC. Desiccation resistance among subpopulations of *Anopheles gambiae* s.s. from Selinkenyi, Mali. J Med Entomol. 2009 Mar;46(2): 316-20. PubMed PMID: 19351082. Epub 2009/04/09. eng.

[69] Gimonneau G, Pombi M, Choisy M, Morand S, Dabire RK, Simard F. Larval habitat segregation between the molecular forms of the mosquito *Anopheles gambiae* in a rice field area of Burkina Faso, West Africa. Med Vet Entomol. 2012 Mar;26(1):9-17. PubMed PMID: 21501199. Pubmed Central PMCID: PMC3140611. Epub 2011/04/20. eng.

[70] Sanford MR, Demirci B, Marsden CD, Lee Y, Cornel AJ, Lanzaro GC. Morphological differentiation may mediate mate-choice between incipient species of *Anopheles gambiae* s.s. PLoS One. 2011;6(11):e27920. PubMed PMID: 22132169. Pubmed Central PMCID: PMC3221689. Epub 2011/12/02. eng.

[71] Diabate A, Dao A, Yaro AS, Adamou A, Gonzalez R, Manoukis NC, et al. Spatial swarm segregation and reproductive isolation between the molecular forms of

Anopheles gambiae. Proc Biol Sci. 2009 Dec 7;276(1676):4215-22. PubMed PMID: 19734189. Pubmed Central PMCID: PMC2821344. Epub 2009/09/08. eng.

[72] Manoukis NC, Diabate A, Abdoulaye A, Diallo M, Dao A, Yaro AS, et al. Structure and dynamics of male swarms of *Anopheles gambiae*. J Med Entomol. 2009 Mar;46(2): 227-35. PubMed PMID: 19351073. Pubmed Central PMCID: PMC2680012. Epub 2009/04/09. eng.

[73] Lehmann T, Licht M, Elissa N, Maega BT, Chimumbwa JM, Watsenga FT, et al. Population structure of *Anopheles gambiae* in Africa. J Hered. 2003 Mar-Apr;94(2):133-47. PubMed PMID: 12721225. Epub 2003/05/02. eng.

[74] Slotman MA, Reimer LJ, Thiemann T, Dolo G, Fondjo E, Lanzaro GC. Reduced recombination rate and genetic differentiation between the M and S forms of *Anopheles gambiae* s.s. Genetics. 2006 Dec;174(4):2081-93. PubMed PMID: 17057242. Pubmed Central PMCID: PMC1698612. Epub 2006/10/24. eng.

[75] Stump AD, Fitzpatrick MC, Lobo NF, Traore S, Sagnon N, Costantini C, et al. Centromere-proximal differentiation and speciation in *Anopheles gambiae*. Proc Natl Acad Sci U S A. 2005 Nov 1;102(44):15930-5. PubMed PMID: 16247019. Pubmed Central PMCID: PMC1276105. Epub 2005/10/26. eng.

[76] Turner TL, Hahn MW, Nuzhdin SV. Genomic islands of speciation in *Anopheles gambiae*. PLoS Biol. 2005 Sep;3(9):e285. PubMed PMID: 16076241. Pubmed Central PMCID: PMC1182689. Epub 2005/08/04. eng.

[77] Turner TL, Hahn MW. Locus- and population-specific selection and differentiation between incipient species of *Anopheles gambiae*. Mol Biol Evol. 2007 Sep;24(9):2132-8. PubMed PMID: 17636041. Epub 2007/07/20. eng.

[78] Wu CI. The genic view of the process of speciation. J Evol Biol. 2001;14:851-65.

[79] Wu CI, Ting CT. Genes and speciation. Nat Rev Genet. 2004 Feb;5(2):114-22. PubMed PMID: 14735122. Epub 2004/01/22. eng.

[80] Noor MA, Grams KL, Bertucci LA, Reiland J. Chromosomal inversions and the reproductive isolation of species. Proc Natl Acad Sci U S A. 2001 Oct 9;98(21):12084-8. PubMed PMID: 11593019. Pubmed Central PMCID: PMC59771. Epub 2001/10/11. eng.

[81] Rieseberg LH. Chromosomal rearrangements and speciation. Trends Ecol Evol. 2001 Jul 1;16(7):351-8. PubMed PMID: 11403867. Epub 2001/06/14. Eng.

[82] Turner TL, Hahn MW. Genomic islands of speciation or genomic islands and speciation? Mol Ecol. 2010 Mar;19(5):848-50. PubMed PMID: 20456221. Epub 2010/05/12. eng.

[83] Hahn MW, White BJ, Muir CD, Besansky NJ. No evidence for biased co-transmission of speciation islands in *Anopheles gambiae*. Philos Trans R Soc Lond B Biol Sci. 2012

Feb 5;367(1587):374-84. PubMed PMID: 22201167. Pubmed Central PMCID: PMC3233708. Epub 2011/12/28. eng.

[84] Slotman MA, Tripet F, Cornel AJ, Meneses CR, Lee Y, Reimer LJ, Thiemann TC, Fondjo E, Fofana A, Traoré SF, Lanzaro GC. Evidence for subdivision within the M molecular form of *Anopheles gambiae*. Mol Ecol. 2007;16(3):639-49.

Chapter 7

Advances and Perspectives in the Study of the Malaria Mosquito *Anopheles funestus*

Ibrahima Dia, Moussa Wamdaogo Guelbeogo and Diego Ayala

Additional information is available at the end of the chapter

http://dx.doi.org/10.5772/55389

1. Taxonomy, biology and distribution of the species within the Funestus Group

1.1. Introduction

Anopheles funestus Giles, 1900 is considered one of the most proficient malaria vectors worldwide [1]. It thrives in a wide range of habitats through the Afrotropical Region. Largely neglected with regard to its counterpart *Anopheles gambiae, An. funestus* cannot be ignored in any comprehensive control program aiming at the eradication of malaria from the African continent. Its transmission role goes beyond that of secondary vector, surpassing *An. gambiae* in many parts of Africa [2]. One of the main reasons of this inattention is the difficulty of adapting this species to standard insectary conditions, despite noteworthy molecular and epidemiological advances over the past three decades. Currently, substantial evidence shows that a group of species belongs to the taxon "*An. funestus*", with different morphological, behavioural and epidemiological characteristics.

1.2. The Funestus Group

The term "Funestus Group" was first coined in its strictest sense by Gillies and De Meillon [3] to designate a group of species morphologically close to *An. funestus*. Seventy years after the first description of *An. funestus sensu stricto* (hereafter *An. funestus*) by Giles in 1900, Mick Gillies and Botha De Meillon developed a new classification based on larva, pupa and adult stages. In fact, first suspicions of the existence of heterogeneity within *An. funestus* populations came from the early 1930's [4, 5]. They stated, based on larval studies, the presence of '*varieties*', most of them were subsequently recognized as species within the group. These species showed minor or no morphological differences at adult stage. They were then classified under the Funestus Group and their recognition was based on the identification of eggs, larvae or pharyngeal armature [3]. However, in Southern and Eastern Africa, several populations of outdoors resting mosquitoes were distinguishable from *An. funestus* by small morphological characters at the adult stage, while the larva were indistinguishable. These taxonomical observations were later confirmed by cytogenetic studies as different species of *An. funestus* [6-8].

Given the laborious nature of morphological and cytogenetic techniques, several studies were undertaken for the research of simple and useful molecular identification tools [9-12]. These techniques have the advantage to be applicable to all developmental stages. On the basis of morphological [13, 14] and molecular studies [15, 16], the status and position of each species within the Funestus Group was revisited. It is now accepted that *An. funestus* belongs to a group composed of five subgroups of which 3 groups containing 13 species are present in the Afrotropical region (Table 1) [17].

		African species of the Funestus Group		
Subgroup	**Species**	**Geographical distribution**	**Host preference**	**Vector role**
Funestus	*An. funestus*	continental	anthropophilic	major
	An. funestus-like	local	unknown	unknown
	An. aruni	local	unknown	unknown
	An. confusus	regional	zoophilic	unknown
	An. parensis	regional	unknown	minor
	An. vaneedeni	local	unknown	unknown
	An. longipalpis type C	local	zoophilic	unknown
Minimus	*An. leesoni*	continental	zoophilic	minor
	An. longipalpis type A	local	zoophilic	unknown
Rivulorum	*An. rivulorum*	continental	zoophilic	minor
	An. rivulorum-like	local	unknown	unknown
	An. brucei	local	unknown	unknown
	An. fuscivenosus	local	unknown	unknown

Table 1. Summary of ecological characteristics of Funestus Group in Africa.

1.3. Geographical distribution

Among the species of the Funestus Group, *An. funestus*, *An. leesoni* and *An. rivulorum* exhibit the widest distribution. They are traditionally represented throughout the entire sub-Saharan Africa [1, 3]. Figure 1 presents the predicted distribution of these species [11, 12]. *Anopheles funestus* is found virtually all across the continent (Fig. 1A). Being predominantly a savannah mosquito [18], this malaria vector is present in many other areas, such as high altitude zones (900 m in Madagascar [19], 1400 m in Central Africa [20] and up to 2000 m in Kenya [21]) and forested areas of West and Central Africa [18, 22-25]. Moreover, it can inhabit extreme dry conditions in the Sahel, when suitable breeding place are available, such as human-made irrigation zones [26, 27]. On the other hand, *An. funestus* is scarce or completely absent along the coast [18]. *Anopheles funestus* disappeared from several parts of Africa after adverse climatic conditions (i.e recurrent droughts) and/or vector control programs [28]. Unfortunately, this mosquito gradually re-emerged once control measures stopped or suitable environmental conditions re-appeared [29-32], evidencing its extraordinary environmental plasticity and dispersion ability.

The other species of the group exhibit locally defined distribution (Fig. 1B, C). *Anopheles parensis, An. confusus* and *An. aruni* are localized in East Africa [33, 34]. In West and Central Africa, we find *An. rivulorum*-like and *An. brucei* [11, 12]. Finally, in Southern Africa, we find *An. vaneedeni, An. parensis* again, *An. fuscivenosus, An. funestus*-like and *An. longipalpis* types A (South Africa) and C (Zambia) [1, 35, 36]. Certainly, these records are based on sampling efforts, and we might expect changes in the number of species within the group as well in their distribution.

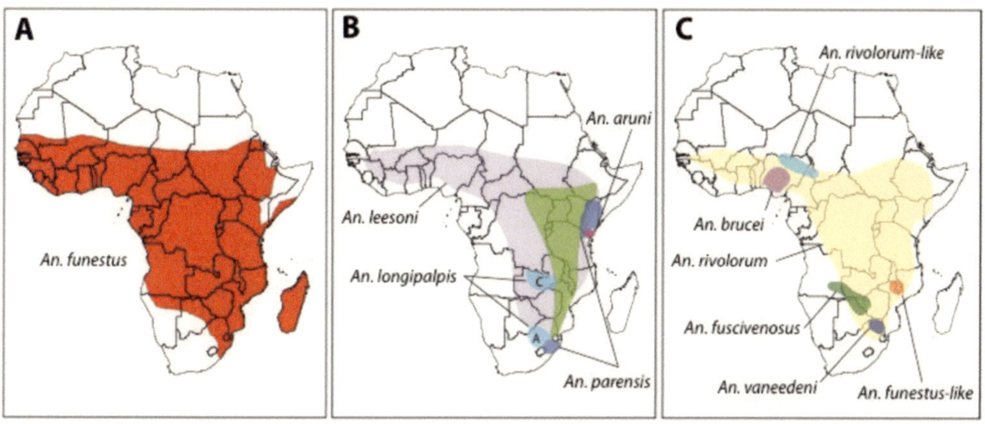

Figure 1. Distribution of the 13 species of the Funestus Group in Africa, A: *Anopheles funestus*, (modified from [37]); B: *An. leesoni*, *An. longipalpis* (type A and C), *An. aruni* and *An. parensis* (Courtesy of Dr. S. Manguin), C: *An. rivolorum, An. rivolorum-like, An. funestus-like, An. vaneedeni, An. fuscivenosus* and *An. brucei* (Courtesy of Dr. S. Manguin).

1.4. Breeding place

Anopheles funestus breeds in natural/artificial permanent and semi-permanent water bodies with floating or emerging vegetation. However, in areas with both vegetation types, this mosquito prefers the latter one [3]. Natural breeding occurs in edges of swamps, in weedy and grassy parts of rivers, streams, furrows, ditches and ponds. The presence of vegetation is crucial for mosquito breeding (Fig 2. A-C). Mainly because aquatic stages have a marked preference for shaded habitats and can barely survive in water bodies directly exposed to sunlight. Artificial breeding opportunities include rice fields, wells and domestic water-containers [3]. The main limiting factors to their development include salinity, extreme

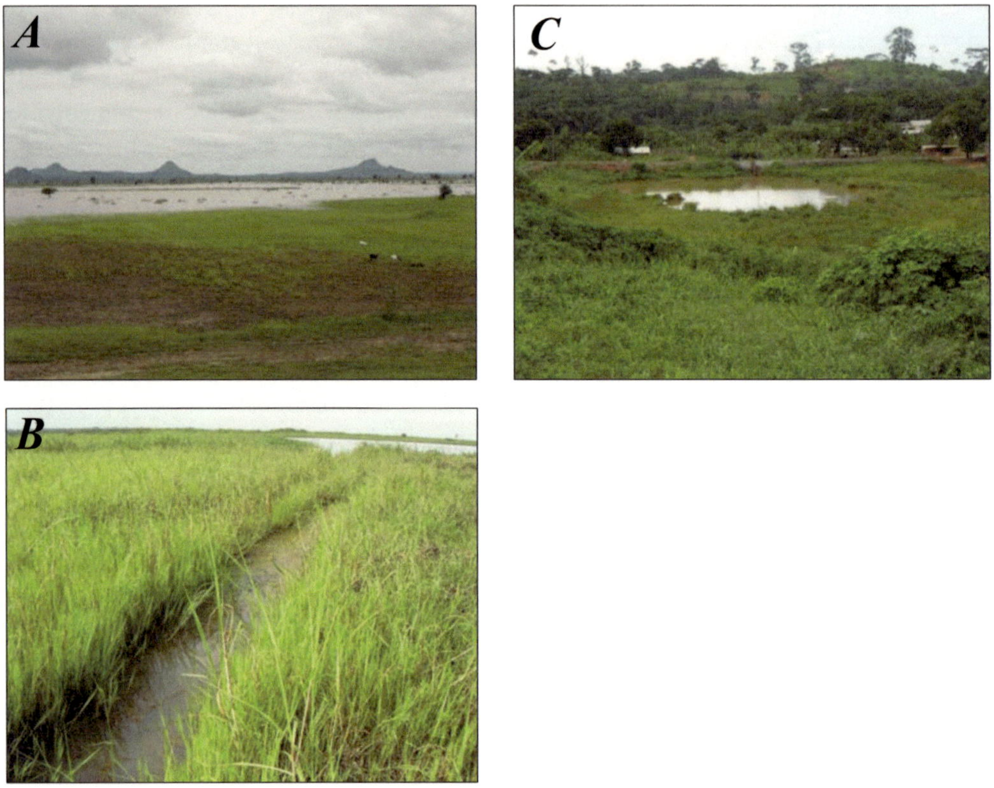

Figure 2. Breeding sites of *Anopheles funestus* (Photos D. Ayala, Cameroon). *A:* Pitoa (Cameroon) is situated in the northern dry savannah, close to a permanent human-made lake, which provides a year-round breeding site for *An. funestus*. *B:* Tibati (Cameroon) is located in the central highlands of the country. *Anopheles funestus* breeds year-round in the lake, which provides shaded areas thanks to the lake vegetation. *C:* Mfou (Cameroon) is situated in the southern rainforest, in the surroundings of Yaoundé. The artificial water-body provides an excellent breeding site for *An. funestus*, making it the major vector of the village.

temperatures and sometimes, heavy rains. For the other species within the Funestus Group, the biology of aquatic stages is poorly understood. The larva of *An. leesoni*, *An. rivulorum* and *An. vaneedeni* are often found in association with those of *An. funestus*. In Kenya, *An. rivulorum* replaced *An. funestus* in rice fields after indoor residual spraying [38]. The presence of vegetation appears to be essential too. These breeding sites are represented generally by slow-moving backwaters of grassy rivers and tide pools. In western Kenya, larva of *An. rivulorum* were recently found in hyacinth water protected by trees [39]. Similarly, *An. parensis* develops in permanent swamps and ponds between the reeds and the emergent vegetation. However, *An. parensis* is a species of stagnant water that has never been found in rivers. The larva were always collected in marshes, temporary and permanent ponds, among reeds and emerging vegetation [1, 3]. *Anopheles aruni* breeds in ponds, rice fields or ditches near human habitations. Larva of *An. brucei* were found in streams of forested river beds. *Anopheles confusus*, on the other hand, breeds in the vegetation of the edges of slow flowing rivers. *Anopheles longipalpis* prefers relatively calm water with abundant aquatic vegetation on the banks of fast-flowing rivers [3]. In many occasions, breeding places are very similar to *An. funestus*. Unfortunately, no information exists about breeding places for *An. fuscivenosus*, *An. rivulorum*-like and *An. funestus*-like [1, 3, 36, 40].

1.5. Resting behaviour and host feeding preference: Their impact on vector capacity

Despite the morphological similarities that exist between members of the group, these species show extreme behavioural differences that affect their vectorial capacities. To date, all malaria transmission studies have shown that *An. funestus* is the main malaria vector in the group, with infection rates up to 11% [41] and exceptionally 50% [42]. *Anopheles funestus* has late-night biting patterns, commonly between midnight and the early hours of the morning [22, 43, 44]. It is also the most endophilic and anthropophilic member of the Funestus Group [45-47]. In savanna areas where its breeding sites are rain-dependant, *An. funestus* follows in peak abundance its counterpart *An. gambiae*, therefore extending malaria transmission from the beginning to the first part of the dry season [48, 49]. Overall, *An. funestus* shows fairly consistent host feeding preferences (human) and resting behaviour (indoor) throughout its entire range. However, behavioural differences linked to chromosomal polymorphisms have been documented. For instance, Lochouarn *et al.* [50] reported a west-east gradient of human to animal biting preference, corresponding to chromosomal polymorphisms that also follow this cline. In Burkina Faso, different chromosomal inversion combinations (chromosomal forms, see below) were associated with different resting and biting activities [42]. These studies showed that carriers of inverted arrangements on the arm 2R and 3R feed predominantly on humans (anthropophilic) and rest inside dwellings, while the standard counterpart exhibit higher levels of zoophily and exophily (Guelbeogo, pers. Comm.). In Madagascar, the carriers of inverted arrangements 3Ra and 3Rb were less anthropophilic than carriers of standard arrangements [51]. In Senegal, the population of mosquitoes with inverted arrangements 3Ra and 3Rb was also more zoophilic. However, this heterogeneity in host preference might also be related to specific local conditions, such as host availability [52] or indoor microclimatic conditions (i.e. humidity).

The other species of the group are mainly zoophilic, but can occasionally feed on humans [3]. *Anopheles rivulorum* has been incriminated as a malaria vector in Tanzania [53]. Indeed, this species was found naturally infected by *Plasmodium falciparum*. However, this species is mainly zoophilic (77% animal hosts) and shows a lower longevity compared to *An. funestus*. Positive infected specimens of *An. rivulorum* were also observed in coastal Tanzania by Temu et al. [54]. This study also found positive specimens of *An. leesoni* and *An. parensis* to *P. falciparum*, suggesting a secondary role of these mosquitoes in malaria transmission. *Plasmodium falciparum* infected *An. parensis* specimens were also observed during an entomological study in South Africa using an Enzyme-Linked Immunosorbent Assay (ELISA) [55]. *Anopheles vaneedeni* feeds rarely on humans outdoors (1.22%). Although experimentally infected with *P. falciparum* in the laboratory, it has never been found involved in transmission in natural conditions [56]. *Anopheles longipalpis* has never been involved in malaria transmission [1, 3, 57]. In East Africa (Tanzania and Ethiopia), different authors have reported human feeding behaviour of *An. longipalpis* from indoor and outdoor collections [58-60]. Recently, Kent et al., [57] reported that even when found in large numbers resting indoors together with *An. funestus* in Zambia, *An. longipalpis* remains predominantly zoophilic.

2. Insecticide susceptibility and vector control

Because of its highly anthropophilic and endophilic behaviour, *An. funestus* has been an "easy" target in malaria control programs (i.e. insecticide treated materials or indoor residual spraying). *Anopheles funestus* has developed insecticide resistance in many parts of the African continent [61-64]. To date, *An. funestus* has been shown resistant to pyrethroids, carbamates and DDT. The first documented reports on insecticide resistance in this malaria mosquito (mainly to BHC, dieldrin, and malathion) were in West Africa (Mali, Ghana, Benin), Central Africa (Cameroon) and East Africa (Kenya), following vector control programs [65-68]. Recent studies have shown that dieldrin resistance is still high in *An. funestus* populations from Burkina Faso, despite the fact that this insecticide is no longer used in public health [47]. In agreement with Burkina Faso results, Wondji et al. [69] documented *An. funestus* resistant populations to dieldrin in Cameroon due to the remaining presence of Rdl^R target-site mutation. With regard to pyrethroids, resistant *An. funestus* populations were first detected in Southern Africa, being at the origin of the malaria outbreaks in the late 1990's [31, 62]. Pyrethroid resistant populations for this mosquito were also reported in Ghana, West Africa, combined with carbamate resistance [70]. Altogether, it is now clearly established that *An. funestus* populations in Africa show resistance to at least the 4 insecticide classes recommended for vector control by WHO.

During the last decade, efforts have been made in order to unravel the molecular mechanisms involved in insecticide resistance. The mechanisms discovered involve insecticide detoxification by one or multiple metabolic pathways mediated by glutathione S-transferases (GST), monooxygenases and/or esterases [61, 71-73]. No evidence for the presence of L1014F *kdr* mutation or G119S *Ace-1* mutation has been detected in *An. funestus* [63, 64, 71, 72]. However, a multiple insecticide resistance profile has been recently observed in Benin [74]. Insecticide resistance is an threat to effective malaria control. With the advent of malaria control program through the use of LLINs (Long Lasting Insecticidal Nets) and IRS (Indoor Residual Spraying), the presence of insecticide resistant populations should be carefully monitored. It would improve the implementation and management of current and future malaria vector control programs in Africa. In this context, a novel approach using the pyrrole insecticide chlorfenapyr against pyrethroid resistant *An. funestus* populations has led to valuable results [75]. An important challenge for the study of molecular mechanisms of insecticide resistance is the development and maintenance of laboratory colonies. To date, only two colonies are currently maintained at insectarium conditions, coming from southern Africa [76], although, some progress has been made and new strains have been established in Burkina Faso (Sagnon *et al.*, pers. comm.).

3. Molecular tools

3.1. Introduction

In 2002, the genome of *An. gambiae* s.s. was publicly released [77]. This event had a very large impact on the better understanding of the complexity of the malaria system. Furthermore, the publication of the *An. gambiae* genome brought with itself a rapid development of new genetic tools, from molecular markers (i.e. SNPs chips, microarrays, microsatellites, etc) to transgenic mosquitoes, for instance. To date, no other malaria mosquito genome has been released but progress has been made, and soon (2013), the release of several *Anopheles* genomes, including *An. funestus* [78], is expected.

Three inherent characteristics of *An. funestus*, have hampered the study of this mosquito at the molecular level. First, its "eternal" role as second important malaria vector. For decades, *An. funestus* has been neglected with regard to its well-studied congener *An. gambiae*. With virtually the same geographical distribution as *An. gambiae* across the African continent, *An. funestus* has been many times overruled because its mosaic-like presence (see previous section in this chapter). However, its major role in malaria transmission has been evidenced throughout the continent, surpassing in a number of locations *An. gambiae* and *An. arabiensis* [2] in many places. Second, the extreme difficulties to breed *An. funestus* in standard insectary conditions. To date, as mentioned earlier in this chapter, there exist only two colonies of *An. funestus* with published records: FANG and FUMOZ (and its pyrethroid resistance counterpart FUMOZ-R), originating from Angola and Mozambique, respectively [76, 79]. Both colonies have been recurrently used in insecticide resistance studies of *An. funestus* [74, 79, 80]. Indeed, it is one of these colonies (FUMOZ), which has been elected as reference *An. funestus* genome for sequencing [78]. Unfortunately and besides the numerous efforts in many parts of Africa, only one new colony has been colonized (Sagnon *et al.*, pers. comm.). Third, polytene chromosomes of this species exhibit a poor quality in comparison with *An. gambiae* [7]. The assembly of the *An. gambiae* genome was primarily based on techniques, which required the identification of probes through polytene chromosomes [77]. Although polytene chromosomes are readable, as several studies assert, however, the effort involved is very high and the rate of success, significantly lower.

Despite these challenges, and the lack of a publicly available *An. funestus* genome, several noteworthy molecular and genetic advances have been reached in this malaria mosquito during the last decade. These advances have been inspired by those previously achieved in *An. gambiae*. Particularly, we can distinguish two fields: molecular markers and expression profiling analysis.

3.2. Molecular markers

In the late 70's and beginning of the 80's, several studies revealed the importance of chromosomal inversions as genetic markers to differentiate species within the Funestus Group [6, 7]. These results mirrored those obtained in the *An. gambiae* complex [81, 82]. But, we had to wait until the end of the 90's and the past decade to settle the role of the chromosomal inversions in local adaptation and speciation within *An. funestus* populations [42, 52, 83-86]. Despite its evident interest, the technical demands of traditional karyotype analysis, the low rate of success in chromosome preparations, and the sex- and stage-specific limitations, have hampered the proliferation of this kind of studies. Nowadays, the new advances in molecular karyotyping in *An. gambiae* (based on quick, low-cost and convenient PCR reactions) have re-launched an interest in this field [87, 88]. Together with new high-throughput technology, the *An. funestus* genome will undoubtedly open new possibilities to develop molecular karyotyping in this mosquito.

Chromosome	Locus	Accession number	Forward primer	Reverse primer	Allele size
Chr. X	FUNE	AY6009	GACCGGTTCTGGTATCGTC	ATCGAGTCACCCAATTCTCC	136–154
	FUNQ	AY6021	GCAAACTGCTAGTAAATGTTTCC	*ACACAACGCCACCACTATGA	84–98
Chr. 2	AFND6	AF171036	GCTTCTTCTCCCCTAATCTG	TCCTGCTTTTTAGTTTGTCG	184–212
	AFUB15	AY029722	GATGCCGGGAGTAATAGCAA	AGACAGCCCGTAGAACGGTA	155–191
	AFND2	AF171032	ATAAACCCGTCCATTCCCTT	CCTATGATTCGCTCCTGACA	131–151
	AFND32	AY291367	GAAGCATTTTGGGTTAGACTC	GCAGTTGTTTACCTTTCACTG	103–121
	AFUB14	AY029721	ATCAGTGCTCCTCCACATCC	CGTGGTTGGCAATGTTACTG	152–188
	AFND17	AF171047	AAAACGCCACAAAGAGCAC	CGGGTCAAATTCTACCGTAAG	129–157
	AFUB4	AY029711	CTATCAGCAGCCGCCACA	GATGCCGATGAGGAATGTTG	183–192
	AFUB25	AY029723	GTGGAAACGGTGGTACTGT	CGCCATGTAGCTAGGGTTTG	212–224
	AFUB10	AY029717	TGTCCATGTACAACCGCAAC	TTCTCCAGCATCATCAGCAC	195–210
	AFND37	AY291373	GATCGATACAATAAGTGTAGAAATAAT	TCACGATGTGCAACCTATAA	161–189
	AFUB30	AY029737	GCCAGTTTGCAGAACCAAAT	CTGCTGCTGATGTTGCTGAT	154–163
	AFUB7	AY029714	ATGGGACGATGGATTACCAA	GCCAGTTTGCAGAACCAAAT	220–223
	AFUB16	AY029723	CGTGGATGGCAATGTTACTG	TGCGACTTATCAGTGCTCCT	179–209
Chr. 3	AFND21	AF171051	CCGCACACCAACTTACACTC	TGGCGTGGGATTAAATAGG	96–104
	AFUB13		GACTTCCGCCACAGAACATC	CTCAGGCTCGCAGTAGGAGT	207–210
	AFND19	AF171049	CAGAACCACTTCGATTCAAC	CCTGCACTCAGAAACACAC	172–205
	FUND	AY6008	GCTAACTACTCCGAAGCGCT	GATCGCAAAACTTCCGGTT	145–177
	FUNI	AY6013	*GCAACTAAGCTGGGACAGGA	GCATCTAACCCTGCTGCTT	181–197
	AFND3	AF171033	ACGACTGTAACCACAACACC	TAGTAGCGAAGGCGAAAGAT	171–195
	FUNF	AY6010	CCTTCAGTTTCGATTGGCG	AATAAGATGCGACCGTGGC	104–118
	AFND10	AF171040	TTTTTTCTTCCCGTGTTGC	TACCATTTGATTACAGCGCC	114–146
	AFUB17	AY029724	GAAAACCGTACGAACGATGG	TGCGACAGTAGCACAGGGTA	187–196
	AFUB1	AY029708	CAGCAGCAGCAGCAACAG	GACGTTAGCATCTCCACCAG	266–269
	AFUB12	AY029719	TGGGGAACTGGTCGTTAGAG	CTGGTGATGGGATTGAGGAT	152–158
	FUNK	AY6015	GCGCTTCCGCAAACATAC	ACTCACACCCCATTCTTGTG	184–202
	263B12		AGTGCGTCAGAGTTTGAA	TCGATTGATGGCGATGATAA	230–242
	261H03		CGCTCAAACTGAAAGCGATA	GGATGCGGAGATGATGTTGT	208–220
	263A06		CGTTCGGTTTCGCTAACTGT	CGTTCTATTTCGGGGTGTGT	210–220
Unknown	AFUB21	AY029728	*AACGCAGCAGTGGAGAGAAT	AACACCAACCCTTGTTGTGC	224–230
	AFND30	AY291369	GCCAGTTTGCAGAACCAAAT	CTGCTGCTGATGTTGCTGAT	81–107

Table 2. Summary of microsatellite loci in *An. funestus* modified from Wondji et al. [89].

In *An. funestus*, several genes have been recurrently involved in genetic studies: three nuclear genes (ITS1, ITS2 and D3) and another three mitochondrial genes (COI, COII and ND5). Nuclear genes have been involved in species differentiation within the Funestus Group [15, 16], while mitochondrial genes revealed signatures of incipient speciation between populations of Burkina Faso [85]. Another kind of molecular markers, Single Nucleotide Polymorphisms (SNPs), have been recently developed in this malaria mosquito. Wondji et al. [79]

reported a genome-wide set of SNP markers from 50 genes. A total of 494 SNPs were identified, which were added to 15 SNPs previously discovered by analyzing sequence traces of 11 physically mapped DNA fragments of cytochrome P450s of *An. funestus*. However, to date, microsatellites are the most frequently employed molecular markers in *An. funestus* [89-92]. Seventy-five microsatellites have been developed, although, only 32 were successfully revisited by Wondji et al [89] (Table 2). They are widely distributed across the *An. funestus* genome. They have allowed the analysis of population genetic structure, gene flow and demographic events across Africa [93], from Senegal [40], Cameroon [83, 86], Kenya [94] to Madagascar [95], revealing important signatures of local adaptation, dispersion or speciation.

These molecular markers have been key in numerous advances. For instance, SNPs and microsatellites allowed to Wondji and co-workers to explore the genetic basis of insecticide resistance in this malaria vectors [79]. Several genes including the P450 cytochrome (CYP6P9a and CYP6P9b) were associated to DDT resistance by Quantitative Trait Loci (QTL) analysis using both markers [72]. The role of microsatellites in population genetic studies is discussed in other sections of this chapter (see below). Despite, we are still far from the molecular advances carried out on *An. gambiae*. For instance, in *An. funestus* 75 microsatellite loci have been identified, compared to 300 in *An. gambiae*. With regards to SNPs, 509 have been reported in *An. funestus* [79, 89], compared to 400,000 in *An. gambiae* [80].

3.3. Expression profiles

Considering the lack of *An. funestus* genome, transcriptome analysis appeared as a suitable alternative to whole genome sequencing. This technique is significantly cheaper and provides important information at the gene transcript level. Moreover, it provides valuable molecular tools for the analysis of gene expression evolution and comparative analysis among other Culicidae members, such as *An. gambiae, Ae. aegypti* or *Cx. pipiens*.

In 2007, Calvo et al., [96] investigated salivary gland genes from 916 cDNA clones coming from adult females. This study debuted the analysis of transcripts in this mosquito, providing important clues about the evolution of salivary gland proteins in blood feeding insects and Culicidae. In particular, a 30 KDa allergen family and several *mucins* were exclusively found in *Culicidae* when compared to *Aedes albopictus, Aedes aegypti* and *Culex pipiens quinquefasciatus*. Moreover, ten proteins and peptide families were only found in *Anopheles* when included in the analysis *An. gambiae, Anopheles stephensi* and *Anopheles darlingi*. Later, two new studies emerged with the aim to analyze the transcriptome evolution and differences in expression profile between insecticide susceptible and resistant phenotypes of *An. funestus*, respectively [80, 97]. While, Serazin et al. [97] used SANGER sequencing technology for this purpose, Gregory et al. [80] employed *de novo* expression profiling by 454 pyrosequencing. In general, these two studies were largely complementary and boosted the available genetic information in *An. funestus*. However, 454 pyrosequencing allowed parallel DNA sequencing and increased sequencing depth and genome coverage. For instance, Gregory et al. [80] improved the number of ESTs (Expressed Sequence Tags) from 2,846 [97] to 18,103 contigs. Regarding comparative analysis with other mosquitoes, both studies agreed on the fact that the highest similarity pattern remains with *An. gambiae*. Interestingly, the mean percentage of similarity differs drastically between functional groups. Two groups of housekeeping functions show the highest amino acid sequence conservation: protein synthesis and degradation. On the other hand, three groups of interest patently showed very low similarity scores, suggesting accelerated rates of evolution. These three functional categories – salivary, immunity and extracellular structures – may be driven by environmental selection pressures. For instance, selective pressures imposed by parasites could explain both the highest genetic variability and the lowest conservation of immune genes between *An. funestus and An. gambiae.* Alternatively, *de novo* 454 sequencing offered the opportunity to identify new SNPs. In this sense, 31,000 potential SNPs were discovered over 4.579 Mb of sequence, meaning one SNP every 70 bp [80]. Thus, expression profile studies led to identify genes under selective pressures (i.e. insecticide resistance, immunity genes) and might generate new functional genomic tools (i.e. microarrays or SNP platforms) while we wait for future genomic sequencing of *An. funestus*.

4. Population genetic structure across Africa

4.1. Introduction

In malaria mosquitoes, population genetics have been revealed as an excellent tool for implementation of vector control programs. The study of gene flow among vector populations allows the analysis of mosquitoes' movement in natural populations, and therefore, how those populations are segregated. They can, for instance, assist to follow the expansion of genes of interest, such as those that confer insecticide resistance [98], or potentially help to introduce transgenic mosquitoes, refractory to parasite infection [99, 100]. On the other hand, these population genetic studies might be useful to investigate the genetic basis of speciation and/or local adaptation processes. They evidence a considerable importance in vector control measures [101].

The biology of *An. funestus* has supported several "*a priories*" about its population structure in natural conditions. As mentioned previously in this chapter, this malaria mosquito mainly breeds in permanent or semi-permanent water bodies, such as rice fields, swamps or artificial lakes, always linked to human presence (see above). Moreover, this mosquito has exhibited a very slow recolonization power of those areas treated with insecticide. Both characteristics have led to assume the population subdivision of *An. funestus*. In this section, we will discuss the population structure of this malaria vector across Africa as revealed by two types of markers: chromosomal inversions and molecular markers.

4.2. Cytogenetic studies

The study of chromosomal rearrangements – cytogenetics – of *An. funestus* debuted early in the 1980's [6, 7], preceded by the success of this kind of studies in its congener *An. gambiae* [81, 82, 102]. It allowed differentiating members of the Funestus Group, avoiding the challenging interpretation of taxo-morphological rules. Green & Hunt [7] and Green [6] showed differences in the chromosomal polymorphism within the species of the group. As in *An. gambiae,* several chromosomal inversions were species-specific, while other inversions were polymorphic in some species and fixed in others. Although, other cytogenetic studies appeared in the meantime, we had to wait until 2001 when Sharakhov et al. [103] finally established the chromosome map of this species (Fig. 2), based on comparisons to the *An. gambiae* map [102].

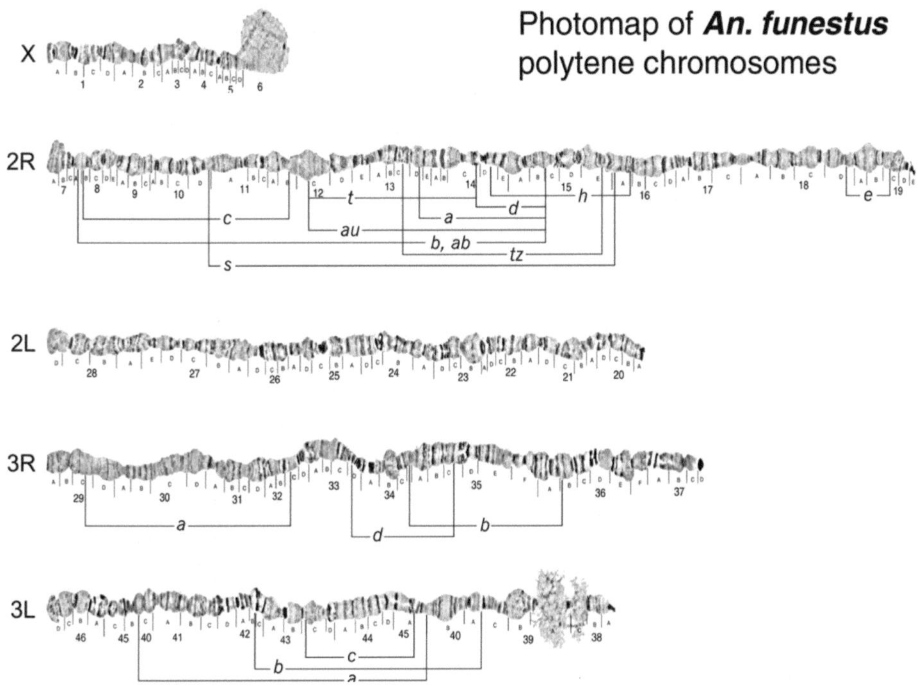

Figure 3. Chromosome map of *An. funestus*

For its predominant role as malaria vector and its wide geographical distribution across sub-Saharan Africa, *An. funestus* has been the most studied species of the group, although greatly exceeded by the studies in *An. gambiae* [82, 104, 105]. Seventeen chromosomal inversions have been recognized, with specific distribution through the African continent [6]; [52]; [84, 106-108]; (D. Ayala pers. comm.). Among them, four inversions are found all across the continent (2Ra, 3Ra, 3Rb, 3La), while others have a regional distribution (i.e. 2Rt in West Africa or 2Rh in South and Central Africa), or a very localized distribution (2Rd in the southern forested areas of Cameroon). These distributional patterns could be due to environmental selection, demographic effects or historical events [109].

Chromosomal inversions have been widely implicated in the process of speciation and local adaptation in a wide range of animals and plants [110, 111]. In recent years, studies on the chromosome composition of the populations of *An. funestus* were conducted in several African countries. These results showed a great complexity with different trends. In Burkina Faso, a deficit of heterozygotes and linkage disequilibrium among some rearrangements, led Costantini et al. [42] to identify two chromosomal forms: Kiribina and Folonzo, with a certain parallelism with the chromosomal forms of *An. gambiae* from Mali [104, 112]. These two forms are also differentiated at the ecological level. While Kiribina appears better adapted to arid conditions, Folonzo inhabits more humid habitats [84, 113]. The presence of these two chromosomal forms was not observed in other countries such as Angola, Madagascar or Kenya [108, 114] (LeGoff, pers. comm.). Nevertheless, deficits of heterozygotes were also detected, particularly in inversions of the 3R and 3L arm, in some areas of Cameroon and Senegal [52, 83, 86, 115]. These studies did not show a clear division between the "chromosomal forms from Burkina Faso", rather a non-random distribution of chromosomal inversions and their frequencies through different habitats and environments. This fact suggests that most inversions frequencies in *An. funestus* do not follow a neutral pattern. Ayala et al. [86] observed a sharp contrast between population structure measured at neutral microsatellite markers and at chromosomal inversions. Microsatellite data detected only a weak signal of population structure due to distance among geographical zones in Cameroon, as previously described by Cohuet et al. [83]. By contrast, strong differentiation among habitats was revealed by chromosomal inversions, strongly suggesting a role of environmental selection in shaping their distribution. Moreover, in the same study, there was no apparent difference between microsatellite loci (F_{ST} estimates) lying within and outside polymorphic chromosomal inversions [86].

4.3. Molecular markers

The first assays to characterize wild populations of this mosquito were based on mitochondrial (Internal Transcribed Spacer 2, ITS2) and ribosomal DNA (cytochrome b gene, cyt-b) [116]. The results did not show any differentiation between chromosomal forms previously described by Costantini [42], rather one panmictic population. At the beginning of this century, new microsatellite markers were developed, which allowed more precise studies [89-92]. At the country scale, the results have evidenced a general trend to only one population, with a slight but significant isolation by distance. In Kenya, Braginets et al. [94] did not find any population genetic structure throughout the country, however, an important sub-division due to Rift Valley was found. A similar pattern was already observed in *An. gambiae* [117]. In Madagascar, Ayala et al. [95] did not find a population structure at the island level, rather a correlation between genetic and geographic distance across vector populations. In Senegal, Cohuet et al. [40] also showed genetic differentiation due to distance, without a clear relationship between "Burkina Faso chromosomal forms" and genetic data.

Similar results were obtained in Cameroon, where for the first time, a latitudinal cline across different environments was analyzed [83, 86]. As in previous studies, genetic differentiation among populations might be explained by isolation by distance. On the other hand, in Burkina Faso, Michel et al. [85] showed a genetic divergence between chromosomal forms on the basis of five microsatellite markers and sequence of a mitochondrial gene (ND-5). These results validated in some extend those precluded by Costantini et al. [42] and Guelbeogo et al. [84]. Unfortunately, they still remain restricted to Burkina Faso, similarly to chromosomal forms of *An. gambiae* in West Africa [118]. In recent years, several population genetic studies have been conducted at the sub-region and/or continental scale. Temu et al. [119], showed a similar pattern to the other studies at the country level for five countries in Eastern and Southern

Africa: the genetic distance limited the gene flow among populations and promoted genetic differentiation among populations. A comprehensive study using samples across the continent provided important findings [93]. *Anopheles funestus* was subdivided into three large blocks: West Africa, East Africa and Central Africa [120, 121]. This subdivision was roughly similar than that observed in *An. gambiae* across Africa [122]. Despite these results and the unquestionable accuracy of the analysis, the question about the incipient speciation of *An. funestus*, still remains to be elucidated.

The very rapid pace of development of genetic and molecular tools will allow characterizing *An. funestus* populations in a very detailed fashion. New molecular tools, such as SNP chip, RAD-tag or DNA microarrays, will certainly contribute to a better understanding of the biology of this mosquito. The expected *An. funestus* genome sequencing will undoubtedly boost new advances in order to elucidate a variety of biological processes involved in local adaptation, speciation, parasite transmission or the immunity system among others. It will also enable comparative studies with other anopheline species, particularly, *An. gambiae*.

5. Conclusion

During the last decade, we have seen how new molecular advances have elevated *An. gambiae* to the level of model species with regard to the number of data and tools available. *Anopheles funestus* is still far from this point. Undoubtedly, it is one of the major and more deadly malaria vectors worldwide. Its capacity to adapt to a wide range of ecological settings coupled with the appearance of insecticide resistance highlight the importance for studying this mosquito. However, the extreme difficulty to establish colonies in insectary conditions has hindered its study. Now, its upcoming genome sequencing and the availability of new molecular tools preclude a promising future for the study of this malaria mosquito.

The *An. funestus* geographical distribution mirrors *An. gambiae*'s across the whole African continent, with presumably similar environmental pressures. This mosquito exhibits a large number of chromosomal and genetic polymorphisms. Furthermore, it belongs to a group of morphologically undistinguishable species. This malaria mosquito is suspected to be at the heart of an ongoing speciation process, as its congener *An. gambiae*. Once the new techniques and vector control strategies have achieved their goals in *An. gambiae, An. funestus* will become the new target for succeeding malaria control programs. Moreover, the parallel study between both species will help to elucidate the ecological and genetics mechanisms involved in many biological processes from immunity system to local adaptation or speciation.

In this chapter, we revisited the *state-of-the-art* of this malaria mosquito as well as the other species of the Funestus Group. Detailed descriptions were provided on their biology, role in malaria transmission and insecticide resistance status. We examined the new genomic advances and how they can be useful for improving vector control strategies. To sum up, we strongly believe that a general knowledge about this mosquito is essential for the success of its control and the ultimate aim to reduce the malaria burden in Africa.

Author details

Ibrahima Dia[1], Moussa Wamdaogo Guelbeogo[2] and Diego Ayala[3]

*Address all correspondence to: dia@pasteur.sn; guelbeogo.crnfp@fasonet.bf; diego.ayala.g@gmail.com

1 Medical Entomology Unit, Institut Pasteur de Dakar, Dakar, Senegal

2 Centre National de Recherche et de Formation sur le Paludisme, Ouagadougou, Burkina Faso

3 UMR 224 MIVEGEC/BEES, Institut de Recherche pour le Développement, Montpellier, France

References

[1] Gillies MT, Coetzee MC. A Supplement to the Anophelinae of Africa South of the Sahara (Afrotropical region). Johannesburg: The South African Institute for Medical Research; 1987.

[2] Coetzee M, Fontenille D. Advances in the study of *Anopheles funestus*, a major vector of malaria in Africa. Insect Biochem Mol Biol. 2004 Jul;34(7):599-605.

[3] Gillies MT, de Meillon B. The anophelinae of Africa, south of the Sahara. Johannesburg: The South African Institute for Medical Research; 1968.

[4] Evans AM, Leeson HS. The Funestus Series of *Anopheles* in Southern Rhodesia with descriptions of a new variety. Annals of Tropical Medicine and Parasitology. 1935;29:33-47.

[5] Evans AM, Symes CB. *Anopheles funestus* and its allies in Kenya. Annals of Tropical Medicine and Parasitology. 1937;31:105-12.

[6] Green CA. Cladistic analysis of mosquito chromosome data *Anopheles* (*Cellia*) *Myzomyia*. The journal of heredity. 1982;73(1):2-11.

[7] Green CA, Hunt RH. Interpretation of variation in ovarian polytene chromosomes of *Anopheles funestus* Giles, *Anopheles parensis* Gillies, and *Anopheles aruni*. Genetica. 1980;51(3):187-95.

[8] Pape T. Cladistic analyses of mosquito chromosome data in *Anopheles* subgenus *Cellia* (Diptera: Culicidae). Mosquito Systematics. 1992;24:1-11.

[9] Koekemoer LL, Kamau L, Hunt RH, Coetzee M. A cocktail polymerase chain reaction assay to identify members of the *Anopheles funestus* (Diptera: Culicidae) group. Am J Trop Med Hyg. 2002 Jun;66(6):804-11.

[10] Koekemoer LL, Lochouarn L, Hunt RH, Coetzee M. Single-strand conformation polymorphism analysis for identification of four members of the *Anopheles funestus* (Diptera: Culicidae) group. J Med Entomol. 1999 Mar;36(2):125-30.

[11] Cohuet A, Simard F, Toto JC, Kengne P, Coetzee M, Fontenille D. Species identification within the *Anopheles funestus* group of malaria vectors in Cameroon and evidence for a new species. Am J Trop Med Hyg. 2003 Aug;69(2):200-5.

[12] Hackett BJ, Gimnig J, Guelbeogo W, Costantini C, Koekemoer LL, Coetzee M, et al. Ribosomal DNA internal transcribed spacer (ITS2) sequences differentiate *Anopheles funestus* and *An. rivulorum* and uncover a cryptic taxon. . Insect Molecular Biology 2000;9:369–74.

[13] Harbach RE. The classification of genus *Anopheles* (Diptera: Culicidae): a working hypothesis of phylogenetic relationships. Bull Entomol Res. 2004 Dec;94(6):537-53.

[14] Harbach RE. Review of the internal classification of the genus *Anopheles* (Diptera: Culicidae): the foundation for comparative systematics and phylogenetic research. Bull Entomol Res. 1994;84:331-42.

[15] Garros C, Harbach RE, Manguin S. Systematics and biogeographical implications of the phylogenetic relationships between members of the Funestus and Minimus groups of *Anopheles* (Diptera: Culicidae). J Med Entomol. 2005 Jan;42(1):7-18.

[16] Garros C, Harbach RE, Manguin S. Morphological assessment and molecular phylogenetics of the Funestus and Minimus groups of *Anopheles* (*Cellia*). J Med Entomol. 2005 Jul;42(4):522-36.

[17] Harbach RE. Mosquito Taxanomic Inventory, http://mosquito-taxonomic-inventory.info/, accessed on November 2012. 2012 [cited 2012]; Available from: http://mosquito-taxonomic-inventory.info/.

[18] Ayala D, Costantini C, Ose K, Kamdem G, Antonio-Nkondjio C, Agbor J-P, et al. Habitat suitability and ecological niche profile of major malaria vectors in Cameroon. Malar J. 2009;8(1):307.

[19] Andrianaivolambo L, Domarle O, Randrianarivelojosia M, Ratovonjato J, Le Goff G, Talman A, et al. Anthropophilic mosquitoes and malaria transmission in the eastern foothills of the central highlands of Madagascar. . Acta Tropica. 2010;116(3):240-5.

[20] Tchuinkam T, Simard F, Lele-Defo E, Tene-Fossog B, Tateng-Ngouateu A, Antonio-Nkondjio C, et al. Bionomics of Anopheline species and malaria transmission dynamics along an altitudinal transect in Western Cameroon. BMC Infectious Diseases. 2010 May;10.

[21] Okara RM, Sinka ME, Minakawa N, Mbogo CM, Hay SI, Snow RW. Distribution of the main malaria vectors in Kenya. Malar J. 2010;9:69.

[22] Oyewole I, Awolola T, Ibidapo C, Oduola A, Okwa O, Obansa J. Behaviour and population dynamics of the major anopheline vectors in a malaria endemic area in southern Nigeria. Journal of Vector Borne Diseases 2007;44: 56–64.

[23] Betsi AN, Tchicaya ES, Koudou BG. Forte prolifération de larves d'*An. gambiae* et *An. funestus* en milieux rizicoles irrigués et non irrigués dans la région forestière ouest de la Côte-d'Ivoire. Bulletin de la Société de Pathologie Exotique. 2010;105(3):220-9.

[24] Adja AM, N'goran EK, Koudou BG, Dia I, Kengne P, Fontenille D, et al. Contribution of *Anopheles funestus*, *An. gambiae* and *An. nili* (Diptera: Culicidae) to the perennial malaria transmission in the southern and western forest areas of Côte d'Ivoire. Annals of Tropical Medicine and Parasitology. 2011;105(1):13-24.

[25] Tanga MC, Ngundu WI, Judith N, Mbuh J, Tendongfor N, Simard F, et al. Climate change and altitudinal structuring of malaria vectors in south-western Cameroon: their relation to malaria transmission. Transactions of the Royal Society of Tropical Medicine and Hygiene 2010;104(7):453-60.

[26] Konate L, Diop A, Sy N, Faye MN, Dieng Y, Izri A, et al. Come back of *A. funestus* in Sahelian Senegal. Lancet. 2001;358:336.

[27] Labbo R, Fouta A, Jeanne I, Ousmane I, Duchemin JB. *Anopheles funestus* in Sahel: new evidence from Niger. Lancet. 2004 363:660-1.

[28] Mouchet J, Faye O, Julvez J, Manguin S. Drought and malaria retreat in the Sahel, West Africa. Lancet. 1996; 348 (9043):1735-6.

[29] Elissa N, Karch S. Re-emergence of *Anopheles funestus* and its possible effect on malaria transmission on Mayotte Island, Indian Ocean. Journal of the American Mosquito Control Association. 2005;21(4):472-3.

[30] Fontenille D, Rakotoarivony I. Reappearance of *Anopheles funestus* as a malaria vector in the Antananarivo region, Madagascar. Transactions of the Royal Society of Tropical Medicine and Hygiene. 1988;82(4):644-5.

[31] Hargreaves K, Koekemoer LL, Brooke BD, Hunt RH, Mthembu J, Coetzee M. *Anopheles funestus* resistant to pyrethroid insecticides in South Africa. Med Vet Entomol. 2000 Jun;14(2):181-9.

[32] Dia I, Samb B, Konate L, Fontenille D. Population structure of newly established *Anopheles funestus* populations in the Senegal River basin using paracentric chromosomal inversions. Acta Tropica. 2010;115:90-4.

[33] Muturi EJ, Kamau L, Jacob BG, Muriu S, Mbogo CM, Shililu J, et al. Spatial distribution, blood feeding pattern, and role of *Anopheles funestus* complex in malaria transmission in central Kenya. Parasitology Research. 2009;105(4):1041-6.

[34] Kamau L, Munyekenye GO, Koekemoer LL, Hunt RH, Coetzee M. A survey of the *Anopheles funestus* (Diptera: Culicidae) group of mosquitoes from 10 sites in Kenya with special emphasis on population genetic structure based on chromosomal inversion karyotypes. Journal of Medical Entomology. 2003 Sep;40(5):664-71.

[35] Spillings BL, Brooke BD, Koekemoer LL, Chiphwanya J, Coetzee M, Hunt RH. A New Species Concealed by *Anopheles funestus* Giles, a Major Malaria Vector in Africa. Am J Trop Med Hyg. 2009;81(3):510–5.

[36] Koekemoer LL, Misiani EA, Hunt RH, Kent RJ, Norris DE, Coetzee M. Cryptic species within *Anopheles longipalpis* from southern Africa and phylogenetic comparison with members of the *An. funestus* group. Bulletin of entomological research. [Research Support, Non-U.S. Gov't]. 2009 Feb;99(1):41-9.

[37] Sinka ME, Bangs MJ, Manguin S, Coetzee M, Mbogo CM, Hemingway J, et al. The dominant *Anopheles* vectors of human malaria in Africa, Europe and the Middle East: occurrence data, distribution maps and bionomic precis. Parasites & Vectors. 2010 Dec 3;3.

[38] Abou-Nasr A. Entomological problems facing malaria eradication in Africa (Uganda). Bulletin Society entomology Egypte. 1970;53: 97-107.

[39] Minakawa N, Dida GO, Sonye GO, Futami K, Njenga SM. Malaria Vectors in Lake Victoria and Adjacent Habitats in Western Kenya. PLoS One 2012;7, e 32725

[40] Cohuet A, Dia I, Simard F, Raymond M, Fontenille D. Population structure of the malaria vector *Anopheles funestus* in Senegal based on microsatellite and cytogenetic data. Insect Molecular Biology. 2004 Jun;13(3):251-8.

[41] Shiff CJ MJ, Hall T, Hunt RH, Lyimo S, Davis JR. . Malaria infection potential of anopheline mosquitoes sampled by light trapping indoors in coastal Tanzanian villages. Medical and Veterinary Entomology. 2005;9:256–62.

[42] Costantini C, Sagnon N, Ilboudo-Sanogo E, Coluzzi M, Boccolini D. Chromosomal and bionomic heterogeneities suggest incipient speciation in *Anopheles funestus* from Burkina Faso. Parassitologia. 1999 Dec;41(4):595-611.

[43] Oyewole I, Awolola T. Impact of urbanisation on bionomics and distribution of malaria vectors in Lagos, southwestern Nigeria. J Vector Borne Dis 2006;43 173-8.

[44] Robert V, Le Goff G, Andrianaivolambo L, Randimby F, Domarle O, Randrianarivelojosia M, et al. Moderate transmission but high prevalence of malaria in Madagascar. Int J Parasitol 2006;36:1273-81.

[45] Awolola T, Oyewole I, Koekemoer L, Coetzee M. Identification of three members of the *Anopheles funestus* (Diptera: Culicidae) group and their role in malaria transmission in two ecological zones in Nigeria. Trans R Soc Trop Med Hyg 2005;99:525-31.

[46] Antonio-Nkondjio C, Kerah CH, Simard F, Awono-Ambene P, Chouaibou M, Tchuinkam T, et al. Complexity of the malaria vectorial system in Cameroon: contri-

bution of secondary vectors to malaria transmission. Journal of Medical Entomology. 2006 Nov;43(6):1215-21.

[47] Dabire KR, Baldet T, Diabate A, Dia I, Costantini C, Cohuet A, et al. *Anopheles funestus* (Diptera: Culicidae) in a humid savannah area of western Burkina Faso: bionomics, insecticide resistance status, and role in malaria transmission. J Med Entomol. 2007 Nov;44(6):990-7.

[48] Fontenille D, Lochouarn L, Diagne N, Sokhna C, Lemasson JJ, Diatta M, et al. High annual and seasonal variations in malaria transmission by anophelines and vector species composition in Dielmo, a holoendemic area in Senegal. Am J Trop Med Hyg. 1997 Mar;56(3):247-53.

[49] Dia I, Diop T, Rakotoarivony I, Kengne P, Fontenille D. Bionomics of *Anopheles gambiae* Giles, *An. arabiensis* Patton, *An. funestus* Giles and *An. nili* (Theobald) (Diptera: Culicidae) and transmission of *Plasmodium falciparum* in a Sudano-Guinean zone (Ngari, Senegal). J Med Entomol. 2003 May;40(3):279-83.

[50] Lochouarn L, Dia I, Boccolini D, Coluzzi M, Fontenille D. Bionomical and cytogenetic heterogeneities of *Anopheles funestus* in Senegal. Transactions of the Royal Society of Tropical Medicine and Hygiene. 1998 Nov-Dec;92(6):607-12.

[51] Boccolini D, Rakotoson R, Ralisoa O, Sabatini A, Randrianarisoa E, Coluzzi M. Polimorfismo cromosomico di *Anopheles funestus* in Madagascar. Parassitologia. 1992; 34:14-5.

[52] Dia I, Lochouarn L, Boccolini D, Costantini C, Fontenille D. Spatial and temporal variations of the chromosomal inversion polymorphism of *Anopheles funestus* in Senegal. Parasite. 2000 Sep;7(3):179-84.

[53] Wilkes TJ, Matola YG, Charlwood JD. *Anopheles rivulorum*, a vector of human malaria in Africa. Medical and Veterinary Entomology. 1996 Jan;10(1):108-10.

[54] Temu EA, Minjas JN, Tuno N, Kawada H, Takagi M. Identification of four members of the *Anopheles funestus* (Diptera: Culicidae) group and their role in *Plasmodium falciparum* transmission in Bagamoyo coastal Tanzania. Acta Trop. 2007 May;102(2): 119-25.

[55] Mouatcho JC, Hargreaves K, Koekemoer LL, Brooke BD, Oliver SV, Hunt RH, et al. Indoor collections of the *Anopheles funestus* group (Diptera: Culicidae) in sprayed houses in northern KwaZulu-Natal, South Africa. Malar J. [Research Support, Non-U.S. Gov't]. 2007;6:30.

[56] De Meillon B. Observations on a species of the *Anopheles funestus* subgroup, a suspected exophilic vector of malaria parasites in north-eastern Transvaal, South Africa. Mosquito News. 1977;37:657-61.

[57] Kent RJ, Coetzee M, Mharakurwa S, Norris DE. Feeding and indoor resting behaviour of the mosquito *Anopheles longipalpis* in an area of hyperendemic malaria trans-

mission in southern Zambia. Medical and Veterinary Entomology. [Research Support, N.I.H., Extramural Research Support, Non-U.S. Gov't]. 2006 Dec;20(4): 459-63.

[58] Adugna N, Petros B. Determination of the human blood index of some anopheline mosquitos by using ELISA. Ethiop Med J. [Research Support, Non-U.S. Gov't]. 1996 Jan;34(1):1-10.

[59] Smith A. The Transmission of Bancroftial Filariasis on Ukara Island, Tanganyika. II. —The Distribution of Bancroftial Microfilaraemia compared with the Distribution of Hut-haunting Mosquitos and their Breeding Places. Bulletin of Entomological Research. 1955;46:437-44.

[60] Smith A. Observations on the man-biting habits of some mosquitoes in the South Pare area of Tanganyika. East Africa Medical Journal 1961;38:246.

[61] Brooke BD, Kloke G, Hunt RH, Koekemoer LL, Temu EA, Taylor ME, et al. Bioassay and biochemical analyses of insecticide resistance in southern African *Anopheles funestus* (Diptera: Culicidae). Bull Entomol Res. 2001 Aug;91(4):265-72.

[62] Casimiro S, Coleman M, Mohloai P, Hemingway J, Sharp B. Insecticide resistance in *Anopheles funestus* (Diptera: Culicidae) from Mozambique. J Med Entomol. 2006 Mar; 43(2):267-75.

[63] Cuamba N, Morgan JC, Irving H, Steven A, Wondji CS. High level of pyrethroid resistance in an *Anopheles funestus* population of the Chokwe district in Mozambique. PLoS ONE. 2010 Jun;5(6), e11010.

[64] Morgan JC, Irving H, Okedi LM, Steven A, Wondji CS. Pyrethroid resistance in an Anopheles funestus population from Uganda. PLoS One. 2010;5(7), e11872.

[65] Hamon J, Sales S, Venard P, Coz J, Brengues J. The presence in southwest Upper Volta of populations of *Anopheles funestus* Giles resistant to dieldrin. Médecine Tropicale. 1968;28:221-6.

[66] Brown AWA. Insecticide resistance in mosquitoes: a pragmatic review. Journal of the American Mosquito Control Association 1986;2:123–40.

[67] Toure YT. Etude de la sensibilité d'*Anopheles funestus* et d'*Anopheles gambiae* sensu lato aux insecticides dans une zone mrale de savane soudanienne an Mali. Cahiers ORSTOM serie Entomologie médicale et Parasitology. 1982;20(2):125-31.

[68] Service MW. A taxonomic study of *Anopheles funestus funestus* Giles (Diptera: Culicidae) from southern and northern Nigeria, with notes on its varieties and synonyms. Proceedings of the Royal Entomological Society of London. 1960;29:77–84.

[69] Wondji CS, Dabire RK, Tukur Z, Irving H, Djouaka R, Morgan JC. Identification and distribution of a GABA receptor mutation conferring dieldrin resistance in the malaria vector *Anopheles funestus* in Africa. Insect Biochem Mol Biol. 2011;41(7):484-91.

[70] Coetzee M, van Wyk P, Booman M, Koekemoer LL, Hunt RH. Insecticide resistance in malaria vector mosquitoes in a gold mining town in Ghana and implications for malaria control. . Bulletin de la Société de Pathologie Exotique. 2006;99(5):400-3.

[71] Okoye PN, Brooke BD, Koekemoer LL, Hunt RH, Coetzee M. Characterisation of DDT, pyrethroid and carbamate resistance in *Anopheles funestus* from Obuasi, Ghana. . Transactions of the Royal Society of Tropical Medicine and Hygiene 2008;102 (6):591-8.

[72] Wondji CS, Irvin H, Morgan J, Lobo NF, Collins FH, Hunt RH, et al. Two duplicated P450 genes are associated with pyrethroid resistance in *Anopheles funestus*, a major malaria vector. Genome Research. 2009;19(3):452–9.

[73] Matambo TS, Paine MJ, Coetzee M, Koekemoer LL. Sequence characterization of cytochrome P450 CYP6P9 in pyrethroid resistant and susceptible *Anopheles funestus* (Diptera: Culicidae). Genetics and Molecular Research. 2010;9(1):554-64.

[74] Djouaka R, Irving H, Tukur Z, Wondji CS. Exploring Mechanisms of Multiple Insecticide Resistance in a Population of the Malaria Vector *Anopheles funestus* in Benin. PLoS One 2011;11:e27760

[75] Oliver SV, M.L. K, Wood OR, Coetzee M, Rowland M, Brooke BD. Evaluation of the pyrrole insecticide chlorfenapyr against pyrethroid resistant and susceptible *Anopheles funestus* (Diptera: Culicidae). Tropical Medicine and International Health. 2010;15(1):127-31.

[76] Hunt RH, Brooke BD, Pillay C, Koekemoer LL, Coetzee M. Laboratory selection for and characteristics of pyrethroid resistance in the malaria vector *Anopheles funestus*. Med Vet Entomol. 2005 Sep;19(3):271-5.

[77] Holt RA, Subramanian GM, Halpern A, Sutton GG, Charlab R, Nusskern DR, et al. The genome sequence of the malaria mosquito *Anopheles gambiae*. Science. 2002;298(5591):129.

[78] Besansky N, Genome analysis of vectorial capacity in major *Anopheles* vectors of malaria parasites. [database on the Internet]. Vectorbase [http://www.vectorbase.org]. 2008. Available from: http://www.vectorbase.org.

[79] Wondji CS, Morgan J, Coetzee M, Hunt RH, Steen K, Black WCt, et al. Mapping a quantitative trait locus (QTL) conferring pyrethroid resistance in the African malaria vector *Anopheles funestus*. BMC Genomics. 2007;8:34.

[80] Gregory R, Darby AC, Irving H, Coulibaly MB, Hughes M, Koekemoer LL, et al. A De Novo Expression Profiling of *Anopheles funestus*, Malaria Vector in Africa, Using 454 Pyrosequencing. PLoS ONE. 2011;6, e 17418.

[81] Coluzzi M, Sabatini A, Petrarca V, Di Deco MA. Behavioural divergences between mosquitoes with different inversion karyotypes in polymorphic populations of the *Anopheles gambiae* complex. Nature. 1977 Apr 28;266(5605):832-3.

[82] Coluzzi M, Sabatini A, Petrarca V, Dideco MA. Chromosomal differentiation and adaptation to human environments in the *Anopheles gambiae* complex. Transactions of the Royal Society of Tropical Medicine and Hygiene. 1979;73(5):483-97.

[83] Cohuet A, Dia I, Simard F, Raymond M, Rousset F, Antonio-Nkondjio C, et al. Gene flow between chromosomal forms of the malaria vector *Anopheles funestus* in Cameroon, Central Africa, and its relevance in malaria fighting. Genetics. 2005 Jan;169(1): 301-11.

[84] Guelbeogo WM, Grushko O, Boccolini D, Ouedraogo PA, Besansky NJ, Sagnon NF, et al. Chromosomal evidence of incipient speciation in the Afrotropical malaria mosquito *Anopheles funestus*. Medical and Veterinary Entomology. 2005 Dec;19(4):458-69.

[85] Michel AP, Guelbeogo WM, Grushko O, Schemerhorn BJ, Kern M. Molecular differentiation between chromosomally defined incipient species of *Anopheles funestus*. Insect Molecular Biology. 2005;14:375-87.

[86] Ayala D, Fontaine MC, Cohuet A, Fontenille D, Vitalis R, Simard F. Chromosomal inversions, natural selection and adaptation in the malaria vector *Anopheles funestus* Mol Biol Evol. 2011;28(1):745–58.

[87] White BJ, Santolamazza F, Kamau L, Pombi M, Grushko O, Mouline K, et al. Molecular karyotyping of the 2La inversion in *Anopheles gambiae*. Am J Trop Med Hyg. 2007 Feb;76(2):334-9.

[88] Lobo N, Sangare D, Regier A, Reidenbach K, Bretz D, Sharakhova M, et al. Breakpoint structure of the *Anopheles gambiae* 2Rb chromosomal inversion. Malar J. 2010;9(1):293.

[89] Wondji CS, Hunt RH, Pignatelli P, Steen K, Coetzee M, Besansky N, et al. An integrated genetic and physical map for the malaria vector *Anopheles funestus*. Genetics. 2005 Dec;171(4):1779-87.

[90] Sinkins SP, Hackett BJ, Costantini C, Vulule J, Ling YY, Collins FH, et al. Isolation of polymorphic microsatellite loci from the malaria vector *Anopheles funestus*. Molecular Ecology. 2000 Apr;9(4):490-2.

[91] Cohuet A, Simard F, Berthomieu A, Raymond M, Fontenille D, Weill M. Isolation and characterization of microsatellite DNA markers in the malaria vector *Anopheles funestus*. Molecular Ecology Notes. 2002;2(4):498-500.

[92] Sharakhov I, Braginets O, Grushko O, Cohuet A, Guelbeogo WM, Boccolini D, et al. A microsatellite map of the African human malaria vector *Anopheles funestus*. Journal of Heredity. 2004 Jan-Feb;95(1):29-34.

[93] Michel AP, Ingrasci MJ, Schemerhorn BJ, Kern M, Le Goff G, Coetzee M, et al. Rangewide population genetic structure of the African malaria vector *Anopheles funestus*. Molecular Ecology. 2005 Dec;14(14):4235-48.

[94] Braginets OP, Minakawa N, Mbogo CM, Yan G. Population genetic structure of the African malaria mosquito *Anopheles funestus* in Kenya. Am J Trop Med Hyg. 2003 Sep;69(3):303-8.

[95] Ayala D, Goff GL, Robert V, de Jong P, Takken W. Population structure of the malaria vector *Anopheles funestus* (Diptera: Culicidae) in Madagascar and Comoros. Acta Tropica. 2006 Mar;97(3):292-300.

[96] Calvo C, Dao A, Pham VM, Ribeiro JMC. An insight into the sialome of *Anopheles funestus* reveals an emerging pattern in anopheline salivary protein families. Insect Biochem Mol Biol. 2007;37:164-75.

[97] Serazin AC, Dana AN, Hillenmeyer ME, Lobo NF, Coulibaly MB, Willard MB, et al. Comparative Analysis of the Global Transcriptome of *Anopheles funestus* from Mali, West Africa. PLoS ONE. 2009;4(11), e 7976.

[98] Pinto J, Lynd A, Vicente JL, Santolamazza F, Randle NP, Gentile G, et al. Multiple origins of knockdown resistance mutations in the Afrotropical mosquito vector *Anopheles gambiae*. PLoS ONE. 2007;2(11):e1243.

[99] Marrelli MT, Li CY, Rasgon JL, Jacobs-Lorena M. Transgenic malaria-resistant mosquitoes have a fitness advantage when feeding on *Plasmodium*-infected blood. Proceedings of the National Academy of Sciences of the United States of America. 2007;104(13):5580-3.

[100] Boete C. Malaria parasites in mosquitoes: laboratory models, evolutionary temptation and the real world. Trends Parasitol. 2005 Oct;21(10):445-7.

[101] Enayati A, Hemingway J. Malaria Management: Past, Present, and Future. Annu Rev Entomol. [Review]. 2010;55:569-91.

[102] Coluzzi M. Spatial distribuion of chromosomal inversions and speciation in anopheline mosquitoes. In: C B, editor. Mechanisms of Speciation. New York: Alan R Liss; 1982. p. 113-5.

[103] Sharakhov IV, Sharakhova MV, Mbogo CM, Koekemoer LL, Yan G. Linear and spatial organization of polytene chromosomes of the African malaria mosquito *Anopheles funestus*. Genetics. 2001 Sep;159(1):211-8.

[104] Coluzzi M, Petrarca V, Di Deco MA. Chromosomal inversion intergradation and incipient speciation in *Anopheles gambiae*. Bollettino di Zoologia. 1985;52:45-63.

[105] Pombi M, Caputo B, Simard F, Di Deco MA, Coluzzi M, Della Torre A, et al. Chromosomal plasticity and evolutionary potential in the malaria vector *Anopheles gambiae* sensu stricto: insights from three decades of rare paracentric inversions. BMC Evol Biol. 2008 Nov 10;8(1):309.

[106] Boccolini D, Sabatini A, Sanogo E, Sagnon N, Coluzzi M, Costantini C. Chromosomal and vectorial heterogeneities in *Anopheles funestus* from Burkina Faso, West Africa. Parassitologia. 1994;36:20.

[107] Boccolini D, Sagnon N, Toure Y. Chromosomal polymorphism in *Anopheles funestus* and description of new inversions in Burkina Faso and Mali. Parassitologia. 1998;40:14.

[108] Kamau L, Hunt R, Coetzee M. Analysis of the population structure of *Anopheles funestus* (Diptera: Culicidae) from western and coastal Kenya using paracentric chromosomal inversion frequencies. J Med Entomol. 2002 Jan;39(1):78-83.

[109] Endler JA. Geographic Variation, Speciation, and Clines. May RM, editor. Princetown, New Yersey: Princetown University Press; 1977.

[110] Hoffmann AA, Sgro CM, Weeks AR. Chromosomal inversion polymorphisms and adaptation. Trends Ecol Evol. 2004 Sep;19(9):482-8.

[111] Hoffmann AA, Rieseberg LH. Revisiting the impact of inversions in evolution: from population genetic markers to drivers of adaptive shifts and speciation? Annu Rev Ecol Evol Syst. 2008;39(1):21-42.

[112] Coluzzi M, Sabatini A, della Torre A, Di Deco MA, Petrarca V. A polytene chromosome analysis of the *Anopheles gambiae* species complex. Science. 2002;298:1415.

[113] Guelbeogo WM, Sagnon N, Grushko O, Yameogo MA, Boccolini D, Besansky NJ, et al. Seasonal distribution of *Anopheles funestus* chromosomal forms from Burkina Faso. Malar J. 2009 Oct;8, 239.

[114] Boccolini D, Carrara GC, Dia I, Fortes F, Cani PJ, Costantini C. Chromosomal differentiation of *Anopheles funestus* from Luanda and Huambo Provinces, western and central Angola. Am J Trop Med Hyg. 2005 Dec;73(6):1071-6.

[115] Dia I, Boccolini D, Antonio-Nkondjio C, Costantini C, Fontenille D. Chromosomal inversion polymorphism of *Anopheles funestus* from forest villages of South Cameroon. Parassitologia. 2000 Dec;42(3-4):227-9.

[116] Mukabayire O, Boccolini D, Lochouarn L, Fontenille D, Besansky NJ. Mitochondrial and ribosomal internal transcribed spacer (ITS2) diversity of the African malaria vector *Anopheles funestus*. Mol Ecol. 1999 Feb;8(2):289-97.

[117] Lehmann T, Besansky NJ, Hawley WA, Fahey TG, Kamau L, Collins FH. Microgeographic structure of *Anopheles gambiae* in western Kenya based on mtDNA and microsatellite loci. Mol Ecol. 1997 Mar;6(3):243-53.

[118] Favia G, della Torre A, Bagayoko M, Lanfrancotti A, Sagnon N, Toure YT, et al. Molecular identification of sympatric chromosomal forms of *Anopheles gambiae* and further evidence of their reproductive isolation. Insect Molecular Biology. 1997 Nov; 6(4):377-83.

[119] Temu EA, Hunt RH, Coetzee M. Microsatellite DNA polymorphism and heterozygosity in the malaria vector mosquito *Anopheles funestus* (Diptera: Culicidae) in east and southern Africa. Acta Trop. 2004 Mar;90(1):39-49.

[120] Garros C, Koekemoer LL, Kamau L, Awolola TS, Van Bortel W, Coetzee M, et al. Restriction fragment length polymorphism method for the identification of major African and Asian malaria vectors within the *Anopheles funestus* and *An. minimus* groups. The American journal of tropical medicine and hygiene. [Research Support, Non-U.S. Gov't]. 2004 Mar;70(3):260-5.

[121] Koekemoer LL, Kamau L, Garros C, Manguin S, Hunt RH, Coetzee M. Impact of the Rift Valley on restriction fragment length polymorphism typing of the major African malaria vector *Anopheles funestus* (Diptera: Culicidae). Journal of Medical Entomology. [Comparative Study Research Support, Non-U.S. Gov't]. 2006 Nov;43(6):1178-84.

[122] Lehmann T, Licht M, Elissa N, Maega BT, Chimumbwa JM, Watsenga FT, et al. Population Structure of *Anopheles gambiae* in Africa. Journal of Heredity. 2003 Mar-Apr; 94(2):133-47.

Chapter 8

Highlights on *Anopheles nili* and *Anopheles moucheti*, Malaria Vectors in Africa

Christophe Antonio-Nkondjio and Frédéric Simard

Additional information is available at the end of the chapter

http://dx.doi.org/10.5772/55153

1. Introduction

Anopheles nili Theobald 1904 and *An. moucheti* Evans 1925 are major human malaria vectors in forested and humid savannah areas of West and Central Africa [1]. Yet, they remain critically understudied and basic knowledge on their biology, ecology and genetics is crucially lacking [2]. To date, most studies of African malaria vectors have focused on *An. gambiae, An. arabiensis,* and *An. funestus,* in part, because molecular and cytogenetic tools for characterizing population structure, ecological adaptation, and taxonomic status of other species have been lacking until recently. Further, no laboratory colony is available for experimental work involving these neglected species. This gap in knowledge needs to be addressed for successful implementation of global strategies for malaria elimination and eradication in the Afrotropical region [3].

Recent studies of the ecological niche profile of major African malaria vectors demonstrated that the habitats of *An. gambiae, An. arabiensis*, and *An. funestus* have more overlap with each other than with the habitat of *An. nili* and *An. moucheti* [4-7]. This results in an unusual geographic distribution of *An. nili* and *An. moucheti* (Figure 1), revealing their crucial role in malaria transmission in forested and degraded forest areas of equatorial Africa [8-13]. Unique aspects of ecological adaptation and behaviour can, in part, explain the increased vectorial capacity of the species in these environments and might protect them from conventional vector control tools targeting highly endophilic and endophagic mosquito species [3, 14]. Moreover, the recent findings of circulation of *Plasmodium falciparum* along with other *Plasmodium* species in great apes and monkeys [15-17] raise concerns about pathogen transfer between humans and primates and further highlight the need to improve our knowledge of forest malaria vectors.

In this chapter, we review knowledge gained so far on mosquitoes from *An. moucheti* and closely related species, as well as the *An. nili* complex. We highlight specific bionomical, ecological and genetic attributes that distinguish these species from the most well-known major African malaria vectors, providing opportunities for further research on neglected aspects of vector biology and control.

2. *Anopheles moucheti* and closely related species

Anopheles moucheti belongs to the series Myzomyia and closely resembles *Anopheles marshallii* Theobald of the Marshallii complex. This close morphological similarity resulted in *An. moucheti* being initially considered a variety of *An. marshallii* before it was raised to the rank of full species on the basis of morphological and bionomic differences [18]. However the taxonomic status of *An. moucheti* has been subject to several interpretations during the past decades. Based on morphological similarities between *An. bervoetsi* and *An. moucheti nigeriensis*, *Anopheles moucheti* was later considered by Brunhes *et al.* [19] as a group consisting of three morphological forms, namely *An. moucheti moucheti* (referred to as the type form), *An. moucheti bervoetsi* and *An. moucheti nigeriensis* distinguishable by slight morphological characters present at the adult and/or at the larval stages [2, 19, 20]. In their classification, Brunhes *et al.* [19] referred to *An. bervoetsi* as a subspecies of *An. moucheti* while they suggested to put in synonymy *An. m. nigeriensis* and the type form. Genetic analysis conducted subsequently provided evidences against any taxonomic value for this morphological classification [21-23]. Recent classification by Harbach [24] recognizes *An. moucheti* and *An. bervoetsi* as formal species while *An. m. nigeriensis* is considered as a morphological variant within *An. moucheti*.

Anopheles moucheti is widely distributed across West and Central Africa (Figure 2) whereas the two other taxa have only been reported so far from their type locality in Nigeria near Lagos (06°27′N; 03°24′E) for *An. moucheti nigeriensis* and in Tsakalakuku (06°34′S; 17°35′E) in the Democratic Republic of Congo (DRC) for *An. bervoetsi* [18].

Anopheles moucheti is among the most important human malaria vectors in the equatorial forest region of Africa, particularly in villages situated along slow moving rivers or streams where its larvae develop in and around floating vegetation and debris (Figure 3) [4, 5]. Larval collections to assess ecological factors influencing *An. moucheti* distribution across river networks in south Cameroun showed that *An. moucheti* larvae are frequently associated with lentic rivers, low temperatures and the abundance of aquatic vegetation at the edge of the river (Figure 4) [5]. Increased urbanization and deforestation as well as lower-scale landscape modification such as river banks cleaning for gardening and/or recreational purposes were shown to be highly detrimental to the species, fostering changes in the malaria vector system composition with a higher prevalence of *An. gambiae*, taking the lead over *An. moucheti* [9]. Insecticide susceptibility tests conducted on several populations from South Cameroon in 2007 indicated that *An. moucheti* is fully susceptible to DDT, permethrin and deltamethrin (Etang *et al.*, unpublished data).

In rural villages situated in deep forest areas, *An. moucheti* usually is the major vector of *Plasmodium*, and quite often the only one maintaining a high level of malaria endemicity in humans. Natural infection rates in the range 1–3% are commonly reported in wild females,

http://dx.doi.org/10.5772/55153

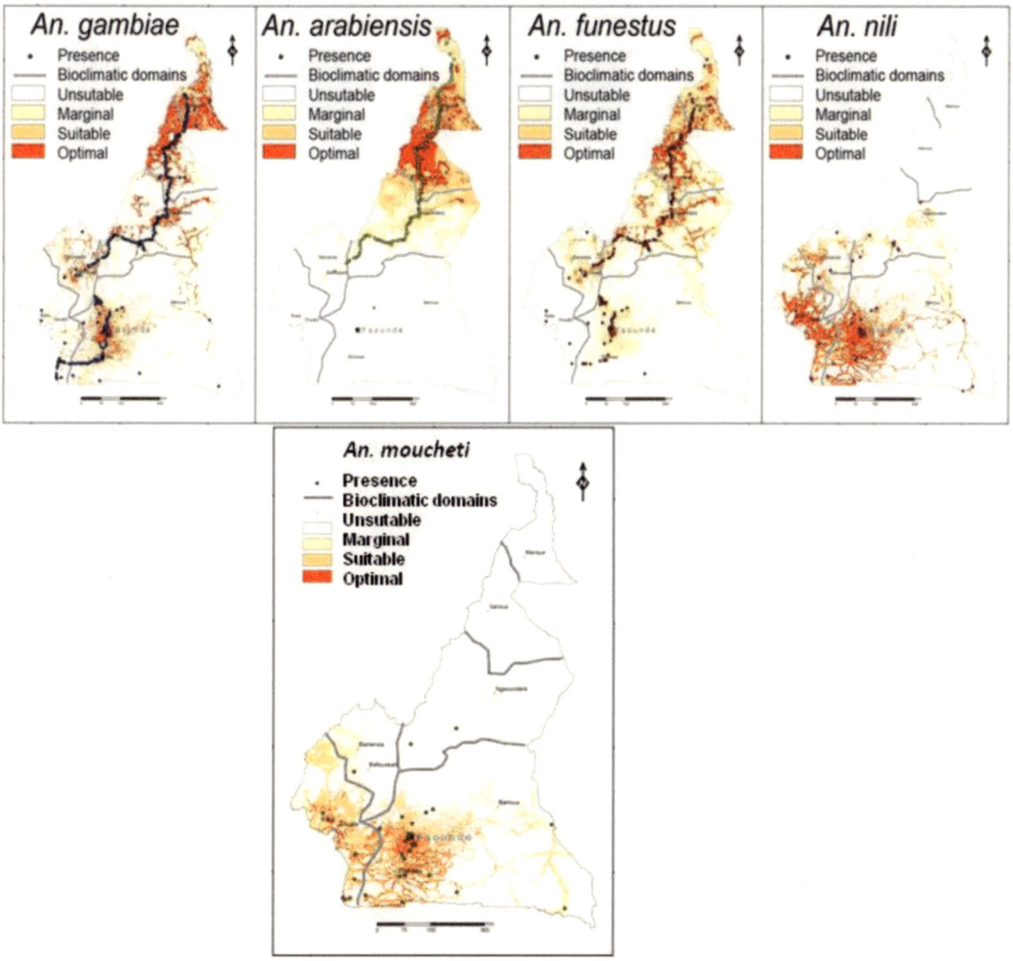

Figure 1. Habitat suitability maps for the five major malaria vectors in Cameroon. A/ *Anopheles gambiae*, *An. arabiensis*, *An. funestus*,, *An. nili*, *An. moucheti*. Different colors identify four classes of habitat quality including optimal (red), suitable (orange), marginal (yellow) and unsuitable habitat (white). Figure drawn from Ayala *et al.*, 2009 [4].

sustaining annual entomological inoculation rates (EIR) reaching up to 300 infective bites/human/year [27, 28]. As such, the species has been incriminated in malaria transmission in a number of countries in Central Africa, including Nigeria [29], Cameroon[28, 30], Gabon [31, 32], Equatorial Guinea [10, 11], Congo [18], the DRC [18] and Uganda [18]. In these settings, *An. moucheti* frequently bites indoors and high densities of blood-fed females can be collected resting indoors, over 95% of which had taken their blood meal on humans demonstrating strong anthropophily. However, high mosquito densities might also be collected far from any human settlements, indicating a probable zoophilic behaviour in some forest populations [33, 34].

Anopheles bervoetsi has only been reported so far from its type locality and surrounding villages in the DRC. Larvae are found in small rivers sheltered by forest galleries that wind through the valleys in a hilly landscape. Adults are highly anthropophilic and preferentially bite

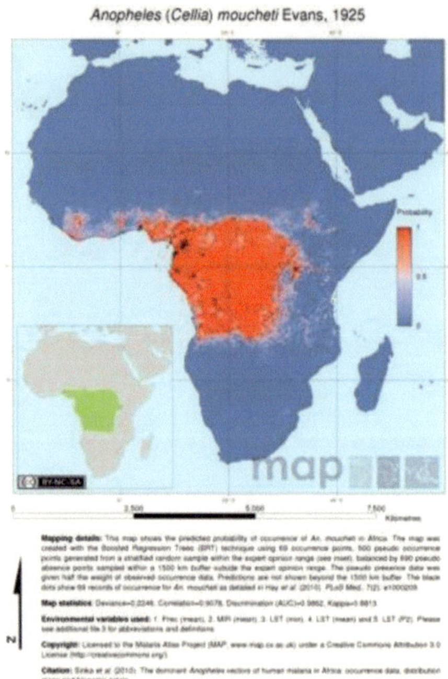

Figure 2. Map of the predicted probability of occurrence of *Anopheles moucheti* in Africa (redrawn from [25]). Black dots represent 69 records of occurrence for *An. moucheti* as described in Hay et al. [26].

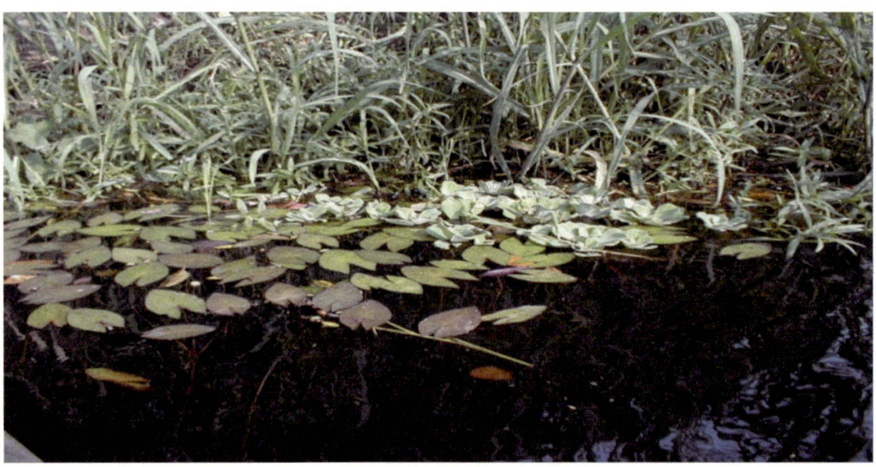

Figure 3. A typical breeding site for *Anopheles moucheti* larvae along river Nyong in southern Cameroon.

outdoors. However, it can be collected biting and resting indoors when abundance is high at the end of the rainy season (Antonio-Nkondjio et al. unpublished data). Biting occurs at night with a peak of activity usually recorded in the second part of the night. A recent study reported three specimens found infected by *Plasmodium falciparum* out of 237 tested by ELISA, confirming its role in malaria parasites transmission [35].

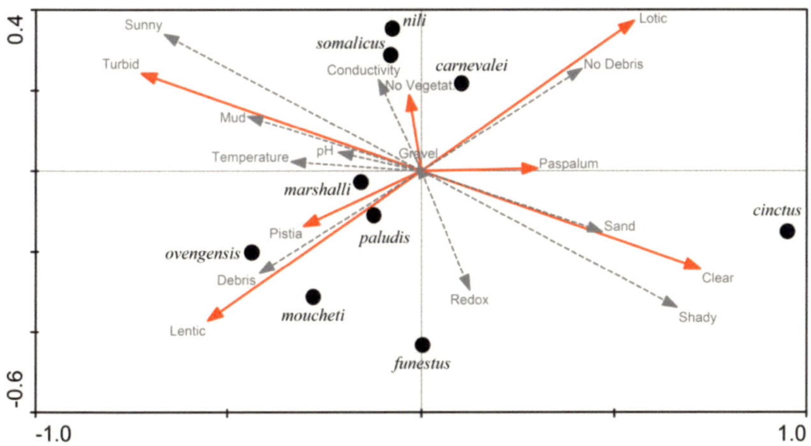

Figure 4. Canonical Correspondence Analysis (CCA) diagram showing the ordination of anopheline species along the first two axes and their correlation with environmental variables. The first axis is horizontal, second vertical. Direction and length of arrows shows the degree of correlation between mosquito larvae and the variables. Figure drawn from Antonio-Nkondjio *et al.*[5].

Anopheles m. nigeriensis is considered as a synonym to *An. moucheti*, due to the absence of reliable morphological differences at the adult and larval stages between the two morphs [19, 24]. Nothing is known of the species bionomics. The only report of its implication in malaria parasites transmission is from Baber and Olinger in 1931 ([18], *loc. cit.*) who reported 1 in 87 mosquitoes infected with sporozoites. Collections conducted in its type locality in 2005 reported few specimens (<10, Antonio-Nkondjio and Simard, unpublished data), probably reflecting habitat deterioration due to the expansion of the urban domain around Lagos.

From morphological analysis (Figure 5), it appears that the type form could display high morphological variation with variants similar to *An. m. nigeriensis* and *An. bervoetsi*. However, genetic investigations and the follow-up of morphological diversity in the progeny of field collected gravid females demonstrated that a single taxon was represented, at least in Cameroon [21]. Population genetic investigations using a set of ten microsatellite markers [36] further strengthened this view, revealing genetic homogeneity between natural populations of *An. moucheti* in South Cameroon and throughout Central Africa, including Uganda and the DRC [36, 37]. Studies comparing sequence variations in nuclear (rDNA Internal Transcribed Spacer 1, ITS2 and the D3 domain of the 28S ribosomal subunit) and mitochondrial (cytochrome b) DNA regions were also concordant, depicting a low level of genetic diversity and differentiation between specimens from Cameroon, Uganda and the DRC and confirming the high genetic homogeneity of *An. moucheti* populations throughout Central Africa [23]. However, when mosquito samples collected from the type localities of *An. bervoetsi* and *An. m. nigeriensis* were included in the analyses, sequence differences were detected between the three taxa, similar in degree to the differences found previously between sibling species within other anopheline groups or complexes [23]. An allele specific PCR assay based on sequence differences in the rDNA ITS1 region was developed to allow rapid identification of each of these three genetic lineages (Figure 6) [23]. Microsatellite analysis further demonstrated significant genetic differentiation between *An. bervoetsi* populations form the DRC and *An. moucheti* populations from Cameroon, suggesting that they represent two different species [35]. In light of accumulating evidences (morphological, behavioral and genetic differences) this taxa was raised to the rank of full species and named *An. bervoetsi* [35] [24]. Yet the issue of the taxonomic status of *An. m. nigeriensis* remains unresolved. It might still be considered as a variant of *An. moucheti* to be further studied.

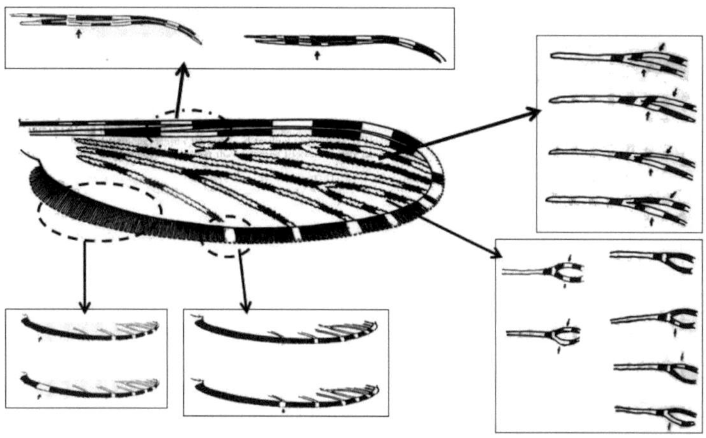

Figure 5. Morphological variations on the wing of *An. moucheti*.

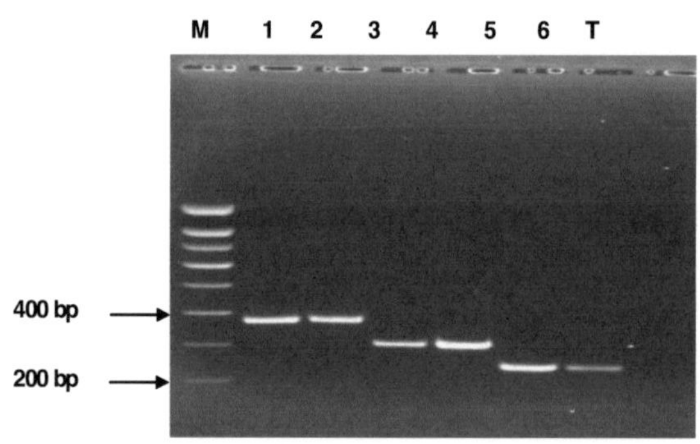

Figure 6. An agarose gel stained with ethidium bromide revealing size differences in the PCR amplification products discriminating *An. moucheti* and closely related species: *An. bervoetsi* (lanes 1 and 2), *An. moucheti* (lanes 3 and 4) and *An. m. nigeriensis* (lanes 5 and 6). Figure from Kengne *et al.*, 2007 [23]

3. Anopheles nili complex

Important morphological, ecological and behavioral differences among natural populations of *Anopheles nili* from sub-Saharan Africa suggested the existence of several taxonomic units and resulted in the description of four formal species, namely: *Anopheles nili sensu stricto*, *An. somalicus*, *An. carnevalei* and *An. ovengensis* [20, 21]. Morphologically, these four species are very close from one another, differing only through subtle morphological characters present at the adult and/or at the larval stages (Figure 7) [18, 38, 39]. Apart from *An. somalicus*, which is zoophilic and was never incriminated in human malaria transmission, the three other members of the complex are highly anthropophilic and are vectors of malaria.

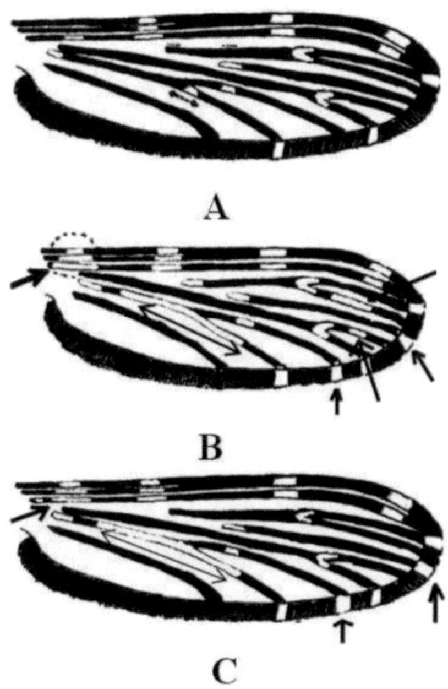

Figure 7. Morphological differences between members of the *An. nili* complex. A: wing of *An. nili* and *An. somalicus*, B: wing of *An. carnevalei*, C: wing of *An. ovengensis*.

Anopheles nili s.s. is among the most important malaria vectors in sub-Saharan Africa. It has a wide geographic distribution range spreading across most of West, Central and East Africa mainly populating humid savannas and degraded rainforest areas (Figure 8) [1, 4, 20, 40]. Larvae thrive at the sunny edge of fast running streams and rivers, where floating vegetation and debris provide suitable shelters (Figure 9) [32]. Forest populations are usually highly anthropophilic and feed regularly indoors whereas savanna populations are more exophilic and exophagic [12, 28]. Despite feeding preferentially on humans, this mosquito can be, at times highly zoophilic [41]. *Anopheles nili* is usually responsible for a high nuisance to humans in villages along rivers, and abundance rapidly decreases within a few kilometers from the breeding sites [42]. It is also present at the periphery of urban areas.

The prevalence of *Plasmodium* infections in wild females typically ranges between 1 and 3%and transmission rate reaching 200 infective bites/human/year have been reported in the literature for *An. nili* [12, 13, 28, 43]. Reports on its epidemiological role in East Africa however, are scarce, dating back to the 1970s [18, 44]. There is no published record available for insecticide susceptibility in *An. nili* populations, although unpublished results from South Cameroon suggest full susceptibility to DDT and pyrethroids (permethrin and deltamethrin) using the diagnostic doses recommended for assessing *An. gambiae* populations (Etang *et al.*, unpublished data). The analysis of key ecological factors associated with the distribution of An. nili larvae across 24 hydrographic networks in Cameroon showed that *An. nili* distribution conforms to that of a generalist species which is adapted in exploiting a variety of environmental conditions (Figure 4).

Anopheles carnevalei and *An. ovengensis* are mainly distributed in deep forest areas where they take over *An. nili s.s.* in this environment [4, 41]. *Anopheles carnevalei* has been reported so far only from Côte d'Ivoire, Cameroon and Equatorial Guinea [10, 11, 38]. It is rarely collected resting indoors and bites more frequently outdoors [12]. This mosquito is mostly zoophilic although it regularly feeds on humans in villages situated close to its breeding sites. Interestingly, although biting activity can be detected all night long, man-biting activity peaks early in the evening, between 6-7 PM, when inhabitants traditionally meet at the river for domestic and body care activities [12]. Studies conducted in Cameroon and Equatorial Guinea reported infection rates *circa* 1% in Cameroon [12, 28], raising up to 24% when using PCR-based protocols for parasite detection in specimens from Equatorial Guinea [10].

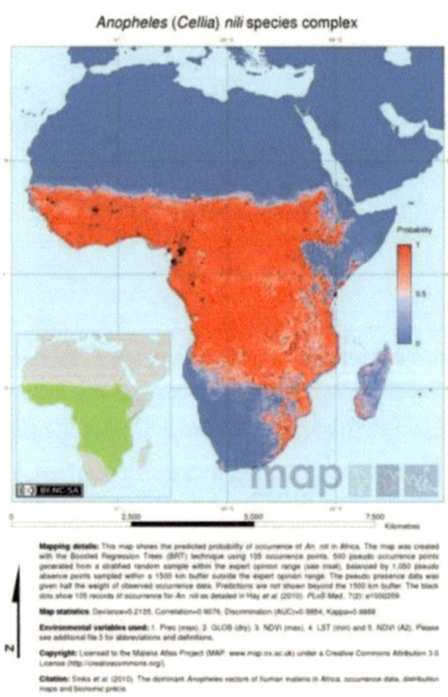

Figure 8. Map of the predicted probability of occurrence of *Anopheles nili* complex in Africa [25]. Black dots represent 105 records of occurrence for *An. nili* complex as described in Hay et al. [26].

Anopheles ovengensis, the most recently described species of the *An. nili* complex, is highly anthropophilic, and bites and rests frequently outdoors [39]. However, studies conducted in Equatorial Guinea reported high densities collected by window exit traps indicating some degree of endophagic and endophilic behavior [11]. *Anopheles ovengensis* usually displays high

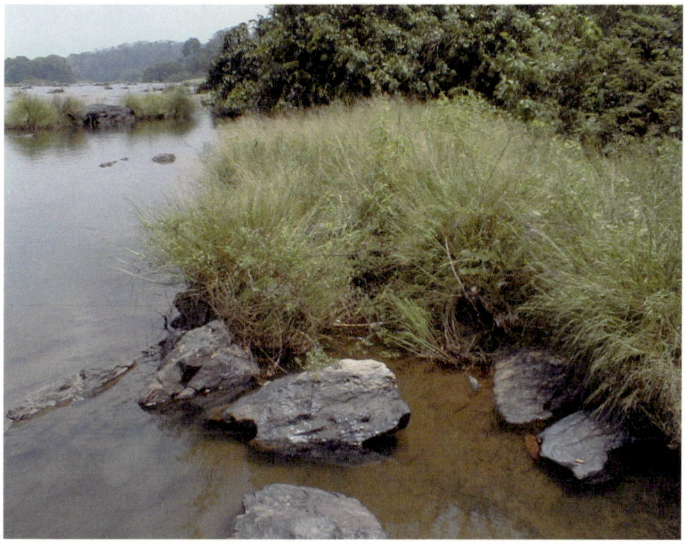

Figure 9. A typical breeding site for *An. nili* along the river Sanaga in South Cameroon.

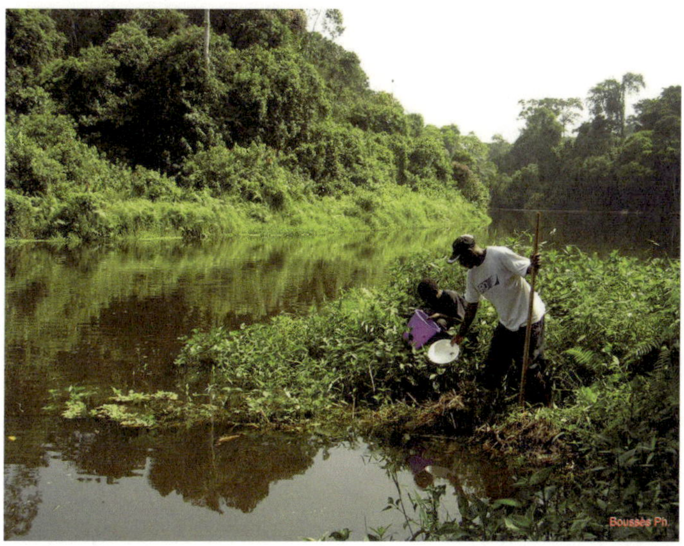

Figure 10. A typical breeding site for *An. ovengensis* along river Njoh in South Cameroon (Photo: P Bousses, IRD/MIVE-GEC).

biting rates for humans, ranging from 50 to 300 bites/man/night along rivers where its larvae develop (Figure 10). Infection rates by *P. falciparum* ranges between 0.4 to 4.4% in specimens from Cameroon [39] and in Equatorial Guinea [11]. Larvae are often found in sympatry with those of *An. moucheti* with whom it shares most of its distribution area. The distribution range of the species probably extends further East, throughout the Congolese forest basin but this has not been investigated yet.

Anopheles somalicus is strictly zoophilic. At the adult stage, *An. somalicus* closely resembles *An. nili* from which it can be morphologically separated at the larval stage only [18]. Adults are rarely recorded in villages although larvae are always found in sympatry with those of *An. nili* [5]. Nothing is known of its bionomics. According to Gillies and De Meillon [18] its distribution range includes Sierra Leone, Guinea, Burkina Faso, Ivory Coast, Cameroon, Somalia and Tanzania.

Genetic studies conducted on the *An. nili* complex using various molecular markers confirmed the high genetic heterogeneity among its members [2]. Multilocus enzyme analysis of the genetic variability detected species-specific alleles and large differences in shared allele frequencies among species of the complex collected in South Cameroon [45]. Analysis of sequence polymorphism in the rDNA ITS2 region estimated genetic distances in the range of 0.11-0.25 between the four species [46]. This heterogeneity in ITS2 DNA sequences was further used to develop a PCR-based protocol for molecular identification of the different species within the complex (Figure 11) [46]. These data provided support for the recent taxonomic classification within the *An. nili* complex [24].

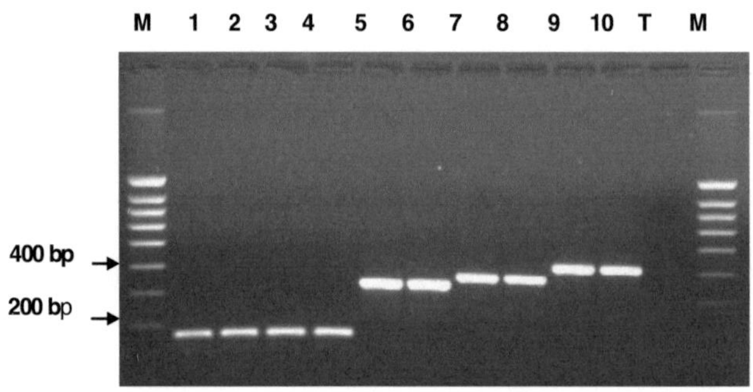

Figure 11. An agarose gel stained with ethidium bromide revealing size differences in the PCR amplification products discriminating between members of the *An. nili* complex: *An. nili* (lanes 1 to 4), *An. somalicus* (lanes 5 and 6), *An. ovengensis* (lanes 7 and 8) and *An. carnevalei* (lanes 9 and 10). Figure from Kengne *et al.*, 2003 [46].

Microsatellite loci were developed in 2003 to allow for more in-depth population genetics investigations [47]. A first comprehensive study explored the level of genetic variability and differentiation between nine populations of *An. nili* distributed in West and central Africa, including samples from Senegal, Ivory Coast, Burkina Faso, Nigeria, Cameroon and the DRC using a set of 11 microsatellite markers and sequence variation in four genes within the nuclear rDNA subunit (ITS2 and D3) and mtDNA (COII and ND4). High genetic homogeneity was revealed among *An. nili* populations distributed from Senegal to Cameroon, suggesting shallow population substructure throughout the humid savannas of West Africa, in agreement with a weak effect of geographic distance [48]. However, the population sampled in DRC was highly significantly differentiated from the core of West African populations (F_{ST}>0.118, P<0.001), and all individuals segregated into a single genetic cluster separated from all other West African populations in Bayesian cluster analysis (Figure 12). Sequence variation in mtDNA genes matched these results, whereas low polymorphism in rDNA genes prevented detection of any population substructure at this geographical scale in savannah populations [48]. Extensive allele sharing between populations and homogeneity across microsatellite loci in the level of genetic differentiation suggested that enhanced genetic drift in the DRC population, rather than selection was responsible for the observed pattern.

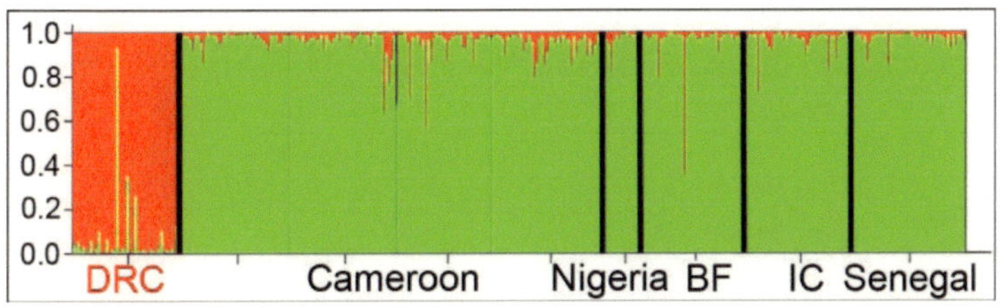

Figure 12. Bayesian genetic cluster analysis of microsatellite allele frequencies in *An. nili s.l.* populations. Genetic homogeneity within savannah populations of *An. nili s.s.* from West/Central Africa and high genetic drift in the DRC population.

In Cameroon, the pattern of genetic differentiation was explored among species within the *An. nili* complex and between populations of *An. nili* collected in different ecological settings including the deep evergreen forest, deforested areas and savannah areas. The average observed heterozygosity varied from 0.359 for *An. ovengensis* to 0.661 for *An. nili s.s.* and mean pairwise F_{ST} over all loci varied from 0.281 (between *An. nili* and *An. carnevalei*) to 0.416 (between *An. somalicus* and *An. ovengensis*) and were highly significant (P<0.0001) [45]. The limited number of loci which could readily amplify and the high proportion of loci departing from Hardy-Weinberg equilibrium in samples collected from the deep forest region suggested the presence of new taxonomic units in this area. Up to seven clusters could be identified in *An. nili* after processing Bayesian cluster analysis (Figure 13). Two of these clusters were specific for *An. nili* populations collected in the East Cameroon forest area, suggesting that *An. nili* from East Cameroon may consist of four new taxa. Data obtained from microsatellites analysis were consistent with the high genetic distance measured with rDNA and mtDNA genes [49].

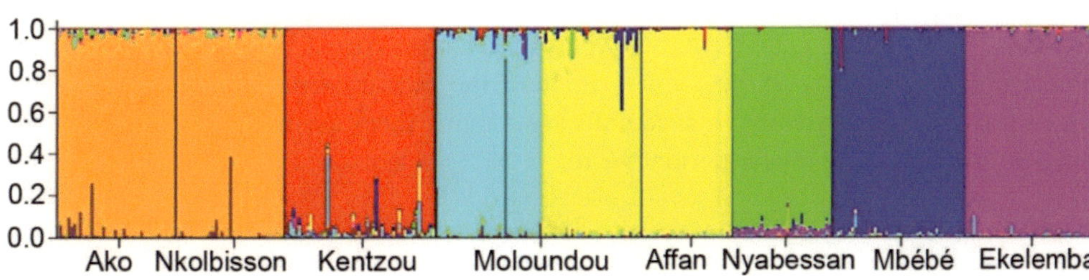

Figure 13. Bayesian genetic cluster analysis of microsatellite allele frequencies in *An. nili s.l.* populations. Genetic heterogeneity between forest populations of *An. nili s.l.* in South Cameroon showing genetic clustering of *An. carnevalei* (yellow), *An. ovengensis* (green), *An. somalicus* (dark blue) and the four genetic clusters suggesting further taxonomic subdivision within *An. nili s.s.* in this area.

Recently, cytogenetic analysis depicted a physical chromosome map for *An. nili* upon which nine microsatellite markers could be mapped (Figure 14) [50, 51]. Chromosomal arm homology with *An. gambiae* was assessed by fluorescent *in situ* hybridization of DNA probes which established that chromosomes X, 2R and 3R are homologous between the two species, while the 2L arm of *An. gambiae* corresponds to the 3L arm of *An. nili*, and vice versa [50]. Preliminary analysis of chromosomal polymorphism in natural *An. nili* populations from Burkina Faso and Cameroon demonstrated that two polymorphic inversions, named 2R*b* and 2R*c*, are often present simultaneously on the right arm of chromosome 2 [50, 51].

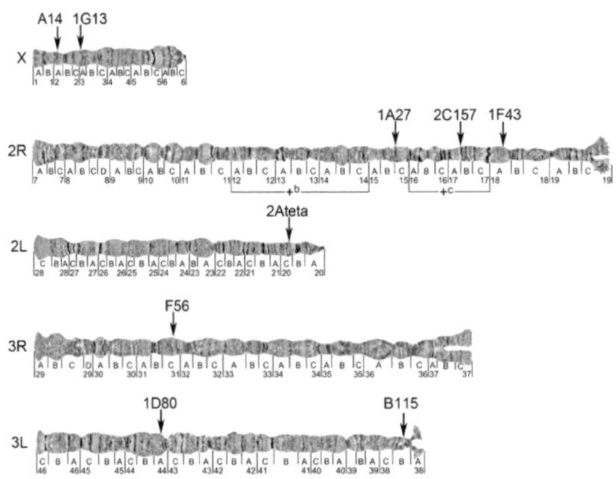

Figure 14. Physical chromosome map of *An. nili* showing the cytological location of the nine microsatellite markers mapped on polytene chromosomes (arrows). Two chromosomal inversions are indicated by brackets. Figure from Peery *et al.*, 2011 [51].

Frequencies of inverted and standard 2R*b* variants were almost equal in the savannah areas of Burkina Faso, albeit with strong deficit in heterozygotes (Fis=+0.603, P<0.0001). In forest areas of Cameroon, only the standard arrangement was found. It is postulated that this inversion may be involved in local ecological or behavioral adaptation in *An. nili* [50]. Inversion 2R*c* occurred at high frequency in Burkina Faso (83%) while its frequency was only 0.6% in samples from Cameroon, suggesting its involvement in ecogeographic cline from dry to more humid environments. Because *An. nili* is a forest-savannah transition species, polymorphic inversions could provide genetic plasticity that allowed its expansion into dry savannah and deforested areas of central Africa, where most of the human population is present. High frequencies of these inversions in savannah areas make them useful markers for studying ecological adaptations of this important vector.

4. Conclusion

Most of the work on malaria vectors has been conducted in the savannah environment, whereas principal vectors and their roles in malaria transmission in the immense African rainforest have barely been explored. Therefore, data are crucially lacking for a large part of Africa where malaria transmission is both intense and permanent throughout the year. Recent results demonstrated high levels of differentiation between populations/species of *An. moucheti* and the *An. nili* complex over short geographic distances within the forest block but not in the savannah. These data suggest that, unlike other major vectors, these mosquitoes originated and speciated in the equatorial forest. Because malaria elimination in forested areas is most difficult, detailed understanding of the genetic structure, gene flow, and species diversity of malaria vectors is important. Original information gained on the genetic structure of *An. moucheti* and *An. nili* can further be used to investigate genes for a signature of selection to uncover the genetic mechanisms of ecological adaptations, speciation, and susceptibility to *Plasmodium*, within a comparative framework that will use information available for other major human malaria vectors. Furthermore, because some species/populations within *An. moucheti* and the *An. nili* complex are highly exophagic/exophilic and can bite man as well as other vertebrates in remote areas, they are likely candidates for acting as bridge vectors, providing opportunities for wildlife pathogens to cause zoonosis in humans. These findings raise a concern in the light of recent reports confirming the circulation of various *Plasmodium* species, including strains of *P. falciparum*, in chimpanzees, gorillas, and guenons in the equatorial forest region [52].

Acknowledgements

Part of the work reported in this manuscript was supported by grants no. A00942, A20727, A60347 from the UNDP/World Bank/WHO Special programme for Research and Training in Tropical Diseases (TDR) to C.A.N, a Wellcome Trust Intermediate Fellowship in Public Health and Tropical Medecine (WTO86423MA) to CAN, the NIH grant R21 AI079350, the Pal+ programme from the French Ministry of Research and the French Institut de Recherche pour le Développement (IRD/MIVEGEC).

Author details

Christophe Antonio-Nkondjio[1,2*] and Frédéric Simard[3]

*Address all correspondence to: antonio_nk@yahoo.fr

1 Laboratoire de Recherche sur le Paludisme, Organisation de Coordination pour la lutte Contre les Endémies en Afrique Centrale (OCEAC), Yaoundé, Cameroon

2 Faculty of Health Sciences University of Bamenda, Bambili, Cameroon

3 Institut de Recherche pour le Développement (IRD), UMR IRD -CNRS 5290-Université de Montpellier 1-Université de Montpellier 2 MIVEGEC (Maladies Infectieuses et Vecteurs : Ecologie, Génétique, Evolution et Contrôle), Montpellier Cedex 5, France

References

[1] Mouchet J, Carnevale P, Coosemans M, Julvez J, Manguin S, Richard-Lenoble D, Sircoulon J: Biodiversité du paludisme dans le monde: Paris: John Libbey Eurotext; 2004.

[2] Fontenille D, Simard F: Unravelling complexities in human malaria transmission dynamics in Africa through a comprehensive knowledge of vector populations. *Comp Immun Microbiol Infect Dis* 2004, 27:357 - 375.

[3] malERA Consultative Group on Vector Control: A research agenda for malaria eradication: vector control. *PLoS Med* 2011, 25(8):e1000401.

[4] Ayala D, Costantini C, Ose K, Kamdem G, Antonio-Nkondjio C, Agbor J, Awono-Ambene P, Fontenille D, Simard F: Habitat suitability and ecological niche profile of major malaria vectors in Cameroon. *Malar J* 2009, 8:307.

[5] Antonio-Nkondjio C, Ndo C, Costantini C, Awono-Ambene H, Fontenille D, Simard F: Distribution and larval habitat characterization of *Anopheles nili* and *An. moucheti* along river networks in south Cameroon. *Acta Trop* 2009, 112:270 - 276.

[6] Moffett A, Shackelford N, Sarkar S: Malaria in Africa: vector species' niche models and relative risk maps. *PLoS ONE* 2007, 2:e824.

[7] Sinka M, Bangs M, Manguin S, Rubio-Palis Y, Chareonviriyaphap T, Coetzee M, Mbogo C, Hemingway J, Patil A, Temperley W *et al*: A global map of dominant malaria vectors. *Parasites & Vectors* 2012, 5(1):69.

[8] Antonio-Nkondjio C, Awono-Ambene H, Toto J, Meunier J, Zebaze-Kemleu S, Nyambam R, Wondji C, Tchuinkam T, Fontenille D: High malaria transmission intensity in sub-urban area of Yaounde: the capital city of Cameroon. *J Med Entomol* 2002, 39:350 - 355.

[9] Antonio-Nkondjio C, Simard F, Awono-Ambene P, Ngassam P, Toto J, Tchuinkam T, Fontenille D: Malaria vectors and urbanization in the equatorial forest region of south Cameroon. *Trans R Soc Trop Med Hyg* 2005, 99:347 - 354.

[10] Cano J, Descalzo M, Moreno M, Chen Z, Nzambo S, Bobuakasi L, Buatiche J, Ondo M, Micha F, Benito A: Spatial variability in the density, distribution and vectorial capacity of anopheline species in a high transmission village (Equatorial Guinea). *Malar J* 2006, 23:21.

[11] Ridl F, Bass C, Torrez M, Govender D, Ramdeen V, Yellot L, Edu A, Schwabe C, Mohloai P, Maharaj R *et al*: A pre-intervention study of malaria vector abundance in Rio Muni, Equatorial Guinea: their role in malaria transmission and the incidence of insecticide resistance alleles. *Malar J* 2008, 7:194.

[12] Awono-Ambene P, Antonio-Nkondjio C, Toto J, Ndo C, Etang J, Fontenille D, Simard F: Epidemological importance of the *Anopheles nili* group of malaria vectors in equatorial villages of Cameroon, Central Africa. *Sci Med Afr* 2009, 1:13 - 20.

[13] Carnevale P, Le Goff G, Toto J, Robert V: *Anopheles nili* as the main vector of human malaria in villages of southern Cameroon. *Med Vet Entomol* 1992, 6:135 - 138.

[14] Takken W, Knols B: Malaria vector control: current and future strategies. *Trends Parasitol* 2009, 25:101 - 104.

[15] Prugnolle F, Durand P, Neel C, Ollomo B, Ayala D, Arnathau C, Etienne L, Mpoudi-Ngole E, Nkoghe D, Leroy E *et al*: African great apes are natural hosts of multiple related malaria species, including *Plasmodium falciparum*. *Proc Natl Acad Sci U S A* 2010, 107:1458 - 1463.

[16] Prugnolle F, Ollomo B, Durand P, Yalcindag E, Arnathau C, Elguero E, Berry A, Pourrut X, Gonzalez J, Nkoghe D *et al*: Africa monkeys are infected by *Plasmodium falciparum* nonhuman primate-specific strains. *Proc Natl Acad Sci U S A* 2011, 108:11948 - 11953.

[17] Duval L, Fourment M, Nerrienet E, Rousset D, Sadeuh S, Goodman S, Andriaholinirina N, Randrianarivelojosia M, Paul R, Robert V *et al*: African apes as reservoir of *Plasmodium falciparum* and the origin and diversification of the *Laverania* subgenus. *Proc Natl Acad Sci U S A* 2010, 107:10561 - 10566.

[18] Gillies M, De Meillon B: The Anophelinae of Africa South of the Sahara. *South Africa Institute of Medical Research Johannesburg, South Africa* 1968.

[19] Brunhes J, Le Goff G, Manga L, Geoffroy B: *Anopheles* afro-tropicaux. IV - Mise au point sur les espèces et sous-espèces du groupe *Anopheles* (Cellia) *moucheti*; rehabilitation d'*An.* (C.) *multicinctus* et d'*An.* (Cellia) *garnhami* basilewskyi. *Annales de la Société Entomologique de France* 1998, 34:397 - 405.

[20] Gillies M, Coetzee M: A supplement to the Anophelinae of Africa south of the Sahara (Afrotropical region). *Pub South Afr Inst Med Res* 1987, 55:143.

[21] Antonio-Nkondjio C, Simard F, Cohuet A, Fontenille D: Morphological variability in *Anopheles moucheti* is not indicative of speciation: evidences from sympatric south Cameroon populations. *Infect Genet Evol* 2002, 2:69 - 72.

[22] Fontenille D, Cohuet A, Awono-Ambene H, Antonio-Nkondjio C, Wondji C, Kengne P, Dia I, Boccolini J, Duchemin J, Rajaonarivelo V *et al*: Systématique et biologie des anophèles vecteurs de *Plasmodium* en Afrique, données récentes. *Med Trop* 2003, 63:247 - 253.

[23] Kengne P, Antonio-Nkondjio C, Awono-Ambene H, Simard F, Awolola T, Fontenille D: Molecular differentiation of three closely related members of the mosquito species complex *Anopheles moucheti*, by mitochondrial and ribosomal DNA polymorphism. *Med Vet Entomol* 2007, 21:177 - 182.

[24] Harbach R: *Anopheles* classification. Mosquito Taxonomic Inventory. *http://mosquito-taxonomic-inventoryinfo/* 2012.

[25] Sinka M, Bangs M, Manguin S, Coetzee M, Mbogo C, Hemingway J, Patil A, Temperley W, Gething P, Kabaria C *et al*: The dominant *Anopheles* vectors of human malaria in Africa, Europe and the Middle East: occurrence data, distribution maps and bionomic precis. *Parasit Vectors* 2010, 3:117.

[26] Hay S, Sinka M, Okara R, Kabaria C, Mbithi P, Tago C, Benz D, Gething P, Howes R, Patil A *et al*: Developing global maps of the dominant *Anopheles* vectors of human malaria. *PLoS Med* 2010, 7:e1000209.

[27] Njan Nloga A, Robert V, Toto J, Carnevale P: *Anopheles moucheti*, vecteur principal du paludisme au sud-Cameroun. *Bulletin de Liaison et de Documentation de l'OCEAC* 1993, 26:63 - 67.

[28] Antonio-Nkondjio C, Kerah C, Simard F, Awono-Ambene H, Mouhamadou C, Tchuinkam T, Fontenille D: Complexity of malaria vectorial system in Cameroon: contribution of secondary vectors to malaria transmission. *J Med Entomol* 2006, 43:1215 - 1221.

[29] Awolola T, Okwa O, Hunt R, Ogunrinade A, Coetzee M: Dynamics of malaria vector populations in coastal Lagos, south-western Nigeria. *Ann Trop Med Parasitol* 2002, 96:75 - 82.

[30] Njan Nloga A, Robert V, Toto J, Carnevale P: *Anopheles moucheti*, vecteur principal du paludisme au sud-Cameroun. *Bull Liais Doc OCEAC* 1993, 26:63 - 67.

[31] Elissa N, Karch S, Bureau P, Ollomo B, Lawoko M, Yangari P, Ebang B, Georges A: Malaria transmission in a region of savanna-forest mosaic, Haut-Ogooue, Gabon. *J Am Mosq Control Assoc* 1999, 15:15 - 23.

[32] Sylla E, Kun J, Kremsner P: Mosquito distribution and entomological inoculation rates in three malaria-endemic areas in Gabon. *Trans R Soc Trop Med Hyg* 2000, 94:652 - 656.

[33] Njan Nloga A: Bioécologie et rôle vecteur du paludisme d'*Anopheles moucheti* à Ebogo au Cameroun. *Thèse de doctorat Université de Montpellier II Sciences et Techniques du Languedoc* 1994:233p.

[34] Livadas G, Mouchet J, Gariou J, Chastang R: Peut-on envisager l'eradication du paludisme dans la region forestiere du Sud-Cameroun? *Revista di Malariologia* 1958, 37:229 - 256.

[35] Antonio-Nkondjio C, Ndo C, Kengne P, Mukwaya L, Awono-Ambene H, Fontenille D, Simard F: Population structure of the malaria vector *Anopheles moucheti* in the equatorial forest region of Africa. *Malar J* 2008, 7:120.

http://dx.doi.org/10.5772/55153

[36] Antonio-Nkondjio C, Ndo C, Awono-Ambene H, Ngassam P, Fontenille D, Simard F: Population genetic structure of the malaria vector *An. moucheti* in south Cameroon forest region. *Acta Trop* 2007, 101:61 - 68.

[37] Annan Z, Kengne P, Berthomieu A, Antonio-Nkondjio C, Rousset F, Fontenille D, Weill M: Isolation and characterisation of polymorphic microsatellite markers from the mosquito *Anopheles moucheti,* malaria vector in Africa. *Mol Ecol Notes* 2003, 3:56 - 57.

[38] Brunhes J, LeGoff G, Geoffroy B: Afro-tropical anopheline mosquitoes: description of three new species: *Anopheles carnevalei* sp. nov., *An. hervyi* sp. nov and *An. dualaensis* sp. nov., and resurrection of *An. rageaui* Mattingly and Adam. *J Am Mosq Control Assoc* 1999, 15:552 - 558.

[39] Awono-Ambene H, Kengne P, Simard F, Antonio-Nkondjio C, Fontenille D: Description and bionomics of *Anopheles* (Cellia) *ovengensis* (Diptera: Culicidae), a new malaria vector species of the *Anopheles nili* group from south Cameroon. *J Med Entomol* 2004, 41:561 - 568.

[40] Okara R, Sinka M, Minakawa N, Mbogo C, Hay S, Snow R: Distribution of the main malaria vectors in Kenya. *Malar J* 2010, 9:69.

[41] Antonio-Nkondjio C, Meunier J, Awono-Ambene H, Fontenille D: La présence de bovins comme hôte alternatifs peut elle modifier le comportement trophique des vecteurs du paludisme en zone de forêt ? *Sciences et Médecines d'Afrique* 2009, 1:7 - 12.

[42] Le Goff G, Carnevale P, Robert V: Low dispersion of anopheline malaria vectors in the African equatorial forest. *Parasite* 1997, 2:187 - 189.

[43] Adja A, N'goran K, Kengne P, Koudou G, Toure M, Koffi A, Tia E, Fontenille D, Chandre F: Transmission vectorielle du paludisme en savane arborée à Ganse en Cote d'Ivoire. *Med Trop* 2006, 66:449 - 455.

[44] Krafsur E: *Anopheles nili* as a vector of malaria in a lowland region of Ethiopia. *Bulletin of the World Health Organization* 1970, 42:466 - 471.

[45] Awono-Ambene H, Simard F, Antonio-Nkondjio C, Cohuet A, Kengne P, Fontenille D: Multilocus enzyme electrophoresis supports speciation within the *Anopheles nili* group of Malaria vectors in Cameroon. *Am J Trop Med Hyg* 2006, 75:656 - 658.

[46] Kengne P, Awono-Ambene H, Antonio-Nkondjio C, Simard F, Fontenille D: Molecular identification of the *Anopheles nili* group African malaria vectors. *Med Vet Entomol* 2003, 17:67 - 74.

[47] Berthomieu A, Kengne P, Awono-Ambene H, Raymond M, Fontenille D, Weill M: Isolation and characterization of microsatellite DNA markers in the malaria vector *Anopheles nili*. *Mol Ecol Notes* 2003, 3:392 - 393.

[48] Ndo C, Antonio-Nkondjio C, Cohuet A, Ayala D, Kengne P, Morlais I, Awono-Ambene P, Couret D, Ngassam P, Fontenille D *et al*: Population genetic structure of the malaria vector *Anopheles nili* in sub-Saharan Africa. *Malaria Journal* 2010, 9(1):161.

[49] Ndo C: Bioécologie et structure génétique des populations d'*Anopheles moucheti* sl et d'*Anopheles nili* vecteurs majeurs du paludisme en Afrique subsaharienne. *Thèse de Doctorat PhD Faculté des Sciences Université de Yaoundé I Cameroun* 2011:286p.

[50] Sharakhova M, Antonio-Nkondjio C, Xia A, Ndo C, Awono-Ambene H, Simard F, Sharakhov I: Cytogenetic map for *Anopheles nili*: Application for population genetics and comparative physical mapping. *Infection, Genetics and Evolution* 2010, 11:746 - 754.

[51] Peery A, Sharakhova M, Antonio-Nkondjio C, Ndo C, Weill M, Simard F, Sharakhov I: Improving the population genetics toolbox for the study of the African malaria vector *Anopheles nili*: microsatellite mapping to chromosomes. *Parasites & Vectors* 2011, 4:202.

[52] Liu W, Li Y, Learn G, Rudicell R, Robertson J, Keele B, Ndjango J, Sanz C, Morgan D, Locatelli S *et al*: Origin of the human malaria parasite *Plasmodium falciparum* in gorillas. *Nature* 2010, 467(7314):420 - 425.

Chapter 9

The Dominant Mosquito Vectors of Human Malaria in India

Vas Dev and Vinod P. Sharma

Additional information is available at the end of the chapter

http://dx.doi.org/10.5772/55215

1. Introduction

In India malaria endemicity is characterized by diverse ecology and multiple disease vector species [1]. In the Southeast Asian region, India alone contributes to nearly 80% of malaria cases with the largest population of the world living at risk of malaria. In 2011, India reported 1.3 million confirmed malaria cases and 753 attributable deaths, but estimated cases and deaths are 10 to 20 times more [2,3]. Of the two *Plasmodium* prevalent in India, *Plasmodium falciparum* incidence has not declined significantly although *P. vivax* has resulting in the rising trend of the former parasite to presently contributing ~50% of the reported cases. Distribution and spread of chloroquine resistance and emergence of multi-drug resistant strains may have contributed to this phenomenon [4]. Even though transmission intensities across India are low-to-moderate, disease remains geographically entrenched in poor marginalized population groups particularly living in remote/ forest fringe/ tribal belts of eastern, central and north-eastern states for contributing >65% of malarial episodes [5,6].

Mosquito fauna is rich in the tropical climate with numerous and diverse breeding resources [7]. Of 58 anophelines in India, only six taxa are major malaria vectors with regional distribution (Figure 1). *Anopheles culicifacies s.l.* is the vector of rural malaria in the country and generates about 65% of cases annually. *An. fluviatilis s.l.* is found in the plains and foothills breeding in streams contributing 15% of malaria cases, *An. minimus* breeds in streams of foothills of the northeast, *An. dirus s.l.* is found in jungles of northeastern states, *An. sundaicus* is found in Andaman and Nicobar islands and breeds in brackish water, and *An. stephensi* is the well known vector species of urban malaria. All these mosquito species except *An. stephensi* have been characterized as species complexes with number of morphologically indistinguishable sibling species which vary for their role in malaria transmission [8].

India is experiencing rapid ecological changes owing to population explosion, urbanization, development projects, deforestation and human migration affecting mosquito ecology and disease transmission. In the recent past, significant progress has been made in understanding the genetics and bionomics of the disease vectors, and in the development of newer control tools to strengthen primary healthcare services specific to India [9-14]. In this chapter we shall restrict systematic review on dominant *Anopheles* vectors of human malaria and their current bionomics to help develop malaria-risk maps for strengthening malaria control for sustainable interventions with ultimate goal of malaria elimination.

2. *Anopheles (Cellia) culicifacies* Giles species complex

Anopheles culicifaciess.l. is widely distributed in India and has been recorded in all mainland zones including Kashmir and high elevations in the Himalayas (up to 3000 meters) except islands of Andaman & Nicobar and Lakshadweep [7,8,11]. It is the most important vector in plains of rural India contributing 60-70% of reported cases annually [15]. Success stories in malaria control during 1950-1960, and malaria resurgence in the 1970s deal primarily with the control of *An. culicifacies s.l.* Biology and genetics of *An. culicifacies* has been extensively studied in India [16-17], and presently characterized to be a species complex with five informally designated species A, B, C, D and E. These five sibling species are spread across India with distinct biological characteristics and role in malaria transmission (Table 1).

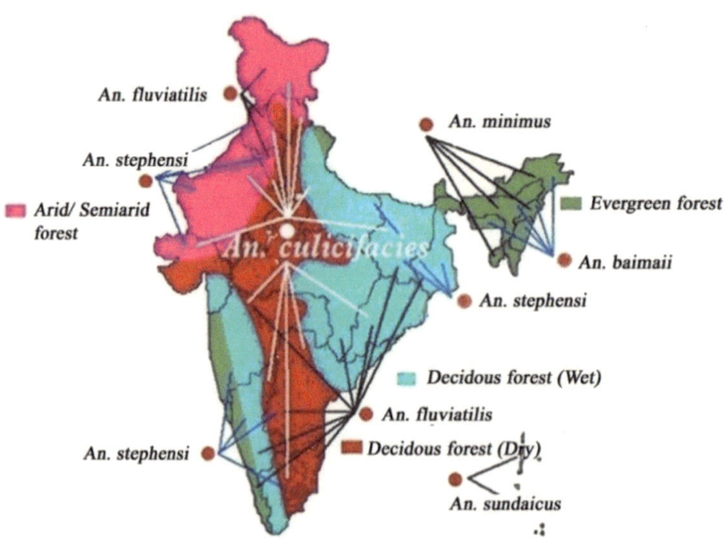

Figure 1. Map of India showing distribution of major malaria vectors in relation to physiogeographic regions encompassing evergreen tropical forest (wet zone receiving rainfall >200 cm), deciduous wet forest (monsoon forests receiving rainfall 100-200 cm), deciduous dry forest (scrub forest receiving rainfall 50-100 cm), and desert forest (arid and semi-arid area receiving rainfall <50 cm) annually.

Sibling species were initially characterized by species specific diagnostic fixed paracentric inversions readable in polytene chromosomes suggestive of pre-mating barriers in field populations [18-24], and further substantiated by number of techniques including post-zygotic isolation mechanisms in laboratory conditions [25], mitotic karyotype Y- chromosome polymorphism [26-28], gene enzyme variation [29], cuticular hydrocarbon profiles [30], and species specific DNA probes [31]. Recently, PCR-based diagnostic assays were developed for sequencing 28S-D3 domain [32], ITS2-PCR-RFLP [33], rDNA ITS2 region [34], which grouped *An. culicifacies* sibling species into two distinct groups namely Group I (species A/D) and Group II (species B/C/E). In another assay from COII region, A/D specific primers distinguished species A and D, and B/C/E specific primers distinguished B, C and E [35]. More recently, a multiplex PCR–based diagnostic assay using D2 domain of 28S rDNA has been reported which can consistently and accurately discriminate members of the species complex forming two unambiguous monophyly clades of species A/D (Group I) and species B/C and E (Group 2) which were supported by strong bootstrap values [36].

Characteristic	Sibling species				
	A	B	C	D	E**
Inversion genotype	$X+^{a}+^{b}$; $2+g^{1}+h^{1}$; $+i^{1}/i^{1}$	Xab; $2g^{1}+h^{1}$	Xab; $2+g^{1}h^{1}$	$X+^{a}+^{b}$; $2i^{1}+h^{1}$	Xab; $2g^{1}+h^{1}$;
Anthropophilic Index (%)	0-4	0-1	0-3	0-1	80
Biting activity (Peak biting activity)	All night (2200-2300 h)	All night (2200-2300 h)	All night (1800-2100 h)	Till midnight (1800-2100 h)	No data
Vector potential	Moderate	Poor	Moderate	Moderate	High
Sporozoite infection rate (%)	0.51	0.04	0.3	0.4	20
Breeding preferences	Rainwater, clean irrigation water	Riverine ecology	Rainwater, clean irrigation water	Rainwater, clean irrigation water	Riverine ecology
Rate of development of resistance					
DDT	Slow (9-10 yr)	Fast (4-5 years)	Fast (4-5 years)	No data	No data
Malathion	Slow (9-10 yr)	Medium (6-7 years)	Fast (4-5 years)	No data	No data
Pyrethroids	No data	Medium (6-7 years)	Medium (6-7 years)	No data	No data

*Source Reference No. 16, 37. **In Rameshwaram island of Tamilnadu

Table 1. Inversion genotype and biological characteristics of *Anophelesculicifacies* sibling species complex in India*

The distribution, relative abundance and predominance of sibling species (but not exclusive) is given in Figure 2. Among its sibling species, species B is the most predominant throughout the country and occurs sympatrically in most areas with predominance of species A in the north and species B in the south [37]. In eastern Uttar Pradesh, north Bihar and northeastern states, species B is either predominant or the only prevalent species. Species B and C are sympatric in western and eastern India. Species D is sympatric with species A and B in northwestern region, and with species A, B and C in central southern India. Species E is sympatric with species B in southern Tamilnadu including Rameshwaram islands. The proportions of sibling species, however, varied in different geographical zones and seasons, e.g., in Alwar (state of Rajasthan), species B proportions increased in post-monsoon months; whereas proportions of species D remained the same throughout the year and density of species C remained very low [38].

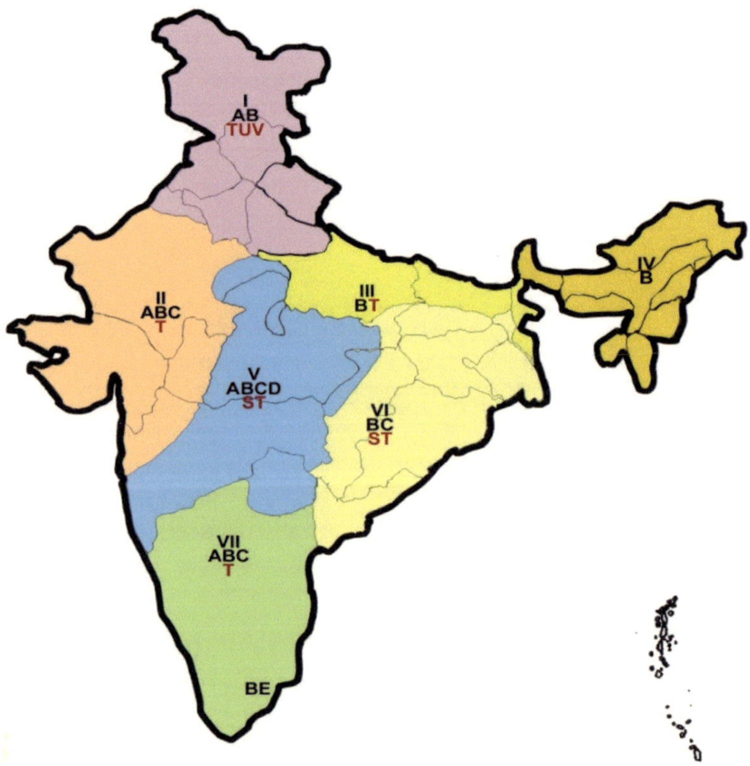

Figure 2. Map of India showing geographical distribution of predominant sibling species of *Anopheles culicifacies* complex (A,B,C,D,E) and *An. fluviatilis* complex (S,T,U, form V), and stratification (Divisions I –VII) for suggested vector control options. For control of *An. culicifacies* malaria vectors in Division I & III: No routine vector control is necessary except for treatment of imported cases of malaria; Division II: Insecticide spraying based on susceptibility status of *An. culicifacies* species A or C; Division IV: DDT spraying to continue; Division V–VII: Insecticide spraying based on susceptibility status of *An. culicifacies* species C. For control of *An. fluviatilis* malaria vectors, even though DDT remains the insecticide of choice, in areas where it is sympatric with *An. culicifacies,* insecticide spraying used for control of latter should be applied. Source Reference No. 37.

All member sibling species of the *An. culicifacies* complex are predominantly zoophilic except species E, and rest indoors in human dwellings and cattle sheds [39]. All are night biting species with different peak biting activity (Table 1). The main strategy for malaria control in areas of *An. culicifacies* distribution is by indoor spraying of residual insecticides chosen based on their susceptibility status in the given region. Presently, *An. culicifacies* has developed resistance to most insecticides in use including malathion (except certain areas) leaving the only option of pyrethroid use for which there are already reports of increased tolerance [40-45]. Molecular characterization revealed a low frequency of the *kdr* allele (mostly in heterozygous condition) in field populations that were resistant to DDT and pyrethroids [46,47]. Based on the geographical distribution of sibling species, the country is now stratified into seven divisions for benefit of prioritizing control options, e.g., for division I and III, no routine control interventions are required, whereas for divisions II, IV - VII, insecticide spraying is necessary based on susceptibility status against the dominant vector species (Figure 2).

An. culicifacies is indeed a prolific breeder and breeding sites are numerous including riverbed pools, rain water collections (Figure 3), streams, rice-fields, seepage water, borrow pits, irrigation channels, etc [7,11]. It has been incriminated by detection of gut and salivary gland infections by numerous independent investigators across its range of distribution throughout India [7]. Further studies using immunoradiometric analysis revealed that sibling species A, C, D and E are vectors of *Plasmodium vivax* and *P. falciparum* malaria, and species B is non-vector or poor vector [48]. Among these, species E was observed to be highly anthropophilic in Rameswaram islands of Tamilnadu [49]. These observations were further supported by comparative reproductive fitness for which sibling species B was observed to be less fit than species A and C of the complex as well as susceptibility to malaria sporogony [50-52].

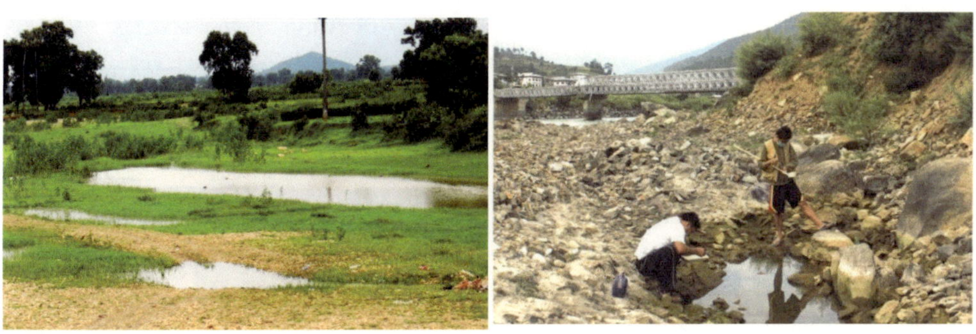

Figure 3. Breeding habitats of *Anopheles culicifacies* (left – rain water pools; right – river bed pools). Courtesy: N. Nanda and R. Namgay.

However, more information on distribution and bionomics of species E is deemed necessary to substantiate its distribution range and role in malaria transmission in India. In addition, understanding population structure of *An. culicifacies* in adjoining countries is also warranted for effective interventions to check spread of drug-resistant malaria across borders. Additional data on crossing experiments between sibling species to demonstrate post-zygotic isolation and existence of possible morphological differences would help name the individual species formally similar to other well defined species complexes of *An. dirus* and that of *An. maculatus* [8,10]. *An. culicifacies* is indeed a fast invading species in areas hitherto with low density (deforested pockets in Northeast India), and its control has become a formidable challenge with its sibling species developing multiple resistance including pyrethroids (42-45). Regional control strategy would require monitoring the insecticide susceptibility status periodically for any given area that qualifies for residual spraying for effective control of *An. culicifacies* malaria vectors.

3. *Anopheles (Cellia) fluviatilis* James species complex

Anopheles fluviatilis s.l. is widespread in mainland India and is considered to be an important vector in hills and foothills contributing ~15% of reported cases annually [1]. It has been extensively studied and recognized a species complex comprising three sibling species, i.e., S, T, U and a form 'V' based on cytotaxonomic study for fixed chromosomal inversions readable in the polytene chromosomes arm 2 [7-11,53]; differentiation of S and T, however, not possible due to diagnostic inversion polymorphism but can be characterized by distinct biological characteristics and regional distribution (Table 2). Earlier reports of existence of X and Y sibling species in *An. fluviatilis* based on rDNA-ITS2 polymerase chain reaction assay subsequently correlated X with sibling species S, and Y with T based on chromosomal data [54,55]. To substantiate these observations, robust molecular techniques now have been developed which distinguish sibling species S, T and U unequivocally based on differences in nucleotide sequences within the D3 domain of 28S rDNA [56]. However, contrary to observations of Garros et al [57] and Chen et al [58] on conspecificity of An. *fluviatilis* species S with *An. harrisoni* (species C of *An. minimus*), Indian population of these two species were observed to be distantly related and did not merit synonymy based on pair-wise distance and phylogenetic inferences using ITS2 sequences [59].

Sibling Species**	Inversion genotypes on Chromosome arm 2	Mosquito densities (per person hour)	Feeding preference	Preferred adult habitat	Prevalence	
					Ecotype	Endemicity
S	+q'+r'	Low to Moderate (1-40)	Anthropophilic	Human dwellings	Hilly forests & foothills	Hyperendemic
T	q'+r'	High (up to 200)	Almost totally zoophilic	Cattle sheds	Foothills & plains	Hypo - mesoendemic
U	+q'r'					

*Source Reference No. 37, **Distribution, bionomics and biology of new sibling form 'V' is being investigated

Table 2. Inversion genotype and biological characteristics of *Anopheles fluviatilis* sibling species complex in India*

Sibling species S is highly anthropophilic and responsible for maintaining hyperendemic malaria predominantly in state of Odisha (formerly Orissa), eastern India [60]. It prefers to rest indoor human dwellings and have been incriminated and proven to be an efficient vector in areas of its distribution [61,62]. Sibling species T is widely distributed but is largely zoophilic and rests in cattle sheds [63]. Sibling U holds similar characteristics but has limited distribution range presently restricted to northern India. Chen et al [58] documented three haplotypes in species T (designated T1, T2, Y) with its distribution in India, Nepal, Pakistan and Iran implicating the existence of additional taxa within the An. *fluviatilis* species complex provisionally designated as 'V form' in India, and the same has recently been recorded in district Hardwar, Uttarakhand state of North India [63]. Both sibling species T and U are held very close with similar biological characteristics and there exists possibility of hybridization in some areas. Even though both siblings species are poor vectors but have shown inherent ability to support normal sporogony in laboratory feeding experiments [64].

Preferred breeding habitats are seepage water streams with perceptible flow of water, river margins, irrigation channels, shallow wells, terraced rice fields along foothills etc [7,11,65]. Peak biting activity occurs between 20:00 to 24:00 hours but it may vary in different seasons and locations. Both *An. fluviatilis* species S and *An. minimus* share similar resting and breeding habitats and are efficient vectors in their respective zones of distribution [66]. Both are subject to misidentification due to morphological variation to the extent that the earlier records of prevalence and seasonal abundance of *An. fluviatilis* in northeast India have now been proven to be hypermelanic variant of *An. minimus* s.s.by molecular assays [67].

For control of *An. fluviatilis*, the choice of insecticide should be based on the susceptibility status of prevalent sibling of *An. culicifacies* in endemic areas where species of both complexes share similar indoor resting behavior and sympatric distribution records (Figure 1). More investigations are, however, warranted for precise distribution of different sibling species of this complex especially in areas hitherto unexplored, particularly 'form V' and its role in malaria transmission. Similar to *An. culicifacies* species complex, there is dearth of data for morphological differentiation and crossing experiments to distinguish member sibling species enabling binomial nomenclature.

4. *Anopheles (Cellia) minimus* Theobald species complex

Anopheles minimus s.l. is considered to be the predominant malaria vector in the oriental region [68]. It is a major vector in sub-Himalayan foothills of eastern and northeastern region of India. In the pre-DDT era (1940s), it was extensively studied in Assam and Bengal for its bionomics and control, and it was widely incriminated across its range of distribution [69-74]. With the advent of DDT and large scale application for residual spraying to control, *An. minimus* disappeared from Terai of Uttarakhand (formerly Uttar Pradesh), eastern Odisha, northeastern states and Nepal [75,76]. Subsequently besides *An. dirus s.l.*, *An. philippinensis* was implicated in malaria transmission in northeastern region of India [77]. However, return of malaria required containment of persistent transmission and spread of drug-resistant malaria.

Towards this objective, systematic investigations were initiated *denovo* during 1980s to incriminate vectors of malaria and to ascertain their relative importance [78,79].

Consequently, systematic studies by independent investigators revealed the reappearance of *An. minimus* in vast areas of northeast. *An. minimus* was re-incriminated in almost all states of the northeast India except in Terai area of Uttarakhand (North India) where it did not return [80-86]. It is only recently that *An. minimus* has been reported to have resurfaced in Odisha (eastern India) after a lapse of 45 years and were observed to be abundant sharing *An. fluviatilis* habitats, and both vectors were incriminated [87,88]. It is presently the most efficient vector in foothill valley areas of northeastern states accounting for nearly 50% reported cases in the region annually, and responsible for focal disease outbreaks characterized by high rise in cases and attributable deaths [89-94]. *An. minimus* is the predominant vector in rice-growing foothill valley areas, and it supplements transmission in forest fringe areas (adjoining to undisturbed forest reserve) predominated by *An. baimaii* [95].

Ever since initial recognition of *An. minimus* as species complex for its three morphological forms [96] and subsequent characterization by population genetic evidence for two isomorphic species [97], *An. minimus s.l.* has been identified to a species complex comprising three formally named species, *An. minimus s.s.* (species A), *An. harrisoni* Harbach & Manguin (species C), and *An. yaeyamaensis* Somboon & Harbach (species E) with distinct bionomical characteristics and distribution [98-101]. The natural distribution range of these species is given in Figure 4. Even though based on classical taxonomy, three designated species are difficult to distinguish due to overlapping morphological characters, yet these can be identified reliably by number of molecular assays [102-107].

Based on DNA sequences of internal transcribed spacer 2 (ITS2) and D3 domain of 28S rDNA (28S-D3) of morphologically identified *An. minimus s.l.* across Indian states of Assam, Arunachal Pradesh, Meghalaya and Nagaland [108] and that of Odisha [87], it has now been clearly established that these populations are indeed *An. minimus* (species A), whereas *An. harrisoni* and *An. yaeyamaensis* are not recorded from India. Correct identification of *An. minimus* is further complicated by the existence of morphological variants which closely resemble *An. varuna* and *An. fluviatilis s.l.*, and these species share similar distribution range and habitats. In northeast India, morphologically identified populations of *An. fluviatilis s.l.* (formerly designated species U based on polytene chromosome banding pattern) have now been genetically characterized as the hypermelanic seasonal variant of *An. minimus* prevalent during cooler months [67]. The ITS2 and 28S-D3 rDNA sequences of morphologically identified *An. fluviatilis* populations of from Assam were observed homologous to that of *An. minimus s.s.* and different from that of any member of the *An. fluviatilis* complex.

An. minimus is primarily an endophilic and endophagic species with a strong predilection for human host for blood meal [85]. It is a perennial species with seasonal peak density during April to August (wet season), and is the most predominant collection in human bait landing catches (13.7 per person/night) with peak biting activity during 01:00–04:00 hours. It has been incriminated in all months of the year (sporozoite infection rate 3.31%) but relative abundance and entomologic inoculation rates (EIRs) vary across malaria endemic districts [85,109]. The relative abundance and risk of malaria is high in localities near to breeding habitat (<1km) suggestive of poor flight range (Figure 5). *An. minimus* breeding were primarily recorded in perennial seepage water foothill streams with grassy margins in all seasons but occasionally recorded in paddy field water pools with perceptible flow of water [110].

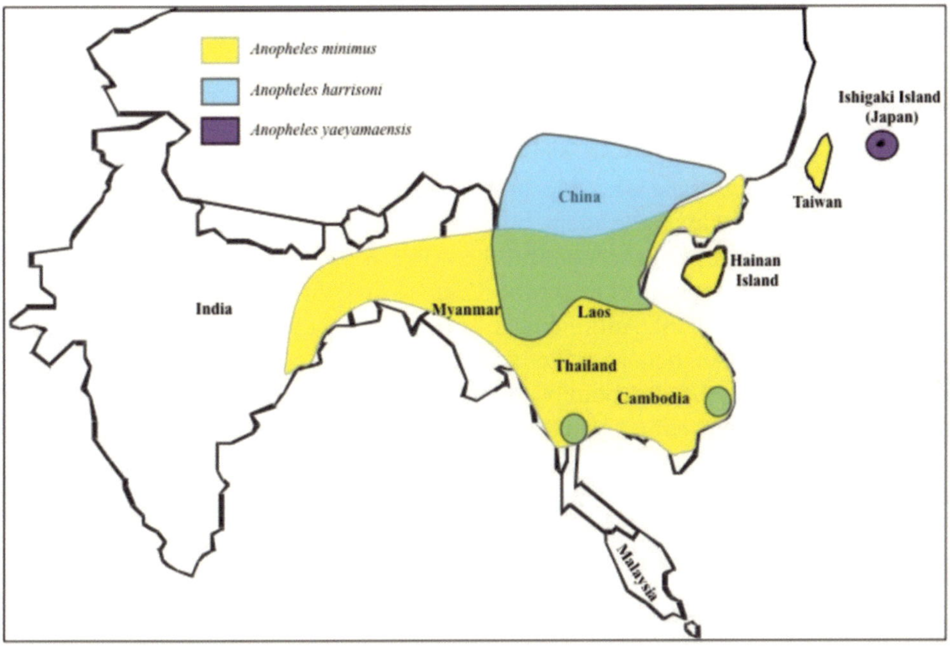

Figure 4. Distribution map of member species of the *Anopheles minimus* complex in Southeast Asia based on molecular identification (Courtesy: Dr. S. Manguin). *An. minimus* has wide distribution extending from East India to Northeast and eastwards to China including Taiwan, and occurs in sympatry with *An. harrisoni* over large areas in southern China, Vietnam, Laos and Thailand. *An. yaeyamaensis* is restricted to Ishigaki island of Ryukyu Archipelago of Japan.

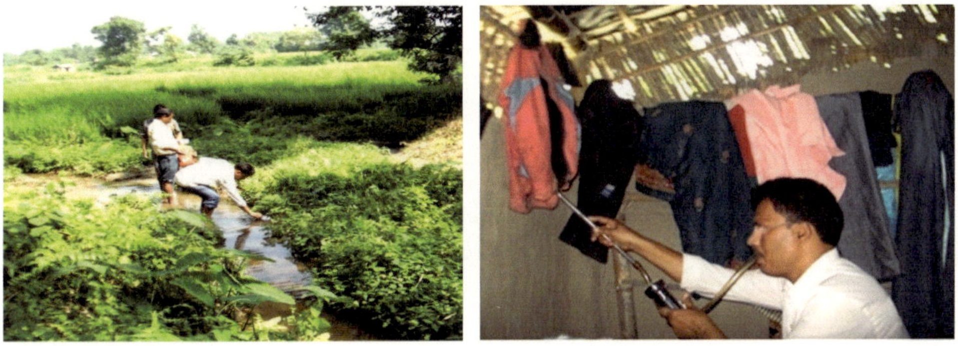

Figure 5. Breeding and resting habitats of *Anopheles minimus* (left- seepage water foothill streams are preferred breeding habitat; right – mud house with thatched roofing located often adjacent to breeding resource is the ideal resting habitat for which relative risk of malaria is high).

An. minimus is susceptible to DDT despite decades of insecticide residual spraying (IRS) by virtue of its physiological resistance and high behavioral plasticity [93]. It avoids resting indoors and instead establishes extra-domiciliary transmission only to return to original habitat after 10 to 12 week post-spray. With the introduction of pyrethroid coated/ incorporated long-lasting insecticidal nets (LLINs) and enhanced population coverage in high-risk areas, the populations of *An. minimus* are once again fast diminishing particularly in broken forest reserve erstwhile domains of this anthropophilic species [111-113]. The niche thus vacated is being accessed by *An. culicifacies* populations which are tolerant to multiple insecticides posing a new challenge for effective vector control and associated transmission (unpublished observations).

It is suggested that in areas with *An. minimus* and *An. fluviatilis* sympatric populations, viz., Odisha and West Bengal, there is need to apply integrated vector management for sustainable interventions [114,115]. Given the adaptability of *An. minimus* to varied environments, there is continued need to monitor its bionomical characteristics in the changing ecological context due to rapid socio-economic development and diminishing malaria transmission in erstwhile areas of high receptivity [116]. Additional data are warranted for analyses of mitotic karyotypes, polytene chromosome maps and cross-breeding experiments which may of diagnostic importance. Equally important would be to understand the population dynamics of member species of the *An. minimus* complex in the adjoining countries of Myanmar, Bangladesh and Bhutan for developing cross-border initiative to institute appropriate interventions to contain drug-resistant malaria.

5. *Anopheles (Cellia) dirus* Peyton & Harrison species complex

Anopheles dirus s.l. comprises eight sibling species, seven of which have been formally named, i.e., *An. dirus s.s.* (species A), *An. cracens* (species B), *An. scanloni* (species C), *An. baimaii* (species D), *An. elegans* (species E), *An. nemophilous* (species F), *An. takasagoensis,* and a cryptic species tentatively designated as *An.* aff. *takasagoensis* (Figure 6). Each of the seven named species has morphological description (117), distribution range and have varied epidemiological significance in Southeast Asia [10,118], whereas the eighth species, reported in northern Vietnam, is morphological similar but phylogenetically distant from both *An. dirus* and *An. takasagoensis* [119]. All these sibling species except *An.* aff. *takasagoensis* have been well characterized by a number of techniques including cross-mating experiments, karyotypic studies, polytene chromosome banding patterns, gene enzyme variation, DNA probes and egg morphology (8,10,120-122]. In addition, PCR assays have been developed based on ITS2 sequences and SCAR (sequence characterized amplified region) based PCR which distinguishes five of its member species unambiguously [123,124]. Further investigations, however, are warranted to characterize *An.* aff. *takasagoensis* to formally name this as valid species of the *An. dirus* species complex.

Among these member species, only *An. baimaii* and *An. elegans* are prevalent in India with distinct distribution range and epidemiological significance [8]. *An. baimaii* is widely abundant in northeastern states and is an efficient vector of human malaria contributing the remaining 50% of reported cases in the region annually [1]. It has been widely incriminated across northeastern states (sporozoite infection rate 1.9%) and its neighboring countries associated with transmission of drug-resistant malaria [125-132]. In earlier records what was initially described as *An. balabacensis balabacensis* and later *An. dirus* (species D) in India are now referred as *An. baimaii* for all purposes. *An. baimaii* is very closely related to *An. dirus*, populations of both species are of significance in understanding evolution and history of expansion in geological time scale [133,134].

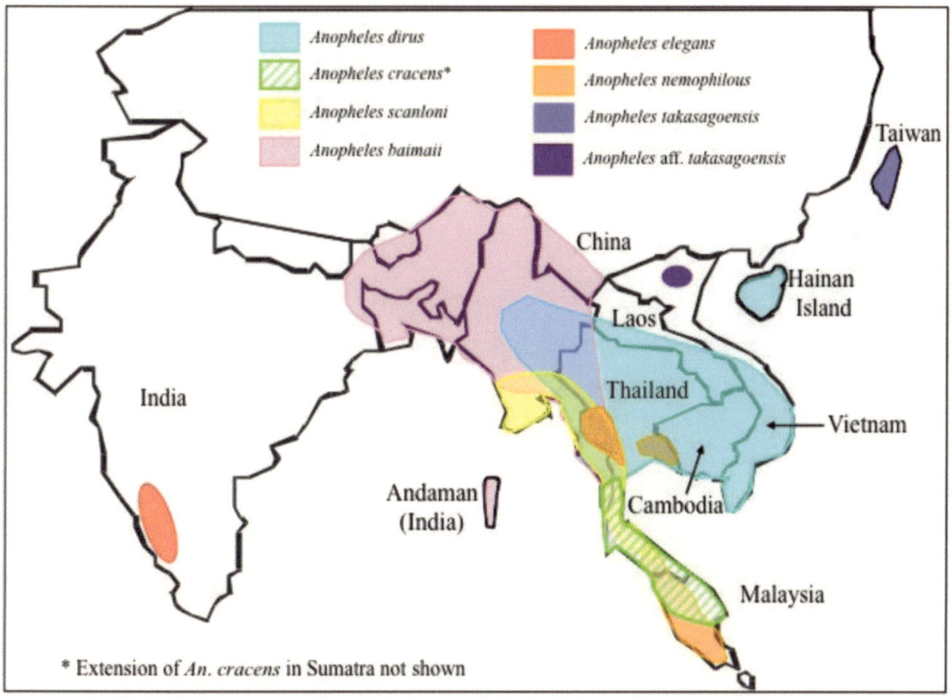

Figure 6. Distribution map of member species of the *Anopheles dirus* complex in Southeast Asia (Courtesy: Dr. S. Manguin). *An. dirus* has a wide distribution in eastern Asia including Myanmar, Thailand, Cambodia, Laos, Vietnam and Hainan Island. *An. cracens* occurs in southern Thailand, peninsular Malaysia and Sumatra (Indonesia). *An. scanloni* distribution is restricted along border of southern Myanmar and western Thailand. *An. baimaii* distribution extends from southwest China to northeast India through western Thailand, Myanmar, Bangladesh and Andaman Islands (India). *An. elegans* distribution is restricted to hilly forests of southwestern India. *An. nemophilous* has a patchy distribution along Thai-Malaya peninsula and Thai border with Myanmar and Cambodia. *An. takasagoensis* is restricted to Taiwan and *An.* aff. *takasagoensis* has recently been reported from northern Vietnam.

An. baimaii is a forest dweller and actively transmits malaria during monsoons in forest fringe population groups particularly along inter-state and inter-country border areas (Figure 7). It is a hygrophilic species (flight range <1km) and demonstrates phenomenon of 'horizontal' pulsation, i.e., population expansion from 'mother foci' in deep forests to periphery during monsoons (June–October) and then retracting to 'mother foci' in dry seasons (November–

March) accounting for its high and low prevalence in respective season, and 'vertical' pulsation for its ability to feed on alternate host to humans in the changing environmental conditions [135]. It is a highly anthropophilic species for its predilection to human host and bites throughout night both indoors and outdoors (36.1 bites/person/night) with peak infective biting activity during second quartile (21:00–24:00) of the night hours [136,137]. The relative risk of infective bite, however, was estimated to be much greater in the post-monsoon season. It is largely an exophilic species and breeds in a variety of habitats in forest including small transient pools, elephant foot prints [138]. It is highly susceptible to all residual insecticides but avoids contact with sprayed surfaces making vector control a difficult proposition [139].

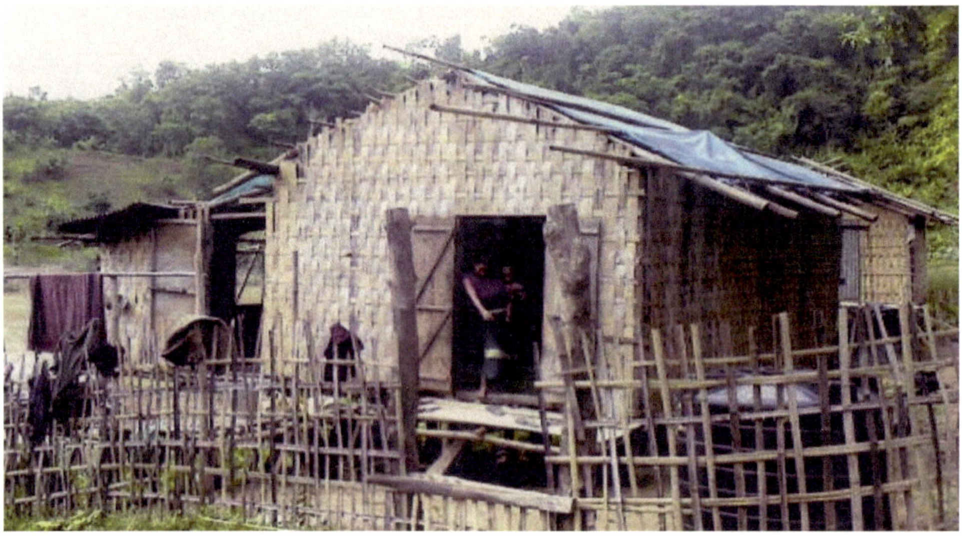

Figure 7. A typical housing structure receptive for *Anopheles baimaii* transmitted malaria located along Indo-Bangladesh border in northeast India

Even though populations of *An. baimaii* from northeast India had high genetic diversity, these populations were genetically distinct from those of the adjoining countries of Bangladesh, Myanmar and Thailand suggesting significant barrier to gene flow [140]. However, there was no significant genetic differentiation between populations of northeast (except for population in the Barail hill range of northeast), thus be considered one entity for implementation of control interventions [141]. Yet owing to continued deforestation and possible disruption of gene flow between populations, there is possibility of existence of another taxon tentatively designated as 'species x' which call for additional investigations. *An. baimaii* is also known to inhabit forests of Andaman and Nicobar islands but there is dearth of data on population genetic structure and role in malaria transmission. *An. elegans* is exclusively found in south-western India but there is no evidence of its role in malaria transmission [8].

6. *Anopheles (Cellia) sundaicus* (Rodenwaldt) species complex

Anopheles sundaicuss.l. is an important vector of malaria throughout its range of distribution in the oriental region (Figure 8). It is currently a complex of four species, i.e., *An. sundaicus s.s.*, *An. epiroticus* Linton & Harbach (formerly species A), *An. sundaicus* species D and *An. sundaicus* species E [8,10,13,14,142,143]. In India, it has disappeared from the mainland eastern coastal belt of West Bengal and Orissa except small focus in the Kutch area of Gujarat [144], and is widely prevalent in Andaman and Nicobar islands populations of which have been characterized to be cytotype species D [145-147]. It is largely a brackish water species and breeds in a variety of habitats including swamps, salt water lagoons, creeks, pits along embankments but breeding in fresh water collections has also been recorded. Molecular characterization of cytotype D, however, did not reveal any difference between fresh water and brackish water populations but were different from *An. epiroticus* of Vietnam and *An. sundaicus s.s* from Borneo, Malaysia [148].

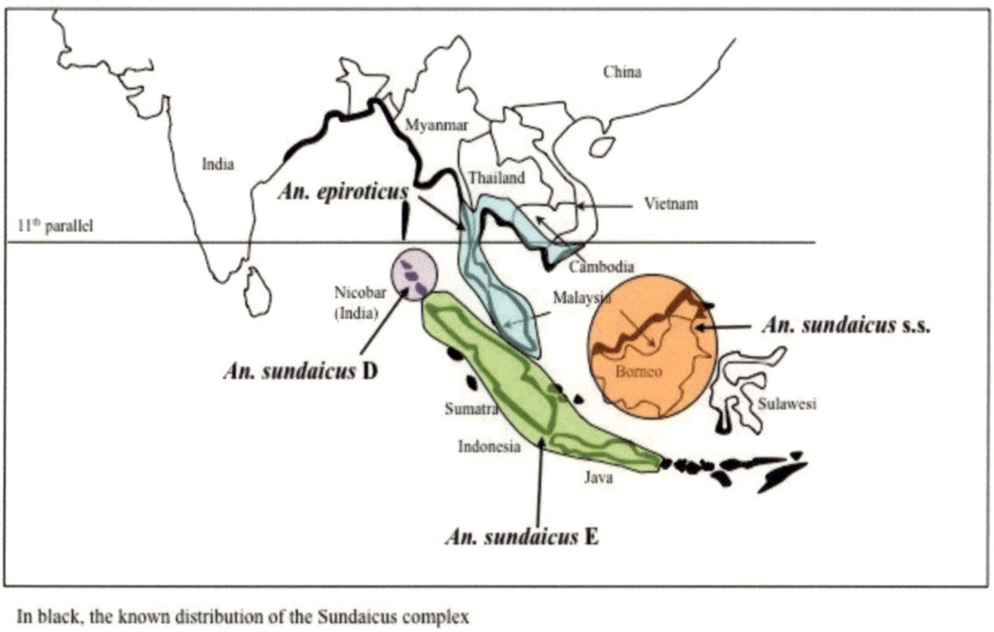

Figure 8. Distribution map of the four member species of the *Anopheles sundaicus* complex in Southeast Asia (Courtesy: Dr. S. Manguin). *An. sundaicus s.s.* is distributed along the coast of Borneo. *An. epiroticus* occurs in coastal brackish water sites extending from southern Vietnam to peninsular Malaysia. *An. sundaicus* species E occurs in Sumatra and Java (Indonesia). *An. sundaicus* species D distribution is restricted to Andaman and Nicobar islands in India.

In Andaman and Nicobar islands, *An. sundaicus* is predominantly zoophilic except for indoor resting populations in human dwellings which had a significantly higher predilection for human host [149]. The relative abundance is reported to be higher in monsoon and post-monsoon months, populations of which rest both indoors and outdoors [149,150]. Biting activity occurred all through the night but peak biting was during 21:00 till 04:00 hours. The species is susceptible to DDT and malathion. It is possible that given the richness of fauna of evergreen equatorial forest in the Andaman and Nicobar group of islands, additional sibling species of the *An. sundaicus* complex do exist with distinct bionomical characteristics, thus additional investigations are warranted for formulating appropriate control interventions [151].

7. *Anopheles (Cellia) stephensi* Liston – A complex of variants

Anopheles stephensi is an important vector of urban malaria and has been widely incriminated in most metropolitan cities by detection of gland and gut infections [7]. It is not considered a species complex but instead comprises three ecological variants, i.e., 'type form', 'intermediate form' and variety '*mysorensis*' characterized by egg morphometrics [152-154]. The 'type form' is an efficient vector of malaria in urban areas, and the variety '*mysorensis*' is largely zoophilic and has no role in malaria transmission [155-157]. The 'intermediate form' is typically recorded in rural and peri-urban localities but its role in malaria transmission is not known. The existence of ecological variants is further evidenced by Y–chromosome variation [158], spiracular index [159], and frequencies of inversion polymorphism in urban and rural populations in range of its distribution [160,161]. However, results of cross-mating experiments were variable ranging from infertility to reduced fertility [162,163] as opposed to full compatibility between populations [152].

An. stephensi is prevalent throughout the year but most abundant during months of rainfall (June–August) which coincides with the transmission period. In urban areas, it is generally endophilic and endophagic and breeds in domestic containers, building construction sites, overhead tanks, underground cement tanks, and evaporator coolers [155,164]. It is largely the 'type form' that is responsible for malaria outbreaks in urban areas related to construction projects and associated tropical aggregation of labor from malaria endemic areas. It is a thermophilic species and has longer flight range, and maintains a high degree of contact with human population [151]. In rural areas it is predominantly a zoophilic species and rests outdoors in cattle sheds, barracks, poorly constructed houses, and breeds in fresh water ponds, stream beds, seepage canals, wells etc. Peak biting activity is recorded between 22:00 to 24:00 hours but varies seasonally in different localities [7,165]. It is an invasive species and enters new towns and settlements.

The species is resistant to multiple insecticides but indoor residual spraying is not used for control. Instead recommended control measures are (i) source reduction, (ii) minor engineering interventions (iii) anti-larval methods including chemical and biological larvicides, (iv) application of larvivorous fish, i.e., guppy and gambusia, (v) aerosol space spraying for control of adult vector populations, (vi) legislative bylaws for preventing mosquito breeding [2]. In the face of rapid urbanization, unplanned growth and mushrooming of urban slums, rationed water supply and unsafe water storage practices; urban malaria is a growing problem presently accounting for >10% reported malaria cases in the country [166]. Overall, malaria cases in the rural and urban areas are grossly underestimated due to scanty surveillance and unreliable laboratory services.

8. Prospects of vector control and research priorities

India has about a billion population at risk of malaria and accounts for the highest disease burden in Southeast Asia for estimated loss of disability adjusted life years [3,6]. Malaria transmission is complex due to multi-species co-existence and variable species dominance and bionomical characteristics [13,14]. Although, transmission trends seem to be declining (Figure 9), National Vector Borne Disease Vector Control Programme (NVBDCP) is faced with new emerging challenges. Some of these are (i) multiple insecticide resistance against target disease vector mosquito species, (ii) emerging multi-drug resistance and steadily rising proportions of *P. falciparum,* (iii) shortage of antimalarial drugs and insecticides, and (iv) human resource attrition of skilled personnel to meet the future challenges.

Indoor residual spraying (IRS) for vector control has become less effective and operationally difficult proposition [9,94]. In addition, ecological driven changes, population migration across borders, deforestation, developmental projects, and poor infrastructure have led to the opportunities for vector proliferation and increased malaria receptivity. Due to poor community acceptance for IRS and spray coverage of target population groups [167], India has embarked upon large scale implementation of Insecticide-treated netting materials / long-lasting insecticidal nets (LLINs) prioritizing high-risk population in malaria endemic states/ districts. Disease transmission trends are declining in beneficiary population groups (formerly intractable high-risk areas); hence it is the right time to siege the opportunity for up scaling LLIN based intervention coupled with appropriate drug policy in place to combat the malaria illness and preventing spread of drug-resistant malaria [112,113,168-170]. It is worrisome, however, that the LLINs presently in use employ only pyrethroids, and *An. culicifacies* that is multi-resistant, is fast invading new territories making a malaria control a complex enterprise. What would be tantamount to vector control is the management of insecticide resistance for increased duration of its efficacy against target disease vector species by strategic application, insecticide rotation and mosaic application, and integrating bio-environmental approaches which should all be considered [171,172]. These approaches combined with environment management methods which are situation-specific and community-based would yield long term dividend for sustainable vector control [173,174]. Among alternate methods of vector control, large scale application of larvivorous fish, i.e., *Poecilia reticulata* and *Gambusia affinis* have been proven to be effective against *An. culicifacies* transmitted malaria in South Indian state of Karnataka [175,176], and inspired by the success story as role model, other malaria endemic states are also contemplating incorporating this method as component of the integrated approach for vector control [177].

Besides dominant proven vector species, sporadic gut/ gland infections have also been recorded in *An. maculatus s.l., An. annularis s.l., An. nivipes/philippinensis,* and *An. subpictus s.l.* substantiated by variable levels of anthropophily and detection of circumsporozoite proteins [8,69,77,109,178,179]. These mosquito species, however, are considered of lesser significance for their role in malaria transmission except in areas reporting diminishing population densities of dominant vector species. Among these, *An. maculatus,* has been investigated in depth for spatial distribution and molecular characterization of its member species for possible role in malaria transmission specific to northeast India [180]. Of the nine formally named species of *An. maculatus* complex [181], six species namely, *An. pseudowillmori* and *An. maculatus* (most abundant), and *An. willmori, An. sawadwongporni, An. rampae, An. dravidicus* (restricted distribution) have been recorded to exist in northeast region; none of these, however, found positive for human malaria parasite [180]. Of the five species in the *Anopheles annularis* group of mosquito species, *An. annularis, An. nivpipes, An. philippinensis* and *An. pallidus* are widely prevalent in India. Among these, *An. annularis* comprises two cryptic species provisionally designated as species A and B with variable distribution records [182]. It has been incriminated in certain localities but it is a predominantly zoophilic species [183]. *An. nivipes* and An. *philippinensis* are morphologically very similar, yet can be characterized by cytogenetic and molecular techniques [184-186]. Both are also predominantly zoophilic. *An. subpictus* that is widely abundant in mainland India has been characterized to be complex of four sibling species provisionally designated as A, B, C and D identified by distinctive morphology, species specific diagnostic inversion genotypes and breeding characteristics [8,187]. It has been incriminated in coastal villages of South India, Central India, and Sri Lanka but additional investigations are warranted for distribution of individual sibling species and role in malaria transmission [188-190].

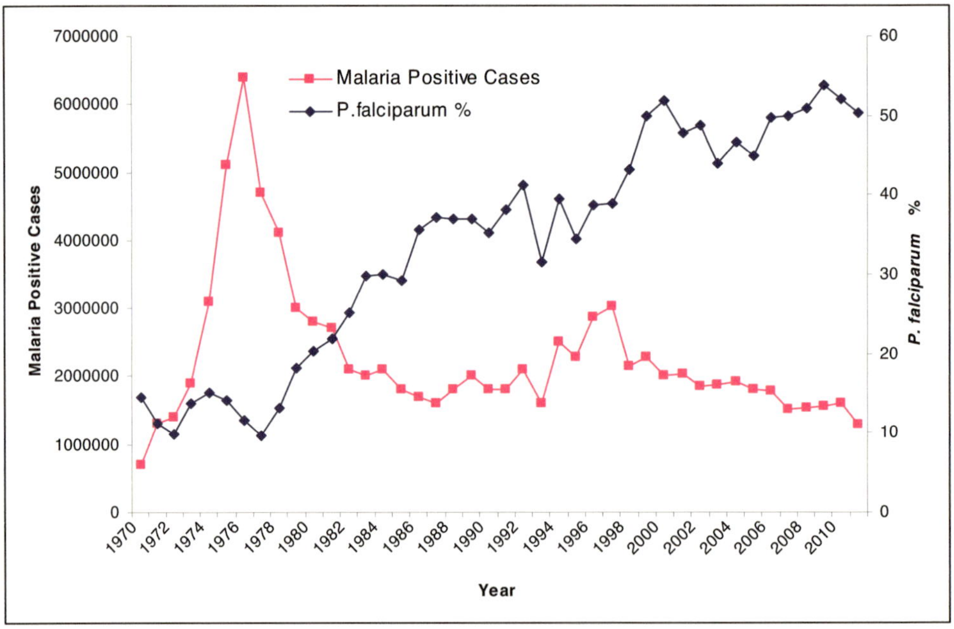

Figure 9. Malaria cases in India (1970-2011) recorded by the Directorate of National Vector Borne Disease Control Programme (NVBDCP). Cases started rising in 1970, reporting 6.45 million cases in 1976 and following the implementation of the Modified Plan of Operation in 1977, malaria cases declined but mainly *Plasmodium vivax* malaria due to its sensitivity to chloroquine. Beginning 2005 with increased allocation of resources for strengthening interventions, cases are gradually declining. *Plasmodium falciparum* proportions, however, that was about 10% in 1977, has risen to about 50% and the parasite has become mono to multi-drug resistant (data source: NVBDCP).

http://dx.doi.org/10.5772/55215

In moving forward for achieving ambitious goal of malaria elimination in feasible districts/ states, lot more needs to be accomplished in understanding vector bionomics in the altered ecology. The future priority area should include developing malaria-risk maps for focused interventions, ecological succession of disease vector species, monitoring insecticide resistance, cross-border initiative with neighboring countries for data sharing and coordinated control efforts, development of evidence-based newer tools for vector control, strengthening health systems for improved surveillance and monitoring, and universal access to malaria treatment and prevention which would help meeting the Millennium Development Goal in reducing malaria morbidity and mortality by 2015 [191-193].

9. Conclusions

During the past decade, there has been significant progress in development of molecular techniques in identification of sibling species of the dominant mosquito vector taxa, understanding their bionomical characteristics and role in malaria transmission in India. Among these, for *An. culicifacies* and *An. fluviatilis* which account for nearly 80% of malaria cases, vector control strategy has been formulated for judicious application of insecticide and saving operational costs. In the changing ecological context, *An. culicifacies* that is fast invading new territories is reportedly developing resistance to multiple insecticides including pyrethroids and inter-alia rising proportions and spread of multi-drug resistant *P. falciparum* malaria are some of the major concerns which call for continued research efforts for newer interventions that are evidence-based, community oriented and sustainable. Future priority area of research in vector control should include developing malaria-risk maps for focused interventions, monitoring insecticide resistance, cross-border initiative with neighboring countries for data sharing and coordinated control efforts for achieving substantial transmission reduction, and help check spread of drug-resistant malaria.

Abbreviations used

DDT: Dichloro-diphenyl-trichloroethane; rDNA: Ribosomal deoxyribonucleic acid; ITS2: Internal Transcribed Spacer 2; PCR: Polymerase Chain Reaction; RFLP: Restricted Fragment Length Polymorphism; CO II: Cytochrome Oxidase II; IRS: Indoor Residual Spray; LLIN: Long-lasting Insecticidal Net; MPO: Modified Plan of Operation; NVBDCP: National Vector Borne Disease Control Programme.

Acknowledgements

We are thankful to Drs. T. Adak, K. Raghavendra, O.P. Singh, N. Nanda, A. Das, A. Kumar, S.K. Ghosh for access to the valued literature and consultations. We are also indebted to Dr.

S. Manguin for encouragement and advice for development of the manuscript. This submission has been approved by the Institute Publication Screening Committee and bears the approval No. 022/2012.

Author details

Vas Dev[1*] and Vinod P. Sharma[2]

*Address all correspondence to: mrcassam@hotmail.com

1 National Institute of Malaria Research (Field Station), Guwahati, Assam, India

2 Centre for Rural Development & Technology, Indian Institute of Technology, New Delhi, India

References

[1] Sharma VP. Fighting malaria in India. Current Science 1998;75: 1127-40.

[2] National Vector Borne Disease Control Programme. Government of India. http://www.nvbdcp.gov.in (accessed 25 June 2012).

[3] Dhingra N, Jha P, Sharma VP, Cohen AA, Jotkar, RM, Rodriguez PS, Bassani DG, Suraweera W, Laxminarayan R, Pet R. Adult and child malaria mortality in India: a nationally representative mortality study. Lancet 2010;376: 1768-74.

[4] Shah NK, Dhillon GPS, Dash AP, Arora U, Meshnick SR, Valecha N. Antimalarial drug resistance of *Plasmodium falciparum* in India: changes over time and space. Lancet 2011;11: 57-64.

[5] Narain JP. Malaria in the South-East Asia: Myth & the reality. Indian Journal of Medical Research 2008;128: 1-3.

[6] Kumar A, Valecha N, Jain T, Dash AP. Burden of malaria in India: Retrospective and prospective view. American Journal of Tropical Medicine and Hygiene 2007;77: 69-78.

[7] Nagpal BN, Sharma VP. Indian Anophelines. Oxford & IBH Publishing Co. Pvt. LTD., 1995; New Delhi (ISBN 81-204-0929-9), p416.

[8] Subbarao SK. Anopheline Species Complexes in South-East Asia. World Health Organization. Technical Publication, SEARO No. 18, 1998. p82.

[9] Raghavendra K, Barik TK, Reddy BPN, Sharma P, Dash AP. Malaria vector control: from past to future. Parasitology Research 2011;108: 757-79.

[10] Manguin S, Garros C, Dusfour I, Harbach RE, Coosemans M. Bionomics, taxonomy, and distribution of the major malaria vector taxa of *Anopheles* subgenus Cellia in Southeast Asia: An updated review. Infection, Genetics and Evolution 2008;8: 489-503.

[11] Rao, TR. The Anophelines of India 1984. Indian Council of Medical Research, New Delhi.

[12] Dash AP, Adak T, Raghavendra K, Singh OP. The biology and control of malaria vectors in India. Current Science 2007;92: 1571-8.

[13] Sinka ME, Bangs MJ, Manguin S, Chareonviriyaphap T, Patil AP, Temperley WH, Gething PW, Elyazar IRF, Kabaria CW, Harbach RE, Hay SI. The dominant *Anopheles* vectors of human malaria in the Asia-Pacific region: occurrence data, distribution maps and bionomic précis. Parasites & Vectors 2011; 4:89

[14] Sinka ME, Bangs MJ, Manguin S, Rubio-Palis Y, Chareonviriyaphap T, Coetzee M, Mbogo CM, Hemingway J, Patil AP, Temperley WH, Gething PW, Kabaria CW, Burkot TR, Harbach RE, Hay SI. A global map of dominant malaria vectors. Parasites & Vectors 2012; 5:69

[15] Sharma VP. Re-emergence of malaria in India. Indian Journal of Medical Research 1996;103: 26-45.

[16] Sharma VP. Vector genetics in malaria control. In: Dronamraju KR and Paolo A. (eds.) Malaria: Genetics and Evolutionary Aspects, Springer, New York, 2006; p147-167. (doi:10.1007/0-387-28295-5_7).

[17] Barik TK, Sahu B, Swain V. A review on *Anopheles culicifacies*: from bionomics to control with special reference to Indian subcontinent. Acta Tropica 2009;109: 87-97.

[18] Green CA, Miles SJ. Chromosomal evidence for sibling species of the malaria vector *Anopheles* (*Cellia*) *culicifacies* Giles. Journal of Tropical Medicine and Hygiene 1980;83: 75-8.

[19] Subbarao SK, Adak T, Sharma VP. *Anopheles culicifacies* sibling species distribution and vector incrimination studies. Journal of Communicable Diseases 1980;12: 102-4.

[20] Subbarao SK, Vasnatha K, Adak T, Sharma VP. *Anopheles culicifacies* complex: evidence for a new sibling species C. Annals of Entomological Society of America 1983;76: 985-8.

[21] Subbarao SK, Adak T, Sharma VP. Cytotaxonomy of certain malaria vectors of India. In: Service MW (ed.). Biosystematics of haematophagous insects 1988, Clarendon Press, Oxford. p25-37.

[22] Subbarao SK. The *Anopheles culicifacies* complex and control of malaria. Parasitology Today 1988;4(3): 72-5.

[23] Saguna SG, Tewari SC, Mani TR, Hiriyan J, Reuben R. A cytogenetic description of a new species of the *Anopheles culicifacies* complex. Genetica 1989;78: 225-30.

[24] Vasantha K, Subbarao SK, Sharma VP. *Anopheles culicifacies* complex: population cytogenetic evidence for species D (Diptera: Culicidae). Annals of Entomological Society of America 1991;84: 531-6.

[25] Subbarao SK, Vasantha K, Sharma VP. Studies on the crosses between the sibling species of the *Anopheles culicifacies* complex. Journal of Heredity 1988;79: 300-3.

[26] Vasantha K, Subbarao SK, Adak T, Sharma VP. Karyotypic variations in *Anopheles culicifacies* complex. Indian Journal of Malariology 1982;19: 27-32.

[27] Vasantha K, Subbarao SK, Adak T, Sharma VP. *Anopheles culicifacies*: mitotic karyptype of species C. Indian Journal of Malariology 1983;20: 161-2.

[28] Adak T, Kaur S, Wattal S, Nanda N, Sharma VP. Y–chromosome polymorphism in species B and C of *Anopheles culicifacies* complex. Journal of American Mosquito Control Association 1997;13(4): 379-83.

[29] Adak T, Subbarao SK, Sharma VP, Rao SRV. Lactate dehydrogenase allozyme differentiation of species in the *Anopheles culicifacies* complex. Medical and Veterinary Entomology 1994;8: 137-40.

[30] Milligan PJM, Phillip A, Molyneux DH, Subbarao SK, White GB. Differentiation of *Anopheles culicifacies* Giles (Diptera: Culicidae) sibling species by analysis of cuticular components. Bulletin of Entomological Research 1986;76: 529-37.

[31] Gunasekera MB, de Silva BGDNK, Abeyewickreme W, Subbarao SK, Nandadasa HG, Karunayayke EH. Development of DNA probes for the identification of sibling species A of the *Anopheles culicifacies* (Diptera; Culicidae) complex. Bulletin of Entomological Research 1995;85: 345-53.

[32] Singh OP, Goswami G, Nanda N, Raghavendra K, Chandra D, Subbarao SK. An allele-specific polymerase chain reaction assay for the differentiation of members of *Anopheles culicifacies* complex. Journal of Biosciences 2004;29: 275-80.

[33] Goswami G, Raghavendra K, Nanda N, Gakhar SK, Subbarao SK. PCR-RFLP of mitochondrial cytochrome oxidase subunit II and ITS2 of ribosomal DNA markers for the identification of members of the *Anopheles culicifacies* complex (Diptera: Culicidae). Acta Tropica 2005;95: 92-9.

[34] Manonmani AM, Sadanandane C, Sahu SS, Mathivanana A, Jambulingam P. rDNA-ITS2-PCR assay for grouping the cryptic species of *Anopheles culicifacies* complex (Diptera: Culicidae). Acta Tropica 2007;104: 72-7.

[35] Goswami G, Singh OP, Nanda N, Raghavendra K, Gakhar SK, Subbarao SK. Identification of all members of the *Anopheles culicifacies* complex using allele-specific poly-

merase chain reaction assays. American Journal of Tropical Medicine and Hygiene 2006;75: 454-60.

[36] Raghavendra K, Cornel AJ, Reddy BPN, Colins FH, Nanda N, Chandra D, Verma V, Dash AP, Subbarao SK. Multiplex PCR assay and phylogenetic analysis of sequences derived from D2 domain of 28S rDNA distinguished members of the *Anopheles culicifacies* complex into two groups, A/D and B/C/E. Infection Genetics and Evolution 2009; 9(2): 271-7.

[37] National Institute of Malaria Research. *Anopheles culicifacies* and *An. fluviatilis* complexes and their control. Technical Report series No. NIMR/TRS/2009-Jan/02, New Delhi, India.

[38] Subbarao SK, Vasnatha K, Adak T, Sharma VP. Seasonal prevalence of sibling species A and B of the taxon *Anopheles culicifacies* in villages around Delhi. Indian Journal of Malariology 1987;24: 9-15.

[39] Joshi H, Vasantha K, Subbarao SK, Sharma VP. Host feeding patterns of *Anopheles culicifacies* species A and B. Journal of American Mosquito Control Association 1988;4: 248-51.

[40] Subbarao SK, Vasantha K, Sharma VP. Response of *Anopheles culicifacies* sibling species A and B to DDT and HCH in India: implications in malaria control. Medical and Veterinary Entomology 1998;2: 219-23.

[41] Raghavendra K, Vasantha K, Subbarao SK, Pillai MKK, Sharma VP. Resistance in *Anopheles culicifacies* sibling species B and C to malathion in Andhra Pradesh and Gujarat States, India. Journal of American Mosquito Control Association 1991;7: 255-9.

[42] Singh OP, Raghavendra K, Nanda N, Mittal PK, Subbarao SK: Pyrethroid resistance in *Anopheles culicifacies* in Surat district, Gujarat, India. Current Science 2002;82: 547-50.

[43] Bhatt RM, Sharma SN, Barik TK, Raghavendra K. Status of insecticide resistance in malaria vector, *Anopheles culicifacies* in Chattisgarh state, India. Journal of Vector Borne Diseases 2012;49: 36-8.

[44] Mishra AK, Chand SK, Barik TK, Dua VK, Raghavendra K. Insecticide resistance status in *Anopheles culicifacies* in Madhya Pradesh, Central India. Journal of Vector Borne Diseases 2012;49: 39-41.

[45] Singh RK, Mittal PK, Gourshettiwar MP, Pande SJ, Dhiman RC. Susceptibility of malaria vectors to insecticides in Gadchiroli district (Maharashtra), India. Journal of Vector Borne Diseases 2012;49: 42-4.

[46] Singh OP, Bali P, Hemingway J, Subbarao SK, Dash AP, Adak T. PCR-based methods for the detection of LI0I4 kdr mutation in *Anopheles culicifacies* sensu lato. Malaria Journal 2009;8:154 (doi:10.1186/1475-2875-8-154).

[47] Hoti SL, Vasuki V, Jambulingam P, Sahu SS. kdr allele-based PCR assay for detection of resistance to DDT in *Anopheles culicifacies* sensu lato Giles population from Malkangiri District, Orissa, India. Current Science 2006;91: 658-61.

[48] Subbarao SK, Adak T, Vasnatha K, Joshi H, Raghavandra K, Cochrane AH, Nussenzweig RS, Sharma VP. Susceptibility of *Anopheles culicifacies* species A and B to *Plasmodium vivax* and *Plasmodium falciparum* as determined by immunoradiometric assay. Transactions of the Royal Society Tropical Medicine and Hygiene 1988;82: 394-7.

[49] Kar I, Subbarao SK, Eapen A, Ravindran J, Satyanarayana TS, Raghavendra K, Nandan N, Sharma VP. Evidence for a new malaria vector species, species E, within the *Anopheles culicifacies* complex (Diptera: Culicidae). Journal of Medical Entomology 1999;36(5): 595-600.

[50] Sharma A, Parasher H, Singh OP, Adak T. Species B of *Anopheles culicifacies* (Diptera: Culicidae) is reproductively less fit than species A and C of the complex. Acta Tropica 2009;112: 316-9.

[51] Adak T, Kaur S, Singh OP. Comparative susceptibility of different members of the *Anopheles culicifacies* complex to *Plasmodium vivax*. Transactions of the Royal Society of Tropical Medicine and Hygiene 1999;93: 573-7.

[52] Kaur S, Adak T, Singh OP. Susceptibility of species A, B, C of *Anopheles culicifacies* complex to *Plasmodium yoelii yoelii* and *Plasmodium vinckei petteri* infections. Journal of Parasitology 2000;86: 1345-8.

[53] Subbarao SK, Nanda N, Vasantha K, Dua VK, Malhotra MS, Yadav RS, Sharma VP. Cytogenetic evidence for three sibling species in *Anopheles fluviatilis*. Annals of Entomological Society of America 1994;87: 116-21.

[54] Manonmani A, Townson H, Adeniran T, Jambulingam P, Sahu S, Vijatkumar T. rDNA-ITS2 polymerase chain reaction assay for the sibling species of *Anopheles fluviatilis*. Acta Tropica 2001;78: 3-9.

[55] Manonmani A, Nanda N, Jambulingam P, Sahu S, Vijaykumar T, Vani JR, Subbarao SK. Comparison of polymerase chain reaction assay and cytotaxonomy for identification of sibling species of *Anopheles fluviatilis* (Diptera: Culicidae). Bulletin of the Entomological Research 2003;93: 169-71.

[56] Singh OP, Chandra D, Nanda N, Raghavendra K, Sunil S, Sharma SK, Dua VK, Subbarao SK. Differentiation of members of the *Anopheles fluviatilis* species complex by an allele-specific polymerase chain reaction based on 28S ribosomal DNA sequences. American Journal of Tropical Medicine and Hygiene 2004;70; 27-32.

[57] Garros C, Harbach RE, Manguin S. Morphological assessment and molecular phylogenetics of the Funestus and Minimus Groups of *Anopheles* (*Cellia*). Journal of Medical Entomology 2005;42: 522-36.

[58] Chen B, Butlin RK, Pedro PM, Wang XZ, Harbach RE. Molecular variation, systematics and distribution of the *Anopheles fluviatilis* complex in southern Asia. Medical and Veterinary Entomology 2006;20: 33-43.

[59] Singh OP, Chandra D, Nanda N, Sharma SK, Htun PT, Adak T, Subbarao SK, Dash AP. On the conspecificity of *Anopheles fluviatilis* species S with *Anopheles minimus* C. Journal of Biosciences 2006;31: 671-7.

[60] Nanda N, Joshi H, Subbarao SK, Yadav RS, Shukla RP, Dua VK, Sharma VP. *Anopheles fluviatilis* complex: host feeding patterns of species S, T and U. Journal of American Mosquito Control Association 1996;12: 147-9.

[61] Gunasekaran K, Sahu SS, Parida SK, Sadanandane C, Jambulingam P, Das PK. Anopheline fauna of Koraput district, Orissa state with particular reference to transmission of malaria. Indian Journal of Medical Research 1989;89: 340-43.

[62] Nanda N, Yadav RS, Subbarao SK, Joshi H, Sharma VP. Studies on *Anopheles fluviatilis* and *Anopheles culicifacies* sibling species in relation to malaria in forested hilly and deforested riverine ecosystems in northern Orissa, India. Journal of the American Mosquito Control Association 2000;16: 199-205.

[63] Sharma SK, Nanda N, Dua VK, Joshi H, Subbarao SK, Sharma VP. Studies on the bionomics of *Anopheles fluviatilis* sensu lato and the sibling species composition in the foothills of Shiwalik range (Uttar Pradesh), India. Southeast Asian Journal of Tropical Medicine and Public Health 1995;26: 566-72.

[64] Adak T, Singh OP, Das MK, Wattal S, Nanda N. Comparative susceptibility of three important malaria vectors *Anophele stephensi*, *Anopheles fluviatilis* and *Anopheles sundaicus* to *Plasmodium vivax*. Journal of Parasitology 2005;91: 79-82.

[65] Sahu SS, Parida SK, Sadanandane C, Gunasekaran K, Jambulingam P, Das PK. Breeding habitats of malaria vector *Anopheles fluviatilis*, *Anopheles annularis*, and *Anopheles culicifacies* in Koraput district. Orissa. Indian Journal of Malariology 1990;27: 209-16.

[66] Dev V, Phookan S. Epidemiology and control of malaria in the Brahmaputra Valley of Assam. In: Advances in Medical & Human Welfare (ed., SC Goel), The UP Zoological Society, Muzaffar Nagar 251001 India, 1998. p 59-65.

[67] Singh OP, Nanda N, Dev V, Bali P, Sohail M, Mehrunnisa A, Adak T, Dash AP. Molecular evidence of misidentification of *Anopheles minimus* as *Anopheles fluviatilis* in Assam (India). Acta Tropica 2010;113: 241-4.

[68] Garros C, Bortel WV, Trung HD, Coosemans M, Manguin S. Review of the Minimus Complex of *Anopheles*, main malaria vector in Southeast Asia: from taxonomic issues to vector control strategies. Tropical Medicine and International Health 2006;11: 102-14.

[69] Viswanathan DK, Das S, Oommen AV. Malaria carrying anophelines in Assam with special reference to the results of twelve months dissections. Journal of the Malaria Institute of India 1941; 4: 297-306.

[70] Muirhead Thomson RC. Studies on the behaviour of *Anopheles minimus*. The behavious of adult in relation to feeding and resting in houses. Journal of the Malaria Institute of India 1941;4: 217-45.

[71] Senior White RA, Ghosh AR, Rao VV. On the adult bionomics of some Indian Anophelines with special reference to malaria control by pyrethrum spraying. Journal of Malaria Institute of India 1945;6: 129-215.

[72] Misra BG, Dhar SK. Malaria in Tripura State. Indian Journal of Malariology 1955; 9: 111-23.

[73] Misra BG. Malaria in northeast Frontier Agency (India). Indian Journal of Malariology 1956;10: 331-47.

[74] Gilroy AB. Malaria control on tea estates in Assam 1947-56. Indian Journal of Malariology 1958;12: 157-64.

[75] Chakrabarti AK, Singh NN. The probable cause of disappearance of *Anopheles minimus* from the Terai area of Nainital district of UP. Bulletin of the National Society of India for Malaria and other Mosquito-borne Diseases 1957; 5: 82-5.

[76] Parajuli MB, Shreshta SL, Vaidya RG, White GB. National wide disappearance of *Anopheles minimus* Theobald 1901, previously the principal malaria vector in Nepal. Transactions of the Royal Society of Tropical Medicine and Hygiene 1981;75: 603.

[77] Rajagopal R. Studies on persistent transmission of malaria in Burnihat, Meghalaya. Journal of Communicable Diseases 1976; 8: 235-45.

[78] Ray AP, Narasimham MVVL, Kondrashin AV, Bill AK. *P. falciparum* Containment Programme, Ten years of operation in India (1978-1988). PfCP/ Directorate of NMEP/ WHO/SIDA, Delhi 1988; p 290.

[79] Dev V. Integrated disease vector control of malaria: a success story based in Assam, northeastern India. ICMR Bulletin 2009;39: 21-8.

[80] Kareem MA, Singh YK, Bhatnagar VN, Dass M. A preliminary report on entomological studies under PFCP in Zone-1. Journal of Communicable Diseases 1983;15: 207-8.

[81] Das SC, Baruah I. Incrimination of *Anopheles minimus* Theobald and *Anopheles balabacensis balabacensis* Baisas (*A. dirus*) as malaria vectors in Mizoram. Indian Journal of Malariology 1985; 22: 53-5.

[82] Dutta P, Baruah BD. Incrimination of *Anopheles minimus* Theobald as vector of malaria in Arunachal Pradesh. Indian Journal of Malariology 1987; 24: 159-162.

[83] Wajihullah, Jana B, Sharma VP. *Anopheles minimus* in Assam. Current Science 1992;63: 7–9.

[84] Dev V, Sharma VP. Persistent transmission of malaria in Sonapur PHC, Kamrup District, Assam. Journal of Parasitic Diseases 1995;19: 65–8.

[85] Dev V. *Anopheles minimus*: Its bionomics and role in the transmission of malaria in Assam, India. Bulletin of the World Health Organization 1996;74: 61-6.

[86] Prakesh A, Mohapatra PK, Srivastava VK. Vector incrimination in Tamulpur primary health centre, district Nalbari, lower Assam during malaria outbreak 1995. Indian Journal of Medical Research 1996;103: 146-9.

[87] Jambulingam P, Sahu SS, Manonmani A. Reappearance of *Anopheles minimus* in Singhbum hills of East-Central India. Acta Tropica 2005; 96: 31-5.

[88] Sahu SS, Gunasekaran K, Vanamail P, Jambulingam P. Seasonal prevalence and resting behaviour of *Anopheles minimus* Theobald & *An. fluviatilis* James (Diptera: Culicidae) in east-central India. Indian Journal of Medical Research 2011;133: 655-61.

[89] Dev V. Malaria survey in Tarajulie Tea Estate and adjoining hamlets in Sonitpur district, Assam. Indian Journal of Malariology 1996;33: 21-9.

[90] Gogoi SC, Dev, V. Phookan S. Morbidly and mortality due to malaria in Tarajulie tea estate, Assam, India. Southeast Asian Journal Tropical Medicine Public Health 1996;27: 526-9.

[91] Dev V, Ansari MA, Hira CR, Barman K. An outbreak of *P. falciparum* malaria due to *Anopheles minimus* in Central Assam. Indian Journal of Malariology 2001;38: 32-8.

[92] Dev V. Hira CR, Rajkhowa MK. Malaria - attributable morbidly in Assam, northeastern India. Annals of Tropical Medicine & Parasitology 2001;95: 789-96.

[93] Dev V, Bhattacharyya PC, Talukdar R. Transmission of malaria and its control in the Northeastern Region of India. Journal of Association of Physicians of India 2003;51: 1073-76.

[94] Dev V, Sharma VP, Hojai D. Malaria transmission and disease burden in Assam: challenges and opportunities. Journal of Parasitic Diseases 2009;33: 3-12.

[95] Prakash A, Mohapatra PK, Bhattacharyya DR, Sharma CK, Goswami BK, Hazarika NC, Mahanta J. Epidemiology of malaria outbreak (April/May, 1999) in Titabor Primary Health Centre, district Jorhat (Assam). Indian Journal of Medical Research 2000;111: 121-6.

[96] Sucharit S, Komalamisra N, Leemingsawat S, Apiwathnasorn C, Thongrungkiat S. Population genetic studies on the *Anopheles minimus* complex in Thailand. Southeast Asian Journal of Tropical Medicine and Public Health 1988;19: 717-23.

[97] Green CA, Gass RF, Munstermann LE, Baimai V. Population-genetic evidence for two species in the *Anopheles minimus* in Thailand. Medical and Veterinary Entomology 1990;4: 25-34.

[98] Harbach RE. The classification of genus *Anopheles* (Diptera: Culicidae). A working hypothesis of phylogenetic relationships. Bulletin of Entomological Research 2004;94: 537-53.

[99] Harbach RE, Parkin E, Chen B, Butlin RK. *Anopheles* (*Cellia*) *minimus* Theobald (Diptera: Culicidae): neotype designation, characterization, and systematics. Proceedings Entomological Society of Washington 2006;108:198-209.

[100] Harbach RE, Garros C, Manh ND, Manguin S. Formal taxonomy of species C of the *Anopheles minimus* sibling species complex (Diptera: Culicidae). Zootaxa 2007;1654: 41-54.

[101] Somboon P, Rory A, Tsuda Y, Takagi M, Harbach RE. Systematics of *Anopheles* (*Cellia*) *yaeyamaensis* sp. n., alias species E of the *An. minimus* complex of southeastern Asia (Diptera: Culicidae). Zootaxa 2010;2651: 43-51

[102] Van Bortel W, Trung HD, Manh ND, Roelands P, Verle P, Coosemans M. Identification of two species within the *Anopheles minimus* complex in northern Vietnam and their behavioural divergences. Tropical Medicine and International Health 1999;4: 257-65.

[103] Sharpe RG, Harbach RE, Butlin RK. Molecular variation and phylogeny of members of the Minimus group of *Anopheles* subgenus *Cellia* (Diptera: Culicidae). Systematic Entomology 2000;25: 263-72.

[104] Kengne P, Trung HD, Baimaii, V, Cooseman M, Manguin S. A multiplex PCR-based method derived from random amplified polymorphic DNA (RAPD) marker for the identification of species of the *Anopheles minimus* group in Southeast Asia. Insect Molecular Biology 2001;10: 427-35.

[105] Garros C, Koekemoer LL, Coetzee M, Coosemans M, Manguin S. A single multiplex assay to identify major malaria vectors within the African *Anopheles funestus* and the Oriental *Anopheles minimus* groups. American Journal Tropical Medicine Hygiene 2004;70: 583-90.

[106] Garros C, Koekemoer LL, Kamau L, Awolola TS, Van Bortel W, Coetzee M, Coosemans M, Manguin S. Restriction fragment length polymorphism method for the identification of major African and Asian malaria vectors within the *Anopheles funestus* and *An. minimus* groups. American Journal Tropical Medicine Hygiene 2004;70: 260-5.

[107] Phuc HK, Ball AJ, Son L, Hanh NV, Tu ND, Lien NG. Verardi A, Townson H. Multiplex PCR assay for malaria vector *Anopheles minimus* and four related species in the

Myzomyia series from Southeast Asia. Medical and Veterinary Entomology 2003;17: 423-8.

[108] Prakash A, Walton C, Bhattacharyya, DR, Loughlin SO, Mohapatra PK, Mahanta J. Molecular characterization and species identification of the *Anopheles dirus* and *An. minimus* complexes in north-east India using r-DNA ITS2. Acta Tropica 2006;100: 156-61.

[109] Dev V, Phookan S, Sharma VP, Anand SP. Physiographic and entomologic risk factors of malaria in Assam, India. American Journal Tropical Medicine Hygiene 2004;71: 451–6.

[110] Dev V. Breeding habitats of Anopheline mosquitoes in Assam. Indian Journal of Malariology 1994;31: 31-4.

[111] Jana-Kara B, Jihullah WA, Shahi B, Dev V, Curtis CF, Shrama VP. Deltamethrin impregnated bed nets against *Anopheles minimus* transmitted malaria in Assam, India. Journal of Tropical Medicine and Hygiene 1995;98: 73-83.

[112] Dev V, Raghavendra K, Barman, K, Phookan S, Dash AP. Wash-resistance and field efficacy of Olyset net, a permethrin incorporated long-lasting insecticidal netting against *Anopheles minimus* transmitted malaria in Assam, Northeastern India. Vector-Borne and Zoonotic Diseases 2010;10: 403-10.

[113] Dev V, Raghavendra K, Singh SP, Phookan S, Khound K, Dash AP. Wash resistance and residual efficacy of long-lasting polyester netting coated with alpha-cypermethrin (Interceptor) against malaria-transmitting mosquitoes in Assam, northeast India. Transactions of the Royal Society of Tropical Medicine and Hygiene 2010;104: 273–8.

[114] Dixit J, Srivastava H, Sharma M, Das MK, Singh OP, Raghavendra K, Nanda N, Dash AP, Saksena DN, Das A. Phylogenetic inference of Indian malaria vectors from multilocus DNA sequences. Infection, Genetics and Evolution 2010;10: 755-63.

[115] Dixit J, Srivastava H, Singh OP, Saksena DN, Das A. Multilocus nuclear DNA markers and genetic parameters in an Indian *Anopheles minimus* population. Infection, Genetics and Evolution 2011;11: 572-9.

[116] Srivastava A, Nagpal BN, Sexena R, Dev V, Subbarao SK. Prediction of *Anopheles minimus* habitat in India – a tool for malaria management. International Journal of Geographical Information Science 2005;19: 91-7.

[117] Sallum MA, Peyton EL, Wilkerson RC. Six new species of the *Anopheles leucosphyrus* group, reinterpretation of *An. elegans* and vector implications. Medical and Veterinary Entomology 2005;19: 158-99.

[118] Obsomer V, Defoumy P, Coosemans M. The *Anopheles dirus* complex: spatial distribution and environmental drivers. Malaria Journal 2007;6.

[119] Takano KT, Nguyen NTH, Nguyen BTH, Sunahara T, Yasunami M, Nguyen MD, Takag M. Partial mitochondrial DNA sequences suggest the existence of a cryptic spe-

cies within the Leucosphyrus group of the genus *Anopheles* (Diptera: Culicidae), forest malaria vectors, in northern Vietnam. Parasites & Vectors 2010; 3:41.

[120] Baimai V, Andre RG, Harrison BA, Kijchalao U, Panthusiri L. Crossing and chromosomal evidence for two additional sibling species within the taxon *Anopheles dirus* Peyton and Harrison (Diptera: Culicidae) in Thailand. Proceedings of the Entomological Society of Washhington 1987;89: 157-66.

[121] Green CA, Munstermann LE, Tan SG, Panyim S, Baimai V. Population genetic evidences for species A, B, C, and D of the *Anopheles dirus* complex in Thailand and enzyme electromorphs for their identification. Medical and Veterinary Entomology 1992;6: 29-36.

[122] Hii JLK. Involvement of the X-chromosome in hybrid male sterility from crosses between species A and species B of the taxon *Anopheles dirus*. Mosquito News 1984;44: 192-96.

[123] Walton C, Handley JM, Kuvangkadilok C, Collins FH, Harbach RE, Baimai V, Butlin RK. Identification of five species of the *Anopheles dirus* complex from Thailand, using allele-specific polymerase chain reaction. Medical and Veterinary Entomology 1999;13: 24-32.

[124] Manguin S, Kengne P, Sonnier L, Harbach RE, Baimai V, Trung HD, Coosemans M. SCAR markers and multiplex PCR-based identification of isomorphic species in the *Anopheles dirus* complex in Southeast Asia. Medical and Veterinary Entomology 2002;16: 46-54.

[125] Clark RHP, Choudhry MA. Observations on *Anopheles leucosphyrus* in Digboi area of upper Assam. Journal of Malaria Institute of India 1941;4: 103-07.

[126] Sen SK, John VM, Krishnan KS, Rajagopal R. Studies on malaria transmission in Tirap district, Arunachal Pradesh (NEFA). Journal of Communicable Diseases 1973;5: 98-110.

[127] Rajagopal R. Role of *Anopheles balabacensis balabacensis* in the transmission of malaria in Assam. Journal of Communicable Diseases 1979;10: 71-4.

[128] Dutta P, Bhattacharyya DR, Sharma CK, Dutta LP. The importance of *Anopheles dirus* (*Anopheles balabacensis*) as a vector of malaria in northeast India. Indian Journal of Malariology 1989;26: 95-101.

[129] Das SC, Baruah I. Incrimination of *Anopheles minimus* Theobald and *Anopheles balabacensis balabacensis* Baisas (*An. dirus*) as malaria vectors in Mizoram. Indian Journal of Malariology 1985;22: 53-5.

[130] Prakash A, Bhattacharyya DR, Mohapatra PK, Mahanta J. Seasonal prevalence of *Anopheles dirus* and malaria transmission in a forest fringed village of Assam, India. Indian Journal of Malariology 1997; 34: 117-25.

[131] Das NG, Talukdar PK, Kalita J, Baruah I, Sribastava RB. Malaria situation in forest-fringed villages of Sonitpur district (Assam), India bordering Arunachal Pradesh during an outbreak. Journal of Vector Borne Disease 2007;44: 213-8.

[132] Rosenberg R, Maheswary NP. Forest malaria in Bangladesh. II. Transmission by *Anopheles dirus*. American Journal of Tropical Medicine and Hygiene 1982;31: 183-91.

[133] O'Loughlin SM, Okabayashi T, Honda M, Kitazoe Y, Kishino H, Somboon P, Sochantha T, Nambanys S, Saikia PK, Dev V, Walton C. Complex population history of two *Anopheles dirus* mosquito species in Southeast Asia suggests the influence of Pleistocene climate rather than human-mediated effects. Journal of Evolutionary Biology 2008;21: 1555-69.

[134] Morgan K, Linton Y-M, Somboon P, Saikia P, Dev V, Socheat D, Walton C. Inter-specific gene flow dynamics during the Pleistocene-dated speciation of forest-dependent mosquitoes in Southeast Asia. Molecular Ecology 2010;19: 2269–85

[135] Kondrashin AV, Jung RK, Akiyama J. Ecological aspects of forest malaria in Southeast Asia. In: (eds, Sharma VP and Kondrashin AV) Forest malaria in Southeast Asia, Proceedings of an Informal Consultative Meeting. WHO/MRC, New Delhi 1991. p1-28.

[136] Dutta P, Bhattacharyya DR, Khan SA, Sharma CK, Mahanta J. Feeding pattern of *Anopheles dirus*, the major vector of forest malaria in North-east India. Southeast Asian Journal of Tropical Medicine and Public Health 1996;27: 378-81.

[137] Prakash A, Bhattacharyya DR, Mohapatra PK, Mahanta J. Malaria transmission risk by the mosquito *Anopheles baimaii* (formerly known as *An. dirus* species D) at different hours of the night in North-east India. Medical and Veterinary Entomology 2005;19: 423-7.

[138] Dutta P, Khan SA, Bhattacharyya DR, Khan AB, Sharma CK, Mahanta J. Studies on the breeding habitats of the vector mosquito *Anopheles baimaii* and its relationship to malaria incidence in Northeastern region of India. EcoHealth 2010;7: 498-506.

[139] Prakash A, Bhattacharyya DR, Mohapatra PK, Mahanta J. Insecticide susceptibility status of *Anopheles dirus* in Assam. Journal of Communicable Diseases 1998;30: 62.

[140] Sarma DK, Prakash A, O'Loughlin SM, Bhattacharyya DR, Mohapatra PK, Bhattacharjee K, Das K, Singh S, Sarma NP, Ahmed GU, Walton C, Mahanta J. Genetic population structure of the malaria vector *Anopheles baimaii* in north-east India using mitochondrial DNA. Malaria Journal 2012;11: 76.

[141] Prakash A, Sarma DK, Bhattacharyya DR, Mohapatra PK, Bhattacharjee, K, Das K, Mahanta J. Spatial distribution and r-DNA second internal transcribed spacer characterization of *Anopheles dirus* (Diptera: Culicidae) complex species in north-east India. Acta Tropica 2010;114: 49-54.

[142] Dusfour I, Blondeau J, Harbach RE, Vythilingham I, Baimai V, Trung HD, Sochanta T, Bangs MJ, Manguin S. Polymerase chain reaction identification of three members

of the *Anopheles sundaicus* (Diptera: Culicidae) complex, malaria vectors in Southeast Asia. Journal of Medical Entomology 2007; 44: 723-31.

[143] Dusfour I, Michaux JR, Harbach RE, Manguin S. Speciation and phylogeography of the Southeast Asian *Anopheles sundaicus* complex. Infection, Genetics and Evolution 2007;7: 484-93.

[144] Singh N, Nagpal BN, Sharma VP. Mosquitoes of Kutch, Gujarat. Indian Journal of Malariology 1985; 22: 17-20.

[145] Nagpal BN, Kalra NL. Malaria vectors of India. Journal of Parasitic Diseases 1997; 21: 105-12.

[146] Das MK, Nagpal BN, Sharma VP. Mosquito fauna and breeding habitats of anophelines in Car Nicobar Island, India. Indian Journal of Malariology 1998; 35:197-205.

[147] Nanda N, Das MK, Wattal S, Adak T, Subbarao SK. Cytogenetic characterization of *Anopheles sundaicus* (Diptera: Culicidae) population from Car Nicobar island, India. Annals of Entomological Society of America 2004;97: 171-6.

[148] Alam MT, Das MK, Ansari MA, Sharma YD. Molecular identification of *Anopheles* (*Cellia*) *sundaicus* from the Andaman and Nicobar islands of India. Acta Tropica 2006;97: 10-18.

[149] Kumari R, Joshi H, Giri A, Sharma VP. Feeding preferences of *Anopheles sundaicus* in Car Nicobar Islands. Indian Journal of Malariology 1993; 30: 201-6.

[150] Kumari R, Sharma VP. Resting and biting habits of *Anopheles sundaicus* in Car Nicobar Islands. Indian Journal of Malariology 1994; 31: 103-4.

[151] Kalra NL. Forest malaria vectors in India: Ecological characteristics and epidemiological implications. In: Proceedings of an Informal Consultative Meeting WHO/MRC 18-22 February 1991(Eds. VP Sharma and AV Kondrashin, New Delhi), p93-114.

[152] Subbarao SK, Vasnatha K, Adak T, Sharma VP, Curtis CF. Egg-float ridge number in *Anopheles stephensi*: ecological variation and genetic analysis. Medical and Veterinary Entomology 1987;1: 265-71.

[153] Sweet WC, Rao BA. Races of *Anopheles stephensi* Liston 1901. Indian Medical Gazette 1937;72: 665-74.

[154] Rao BA, Sweet WC, Subba Rao AM. Ova measurements of *Anopheles stephensi* type and *Anopheles stephensi* var. *mysorensis*. Journal of Malaria Institute of India 1938;1: 261-6.

[155] Sharma SN, Subbarao SK, Choudhury DS, Pandey KC. Role of *An. culicifacies* and *An. stephensi* in malaria transmission in urban Delhi. Indian Journal of Malariology 1993;30: 155-68.

[156] Chakraborty S, Ray S, Tandon N. Seasonal prevalence of *Anopheles stephensi* larvae and existence of two forms of the species in an urban garden in Calcutta City. Indian Journal of Malariology 1998;35: 8-14.

[157] Ghosh SK, Tiwari S, Raghavendra K, Sathyanarayan TS, Dash AP. Observations on sporozoite detection in naturally infected sibling species of the *Anopheles culicifacies* complex and variant of *An. stephensi* in India. Journal of Biosciences 2008;33: 333-6.

[158] Saguna SG. Y-chromosome dimorphism in the malaria vector *Anopheles stephensi* from south India. Medical and Veterinary Entomology 1992; 6: 84-6

[159] Nagpal BN, Srivastava A, Kalra NL, Subbarao SK. Spiracular indices in *Anopheles stephensi*: a taxonomic tool to identify ecological variants. Journal of Medical Entomology 2003;40: 747-9.

[160] Saguna SG. Inversion (2) R1 in *Anopheles stephensi*, its distribution and relation to egg size. Indian Journal of Medical Research 1981;73 (Supplement): 124-8.

[161] Mahmood F, Sakai RK. Inversion polymorphism in natural populations of *Anopheles stephensi*. Canadian Journal of Genetics and Cytology 1984;26: 538-46.

[162] Sweet WC, Rao BA, Subba Rao AM. Cross-breeding of *Anopheles stephensi* type and *An. stephensi* var. *mysorensis*. Journal of Malaria Institute of India 1938;1: 149-54.

[163] Rutledge LC, Ward RA, Bickely WE. Experimental hybridization of geographic strains of *Anopheles stephensi* (Diptera: Culicidae). Annals of Entomological Society of America 1970;63: 1024-30.

[164] Sumodan PK, Kumar A, Yadav RS. Resting behavior and malaria vector incrimination of *Anopheles stephensi* in Goa, India. Journal of the American Mosquito Control Association 2004;20: 317-8.

[165] Korgaonkar NS, Kumar A, Yadav RS, Kabadi D, Dash AP. Mosquito biting activity on humans and detection of *Plasmodium falciparum* infection in *Anopheles stephensi* in Goa, India. Indian Journal of Medical Research 2012;135: 120-6.

[166] Akhtar R, Dutt AK, Wadhwa V. Malaria resurgence in urban India: lessons from health planning strategies. In: Malaria in South Asia, eradication and resurgence during the second half of the twentieth century. (eds. R Akhtar, AK Dutt, V. Wadhwa), Springer, New York; 2010. p141-155. DOI 10.1007/978-90-481-3358-1_8.

[167] Prasad H. Evaluation of malaria control programme in three selected districts of Assam, India. Journal of Vector Borne Diseases 2009;46: 280-7.

[168] Dev V. Long-lasting insecticidal nets for malaria control. Current Science 2009;97: 469-70.

[169] Dev V. Rolling back malaria initiative in India. Transactions of the Royal Society of Tropical Medicine and Hygiene 2009;103: 210.

[170] Dev V. Malaria recession and the way forward. Current Science 2010;99: 1507–9.

[171] World Health Organization. Global Plan for Insecticide Resistance Management in Malaria Vectors (GPIRM). http://www.who.int/malaria/vector_control/ivm/gpirm (Accessed 02 July 2012).

[172] Sharma SK, Upadhyay AK, Haque MA, Tyagi PK, Kindo BK. Impact of changing over of insecticide from synthetic pyrethroids to DDT for indoor residual spray in malaria endemic area of Orissa, India. Indian Journal of Medical Research 2012;135: 382-8.

[173] Sharma RC, Gautam AS, Bhatt RM, Gupta DK, Sharma VP. The Kheda malaria project: the case for environmental control. Health Policy and Planning 1991;6 (3): 262-70.

[174] Beier JC, Keating J, Githure JI, Macdonald MB, Impoinvil DE, Novak RJ. Integrated vector management for malaria control. Malaria Journal 2008; 7 (Suppl1): S4 doi: 10.1186/1475-2875-7-S1-S4.

[175] Ghosh SK, Tiwari SN, Sathyanarayan TS, Sampath TR, Sharma VP, Nanda N, Joshi H, Adak T, Subbarao SK. Larvivorous fish in wells target the malaria vector sibling species of the *Anopheles culicifacies* complex in villages in Karnataka, India. Transactions of the Royal Society of Tropical Medicine and Hygiene 2005; 99: 101-5.

[176] Ghosh SK, Satyanarayan T, Ojha VP. A renewed way of malaria control in Karnatka, South India. Frontiers in Physiology 2012;3: 1-3.

[177] Dev V, Dash AP, Hojai D. Fishing out malaria in Assam, northeastern India: hope or hype? Transactions of the Royal Society of Tropical Medicine and Hygiene 2008;102: 839-40.

[178] Prakash A, Bhattacharyyya DR, Mohapatra PK, Mahanta J. Role of the prevalent *Anopheles* species in the transmission of *Plasmodium falciparum* and *P. vivax* in Assam state, north-eastern India. Annals of Tropical Medicine and Parasitology 2004;98: 559-68.

[179] Dhiman S, Bhola RK, Goswami D, Rabha B, Kumar D, Baruah I, Singh L. Polymerase chain reaction detection of human host preference and *Plasmodium* parasite infections in field collected potential malaria vectors. Pathogens and Global Health 2012; 106: 177-180.

[180] Singh S, Prakash A, Yadav RNS, Mohapatra PK, Sarma NP, Sarma DK, Mahanta J, Bhattacharyya DR. *Anopheles* (*Cellia*) *maculatus* group: Its spatial distribution and molecular characterization of member species in north-east India. Acta Tropica 2012; 124: 62-70.

[181] Harbach RE. Mosquito Taxonomy Inventory. (http://www.mosquito-taxonomy-inventory.info/) accessed 23 September 2012.

[182] Alam MT, Das MK, Dev V, Ansari MA, Sharma YD. Identification of two cryptic species in the *Anopheles* (*Cellia*) *annularis* complex using ribosomal DNA PCR-RFLP. Parasitology Research 2007; 100:943-48.

[183] Dash AP, Bendley MS, Das AK, Das M, Dwivedi SR. Role of *Anopheles annularis* as a vector of malaria in island of Orissa. Journal of Communicable Diseases 1982; 14: 224.

[184] Subbarao SK, Vasantha K, Nanda N, Nagpal BN, Dev V, Sharma VP. Cytotaxonomic evidence for the presence of *Anopheles nivipes* In India. Journal of the American Mosquito Control Association 2000;16: 71-4.

[185] Alam MT, Das MK, Dev V, Ansari MA, Sharma YD. PCR-RFLP method for the identification of four members of the *Anopheles annularis* group of mosquitoes (Diptera: Culicidae). Transactions of the Royal Society of Tropical Medicine and Hygiene 2007;101: 239-44.

[186] Bhattacharyya DR, Prakash A, Sarma NP, Mohapatra PK, Singh S, Sarma DK, Kalita MC, Mahanta J. Molecular evidence of involvement of *Anopheles nivipes* (Diptera: Culicidae) in the transmission of *Plasmodium falciparum* in north-east India. Annals of Tropical Medicine and Parasitology 2010; 104: 331-36.

[187] Suguna SG, Gopal Rathinam K, Rajavel AR, Dhanda V. Morphologcial and chromosomal description of new species in the *Anopheles subpictus* complex. Medical and Veterinary Entomology 1994; 88-94.

[188] Panicker KN, Geetha Bai M, Bheema Rao US, Viswam K, Suryanaryanmurthy U. *Anopheles subpictus* vector of malaria in coastal villages of Southeast India. Current Science 1981; 50: 694-5.

[189] Kulkarni SM. Detection of sporozoites in *Anopheles subpictus* in Bastar district, Madhya Pradesh. Indian Journal of Malariology 1983; 20: 159-60.

[190] Amerasinghe PH, Amerasinghe FP, Wirtz RA, Indrajith NG, Somapala W, Pereira LR, Rathnayake AMS. Malaria transmission by *Anopheles subpictus* (Diptera: Culicidae) in a new irrigation project in Sri Lanka. Journal of Medical Entomology 1992; 29: 577-81.

[191] John TJ, Dandona L, Sharma VP, Kakkar M. Continuing challenge of infectious diseases in India. Lancet 2011;377: 252-69.

[192] Dash AP, Valecha N, Anvikar AR, Kumar A. Malaria In India: Challenges and opportunities. Journal of Biosciences 2008;33: 583-92.

[193] World Health Organization. World Malaria Report 2011. http://www.who.int/malaria/world_malaria_report_2011. (accessed 02 July 2012).

Chapter 10

Vector Biology and Malaria Transmission in Southeast Asia

Wannapa Suwonkerd, Wanapa Ritthison,
Chung Thuy Ngo, Krajana Tainchum,
Michael J. Bangs and
Theeraphap Chareonviriyaphap

Additional information is available at the end of the chapter

http://dx.doi.org/10.5772/56347

1. Introduction

There are two primary geographical divisions within an area collectively called Southeast Asia, Mainland SEA and Maritime SEA. Mainland SEA includes Cambodia, Lao PDR, Myanmar, Thailand, Vietnam and Peninsular Malaysia. The first five countries including Yunnan Province, southern China is referred to as the Greater Mekong Subregion (GMS). Maritime SEA consists of Eastern Malaysia (Sarawak and Sabah States located on Borneo Island), Brunei Darussalam, Indonesia, Philippines, Singapore and East Timor (Timor-Leste). Most of these areas are at risk for a variety of vector-borne diseases, especially malaria, one of the most important diseases transmitted by mosquitoes in the genus *Anopheles*.

Despite over 100 years of scientific investigation, malaria remains the leading cause of death among children living in Sub-Saharan Africa and every year is responsible for more than 200 million clinical infections worldwide. The World Malaria Report in 2011 estimated that the number of malaria cases rose from 233 million in 2000 to 244 million in 2005 then dropped to 225 and 219 million in 2009 and 2010, respectively [1, 2].However, mortality from malaria has decreased by over 26% globally since 2000 due to the increased availability of long-lasting insecticide-treated nets, indoor residual spraying, and better access to diagnostic and effective treatment using artemisinin-based therapies (ACTs) [3]. In Thailand, the malaria incidence has markedly decreased over the past 60 years in response to organized malaria control programs [4, 5] and other countries like Vietnam have made great strides in reducing both incidence and mortality in recent decades [6,7]. During the past two decades, significant reduction in malaria cases has also been reported in Cambodia, Laos, and eastern Malaysia, [8, 9,10]. During this same period, Myanmar and East Timor reported either no change or an increase in the number of cases; however the coverage of control activities appeared to be limited in relation to the total population at risk. The confirmed malaria cases in Myanmar increased by more than 16-fold between 2000 and 2009, primarily the result of an increased availability of parasitological diagnosis by both microscopy and RDTs [1, 9, 10]. Several countries have advanced a great deal in tackling malaria transmission and providing ready access to diagnosis and treatment using artemisinin-based combination therapies (ACTs) against *Plasmodium falciparum,* the most deadly form of malaria parasite, with treatment success >90% of cases. However, resistance to artemisinin-based compounds has already emerged along the Thai-Cambodia border, a similar pattern of resistance that begun with chloroquine, followed by sulfadoxine-pyrimethamine and mefloquine, common drug treatments used in malaria control years ago [11,12].

Malaria transmission continues with high risk in refractory foci, especially areas near the international borders between countries, such areas are commonly associated with rural, forested, undeveloped and sylvan environments compounded by frequent uncontrolled human population movement across shared borders for economic and socio-political reasons [13,14,15,16,17,18]. Other contributing epidemiological factors have either maintained or even enhanced transmission potential in certain areas including various factors that contribute to malaria mosquito vector distribution, vector competency and capacity for transmission, bionomics, adult behavior, and abundance. Contributing factors also include physical and topographical changes such as new development projects including dam and road construction, mining, reforestation, deforestation and commercial plantations (e.g., rubber, palm oil). Deforestation is particularly severe and widespread in Southeast Asia, the highest relative rate of deforestation of any major tropical region in the world. By year 2100, it is estimated that over three quarters of the original forests and up to 42% of the associated biodiversity will result in massive species declines and outright extinctions [19].

Outdoor transmission and biting immediately after dusk and early morning hours continue to pose a major prevention and control challenge. Additionally, population movement and congregation increase the likelihood of exposure to malaria and reintroduction of transmission in receptive areas. To understand malaria risk in an area, the *Anopheles* fauna and bionomics of the important species including those composed of complexes must be better understood. Unfortunately, there are only a few recent studies in each country which cannot provide a complete picture on malaria vectors in this region. Because the accurate identification of vector species and knowledge of their ecology and behavior is essential for epidemiologic studies and the design and implementation of vector control strategies, a major challenge in most countries in the region is the lack of trained entomologists and budgets supporting essential field and laboratory work. Our aim in this chapter is to provide an overview on the malaria vectors of the Greater Mekong Subregion, in which 6 countries are reviewed. Thailand represents the epicenter of the Mekong countries from northwest to southwest (Myanmar), the eastern border (Cambodia & Vietnam), northeast (Lao PDR) and the southern border (Malaysia). The focus will be on reviewing the current malaria transmission in relation to the various malaria vectors, with an emphasis on the geographic variation, vector biology and ecology of each species and how these factors promote malaria transmission in the region.

2. Malaria transmission and primary vectors in mainland Southeast Asia

Review of mosquito biogeography has shown that the greatest mosquito biodiversity occurs in the SEA region and the Neotropics, with high species richness in Indonesia, Malaysia and Thailand [20, 21, 22]. The basic malaria transmission equation (model) indicates a positive correlation between vector density (and life span) in relation to attack on humans and number of malaria cases; however, even small changes in vector density can result in substantial changes in the proportion of humans infected [23]. This is more apparent in areas of relatively lower transmission than those with stable high attack rates. Malaria stability over time is generally greater in areas with highly efficient vector(s) and those having multiple primary vector species present throughout the year or alternating activity patterns based on seasonal changes and local conditions. However, the primary inter-dependent relationship between Human – Vector – Pathogen is influenced by a fourth set of factors, namely demography (human placement and movement), numerous environmental factors, landscape (vector habitat), socioeconomic conditions, that can greatly impact malaria transmission in each country and specific locations (foci) [24, 25, 26, 27, 28, 29, 30,16]. In general, SEA is faced with a complex vector system whose members are difficult to distinguish morphologically that often include a diverse array of non-vectors, potential vectors and malaria vectors [31, 32]. As members of a species complex usually exhibit significant behavioral differences, understanding the biological, behavioral and ecological characteristics of each species will be relevant to the epidemiology and disease control methods used. Three main malaria vectors are recognized on the SEA mainland: *Anopheles dirus* sensu lato (s.l.) (Dirus Complex), *An. minimus* s.l. (Minimus Complex), *An. sundaicus* s.l. (Sundaicus Complex). The Minimus Complex comprises of three sibling species; *An. minimus* (formerly species A), *An. harrisoni* (species C) and *An. yaeyamaensis* (species E). Whereas the latter species is found only in Japan, *An.minimus* and *An. harrisoni* have a broad distribution in SEA and are known vectors of malaria throughout their respective distributions [33, 34]. *An. minimus* s.l. is widespread in the hill forested areas, utilizing mainly margins of slow running streamsunder partial shade and grassy margins [35, 36, 37, 38, 7, 34].

In these forested areas of SEA, malaria transmission can be perennial because of the presence of both *An. dirus* s.l. during rainy season and *An. minimus* s.l. during the drier periods of the year. The Dirus Complex currently includes eight species [39, 40]. Among them two main malaria vectors, *An. dirus* and *An. baimaii* which are considered forest and forest-fringe malaria vectors with an anthropophilic and exophagic behaviors. Their reproduction takes place in and near forested areas (primary and secondary evergreen, deciduous and bamboo forests) with plentiful rain water pools, puddles, as well as artificial containers. Both species are also found in dense mono-agricultural environments, in particular rubber, fruit, and manioc/cassava plantations [18, 32, 33, 41, 42]. One of the factors that make *An. dirus* an important and efficient malaria vector is its strong attraction to humans [32, 43]. The Sundaicus Complex comprises 4 members, however only *An. epiroticus* is reported on the SEA mainland [44]. These four species are coastal vectors, developing primarily in brackish water while some populations can exist in freshwater habitats. *An. epiroticus,* has adapted to a diverse array of biotopes, but also share some common features such as brackish water (optimum 1-7 g NaCl/litre), moderate sun exposure, stagnant or slightly moving water, with floating green algae and presence of vegetation [44, 45]. *Anopheles epiroticus* exhibits both endo- and exophagy while being mainly endophilic and anthropophilic in resting and feeding preference, respectively, although both exophily and zoophily have also been demonstrated [7, 32, 46].

New insights into malaria vectors, in terms of vector bionomics and malaria transmission, are detailed within each country and are framed by the inherent complexity of the epidemiology and the current challenges faced in SEA for implementation of appropriate vector control as one of the key approaches of integrated control for eventual malaria elimination in the region.

2.1. Cambodia

2.1.1. Overview

The Kingdom of Cambodia covers an area of approximately 181,000 km² with 15 million inhabitants, comprised mainly of ethnic Khmer (90%), along with Vietnamese, Chinese and other minorities. This country is bounded on the north by Thailand and Lao PDR, on the east and southeast by Vietnam, and on the west by Thailand and the Gulf of Thailand. Much of the country's topography consists of rolling plains. Dominant geo-physical features include the large, centrally located, Tonle Sap (Great Lake) and the Mekong River, which traverses the entire country from north to south. The climate is monsoonal and has marked wet and dry seasons of relatively equal length. Both ambient air temperatures and relative humidity generally are high throughout the year. Forest covers about two-thirds of the country, but it has been degraded in the more readily accessible areas by burning (slash-and-burn agriculture), and by traditional shifting agricultural practices. Approximately 44% of the population live in high malaria risk areas among which approximately half (~3 million people) live in or around forested areas where there is potentially intense transmission [2]. *Plasmodium falciparum* is the dominant malaria infection reported (63%) followed by *P. vivax* [3]. Between 2001-2009, the number of reported cases detected by the official health system in Cambodia (confirmed cases by MOH) fell from 121,612 to 80,644 and further declined to 44,659 in 2010 [47, 1]. The main provinces with endemic malaria are Battambang, Kampong Speu, Pursat, Peah Vihear, Mondulkiri, Rattanakiri, Pailin and Siem Reab [10, 48]. Malaria transmission is seasonal with a peak occurring during May–July and October–November in the forested and forest-fringe areas of the north, west and northeast, and also in the rubber plantations located in the east and northeast parts of the country. In the rice growing areas of the south and central regions, transmission is typically low or non-existent. There is no reported endemic transmission in urban areas. Low intensity transmission is found focally in coastal areas. Malaria incidence is highest in the eastern provinces of Mondulkiri and Rattanakiri where the disease disproportionately affects ethnic minorities and migrants [8]. According to the Health Management Information System (HMIS), confirmed malaria cases is predominantly observed in males aged 15-49 years (51%), and regarded an occupational risk [49]. Because of the decades long civil war, including the brutal genocide in the 1970's and systematic destruction of infrastructure under the Khmer Rouge regime, Cambodia was left with a very limited health infrastructure and capacity, particularly in rural areas. In recent years, this situation has seen a remarkable rebound, with the public sector providing the majority of diagnosis and treatment through both community-based and government health centers. Over the last decade, many of Cambodia's key health indicators have improved dramatically with the increased resources. Universal diagnostic testing for malaria, primarily using malaria microscopy and Rapid diagnostic test (RDTs) formats, is now common practice in the majority of Cambodian public sector facilities [50]. In addition, with both Global Fund against HIV/AIDS, Tuberculosis and Malaria and USAID support, village malaria workers and mobile malaria workers have been trained and equipped with RDTs and artemisinin-based combination treatments (ACTs) to more accurately diagnose and effectively treat malaria, thereby improving access to these services in remote rural communities. In spite of this, the quality of malaria microscopy in many facilities is regarded sub-optimal, particularly in remote locations. In facilities where both microscopy and RDTs are available, the staff prefers using RDTs because of the ease of use. Additionally, the majority of persons with fever are reported to go to private sector providers where the availability of high-quality diagnostic testing is limited and where there is a financial incentive to provide treatment (sometimes outdated, ineffective chemotherapies) to a patient with a negative test. Another challenge is that an increased prevalence of *Plasmodium vivax* would have implications on the severity of illness, risk of death, and provision of optimal drug therapies to eliminate latent, relapsing forms of the parasite; therefore identifying the parasite species is crucial for case management [51]. Further progress in reducing the burden of the disease will require improved access to reliable diagnosis and effective treatment of both blood-stage and latent parasites and more detailed characterization of the epidemiology, morbidity and economic impact of vivax malaria.

2.1.2. Malaria vectors and biodiversity of Anopheles *in Cambodia*

In 1975, the list of anophelines known from Cambodia was revised to include 37 species [52]. Between 1959-1963, *An. dirus* s.l., *An. minimus* s.l., *An. maculatus* and *An. sundaicus* s.l. were reported as main malaria vectors in Cambodia [53, 34]. However, there has been no record of entomology activities in the following 25 years due to socio-political issues in the country. In 1997, two years of vector surveys reported 19 and 25 species of anopheline mosquitoes in Kompong Speu and Kratie Provinces, respectively in which *An. dirus* s.l, *An. minimus* s.l and *An. maculatus* were included [53]. With molecular techniques having been developed for identifying members within the species complexes, a significant increase of anopheline species have been recorded in Cambodia. *An. minimus* has been the only species of the Minimus Complex recorded in Cambodia [54, 55, 31]. *An. minimus* was recorded as a late evening biter and more anthropophilic where cattle were scarce with the ratio of indoor to outdoor human landing collections ranging between 0.62 and 7.95 [32]. *Anopheles* specimens were found sporozoite positive by ELISA tests for the detection of circumsporozoite protein (CSP) of *Plasmodium falciparum* and *P. vivax* [7, 32]. Distribution and abundance of this primary malaria vector has changed in response to land-use modifications, deforestation, climate change, and

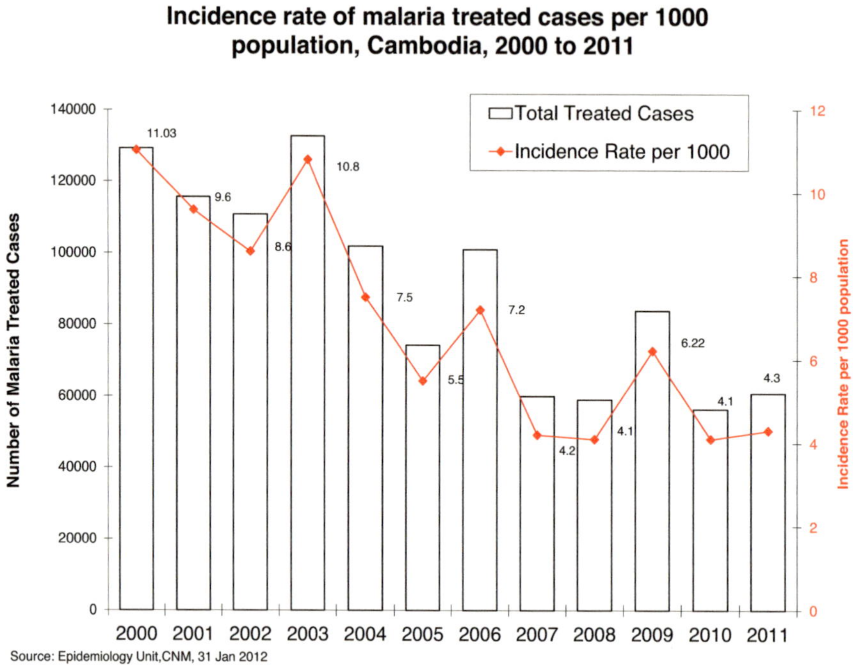

Figure 1. Malaria Incidence Rate per 1,000 population (solid line) and a total treated cases (bar) in Cambodia between 2000 and 2011. Source: Meeting on Outdoor Malaria Transmission in the Mekong Countries for 13 countries during 12-13 March 2012, Bangkok, Thailand. [http://www.rbm.who.int/partnership/wg/wg_itn/ppt/ws2/m4SivSovannaroth.pdf.]

possibly due to insecticides used as part of vector control in malaria endemic areas [35, 34, 38, 27, 56, 41, 57]. The Dirus Complex in Cambodia is represented by *An. dirus* only which plays an important role in malaria transmission [31] with CSP rates having been reported above 1% [7]. *An. sundaicus* s.l. has been recorded along the southern coastal areas of Cambodia [58] and later identified as *An. epiroticus* (*An. sundaicus* A). Larvae of *An. epiroticus* are found in large open stagnant brackish water areas, sunlit pools, and often occurring in distinct foci along the coast [59]. In Cambodia, suspected and potential malaria vectors include *An. annularis* s.l., *An. barbirostris* s.l, *An. culicifacies* B although this latter species is mostly considered as a poor or non-vector (collected in Rattanakiri Province, northeast of Cambodia), *An. nivipes*, *An. philippinensis*, *An. sinensis*, and *An. subpictus* s.l. [54, 60]. Within the Maculatus Group, a recent study recorded for the first time *An. sawadwongporni* in the Kampong Spoe Province [31], yet its vector status in Cambodia is unknown. The Subpictus Complex has a coastal distribution in southern Cambodia [59].

2.1.3. Distribution of malaria vectors and behavior of Anopheles *species in Cambodia*

Forest cover is a very strong determinant of malaria risk. In SEA, forest malaria remains a big challenge for malaria control and in Cambodia malaria risk has increased within 2 to 3 km from the forest border. It is important to note that forest-related malaria covers a wide epidemiological spectrum regard varying vector species and bionomics, human demographics and behavior and control [61]. In Cambodia, malaria transmission is closely associated with two primary malaria vectors that inhabit the forest and forest fringe, *An.dirus* which inhabits predominantly forested areas, and *An. minimus*, a relatively less efficient malaria vector, that occurs in and around rice fields near the forest fringe [7,34,31]. *An. dirus, An. minimus* and *An. maculatus* are mainly outdoor biters [32]. This exophagic tendency of vectors is associated with the persistence of malaria transmission among populations with outdoor activities during night time. Intraspecific behavior differences have been observed among different populations of *Anopheles* species. However, in Cambodia, *An. dirus* has shown a higher degree of anthropophily than other malaria vector species [32]. The inoculation rate of *An. dirus* has been recorded over 1% in Rattanakiri Province indicating this species is a very efficient vector and plays an important role for perennial malaria transmission [7]. *Anopheles minimus* has been found less anthropophilic, preferentially attacking animals more than humans, whereas *An. dirus* showed a higher degree of anthropophily and early biting before 22.00 hr [32]. The host and temporal feeding patterns of malaria vectors are important factors in determining the vector status of *Anopheles* species, both influenced by host availability and location (indoors or outside)[62]. The abundance of malaria vectors in Cambodia is site-specific, for example in Pailin Province, among the three main malaria vectors, *An.minimus* (67.2%) was found more predominant than *An. maculatus* (20.6%) and *An. dirus* (9.9%), while in Pursat Province, 52% of the vector species were *An. dirus*, probably influenced by the suitability of the local environmental conditions and topography [63].

The current vector control methods against indoor feeding and resting vectors include indoor residual spraying (IRS) and insecticide-treated nets (ITNs), but where the vectors primarily feed and rest outdoors, these vector control methods are ineffective, except possibly in those cases where the insecticide used has a high spatial repellent effect [64, 65]. A recent study showed a nearly 45% reduction of blood feeding *An. minimus* in two villages after introduction of long-lasting insecticide-treated hammocks (LLIH) in study sites in Pailin and Pursat Provinces [63]. The obvious risk of regular insecticide use is the development of insecticide resistance in the vector populations. However, so far insecticide resistance has not been a major problem for the primary malaria vectors, *An. dirus* and *An. minimus*. Both species remain susceptible to permethrin, only one site study in Cambodia found *An. dirus* DDT resistant, but this was only based on 23 specimens tested [56]. *Anopheles epiroticus* remains susceptible to permethrin but shown some evidence of possible deltamethrin resistance. The monitoring of the susceptibility status of *Anopheles* to insecticides should be performed regularly as this provides essential information for the correct choice of insecticide to be most effective in vector control. Most studies suggest that ITNs can provide a fair degree of protection if properly used [66, 63, 67, 68, 69]. Therefore, Cambodia has actively distributed ITNs to many at-risk populations. Overall, ITNs ownership improved from 43% in high risk areas in 2007 to 75% in 2011 [63, 3]. Cambodia has recently drafted a new strategic plan following the Prime Minister's announcement that Cambodia's goal would be to eliminate malaria by 2025 [70, 48].

2.1.4. *Implication of changing social and environment conditions on vectors and transmission*

Environmental factors can have a pronounced impact on the distribution and behavior of malaria vectors [71]. *Anopheles dirus* occurs in forest areas but has an ability to adapt to changing environmental conditions from natural forest habitats to cultivated forests, such as rubber and tea plantations and various types fruit orchards [72, 73, 27]. Deforestation is one of the most potent factors either promoting or reducing infectious diseases, in particular malaria in SEA [74, 75, 57]. Deforestation is caused by a wide variety of human activities, including logging, land clearance for agricultural development, transmigration programs, road construction, mining and hydropower development [76, 77]. Globally, estimates of deforestation range from 36,000-69,000 km^2/year. Deforestation in SEA has been extensive with the mean annual rate of deforestation of 0.71 to 0.79% of land cover and is higher than reported in Latin America (0.33%-0.51%) or Africa (0.34%-0.36%) [78].The forest vector species that transmit malaria are among the most sensitive to environmental changes [27]. The extensive clearing of forests has had enormous impact on local natural ecosystems, in particular dramatically altering micro-climates by reducing shade, humidity, and rainfall patterns [38, 79]. For anopheline species that use shaded water bodies, deforestation can reduce larval habitats, thus their propagation and adult densities [38]. In Cambodia, the forest area was reduced from 93,000 km^2 in 2003 to 66,959 km^2 in 2005 [57], and this possibly has had a direct influence on the richness of anopheline mosquito fauna including some malaria vectors.

2.2. Lao People Democratic Republic (Lao PDR, Laos)

2.2.1. *Overview*

Lao PDR is a land-locked country, which borders five countries, China, Vietnam, Cambodia, Thailand and Myanmar, respectively. Most of the western border of Laos is demarcated by the Mekong River, which is an important artery for transportation and commerce. Two-thirds of Laos is covered by primary and secondary forests with a mountainous landscape and an abundance of rivers and natural resources which remain intact. The country has a tropical climate with high humidity throughout the year. The Mekong has not been an obstacle but a facilitator for communication between Laos and northeast Thai society (same people, same language) reflecting the close contact that has existed along the river for centuries.

Malaria is considered endemic throughout the country, but intensity of transmission is known to vary between different ecological zones; from relatively low transmission in the plains near the Mekong River and in areas of high altitude, to intense transmission in more remote, hilly and forested areas. Malaria has long been a leading cause of mortality and morbidity in the country. Transmission of malaria is perennial, but with large seasonal and regional variations. Peak transmission occurs between May and October, coinciding with the hot and rainy season. Malaria is also a problem in the dry season in certain areas of Laos [80]. In 1992, *P. falciparum* was the predominant species accounting for 95% of all recorded malaria cases [81] and remains so with 93% of all reported cases [3] representing leading cause of morbidity and mortality in Laos. A field survey for malaria prevalence in southern Laos using molecular-based parasite detection assay showed that mixed species infections were common with all 4 human plasmodia species detected among 23.1% of positive samples [82]. A recent national survey of the malaria distribution revealed that approximately 41% of the country's population is living in areas of no malaria transmission, particularly large areas in the central regions of the country while malaria incidence of more than 1 per 1,000 population is occurring in seven provinces, Saravane, Savannakhet, Sekong, Attapeu, Champasack, Khammouan, Phongsaly, collectively representing 36% of the Lao population [3, 69]. Significant reductions have been reported following investments in malaria control, in particular the large-scale introduction of artemi sinin-based combination therapy (ACT) beginning in 2004, ITNs introduced in 2000, and IRS in 2010, in conjunction with socio-economic and environmental changes [3]. In 2008, only 11 deaths among 18,743 confirmed malaria cases were reported (population ~6 million), compared with 600 deaths and 70,000 confirmed cases in 1997 (Center for Malariology, Parasitology and Entomology [CMPE] unpublished data). However, malaria still continues to be a serious public health problem in some focal areas such as remote areas in southern Laos [8].

Between 2005 and 2008, the National Malaria Control Programme introduced a new strategy to improve case management at the community level, which involved training of 12,404 village health volunteers (VHVs) in 6,202 villages in the use of *P. falciparum*-specific malaria rapid diagnostic tests and to guide administration of ACT to infected patients. The VHVs represent the most peripheral level of the public health care system in Laos. Volunteers are selected by villagers and a village committee to provide primary health care services, including diagnosis and management of respiratory diseases, diarrhea, and uncomplicated malaria. Activities also include performing health education, assist in vaccination campaigns, and report morbidity and mortality data to the local health center or the district health office [69]. In Laos, insecticide-impregnated bednets have been reported to reduce malaria transmission successfully [68]. Much of the support has focused on the distribution of ITNs. The CMPE is now in the process of scaling up bed net coverage with a projected target of 3.6 million units reaching the most vulnerable ethnic minority groups, other persons at risk, and together with implementing appropriate diagnosis and effective treatment programs. Improving access to effective malaria treatment has become one of the greatest challenges. In recent years, artemisinin-derivative combination therapy (ACT; artemether-lumefantrine) has been adopted as the first-line treatment for uncomplicated malaria in many countries including Lao [83, 84, 85]. Recent data has shown that 89% of patients with malaria received a parasitological-confirmed diagnosis and were treated with an ACT [69, 86]. Furthermore, as the government public health system in Laos provides the vast bulk of primary health care, a private system for health access is growing, especially in the peripheral areas.

2.2.2. Malaria vectors and biodiversity of Anopheles *in Laos*

South-East Asia is one of the world's richest regions in terms of biodiversity. The species distribution and factors shaping it are not well understood, yet essential for identifying conservation priorities for the region's highly threatened flora and fauna. Several malaria vectors belong to sibling species that may greatly differ in their biology, behavior and other characteristics of epidemiological importance, such as resistance to insecticides. The sibling

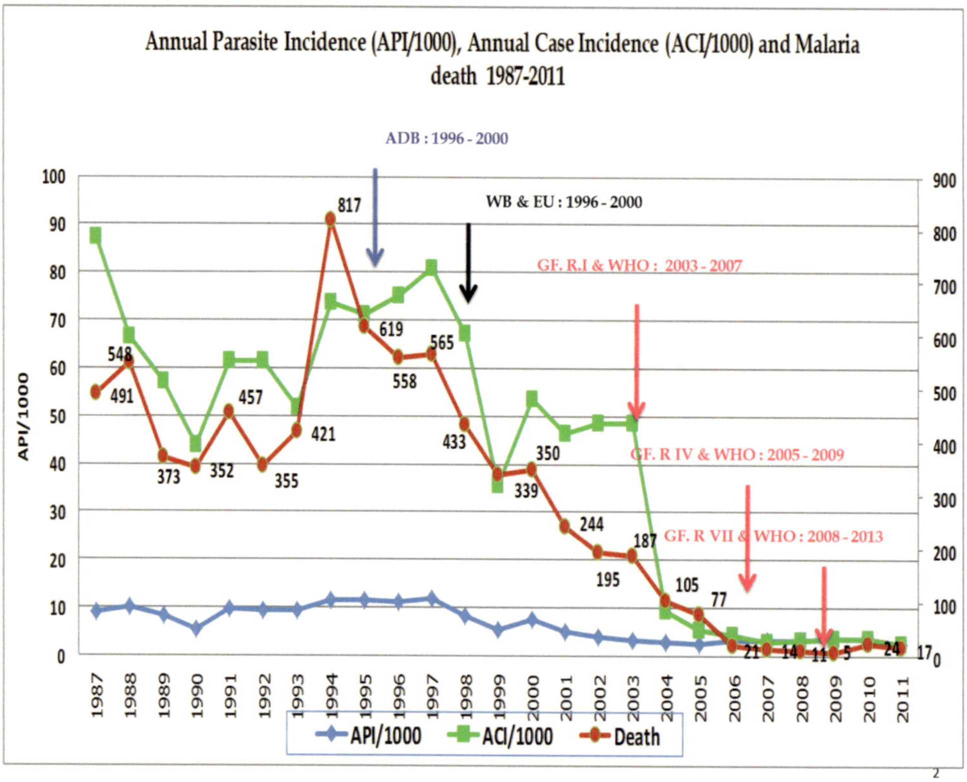

[http://www.rbm.who.int/partnership/wg/wg_itn/ppt/ws2/m4LaoPDR.pdf.]

Figure 2. Annual Parasite Incidence (API/1,000 population), Annual Case Incidence (ACI/1,000 population) and malaria deaths in Laos from 1987 to 2011. Source: Meeting on Outdoor Malaria Transmission in the Mekong Countries for 13 countries during 12-13 March 2012, Bangkok, Thailand.

species have been described as having individual distribution patterns depending on the landscape and seasonal environmental changes.

There are four recognized malaria vectors in Laos: *An. dirus, An. minimus s.l., An. maculatus s.l.*, and *An. jeyporiensis*. Among these *An. dirus* and *An. minimus* are considered the primary vector species. The anopheline situation in Laos is regarded as complex because of taxonomic and ecological variations that affect malaria transmission in the country [80,86]. *Anopheles minimus* and *An. harrisoni* are known to occur largely in sympatry (i.e., occurring together in the same area) in northern Laos [34]. Anopheline abundance and species composition are site-specific and can vary throughout the year depending on conditions. A mosquito survey in Khammouane in 1996 and 1999-2000 found 19 and 28 different anopheline species, respectively. Studies have shown that the vectorial capacity (a transmission probability index) of *An. dirus* was 0.009-0.428, while *An. minimus* s.l was 0.048-0.186, *An. vagus, An. philippinensis, An. nivipes* were predominant species but mostly zoophilic [87, 88]. Three other species belonged to *An. maculatus* Group, including *An. notanandai, An. sawadwongporni*, and *An. willmori* along with *An. hodgkini* (Barbirostris Subgroup), a species reported for first time in Khammouane Province [88]. In 1999, an entomological survey covering 8 provinces, found that out of 19 anopheline species collected, *An. aconitus* was the predominant one, especially in the month of December, yet only 3 species, *An. dirus, An. maculatus* s.l. and *An. minimus* s.l. were found infected with malaria oocysts [86]. In 2000-2001, 16 anopheline species from Sekong Province were captured with only *An. dirus, An. maculatus* s.l. and *An. jeyporiensis* found positive for human malaria sporozoites [89]. *Anopheles dirus* was found to be the primary vector and sporozoite rates were highest during the transitional dry season. Two years of mosquito surveys, from 2002-2004, were conducted in Attapeu, the southern-most province bordering Vietnam and Cambodia, and a town located in a large valley surrounded with forest. It is one of the endemic malaria provinces which documented 8,945 mosquitoes belonging to 14 genera and 57 species, of which 21 species were *Anopheles*. Maculatus Group, *An. sawadwongporni* and *An. notanandai,* were found in large numbers but only *An. minimus* was found malaria sporozoite positive [90, 91]. There is very limited information about adult behavior and breeding habitats of anophelines in Laos. Recently, information has also been provided on non-vector species, for example, *An. annularis* s.l., *An. philippinensis,* and *An. sinensis* [60].

2.2.3. Distribution of malaria vectors and behavior of Anopheles *in Laos*

An. minimus s.l. is widespread in the country and has been identified in all malaria endemic provinces in Laos. It primarily breeds in slow running streams closely associated with forested hilly areas, irrigation ditches, and rice fields. The mosquito feeds predominantly on humans but also on cattle and other animals and is regarded as primarily endophagic and endophilic. A recent study found both *An. minimus* and *An. harrisoni* present in northern Laos [56]. While *An. dirus* is most common in the central and southern parts of the country, it is considered rare in the north. *Anopheles dirus* is the most important malaria vector in the southern part of Laos. It breeds preferentially in stagnant and shaded waters (e.g. hoof prints, small rain-fed ground pools) in the rainforest, forested foothills and agricultural plantations, but has also been found to breed in scrub lands with lower vegetation. Population densities for this species typically increase during the wet season of the year while also having higher sporozoite infective rates at the end of the rainy season [89, 90]. The species is predominantly anthropophilic making it an ideal vector, but it will also feed on domestic animals with an indoor: outdoor blood feeding ratio of 1.6 [90]. The biting cycle of *An. dirus* has been documented to begin early evening, from 19:00 and remaining active through the night until 06:00, with peak activity around 22:00 [90, 92].

2.2.4. Implications of changing social and environment conditions on vector and transmission

Anopheles dirus is the most capable and dangerous malaria vector in Laos, particularly in southern Laos associated with forest-related habitats. This species has also become well adapted to human-induced environmental change, for example utilization of disturbed scrub areas containing low standing vegetation [90]. Laos' national forest coverage has dropped from 70% in 1940, at around 17 million hectares, to 41% in 2001, when a ban on timber exports was enacted, yet illegal deforestation has remained rampant over the past decade. From 2002 to

2010, central Laos's forestry cover decreased by 3.5%, while 9% of the southern forests disappeared [(http://www.nationmultimedia.com/home/Laos-to-increase-forest-cover-age-30145391html (December 2010)]. The government plans to increase forestry cover in Laos to 65% by 2015 and 70% by 2020 (The National Assembly, seventh five-year economic plan for 2011-2015). The current reforestation programmes have concentrated on allowing investments in large rubber plantations in Laos' border regions with southern China and Vietnam. For example, 10,000 hectares have been allocated for rubber plantation development in one area, and this has attracted populations from the Laos highlands to migrate to the plains, especially in Sanamxay District, to work in the rubber and sugar cane plantations. From October to December 2011, a total of 11,833 persons tested for malaria found 3,091 infected as reported from all facilities in the area including Attapeu Province villages. Up to the end of January 2012, 8 deaths due to malaria were reported from Attapeu.This outbreak of malaria has been attributed to the large scale development projects in the province, mainly concentrated in Phuvong and Sanamxay Districts, and the resulting population movements into the areas. In Phuvong District, extensive land clearing for Nam Kong 2 and 3 hydroelectric dams have been completed with dam construction beginning in 2013. The surge in logging activities associated with land clearing, primarily for the prized 'MaiKhayung' (rosewood), has attracted both local populations as well as people from other provinces to Attapeu. Most malaria patients admitted to provincial and district hospitals have been from other provinces or neighboring countries. In Phuvong District, from October to December 2011, 68% of the non-local malaria cases were from Vietnam and approximately 10% of cases were seen in children under the age of 5 years. This should be the lesson for other neighboring malaria-endemic provinces of Savannakhet, Saravane, Sekong and Champasack in southern Laos, where significant development projects are also planned, as well as other neighboring countries that are either initiating, planning or contemplating major development projects that would create extensive environment changes to design strategies to prevent or mitigate the occurrence of disease outbreaks as a result.

2.3. Malaysia

2.3.1. Overview

The Federation of Malaysia, a federal constitutional monarchy in Southeast Asia, consists of thirteen states and three federal territories and has a total landmass of 329,847 km^2 separated by the South China Sea into two similarly sized areas, Peninsular Malaysia located on mainland SEA and Malaysian Borneo. National borders are shared with Thailand, Indonesia, and Brunei, and maritime borders exist with Singapore, Vietnam, and the Philippines. Malaysia is a multiracial country consisting of Malays, Chinese, Indians, Ibans, Kadazans and smaller ethnic groups with total population of approximately 28.3 million [93]. Several vector-borne diseases remain serious concerns in Malaysia, including malaria.

During the 1960s, the number of malaria cases were estimated at 300,000 annually before the Malaria Eradication Program (MEP) was launched. The program was successful in dramatically reducing malaria transmission with number of cases decreasing from 181,495 at the start of MEP in 1967 to 44,226 cases at the end of the program in 1980. In 1983, the country changed strategy to one focused on 'control' by adopting the Malaria Control Program (MCP). The MCP continued the fight against malaria before reorganizing to the Vector-Borne Disease Control Program (VBDCP) in 2010. The key objective of the current program is to continue the reduction of malaria morbidity and mortality and to prevent the recurrence of malaria in non-endemic areas. The VBDCP also includes activities for the prevention and control of other vector-borne diseases like dengue fever and lymphatic filariasis [94, 95]. The MCP activities had been successful in reducing the number of malaria cases in Malaysia from 48,007 cases in 1986 to 7,010 cases in 2009 [96, 97].

Currently, malaria is still one of the most important vector-borne diseases in the country, primarily in Malaysian Borneo (Sarawak and Sabah states), although only 4% of the population is living in areas within active malaria transmission foci [3]. These refractory areas are partly attributed to anti-malarial drug resistance, insecticide resistance and cross border migration. In 2005, there were almost two million legal migrant workers in Malaysia. Most of these foreigners came from malaria endemic countries, a majority being from Indonesia (68.9%), followed by Nepal (9.9%), India (6.9%) and Myanmar (4.6%) [98,99]. In addition, the risk of malaria is high among the aboriginal groups such as Orang Asli, who lived in the interior of Peninsular Malaysia in remote hilly, cleared jungle areas [96]. In 2009, 7,010 malaria cases were reported in the country with approximately 57.2% of cases occurring in Sabah, 26% in Sarawak and 16.8% in Peninsular Malaysia. Most cases were caused by *Plasmodium vivax* (48.15%), followed by *P. falciparum* (26.75%), *P. knowlesi* (13.01%), *P. malariae* (8.37%) and mixed species infections (3.68%) [97,2]. *Plasmodium knowlesi* has more recently been recognized as an important zoonotic malaria species in eastern Malaysia (Borneo) and outbreaks have been found primarily in Borneo, Sarawak and Sabah and West Malaysia, [100] as well as other countries in SEA (see the Chapter by Vythilingam & Hii). In Malaysia, *An. latens* and *An. cracens* (both members of the *An. leucosphyrus* Subgroup) have been incriminated as vectors of *P. knowlesi* [101, 102, 103].

Malaysia has launched a national vector control program to include use of targeted indoor residual spraying (IRS), ITN distribution, artemisinin-based combination anti-malarial drugs, larviciding aquatic habitats harboring immature stages of vector species, environmental management measures, and personal protection methods [104]. After years of insecticide use to control vectors, development of physiological resistance to insecticides has been detected in some malaria vectors. Hii (1984) reported that *An. balabacensis* was tolerant to DDT and years later that several other anopheline species had also developed resistance to DDT and permethrin [105].

2.3.2. Malaria vectors in Malaysia

Seventy-five species of *Anopheles* have been recorded in the country, only 9 of which are reported as malaria vectors to include *An balabacensis* and *An. latens* (both Leucosphyrus Complex), *An. cracens* (Dirus Complex), *An. maculatus* (Maculatus Group), *An. letifer*, *An. campestris*, *An. sundaicus* and *An. epiroticus* (both Sundaicus Complex), *An. donaldi*, and *An. flavirostris* [96]. Each species is considered a malaria vector in various areas of the country, sometimes existing in sympatry (Table 1).

Anopheline species	Peninsular Malaysia	Sarawak and Sabah
An. balabacensis		+
An. campestris	+	
An. cracens (=*An. dirus* B)	+	
An. donaldi	+	+
An. flavirostris		+
An. letifer	+	+
An. latens (=*An. leucosphyrus* A)		+
An. maculatus	+	+
An. epiroticus/*An. sundaicus*	+	+

Table 1. Anopheline vectors in Malaysia [33,59]

Anopheles maculatus is within a species group that comprises at least nine genetically-related species [39]. Historically, *An. maculatus* has been the principal vector of malaria in West Malaysia, particularly in hilly areas not covered with dense forest [106,107,108]. This species prefers to breed in pools formed along the still banks of rivers and small streams. The larval breeding habitats include shallow pools (5-15cm depth) of clear water, with muddy substrate and plants or flotage [109]. In Borneo, this species appears to be more zoophilic and is not regarded a malaria vector of any importance [106].

Anopheles campestris belongs to the Barbirostris Subgroup (subgenus *Anopheles*) and is a potential vector of malaria and filariasis, particularly along the west coast of Peninsular Malaysia [110]. The larvae commonly breed in rice fields, burrow pits, stagnant ditches in coconut plantations, earthen wells, and sometimes in slightly brackish water [111]. Reid (1968) reported that this species could be found in deep water with some vegetation and light shade. Adults are generally anthropophilic, will enter houses to blood feed and rest.

Anopheles cracens (formerly *An. dirus* species B), is a member of the Dirus Complex, found exclusively in the Thai-Malaysian peninsular area of mainland SEA. *An. cracens* is the vector of *P. knowlesi* in Kuala Lipis of peninsular Malaysia [102]. Larvae typically inhabit small, usually temporary, shaded bodies of fresh, stagnant water, including ground pools, puddles, animal footprints, and wells. This species is found in hilly and mountainous areas containing primary or secondary evergreen and deciduous forests, bamboo, and fruit and rubber plantations [112, 113, 114].

Anopheles letifer larvae prefer to breed in stagnant dark-brown (often acidic) water found in peat swamps, especially in jungle clearings along forest edges, with or without shade. Oil palm cultivation areas are also habitats for *An. letifer* associated with open and blocked swamps [115]. In peninsular Malaysia, *An. letifer* is regarded a vector of human malaria and Bancroftian filariasis [106, 96, 116], particularly at low elevations on the coastal plains.

Anopheles epiroticus (formerly *An. sundaicus* species A) and *An. sundaicus* s.s. are members of the Sundaicus Complex [117] and considered important vectors of malaria in coastal areas [106, 118, 44]. In Peninsular Malaysia, *An. epiroticus* occurs mostly along coastal areas while *An. epiroticus* is found in Sarawak (Borneo) [46]. The immature stages are typically found in sunlit pools of brackish water, containing filamentous and floating algal mats, and sparse vegetation. Particularly favorable habitats include ponds, swamps, lagoons, open mangrove, rock pools and abandoned or poorly maintained coastal shrimp and fish ponds [46]. Adults rest by day both outdoors and indoors and readily bite people indoors. Sporozoite rates can often be relatively low but are compensated by large adult densities [106].

Anopheles donaldi is one of the primary malaria vectors in Sarawak with a reported sporozoite rate of 0.23% [119]. This species prefers small streams and ground pools, containing clean and shaded fresh water, occasionally rice fields and open marshlands [106,115]. The adults are found in forest fringes in hilly areas and near tree-covered swamps in the lowlands [106]. *Anopheles balabacensis*, a member of the Leucosphyrus Complex,is regarded as the main vector of malaria in Sabah [120,111]. This species occurs in forested area of Malaysian Borneo (eastern Sarawak and Sabah). The immature stages are principally found in shaded temporary pools of stagnant fresh water, including ground puddles, animal footprints, wheel tracks, ditches and rock pools [59]. In addition, *An. balabacensis* is also a vector of *Wuchereria bancrofti* responsible for lymphatic filariasis [121,116]. In most areas, this species is very anthropophilic and will readily enter houses to blood feed.

Anopheles flavirostris is a malaria vector in Sabah along the eastern coast [111] belonging to the Minimus Subgroup [122]. This species demonstrates anthropophilic and endophagic behaviors in Sabah [121]. Characteristically, *An. flavirostris* larvae are found in clear, slow-moving freshwater stream habitats that are partly shaded by over hanging vegetation and margins containing emergent plants or grasses [123]. *Anopheles latens* (formerly *An. leucosphyrus* A), a member of the Leucosphyrus Group, is a primary vector of human malaria in Sarawak. Additionally, *An. latens* also transmits the monkey malaria parasite, *P. knowlesi* to humans in Sarawak [101]. Like all members in the group, this is a forest mosquito and larval habitats of *An. latens* are primarily found in shaded, temporary ground pools, small pools on margins of forest streams, and natural containers of clear or turbid water in forested areas [59]. In Sarawak, [124] this species was commonly found in shaded pools, a forest stream and swampy patches. Adults will enter houses in the evening to bite, generally delaying activity until after 2200 hr.

2.3.3. Effects of changing environmental conditions on malaria vectors and transmission

In Malaysia, malaria transmission appears more strongly associated with land development rather than water development projects [125]. Land use changes, such as deforestation, increased urbanization and agriculture can directly impact mosquito abundance, species biodiversity, biting behavior, and vector competence [77]. For example, the effect of forest clearance for rubber plantations exposes land and streams to direct sunlight and thus increased and expanded the available breeding habitats for *An. maculatus*, which further led to a marked increase in the incidence and severity of malaria [126]. Vythilingam et al. [119] found that *An. donaldi* appears to have replaced *An. balabacensis* as the main vector in Kinabatangan of Sabah as a result deforestation and malaria control activities. Similarly, the clearing of mangroves and swamps for fish aquaculture or mining resulted in an increase in suitable larval habitats of filariasis vectors and *An. epiroticus* followed by malaria outbreaks [76,119, 127].

2.4. Myanmar

2.4.1. Overview

Myanmar (formerly Burma) has a total land area of 678,500 km^2. The extent of border areas with the 5 surrounding countries include 193 km with Bangladesh; 2,185 km with China; 1,463 km with India; 1,800 km with Thailand, and a relatively small stretch with Laos. Administratively, the nation is divided into 14 states and divisions, 65 districts, 325 townships. The climate is tropical with the southwest monsoon occurring from June to September and a northeast monsoon from December to April.

Migration across international borders through specific points of entry from Myanmar includes, Tachilek, Myawaddy and Kawthaung, Thailand; Muse, Namkhan and Khukok, China; Tamu, India; and Maungdaw, Bangladesh. There are also other less important points of entry into Thailand where Thai and Burmese citizens normally need only a valid border pass to cross at official check points. At Mae Sai, approximately 60,000 Thais and 30,000 Burmese nationals crossed the border in 1997. That is one important reason why malaria morbidity and mortality along the Thai-Myanmar border is especially high and refractory to most control methods [127] and why the disease peaked in intensity between 1988 and 1991 [128].

Malaria is a severe public health problem in Myanmar, in particular along parts of international borders [129]. Confirmed malaria cases in Myanmar increased from 120, 029 in 2000 to 447,073 cases in 2008. The 2009 World Malaria Report (WMR) stated that Myanmar (Burma), with a population of over 50 million, had 17% of all malaria cases recorded in Southeast Asia, the highest percentage in the region [47]. There were 400,000 confirmed malaria cases in the country and about 1,100 deaths due to malaria in 2008, occurring in 284 out of 324 townships [85].

In 2008, Chin State reported the highest morbidity rate of 44.7 per 1,000 inhabitants, whereas the highest number of malaria cases was reported in the Rakhine State, followed by Sagaing State (Figure 4) [130,131].

Generally, malaria transmission peaks just before and after the monsoon rains which normally occur between June and September. The populations most at risk include: 1) people who live or migrate into high malaria risk areas, especially along the borders; 2) international migrants or laborers involved in mining, agriculture (e.g., rubber plantations), the construction of dams, roads, and irrigation projects; 3) those who farm or related work near or in forests and along forest fringes such as wood and bamboo cutters; 4) pregnant women and children under five years old; and 5) ethnic minorities residing in more remote areas with poorer access to primary health care. Out of a total population of 60 million, the proportion of residents living under some degree of malaria risk or none is as follows: high risk 37%, low risk 23% and no risk 40% [3]. Overall 36 townships had higher than 4% mortality in cases diagnosed [132]. Significant numbers of ethnic minorities (approximately 100,000) live in semi-permanent refugee camps

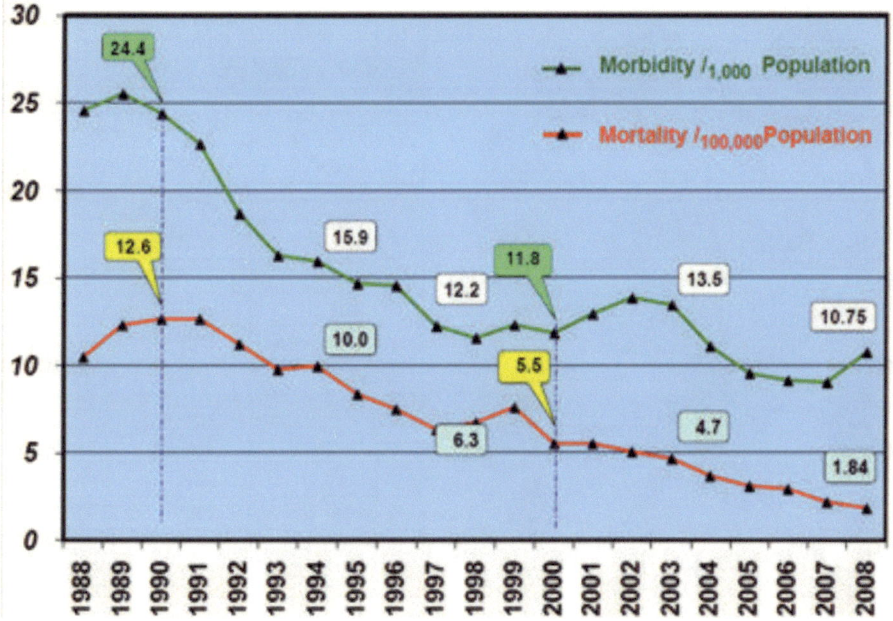

Figure 3. Malaria morbidity and mortality rate in Myanmar during 1988-2008. (http://www.actmalaria.net/home/vector_control.php#base)

along the Thai-Myanmar border where malaria transmission is rampant. The Thai government's policy is to eventually repatriate Shan and other minorities back to Myanmar.

All four species of human plasmodia (*P. falciparum, P. vivax, P. malariae* and *P. ovale*), exist in Myanmar. In 2008, the NMCP Myanmar reported 391,461 *P. falciparum* cases (87.6% of all malaria infections) followed by *P. vivax* at 52,256 (11.7%), while *P. malariae* and *P. ovale* were seen in only 283 and 5 cases, respectively. Currently, *P. falciparum* is still the predominate species at 68% of all cases detected [3]. Additionally, one human infection with *P. knowlesi* was found in a Burmese worker at Ranong Province of Thailand. This zoonotic infection may have been acquired in Kawthoung District, Myanmar, a district close to Ranong Province [133]. *Plasmodium falciparum* resistance to antimalarial drugs is a primary concern in the country. Chloroquine and sulfadoxine-pyrimethamine (S-P) resistance at various levels is now common. Also, well documented report of resistance in small case series has appeared. Resistance to chloroquine by *P. vivax* has been reported [134,135].

2.4.2. Malaria vectors and species diversity

Due to Myanmar's diverse geography, there is a relatively large number of dominant malaria vector species. Out of 36 *Anopheles* species distributed in the country, 10 species at 16 locations have been found infected with malarial parasites [136]. In Myanmar, the primary vectors responsible for the majority of infections are *An. dirus* s.l. and *An. minimus* s.l. [59]. Other anopheline species, predominantly zoophilic feeders, may also, under ideal conditions, feed

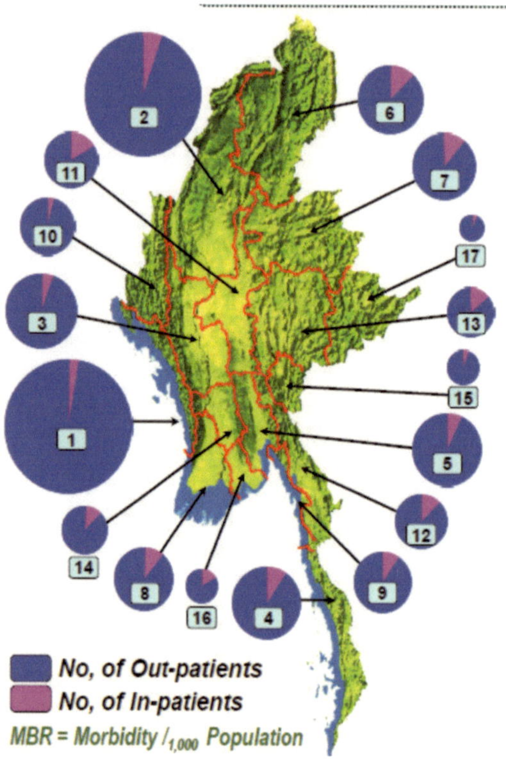

Sr	S/D	Malaria Cases	Country %	Morbidity Rate
1	Rakhine	138377	21.8%	42.04
2	Sagaing	116080	18.3%	18.12
3	Magway	42886	6.8%	7.77
4	Tanintharyi	40141	6.3%	15.86
5	Bago (E)	39649	6.3%	11.62
6	Kachin	35811	5.6%	23.18
7	NSS	33245	5.2%	12.96
8	Ayeyarwady	30209	4.8%	3.72
9	Mon	27729	4.4%	9.14
10	Chin	24921	3.9%	44.72
11	Mandalay	24205	3.8%	2.95
12	Kayin	22053	3.5%	12.37
13	SSS	19247	3.0%	8.60
14	Bago (W)	17261	2.7%	6.64
15	Kayah	8896	1.4%	26.64
16	Yangon	8590	1.4%	1.25
17	ESS	4980	0.8%	5.55
Others S/D total		495903	78.2%	8.90
Grand Total		634280	100.0%	10.75

Figure 4. Malaria morbidity rate in States/Divisions of Myanmar in 2008. (http://www.actmalaria.net/home/vector_control.php#base)

on man [137,138]. These secondary vectors include *An. aconitus, An.annularis* s.l., *An. culicifacies* s.l., *An. sinensis, An. jeyporiensis, An. maculatus* s.l., *An. philippinensis,* and *An. sundaicus* s.l. [136].

2.4.3. Anopheline behavior

Much of the recent work on anopheline bionomics and distribution in Myanmar is attributed to Oo et al. [113, 136] herein. *Anopheles baimaii* is the most common species of the Dirus Complex present in Myanmar, which is also the primary vector species in neighboring Bangladesh [113]. Highest numbers of immature stages were collected during the pre- and post-monsoon periods, while the lowest numbers were seen during the cool-dry and hot-dry months. The larvae were found in rock pools along the banks of thickly shaded streams and in cut bamboo stumps. Adults of this species are plentiful in the monsoon months with a peak densities occurring during September and October. *An. dirus* s.l. was also found daytime resting in the crevices and vegetation around the inner walls of domestic wells and on the underside of banana leaves. Adult behavior indicated this species highly exophilic and it will bite both humans and cattle. A previous study [139] has reported a higher zoophilic tendency despite the breeding sites being found very near human dwellings. Outdoor biting peak has been shown to occur between 21:00 and 03:00 hr. [139]. The results of the dissection both of midgut and salivary glands together for determination of natural infection rates in different localities ranged from 0.4 to 2.8%. The highest infection rate for midgut dissection was 0.4 % (1/250) and salivary gland dissection 2.4% (6/250).

For *An. minimus* s.l., adult densities vary seasonally, although it is also abundant throughout the entire year in many locations [136]. The highest prevalence of *An. minimus* s.l. occurs during the post-monsoon months of October to December. Adults prefer to rest in houses and cattle sheds during daytime. The preference of *An. minimus* s.l. for human blood is well documented during different periods of the year and various locations. Even when cattle are present, only a small proportion of mosquitoes appear to deviate from biting humans. *Anopheles minimus* s.l. feeds mainly during the early hours of the evening, beginning before 21:00 hr and peaking in activity just before or after midnight. However, when adult densities are high, *An. minimus* s.l. populations will bite throughout the night (both outdoors and indoors) with greater activity during the first quarter of the evening and a gradual decrease in biting till dawn (06:00 hr). The infection rate both in midgut and salivary glands has been reported to vary between 1.1-3.0%. *Anopheles minimus* s.l. is primarily a mosquito of hilly regions, low rolling foothills to narrow river valleys in more mountainous areas; it has not been recorded in locations over 915 m above sea level. When found in lowland plains, it is always in association with irrigation systems.

Anopheles aconitus is a secondary vector in certain localities and is a fairly abundant species from October to February, peaking in November [136]. From March to September it is very seldom seen. *An. aconitus* is more commonly seen in hilly tracts, foothills and also in the plains of central and southern Myanmar closely associated with active rice cultivation. Only a few *An. aconitus* females are found resting in houses or stables during daytime preferring to rest outdoors in scrub and other locations. *An. aconitus* appears to prefer cattle for blood meals, although it will bite humans if cattle are not available or very limited in number. It is active in the early evening, biting as early as 18:00 hr, with very little activity after 01:00 hr. *An. aconitus* had a 0.2% (1/350) infection rate [136].

An. annularis s.l. has been found in few localities with high adult densities. Stagnant water with thick grassy edges in permanent ponds, ground pits, tanks, swamps, stagnant drains and rice fields are common larval habitats of *An. annularis*. Its abundance varies according to rainfall patterns. In coastal areas with heavy rainfall (between 3,800 mm to 5,150 mm annually), *An. annularis* densities typically increase from October to January. This species appears to preferentially feed on cattle with a far greater proportion (80-90%) of biting activity seen during the first half of the night (18:00-24:00 hr). The midgut dissection records on *An. annularis* have seen 0.1-0.2% (350-700 samples) plasmodia infection rates [136].

An. culicifacies s.l. is a suspected malaria vector in central Myanmar, especially in irrigated areas. The larval stage of this species breeds in fresh (unpolluted) water and also in artificial water containers and unused swimming pools. *An. culicifacies* is more abundant in August and September, dropping of in October and virtually none from November to March. Adults prefer to rest in cattle sheds and houses during the day, but it may take shelter in paddy-sheds, stacked fire-wood and piles of straw near the stables and outside houses. *Anopheles culicifa-*

cies is primarily a cattle feeder with generally far fewer numbers attacking humans.This species feeds mostly around midnight with very few biting after 03:00 hr. Midgut infections (with oocysts present) have been recorded at 1.83% (6 infections from 328 examined mosquitoes) [136].

When adult densities are high, *An. sinensis* is a secondary vector along the Myanmar-China border. Larvae are predominately found in stagnant waters and rice fields. This species was found from July to December with a peak in August. It is predominantly zoophilic, preferring cattle over humans. Very few have been caught biting humans at night. The peak biting activity of *An. sinensis* is during the first half of the evening beginning at 18.00 hr. In Shan State, along the Myanmar-China border, 300 specimens of *An. sinensis* were examined of which 2.3% (6/300) were found malaria infected [139]. *Anopheles jeyporiensis* is regarded a secondary vector on the Myanmar-China and Myanmar-Bangladesh borders when adult densities are high. Immature stages are mainly found along margins of slow-moving streams and channels with grassy edges and often sympatric with larvae of *An. aconitus*. Rice fields are also attractive breeding sites for *An. jeyporiensis* when uncultivated or early stages of plant growth but become unfavorable as the plants increase in height. Adults are normally abundant during the pre-monsoon period of March and April. They will feed on both humans and cattle. The peak biting period has been recorded from 23:30 to 03:00. On the Myanmar-Bangladesh border (Rakhine State), 500 specimens of *An. jeyporiensis* were dissected with four having sporozoite-infected salivary glands (0.8% infection rate). On the Myanmar-China border (Shan State), 500 specimens of *An. jeyporiensis* were dissected with a 1.2% (6/500) infection rate.

An. maculatus s.l. has been reported as a primary vector, especially in Tanintharyi Division, and elsewhere as a secondary vector depending on the location. The greatest density of this species in nearly all areas where it occurs is during January (cold dry season). Numbers start to increase at the end of southwest monsoon period in early October and relatively rare during the two annual monsoon seasons.There is only one exception, in Mandalay Division, where *An. maculatus* has been recorded in large numbers during September, at the end of the rainy season. It has not been recorded resting indoors during the day, even though many houses in the foothill areas are semi-enclosed. However, at times of peak densities, *An. maculatus* can be collected in cattle sheds. This species member feeds on both humans and various animals, mainly during the first half of the night beginning at 18:00 hr. The midgut dissections have shown a 0.5% (1/180) infection rate. *Anopheles maculatus* is primarily recorded from forested foothills, around deep forest camps and in mountainous areas at 1, 200m above sea level and typically not found in low lying areas far from foothill environments.

Anopheles philippinensis is a vector of minor importance near the Myanmar-Bangladesh border. This species was not found resting in houses and cattle sheds during daytime and presumably selects natural sites outdoors. *An. philippinensis* has only been found resting in houses during morning collections. *An. philippinensis* is a zoophilic species and feeds mainly on cattle. In areas where cattle are either scarce or absent, this species will readily feed on man. In Innwaing Village (Mawlamyine Township, Mon State) and Patheingyi Township *An. philippinensis* has been reported in large numbers during the post-monsoon months from September to November [136].

An. sundaicus s.l. is a secondary vector restricted to coastal areas where larval habitats are-mainly located in sunlit lagoons, natural fresh and brackish water impoundments and back-up streams, often with dense aquatic vegetation (floating algal mats), and brackish water seepage areas. The seasonal abundance of *An. sundaicus* s.l. often increases between May and July and again in October to February. This species was recorded in moderate numbers from houses and cattle sheds from daytime collections. They feed on both human and cattle. In Chaungthar and Seikgyi areas in Ayeyarwady Division, *An. sundaicus* s.l. had a 0.4 % midgut infection rate (1 oocyst positive /220 sampled and 1 positive per 230, respectively). Along the Myanmar-Bangladesh border in Rakhine State, a total of 202 specimens were dissected from which 0.5% had positive salivary gland infections [136].

Myanmar's national malaria control program aims to achieve the WHO Millennium Development Goal of halting the increase in malaria cases by 2015 and significantly reversing the incidence of malaria thereafter. The principle method for malaria vector control in malaria endemic areas of Myanmar relies on the application of ITNs distribution and case management [3]. Biological control using two predacious 'top minnow' fish species, *Poecilia reticulata* and *Aplocheilus panchax* are also effective in certain aquatic habitats and when the correct conditions merit. Inter-sector cooperation, community participation and health education are also part of this integrated approach to reducing disease transmission [131]. Although insecticides are an important component of malaria control operations in Myanmar there is lack information on the status of insecticide resistance in key vector species [12]. Information from the NMCP showed insecticide resistance present in anopheline mosquitoes from Rakhine State. In 2009, both *An. annularis* s.l. and *An. barbirostris* were found resistant to 4% DDT, and *An. barbirostris* was also resistant to 0.25% permethrin, while both species were susceptible to 5% malathion and 0.05% deltamethrin [132]. Although the threat of malaria must be targeted at the local and regional level, especially in the remaining conflict areas of eastern Myanmar, the government does not yet conduct extensive malaria control programmes in many areas in need [140].

2.4.4. *Effects of changing environmental conditions on malaria vectors and transmission*

Since Nay Pyi Taw, the new administrative capital of Myanmar was opened in November 2005 to include relocation of all government ministries approximately 320 km north of Yangon. This major infrastructural change has had a major impact on the land-use characteristics in the area with new buildings a connecting train network, roads and other projects. [85]. Land-use changes could create ideal new habitats ideal for mosquito propagation, the extension or reduction of a vector's distribution, and modify the composition of the mosquito vectors in an area [141]. *An. dirus* s.l. and *An. minimus* are the major malaria vectors in the hilly regions of Myanmar. There is a profound lack of information about the effects of environmental changes on malaria vectors in Myanmar. Currently there are only a few publications that describe [77, 142, 75] the effects of major infrastructural projects (e.g., dam construction), deforestation, vegetation replacement, increased in human population density and movement, modified topography and hydrological characteristics that can affect the epidemiology of malaria and risk of transmission.

Myanmar is the country where the malaria situation is still poorly understood and well-organized control programs remain lacking in many areas of the country. Current and available information is generally lacking and operational research limited to better assess the epidemiology throughout the country. Both published literature and unpublished departmental reports by the Department of Medical Research (DMR) and Department of Vector Borne Disease Control (VBDC) are regarded as inadequate to address managing an effective malaria control program.

2.5. Thailand

2.5.1. Overview

Thailand is the world's fifty-first largest country in terms of total land area (513,120 km^2), and a total population of nearly 67 million people. Thailand shares national boundaries with Myanmar on the west and north, Laos on the north and east, Cambodia on the east, and Malaysia in the south. Gem mining, hunting, logging, agriculture, road construction and other economic activities along Thailand's border areas attract many migrant workers from neighboring countries. The constant movement of workers and the transient, often poorly constructed dwellings they occupy facilitates cross-border transmission of malaria and complicates efforts to control it, making it one of the most serious vector-borne diseases in these areas.

Despite decades of success in reducing the number of cases of malaria in the country, the disease remains a major cause of morbidity and mortality. Approximately 32 million people in Thailand's border areas (50% of the Thailand's population) are at risk of contracting malaria. All four malaria parasites are present with the most common being *P.vivax* with 60% of all reported infections in 2011 [3]. Since 1997, *P. falciparum* and *P. vivax* infections have been recorded at near equal prevalence [70] (Figure 5). The under-developed border areas between Thailand and eastern Myanmar remain the worst affected area for continuing transmission [1, 2]. Non-immune workers who migrate across the international border remain the most susceptible and vulnerable populations. The constant movement of this population involved in gem mining, logging, agriculture, construction and other pursuits, has helped to increase the spread of multi-drug resistant *P. falciparum* malaria in the area and region. Serious outbreaks of malaria have taken place in high risk areas along the Thai-Myanmar border, especially in Kanchanaburi and Tak Provinces [70,143]. In four southern provinces of Thailand, malaria cases have risen to nearly 4,000 per year in the areas bordering Malaysia where social conflict and a local insurgency have greatly complicated control efforts [70]. At the same time, a rapid increase of rubber plantations in northeastern Thailand has become a major concern because of the potential for the reemergence of malaria [144]. Several major malaria vectors, mainly *Anopheles dirus* s.l., *An. maculatus* s.l., and *An. minimus* s.l., can adapt and utilize rubber plantations in place of more typical habitats like hill environments and natural forests [4]. Careful attention and monitoring to land use changes along with climatic and other environmental changes is essential to help prevent or delay the reemergence of malaria in receptive areas.

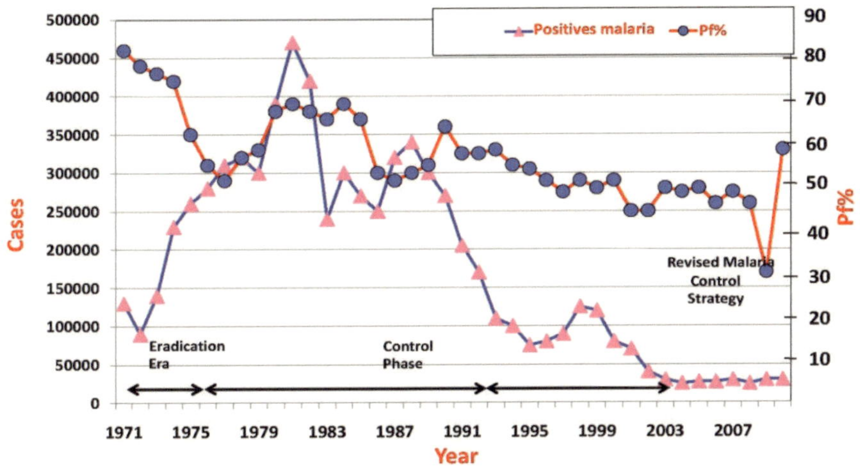

Figure 5. Trends of malaria in Thailand between 1971 and 2010.'Positives' refer to all malaria cases, "Pf" = *P. falciparum* infections only. (http://www.searo.who.int/en/Section10/Section21/Section340_4027.htm).

Based on recorded malaria surveillance activities in Thailand from 1971 to 2011, the peak of malaria cases was seen in 1981 with the total of 473,210 infections, and has since declined thereafter despite another rise in case load seen in 1988 (349,291 infections). In general, from 1988 to 2010, malaria has declined significantly [143, 70]. Despite the significant achievements in malaria control in Thailand over the past five decades, between 25,000 and 35,000 confirmed malaria cases still occur annually [70]. There were 32,502 confirmed cases of malaria in 2010, a decrease of 61.2% compared to 2000. Mortality has also dramatically declined, dropping from 625 in 2000 to 80 in 2010, a decrease of 87.2%. The decline in malaria cases has been attributed to the effective implementation of selective and targeted indoor residual spray of homes and treated netting as vector control measures. Reduction of malaria in Thailand is also the consequence of expanded programs and access to prompt diagnosis and treatment in rural areas as well as an active disease surveillance program.

2.5.2. Malaria vectors and species diversity

Approximately 73 *Anopheles* species are recognized in Thailand. Members within the Leucosphyrus Group, the Maculatus Group and the Minimus Complex are recognized as the most important malaria vectors in the country [145,146,147,148,149]. Molecular techniques based on polymerase chain reaction (PCR) technology have allowed important malaria vectors comprised of sibling species to be correctly identified [33,59]. Within the Dirus Complex, *An. baimaii* and *An. dirus* are considered to be primary malaria vectors in Thailand [149]. Both are forest and forest-fringe inhabiting mosquitoes that are considered highly anthropophilic [150,112,149]. However, a recent study showed a significantly greater number of *An. dirus* and *An. baimaii* collected from cattle-baited traps as compared to human-landing collections, demonstrating that both species could also show strong zoophilic behavior [151].

Among the members of the Maculatus Group, seven known species have been reported in Thailand, including *An. maculatus, An. sawadwongporni, An. dravidicus, An. notanandai, An. willmori, An. pseudowillmori,* and *An. rampae* [152,153,154,155,147,149,156]. *Anopheles maculatus* and *An. pseudowillmori* has been implicated as important malaria vectors in southern and western Thailand, respectively [145, 147, 149]. *Anopheles sawadwongporni* is a common species often found in high density throughout Thailand, especially along the border provinces with Myanmar and Malaysia [157]. Based on feeding behavior and the natural infection rate detected in this species, *An. sawadwongporni* appears to be a malaria vector in Thailand [16,158,149]. Plasticity in trophic behavior and host preferences over the geographical range of members of this group have been reported [159,153,160]

An. minimus is also an important vector of malaria and is widespread throughout Thailand [161]. Its sibling species, *An. harrisoni* (formerly *An. minimus* C) appears restricted to only two districts of Kanchanaburi Province, western Thailand, where it also occurs in sympatry with *An. minimus* [162]. *Anopheles harrisoni* was previously collected from Mae Sot in Tak Province and Mae Rim in Chiangmai Province, northern Thailand, but no clear confirmation was made at the time [149].

Several other potential secondary or incidental vectors of malaria are also present in Thailand. These mosquitoes can have a close association with humans and include *An. barbirostris* s.l. and *An. epiroticus* (Sundaicus Complex) [163]. Within the *An. barbirostris* Subgroup, *An. campestris* is incriminated as a potential vector of *P. vivax* in Thailand [164]. Additionally, under the correct conditions *An. karwari, An. philippinensis* and *An. tessellatus* are also considered to be potential malaria vectors in Thailand. Recently, *An. cracens* (Dirus Complex) and *An. latens* (Leucosphyrus Complex) have been shown natural vectors of *P. knowlesi* in the south of Thailand [165,166,163]. A list of known and potential malaria vector species in Thailand is provided in Table 2.

***Anopheles* species**	**Vector in Thailand**	**Vector in neighboring countries**	**Vector of *Plasmodium knowlesi* in Thailand**
Anopheles dirus	+	+	-
Anopheles baimaii	+	-	-
Anopheles cracens	-	-	+
Anopheles minimus	+	+	-
Anopheles maculatus	+	+	-
Anopheles pseudowillmori	+	-	-
Anopheles sawadwongporni	+	-	-
Anopheles epiroticus	+	+	-
Anopheles campestris	+	-	-
Anopheles latens	-	-	+

+: malaria vector, -: not recorded as vector

Table 2. Known and potential malaria vector species in Thailand [163].

2.5.3. *Anopheline behavior*

Knowledge of mosquito behavior is of paramount importance to understand the epidemiology of disease transmission and apply effective vector control. Details on mosquito biology, especially blood feeding activity and host preference of a defined species within its particular group or complex is essential to help identify their respective role in disease transmission in specific areas and help vector control operators to design the most appropriate strategy to reduce biting densities. Numerous observations on biting cycles and host preference of the three complexes/group, *An. dirus, An. minimus,* and *An. maculatus*, have been conducted in Thailand [167, 168, 169, 170, 171, 172]. However, nearly all previous ecological and behavior studies were based on species populations identified by morphological characters only. Studies on vectors have recognized additional *Anopheles* species within species complexes in Thailand [150, 173, 161, 149]. Infrastructure development and deforestation along the national borders with other countries in the past two decades has led to a significant reduction in malaria incidence, yet many malaria vectors have apparently and successfully adapted to the environmental changes. Using molecular approaches enables investigators to describe the trophic behavior of each species within a complex. For example, the different biting activities of *An. minimus* and *An. harrisoni* were described from two malaria endemic areas of Tak [143] and Kanchanaburi [174] provinces, respectively. Recently, the biting activity and host preference of *An. dirus* and *An. baimaii* have been described from Kanchanaburi [151]. More meaningful investigations on population biology, bionomics and blood feeding activity of sympatric sibling species within medically important complexes can now be conducted with greater accuracy.

2.5.4. *Effects of changing environmental conditions on malaria vectors and transmission*

Most insect species are generally very sensitive to changes in climatic and environmental conditions, such as ambient temperature, relative humidity, wind speed, and rainfall. The natural environment imposes significant constraints on insect populations [175, 176]. Among the blood-sucking species in the forest-type habitat that transmit diseases to humans, mosquitoes are found to be susceptible to environmental/climatic modifications [144]. Longevity (survival), population density, and ecological distribution of any mosquito can be dramatically influenced by small changes in environmental conditions, and the availability of suitable hosts, larval habitats and adult resting sites. Changes in environmental conditions are directly influenced by modification and increased land use, such as conversion of rice fields to rubber plantations, forested areas to urbanized environments. Human activities are of major concern in changing the patterns of vector-borne diseases. For example, in 1988 a major malaria outbreak along the Thai-Cambodia border was due to transient employment opportunities from gem mining activities with almost 60,000 malaria cases detected in this population [4]. Similarly, between 1998 and 2000 an outbreak of malaria occurred at Suan Ping Village, Ratchaburi Province, western Thailand, in another gem mining area where most of the work force was recruited from Myanmar. This outbreak clearly showed that the man-made activity and population movement could be a significant factor in contributing to disease transmission.

In the past three decades, rubber plantations have expanded in most SEA countries, including Thailand. Although Thailand is known as a significant producer of natural rubber, these plantations were generally restricted to southern Thailand. Recently, rubber trees have been planted in the east and northeastern parts of the country. Rubber plantations placed in once forested hill areas provide potential habitats for several primary malaria vectors such as *An. dirus* and *An. maculatus,* two commonly found vectors in southern Thailand [161]. Recent rubber plantation expansion in the northeast has also opened more job opportunity for migrant workers from neighboring countries. Lacking sufficient labor resources in Thailand, over one million registered migrant workers from neighboring countries have entered the country since 2004 [144]. This has undoubtedly resulted in trans-border movement of malaria into Thailand with the potential of re-introduction of transmission in once malaria-free areas and malaria resurgence and outbreaks in more vulnerable environments.

In summary, efforts are being directed to strengthen malaria control activities along the international borders of Thailand. The problem of border malaria due to inter-country human population movement, both legal and not, is known to greatly complicate the control efforts. In addition, land use modifications have a great influence on vector-borne disease transmission. Careful attention to land use changes along with the climatic and environmental changes is needed to help predict and prevent the reemergence of malaria in all areas of Thailand. Effective collaborative efforts between neighboring countries with trans-border malaria have to be implemented to mitigate continued high malaria transmission in these sensitive areas of the country.

2.6. Vietnam

2.6.1. Overview

Vietnam has a land area of 331,690 km^2, and 4,550 km long with a total population of approximately 88.2 million [177].) This country shares borders with China in the north, Laos and Cambodia in the west. Malaria is the most important public health burden. A massive epidemic of 1991 resulted in more than one million cases and 4,600 deaths [178]. After this epidemic, the National Malaria Control Program (NMCP) focussed on malaria as its first public health priority and intensive control activities were implemented to help reduce malaria transmission in the country, including mass drug treatment in high endemic areas, indoor residual insecticide spraying and distribution of insecticide-treated bet nets. The successes of the NMCP have been witnessed in many areas, especially in northern Vietnam where no local malaria cases have been reported and malaria entomological inoculated rate has been nil for many years [6, 7, 32]. While malaria control has been successful in northern Vietnam, malaria continues to be a problem further south, particularly in the hilly-forested areas of central and southern Vietnam, and along the international borders with Cambodia and Lao PDR where frequent human population movements occur [92, 43]. Various ethnic minorities are the populations at greatest risk of malaria, suffering five times more malaria paroxysms than the vast majority of the Vietnamese population [179, 180]. From 2010 to 2011, respectively 36% to 18% of the population were still living in defined high transmission areas, while 54% to 20% were exposed to low transmission and 10% to 63% where in malaria-free, many urbanized, areas [2,3].

All four human malaria parasites and *P. knowlesi* have been reported in Vietnam [181, 182, 183]. Reported malaria cases are mostly due to *P. falciparum* (66%), followed by *P. vivax* (34%), while *P. malariae* and *P. ovale* are seldom recorded [3]. Transmission of zoonotic *Plasmodium knowlesi* has been reported in southern-central Vietnam [184, 185, 186, 187, 188, 189]. *Plasmodium knowlesi* has been found in several *Anopheles* species, especially *An. dirus* considered as the main malaria vector in Vietnam [181, 183].

Insecticide use and mass drug treatment were effective measures for controlling vectors and malaria transmission in Vietnam [190]. However, with decades of insecticide and anti-malarial drug use, both resistance of *Anopheles* to insecticides and malaria parasites to malarial drugs has appeared [191, 192, 56, 193, 194]. Moreover, land use modifications caused by deforestation, expansion of agriculture, conversion from rice to shrimp production, have introduced dramatic changes in mosquito habitats and represent new challenges for malaria control strategies in Vietnam. Although considerable effort has been invested applying malaria control activities following the 1991 epidemic, malaria still ranks as an important public health problem. In 2011, 16, 539 malaria cases (6 deaths) were reported in central and highland areas of Vietnam [195]. There are two periods of the year during which malaria transmission is the highest: (1) from the end of the rainy season to the early dry season (September to January) and (2) from the late dry season to the early rainy season (May to August).The dry and rainy seasons may slightly shift from year to year and the intensity of malaria transmission is also dependent on the geographic area and other variables.

The term "forest malaria" is defined within a specific context of transmission epidemiology and involves several sylvatic vectors such as *An. dirus* [7, 196, 43, 183]. The population at greatest risk of infection are the inhabitants of hilly forested areas, particularly ethnic minorities that have the poorest living standards, low educational background, and where their normal life activities include jungle exploitation and subsistence-level slash and burn cultivation practices [196, 71, 180]. Moreover, in both recovered forests and deforested areas, many workers come to live in rudimentary huts and other shelters during harvest time that afford poor protection against mosquitoes. Population movements between different areas, together with generally poor living conditions expose them to high malaria risk. Indeed, the social-ecological factors such as living in remoted areas and the logistical difficulties in implementing and sustaining control efforts against highly efficient forest vectors favour malaria transmission [17, 196, 18, 197, 26].

After the last local malaria cases were reported in northern Vietnam in 1995, malaria transmission has apparently not returned despite reports that malaria vectors remain common [7, 198, 199]. A study on the health information system on malaria surveillance activities in Vietnam [200] called into question the accuracy of data captured and that there was likely a great underestimation for the actual malarial burden reported during the past decade. By applying spatial-temporal analytical tools to determine the association among social aspects, environmental factors and malaria risk in Vietnam, Bui et al., (2011) suspected that malaria transmission is still occurring in some focal areas of northern Vietnam, therefore, emphasizing that malaria surveillance activities and control capabilities should be sustained to prevent or respond to the reintroduction of malaria in receptive areas.

The prevalence of human malaria and entomological inoculation rates have been reported in several provinces of southern and central Vietnam, such as Binh Thuan, Ninh Thuan, Khanh Hoa, Quang Binh, Binh Phuoc, Dak Nong, Dak Lak, Bac Lieu [7, 181,42, 180, 43, 183, 195].

Area	Population	Population living in the risk area	Malaria cases	Parasite Cases (Confirmed by microscopy)
North	39,723,077	4,498,201	22,598	638
Center	23,695,858	9,071,902	21,557	15,272
South	24,830,313	1,892,751	1,433	522
Total	88,249,248	15,462,854	45,588	16,432

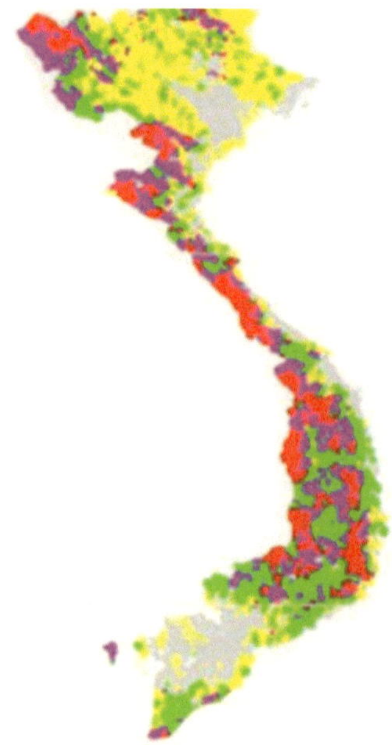

Source: Meeting on Outdoor Malaria Transmission in the Mekong Countries for 13 countries during 12-13 March 2012, Bangkok, Thailand. [http://www.rbm.who.int/partnership/wg/wg_itn/ppt/ws2/m4VuDucChinh.pdf.]

Figure 6. Total population living in risk area, malaria cases and positive cases (confirmed by microscopy) in Vietnam in 2011.

2.6.2. *Biodiversity of* Anopheles *vectors in Vietnam*

In Vietnam, 61 *Anopheles* species have been reported using morphological identification methods [201]. Many species of *Anopheles* from SEA belong to a species complex or group [39]. For species complexes, as often there is either no or unreliable morphological characters to accurately distinguish each sibling species from one another. Therefore, their specific role in malaria transmission remains unclear [202, 203, 40]. The *Anopheles* in Vietnam can be divided into three categories based on their vectorial capacity to transmit malaria: (i) the primary vectors include species in the Dirus (*An. dirus*), Minimus (*An. minimus, An. harrisoni)* and Sundaicus (*An. epiroticus)* Complexes; (ii) secondary or incidental vectors include *An. aconitus, An. jeyporiensis, An. maculatus, An. subpictus, An. sinensis, An. pampanai, An. vagus, An. indefinitus*; and (iii) suspected vectors are *An. interruptus, An. campestris, An. lesteri* and *An. nimpe*. Therefore, 16 (26%) are considered as having some role in malaria transmission in the country.

However, more studies are needed to better define the importance and role of each species, especially secondary and suspected vectors. For example, *An. culicifacies* s.l., an important vector in India, was recently found in Vietnam. However, the species identified was *An. culicifacies* species B of the Culicifacies Complex which is primarily zoophilic and thus regarded as not involved in malaria transmission in the country [54]. In addition, extensive environmental changes have occurred since the 90's, which have modified the *Anopheles* habitats and the presence and prevalence of some species.

2.6.3. Distribution of Anopheles *vectors in Vietnam*

According to Phan (2008), the anopheline fauna in Vietnam has been sorted based on two criteria [204]:

- **Geographically**, clustered into 4 zones: Northern, South Central-Highlands, Southern and Lam Dong (Province in south-central Vietnam within a temperate zone climate).
- **Physio-geographically** by combining the epidemiology of foci and clustered into 7 different zones: (1) Plains with standing water, (2) Low hills with streams, (3) Low mountains-hills and woodlands with streams, (4) Mountains and forests with streams, (5) Northern plateau, (6) High mountains with streams and waterfalls, and (7) Coastal brackish water habitats.

Vectors such as *An. minimus* and *An. dirus* are present in almost all clusters, whereas *An. epiroticus* and *An. subpictus* are vectors restricted along the coast line with varying degrees of brackish water in natural impoundments (e.g., lagoons, blocked coastal streams and small rivers). The SEA distribution of the dominant vector species has recently been well delineated [59]. Many studies have contributed to new insights on the presence, biology and behavior, and distribution of *Anopheles* in Vietnam. The majority of investigations have focused in the central and southern regions where malaria transmission is most endemic. In Ma Noi and Phuoc Binh Communes, a forested area of Binh Thuan Province, central Vietnam, 24 *Anopheles* species were collected between 2004 and 2006. The predominant malaria vectors were *An. dirus* and *An. minimus* s.l. and also included *An. maculatus* s.l., *An. pampanai, An. aconitus, An. annularis* s.l., *An. nigerrimus, An. philippinensis, An. sinensis, An. annandalei, An. argyropus, An. barbumbrosus, An. crawfordi, An. jamesii, An. jeyporiensis, An. monstrosus, An. tessellatus, An. vagus, An. varuna, An. barbirostris, An. kochi, An. nivipes, An. peditaeniatus,* and *An. splendidus* [43].

A nation-wide study to evaluate the status and the distribution of *Anopheles* malaria vectors in four forested regions in northern Vietnam (northern part of the Hai Van Pass) recorded 30 *Anopheles* species, of which, 20 species were collected in primary forests, 21 in secondary growth forests, 16 in woodland or shrub biomes, and 6 species in tidal mangrove zones. Two main malaria vectors were present, *An. minimus* s.l. and *An. dirus*, as well as potential secondary vectors, including *An. aconitus, An. jeyporiensis, An. maculatus, An. subpictus, An. sinensis* and *An. donaldi*, the latter species representing a new country distribution record for Vietnam [205]. Sympatric sibling species, *An. minimus* and *An. harrisoni*, was confirmed in Hoa Binh Province in north-eastern Vietnam [32] as well as 21 other *Anopheles* species near the Son La hydro-electrical dam (Son La Province), including *An. minimus* [199]. This finding showed that even though malaria prevalence in this region is very low, malaria risk still remains and vector control capacity in this region should be sustained to prevent or combat possible malaria outbreaks.

Molecular methods have been developed to resolve identification problems due to overlap in morphological characters among sibling species [206, 207, 208, 55, 209, 210, 211]. The distribution of species that were once morphologically identical has been clarified for many localities.

In Vietnam, *An. minimus* has an extensive north-south distribution, while *An. harrisoni* has a much more patchy occurrence [212]. The presence of *An. minimus* and *An. harrisoni* occurs from northern to south-central regions where they often occur in sympatry [213, 32, 212, 42]. In central Vietnam, an increase in density of *An. harrisoni* has been seen compared to *An. minimus* which also coincided with the wide use of permethrin-treated bed nets in the study village [7,213]. The dominance of *An. harrisoni* was also reported in Quang Binh Province, northern central Vietnam [42].

Out of the 8 species that make up the Dirus Complex, only two occur in Vietnam: *Anopheles dirus*, the main vector found in hilly forested areas [32, 41, 18, 42, 43] and the recently described cryptic species, *An.* aff. *takasagoensis* collected in northern Vietnam [40]. Khanh Phu Commune (Khanh Hoa Province in south-central Vietnam) is a hilly-forested area where malaria transmission is endemic. Twelve *Anopheles* species were captured in this area in which *An. dirus* was the dominant (83.2%) species present [183].

Anopheles epiroticus is considered the main malaria vectors in the southern coastal areas below the 11th parallel. Recent studies have shown extremely low infectious rates for this species [46, 58, 7, 214]. *An. epiroticus* is the only member of the Sundaicus Complex present in Vietnam [58, 117, 32, 44].

Anopheles nimpe (Hycarnus Group) is a recently described species which was discovered along the coastal area of southern Vietnam and is suspected as a malaria vector due to its high attraction to humans [45, 215, 32, 42]. To date, very little else is known about this species.

The Maculatus Group has three representatives present in the country, *An. maculatus, An. sawadwongporni* and *An. rampae* (Form K), with variable distributions and densities based on geographic area [42, 43]. Only *An. maculatus* is regarded as a vector of minor (secondary) importance [45, 204].

2.6.4. Vector habitats and behavior

Anopheles dirus is primarily a forest malaria vector and the main vector species in many cases. However, in Truong Xuan Commune (Quang Binh Province) and Phuoc Chien Commune (Ninh Thuan Province), locations where malaria transmission is still high, *An. dirus* has not been reported infected [18,42], therefore the role of secondary vectors in malaria transmission may be under estimated [32,42,43].

Species of the Minimus Complex are normally found in forested foothills associated with freshwater streams and canals. *Anopheles minimus* has also been found in sunlit and shaded ponds, rock pools, and rice paddies. On the outskirts of Hanoi, along the Red River Delta, *An. minimus* was found to oviposit in artificial containers such as rainwater tanks near houses [204,206,216]. *Anopheles epiroticus* is an important malaria vector along the coast of southern Vietnam and has been commonly found in man-made fish and shrimp ponds. This species has been observed to bite humans throughout the night [32].

Species of the *An. maculatus* Group has been found in hilly forested areas, especially in the recovered forest areas. Their larval habitats are closely associated with stream pools and drying river beds. They are generally zoophilic being more attracted to cattle than humans and tend to bite from early evening to the early morning hours [32, 42, 43].

2.6.5. Implication of changing social and environment conditions on vectors and transmission

Extensive environmental changes have occurred in Vietnam since the 1990's [217], which have modified the *Anopheles* habitats and the presence and prevalence of some species. *Anopheles minimus,* known as an endophilic and fairly anthropophilic vector, is abundant mainly during the dry season that generally lasts from November to April in the south and from November to February in northern Vietnam [7]. The use of indoor insecticide residual spraying has been successfully used to reduce malaria transmission as *An. minimus* has a strong behavioral tendency for biting indoors. However, this adaptable vector has shown marked variations in its behavior from endophilic to exophilic and anthropophilic to zoophilic in northern Vietnam where it was more attracted to cattle and other domestic animals kept near the house [32, 34, 42]. In parallel, insecticide use led to the significant increase in density of *An. harrisoni* in Khanh Phu Commune [213].

Human practices are generating important environmental changes throughout the country, such as deforestation, reforestation, plantations, fish and shrimp ponds replacing rice cultivation, road construction, dams, more intensive slash and burn activities, and so on. Such land use changes have an impact on vector habitats, vector diversity and distribution that could either promote or discourage the propagation of some vector species and therefore impact risk of malaria transmission [199,218]. In urban and rural settings, the expansion of electricity to the more mountainous and remote villages encourages people to remain outdoors for longer periods during night time, thereby increasing risk in this unprotected population of being bitten by the *Anopheles* vectors, especially *An. dirus* which is more likely to be exophagic and exophilic [32,43]. Housing construction has implications on malaria transmission. Houses with open construction (e.g., with uncompleted walls, no doors) allow anthropophilic mosquitoes to easily detect human host attractant stimuli and enter the houses to bite [32]. As standard of living and economic development increase in the country, so will the type and quality of houses thus adding additional barriers to host-seeking vectors.

3. Conclusions

Many years of organized malaria control and research have led to some notable successes in reducing the incidence of malaria in countries located on mainland SEA. However, this disease is still a major health risk in rural and remote communities close to forest and forest fringe areas where socioeconomic conditions remain low, the areas more difficult to -reach, and daily human are closely-related or dependant on the subsistence from forests.

More recent and dramatic changes in the local ecology created by development projects, while aiming to improve the standard of living of the local populations, may have profound and negative effects upon human health and vector-borne diseases. In most countries, deforestation, and reforestation, is one of the most potent factors in relation to emerging and re-emerging infectious diseases. For example, rubber plantations have had the effect of increasing the density of important malaria vectors in Thailand [75]. Southeast Asia has the highest relative rate of deforestation of any major tropical region in the world, and could deplete three quarters of its native forest cover by 2100, effectively removing up to 42% of its fauna and flora biodiversity [19]. Most of the main malaria vectors occurring in mainland SEA are associated with forests, therefore we can anticipate changes in distribution and population densities of malaria vectors, some possibly disappearing while secondary or potential vectors move to exploit the altered habitats to become primary malaria vectors of the future.

Moreover, the expanding exploitation and over utilization of natural resources, together with other forms of economic development can help to improve living conditions, while simultaneously changing the environment in ways that might increase disease transmission risk of malaria or other vector-borne diseases (e.g., dengue). Together with changes in human practices, the adaptation of vector fauna to altered environments, including vector behaviour, might profoundly alter the dynamics of malaria transmission. These are some of the challenges to be raised by all countries in order to reach the goal of malaria elimination by 2015 (Lao PDR), 2020 (Vietnam), 2025 (Cambodia). Clearly there is a need for more studies on *Anopheles* malaria vectors in some countries of SEA, such as Myanmar, where work is now dated. For instance, in order to better control malaria and its vectors, a trans-border network should be organized at the SEA region scale. A better understanding of the mechanisms linking deforestation and development projects with anopheline ecology and malaria epidemiology, and that to contribute to improved health impact assessments in the future, are challenges for further study. Malaria vector control is still predominantly based on the use of insecticides as residual house spraying and bednet impregnation, and still regarded as the most effective way to attack vectors. Yet relatively little work has been done to exploit the behaviour of mosquito vectors as a means of transmission control (e.g., use of spatial repellents to impact outdoor transmission, search of natural substances with insecticide properties respectful of the environment). With expected changes in the distribution and epidemiology of malaria, there will be a critical need to continue to explore and develop new and innovative methods of intervention to complement existing strategies.

Acknowledgements

We would like to thank Dr. Steven Bjorge (World Health Organization, Cambodia) and Prof. Sylvie Manguin (Institut de Recherche pour le Développement (IRD, France) for the critical review of this book chapter. We also thank Vithee Muenworn, Ph.D candidate Kasetsart University for general help. Sincere thanks to Thailand Research Fund (TRF) and Department of Disease Control, MOPH, Thailand for providing financial support over the many fruitful years of entomological research.

Author details

Wannapa Suwonkerd[1*], Wanapa Ritthison[2,5], Chung Thuy Ngo[3,4], Krajana Tainchum[2], Michael J. Bangs[6] and Theeraphap Chareonviriyaphap[2]

*Address all correspondence to: suwannapa@yahoo.com

1 Office of Disease Prevention and Control # 10, Department of Disease Control, Ministry of Public Health, Chiang Mai, Thailand

2 Department of Entomology, Faculty of Agriculture, Kasetsart University, Bangkok, Thailand

3 Institut de Recherche pour le Développement (IRD), Lab. Immuno-Physiopathologie Moléculaire Comparée, UMR-MD3, Université Montpellier, Montpellier, France

4 National Institute of Veterinary Research, Ha Noi, Viet Nam

5 Office of Disease Prevention and Control # 3, Department of Disease Control, Ministry of Public Health, Chonburi, Thailand

6 Public Health & Malaria Control, International SOS, Kuala Kencana, Papua, Indonesia

References

[1] World Health Organization. (2010). World malaria report. Nonserial Publication.World health Organization.pp.274. ISBN 13 9789241564403. Worldatlas.com http://www.worldatlas.com/ webimage/countrys/as.htm

[2] World Health Organization. (2011). World malaria report. Nonserial Publication. World Health Organization. pp.270. ISBN 9789241564403.http://www.int/malaria/world_malaria_report_2011/9789241564403_eng.pdf.

[3] World Health Organization. (2012). World malaria report. Non serial Publication. World Health Organization. pp.260. ISBN ISBN 978 92 4 156453 3. http://www.who.int/malaria/publications/world_malaria_report_2012/en/index.html

[4] Charoenviriyaphap, T.; Bangs, M.J. & Ratanatham, S. (2000). Status of malaria in Thailand. *Southeast Asian Journal Tropical Medicine and Public Health,* Vol. 31, pp. 225-237. ISSN: 0125-1562.

[5] Childs, D.Z.; Cattadori, I.M., Suwonkerd, W., Prajakwong, S. & Boots, M. (2006). Spatiotemporal patterns of malaria incidence in northern Thailand. *Transaction of the Royal Society of Tropical Medicine and Hygiene.* Vol. 100, pp. 623-631. ISSN: 0035-9203.

[6] Verle, P.; Ruyen, N. T., N Huong,. T. N., Be, T., Kongs, A., Van der Stuyft, P., & Coosemans, M. (1998). A simple field test for detecting pyrethroids on impregnated nets. *Tropical Medicine and International Health,*Vol.3, pp. 833-6.

[7] Trung, H. D.; Van Bortel, W., Sochantha, T., Keokenchanh, K., Quang, N. T., Cong, L. D., & Coosemans, M. (2004). Malaria transmission and major malaria vectors in different geographical areas of Southeast Asia. *Tropical Medicine and International Health,* Vol. 9, pp. 230-7.

[8] Delacollette, C.; Souza, C.D., Christophel, E., Thimasarn, K., Abdur, R., Bell, D., Dais,T.C., Gopinath, D., Lu, S., Mendoz, R., Ortega, L., Rastogi, R., Tantinimitkul, C. & Ehrenberg, J. (2009). Malaria trends and challenges in the Greater Mekong subregion, *Southeast Asian Journal of Tropical Medicine and Public Health.*Vol.40, No.4, pp. 674-691. ISSN: 0125-1562.

[9] World Health Organization [WHO], (2010). Malaria: Malaria situation in SEAR countries: Thailand. http://www.searo.who.int/en/Section10/ Section21/Section 40_4027.htm

[10] World Health Organization. (2010). Malaria in the Greater Mekong Sub-region.Regional and Country profiles. SEARO Nonserial Publication.SEARO.pp. 64. ISBN-13 9789290223733.

[11] Anderson, T. J.; & Roper, C. (2005). The origins and spread of antimalarial drug resistance lessons for policy makers. *Acta Tropica,* Vol. 94, pp. 269–280.

[12] Cui, L.; Yan, G., Sattabongkot,J., Cao, Y., Chen, B., Chen, X., Fan, Q., Fang, Q., Jongwutiwesi,S., Parker, D., Sirichaisinthop, J., Kyaw, M.P., Su, X.Z., Yang, H., Yang, Z., Wang, B., Xu, J., Zheng, B., Zhong, D. & Zhou, G. (2012). Malaria in the Greater Mekong Subregion: Heterogeneity and complexity. *Acta Tropica,* Vol. 212, pp. 227-239.ISSN:0001-706X.

[13] Phan, V.T.; Tuy, T.Q., Hung, L.X. & Ngo, L.V. (1998). Epidemiological characteristics of malaria in Vietnam 1992-1997. http://www.ecmalaria.org/mcis/bookl_21.htm.

[14] Sharma, V.P.; & Kondrashin, A.V. (1991).Forest Malaria in Southeast Asia, Proceedings of an Informal Consultative Meeting. *World Health Organization*/Medical Research Council., eds. New.

[15] Tun-Lin, W.; Thu, M.M., Than, S.M. & Mya, M.M. (1995). Hyperendemic malaria in a forested hilly Myanmar village. *Journal of American Mosquito Control Association.* Vol. 11, pp.401-407.

[16] Somboon, P.; Aramrattana, A., Lines, J. & Webber, R., 1998. Entomological and epidemiological investigations of malaria transmission in relation to population movements in forest areas of north-west Thailand. *Southeast Asian Journal of Tropical Medicine and Public Health,* Vol. 29 pp3-9.

[17] Erhart, A.; Thang, N.D., Hung, N.Q., Toi, L.E.V., Hung, L.E.X., Tuy, T.Q., Cong, L.E.D., Speybroeck, N., Coosemans, M. & Alessandro, U.D. (2004). Forest malaria in Vietnam: A challenge for control. *American Journal Tropical Medicine and Hygiene,* Vol. 70, No.2,pp. 110-118. ISSN: 0002-9637.

[18] Sanh, N. H., Van Dung, N., Thanh, N. X., Trung, T. N., Van Co, T., Cooper, R. D. (2008). Forest malaria in central Vietnam. *American Journal of Tropical Medicine and Hygiene,* Vol. 79, pp. 652-654.

[19] Sodhi, N.S.; Koh, L.P., Brook, B.W. & Ng, P.K.L. (2004). Southeast Asian biodiversity: an impending disaster. *Trends in Ecology and Evolution.* Vol. 19, No. 2 (December 2004), pp.654-660.

[20] Gaston, K.J. & Hudson, E. (1994). Regional patterns of diversity and estimates of global insect species richness. *Biodiverstiy and Conservation,* Vol. 3, pp.493-500.

[21] Foley, D.H., Rueda, L.M., Peterson, A.T. & Wilkerson, R.C. (2007). Insight into global mosquito biogeography from country species records. *Journal of Medical Entomology,* Vol. 44, No. 4, pp. 554-567.

[22] Manguin S. & Boëte C. 2011. Global impact of mosquito biodiversity, human vector-borne diseases and environmental change. Chapter 3: *In* The importance of biological interactions in the study of biodiversity, Lopez-Pujol J. (Ed.), InTech open access Publisher, Rijeka, Croatia, 390 p

[23] Anderson R.M; May R.M. (1991). Infectious Diseases of Humans: Dynamics and Control. Oxford, Oxford University Press, pp.757. ISBN 0-19-854599-1.

[24] Mouchet, J.; Manguin, S., Sircoulon, J., Laventure, S., Faye, O., Onapa, A. W., Carnevale, P., Julvez, J., & Fontenille, D. (1998). Evolution of malaria in Africa for the past 40 years: impact of climatic and human factors. *Journal of American Mosquito Control Association,* Vol. 14, pp. 121-30.

[25] Yewhalaw, D., Kassahun, W., Woldemichael, K., Tushune, K., Sudaker, M., Kaba, D., Duchateau, L., Van Bortel, W., Speybroeck, N. (2010). The influence of the Gilgel-Gibe hydroelectric dam in Ethiopia on caregivers' knowledge, perceptions and health-seeking behaviour towards childhood malaria. *Malaria Journal,* Vol. 9, pp. 47.

[26] Bui, H. M., Clements,A. C., Nguyen, Q. T., Nguyen, M. H., Le, X. H., Hay, S. I., Tran,T. H., Wertheim, H. F., Snow, R. W., Horby, P. (2011). Social and environmental

determinants of malaria in space and time in Viet Nam. *Int J Parasitol*, Vol. 41, pp. 109-16.

[27] Suwonkerd, W.; Overgaard, H.J., Tsuda, Y., Prajakwong, S & Takagi, M. (2002). Malaria vector densities in transmissionand non-transmission areas during 23 years and land use in Chiang Mai province, Northern Thailand. *Basic andApplied Ecology*. Vol. 3, No. 3,pp 197-207. ISSN 1439-1791.

[28] Suwonkerd, W.; Yoshio, T., Overgaard, H.J., Chawprom, S.,Tuno, N., Prajakwong, S. & Takagi, M. (2004). Changes in malaria vector densities over a twenty-three year period in Mae Hong Son Province, northern Thailand.*Southeast Asian journal of Tropical Medicine and Public Health*, Vol. 35, No.2, pp.316-324.

[29] Butraporn, P.; Sornmani, S., & Hungsapruek, T. (1986). Social, behavior, housing factors and their interactive effects associated with malaria occurrence in east Thailand. *Southeast Asia Journal of Tropical Medicine and Public Health.* Vol. 17,pp. 386-392.

[30] Butraporn, P.; Prasittisuk, C., Krachaiklin, S. & Chareonjai, P. (1995). Behavior in self-prevention of malaria among mobile population in east Thailand. *Southeast Asia Journal of Tropical Medicine and Public Health.* Vol. 26,pp. 213-218.

[31] Ma, Y.; Vanne, S., Li, S. & Yang, P. (2005). Molecular identification of *Anopheles minimus* sensu lato and *Anopheles dirus* sensu lato (Diptera: Culiciadae) from Kampong Spoe province, Cambodia. *Zootaxa.* Vol. 1028, (August 2005) pp.37-47.

[32] Trung, H. D.; Bortel, W. V., Sochantha, T., Keokenchanh, K., Briet, O. J., & Coosemans, M. (2005). Behavioural heterogeneity of *Anopheles* species in ecologically different localities in Southeast Asia: a challenge for vector control. *Tropical Medicine and International Health*, Vol. 10, pp. 251-262.

[33] Manguin; S.; Garros, C., Dusfour, I., Harbach, R.E., & Coosmans, M. (2008 a). Bionomics, taxonomy, and distribution of the major malaria vector taxa of *Anopheles* subgenus *Cellia* in Southeast Asia: an updated review. *Infectious Genetic Evolution* Vol. 8,pp.489-503.

[34] Garros, C.; Van Bortel, W.,Trung, M., Coosemans, M. & Manguin, S. (2006). Review of the Minimus Complex of *Anopheles*, main malaria vector in Southeast Asia: from taxonomic issues to vector control strategies. *Tropical Medicine and International Health*, Vol.11, No.1, (January 2006), pp,102-114.

[35] Harrison, B.A. (1980). Medical Entomological study XIII. The Myzomyia series of *Anopheles* (*Cellia*) in Thailand, with emphasis on intra-interspecific variations (Diptera: Culiciade). Contribution of the American Entomological Institute. Vol 17, pp. 1-195.

[36] Suwonkerd, W.; Takagi, M., Amg-ung, B. & Prajakwong, S. (1995). Seasonal and spatial distribution of 3 malaria vectors at three mountainous villages in north Thailand.

Japanese Journal Tropical Medicine and Hygiene. Vol 23, No. 3 (August 1995), pp. 183-187.

[37] Foley, D.H.; Rueda, L.M., Peterson, A.T., & Wilkerson, R.C. (2008). Potential distribution of two species in the medically important *Anopheles minimus* complex (Diptera: Culicidae). *Journal of Medical Entomology*, VOl. 45, pp.852-860

[38] Overgaard, H.; Tsuda, Y., Suwonkerd, W.& Takagi, M. (2002). Characteristics of *Anopheles minimus* (Diptera: Culicidae) larval habitat in northern Thailand. *Environmental Entomology*, Vol. 30, pp. 134-141.

[39] Harbach, R. E. (2011). *Anopheles* classification. Mosquito Taxonomic Inventory (http://.mosquito-taxonomic-inventory.info/). accessed on 20 January 2013.

[40] Takano, K. T.; Nguyen, N. T., Nguyen, B. T., Sunahara, T., Yasunami, M., Nguyen, M. D., & Takagi, M. (2010). Partial mitochondrial DNA sequences suggest the existence of a cryptic species within the Leucosphyrus Group of the genus *Anopheles* (Diptera: Culicidae), forest malaria vectors, in northern Vietnam. *Parasite & Vectors* Vol. 3, pp. 41.

[41] Obsomer, V.; Defourny, P., & Coosemans, M. (2007). The *Anopheles dirus* complex: spatial distribution and environmental drivers. *Malaria Journal*, Vol. 6, pp. 26.

[42] Manh, C. D.; Beebe, N. W., Van, V. N., Quang, T. L., Lein, C. T., Nguyen,D. V., Xuan, T. N., Ngoc, A. L., & Cooper, R. D. (2010). Vectors and malaria transmission in deforested, rural communities in north-central Vietnam. *Malaria Journal*, Vol. 9, pp. 259.

[43] Van Bortel, W.; Trung,H. D., Hoi le, X., Van Ham, N., Van Chut, N., Luu, N. D., Roelants, P., Denis, L., Speybroeck, N., D'Alessandro, U., & Coosemans, M. (2010). Malaria transmission and vector behaviour in a forested malaria focus in central Vietnam and the implications for vector control. *Malaria Journal*, Vol. 9: 373.

[44] Dusfour, I. ; Michaux, J. R., Harbach, R. E., Manguin, S. (2007). Speciation and phylogeography of the Southeast Asian *Anopheles sundaicus* complex. *Infectious Genet Evol*, Vol. 7, pp. 484-93.

[45] Nguyen, T. A. (1993). [Malaria in Vietnam.Environment, prevention and treatment]. Bull Soc Pathol Exot 86: 494-9.

[46] Dusfour, I.; Harbach, R.E. & Manguin, S. (2004). Bionomics and systematics of the oriental *Anopheles sundaicus* complex in relation to malaria transmission and vector control. *Am J Trop Med Hyg.* Vol. 71, pp. 518-524. ISSN: 0002-9637.

[47] World Health Organization. (2009). World malaria report. Nonserial Publication. World Health Organization. pp.78. ISBN 9789241563901.http://whqlibdoc.who.int/publications/2009/9789241563901_eng.PDF.

[48] Mekong Malaria Program. Malaria in the Greater Mekong Sub Region: Regional and country profiles. WHO Mekong Malaria Programme. http://www.whothailand.org/

linkFiles/Mekong Malaria Programme MMP Profile.pdf Date Accessed 20 October 2012.

[49] Dysoley, L.; Kaneko, A.. Eto, H., Mita, T.,Socheat, D., Brkman, A., & Kobayakawa, T. (2008). Changing patterns of forest malaria among the mobile adult male population in Chumkiri District, Cambodia. *Acta Tropica.* Vol.106, pp.207-212.

[50] Yeung, S.; Patouillard, E., Allen, H. & Socheat, D. (2011). Socially-marketed rapid diagnostic tests and ACT in the private sector: ten years of experience in Cambodia. *Malaria Journal* Vol.10, (18 August 2011), pp.243.

[51] Socheat, D.; Denis, M.B., Fandeur, T., Zhang, Z., Yang,H., Xu, J., Zhou, X., Phompida, S., Phetsouvanh, R.Lwin, S., Lin,K., Win, T., Than, S.W., Htut, Y., Prajakwong, S., Rojanasirivet, C., Tipmotree, R., Vijaykadga, S., Konchom, S., Cong, L.D., Thien, N.T., Thuan, L.K., Ringwald, P., Schapira, A., Christophel, E., Palmer, K., Abani, P.R., Prasittisuk, C.,Rastogi,R., Monti, F., Urbani, C., Tsuyuoka, R., Hoyer, S., Otega,L., Thimasarn,K., Songchareon, S., Meert, J.p., Gay, F., Crissman, L., ChoMin, N., Wongsrichanalai, C., Darasri, D., Indaratna, K., Singhasivanon, P., Chuprapawan, S., Looareesuwan, S., Supavej, S., Kidson, C, Baimai, V., Yimsamran, S., & Buchachart, K. (2003). Mekong malaria. II update of malaria, multi-drug resistance and economic development in the Mekong region of Southeast Asia. *Southeast Asian Journal Tropical medicine and Public Health.* Vol 34 (suppl 4)., pp. 1-102.

[52] Harrison, B.A.; & Klein, J.M. (1975). A revised list of the *Anopheles* of Cambodia. *Mosquito Systematics.* Vol. 7, pp. 9-12.

[53] Socheath, S.; Seng, C., Rath, T.S., Deesin, V., Deesin, T. & Apiwathanasorn, C. (2000) Study on bionomics of principal malaria vectors in Kratie Province, Cambodia. *Southeast Asian Journal of Tropical Medicine and Public Health,* Vol. 31 (Suppl), pp. 354-7.

[54] Van Bortel, W.; Sochanta, T., Harbach, R. E., Socheat, D., Roelants, P., Backeljau, T., & Coosemans, M. (2002). Presence of *Anopheles culicifacies* B in Cambodia established by the PCR-RFLP assay developed for the identification of *Anopheles minimus* species A and C and four related species. *Medical Veterinary Entomology, Vol.* 16, pp. 329-34.

[55] Garros, C.; Harbach, R. E., &Manguin, S. (2005). Systematics and biogeographical implications of the phylogenetic relationships between members of the Funestus and Minimus groups of *Anopheles* (Diptera: Culicidae). *Journal of Medical Entomology,* Vol. 42, pp. 7-18.

[56] Van Bortel, W.; Trung, H. D., Thuan le, K., Sochantha, T., Socheat, D., Sumrandee, C., Baimai, V., Keokenchanh, K., Samlane, P., Roelants, P., Denis, L., Verhaeghen, K., Obsomer, V., & Coosemans, M. (2008). The insecticide resistance status of malaria vectors in the Mekong region. *Malaria Journal,* Vol. 7: 102.

[57] Guerra, C.; Snow, R.W. & Hay, S.I. (2006). Defining the global spatial limits of malaria transmission in 2005. *Advances in Parasitology.* Vol. 62, pp. 157-179.

[58] Dusfour, I., Linton, Y. M., Cohuet, A., Harbach, R. E., Baimai, V., Trung, H. D., Seng, C. M., Matusop, A., Manguin, S. (2004). Molecular evidence of speciation between island and continental populations of *Anopheles* (*Cellia*) *sundaicus* (Diptera: Culicidae), a principal malaria vector taxon in Southeast Asia. *Journal of Medical Entomology*, Vol. 41, pp. 287-95.

[59] Sinka, M. E.; Bangs, M. J., Manguin, S., Chareonviriyaphap, T., Patil, A. P., Temperley, W. H., Gething, P. W., Elyazar, I. R., Kabaria, C. W., Harbach, R. E. & Hay, S. I. (2011). The dominant *Anopheles* vectors of human malaria in the Asia-Pacific region: occurrence data, distribution maps and bionomic précis. *Parasite & Vectors*, Vol. 4, pp. 89.

[60] World Health Organization, 2007 *Anopheles* species complexes in south and Southeast Asia World Health Organization (WHO) (2007). *Anopheles* species complexes in South and Southeast Asia. SEARO Technical Publication No. 57-102.

[61] Schapiara, A. & Boutsika, K. (2012). Malaria ecotypes and stratification. In D. Rollinson & S.I. Hay, editors: Advances in Parasitology, Vol. 78, Amsterdam: The Netherlands, pp.97-167. (SBN: 978-0-12-394303-30. Elsevir Ltd. Academic Press. URL: http://www. Sciencedirect.com/science/article/pii/B978-0-12-394303-3.00001-3

[62] Klowden, M.J. (1996). Vector behaviour. The biology of disease vectors (eds BJ Beaty & WC Marquardt) University Press of Colorado, Colorado, pp. 34–50.

[63] Sothantha, T.; Bortel, W.V., Savonnaroth, S. Marcotty, T., Speybroeck, N. & Coosemans, M. (2010). Personal protection by long-lasting insecticidal hammocks against the bite of forest malaria vectors. *Tropical Medicine and International Health*. Vol. 15, No. 3, pp. 336-341.

[64] Chareonviriyaphap, T.; Parbaripai, A., Bangs, M.J., Kongmee, M., Sathantriphop, S., Muenvorn, V., Suwonkerd, W. & Akratanakul, P. (2006). Influence of nutritional and physiological status on behavioral responses of *Aedesaegypti* (Diptera: Culicidae) to deltamethrin and cypermethrin. *Journal of Vector Ecology*, Vol. 31, pp. 89-101.

[65] Grieco, J.P.; Achee, N.L., Chareonviriyaphap, T., Suwonkerd, W., Chauhan, K.R., Sardelis, M. & Roberts, D.R. (2007). A new classification system for the actions of IRS chemicals traditionally used for malaria control. *PLoS ONE*, Vol.2, Issue. 8, (August 2008), pp. e716, ISSN 1932-6203.

[66] Sochantha, T.; Hewitt, S.; Nguon, C.; Okell, L.; Alexander, N.; Yeung, S.; Vannara, H.; Rowland, M. & Socheat, D. (2006). Insecticide-treated bednets for the prevention of *Plasmodium falciparum* malaria in Cambodia: a cluster-randomized trial. *Tropical Medicine and International Health*. Vol 11, No. 8 (August 2006), pp.1166-1177.

[67] Kamol-Ratanakul, P.; & Prasittisuk, C. (1992). The effectiveness of permethrin-impregnated bed nets against malaria for migrant workers in easthern Thailand. *The American Journal of Tropical Medicien and Hygiene*. Vol 47. pp. 305-360.

[68] Kobayashi, J.; Phompida, S., Toma, T., Looareensuwan, S., Toma, H., Miyai, I., (2004). The effectiveness of impregnated bed net in malaria control in Laos. *Acta Tropica.* Vol. 89,pp. 299-308.

[69] Jorgensen, P.; Nambanya, S., Gopinath, D., Hongvanthong, B., Luangphengsouk, K., Bell, D., Phompida, S., & Phetsouvanh, R. (2010). High heterogeneity in *Plasmodium falciparum* risk illustrates the need for detailedmapping to guide resource allocation: a new malaria risk map of the Lao People's Democratic Republic. *Malaria Journal* Vol 9, No.1 pp 59. ISSN 1475-2875. URL. http://www.malaria journal.com/content/9/1/266

[70] Ministry of Public Health [MOPH], (2011). Annual Malaria Reports. Malaria Division, Department of Communicable Disease Control. Ministry of Public Health, Thailand.

[71] Manguin, S.; Carnevale, P., Mouchet. J., Coosemans. M. & Julvez, J. (2008b) Biodiversity of malaria in the world. Montrouge, France: *John Libbey Eurotext*. pp. 464. ISSN 2035-3006.

[72] Gingrich, J.B.; Weatherhead, A, Sattabongkot, J., Pilaksiri, C & Wirtz, R.A. (1990). Hyperendemic malaria in a Thai village: dependence of year-round transmission on focal and seasonally circumscribed mosquito (Diptera: Culicidae) habitats. *Journal of Medical Entomology*. Vol 27, pp. 1016-1026.

[73] Rosenberg, R. Andre, R.G., Somchit, L. (1990). Highly efficient dry season transmission of malaria in Thailand. *Transaction Royal of Tropical Medicine and Hygiene*. Vol. 84, pp.22-28.

[74] Vanwambeke, S.O.; Somboon, P, Harbach, R., Isenstadt, M., Lambin, E.F., Walton, K., & Bultin, R. Landscape and land cover factors influence the presence of *Aedes* and *Anopheles* larvae. (2007). *Journal of Medical Entomology.* Vol 44, No. 1, pp.133-144.

[75] Yasuoka, J.; & Levins, R. (2007). Impact of deforestation and agricultural development on anopheline ecology and malaria epidemiology. *American Journal of Tropical Medicine and Hygiene.* Vol. 70, No. 3, pp. 450-460. ISSN 0002-9637.

[76] Walsh, J.F.; Molyneux, D.H. & Birley, M.H. (1993). Deforestation: effects on vector borne disease. *Parasitology,* Vol.106, (Suppl),pp. 55–75.

[77] Patz, J.A.; Graczyk, T.K., Geller, N. & Vittor, A.Y. (2000). Effects of environmental change on emerging parasiticdiseases. *International Journal for Parasitology,* Vol. 30, pp.1395-1405.

[78] Achard, F. Eva, H.D., Stibig, H.J., Mayaux, P., Gallego, J., Richards, T., & Mallingreau, J.P. (2002). Determination of deforestation rates of the world's humid tropical forests. *Science,* Vol. 297, pp. 999-1002.

[79] Reiter, P. (2001). Climate change and mosquito borne disease. *Environmental Health Perspect*. Vol. 109, pp. 141-161.

[80] Kobayashi, J.; Somboon, P., Keomanila, H., Inthavonsa, S., Nambanya,S., Inthakone, S., (2000). Malaria prevalence and a brief entomological survey in a village surrounded by rice fields in Khammouan Province, Lao PDR. *Tropical Medicine and International Health*, Vol. 5, pp.17-21.

[81] Denis, M.B. & Meek, S.R. (1992). Malaria in Cambodia. *Southeast Asian Journal Tropical Medicine and Public Health*, Vol.23 (Suppl 4), pp.23-28. ISSN: 0125-1562.

[82] Toma, T.; Kobayashi,J, Vannachone, B., Nambanya, S., & Wasabe, K. (2001). A field survey on malaria prevalence in southern Laos by polymerase chain reaction assay. *American Journal of Tropical Medicine and Hygiene*, Vol.64, pp. 257-261.

[83] Rattanaxay, P.; Phompida, S. & Kobayashi, J., (2005). A review of malaria situation and its control in Lao PDR. In: Tongol-Rivera, P., Kano, S. (Eds.), Asian Parasitology, vol. 6, Malaria in Asia. The Federation of Asian Parasitologists, Chiba, pp. 85-104. ISSN:4-902971-01-1.

[84] Phommanivong, V.; Thongkham, K., Deyer, G., Rene, J.P., & Barennes, H. (2010). An assessment of early diagnosis and treatment of malaria by village health volunteers in the Lao PDR. *Malaria Journal*, Vol. 9, pp: 347.

[85] World Health Organization. (2008). WHO Mekong Malaria programme, Malaria in the Greater Mekong Subregion: Regional and Country Profiles. *World Health Organization*, New Delhi, pp. 55, ISBN: 978-92-9022-373-1.

[86] Vythilingam, I.; Keokenchan, K., Phommakot, S., Nambanya, S., & Inthakone, S. (2001). Preliminary studies of anopheline mosquitoes in eight provinces in Lao PDR. *Southeast Asian Journal of Tropical Medicine and Public Health*, Vol. 32, No. 1 (March 2001), pp.83-86.

[87] Kobayashi, J.; Nambanya, S., Miyaki, I., Vanachone, B., Manivong, K., Koubouchan, T., Amano, H., Nozaki, H., Inthakone, S., & Sato, Y. (1997). Collection of anopheline mosquitoes in three villages endemic for malaria in Khammouane. Lao PDR. *Southeast Asian Journal Tropical and Public Health*. Vol 28, No. 3. pp. 615-620.

[88] Toma, T.; Miyaki, I, Okasawa, T., Kobayashi, J., Saita, S., Tuzuki, A., Keomanila, H., Nambanya, S., Phompida, S., Uza, M., & Takakura, M. (2002). Entomological surveys of malaria in Khammouane Province, Lao PDR, in 1999-2000. *Southeast Asian Journal of Tropical Medicine and Public Health*, Vol. 33, No. 3, pp. 532-546.

[89] Vythilingam, I.; Phetsouvanh, R., Keokenchanh, K., Yengmala, V., Vanisaveth, V., Phompida, S. & Hakim, S.L. (2003). The prevalence of *Anopheles* (Diptera: Culicidae) mosquitoes in Sekong province, Lao PDR. *Tropical Medicine and International Health*. Vol. 8, No. 6 (June 2003) pp. 525-535.

[90] Sidavong, I; Vythilingam, I., Phetsouvanh, R., Chan, S.T.,Phonemixay, T., Hakim, S.L. & Phompida, S. (2004). Malaria transmission by *Anopheles dirus* in Attapeu Prov-

ince, LAO PDR. *Southeast Asian Journal Tropical Medicine Public Health*. Vol. 35, No. 2 (June 2004). pp. 309-315.

[91] Vythilingam, I.; Sidavong, B., Thim, C.S., PhonemixAY, t., Phompida, S. & Jeffera, J. (2006a). Species composition of mosquitoes of Attapeu province, LAO People's Democratic Repubic. *Journal of American Mosquito Control Association*, Vol 22 No. (March 2006). pp.140-143. ISSN 1046-3607.

[92] Vythilingam, I.; Sidavong, B., Chan, S. T., Phonemixay, T., Vanisaveth, V., Sisoulad, P., Phetsouvanh, R., Hakim, S. L., Phompida, S. (2005b). Epidemiology of malaria in Attapeu Province, Lao PDR in relation to entomological parameters. *Transactions of the Royal Society of Tropical Medicine and Hygiene*, Vol. 99. (August 2005), pp. 833-839. ISSN : 0035-9203.

[93] Department of Statistics, Malaysia. (2010). Population distribution and basic demographic characteristics. 2010. pp. 5.

[94] Ministry of Health (MOH). (2001). Vector-borne Disease Control Programme. Kuala Lumpur: Ministry of Health Malaysia,: pp. 18.

[95] Ali, W.N.; Ahmad, R., Nor, Z.M., Ismail, Z. &Lim, L.H. (2011). Population dynamics of adult mosquitoes (Diptera: Culicidae) in malaria endemic villages of Kuala Lipis, Pahang, Malaysia. *Southeast Asian J Trop Med Public Health*. Vol. 42, pp. 259-67.

[96] Rahman, W.A.; Adanan, C.R. & Abu Hassan, A. (1997). Malaria and *Anopheles* mosquitoes in Malaysia. *Southeast Asian Journal of Tropical Medicine and Public Health*, Vol. 42, pp. 559-605.

[97] Asian Collaborative Training Network for Malaria (ACTMalaria). Country updates Malaysia. Executive Board Meeting 15 –17 March 2010 Luang Prabang, Lao PDR. http://www.actmalaria.net/home/epidemiological_profile.php#base.

[98] Jayakumar, G. (2006). Pre-employment medical examination of migrant workers—The ethical and illegal issues. *Med J Malaysia*, Vol.61, pp. 516-518. ISSN: 0300-5283.

[99] Vijayakumari, K. (2006). Towards an East Asian cooperation framework for migrant labor. Migrant workers in Malaysia: An Overview. http://www.isis.org.my/files/pubs/papers/VK_MIGRATION-NEAT_6Dec06.pdf.

[100] White, N. J. (2008). *Plasmodium knowlesi*: the fifth human malaria parasite. *Clinical Infectious Diseases*, Vol. 46, No. 2, pp. 172–173.

[101] Vythilingam, I.; Tan, C.H., Asmad,M., Chan, S.T.,Lee,K.S. & Singh, B.(2006b). Natural transmission *of Plasmodium knowlesi* to humans by *Anopheles latens* in Sarawak, Malaysia. *Transaction Royal Society of Tropical Medicine and Hygiene,* Vol. 100, pp. 1087–1088.

[102] Vythilingam, I.; Noorazian, Y.M., Huat, T.C., Jiram, A.I., Yusri, Y.M., Azahari, A.H., Norparina, I., Noorrain, A. & Lokmanhakim, S. (2008). *Plasmodium knowlesi* in hu-

mans, macaques and mosquitoes in peninsular Malaysia. *Parasite & Vectors,* Vol. 1, pp.26.

[103] Vythilingam, I. (2012). *Plasmodium knowlesi* and *Wuchereria bancrofti:* Their Vectors and Challenges for the Future. In *Frontiers in Physiology*. Vol.3, pp. 115.

[104] Becker, N.; Petric, D., Zgomba, M., Boase, C., Madon, M., Dahl, C. & Kaiser, A. (2010). Mosquitoes and their control. Springer, London. ISBN-13: 9783540928737.

[105] Seleena, P.; Lee, H.L., Chooi, K.H. & Junaidih, S. (2004). Space spraying of bacterial and chemical insecticidesagainst *Anopheles balabacensis* Baisas for the control of malaria in Sabah, East Malaysia. *Southeast Asian Journal of Tropical Medicine and Public Health*. Vol. 35, No. 1, pp. 68-78.

[106] Reid, J.A. (1968). Anopheline mosquitoes of Malaya and Borneo. *Stud Inst Med Res Malaysia*. Vol 31, pp 520.

[107] Baimai, V.; Kijchalao, U., Rattanarithikul, R. & Green, C.A. (1993). Metaphase karyotypes of *Anopheles* of Thailand and Southeast Asia. II. Maculatus Group, Neocellia Series, subgenus *Cellia. Mosq. Syst*. 25, 116–123. ISSN: 0091-3669.

[108] Vythilingam, I.; Foo, L.C., Chiang, G.L., Inder, S. & Loong, K.P. (1995). The impact of permethrin impregnated bednet on the malaria vector *Anopheles maculatus* (Diptera: Culicidae) in aboriginal villages of Pos Betau Pahang, Malaysia. *Southeast Asian Journal of Tropical Medicine and Public Health,* Vol. 26, pp. 354-7.

[109] Rohani.A.; Wan Najdah, W.M., Zamree, I., Azahari, A.H., Mohd Noor, I., Rahimi, H. & Lee, H.L. (2010).Habitat characterization and mapping of *Anopheles maculatus* (Theobald) mosquito larvae in malaria endemic areas in Kuala Lipis, Pahang, Malaysia. *Southeast Asian Journal of TropicalMedicine andPublic Health*. Vol.41, pp. 821-30.

[110] Miyagi, I. & Toma, T. (2000).The mosquitos of Southeast Asia. In: Ng FSP, Yong HS, eds. Mosquitoes and mosquito-borne diseases. Kuala Lumpur: Academy of Sciences. pp. 1-43.

[111] Chooi, C.K. (1985). Status of malaria vectors in Malaysia. *Southeast Asian J Trop Med Public Healt*.Vol. 16, No.2, pp.133-8.

[112] Baimai, V.; Kijehalao, U., Sawadwongporn, P. & Green, C. A. (1988). Geographic distribution and biting behaviour of four species of the *Anopheles dirus* complex (Diptera: Culicidae) in Thailand. *Southeast Asian. J. Trop. Med. Public Health*. Vol. 19, pp. 151–161.

[113] Oo, T.T.; Storch, V. & Becker, N. (2002). Studies on the bionomics of *Anopheles dirus* (Culicidae: Diptera) in Mudon, Mon State, Myanmar. *Journal of Vector Ecology*. Vol. 27, pp. 44–54. ISSN: 1081-1710.

[114] Prakash, A.; Bhattacharyya, D.R. Mohapatra, P.K., & Mahanta, J. (2002). Physico-chemical characteristics of breeding habitats of *Anopheles dirus* (Diptera: Culicidae) in Assam, India. *Journal Environ. Biol.* Vol. 23, pp. 95–100.

[115] Chang, M.S.; Hii, J., Buttner, P. & Mansoor, F. (1997). Changes in abundance and behaviour of vector mosquitoes induced by land use during the development of an oil palm plantation in Sarawak. *Transactions of the Royal Society of Tropical Medicine and Hygiene.* Vol. 91, pp. 382-386.

[116] Manguin, S.; Bangs, M.J., Pothikasikorn, J. & Chareonviriyaphap, T. (2010). Review on global cotransmission of human *Plasmodium* species and *Wuchereria bancrofti* by *Anopheles* mosquitoes. *Infect. Genet. Evol.* Vol.10, pp. 159–177.

[117] Linton, Y.M.; Dusfour, I, Howard, T.M., Ruiz, L., Nguyen, D.M., Trung, H.D., Sochantha, T., Coosemans, M., & Harbach, R.E. (2005). *Anopheles (Cellia) epiroticus* (Diptera: Culicidae), a new malaria vector species in the Southeast Asian Sundaicus Complex. *Bulletin of Entomological Research.* Vol 95, pp. 329-339

[118] Meek, S.R. (1995). Vector control in some countries of Southeast Asia: comparing the vectors and the strategies. *Ann Trop Med Parasitol.* Vol.89, pp. 135-147. ISSN: 0003-4983.

[119] Vythilingam, I.; Chan, S.T., Shanmugratnam, C., Tanrang, H. & Chooi, K.H. (2005a). The impact ofdevelopment and malaria control activities on its vectors in the Kinabatangan area of Sabah, East Malaysia. *Acta Tropica.* Vol.96, pp. 24-30.

[120] Hii, J.L.K. & Vun, Y.S. (1985). A study of dispersal, survival and adult population estimates of malaria vector, *Anopheles balabacensis* Baisas (Diptera: Culicidae) in Sabah, Malaysia. *Trop Biomed.* Vol. 2, pp. 121-131.

[121] Hii, J.L.K.; Kan, S., Foh. C.K. & Chan, M.K. (1984). *Anopheles (Cellia) balabacensis* Baisas is a vector of *Wuchereria bancrofti* in Sabah, Malaysia. *Transaction Royal Society of Tropical Medicine and Hygene.* Vol. 78, pp. 281-282. ISSN: 0035-9203.

[122] Chen, B.; Butlin, R.K. & Harbach, R.E. (2003). Molecular phylogenetics of the Oriental members of the Myzomyia Series of *Anopheles* subgenus Cellia (Diptera: Culicidae) inferred from nuclear and mitochondrial DNA sequences. *Syst Entomol.* Vol. 28, pp. 57-69.

[123] Wooster, M.T. & Rivera, D (1985). : Breeding point and larval association of anopheline mosquitoes of northwest Mindoro, Philippines. *Southeast Asian Journal of Tropical Medicine and Public Health.* Vol. 16, pp. 59-65.

[124] Colless, D.H. (1956).The *Anopheles leucosphyrus* group. *Trans R Entomol Soc Lond,* Vol. 108, pp. 37-116.

[125] De Las Llagas, L. A. (1985). Impact of ecological changes on *Anopheles* vectors of malaria in some countries of Southeast Asia. Southeast Asian Journal of Tropical Medicine and Public Health, Vol. 16, pp. 146-148. ISSN: 0125-1562.

[126] Cheong, W.H. (1983). Vectors of filariasis in Malaysia. Mak JW, ed. *Filariasis*. Kuala-Lumpur: Institute for Medical Research. *Bulletin* No.19, pp. 37–44.

[127] Kritsiriwuthinan, K. & Ngrenngarmlert, W. (2011). Asymptomatic malaria infections among foreign migrant workers in Thailand. *Asian Pacific Journal of Tropical Medicine*, Vol. 560, pp. 560-563, ISSN: 1995-7645.

[128] Kumar, A.; Chery, L., Biswas,C., Dubhashi, N., Dutta, P., Duaf, V. K., Kacchap, M., Kakati,S., Khandeparkar, A., Kour, D., Mahajan, S.N., Maji, A., Majumder, P., Mohanta, J., Mohapatra, P. K., Narayanasamy, K., Roy, K., Shastri, J., Valecha, N., Vikash, R., Wani, R., White, J. & Rathod, P. K. (2012). Malaria in South Asia: Prevalence and control. *Acta Tropica*, Vol.121, pp. 246– 255.ISSN 0001-706X.

[129] Moon, S.U.; Lee, H.W., Kima, J.Y., Na, B.K., Cho, S. H., Lin, K., Sohn, W. M. & Kim, T. S. (2009). High frequency of genetic diversity of *Plasmodium vivax* field isolates in Myanmar. *Acta Tropica*, Vol. 109. pp. 30-36. ISSN: 0001-706X.

[130] World Health Organization. (2005). Overview of malaria control activities and programme progress: Country profile Myanmar. *World Health Organization*, Geneva, pp. 1-5,

[131] National Malaria Control Programe. (2010). Malaria situation in Myanmar. Myanmar, Yangon, (unpublished).

[132] Ministry of Health. (2010). Myanmar health statistics. Department of Health Planning, Ministry of Health. Yagon. pp.72.

[133] Sermwittayawong, N.; Singh, B., Nishibuchi, M., Sawangjaroen, N. & Vuddhakul. V. (2012). Human *Plasmodium knowlesi* infection in Ranong province, southwestern border of Thailand. *Malaria Journal*, Vol. 11, pp. 11-36. ISSN: 1475-2875.

[134] Than, M.; Kyaw M.P., Soe A.Y, Gyi K.K., Sabai M.& Oo M. (1995). Development of resistance to Chloroquin by *Plasmodium vivax* in Myanmar. *Transactions of the Royal Society of Tropical Medicine and Hygiene*, Vol 89. pp. 307-308.

[135] World Health Organization/ Roll Back Malaria. (2001). The use of antimalaria drugs: Report of an Informal Consultation. *World Health Organization*, Geneva, pp. 1-114.

[136] Oo, T.T.; Storch, V. & Becker, N. (2004). Review of the anopheline mosquitoes of Myanmar. *Journal of Vector Ecology*. Vol. 29, pp21-40, ISSN: 1081-1710.

[137] Paing, M.; A.A. Sebastain, and T. Lin. (1988). Behavior of *Anopheles minimus* in relationship to its role as vector of malaria in a forested foothill area of Burma. *Tropical Biomedicine*, Vol. 5, pp. 161-166.

[138] Paing, M. (1989). Anopheline mosquitoes of Myanmar II. *Anopheles minimus* Theobald, 1901. *Myanmar Health Science Res. Journal*. Vol. 1, pp. 130-134.

[139] Oo, T.T. (2003). The biology and vector competence of the Anopheline mosquitoes of Myanmar with special consideration of *Anopeles dirus*. Doctoral Dissertation, *the Ruperto-Carola University of Heidelberg*, Germany, pp 286.

[140] Lee, C.I.; Smith, L.S., Shwe Oo,E.K., Scharschmidt, B.C., Whichard, E., Thart Kler, T., Lee, J. & Richards, A.K. (2008). Internally displaced human resources for health: villager health worker partnerships to scale up a malaria control programme in active conflict areas of eastern Burma. *Global Public Health,* Vol.0. No.0. pp. 1-13. ISSN: 1744-1692.

[141] Patz, J. A.; & Norris, D. E. (2004). Land use change and human health. In: De Fries, R., Asner, G., & Houghton, R., editors, Ecosystems and land use change, Vol. 153, pp. 344. American Geophysical Monograph Series.

[142] Keiser, J.; Utzinger, J., & Tanner, M. (2005). The effect of irrigation and large dams on the burden of malaria on global and regional scale. *American Journal of Tropical Medicine and Hygiene*, Vol. 72, No. 4, pp. 392-406.

[143] Tisgratog, R.; Tananchai, C., Juntarajumnong, W., Tuntakom, S., Bangs, M.J., Corbel, V., & Chareonviriyaphap, T. (2012). Host feeding patterns and preference of *Anopheles minimus* (Diptera: Culicidae) in a malaria endemic area of western Thailand: baseline site description. *Parasite & Vectors*, Vol. 5, pp. 114.

[144] Petney, T., Sithithaworn, P., Satrawaha, R., Warr, C.G., Andrews, R., Wang, Y.C., Feng, C. (2009). Potential malaria reemergence, northeastern *Thailand. Emerg Infect Dis*, 15: 1330–1331.

[145] Green C.A. : Gass, R.F, Munstermann L.E. & Baimai V. (1990). Population-genetic evidence for two species in *Anopheles minimus* in Thailand. *Med Vet Entomol.*;4(1): 25-34.

[146] Gould, D.J. ; Esah, S. & Pranith, U. (1967). Pelation of *Anopheles aconitus* to malaria transmission in the central plain of Thailand. *Transaction Royal Society of Tropical Medicine Hygiene, Vol.* 31, pp. 441-442.

[147] Green, C.A. ; Rattanarithikul, R., Pongparit, S., Sawadwongporn, P.& Baimai, V. (1991). A newly recognized vector of human malaria parasites in the Oriental region, *Anopheles* (*Cellia*) *pseudowillmori* (Theobald, 1910). *Transaction Royal Society of Tropical Medicine Hygiene*, Vol. 85:, pp. 35-6.

[148] Maheswary, N.P.; Khan, Z., Molla, F.R., & Haq, M.I. (1993). Incrimination of *Anopheles annularis* van der Wulp1854 [sic] as an epidemic malaria vector in Bangladesh. *Southeast Asian J Trop Med Public Health,Vol.* 24, pp.776-778.

[149] Rattanarithikul, R., Harrison, B.A., Harbach, R.E., Panthusiri, P., Coleman, R.E. (2006). Illustrated keys to the mosquitoes of Thailand IV. *Anopheles. Southeast Asian Journal of Tropical Medicine and Public Health,* Vol. 37, pp. 1–128.

[150] Baimai, V.; Andre, R.G., Harrison, B.A., Kijehalao, U. & Panthusiri, L. (1984). Crossing and chromosomal evidence for two additional species within the taxon *Anopheles*

dirus Peyton and Harrison (Diptera: Culicidae) in Thailand. *Proc Entomol Soc Wash,* 89: 157-66.

[151] Tananchai, C.; Tisgratog, R., Juntarajumnong, W., Grieco, J.P., Manguin, S., Prabaripai, A., & Charonviriyaphap, T. (2012). Species diversity and biting activity of *Anopheles dirus* and *Anopheles baimaii* (Diptera: Culicidae) in a malaria prone area of western Thailand. *Parasite & Vectors.* 5, pp. 211.

[152] Green, C.A. ; Baimai, V., Harrison, B.A. & Andre, R.G. (1985). Cytogenetic evidence for a complex of species within the taxon *Anopheles maculatus* (Diptera: Culicidae). *Biol J Linn Soc,* Vol. 24, pp. 321-28.

[153] Rattanarithikul, R., Green, C.A. (1986). Formal recognition of the species of the *Anopheles maculatus* Group (Diptera: Culicidae) occuring in Thailand, including descriptions of two new species and a preliminary key to females. *Mosquito Systematic, Vol.,* 18, pp. 246-78.

[154] Rattanarithikul, R., Harbach, R.E. (1990). *Anopheles maculatus* (Diptera: Culicidae) from the type locality of Hong Kong and two new species of the Maculatus Complex from the Philippines. *Mosquito Systematics, Vol.,* 22, pp. 160-83.

[155] Kittayapong, P. ; Clark, J.M., Edman, J.D., Potter, T.L., Lavine, B.K., & Brooks, M. (1990). Cuticular hydrocarbon differences between the malaria vector and non-vector forms of the *Anopheles maculatus* complex. *Med Vet Entomol,* 4: 405- 3.

[156] Somboon P.; Thongwat, D., Morgan, K. & Walton, C. (2008). Crossing experiment of *Anopheles maculatus* form K and *Anopheles willmori* (James) (Diptera: Culicidae). *Parasitol Research.* Vol. 103(6), pp.1317-22.

[157] Ministry of Public Health [MOPH], (2005). Annual Malaria Reports. Malaria Division, Department of Communicable Disease Control. Ministry of Public Health, Thailand.

[158] Coleman, R.E.; Sithiprasasna, R., Kankaew, P., Kiaattiu,t C., Ratanawong, S., Khuntirat, B. & Sattabongkot, J. (2002). Naturally occurring mixed infection of *Plasmodium vivax* VK210 and *P. vivax* VK247 in *Anopheles minimus* and *An. maculatus* (Diptera: Culicidae) in western Thailand. *J Med Entomol,* 39: 556-559.

[159] Upatham, E.S.; Prasittisuk, C., Ratanatham, S., Green, C.A., Rojanasunan, W., Setakana, P., Theerasilp, N.,Tremongkol, A., Viyanant, V., Pantuwatana, S., & Andre, R.G. (1988). Bionomics of *Anopheles maculatus* complex and their role in malaria transmission in Thailand. *Southeast Asian Journal Tropical Medicine and Public Health,* Vol. 19, pp. 259-269.

[160] Muenworn, V.; Sungvornyothin, S., Kongmee, K., Polsomboon, S., Bangs, M.J., Akrathanakul, P., Tanasinchayakul, S., Prabaripai, A., & Chareonviriyaphap, T. (2008). Biting activity and host preference of the malaria vectors *Anopheles maculatus* and

Anopheles sawadwongporni (Diptera: Culicidae) in Thailand. *Journal of Vector Ecology*, Vol. 34, pp. 62-69.

[161] Baimai, V. (1989). Speciation and species complexes of the *Anopheles* malaria vectors in Thailand. In: Proceedings of the 3rd Conference on Malaria Research, Thailand. pp. 146-62.

[162] Kengluecha, A.; Rongnoparut, P., Boonsuepsakul, S., Sithiprasasna, R., Rodpradit, P., & Baimai, V. (2005). Geographical distribution of *Anopheles minimus* species A and C in western Thailand. *Journal of Vector Ecology*, Vol., 30, pp. 225-230.

[163] Saeung,T. (2012). *Anopheles* (Diptera: Culicidae) species complex in Thailand: identification, distribution, bionomics and malaria-vector importance. *International Journal of Parasitology Research*. Vol. 4, No.1, pp, 75- 82.ISSN: 09753702 & E-ISSN: 0975-9182,

[164] Thongsahuan S.; Baimai, V., Junkum, A., Saeung, A., Min, G.S., Joshi, D., Park, M.H., Somboon, P., Suwonkerd, W., Tippawangkosol, P., Jariyapan, N. & Choochote, W. (2011). Susceptibility of *Anopheles campestris*-like and *Anopheles barbirostris* species complexes to *Plasmodium falciparum* and *Plasmodium vivax* in Thailand. *Mem Inst Oswaldo Cruz*. Vol. 106, No.1, pp. 105-12.

[165] Jongwutiwes, S.; Buppan, P., Kosuvin, R., Seethamchai, S., Pattanawong, U., Sirichaisinthop J. & Putaporntip C. (2011). *Plasmodium knowlesi* malaria in humans and macaques, Thailand. *Emerg. Infectious Disease.*, Vol. 17, pp. 1799-1806.

[166] Putaporntip, C.; Hongsrimuang, T., Seethamchai, S., Kobasa, T., Limkittikul, K., Cui, L., Jongwutiwes, S. (2009). Differential prevalence of *Plasmodium* infections and cryptic *Plasmodium knowlesi* malaria in humans in Thailand. *Journal of Infectious Disease*, Vol. 199, pp. 1143–1150.

[167] Ismail, I.H.A.; Notananda, V., and Schepens, J. (1974). Studies on malaria and response of *Anopheles balabacensis balabacensis* and *Anopheles minimus* to DDT residual spraying in Thailand. Part 1; pre- spraying observations. *Acta Tropica*, Vol. 31, pp. 129-164.

[168] Harbach, R.E. ; Gingrich, J.B., & Pang, L.W. (1987). Some entomological observations on malaria transmission in a remote village in northwestern Thailand. *J Am Mosq Control Assoc*, 3: 296-301.

[169] Ratanatham, S., Upatham, E.S., Prasittisuk, C., Rojanasunan, W., Theerasilp, N., Tremongkol, A., Viyanant, V. (1998). Bionomics of *Anopheles minimus* and its role in malaria transmission in Thailand. *Southeast Asian Journal of Tropical Medicine and Public Health*, Vol. 19, pp.283–289.

[170] Rattanarithikul, R.; Linthicum, K.J., Konish, E. (1996). Seasonal abundance and parity rates of *Anopheles* species in southern Thailand. *Journal of American Mosquito Control Association*, Vol. 12, pp.75–83.

[171] Rwegoshora, R.T.; Sharpe, R.G., Baisley, K.J., Kittayapong, P. (2002). Biting behavior and seasonal variation in the abundance of *Anopheles minimus* species A and C in

Thailand. *Southeast Asian Journal of Tropical Medicine and Public Health*, Vol. 33, pp. 694–701.

[172] Chareonviriyaphap, T.; Prabaripai, A., Bangs, M.J. & Aum-Aung, B. (2003). Seasonal abundance and blood feeding activity of *Anopheles minimus* Theobald (Diptera: Culicidae) in Thailand. *J Med Entomol*, 40: 876–881.

[173] Baimai, V.; Kijehalao, U., Sawadwongporn, P. & Green, C. A. (1988). Geographic distribution and biting behaviour of four species of the *Anopheles dirus* complex (Diptera: Culicidae) in Thailand. *Southeast Asian. J. Trop. Med. Public Health*. Vol. 19, pp. 151–161.

[174] Sungvornyothin, S.; Muenvorn, V., Garros, C., Prabaripai, A., Bangs, M.J., Manguin, S., & Chareonviriyaphap, T. (2006). Trophic behavior and biting activity of the two sibling species of the *Anopheles minimus* complex in western Thailand. *Journal of Vector Ecology*, Vol. 31, pp.252–261.

[175] Patz, J.A., Martens, W.J., Focks. D.A. & Jetten, TH. (1998). Dengue fever epidemic potential as projected by general circulation models of global climate change. *Environ Health Perspect*. Mar Vol 106 No. 3, pp.147-53.

[176] Suwannachote, N.; Grieco, J.P., Achee, N.L., Suwonkerd, W., Wongtong, S., & Chareonviriyaphap, T. (2009). Effects of environmental conditions on the movement patterns of *Aedes aegypti* (Diptera: Culicidae) into and out of experimental huts in Thailand. *Journal of Vector Ecology*, Vol. 34, No.2, pp. 267-275.

[177] Vietnamese Government. (2012). Socialist Republic of Vietnam - Government web portal.

[178] Shuftan, C.; & Le, D. C. (2001). The successful fight against malaria in Vietnam, pp. 30-35, Mekong malaria forum information exchange on malaria control in Southeast Asia. Regional malaria control program in Cambodia, Laos and Vietnam.

[179] Marchand, R.; Tuyen, N. Q., Hoanh, N. Q., & Vien, N. T. (1996). The Khanh Phu malaria research project, pp. 168, Review Meetings 1-2 March 1996. Medical Publishing House 1997, Hanoi.

[180] Grietens, P. K.; Xuan, X. N., Van Bortel, W., Duc, T. N., Ribera, J., Ba Nhat, M. T., Van, K. P., Le Xuan, H., D'Alessandro, U., & Erhart, A. (2010). Low perception of malaria risk among the Ra-glai ethnic minority in south-central Vietnam: implications for forest malaria control. *Malaria Journal*, Vol. 9, pp. 23.

[181] Nakazawa, S.; Marchand, R. P., Quang, N. T., Culleton, R. N., Manh, D., & Maeno, Y. (2009). *Anopheles dirus* co-infection with human and monkey malaria parasites in Vietnam. *International Journal Parasitol*ogy, Vol. 39, pp.1533-1537.

[182] Thang, N. D.; Erhart, A., Hung le, X., Thuan le, K., Xa, N. X., Thanh, N. N., Ky, P. V., Coosemans, M., Speybroeck, N., & D'Alessandro, U. (2009). Rapid decrease of malar-

ia morbidity following the introduction of community-based monitoring in a rural area of central Vietnam. *Malaria Journal,* Vol. 8, pp. 3.

[183] Marchand, R. P.; Culleton, R., Maeno, Y., Quang, N. T., & Nakazawa, S. (2011). Co-infections of *Plasmodium knowlesi, P. falciparum,* and *P. vivax* among humans and *Anopheles dirus* mosquitoes, Southern Vietnam. *Emerg Infect Dis,* Vol.17, pp. 1232-9.

[184] Singh, B.; Kim Sung, L., Matusop, A., Radhakrishnan, A., Shamsul, S. S., Cox-Singh,J., Thomas, A., & Conway, D. J. (2004). A large focus of naturally acquired *Plasmodium knowlesi* infections in human beings. *Lancet,* Vol. 363, pp. 1017-24.

[185] Cox-Singh, J.; & Singh., B. (2008a). Knowlesi malaria: newly emergent and of public health importance? *Trends Parasitol,* Vol. 24, pp. 406-10.

[186] Cox-Singh, J.; Davis, T.M., Lee, K.S., Shamsul, S.S., Matusop, A., Ratnam, S., Rahman, H.A., Conway, D.J., & Singh, B. (2008b). *Plasmodium knowlesi* malaria in humans is widely distributed and potentially life threatening. *Clinical Infectious Diseases,* Vol. 46, No.2, pp. 165-171.

[187] Cox-Singh, J.; Hiu, J., Lucas,S. B., Divis,P. C., Zulkarnaen, M., Chandran, P., Wong, K. T., Adem,P., Zaki, S. R., Singh,B., Krishna, S. (2010). Severe malaria - a case of fatal *Plasmodium knowlesi* infection with post-mortem findings: a case report. *Malaria Journal,* Vol. 9, pp. 10.

[188] Cox-Singh, J. (2009). Knowlesi malaria in Vietnam. *Malaria Journal,* Vol. 8, pp. 269.

[189] Van den Eede, P.; Van, H. N., Van Overmeir, C., Vythilingam, I., Duc, T. N., Hung le, X., Manh, H. N., Anne, J., D'Alessandro, U., & Erhart, A. (2009). Human *Plasmodium knowlesi* infections in young children in central Vietnam. *Malaria Journal,* Vol. 8: 249.

[190] Hung le, Q.; Vries, P. J., Giao, P. T., Nam, N. V., Binh, T. Q., Chong, M. T., Quoc, N. T., Thanh, T. N., Hung, L. N., & Kager, P. A. (2002). Control of malaria: a successful experience from Viet Nam. *Bull World Health Organ* 80: 660-6.

[191] Huong, N. M.; Hewitt, S., Davis, T. M., Dao, L. D., Toan, T. Q., Kim,,T. B., Hanh, N. T., Phuong, V. N., Nhan, D. H., & Cong, L. D. (2001). Resistance of *Plasmodium falciparum* to antimalarial drugs in a highly endemic area of southern Viet Nam: a study in vivo and in vitro. *Trans R Soc Trop Med Hyg,* Vol. 95, pp. 325-9.

[192] Ngo, T.; Duraisingh, M., Reed, M., Hipgrave, D., Biggs, B., & Cowman, A. F. (2003). Analysis of pfcrt, pfmdr1, dhfr, and dhps mutations and drug sensitivities in *Plasmodium falciparum* isolates from patients in Vietnam before and after treatment with artemisinin. *American Journal of Tropical Medicine and Hygiene,* Vol. 68, pp. 350-356.

[193] Van Bortel, W.; Chinh, V. D., Berkvens, D., Speybroeck, N., Trung, H. D., & Coosemans, M. (2009). Impact of insecticide-treated nets on wild pyrethroid resistant *Anopheles epiroticus* population from southern Vietnam tested in experimental huts. *Malaria Journal,* Vol. 8: 248.

[194] Verhaeghen, K.; Van Bortel, W., Trung, H. D., Sochantha, T., & Coosemans, M. (2009). Absence of knockdown resistance suggests metabolic resistance in the main malaria vectors of the Mekong region. *Malaria Journal,* Vol. 8: 84.

[195] IMPEQN. (2012). Statistic data of malaria case in Central Highlands Vietnam. Institute of malaria, parasite and Entomology sub Quy Nhon.

[196] Erhart, A.; Ngo, D. T., Phan, V. K., Ta, T. T., Van Overmeir, C., Speybroeck, N., Obsomer, V., Le, X. H., Le, K. T., Coosemans, M., D'Alessandro, U. (2005). Epidemiology of forest malaria in central Vietnam: a large scale cross-sectional survey. *Malaria Journal,* Vol. 4, pp. 58.

[197] Abe, T.; Honda, S., Nakazawa, S., Tuong, T. D., Thieu, N. Q., Hung le, X., Thuan le, K., Moji, K., Takagi, M., & Yamamoto, T. (2009). Risk factors for malaria infection among ethnic minorities in Binh Phuoc, Vietnam. *Southeast Asian J Trop Med Public Health,* Vol. 40, pp. 18-29.

[198] Nguyen, V. Q. (2005). Chemical methods applicable for the areas with low malarial prevalence in Bac Kan province, pp. 30. NIMPE - Hanoi.

[199] Tran, Q. T. (2005). Epidemiological studies of malaria and the malarial prevention measures, applicable at Son La hydro-electrical areas pp. 50. NIMPE - Hanoi.

[200] Erhart, A; Thang, N. D., Xa, N. X., Thieu, N. Q., Hung, L. X., Hung, N. Q., Nam, N. V., Toi, L. V., Tung, N. M., Bien, T. H., Tuy, T. Q., Cong, L. D., Thuan, L. K., Coosemans, M., and D'Alessandro, U. (2007). Accuracy of the health information system on malaria surveillance in Vietnam. *Transaction Royal Society of Tropical Medicine and Hygiene,* Vol. 101, pp. 216-25.

[201] NIMPE. (2008). Keys to identify of *Anopheles* mosquitoes (Adults-Pupae-Larvae). Department of Entomology, Institute of Malariology, Parasitology and Entomology, Hanoi.

[202] Van Bortel, W.; Harbach, R. E., Trung, H. D., Roelants, P., Backeljau, T., & Coosemans, M. (2001). Confirmation of *Anopheles varuna* in Vietnam, previously misidentified and mistargeted as the malaria vector *Anopheles minimus. American Journal of Tropical Medicine and Hygiene,* Vol. 65, pp. 729-32.

[203] Cuong do, M.; Van, N. T., Tao le, Q., Chau,T. L., Anh le, N., Thanh, N. X., & Cooper, R. D. (2008). Identification of *Anopheles minimus* complex and related species in Vietnam. *Southeast Asian JTrop Med Public Health* 39: 827-31.

[204] Phan, V. T. [ed.] (1998). Epidemiologie du paludisme et lutte antipaludique au Vietnam. Editions Médicales Vietnam, Hanoi.

[205] Vu, D. C. (2006). Distribution of *Anophele*s mosquito and the malarial transmission vector in some forested habitat, located in northern part of Vietnam, pp. 40. NIMPE - Hanoi, Hanoi.

[206] Van Bortel, W.; Trung, H. D., Manh, N. D., Roelants, P., Verle, P., & Coosemans, M. (1999). Identification of two species within the *Anopheles minimus* complex in northern Vietnam and their behavioural divergences. *Tropical Medicine and International Health, Vol.* 4, pp. 257-65.

[207] Walton, C.; Handley, J. M., Kuvangkadilok, C., Collins, F. H., Harbach, R. E., Baimai, V., & Butlin, R. K. (1999). Identification of five species of the *Anopheles dirus* complex from Thailand, using allele-specific polymerase chain reaction. *Medical Veterinary Entomology,* Vol. 13, pp. 24-32.

[208] Garros, C.; Koekemoer, L. L., Kamau, L., Awolola, T. S., Van Bortel, W., Coetzee, M., Coosemans, M., & Manguin, S. (2004). Restriction fragment length polymorphism method for the identification of major African and Asian malaria vectors within the *Anopheles funestus* and *An. minimus* groups. *American Journal of Tropical Medicine and Hygiene,* Vol. 70, pp. 260-265.

[209] Ma, Y.; Li, S., & Xu, J. (2006). Molecular identification and phylogeny of the Maculatus Group of *Anopheles* mosquitoes (Diptera: Culicidae) based on nuclear and mitochondrial DNA sequences. *Acta Tropica,* Vol. 99, pp. 272-80.

[210] Walton, C.; Somboon, P., Harbach, R. E., Zhang, S., Weerasinghe, I., O'Loughlin, S. M., Phompida, S., Sochantha, T., Tun-Lin, W., Chen, B., & Butlin, R. K. (2007a). Molecular identification of mosquito species in the *Anopheles annularis* group in southern Asia. *Medical Vet Entomology,* Vol. 21, pp. 30-35.

[211] Walton, C.; Somboon, P., O'Loughlin, S. M., Zhang, S., Harbach, R. E., Linton, Y. M., Chen, B., Nolan, K., Duong, S., Fong, M. Y., Vythilingam, I., Mohammed, Z. D., Trung, H. D., Butlin, R. K. (2007b). Genetic diversity and molecular identification of mosquito species in the *Anopheles maculatus* group using the ITS2 region of rDNA. *Infectious Genetic Evoluation,* Vol. 7: 93-102.

[212] Garros C., Nguyen C.V., Trung H.D., Van Bortel W., Coosemans M., ManguinS.. (2008). Distribution of *Anopheles* in Vietnam, with particular attention to malaria vectors of the *Anopheles minimus* complex. *Malaria Journal,* Vol 7, pp 11.

[213] Garros, C.; Marchand, R. P., Quang, N. T., Hai, N. S., & Manguin, S. (2005b). First record of *Anopheles minimus* C and significant decrease of *An. minimus* A in central Vietnam. *Journal of American Mosquito Control Association, Vol.* 21, pp. 139-43.

[214] Le, X. H. (2006). Investigating into composition and distribution of *Anopheles* mosquitoes, malarial vectors in the U Minh forest and evaluation of Agnique MMF effectiveness, used in controlling of *An. sundaicus* larvae, pp. 28. NIMPE -Hanoi.

[215] Nguyen, D. M;, Tran, D. H., Harbach, R. E., Elphick, J., & Linton, Y. M. (2000). A new species of the *Hyrcanus* Group of *Anopheles,* subgenus *Anopheles,* a secondary vector of malaria in coastal areas of southern Vietnam. *Journal of American Mosquito Control Association,* Vol. 16, pp. 189-98.

http://dx.doi.org/10.5772/56347

[216] Van Bortel, W.; Trung, H. D., Roelants, P., Backeljau,T., & Coosemans, M. (2003). Population genetic structure of the malaria vector *Anopheles minimus* A in Vietnam. *Heredity (Edinb)*, Vol. 91, pp.487-93.

[217] GSOV. Socio-economic statistics in the first half of 2012 monthly statistical information. General statistic officer of Vietnam, Hanoi.

[218] Ho, V. H. (2008). Baseline survey on malaria and appropriated measures in malarial prevention for migrant population in Dak Glong District - Dak Nong Province. pp. 57. IMPE-Quy Nhon.

Chapter 11

Understanding *Anopheles* Diversity in Southeast Asia and Its Applications for Malaria Control

Katy Morgan, Pradya Somboon and
Catherine Walton

Additional information is available at the end of the chapter

http://dx.doi.org/10.5772/55709

1. Introduction

1.1. Why study *Anopheles* diversity: Relevance for malaria control

The need to understand diversity in *Anopheles* mosquitoes to win the fight against malaria first became apparent with the paradox of 'anophelism without malaria', as it became evident that there is a vast diversity of *Anopheles* species and that not all species transmit malaria [1]. For example, in Europe it was eventually deduced that the mosquito *Anopheles maculipennis* existed as a species complex comprising several species that differed in their breeding, feeding and resting habitats, which resulted not only in differences in malaria epidemiology but also the success or failure of malaria control efforts [2]. This realisation resulted in countless studies around the world to distinguish and characterise *Anopheles* species, often using molecular or chromosomal characters in the absence of reliable morphological characters [3-4]. Such studies have played an invaluable role in improving malaria control and have, in turn, revealed another layer of complexity. This is exemplified most clearly in the *Anopheles gambiae* Complex, which includes several important African malaria vectors. Taxa within the *An. gambiae* Complex can exist as recently diverged species such as *An. gambiae* and *An. arabiensis*, which still have the potential to exchange genes [5]; as incipient species such as the S and M molecular forms, or as genetically divergent locally adapted forms, e.g. adapted to forest or savannah [6]. Recent genomic studies of the *An. gambiae* Complex are revealing patterns of differential divergence and introgression across the genome between species [7-8]; such phenomena are likely to further complicate the definition of species boundaries within *Anopheles* complexes. Differences in characteristics relevant to malaria control may be present at even the subspecific level (e.g. larval habitat and insecticide resistance both within and between the S and M molecular forms [9-11]), demonstrating the need to understand the generation and maintenance of *Anopheles* diversity at all levels.

This chapter focuses on the need to not only characterise species boundaries, ecology and distributions, but also to understand the potential for divergence and the extent of gene flow within and between species of *Anopheles* in Southeast Asia. Southeast Asia is characterised by having numerous vector taxa and epidemiological settings, and though there has been great progress in reducing malaria in Southeast Asia, it has proved difficult or impossible to completely eradicate in many places, e.g. [12-13]. A complete understanding of transmission dynamics in Southeast Asia and the best approach to interrupt them is complicated by several factors, including intraspecific variation in ecology and vector status across species distributions, potential interactions between species in malaria transmission (i.e. the fact that the vectorial capacity of one species may vary depending on the presence of a second vector species), and by the potential for ongoing gene flow between species. In this chapter, we argue that understanding the complexity and diversity of *Anopheles* species in this region and the nature of isolation, ecological variation and gene flow in driving divergence or homogenising variation within and between them is key to a complete understanding of malaria transmission dynamics and our attempts to interrupt it via vector control. This involves determining the historical processes that have driven diversification to understand both current intraspecific and interspecific variation and the potential for future change (e.g. in adaptation to environmental change) that could affect malaria transmission and/or vector control efforts.

2. Diversity of *Anopheles* species across Southeast Asia

This chapter primarily focuses on the diversity of *Anopheles* species in Southeast Asia, which encompasses the geographical area east of India, south of China and west of New Guinea. Southeast Asia is further subdivided into two sub regions: mainland Southeast Asia, comprised of Myanmar, Thailand, Cambodia, Lao People's Democratic Republic, Vietnam and peninsular Malaysia; and insular Southeast Asia, comprised of Indonesia, East Timor, Singapore, East Malaysia, Brunei and the Philippines. However, as many of the vector species found within Southeast Asia, e.g. members of the *An. minimus, An. dirus* and *An. subpictus* Complexes, and Funestus and Maculatus Groups, also overlap into India (particularly northeast India), Sri Lanka and China we have included these regions where relevant in order to achieve a more complete understanding of *Anopheles* diversity in Southeast Asia.

The diversity of Anopheline fauna that exists within Southeast Asia is richer than in any other region of the world [14], and at least 19 species, some of which comprise cryptic species complexes, are known to play some role in malaria transmission [15]. Exactly 50% of the 24 currently recognised *Anopheles* species complexes are found within Asia, which when compared with the 21%, 13%, 13% and 4% found in the Americas, Africa, Australia-Pacific and Europe, respectively, emphasises the complexity of diversity found within the Asian continent [14]. The considerable variation that exists between species in terms of habitat preference and feeding behaviour makes the characterisation of species distributions highly relevant to malaria control efforts. Malaria transmission characteristics and the effectiveness of control efforts such as insecticide treated bednets (ITNs), larvicides, and indoor residual spraying (IRS), will depend to a large extent on the vector species present in a given area [14], and since the effectiveness of a given vector species can be influenced by other species present in the region, malaria transmission dynamics also depend on species composition. Hence considerable effort has been focussed on the stratification of malaria units for effectively targeted malaria control, with the ecological characteristics and geographical distributions of species having particular relevance [16]. In this section we discuss the geographical features that appear to define and limit species distributions, and the relevance of this information for malaria control.

Early attempts for a geographical stratification of malaria units [17] were based on the biogeographical realms of Wallace (1876). However, Wallace's Oriental Realm is largely inappropriate for South Asia and Southeast Asia due to the exceptionally high biodiversity and high heterogeneity of spatial distribution of vectors in this region [14-15]. On a smaller spatial scale there are multiple biogeographical subregions within Southeast Asia, including the biodiversity hotspot regions of IndoBurma, Sundaland, the Philippines and Wallacea ([18]; see figure 1). These hotspots were defined in part on the basis of endemism so it is not surprising that they appear to define the distributions of many malaria vectors, with clear patterns of species turnover apparent at each of the biogeographical boundaries.

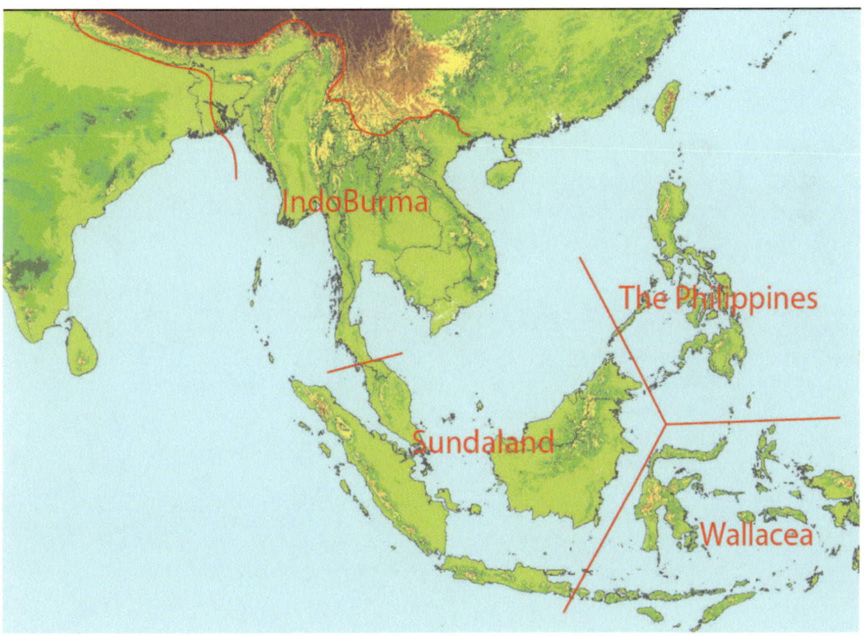

Figure 1. Topological map of Southeast Asia, indicating the four main biogeographical zones as defined by Myers *et al.* (2000) [17].

The first biogeographical boundary that shows a clear association with species distributions is that separating IndoBurma from southwestern Asia (Figure 1). It should be noted that northeast India, although politically part of India, is biogeographically and ecologically aligned with IndoBurma rather than southwestern Asia. The *Anopheles* fauna on either side of this boundary is generally distinct, for example several vector species that are distributed across IndoBurma, including *An. baimaii*, *An. sawadwongporni* and *An. maculatus* (Figures 2 and 3), have distributions that extend little further than this western border. The closely related *An. minimus* and *An. fluviatilis* Complexes show largely parapatric distributions that overlap along the western border of IndoBurma, with the distribution of the *An. minimus* Complex being primarily restricted to IndoBurma and that of the *An. fluviatilis* Complex being mostly limited to southwestern Asia (Figure 4).

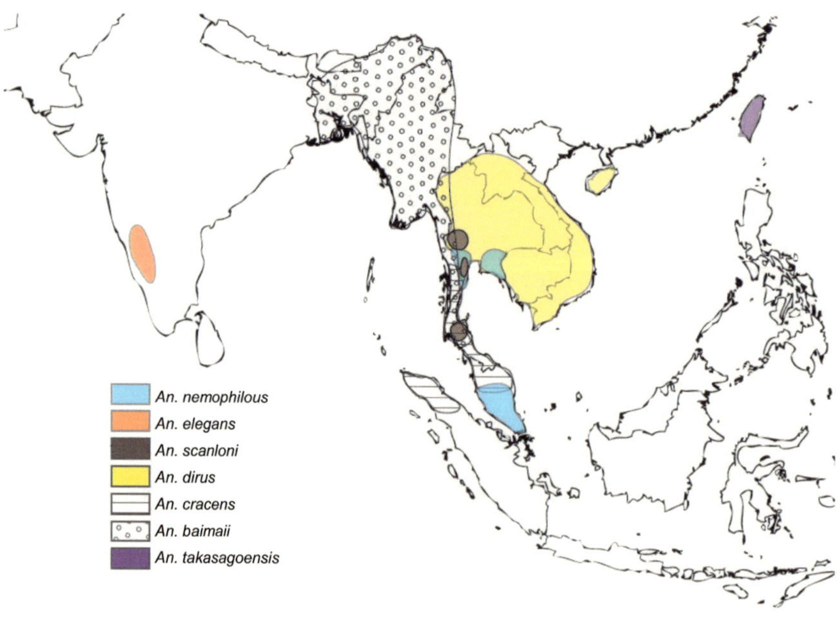

Figure 2. The distribution of species within the *Anopheles dirus* Complex.

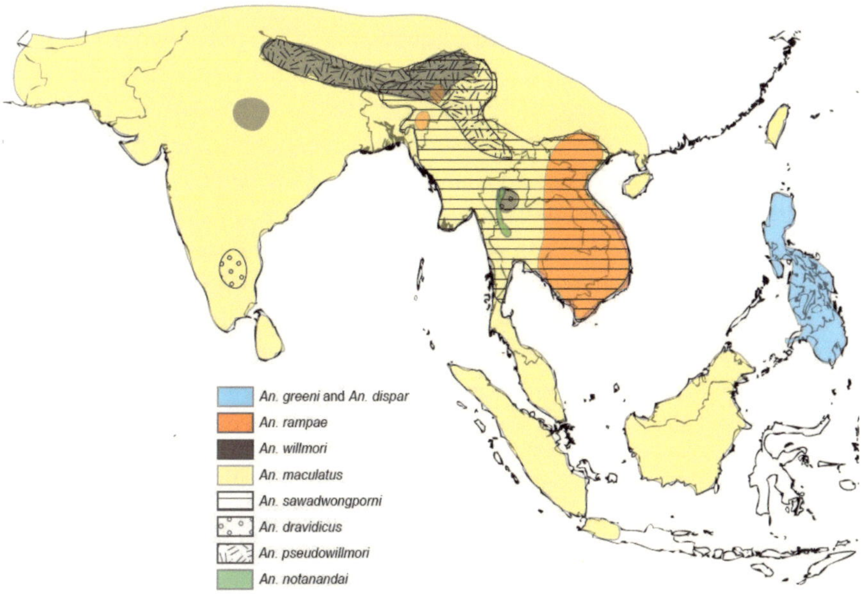

Figure 3. The distribution of species within the Maculatus Group.

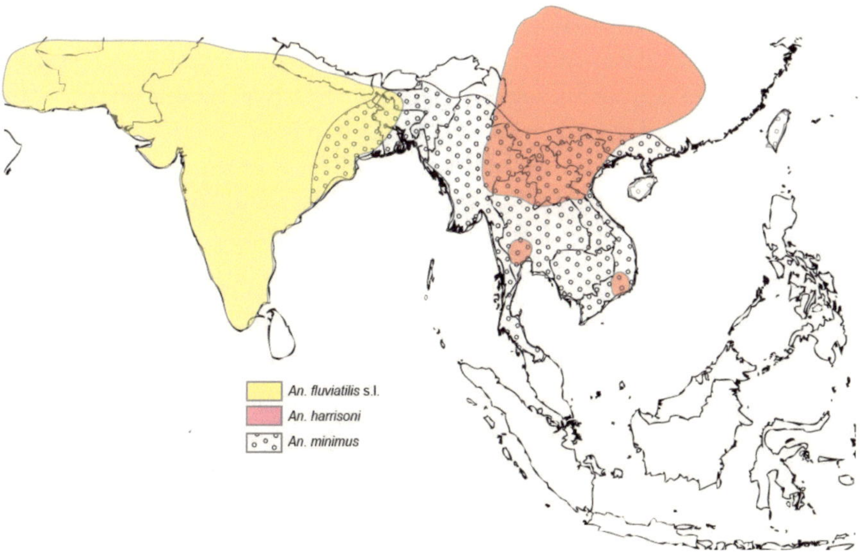

Figure 4. The distribution of species within the Minimus Subgroup (which encompasses the *An. minimus* and *An. fluviatilis* Complexes).

The boundary between the biodiversity hotspot regions of IndoBurma and Sundaland (Figure 1) represents a second major biogeographic transition in Southeast Asia, and is characterised by high species turnover in a number of taxonomic groups (e.g. birds, mammals and reptiles [19-21]). This long-recognised biogeographic transition was first noted by Wallace in 1869, and though its exact position along the Thai-Malay Peninsula is debated, with some dispute as to whether the transition occurs at the Isthmus of Kra (10º30′N) or the Kangar-Pattani line (6-7ºN) further south [22], its biogeographical significance is unquestioned. The transition is associated with dramatic climate and phytological changes. IndoBurma has a very seasonal climate in terms of both temperature and rainfall, whereas that of Sundaland is much more stable, with precipitation levels remaining high throughout the year. Whereas mixed moist deciduous forest is the dominant forest habitat type of IndoBurma, that of Sundaland is perhumid evergreen forest [23-24]. Thus it seems unsurprising that this is a region of high species turnover, as the selective pressures on either side of the Isthmus of Kra biogeographic transition would differ considerably, potentially driving rapid adaptive change and subsequent ecological speciation following the dispersal of taxa from one side to the other.

Again, the majority of *Anopheles* species are limited in distribution to either side of the IndoBurma-Sundaland biogeographical transition. Within the Leucosphyrus Group (which encompasses both the *An. dirus* and *An. leucosphyrus* Complexes), for example, *An. baimaii* and *An. dirus* are found to the north of this biogeographical boundary whereas many other species in the Leucosphyrus Group occur only to the south, with many species spanning from the mainland of peninsular Malaysia into the major islands e.g. *An. macarthuri, An. cracens, An. introlatus* and *An. latens* (Figures 2 and 5). Again, the major vector species of the *An. minimus* Complex, *An. minimus* and *An. harrisoni*, are limited in distribution to IndoBurma, as are the majority of species within the Maculatus Group (Figures 3 and 4). Although there does appear to be species turnover between the mainland and each of the islands (e.g. *An. nemophilous* is found within peninsular Malaysia but on none of the islands (Figure 2); *An. leucosphyrus* is found only on Sumatra (Figure 5)), several species are found on more than one of the major landmasses but are limited to only one of the biogeographical zones (e.g. *An. balabacensis* is found on both Borneo and Java). This suggests that whilst sea barriers play a role in limiting dispersal, the mainland biogeographical transition is clearly important in limiting species distributions despite the lack of such an obvious physical barrier.

The final distinct biodiversity hotspot regions of Southeast Asia are those of Wallacea and the Philippines, each of which harbours a unique assemblage of *Anopheles* species. Although separated from Borneo by only a narrow sea barrier, the Philippines are thought to share few of the major vector species of Southeast Asia. The Minimus Subgroup (which comprises the *An. minimus* and *An. fluviatilis* Complexes) appears not to have colonised the Philippines, and the species within both the *An. leucosphyrus* Complex and the Maculatus Group found in the Philippines (*An. baisasi*, and *An. greeni* and *An. dispar*, respectively) are limited in distribution to these islands (Figures 3 and 5). *An. balabacensis* provides somewhat of an exception, being found on both Borneo and within the Philippines, although its distribution within the Philippines is limited to the small, western islands between Borneo and the major Philippine Island of Luzon (Figure 5). *Anopheles annularis s.l.*, on the other hand, is distributed within the Philippines as well

http://dx.doi.org/10.5772/55709

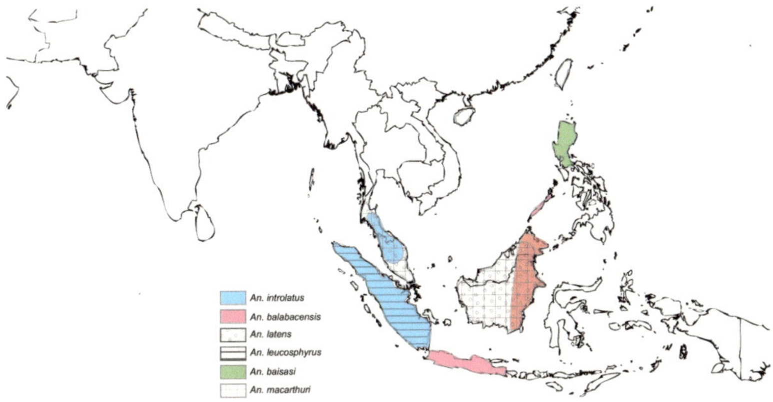

Figure 5. The distribution of species within the *Anopheles leucosphyrus* Complex and *Anopheles macarthuri* of the Leucosphyrus Group

as throughout mainland and insular Southeast Asia, although the limited available evidence suggests that the Philippine populations of this species show strong differentiation from those in other regions of Southeast Asia [25]. As a result of the described species turnover patterns, the subregions differ in terms of major malaria vectors, with the *An. dirus* and *An. minimus* Complexes, and Maculatus Group dominating throughout IndoBurma, the *An. leucosphyrus* Complex dominating within the Sundaic Region, and *An. flavirostris* being the main malaria vector within the Philippines and a major malaria vector within Indonesia [15].

In addition to the divisions between the biogeographic regions discussed above, there are some apparent transitions within biogeographic regions. As previously discussed, there is some distinction between the species composition of each of the major Sundaic Islands and the mainland, although several species within the *An. dirus* and *An. leucosphyrus* Complexes are found on more than one of the landmasses. An apparent distinction in species composition between the landmasses is seen in other taxa from shrike babblers [26] to macaques [27]. Besides this pattern, there is also an apparent distinction within IndoBurma, between the distribution of genetic diversity east and west of the Thai-Myanmar border. The closely related sister species *An. dirus* and *An. baimaii* have parapatric distributions within Southeast Asia, which overlap along this border region (Figure 2). *An. sawadwongporni* and *An. rampae* are a second pair of sister species that show a similar pattern, with *An. rampae* having a primarily easterly distribution, which extends from eastern Thailand towards Vietnam and does not overlap the Thai-Myanmar border (Figure 4). *An. rampae* has, however, recently been recorded at low frequency within northeastern India, suggesting the distribution and population structure of this species warrant further attention [28]. The Thai-Myanmar border region is also the site of a suture zone between highly divergent intraspecific lineages within species including *An. splendidus, An. minimus* and *An. annularis* [29]. The patterns in species distribution discussed throughout this section, with closely related species often falling on either side of biogeographical divisions that lack obvious geographical barriers, clearly indicate a role for vicariance and/or ecology in generating biodiversity within Southeast Asia, as will be discussed later in this chapter.

Although the distributions of the majority of *Anopheles* taxa appear to be defined by biogeographical boundaries, there are some taxa with relatively wide distributions that span many of the biogeographic subregions discussed above. For example, *An. maculatus* is distributed throughout Nepal, Pakistan, Bhutan and India and throughout the IndoBurma (including Taiwan) and Sundaic Regions of Southeast Asia, and *An. vagus* has a similar distribution throughout India, IndoBurma and the Sundaic Region. These species appear to be largely panmictic throughout their distributions [29-30], suggesting an ability to combine high dispersal capacities with generalist habitat requirements.

The distinctiveness of the Anopheline fauna of each of the major biogeographic regions of Southeast Asia, which occurs despite the continuity of landmass between these regions, suggests that ecological factors, such as climate and dominant habitat type, play a key role in defining species distributions. Malaria stratifications based on ecological biomes, such as forest, foothill and urban regions, are therefore especially useful in designating control efforts [16]. The clear ecological similarity between many closely related vector species also suggests a strong conservation of ecological niche. Species within the *An. dirus* and *leucosphyrus* Complexes, for example, show a strong association with forest habitat [31-33]. Thus in the IndoBurma and Sundaic Regions, where species within these complexes are distributed, malaria is often most prevalent in villages that are in close proximity to the forest fringe, and people involved in forest activities are often most at risk [16]. Species within the Minimus Complex, on the other hand, are prevalent within foothill regions and generally breed in slow running streams [31, 33-34], leading to the designation of a 'foothill' malaria stratification. The brackish water tolerant species *An. sundaicus* and *An. epiroticus,* which are also major vectors of malaria throughout Southeast Asia, dominate malaria transmission in coastal regions [35-37]. Thus the characterisation of species relationships, ecology and distributions has clearly facilitated great improvements to malaria control efforts. However, understanding of malaria transmission dynamics is still complicated by the potential for interactions between vector species, variation in vector capacity across a species range, and remaining taxonomical confusion in some groups (e.g. the *An. culicifacies* Complex) (reviewed in [33]). Thus the previously discussed high diversity of cryptic species within Southeast Asia may be one of the factors making malaria difficult to eliminate in parts of Southeast Asia.

3. Processes driving the diversification of the Anopheline fauna of Southeast Asia

3.1. The role of historical environmental change

As discussed in the first section of this chapter, as well as an understanding of extant species distribution and ecology, the characterisation of population dynamics and levels and patterns of gene flow both within and between species is essential, as the effective size and connectivity of populations will influence the speed at which traits relevant to malaria control evolve and spread between them [38]. The release of genetically modified mosquitoes has been proposed for the control of vector populations in Africa [39]; if such approaches were developed for

Southeast Asia, population genetic studies would be necessary to determine the number of genetically modified individuals and release sites needed for a successful program [39-40]. The estimation of levels of contemporary gene flow is greatly complicated, however, by the historical genetic structuring of mosquito populations [41-42]. In order to reliably infer patterns of contemporary gene flow, it is therefore essential that we first gain a thorough understanding of the population history of the *Anopheles* fauna.

As with all organisms, the genetic structuring of *Anopheles* populations through time is likely to have been greatly impacted by the influence of geographical features on patterns of gene flow and dispersal. Geographical barriers such as mountains, rivers or sea can restrict or prevent gene flow between populations, so causing them to become increasingly differentiated from one another due to the processes of neutral genetic drift and differential natural selection [38]. Many of the *Anopheles* taxa of Southeast Asia, including those within the Minimus and the Leucosphyrus subgroups and the Maculatus Group, are forest associated [31]. Hence for these taxa, expanses of open habitat such as grassland or savannah can constitute an important barrier to gene flow and dispersal. In the absence of gene flow, reproductive barriers may accumulate between isolated populations and cause allopatric speciation [43]. Geographical barriers can shift over time, leading to patterns of repeated expansion and contraction in the ranges of species constrained by them. The biogeographical history of Southeast Asia is especially dynamic, featuring tectonic activity [44], substantial sea-level fluctuations, large shifts in the region's landmass configuration [45], and climate-associated fluctuations in the distribution and extent of forest habitat [46-47]. The time-line below indicates the major biogeographic events inferred to have influenced Anopheline diversification from the mid-Miocene onwards (see figure 6).

3.1.1. Miocene (23.0 – 5.3 mya): Dispersal of Pyretophorus series and Myzomyia series from Africa to Asia

The collisions of the Indian, African and Australian plates with Eurasia all had substantial impacts on the landscape and fauna of Southeast Asia. India initially collided with Southeast Asia approximately 50 million years ago (mya), and the subsequent northwards push of the Indian plate resulted in the formation and uplift of the Himalayas [44], forming a geographical barrier between Southeast Asia and the rest of the Asian continent. The second major period of tectonic activity, which involved the uplift of the Himalayas approximately 25mya, coincided with the collision of the African and Eurasian plates. This latter event resulted in the closure of the Tethys Sea and so created a land connection between the continents of Africa and Asia [48]. Although this region is now characterised by arid desert habitat, a corridor of tropical forest is thought to have persisted during the humid periods of the early and mid-Miocene [48]. Combined with low sea-levels, this allowed forest taxa such as the ancestors of the Oriental Myzomyia and Pyretophorus Series to disperse from their African origins into Southeast Asia [49-50]. Increasingly arid conditions and the consequent desertification of East Asia during the late Miocene (6.2 – 5mya) restricted this exchange [48, 51], effectively isolating the forest fauna of Asia and Africa. The Oriental and African taxa within the Myzomyia and Pyretophorus Series form monophyletic groups in both cases (with the exception of the

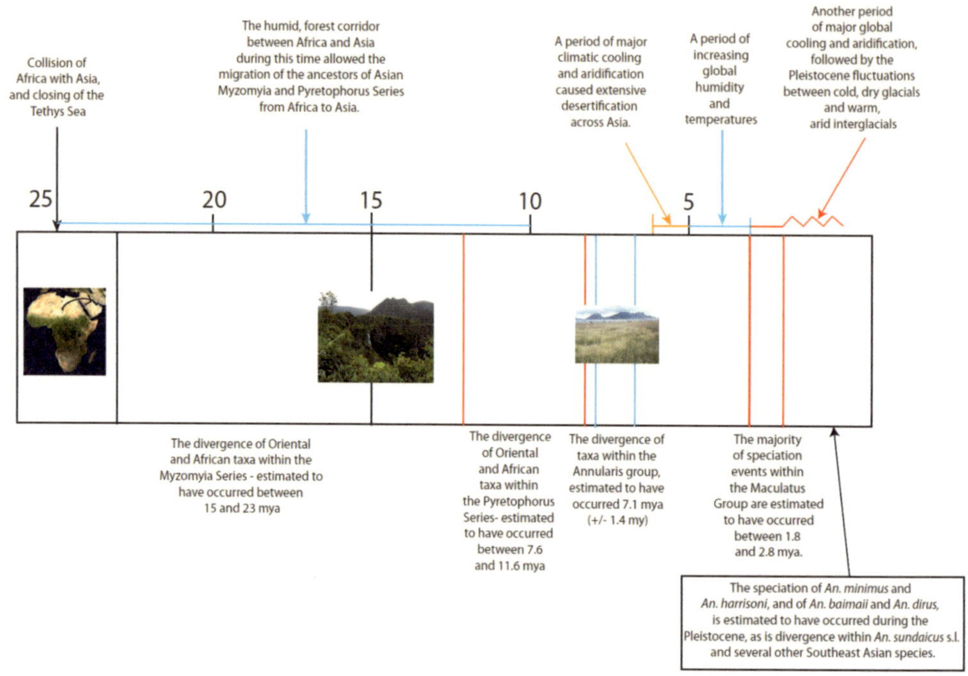

Figure 6. Timeline showing the major biogeographic events inferred to have driven speciation and divergence in the Anopheline fauna of Southeast Asia.

placement of the African species *An. leesoni* within the Oriental Myzomyia clade), and are estimated to have diverged during the late Miocene [49-50]. This suggests that dispersal from Africa to Asia occurred during the humid mid Miocene in both cases, and was followed by the isolation of Asian and African lineages after the late-Miocene expansion of desert across East Asia (Figure 6). As *Anopheles* species rely on water bodies for their larval habitats, desert habitat is likely to pose an extremely effective barrier to dispersal. The close relationship of the African species *An. leesoni* with the Oriental Myzomyia species, from which it is estimated to have diverged just 2-3 mya, is somewhat of a mystery, and suggests some faunal exchange during the mid Pliocene despite the dominance of desert habitat throughout East Asia [49].

3.1.2. Late Miocene and Pliocene (6 – 2mya): Forest fragmentation drives allopatric speciation

The increasingly cool and arid climate responsible for extensive desertification across East Asia during the late Miocene also resulted in the expansion of grassland and savannah habitat across Southeast Asia [52]. The consequent reduction in available *Anopheles* larval habitats likely to have occurred during this time, and the potential consequent fragmentation and isolation of populations in allopatry, is hypothesised to have driven late Miocene speciation (dated to 7.1 mya +/- 1.4 my) within the Neocellia Series Annularis Group [25] (Figure 6). This trend of increasing aridification was reversed during the early Pliocene (5-2.8 mya), which was characterised by increasingly warm and humid conditions, with global temperatures reaching approximately 3°C above current temperatures [53-54]. Tropical forest would have expanded across Southeast Asia during this period, and *Anopheles* habitats would have been more abundant and widespread. A subsequent major climatic transition towards a substantially cooler and more arid climate began approximately 2.8 mya, and culminated in the first of the Pleistocene glacial maxima, 1.8 mya [55]. Once again, tropical forest habitat would have been replaced by large areas of grassland and savannah, fragmenting and isolating populations of forest-dependent *Anopheles* species across Southeast Asia. The consequent divergence of populations in allopatry is thought to have driven speciation within the forest-associated Maculatus Group [25], with contemporary species distributions in this group being fairly distinct (although exhibiting large areas of overlap), and the majority of speciation events dating to within the 2.8-1.8 mya period of major climatic cooling (Figure 6).

3.1.3. Pleistocene (1.8 mya – 11,000 ya): Changes in landmass configuration drive dispersal and divergence within species

During the Pleistocene, the ongoing fluctuations in the extent of forest cover across Southeast Asia were exacerbated by the dramatic impact of glacio-eustatic sea level change on the region's climate [45-46]. These sea-level fluctuations, which involved drops of between 50 and 200 meters during each of the Pleistocene glaciations [56], had a more dramatic effect on the climate and habitats of Southeast Asia than those of any other tropical region [46]. Sea level regressions of 60 meters or more result in the exposure of the Gulf of Thailand, and dramatically reduce the surface area of the South China Sea [45] (Figure 7). This reduction in the surface area of ocean across Southeast Asia would have reduced evaporation from the ocean's surface, and consequently the levels of moisture carried across the mainland by the monsoon rains. Due to the coincidence of periods of reduced sea level with glacial maxima, the reduction in the monsoon moisture content would have been exacerbated by the cool temperature and consequently reduced moisture-carrying capacity of the air [46]. The distribution of forest across Southeast Asia was in turn affected by the reduced precipitation levels, as regions with sufficient moisture to support them shrank [47, 57]. Reconstructions of the dominant habitat types across Southeast Asia during the Last Glacial Maximum (LGM), which are based on palynonlogical and sedimentological data, indicate that tropical forest became restricted to small and isolated pockets, often at intermediate altitudes and at the base of mountains, where precipitation run-off ensured moisture levels remained high enough to support it [58-59]. Substantial areas of forest habitat were replaced by grassland and savannah, although larger areas of forest are thought to have persisted in insular relative to mainland Southeast Asia [47, 57].

The reduction of forest habitat to small and isolated patches would have resulted in the fragmentation of forest-associated *Anopheles* populations, and their subsequent divergence in allopatry through genetic drift and differential local adaptation (see figure 8). The repeated climatic fluctuations during the Pleistocene are thought to have led to repeated cycles of forest fragmentation during the cool and arid glacial periods, and expansion during the warm and humid interglacials. This would have caused associated repeated cycles of *Anopheles* population range reduction and fragmentation, and subsequent divergence of populations in allopatry, followed by range expansion and secondary contact between the now genetically differentiated populations. The 'refuge hypothesis' of Haffer [52] was originally put forward to propose a scenario of increased allopatric speciation driven by such repeated cycles of population divergence during periods of major climatic fluctuation such as that characterising the Pleistocene. This hypothesis has since been frequently discussed in the literature and often contested as an explanation for Pleistocene tropical diversification events, due to evidence that speciation in tropical taxa generally predates the Pleistocene, and that forest habitat was not reduced in tropical regions to the extent originally thought [60-62]. As previously discussed, however, the biogeographical changes within Southeast Asia during the Pleistocene were more severe than in other tropical regions, due to the substantial impact of the sea level changes on the region's climate [45]. The likelihood of allopatric speciation driven by such biogeographical change could therefore be expected to be greater. Indeed, speciation dated to within the Pleistocene has been inferred in both the forest-dependent Leucosphyrus Group [63-64] and the Minimus Subgroup [49], as well as the coastal *An. sundaicus* Complex [65], and has been attributed to the repeated isolation of populations following the reduction of forest habitat and on sea-level fluctuations, respectively, across mainland Southeast Asia during glacial periods [25, 49].

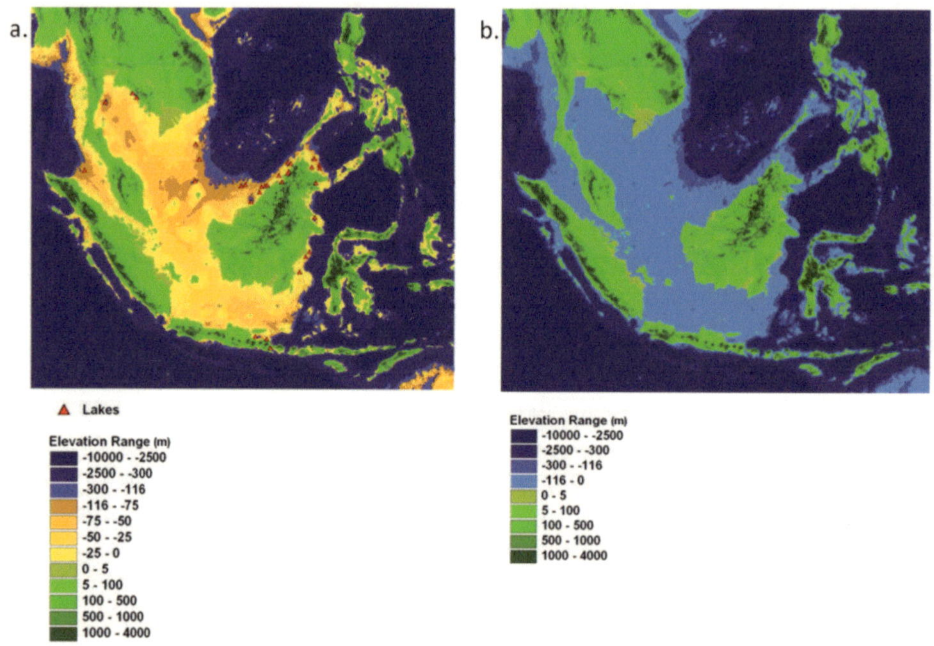

Figure 7. Maps showing the IndoBurma and Sundaic Regions of Southeast Asia, a. 21 kya, the Last Glacial Maximum (LGM), when sea levels were 116 m below the current level, and b. 6.07 kya, when sea levels were the same as at present. Figures taken from [66]).

The evidence for allopatric speciation associated with Pleistocene environmental change is especially strong between the cryptic sister species *An. dirus* and *An. baimaii,* which are classified within the *An. dirus* Complex of the Leucosphyrus Subgroup. As discussed in the previous section, these species are major malaria vectors throughout mainland Southeast Asia, and have a parapatric distribution that overlaps along the Thai-Myanmar border. Although

http://dx.doi.org/10.5772/55709

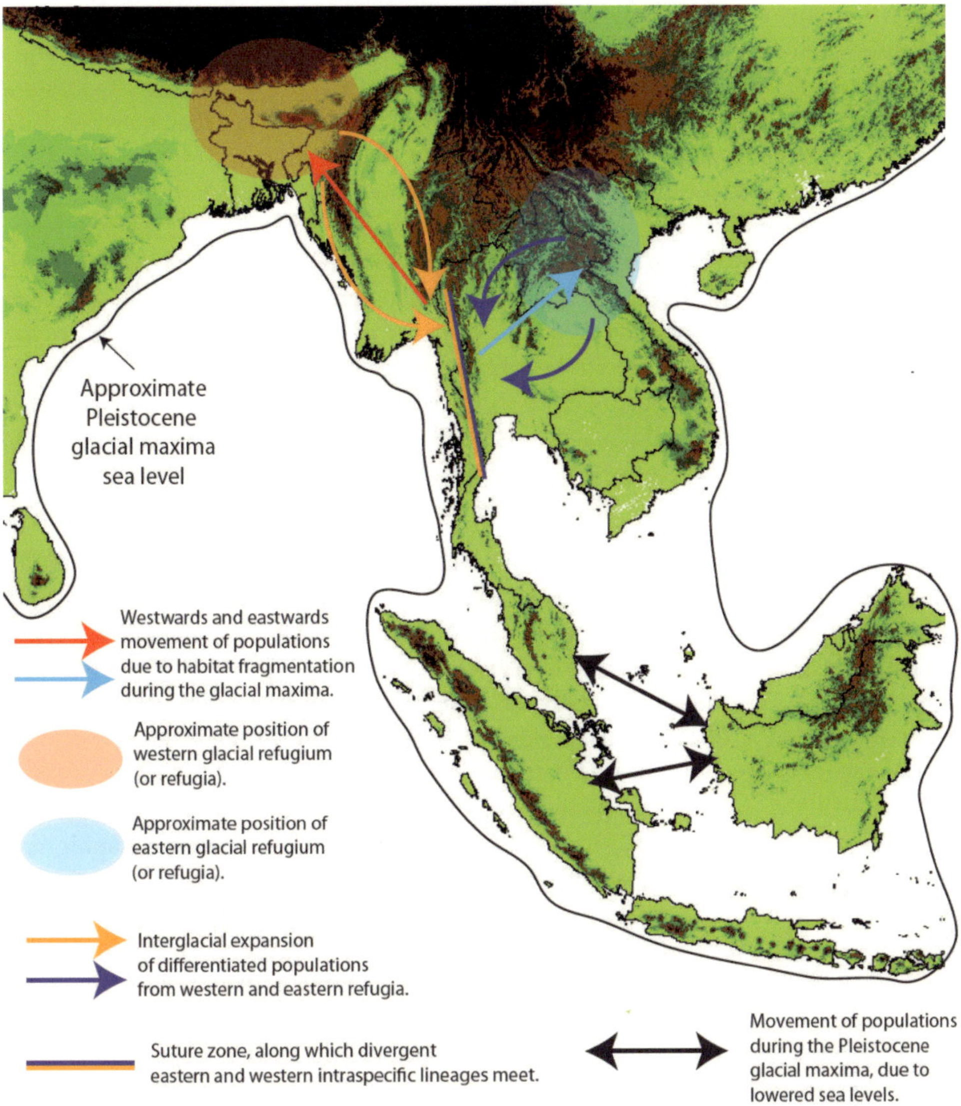

Figure 8. The influence of Pleistocene climatic change on *Anopheles* diversity within Southeast Asia.

characterisation of their divergence is complicated by mitochondrial introgression and consequent widespread haplotype sharing between the species [42, 67], application of an isolation-with-migration model to data from three nuclear genes supported their divergence within the last 1.5 my of the Pleistocene [63]. The east-west divide between the distributions of these species suggests that their common ancestor was restricted to habitat fragments in the west and east of the Southeast Asian mainland, and that the subsequently differentiated lineages expanded from these restricted distributions during the warm and moist interglacials to meet along the Thai-Myanmar border (figure 8) [63].

Although the above examples provide exceptions, the majority of speciation events within the Anopheline fauna of Southeast Asia are estimated to pre-date the Pleistocene [25, 30, 49], and the environmental fluctuations of the Pleistocene appear to have been much more influential in driving divergence and shaping population structure within, rather than between, *Anopheles* species. Patterns of genetic divergence between largely allopatric eastern and western lineages, and signals of Pleistocene population expansion, have been reported within several *Anopheles* species (e.g. *An. minimus* [68]); *An. annularis* and *An. splendidus* [25]). These patterns have generally been attributed to the restriction of populations to isolated forest 'refugia' during the glacial periods, and expansion from these regions during the interglacials (Figure 8). Chen *et al.* [68] investigated this hypothesis further in the forest-associated *An. minimus*, using a modelling approach to compare the hypotheses of a single panmictic population, a stable but spatially structured population, and past fragmentation into eastern and western refugia followed by growth and range expansion. The latter hypothesis was strongly supported, providing further evidence for an evolutionary history shaped by Pleistocene climatic change [68].

Such an influence of Pleistocene climatic change might be expected to be shared across multiple forest-dependent taxa. This hypothesis has been statistically evaluated in several *Anopheles* species, which exhibit varying degrees of forest-dependency, using a comparative phylogeographical approach [29]. Simultaneous divergence of eastern and western lineages within four *Anopheles* species (*An. annularis, An. splendidus, An. minimus* and *An. maculatus*), dated to the mid-Pleistocene and attributed to the similarly-timed restriction of populations to allopatric forest refugia, was strongly supported. Patterns of isolation in allopatry followed by secondary contact across the ranges of these species resulted in the formation of a common suture-zone along the Thai-Myanmar border [29]. Various hypotheses of Pleistocene demographic history were further evaluated using a spatially explicit modelling approach, in which the simulation of demographic and spatial expansions, incorporating environmental information, is followed by the generation of simulated genetic datasets through coalescent theory [69]. Comparison of real to simulated datasets best supported scenarios in which populations were restricted to allopatric eastern and western refugia, before expanding their ranges during the warm and moist interglacials, in all seven species examined (*An. aconitus, An. philippinensis, An. maculatus, An. sawadwongporni, An. annularis, An. baimaii,* and *An. minimus*). Similarly timed population expansions dating to the mid-Pleistocene were inferred in all species, further supporting this scenario [29]. Hence there is substantial evidence supporting a common role of historical environmental change in driving vicariance, and shaping the intraspecific population structure that we see today.

Besides driving divergence between isolated populations, the restriction of populations to refugial regions is also likely to have influenced patterns of genetic diversity across the landscape. The long-term persistence of populations within refugial regions leads to the accumulation of high genetic diversity and population structure. Since only a fraction of the gene pool is generally involved in range expansion, regions that are repeatedly re-colonised following local extinction are expected to harbour substantially lower genetic diversity [70-71]. These predicted patterns can be used to identify potential refugial regions, and in Southeast

http://dx.doi.org/10.5772/55709

Asia have led to the identification of the mountainous regions of northeastern India, northern Myanmar, northern Thailand, southern China and northern Vietnam as potential Pleistocene glacial refugia for *Anopheles* mosquitoes [25, 29, 42, 68, 72]. Indeed, mountain foothills are the most likely regions to support the persistence of forest habitat during cool and arid climatic periods, due to the interception of precipitation by the mountains surrounding them [46]. The prediction and characterisation of these historically driven patterns, of high diversity and spatially structured populations within formal refugial regions and more homogeneous populations in more recently colonised regions, is important if contemporary levels of gene flow are to be reliably estimated and used to predict malaria transmission dynamics.

Although the majority of main *Anopheles* malaria vectors within Southeast Asia show a strong association with forest habitat, this is not true of all species. The influence of historical environmental change on species such as *An. vagus* and *An. sundaicus,* which typically inhabit open habitat and coastal habitat [31, 37, 73], respectively, are likely to have differed substantially from the effects on forest-associated species discussed above. Relative to the majority of forest-associated species, *An. vagus* shows relatively little population structure, and appears to be a single, widespread and highly diverse species that is distributed throughout the biogeographic realms of IndoBurma, Sundaland and the Philippines. The expanse of the open grassland habitat favoured by this species throughout much of the Pleistocene is thought to have facilitated gene flow and dispersal, maintaining population connectivity and homogenising population genetic structure [30]. The Pleistocene evolutionary history of the coastal species *An. sundaicus,* meanwhile, is likely to have been influenced by changes to the landmass configuration, as is discussed below. This illustrates the importance of taking species ecology into account when predicting patterns of historical intraspecific genetic structure across a landscape.

3.1.4. The formation of land-bridges and consequent creation and destruction of dispersal routes during the Pleistocene

Besides substantially influencing climatic conditions across Southeast Asia, the alterations in landmass configuration during the Pleistocene also had a considerable effect on the availability of migration routes across Southeast Asia. The Sunda Shelf is thought to have been dominated by grassland and savannah habitats during periods of exposure, and thus was important in allowing the exchange of open-habitat species such as early hominins and hoofed mammals between the mainland and the Sundaic Islands [56, 74]. Although the open habitat is thought to have acted as a barrier to dispersal of forest-associated taxa between Borneo and Sumatra, the persistence of gallery forests along the major river systems of the Sunda Shelf is thought to have provided narrow dispersal corridors for such taxa [74]. The repeated exposure and submergence of the Sunda Shelf is thought to have promoted allopatric speciation in a number of Sundaic taxa, with periods of dispersal facilitated by the exposure of the Sundaland bridge being followed by the isolation of populations on different landmasses as sea levels rose, e.g. [26, 75]. Although as previously mentioned, there is some species turnover within *Anopheles* between each of the islands and the mainland, several species of the *An. leucosphyrus* Complex are found on more than one land mass. This suggests that the intermittent presence of forest corridors between the mainland and insular regions during the Pleistocene was sufficient to allow some dispersal and gene flow between current land masses [64].

Inferred speciation events within the *An. sundaicus* Complex have also been attributed to patterns of dispersal and isolation driven by the Pleistocene exposure and submergence of sea barriers, with the subsequent isolation and divergence of the nominal species *An. sundaicus, An. sundaicus* E and *An. epiroticus* within Borneo, Sumatra and Java, and mainland Southeast Asia, respectively [65]. These species designations have since been disputed, however, and evidence supporting the existence of only a single, widespread species within the *An. sundaicus* species Complex was presented after more intensive sampling, sequencing of additional markers, and more comprehensive analysis [50]. An alternative scenario of Pleistocene evolutionary history was also presented for this littoral species. Although the current species distribution extends along the coast of mainland Southeast Asia, with the Thai-Malay Peninsula coast connecting that of southern Thailand with Cambodia and Vietnam [31, 37], the exposure of the Sunda Shelf would have eliminated habitat availability through the Gulf of Thailand and isolated populations on the east and west of the glacial insular landmass (Figure 7). This would have limited gene flow between the current coastal regions of Thailand, Cambodia and Vietnam, and facilitated dispersal between the mainland and insular regions. The detection of allopatric eastern and western mitochondrial and nuclear genetic lineages within *An. sundaicus* s.l., the closer relationship of Vietnamese populations with populations from Borneo and Indonesia than with those from Thailand and Myanmar, and the detection of Pleistocene gene flow between Borneo and Vietnam, and between Indonesia and the mainland, strongly support the influence of sea-level changes on the dispersal and population genetics of *An. sundaicus* s.l. [37, 50], although evidence suggests speciation has not resulted in this case.

3.2. Ecological factors

The rich diversity of habitat types and host species available within Southeast Asia is likely to have driven differential local adaptation leading to divergence between ecologically isolated populations and consequent ecological speciation [43]. Characterisation of the bionomics, habitat and feeding preferences of vector species, and of interspecific and intraspecific variation in these traits, is an important step in defining appropriate vector control strategies. Additionally, through the relation of species biology and ecology to phylogenetic relationships we may infer the ecological adaptations that are likely to have driven divergence and speciation, and given rise to the most effective malaria vectors within Southeast Asia. This may also give an indication of the characters that are evolutionarily labile and those that show niche conservatism, which may allow the prediction of how species may respond to anthropogenic change such as urbanisation and an expansion of agriculture. The Leucosphyrus Group provides one example of ecological differentiation between closely related species. This group includes several important vectors of both human and simian malaria, and due to its medical importance, has been well characterised in terms of taxonomy, phylogeny and ecology ([76]; reviewed in [33] and [32]). The mapping of species feeding preferences onto a phylogenetic tree supported two independent host-switching events, each leading to the evolution of anthropophilic taxa from their zoophilic ancestors, which fed on non-human primates in the forest canopy [64]. This switch in host preference is likely to have involved a change in behaviour, from feeding in the forest canopy to feeding on the forest floor, as well as changes in host detection. This host switch was estimated to have occurred during the late Pliocene/ early Pleistocene, which has important implications for human evolution, suggesting that hominins were present within Southeast Asia as early as 2.2 million years ago (mya), and that their arrival shaped the evolution of malaria vectors [64].

As well as the change in host preference, several other ecological adaptations are likely to have driven divergence within the Leucosphyrus Group. The distribution of the group overlaps the biogeographical transition zone that lies between IndoBurma and Sundaland (figure 1;[21]), with the majority of species being limited in distribution to the region either south, or north, of this divide. All basal species are limited in distribution to insular Southeast Asia, suggesting that this region represents the group's ancestral origin [64]. Despite the existence of several species within peninsular Malaysia only two northwards dispersal events into IndoBurma were supported, suggesting that this dispersal required some kind of ecological adaptation. It has been suggested that this may have involved an adaptation specific to the more seasonal climate of Southeast Asia, such as the increased resistance of larvae to desiccation observed in *An. dirus* and *An. baimaii* [32, 64]. Whatever the nature of the ecological adaptation, it is likely to have driven divergence between Indo-Burmese and Sundaic taxa, facilitated the spread of the Leucosphyrus Group throughout mainland IndoBurma, and maintained the distinction between Indo-Burmese and Sundaic species assemblages.

All species within the Leucosphyrus Group show a strong association with tropical forest habitat and are remarkably similar in terms of habitat preference; however *An. scanloni* and *An. nemophilous* do show a unique specialisation to specific habitat types. *An. scanloni* is found in association with limestone karst habitats, whereas *An. nemophilous* is found within mangrove swamp habitats [31], thus specialisation and ecological divergence is likely to have played a role in the history of these species. The divergence of *An. scanloni* from its sister species *An. dirus* occurred despite inferred uni-directional gene flow from *An. scanloni* into *An. dirus* [63]. The uni-directional nature of this gene flow is thought to have resulted from a unique ecological adaptation of *An. scanloni* to limestone karst habitat, which confers a fitness advantage to this species in regions of sympatry with *An. dirus*, reducing hybrid fitness. The accumulation and maintenance of reproductive isolation between *An. scanloni* and *An. dirus* is therefore likely to have been driven by ecological adaptation [63].

The likely involvement of ecological variation in species divergence has also been assessed within the Maculatus Group, within which the phylogenetic mapping of species' altitudinal distribution supported a scenario of ecological speciation through altitudinal replacement[25]. This is a phenomenon in which the distribution of one species replaces that of its sister species along an altitudinal gradient, as populations become adapted to the environmental conditions within their altitudinal zone [77-78]. Species within the Maculatus Group typically lay their eggs within streams or the rock pools associated with them. Various characteristics of these typical larval habitats, such as the water temperature and the speed of water flow, are likely to vary with altitude. Adaptation to these specific larval habitats may therefore have played a role in the ecological divergence of populations at higher altitudes [25].

Whilst ecological differences between species may provide clues as to the factors driving past speciation events, investigation of intraspecific ecological variation within a species range may give an indication of the processes involved in the early stages of ecological divergence and speciation. Variation in traits such as anthropophilic vs. zoophilic, or exophagic vs. endophagic feeding preferences have the potential to greatly influence vector status, and there are several species in which vector status is reported to vary across the range. *Anopheles minimus,* for example, is reported to show strong anthropophily within central Vietnam and Laos, but is more attracted to cattle in northern Vietnam and Cambodia [79]. This behavioural variation is thought to be related to the availability of cattle hosts in a region, and will considerably impact the role of *An. minimus* in malaria transmission. Variation in anthropophily, endophagy, biting cycle and endophily in both *An. dirus* and *An. minimus* across the species' ranges have been related to regional variation in human land-use and habits [79], and may be driving intraspecific adaptive divergence between vector populations. Although it is not currently known whether this variation is the result of phenotypic plasticity or genetic adaptation, any rapid ecological diversification may affect patterns of disease transmission. Thus uncovering the processes involved in the generation of ecological divergence within a species may have considerable relevance for malaria control.

Although several examples of species-specific differences in ecology can be found, there does seem to be considerable ecological similarity between species within each of the major groups, as was discussed earlier in this chapter. All species within the Leucosphyrus Group, for example, show an extremely strong association with forest habitat, laying their eggs within temporary forest pools [31-32]. Although species vary in their feeding preferences, and *An. scanloni* and *An. nemophilous* show previously discussed unique habitat specialism, a number of species within the group show no apparent ecological differentiation from one another. This pattern of apparent 'niche conservatism' is also the case within the Maculatus Group and Minimus Subgroup, with the majority of species within showing preferences for disturbed habitat within forest clearings, and for hilly forest habitats, respectively [31, 80]. It seems surprising that so many apparently ecologically similar species coexist, often with large areas of distributional overlap, and it seems likely that there are subtle ecological differences between species that we are yet to uncover. These ecological differences may involve the bionomics or feeding behaviour of species, and may therefore be of considerable interest in terms of malaria control. The probability of undiscovered ecological differences between species seems especially likely given the fact that methods of cryptic species identification have only recently been developed (e.g. [81-86]), and that early studies of species biology and ecology were marred by incorrect species identifications. Besides the clear direct applications of studies into the biology of *Anopheles* species within Southeast Asia, such studies may shed further light on the role of ecological speciation in the evolutionary history of the region's Anopheline fauna.

4. Gene flow within and between species

The absence or presence of gene flow between populations and species has a considerable impact on the dynamics of malaria transmission, and on the measures used for vector control. In the absence of gene flow, genetic drift and local adaptation result in the genetic differentiation of populations, and potentially in divergence at ecological traits likely to influence malaria transmission [38, 43]. The presence of gene flow, on the other hand, homogenises genetic variation and may lead to the exchange of adaptive and potentially medically relevant alleles between populations. Although the accumulation of reproductive barriers generally restricts gene flow between species, gene flow may still continue across certain genomic regions, creating patterns of differential divergence and introgression across the genome [7, 87-89]. Numerous cases of mitochondrial introgression between *Anopheles* species, including the Southeast Asian malaria vectors *An. dirus* and *An. baimaii* [63, 67], reveal that gene flow between species may be fairly common. The adaptive exchange of the 2La inversion between *An. arabiensis* and *An. gambiae* provides evidence of the phenomenon of gene flow across certain regions of the genome [5, 8, 90-91], and recent advances in next generation sequencing and population genomics have enabled more detailed examination, providing comprehensive examples of interspecific gene flow such as between the purported species *An. gambiae* M and S [92-93], and between the diverged species *An. gambaie* and *An. arabiensis* [7]. An understanding of patterns of contemporary gene flow both within and between species, and of the landscape features that facilitate or restrict this exchange, is of great importance for malaria control efforts. Characterisation of gene flow within and between species will also be relevant to the design of control efforts involving the release of genetically modified mosquitoes, as it will enable prediction of spread of relevant alleles (such as those influencing vectorial capacity) throughout *Anopheles* populations [39].

The dynamic demographic histories of the major malaria vector species, as discussed previously in this chapter, complicate the inference of contemporary gene flow. For example, population bottlenecks and subsequent expansions, which appear to be common in the Anopheline fauna of Southeast Asia (e.g. [29, 42]), can homogenise genetic variation and thus eliminate accumulated genetic diversity between isolated populations, giving false signal of ongoing gene flow [94]. Knowledge of the historical patterns of divergence, range restriction and expansion in *Anopheles* populations, as discussed in previously in the chapter, may provide a baseline from which to study contemporary gene flow. Additionally, whereas to date studies of population structure and gene flow within and between species has been primarily restricted to neutral markers, the increasing availability of next generation sequencing (NGS) data will provide the opportunity to study the exchange of adaptive alleles across landscapes (e.g. [8], see below).

5. Future directions

Despite the wealth of knowledge of *Anopheles* diversity within Southeast Asia, there are many directions that remain to be explored. Firstly, although much is known of the historical dynamics of gene flow and divergence and the climatic and landscape features that have been important in defining those patterns, little is known of the impact of contemporary landscape features on dispersal and gene flow. Such questions may be addressed using a landscape genetics approach, which involves the combination of fine-scale, dense spatial sampling with spatial and environmental information [95-96]. This approach has been successful, for example, in revealing the impact of urbanisation and forest corridors on connectivity in amphibian populations [97], and the impact of major roads on the genetic structure of caribou populations [98]. Such an approach may reveal the impact of phenomena such as deforestation and increased urbanisation on the demography of *Anopheles* populations, information which would be beneficial for predicting the impact of future landscape changes on the origin and spread of adaptive alleles relevant to vector control.

Secondly, the investigation of patterns of population structure at a genomic level remains to be performed in the *Anopheles* taxa of Southeast Asia, and will have many potential applications. As previously discussed in this chapter, intraspecific phenotypic variation such as that reported within *An. dirus* and *An. minimus* [79] may be due to phenotypic plasticity, or may have an underlying genetic adaptive basis. Patterns of divergence at small numbers of neutral loci, while useful in identifying general population genetic patterns, are insufficient to address such issues comprehensively. Genome-wide approaches can, however, facilitate the identification of loci involved in adaptive response to environmental variation, and may reveal associations between adaptive loci and phenotypic traits (e.g.[99-101]). The availability of the *Anopheles gambiae* reference genome [102] provides additional scope for genomic studies using NGS data, enabling annotation of any identified adaptive loci, and the future availability of 13 additional *Anopheles* genomes, including those of several Southeast Asian species, will aid genomic studies even further [103].

Besides gene flow between populations within a species, the possibility of contemporary interspecific gene flow should also be considered. The identification and characterisation of such contemporary gene flow between species will be vitally important in determining whether medically important traits may spread between them. Again, this issue will benefit from a genome-wide approach, as patterns of introgression and divergence will vary across the genome due to the differential influence of selection [7, 87-89]. Genomic studies have been invaluable in characterising divergence and introgression across the genome, and identifying the targets of selection within the genomes of *An. gambiae* M and S forms [8]. For example, in contrast to the *kdr* mutation, which is responsible for pyrethroid resistance to insecticide and is thought to have spread from the S to the M form of *An. gambiae* through introgression [104], different resistance substitutions within the resistance to dieldrin (*rdl*) gene are thought to have evolved independently within *An. gambiae* M and S forms [8]. Genome-wide approaches will enable similar issues to be addressed within recently diverged species pairs such as *An. baimaii* and *An. dirus.*

The possibility of ongoing gene flow or historic introgression between species is also important for the reliable delineation of species boundaries, particularly within complexes of closely related and morphologically identical *Anopheles* species. The importance of selecting appropriate markers for species delineation, and of considering levels of interspecific gene flow has

http://dx.doi.org/10.5772/55709

been recently reviewed [105], and highlights the potential benefits of a genome-wide approach. Questions relating to Anopheline taxonomy and ecology remain to be answered within several of the medically important *Anopheles* groups (including the *An. sundaicus, An. subpictus, An. culicifacies* and *An. fluviatilis* Complexes, for example [33]), and the delineation of species boundaries, resolution of species relationships, development of species identification methods and characterisation of species ecology are still vitally important for the design of more traditional methods of vector control. The usefulness of bed nets in reducing malaria, the identification and control of potential larval habitats within a region, and informing of residents of how to reduce exposure, all rely on detailed information of the species present within a region and of their ecology. Zarowiecki [50] has illustrated the importance of taking a systematic approach to delineating and identifying species and resolving taxomonic relationships, and such an approach should be followed for potentially cryptic species complexes in which taxonomy is still uncertain. Thus taken together, the development of NGS technologies and population genomic analytical methods provides great scope for studies into Anopheles diversity in Southeast Asia, which are likely to considerably benefit both the understanding of malaria transmission dynamics and the effectiveness of vector control.

Author details

Katy Morgan[1], Pradya Somboon[2] and Catherine Walton[3*]

*Address all correspondence to: Catherine.Walton@manchester.ac.uk

1 Max Planck Institute for Developmental Biology, Tuebingen, Germany

2 Department of Parasitology, Faculty of Medicine, Chiang Mai University, Chiang Mai, Thailand

3 Faculty of Life Sciences, University of Manchester, Manchester, UK

References

[1] Fantini B. Anophelism without malaria: an ecological and epidemiological puzzle. Parassitologica 1994; 36: 83-106.

[2] Hackett L.W. and Missiroli A. The natural disappearance of malaria in certain parts of Europe. American Journal of Epidemiology 1931; 13: 57-78.

[3] Collins F.H. and Paskewitz S.M. A review of the use of ribosomal DNA (rDNA) to differentiate among cryptic *Anopheles* species. Insect Molecular Biology 1996; 5: 1-9.

[4] Coluzzi M., Sabatini A., Petrarca V., and Di Deco M.A. Chromosomal differentiation and adaptation to human environments in the *Anopheles gambiae* Complex. Transactions of the Royal Society of Tropical Medicine and Hygiene 1979; 73: 483-497.

[5] Besansky N.J., Krzywinski J., Lehmann T., *et al.* Semipermeable species boundaries between *Anopheles gambiae* and *Anopheles arabiensis*: Evidence from multilocus DNA sequence variation. Proceedings of the National Academy of Sciences 2003; 100: 10818-10823.

[6] Lehmann T. and Diabate A. The molecular forms of *Anopheles gambiae*: A phenotypic perspective. Infection, Genetics and Evolution 2008; 8: 737-746.

[7] Neafsey D.E., Lawniczak M.K.N., Park D.J., *et al.* SNP genotyping defines complex gene-flow boundaries among African malaria vector mosquitoes. Science 2010; 330: 514-517.

[8] Lawniczak M.K.N., Emrich S.J., Holloway A.K., *et al.* Widespread divergence between incipient *Anopheles gambiae* species revealed by whole genome sequences. Science 2010; 330: 512-514.

[9] Torre A.d., Fanello C., Akogbeto M., *et al.* Molecular evidence of incipient speciation within *Anopheles gambiae* s.s. in West Africa. Insect Molecular Biology 2001; 10: 9-18.

[10] Favia G., della Torre A., Bagayoko M., *et al.* Molecular identification of sympatric chromosomal forms of *Anopheles gambiae* and further evidence of their reproductive isolation. Insect Molecular Biology 1997; 6: 377-383.

[11] Appawu M.A., Baffoe-Wilmot A., Afari E.A., Nkrumah F.K., and Petrarca V. Species composition and inversion polymorphism of the *Anopheles gambiae* Complex in some sites of Ghana, West Africa. Acta Tropica 1994; 56: 15-23.

[12] Chareonviriyaphap T., Bangs M.J., and Ratanatham S. Status of malaria in Thailand. Southeast Asian Journal of Tropical Medical Public Health 2000; 31: 225-237.

[13] Trung H.D., Van Bortel W., Sochantha T., *et al.* Malaria transmission and major malaria vectors in different geographical areas of Southeast Asia. Tropical Medicine & International Health 2004; 9: 230-237.

[14] Manguin S. and Boëte C. Global impact of mosquito biodiversity, human vector-borne diseases and environmental change. In: J.L. Pujol (eds), The Importance of Biological Interactions in the Study of Biodiversity. InTech: Winchester, UK.2011 27-50.

[15] Sinka M., Bangs M., Manguin S., *et al.* The dominant *Anopheles* vectors of human malaria in the Asia-Pacific region: occurrence data, distribution maps and bionomic precis. Parasites & Vectors 2011; 4: 89.

[16] Schapira A. and Boutsika K. Chapter 3 - Malaria Ecotypes and Stratification. In: D. Rollinson and S.I. Hay (eds), Advances in Parasitology. Academic Press.2012 97-167.

[17] Macdonald G. Local features of malaria. (eds), The Epidemiology and Control of Malaria. Oxford University Press: London.1957 63-99.

[18] Myers N., Mittermeier R.A., Mittermeier C.G., da Fonseca G.A.B., and Kent J. Biodiversity hotspots for conservation priorities. Nature 2000; 403: 853-858.

[19] Hughes A.C., Satasook C., Bates P.J.J., Bumrungsri S., and Jones G. Explaining the causes of the zoogeographic transition around the Isthmus of Kra: using bats as a case study. Journal of Biogeography 2011; 38: 2362-2372.

[20] Round P.D., Hughes J.B., and Woodruff D.S. Latitudinal range limits of resident forest birds in Thailand and the Indochinese–Sundaic zoogeographic transition. Natural History Bulletin of the Siam Society 2003; 51: 69-96.

[21] Woodruff D.S. and Turner L.M. The Indochinese - Sundaic zoogeographic transition: a description and analysis of terrestrial mammal species distributions. Journal of Biogeography 2009; 30: 569-580.

[22] Woodruff D. Biogeography and conservation in Southeast Asia: how 2.7 million years of repeated environmental fluctuations affect today's patterns and the future of the remaining refugial-phase biodiversity. Biodiversity and Conservation 2010; 19: 919-941.

[23] Hughes J.B., Round P.D., and Woodruff D.S. The Indochinese-Sundaic faunal transition at the Isthmus of Kra: an analysis of resident forest bird species distributions. Journal of Biogeography 2003; 30: 569-580.

[24] Woodruff D.S. Neogene marine transgressions, palaeogeography and biogeographic transitions on the Thai-Malay Peninsula. Journal of Biogeography 2003; 30: 551-567.

[25] Morgan K., O'Loughlin S.M., Mun-Yik F., *et al.* Molecular phylogenetics and biogeography of the Neocellia Series of *Anopheles* mosquitoes in the Oriental Region. Molecular Phylogenetics and Evolution 2009; 52: 588-601.

[26] Reddy S. Systematics and biogeography of the shrike-babblers (*Pteruthius*): Species limits, molecular phylogenetics, and diversification patterns across southern Asia. Molecular Phylogenetics and Evolution 2008; 47: 54-72.

[27] Abegg C. and Thierry B. Macaque evolution and dispersal in insular south-east Asia. Biological Journal of the Linnean Society 2002; 75: 555-576.

[28] Singh S., Prakash A., Yadav R.N.S., *et al. Anopheles* (Cellia) *maculatus* group: Its spatial distribution and molecular characterization of member species in north-east India. Acta Tropica 2012; 124: 62-70.

[29] Morgan K., O'Loughlin S.M., Chen B. , *et al.* Comparative phylogeography reveals a shared impact of Pleistocene environmental change in shaping genetic diversity within nine *Anopheles* mosquito species across the Indo-Burma biodiversity hotspot. Molecular Ecology 2011; 20: 4533-4549.

[30] Zarowiecki M., Walton C., Torres E., *et al.* Pleistocene genetic connectivity in a widespread, open-habitat-adapted mosquito in the Indo-Oriental region. Journal of Biogeography 2011; 38: 1422-1432.

[31] Reid J.A. Anopheline mosquitoes of Malaya and Borneo. Malaysia, Government of Malaysia 1968

[32] Obsomer V., Defourny P., and Coosemans M. The *Anopheles dirus* Complex: spatial distribution and environmental drivers. Malaria Journal 2007; 6: (26).

[33] Manguin S., Garros C., Dusfour I., Harbach R.E., and Coosemans M. Bionomics, taxonomy, and distribution of the major malaria vector taxa of *Anopheles* subgenus *Cellia* in Southeast Asia: An updated review. Infection, Genetics and Evolution 2008; 8: 489-503.

[34] Foley D.H., Rueda L.M., Peterson A.T., and Wilkerson R.C. Potential distribution of two species in the medically important *Anopheles minimus* Complex (Diptera: Culicidae). Journal of Medical Entomology 2008; 45: 852-860.

[35] Brandling-Bennett A.D., Doberstyn E.B., and Pinichpongse S. Current epidemiology of malaria in Southeast Asia. Southeast Asian J Trop Med Public Health 1981; 12: 289-297.

[36] Das M.K., Adak T., and Sharma V.P. Genetic analysis of a larval colour mutant, yellow larva, in *Anopheles sundaicus*. Journal of the American Mosquito Control Association 1997; 13: 203-204.

[37] Dusfour I., Linton Y.-M., Cohuet A., *et al.* Molecular Evidence of Speciation Between Island and Continental Populations of *Anopheles* (*Cellia*) *sundaicus* (Diptera: Culicidae), a principal malaria vector taxon in Southeast Asia. Journal of Medical Entomology 2004; 41: 287-295.

[38] Hartl D.L. and Clark A.G. Principals of population genetics. Sunderland, U.S.A., Sinauer Associates, Inc. 2007.

[39] Riehle M.A., Srinivasan P., Moreira C.K., and Jacobs-Lorena M. Towards genetic manipulation of wild mosquito populations to combat malaria: advances and challenges. Journal of Experimental Biology 2003; 206: 3809-3816.

[40] Hay B.A., Chen C.-H., Ward C.M., *et al.* Engineering the genomes of wild insect populations: Challenges, and opportunities provided by synthetic Medea selfish genetic elements. Journal of Insect Physiology 2010; 56: 1402-1413.

[41] Zellmer A.J. and Knowles L.L. Disentangling the effects of historic vs. contemporary landscape structure on population genetic divergence. Molecular Ecology 2009; 18: 3593-3602.

[42] O'Loughlin S.M., Okabayashi T., Honda M., *et al.* Complex population history of two *Anopheles dirus* mosquito species in Southeast Asia suggests the influence of Pleisto-

cene climate change rather than human-mediated effects. Journal of Evolutionary Biology 2008; 21: 1555-1569.

[43] Coyne J.A. and Orr H.A. Speciation.Sunderland, MA, Sinauer Associates 2004.

[44] Hall R., The plate tectonics of the Cenozoic SE Asia and the distribution of land and sea. 1998, Leiden: Backhuys Publishers. p. 133 - 163.

[45] Voris H.K. Maps of Pleistocene sea levels in Southeast Asia: shorelines, river systems and time durations. Journal of Biogeography 2000; 27: 1153-1167.

[46] Heaney L.R. A synopsis of climatic and vegetational change in Southeast Asia. Climatic Change 1991; 19: 53-61.

[47] White J.C., Penny D., Kealhofer L., and Maloney B. Vegetation changes from the late Pleistocene through the Holocene from three areas of archaeological significance in Thailand. Quaternary International : The record of Human /Climate interaction in Lake Sediments 2004; 113: 111-132.

[48] Janis C.M. Tertiary mammal evolution in the context of changing climates, vegetation, and tectonic events. Annual Review of Ecology and Systematics 1993; 24: 467-500.

[49] Garros C., Harbach R.E., and Manguin S. Systematics and biogeographical implications of the phylogenetic relationships between members of the Funestus and Minimus Groups of *Anopheles* (Diptera: Culicidae). Journal of Medical Entomology 2005; 42: 7-18.

[50] Zarowiecki M. Speciation and species delineation in the Pyretophorus Series of *Anopheles* mosquitoes. University of Manchester PhD thesis 2009.

[51] Guo Z., Peng S., Hao Q., *et al.* Late Miocene–Pliocene development of Asian aridification as recorded in the Red-Earth Formation in northern China. Global and Planetary Change 2004; 41: 135-145.

[52] Haffer J. Speciation in Amazonian forest birds. Science 1969; 165: 131-137.

[53] Chandler M., Rind D., and Thompson R. Joint investigations of the middle Pliocene climate II: GISS GCM Northern Hemisphere results. Global and Planetary Change 1994; 9: 197-219.

[54] Cronin T.M., Kitamura A., Tkeya N., *et al.* Late Pliocene climate change 3.4-2.3 Ma: paleoceanographic record from the Yabuta Formation, Sea of Japan. Palaeogeography, Palaeoclimatology, Palaeoecology 1994; 108: 437-455.

[55] Ravelo A.C., Andreasen D.H., Lyle M., Lyle A.O., and Wara M.W. Regional climate shifts caused by gradual global cooling in the Pliocene epoch. Nature 2004; 429: 263-267.

[56] Tougard C. Biogeography and migration routes of large mammal faunas in South–East Asia during the Late Middle Pleistocene: focus on the fossil and extant faunas

from Thailand. Palaeogeography, Palaeoclimatology, Palaeoecology 2001; 168: 337-358.

[57] Hope G., Kershaw A.P., van der Kaars S., *et al.* History of vegetation and habitat change in the Austral-Asian region. Quaternary International 2004; 118-119: 103-126.

[58] Brandon-Jones D. The Asian Colobinae (Mammalia: Cercopithecidae) as indicators of Quaternary climatic change. Biological Journal of the Linnean Society 1996; 59: 327-350.

[59] Gathorne-Hardy F.J., Syaukani, Davies R.G., Eggleton P., and Jones D.T. Quaternary rainforest refugia in south-east Asia: Using termites (Isoptera) as indicators. Biological Journal of the Linnean Society 2002; 75: 453-466.

[60] Colinvaux P.A., De Oliveira P.E., and Bush M.B. Amazonian and neotropical plant communities on glacial time-scales: The failure of the aridity and refuge hypotheses. Quaternary Science Reviews 2000; 19: 141-169.

[61] Colinvaux P.A., Irion G., Raesaenen M.E., and Bush M.B. Geological and paleoecological data falsify the Haffer & Prance refuge hypothesis of Amazonian speciation. Amazoniana 2001; 16: 609-646.

[62] Mayle F.E., Beerling D.J., Gosling W.D., and Bush M.B. Responses of Amazonian ecosystems to climatic and atmospheric carbon dioxide changes since the last glacial maximum. Philosophical Transactions of the Royal Society B 2004; 359: 499–514.

[63] Morgan K., Linton Y.-M., Somboon P., *et al.* Inter-specific gene flow dynamics during the Pleistocene-dated speciation of forest-dependent mosquitoes in Southeast Asia. Molecular Ecology 2010; 19: 2269 - 2285.

[64] Morgan K. Determining the processes generating biodiversity in Southeast Asia using *Anopheles* mosquitoes. University of Manchester PhD thesis 2009.

[65] Dusfour I., Michaux J.R., Harbach R.E., and Manguin S. Speciation and phylogeography of the Southeast Asian *Anopheles sundaicus* complex. Infection, Genetics and Evolution 2007; 7: 484-493.

[66] Sathiamurthy E. and Voris H.K. Maps of holocene sea level transgression and submerged lakes on the Sunda Shelf. The Natural History Journal of Chulalongkorn University 2006; Supplement 2: 1-43.

[67] Walton C., Handley J.M., Collins F.H., *et al.* Population Structure and Population History of *Anopheles dirus* Mosquitoes in Southeast Asia. Molecular Biology and Evolution 2000; 17: 962-974.

[68] Chen B., Pedro P.M., Harbach R.E., *et al.* Mitochondrial DNA variation in the malaria vector *Anopheles minimus* across China, Thailand and Vietnam: evolutionary hypothesis, population structure and population history. Heredity 2011; 106: 241–252.

[69] Currat M., Ray N., and Excoffier L. SPLATCHE: a program to simulate genetic diversity taking into account environmental heterogeneity. Molecular Ecology Notes 2004; 4: 139-142.

[70] Hewitt G.M. Genetic consequences of climatic oscillations in the Quaternary. Philosofical Transactions of the Royal Society of London, Series B, biological Sciences 2004; 359: 183-195.

[71] Hewitt G.M. Some genetic consequences of ice ages, and their role in divergence and speciation. Biological Journal of the Linnean Society 1996; 58: 247-276.

[72] Chen B., Harbach R.E., and Butlin R.K. Genetic variation and population structure of the mosquito *Anopheles jeyporiensis* in southern China. Molecular Ecology 2004; 13: 3051-3056.

[73] Amerasinghe P.H., Amerasinghe F.P., Konradsen F., Fonseka K.T., and Wirtz R.A. Malaria vectors in a traditional dry zone village in Sri Lanka. The American Journal of Tropical Medicine and Hygiene 1999; 60: 421-9.

[74] Bird M.I., Taylor D., and Hunt C. Palaeoenvironments of insular Southeast Asia during the Last Glacial Period: a savanna corridor in Sundaland? Quaternary Science Reviews 2005; 24: 2228-2242

[75] Ziegler T., Abegg C., Meijaard E., *et al.* Molecular phylogeny and evolutionary history of Southeast Asian macaques forming the *M. silenus* group Molecular Phylogenetics and Evolution 2007; 42: 807-816.

[76] Sallum M.A.M., Foster P.G., Li C., Sithiprasasna R., and Wilkerson R.C. Phylogeny of the Leucosphyrus Group of *Anopheles* (*Cellia*) (Diptera: Culicidae) based on mitochondrial gene sequences. Annals of the Entomological Society of America 2007; 100: 27-35.

[77] Moritz C., Patton J.L., Schneider C.J., and Smith T.B. Diversification of rainforest faunas: an integrated molecular approach. Annual Review of Ecology and Systematics 2000; 31: 533–563.

[78] Norman J.A., Rheindt F.E., Rowe D.L., and Christidis L. Speciation dynamics in the Australo-Papuan *Meliphaga* honeyeaters Molecular Phylogenetics and Evolution 2007; 42: 80-91.

[79] Trung H.D., Bortel W.V., Sochantha T., *et al.* Behavioural heterogeneity of *Anopheles* species in ecologically different localities in Southeast Asia: a challenge for vector control. Tropical Medicine & International Health 2005; 10: 251-262.

[80] Scanlon J.E., Reid J.A., and Cheong W.H. Ecology of *Anopheles* vectors of malaria in the Oriental region. Ent. med., 1968; 6: 237 - 246.

[81] Walton C., Sharpe R.G., Pritchard S.J., Thelwell N.J., and Butlin R.K. Molecular identification of mosquito species. Biological Journal of the Linnean Society 1999; 68: 241-256.

[82] Walton C., Somboon P., O'Loughlin S.M., *et al.* Genetic diversity and molecular identification of mosquito species in the *Anopheles maculatus* group using the ITS2 region of rDNA. Infection, Genetics and Evolution 2007; 7: 93-102.

[83] Walton C., Somboon P., Harbach R.E., *et al.*, Molecular identification of mosquito species in the *Anopheles annularis* group in southern Asia. Medical and Veterinary Entomology 2007; 21: 30-35.

[84] Phuc H.K., Ball A.J., Son L., *et al.* Multiplex PCR assay for malaria vector *Anopheles minimus* and four related species in the Myzomyia Series from Southeast Asia. Medical and Veterinary Entomology 2003; 17: 423-428.

[85] Sharpe R.G., Hims M.M., Harbach R.E., and Butlin R.K. PCR-based methods for identification of species of the *Anopheles minimus* group: allele-specific amplification and single-strand conformation polymorphism. Medical and Veterinary Entomology 1999; 13: 265-273.

[86] Walton C., Handley J.M., Kuvangkadilok C., *et al.* Identification of five species of the *Anopheles dirus* complex from Thailand, using allele-specific polymerase chain reaction. Medical and Veterinary Entomology 1999; 13: 24-32.

[87] Wu C.-I. and Ting C.-T. Genes and speciation. Nature Reviews Genetics 2000; 5: 114-122.

[88] Emelianov I., Marec F., and Mallet J. Genomic evidence for divergence with gene flow in host races of the larch budmoth. Proceedings of the Royal Society of London. Series B: Biological Sciences 2004; 271: 97-105.

[89] Via S. Divergence hitchhiking and the spread of genomic isolation during ecological speciation-with-gene-flow. Philosophical Transactions of the Royal Society of London, Series B: Biological Sciences 2012; 367: 451-460.

[90] Gray E.M., Rocca K.A., Costantini C., and Besansky N.J. Inversion 2La is associated with enhanced desiccation resistance in *Anopheles gambiae*. Malaria journal 2009; 8: 215.

[91] Torre A.D., Merzagora L., Powell J.R., and Coluzzi M. Selective introgression of paracentric inversions between two sibling species of the *Anopheles gambiae* Complex. Genetics 1997; 146: 239–244.

[92] Reidenbach K.R., Neafsey D.E., Costantini C., *et al.* Patterns of genomic differentiation between ecologically differentiated M and S forms of *Anopheles gambiae* in West and Central Africa. Genome Biology and Evolution 2012; 4: 1202-1212.

[93] Weetman D., Wilding C.S., Steen K., Pinto J., and Donnelly M.J. Gene flow–dependent genomic divergence between *Anopheles gambiae* M and S forms. Molecular Biology and Evolution 2012; 29: 279-291.

[94] Marko P.B. and Hart M.W. The complex analytical landscape of gene flow inference. Trends in Ecology & Evolution 2011; 26: 448-456.

[95] Balkenhol N., Gugerli F., Cushman S., *et al.* Identifying future research needs in landscape genetics: where to from here? Landscape Ecology 2009; 24: 455-463.

[96] Storfer A., Murphy M.A., Spear S.F., Holderegger R., and Waits L.P. Landscape genetics: where are we now? Molecular Ecology 2010; 19: 3496-3514.

[97] Emaresi G., Pellet J., Dubey S., Hirzel A., and Fumagalli L. Landscape genetics of the Alpine newt (*Mesotriton alpestris*) inferred from a strip-based approach. Conservation Genetics 2011; 12: 41-50.

[98] Galpern P., Manseau M., and Wilson P. Grains of connectivity: analysis at multiple spatial scales in landscape genetics. Molecular Ecology 2012; 21: 3996-4009.

[99] Hancock A.M., Brachi B., Faure N., *et al.* Adaptation to climate across the *Arabidopsis thaliana* genome. Science 2011; 334: 83-86.

[100] Hohenlohe P.A., Bassham S., Etter P.D., *et al.* Population genomics of parallel adaptation in threespine stickleback using sequenced RAD tags. PLoS Genet 2010; 6: e1000862.

[101] Herrera C.M. and Bazaga P. Population-genomic approach reveals adaptive floral divergence in discrete populations of a hawk moth-pollinated violet. Molecular Ecology 2008; 17: 5378-5390.

[102] Holt R.A., Subramanian G.M., Halpern A., *et al.* The genome sequence of the malaria mosquito *Anopheles gambiae*. Science 2002; 298: 129-149.

[103] Broad Institute. Genome analysis of vectorial capacity in major *Anopheles* vectors of malaria parasites. http://www.broadinstitute.org/annotation/genome/anopheles.1/Info.html (accessed 4 January 2013).

[104] Weill M., Chandre F., Brengues C., *et al.* The kdr mutation occurs in the Mopti form of *Anopheles gambiae* s.s. through introgression. Insect Molecular Biology 2000; 9: 451-455.

[105] Petit R.J. and Excoffier L. Gene flow and species delimitation. Trends in Ecology and Evolution 2009; 24: 386-393.

Chapter 12

The Systematics and Bionomics of Malaria Vectors in the Southwest Pacific

Nigel W. Beebe, Tanya L. Russell, Thomas R. Burkot, Neil F. Lobo and Robert D. Cooper

Additional information is available at the end of the chapter

http://dx.doi.org/10.5772/55999

1. Introduction

1.1. Malaria in the Southwest Pacific

The malaria transmission zone in the southwest Pacific ranges from Indonesia (Papua Province) through Papua New Guinea (PNG) and the Solomon Islands to Vanuatu. The island of Tanna in Vanuatu marks the southern and eastern limit of the region's malaria endemic area. The malaria-free island of Aneityum is the most easterly location where anophelines are found (Fig 1). While northern Australia previously experienced regular outbreaks of malaria, the disease was eliminated in 1962 [1] – although it still experiences sporadic outbreaks following reintroductions of the parasites [2]. Malaria remains the most important vector-borne disease in the region with Indonesian Papua, PNG and the Solomon Islands enduring some of the highest attack rates in the world outside Africa [3].

Malaria is endemic below 1000m, with the degree of endemicity ranging from hypoendemic to holoendemic [4, 5]. Above 1000m malaria tends to be unstable with epidemics of varying degrees of severity [6-8]. Serious control efforts were initiated in the 1950s-1960s as part of the WHO Global Eradication Program, with pilot projects implemented in Papua Province (Indonesia) and PNG (late 1950s) and in the Solomon Islands and Vanuatu (late 1960s). The principal strategy was indoor residual spraying (IRS) with DDT supplemented with mass drug administration of chloroquine [9].

In 1969, the malaria eradication was abandoned in Papua Province and PNG as it was realized that this goal was not attainable – instead, various control programs were introduced. In PNG, IRS continued until 1984, after which little more was done in the way of malaria vector control until the early 1990s, when insecticide treated bed nets (ITNs) were trialed [10] prior to widespread distribution. In the Solomon Islands and Vanuatu, full-scale malaria eradication programs (MEP) commenced in the early 1970s but were also abandoned after three years and replaced with control programs [11]. In both countries pyrethroids replaced DDT in IRS in the early 1990s and ITNs became the main method of control [12]. During the 1990s, malaria was successfully eliminated on Aneityum Island, the most southern island of Vanuatu [13] with mass drug administration as the primary intervention. Recently, renewed efforts at malaria elimination and intensified control were initiated in Tafea Province in Vanuatu and Temotu and Santa Isabel Provinces in the Solomon Islands [14].

1.2. Geography and climate

This work covers the malarious area of the southwest Pacific as it lies within the Australian faunal region (Fig. 1). This region is made up of numerous islands many of which are mountainous (>4000m) with ranges extending to the coasts and drained by river systems over a narrow coastal plain. In New Guinea, the ranges are fragmented by river valleys, creating extensive lowlands comprising flood plains and swamps. Throughout the region, the climate is dominated by two wind systems and by the influence of mountain barriers and the surrounding oceans. From December to April (the wet season), moist northwesterly winds produce the heaviest and most frequent rains. From May to October (the dry season), southeasterly winds prevail and conditions are drier. However during this period substantial rainfall occurs wherever prominent mountain barriers exist. Thus the climate for most of the region is continuous hot/wet with rainfall >2000mm p.a. with rainless periods rarely exceeding four days. Exceptions occur in southern Western Province and around Port Moresby in PNG where the climate is more monsoonal, the dry season is more pronounced, and the rainfall is less (1600-2000mm p.a.) (Fig. 1) [15].

Temperature is not a major climatic factor as there is little seasonality and minimal variation throughout each year in a given elevation. However, elevation exerts the main influence on temperature: in coastal and lowland areas (<500m), the mean temperature is 26°C (max 31°C; min 22°C), while in the highland regions (>500m), the mean temperature is 20°C (max 23°C; min 14°C) [15].

2. Systematics of the malaria vector Groups

The anopheline fauna of the Australian Region is delimited in the west by the Weber Line, which runs through the Moluccas, though there is some incursion east and west of this line by anophelines from the Oriental and Australian Regions (Fig 1 and Table 1). The Australian fauna is highly endemic and most likely of Oriental origin. The malaria vectors in the Australian Region are composed of groups and complexes of closely related, morphologically similar, cryptic or sibling anopheline species. Accurate identification of vector species is essential for interpreting the efficacy of interventions in an area. Since the discovery of cryptic sibling species, the use of morphological characters previously used to identify species has been rendered uncertain. Techniques such as cross-mating, chromosome studies and allozyme

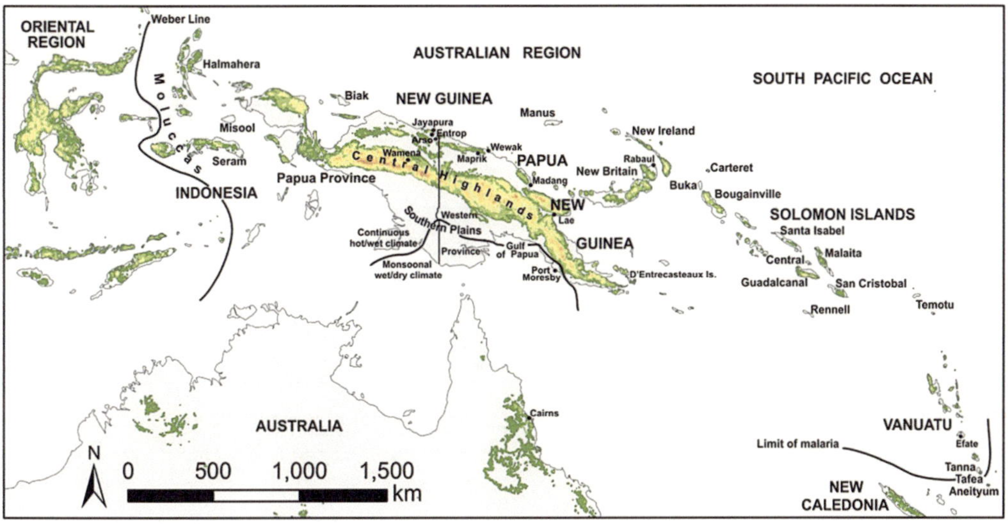

Figure 1. Map of the southwest Pacific region showing regions and sites described in the text. The malaria vectors described in this chapter exist from the Moluccas in the west (approximately at the Weber line) to Vanuatu in the east and south into northern Australia. Note: The green to orange shading represents elevation from 600m to 4,800m.

analysis were initially deployed to resolve the problems of identifying these sibling species, though none of these can match the speed and simplicity of morphological markers which could be applied in the field. Advances in DNA-based technology with high throughput capability during the past two decades allow large and detailed analyses of vector populations. Although more costly and requiring sophisticated laboratory support, methods such as DNA probe hybridization and PCR are both quick, user-friendly and offer advantages in the study of intraspecific differences between species and for phylogenetic studies. Studies of the *Anopheles punctulatus* group of the southwest Pacific provides a prime example of both the application of this technology and how it has progressed.

Because of advances in DNA-based technologies, mosquito taxonomists and systematists can now identify, describe, and classify *Anopheles* biodiversity, in addition to studying and understanding their evolution, distribution, and species' relationships. The practical relevance of such information extends beyond the labeling and ordering of taxa. Studies of malaria transmission reinforce time and again the importance of incorporating an intimate knowledge of *Anopheles* species biology, behavior, and ecology into the design, implementation and evaluation of any successful vector control strategy. Control strategies require information on vector species distribution, their density, and seasonal prevalence as well as data on mating, oviposition, feeding and resting habits, longevity and fecundity, and susceptibility to both parasites and insecticides. Yet measurements of these entomological parameters are only relevant if accurate vector species' identifications are possible. Each species has evolved characteristics that will influence its ability to transmit malaria and its vulnerability to any control strategies depends on these behavioural characteristics. Additionally, systematics and phylogeny can provide useful information on host/parasite evolution, ecological adaptation,

Species, Groups, and Complexes	Moluccas	New Guinea[1]					Solomon Islands	Vanuatu	Vector status
		Monsoo-nal	Hot / wet	High-lands	SCH	NCH			
Subgenus *Anopheles*									
An. bancroftii complex four species A-D		xxx[2]	xxx	xx	xxx	xxx			secondary
An. papuensis				x					non-vector
Subgenus *Cellia*									
An. annulipes complex:									
An. annulipes L		xxx			x				non-vector
An. annulipes M				xxx					non-vector
An. hilli		xxx							possible
An. karwari (Oriental)	xx					xxx			secondary
An. longirostris complex: nine species 1-9			xxx		xxx	xxx			secondary
An. lungae complex:									
An. lungae							xxxx		possible
An. solomonis							xxxx		possible
An. nataliae							xxxx		possible
An. meraukensis		xx							possible
Annovaguinensis		xx							possible
An. punctulatus group:									
An. farauti complex:									
An. farauti	xxx	xxxx	xxxx		xxxx	xxxx	xxxx	xxxx	primary
An. hinesorum	x	xxxx	xxxx	x	xxxx	xxx	xxxx		secondary
An. torresiensis		xx							possible
An. farauti 4			xxx			xxx			secondary
An. farauti 5				x					non-vector
An. farauti 6				xxx					secondary
An. irenicus							xxx		non-vector
An. farauti 8			x						secondary
An. clowi			x			x			non-vector
An. koliensis			xxxx		xxxx	xxxx	x		primary
An. punctulatus			xxxx	xx	xxxx	xxxx	xx		primary
An. sp near *punctulatus*			xx		xx	xx			non-vector
An. rennellensis							x		non-vector
An. subpictus (Oriental)	x	xx	xx		xx	x			possible
An. tessellatus (Oriental)	x		x			x			non-vector

Monsoonal type climate; continuous hot/wet type climate, highlands >300m; SCH: south of the central highlands; NCH: north of the central highlands

xxxx: abundant, xxx: common, xx: uncommon, x: rare

Table 1. The *Anopheles* species currently found in the Australian Region, their distribution and vector status.

and biogeography. The following section outlines our current knowledge of the primary and secondary malaria vectors of the southwest Pacific region.

2.1. The *Anopheles* (*Cellia*) *punctulatus* group

The primary vectors of malaria throughout the southwest Pacific region are members of the *Anopheles punctulatus* group. In 1901 Dönitz described the type form [16], *Anopheles punctulatus*, from the Madang area of PNG, while Laveran described *Anopheles farauti* in Efate, Vanuatu, the following year [17]. Given that the range of the *An. punctulatus* group spans several countries, the early identity and relationship of the members was somewhat confused – a detailed account of this early history is given in Lee et al. [18] and Rozeboom and Knight [19].

Thanks in part to the necessary deployment of Allied defense personnel throughout this region; the taxonomy of this vector group was studied in depth during World War II. Four closely related species were identified – *An. punctulatus* Dönitz, *An. farauti* Laveran, *An. koliensis* Owen and *An. clowi* Rozeboom and Knight – and assembled within the Punctulatus Complex [19].

In 1962, Belkin referred to the group in his taxonomic study of South Pacific mosquitoes [20]. However, this study did not include Irian Jaya, Indonesia (now West Papua/Papua Province) or PNG. Rozeboom and Knight [19] provide descriptions of the original four members of the *An. punctulatus* complex and taxonomic keys for the members of the complex. For adult females, the diagnostic characters used were the black and white scaling patterns on the proboscis and, to a lesser extent, on the wings, palpi, and tarsi. Proboscis morphology readily, but unreliably as was later learned, separated the three most common and widespread members, *An. farauti*, *An. punctulatus*, and *An. koliensis*. *Anopheles farauti* displays an all black scaled labium; *An. punctulatus* has the apical half of the labium extensively pale scaled; and *An. koliensis* has a patch of pale scales, varying in size, on the ventral surface of the apical half of the labium [19]. For *An. clowi*, the tarsi on the fore- and mid-legs were used [19].

Taxonomic and systematic studies of the group were renewed in the 1970's when Bryan showed that cross-mating between two *An. farauti* colonies (from Rabaul in PNG and north Queensland) was incompatible as the species differed by two paracentric inversions [21]. The two species were then called *An. farauti* 1 and *An. farauti* 2. Bryan then collected material from the type locality (Efate, Vanuatu) and identified it as *An. farauti* 1 [22], hereafter referred to as *An. farauti*. Hybridization experiments by Mahon and Miethke in 1982 [23] revealed another species (designated *An. farauti* 3) and also found three sympatric sibling species with no evidence of interbreeding in the Innisfail region south of Cairns in north Queensland. Bryan also confirmed the species status of *An. koliensis* in 1973 by cross-mating experiments [24]. Also in 1973, Maffi described specimens from Rennell Island in the Solomon Islands as belonging to the *An. punctulatus* group [25] and subsequently declared these mosquitoes as a new species, *An. rennellensis* [26]. In the late 1980s, *An. farauti* was identified from the coastal areas around Madang, PNG [27], and Sweeney showed that salt tolerance could be used as a species diagnostic feature [28].

Although proboscis markings are often obvious and easy to detect, proboscis morphology is not a reliable means of distinguishing species in this group. As early as 1945, working in PNG, Woodhill [29] examined the progeny of wild caught females of the "intermediate form" (now called *An. koliensis*) and found both *An. farauti*- and *An. punctulatus*-type proboscis. Similar polymorphisms in this character were also noted by Foley et al. [30] and Cooper et al. [31]. Later morphological studies [32, 33] using specimens from Australia and the Solomon Islands described morphological features for *An. farauti* species and provided preliminary keys. However these keys are problematic as the characters used are both difficult for routine identification and are not 100% accurate. In addition, they were developed using material from a limited range of the species' distributions. Figure 2 and Table 2 summarizes some problems with using proboscis morphology for identifying members of the *An. punctulatus* group.

The *An. punctulatus* group currently consists of 13 species that include: *An. punctulatus, An koliensis, An.* species near *punctulatus, An. clowi, An. rennellensis,* and the members of the *An. farauti* complex: *An. farauti* (formally *An. farauti* 1), *An. hinesorum* (formally *An. farauti* 2), *An. torresiensis* (formally *An. farauti* 3), *An. irenicus* (formally *An. farauti* 7) and *An. farauti* 4-6 and 8 [30, 33-37]. Given that the majority of the 13 species currently known in the *An. punctulatus* group were discovered in the 1990's, a great deal of polymorphism can be presumed to exist in the morphological characters previously used to describe the members of this group. As a consequence, field workers who rely on proboscis morphology should also be using the available molecular tools [30, 31, 38-40] (see Fig. 2 and Table 2).

Species (number identified by PCR)	**Proboscis Type[1] number (%)**		
	farauti	**koliensis**	**punctulatus**
An. farauti (n=1,131)	1,128 (99.7)	0 (0)	3 (0.3)
An. hinesorum (n=1,050)	1,048 (99.8)	1 (0.1)	1 (0.1)
Anfarauti 4 (n=842)	235 (28.0)	472 (56.0)	135 (16.0)
An. koliensis (n=1,223)	151 (12.3)	1,035 (84.7)	37 (3.0)
An. punctulatus (n=676)	4 (0.6)	16 (2.4)	656 (97.0)

farauti - all black scaled labium; *koliensis* - dorsal white patch of scales on the anterior end; *punctulatus*: anterior half all white scaled.

Table 2. Proboscis morphology of five common members of the *Anophelespunctulatus* group from the Australian Region and identified using DNA hybridisation and PCR-RFLP analysis.

The distribution of these species is only beginning to be understood as the group ranges over hundreds of small islands with varying landforms and ecotypes, each island providing opportunities for reproductive isolation and consequent speciation. It is possible that further species may be found when the remote and inaccessible areas of the Moluccas, Indonesian Papua, Papua New Guinea, and the Solomon Islands are more thoroughly surveyed.

2.1.1. *Molecular genetic markers*

After cross-mating experiments revealed post-mating barriers and the presence of the three species designated *An. farauti, An. hinesorum,* and *An. torresiensis* [24], mosquito cytogenetics became a more informative and practical method to study and identify these species. In 1971, Bryan and Coluzzi [21] produced preliminary maps of polytene chromosomes from the salivary glands of 4th instar larvae of *An. farauti* and *An. hinesorum.* Taking *An. farauti* as the standard, *An. hinesorum* differed by a paracentric inversion on each of the left and right arms of chromosome 2 [21]. Mahon [41] found that *An. torresiensis* had the standard arrangement for the autosomes but the X chromosome differed by two inversions. The same author also looked at chromosome maps of *An. punctulatus* and *An. koliensis* and predicted chromosomal relationships among the five species and possible ancestral characters [41].

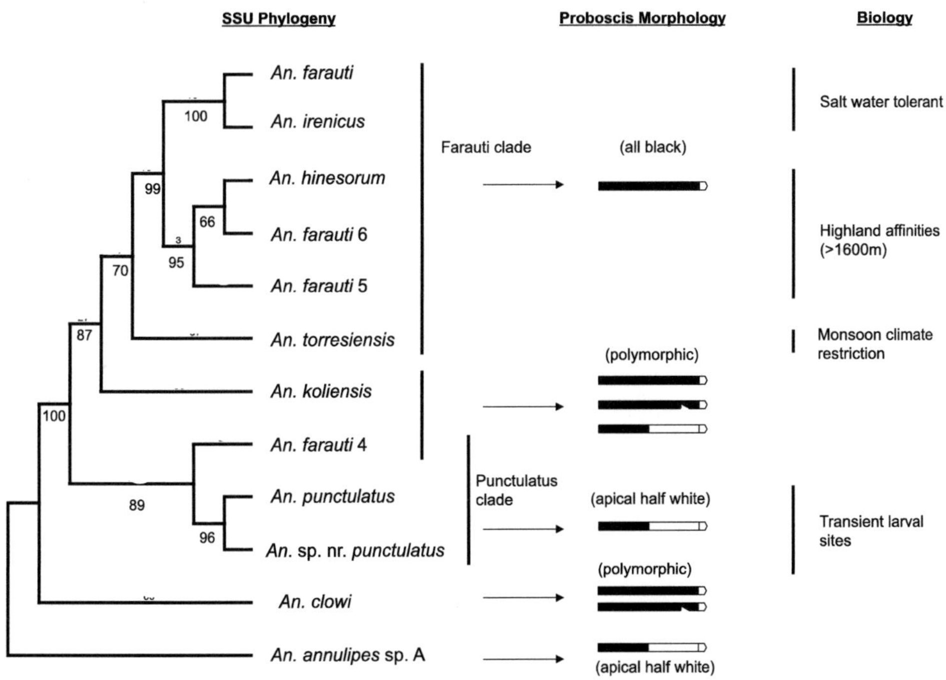

Figure 2. This single most parsimonious phylogenetic tree generated from the structural alignment of the nuclear ssrDNA reveals 11 members of the *An. punctulatus* group with *An. annulipes* sp. A from the *An. annulipes* outgroup. Proboscis morphologies identified from field-collected specimens are displayed to the right and overt biological characteristics are also listed.

2.1.2. Molecular markers

Allozymes: In the 1990's Foley and colleagues [30] executed the first population genetic studies into the group using allozyme electrophoresis methods to show that *An. farauti* specimens from inland areas around Madang were reproductively isolated from the PNG highlands. In doing this, they discovered *An. farauti* 4 from the Madang area and *An. farauti* 5 and 6 from the PNG highlands. Then, also using allozymes, Foley revealed a reproductively isolated *An. farauti*-like species from Guadalcanal in the Solomon Islands and designated it *An. farauti* 7 (now *An. irenicus*) [35]. Furthermore, a population with morphology very like *An. punctulatus* was found in the Western Province of PNG and appeared reproductively isolated; this was named *Anopheles* species near *punctulatus* [34].

To facilitate the identification of the large numbers of field-collected material required for malaria studies, Mahon [42] developed a starch gel allozyme electrophoresis method using two enzymes, lactate dehydrogenase and octanol dehydrogenase. This method was employed to study the distribution of cryptic species of *An. farauti* throughout northern Australia [43, 44]. The allozyme technique was further refined with cellulose acetate electrophoresis by Foley in 1993 [30, 45] to also identify *An. farauti* 4, 5, 6, *An. irenicus*, and *An.* species near *punctulatus* [30, 34, 35]. Thus electrophoretic keys were now available for ten species in the *An. punctulatus* group – excluding the rarely recorded *An. clowi* and *An. rennellensis* [34]. These allozyme markers represent the first molecular tools to identify the members of the *An. punctulatus* group. The requirement of a cold (frozen) chain from the field to the lab to prevent protein degradation of samples was the most limiting feature of this technology.

2.1.3. Species-specific genomic DNA probes

Chromosome banding differences discovered while identifying cryptic species revealed a large variations in the genomic DNA of these species, and suggested possible avenues for producing new technologies for identifying cryptic species. Advances in recombinant DNA technology in the early 1980's enabled the isolation of species-specific repetitive DNA sequences. The use of nucleic acids as characters to identify the members of this group began in 1991 with the development of isotopic DNA probes for the Australian species *An. farauti, An. hinesorum,* and *An. torresiensis* [46]. Genomic DNA probes were developed for use with squash blot techniques for ten species in the *An. punctulatus* group [38, 46, 47]. The "squash blot" (see Fig. 3 for an example) technique requires no DNA extraction; the specimen (or part of specimens) is squashed directly onto the membrane in the presence of a detergent that ruptures the tissue. The liberated DNA then binds to the nylon membrane. Species-specific probes labeled with a reporter molecule such as biotin or ^{32}P hybridize to homologous DNA from the squashed material and are visualized by the reporter molecule [46]. Up to 100 membranes can be probed simultaneously, permitting thousands of field specimens to be identified for a particular species. Over 100,000 species identifications were thereby processed to produce the extensive distribution data generated by Cooper and colleagues [31, 44, 48, 49].

http://dx.doi.org/10.5772/55999

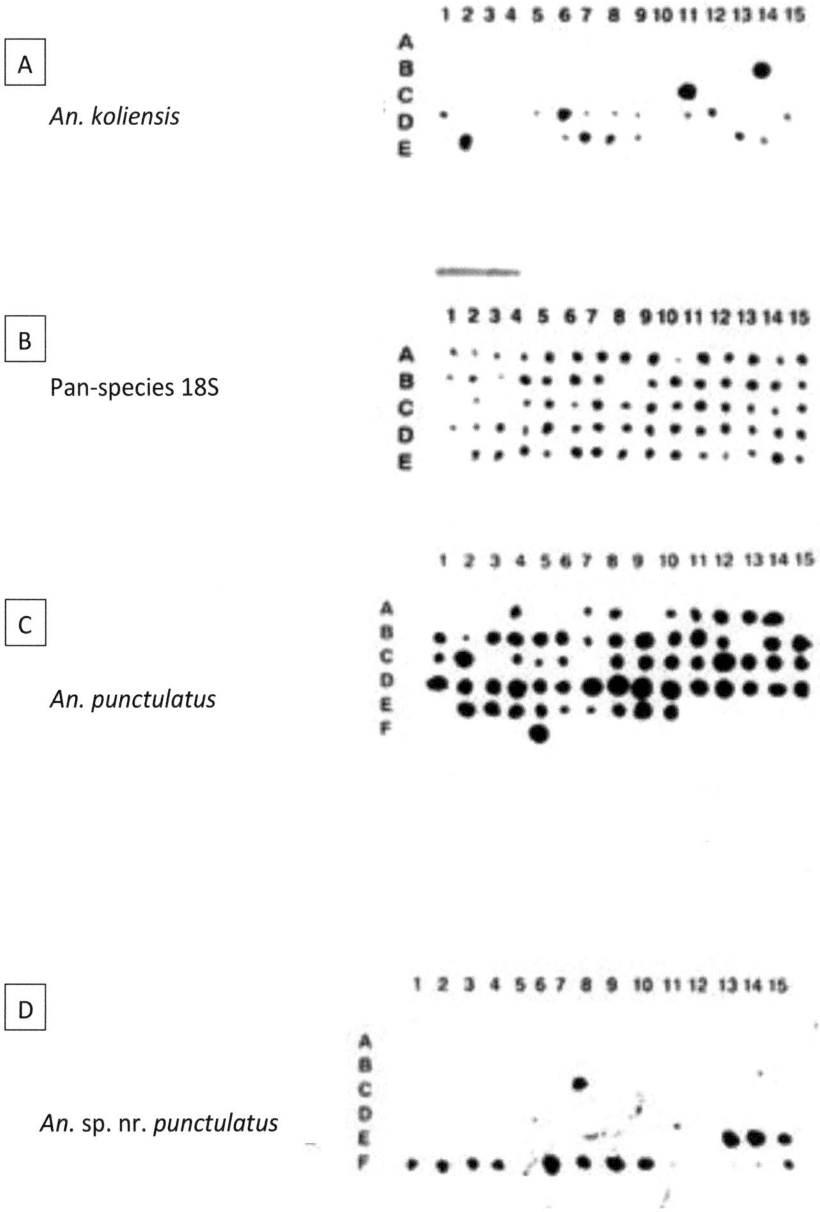

Figure 3. Mosquito squash blots hybridized with species-specific genomic DNA probes labeled with ^{32}P can distinguish cryptic species in the *An. punctulatus* group. **Panel A:** squash blot of mosquitoes morphologically identified as *An. koliensis* and probed with a species-specific probe reveals that only a subset of samples are *An. koliensis* (*An. farauti* 4 made up the other individuals identified as *An. koliensis*). **Panel B:** same blot was stripped and probed with a pan-species rDNA 18S probe that binds to all species revealing the total amount of gDNA on the blot. **Panel C:** mosquitoes identified as *An. punctulatus* are probed with the *An. punctulatus* species-specific probe and **Panel D** is the same blot stripped and reprobed with the *An.* sp. nr *punctulatus* probe.

2.1.4. PCR-based species diagnostics

2.1.4.1. Ribosomal DNA ITS2

The advent of polymerization chain reaction (PCR) for DNA amplification in the late 1980's facilitated technologies for both cryptic species' identification and within-species population studies. The most popular marker for species-specific PCR-based diagnosis has been the rDNA gene family. Despite a lack of understanding of the evolution of this non-Mendelian evolving repetitive gene family, its rapidly evolving transcribed spacers allow a simplistic evaluation of genetic discontinuity within and between species. The internal transcribed spacer 2 (ITS2) region proved the most useful for developing two different species diagnostic tools for identifying *An. punctulatus* group members [40, 50]. In the first PCR-RFLP (restricted fragment length polymorphism) technology, the size of the ITS2 region (~710bp) was identical for all *An. punctulatus* group members and was thus diagnostic for the group; this means that mosquito collections of other (non-*An. punctulatus* group) species can be detected simply as RFLPs of different banding profiles. Digestion of this product with the restriction enzyme *Msp* I generates species-specific DNA fragments for the 11 most abundant and most widely distributed members of this group, *An. farauti, An. hinesorum, An. torresiensis, An. farauti* 4-6, *An. irenicus, An. punctulatus, An.* species near *punctulatus,* and *An. clowi* (Fig. 4). This species-specific PCR-RFLP has been extensively used both independently and alongside genomic DNA probes in species distribution studies of the *An. punctulatus* group [31, 44, 48, 51]. However, more recently, a "Luminex®"-based multiplex ligase detection reaction and fluorescent microsphere-based assay method became available, also based on species-specific ITS2 sequences, and can separate the five common malaria vector species in PNG: *An. punctulatus, An. koliensis, An. farauti, An. hinesorum,* and *An. farauti* 4 [40].

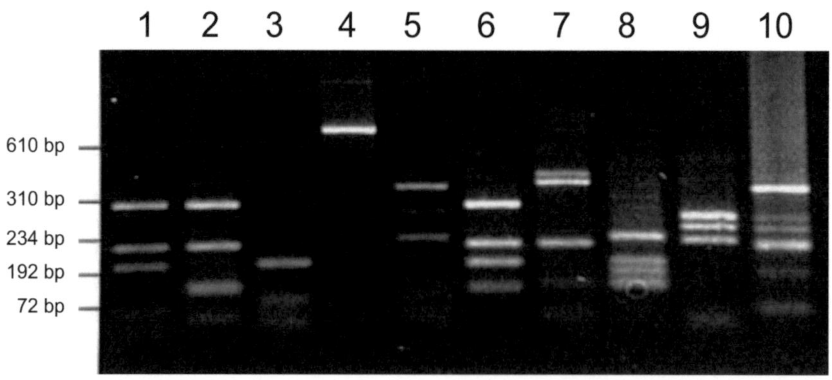

Figure 4. Molecular diagnostic that discriminates over 10 members of the *An. punctulatus* group based on a PCR-RFLP of the ITS2, cut with the restriction enzyme *Msp* I and run out on a 3% agarose gel. Banding profiles are as follows: Lane 1, *An. farauti*; (formally *An. farauti* 1) Lane 2, *An. hinesorum* (formally *An. farauti* 2); Lane 3, *An. torresiensis* (formally *An. farauti* 3); Lane 4, *An. farauti* 4 (contains no restriction site); Lane 5, *An. farauti* 5; Lane 6, *An. farauti* 6; Lane 7, *An. irenicus* (formally *farauti* 7), Lane 8, *An. koliensis*, Lane 9, *An. punctulatus*; Lane 10, *An.* sp. nr. *punctulatus*. Additionally *An. clowi* can be distinguished using this method however *An. farauti* 8 produces the same RFLP profile as *An. farauti*, but is distinguishable by ITS1 RFLP[52].

Analysis of the ITS2 region reveals substantial insertion and deletion events (indels) between species that are probably due to sequence slippage of common, simple, sequence repeat motifs. Interestingly, no ITS2 PCR-RFLP mixed species hybrids have yet been reported, which would be observed as single mosquitoes sharing RFLP profiles of more than one species. The lack of hybrids at the rDNA locus reinforces the species status for members of this group. Additionally evolutionary information about the *An. punctulatus* group has been obtained with studies of the ITS2 region. The undigested ITS2 PCR products from single mosquitoes contain ITS2 sequence copy variants in the multicopy rDNA array and can provide another view on population genetic structure. For example, intraspecific rDNA genotypes of *An. farauti* were found to be geographically structured by the presence of fixed ITS2 copy variants amplified in the PCR [53] (also see Figs. 5, 6, and 7 for examples). Population genetic analyses of *An. farauti* revealed macrogeographic population structure in *An. farauti* throughout the southwest Pacific comprising several distinct genotypes, suggestive of potential barriers to gene flow. Interestingly, only a subset of these geographically structured genotypes were identified at the level of the mitochondrial DNA cytochrome oxidase I (COI) sequence level in a recent population genetic study of this species [54], suggesting that the rDNA array may be a sensitive tool for species-level diagnostics.

While the ITS1 region has not been examined in as much detail as the ITS2, the ITS1 is an informative marker for intraspecific population studies for some *An. punctulatus* group members, separating *An. farauti* into several geographically and climatically distributed genotypes [52, 53]. For example, Fig. 5 shows how the ITS2 and ITS1 can reveal qualitative information on population genetic discontinuities within *An. farauti* where rDNA genotypes could also be identified within and between landmasses reflecting genetic and geographic structure [53]. This phenomena was most likely possible because of the extended time this species existed in a region with natural barriers to gene flow [54].

2.1.5. Evolutionary and phylogenetic studies

Identifying levels of genetic differences among mosquito taxa and the phylogenetic relationships of closely related species allows an understanding of the evolutionary forces acting on mosquito populations. Knowing the evolutionary relationships among vector species can provide insights into understanding the dynamics of disease transmission. Initial attempts to generate a species-level phylogeny of the *An. punctulatus* group were based on the DNA sequence of the rDNA ITS2. However, the large amount of sequence variation between each species appearing as insertion or deletion indels made computer-based sequence alignment difficult, and the resulting systematic trees could not resolve all species in the group [55]. The closely linked ssrDNA (rDNA 18S) structural RNA gene with alignment based on established secondary structures proved more useful for resolving the relatedness of this group [36, 56]. An independent assessment of a 684bp section of the mitochondrial cytochrome oxidase II region [57] found the COII useful in resolving most Australian and Oriental anophelines at the species level, but limited in resolving the known members in the *An. punctulatus* group. However, most phylogenetic studies of the group do consistently reveal two main clades, one containing all the *An. farauti*-like species (all-black proboscis) except *An. farauti* 4, which appears in a second clade with *An. punctulatus* and *An.* species near *punctulatus* (all of which can display a half-black, half-white proboscis) [31, 58] (see Fig. 2 and Table 2). *Anopheles koliensis* is positioned either basal to all species in the COII tree or between the *An. farauti* and *An. punctulatus* clades in the rDNA trees, neither of which branches showed strong support.

The same evolutionary mechanisms that led to the existence of these species have also produced a number of genetically distinct populations within each species that may differ in behaviour and in their potential to transmit malaria parasites. For example, recent investigations have revealed that genotypes of *An. hinesorum* exist in the Solomon Islands that do not appear to bite humans while in other parts of this species' range, there are distinct genetic populations that are anthropophilic and are known to transmit malaria [51, 54, 59]. This study revealed restricted gene flow throughout *An. hinesorum*'s distribution and distinct differences in malaria vectoring potential and demonstrates the importance of detailing how species' populations connect to each other through population genetic studies – particularly in light of the design and efficacy of any control strategy [60].

2.2. *Anopheles* (*Cellia*) *longirostris* complex

The morphospecies *Anopheles longirostris* Brug is widespread throughout the coastal and inland lowland regions of New Guinea. Subsequent analysis of this morphospecies using both mtDNA and the rDNA ITS2 from 70 sites in PNG revealed up to nine distinct species that appear reproductively isolated at the rDNA locus [61]. Most of these putative species also exist as distinct mtDNA COI lineages and have been designated A, B, C1, C2, D, E, F, G, H [61]. Fig. 6 displays the phylogenetic study and molecular diagnostic developed with the same *Msp* I PCR-RFLP method as used for the *An. punctulatus* group. Of note, the species designated C1 and C2 produce the same ITS2 PCR-RFLP banding profile but curiously display different ITS2 copy variant organization. Where C1 is uncommon and extant only in the Western Province of PNG to date, species C2 appears to be the most common and widespread species in the group [61]. Thus the molecular diagnostic discrimination of C1 and C2 may only be problematic south of the central highlands in PNG's Western Province. However, species C1 may exist north of the central highlands. As it is only a recently recognized cryptic species group, little is now known about each species' biology and ecology and malaria transmission potential.

2.3. *Anopheles* (*Cellia*) *lungae* complex

Initially described by Belkin [20], the *An. lungae* group members show a distribution throughout the highly malarious Solomon Islands and Bougainville to the north. Belkin described three distinct morphological forms – *An. lungae, An. solomonis* and *An. nataliae* [20] – and variation among geographical populations was also noted. [20]. The three species have white scaling on the halters which readily separates them from the members of the *An. punctulatus* group which occur in the Solomon Islands [20]. Within the *An. lungae* complex the members can be separated using proboscis morphology though there is some overlap between the species with this character and this method is not reliable. A molecular diagnostic has been developed for the three species based on a *Msp* I digest of the ITS2 (Fig. 7).

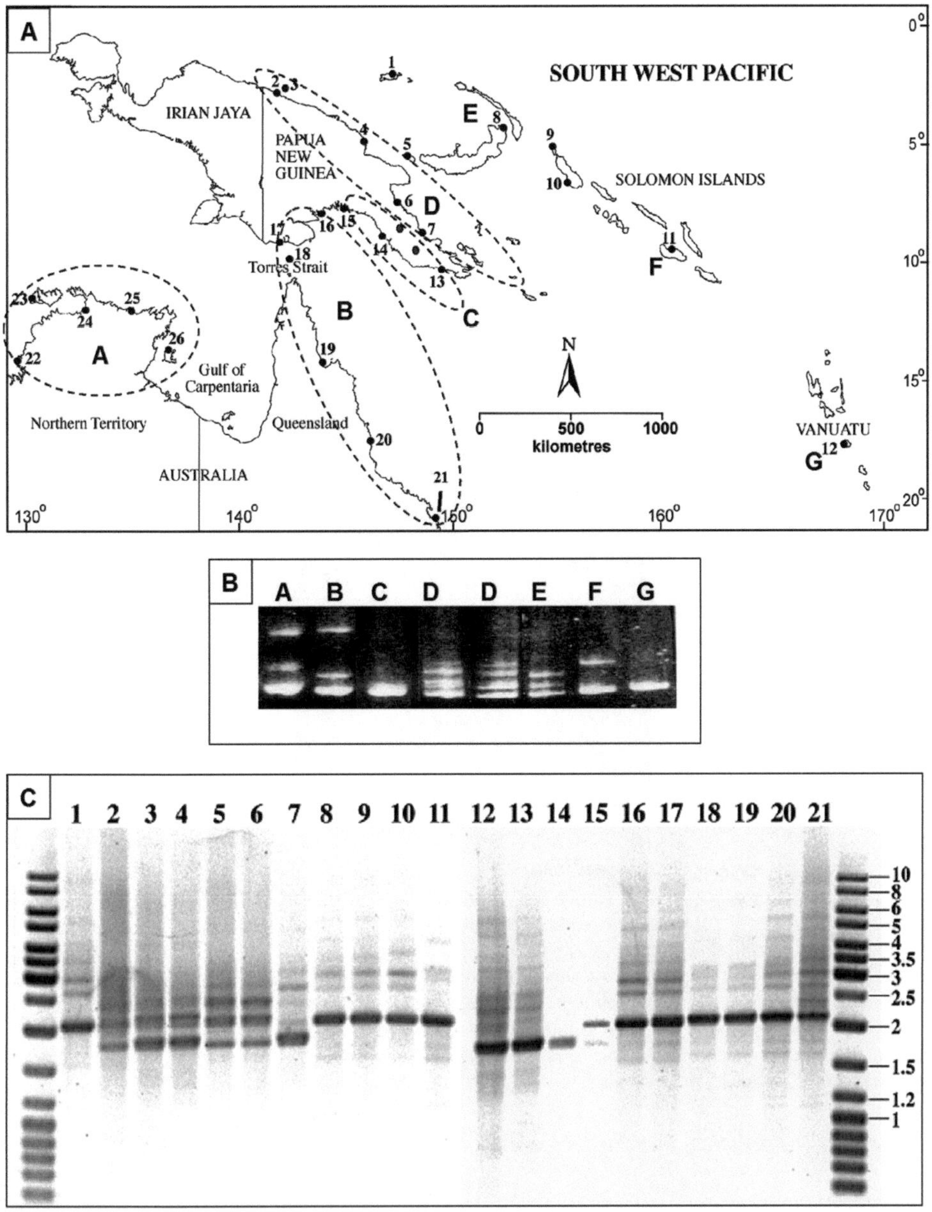

Figure 5. The rDNA genotypes of *An. farauti*. **Panel A** shows a map of southwest Pacific and the 21 *An. farauti* collection sites. Dotted circles represent the distribution grouping of ITS2 PCR heteroduplex profiles (genotypes) that appeared in native acrylamide gels shown in **Panel B** (samples 22-24 not shown). **Panel C** is an agarose gel showing individual *An. farauti* ITS1 PCR products with lanes representing collection sites on Panel A. Intragenomic size variation is evident between collection sites and in most cases individuals showed the same ITS1 and ITS2 heteroduplex profiles, exceptions were found in some sites on the north coast of PNG where rDNA profiles are highly polymorphic. This coastally restricted species shows remarkable rDNA turnover throughout its distribution. Cloning and sequencing ITS2 copy variants revealed no phylogenetic information, however the longer ITS1 (up to 2.5kb) revealed a robust phylogenetic signal resolving genotypes into regions [52].

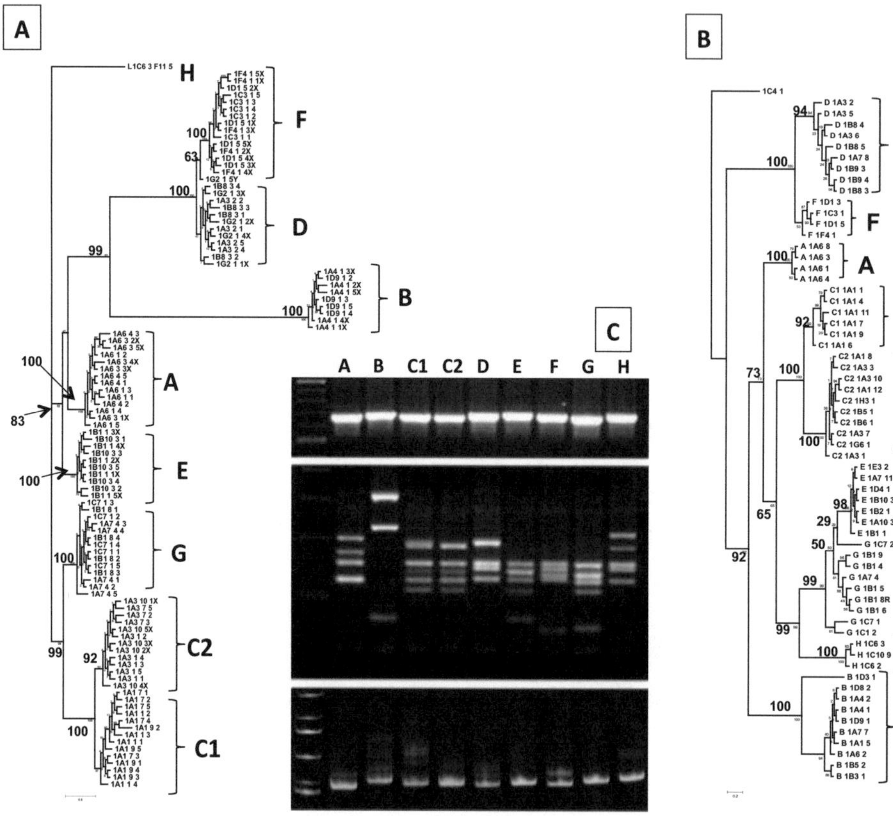

Figure 6. The discovery of nine cryptic species within mosquitoes identified morphologically as *Anopheles longirostris* from PNG. Phylogenetic assessment of *A. longirostris* based on cloned ITS2 DNA sequence from PCR products (**Panel A**) and directly sequenced mtDNA COI PCR products (**Panel B**) reveal nine distinct lineages. Bayesian posterior probabilities (converted to percentage) are shown as branch support values above 70%. **Panel C**: The molecular diagnostic developed revealed nine ITS2 genotypes of *A. longirostris*. Panel C-top, uncut ITS2 PCR products; Panel C-middle, ITS2 PCR products cut with *Msp* I and run through a 3% agarose gel; Panel C-bottom, ITS2 PCR products run through a 7.0% 7 acrylamide gel revealing individuals within interbreeding populations contained fixed copy variants, suggesting reproductive isolation at the rDNA locus. Only the RFLP profile for genotype C showed two distinct heteroduplex profiles (designated C1 and C2) thus revealing the presence of two independently evolving ITS2 genotypes.

2.4. *Anopheles* (*Anopheles*) *bancroftii* group

Two morphological species were initially described in the *Anopheles bancroftii* group based on wing fringe patterns –*Anopheles bancroftii* Giles, and *Anopheles pseudobarbirostris* Ludlow [63] – although some confusion as to the distributions of these two morphotypes existed. The ITS2 PCR-RFLP method using the enzyme *Msp* I identified four distinct ITS2 genotypes designated A, B, C and D [39]. ITS2 DNA sequence analysis of this group revealed intragenomic sequence copy variants existing in individual mosquitoes that assist in the identification of these four ITS2 genotypes (Fig. 8). For example, genotype C could be interpreted as a combination (hybrid) RFLP profile between genotypes A and B, however both DNA sequence analysis and intragenomic ITS2 copy variant studies revealed the presence of four independently evolving

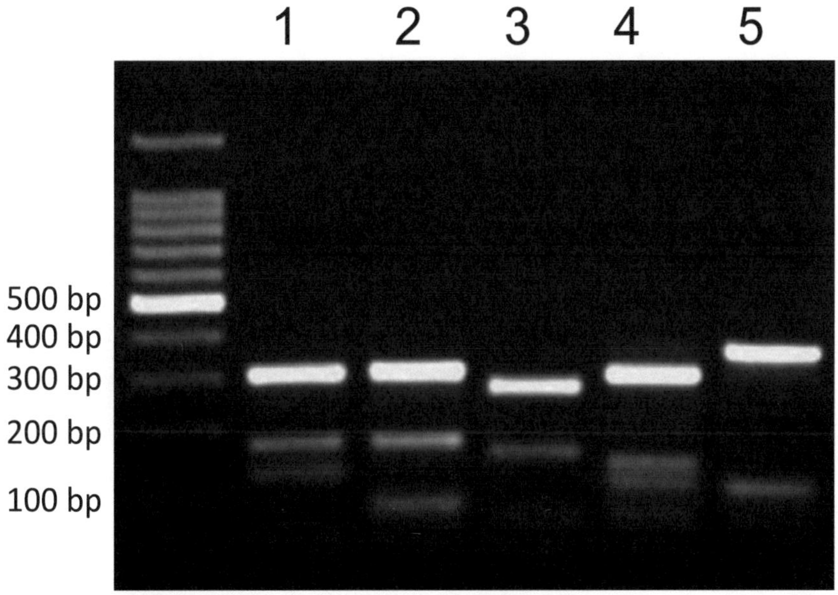

Figure 7. Molecular diagnostic for *Anopheles* species collected in Santa Isabel Province in the Solomon Islands based again on an ITS2 PCR-RFLP using *Msp* I [62]: Lanes 1-2 isomorphic species *An. farauti*, *An. hinesorum*. Lanes 3-5 are cryptic the members of the *Anopheles lungae* complex that exist in the Solomon Island: Lane 3, *An. nataliae*; Lane 4, *An. lungae*; and Lane 5, *An. solomonis*.

ITS2 genotypes with cloned ITS2 sequences showing little phylogenetic information [39]. No correlation was identified with the wing fringe characteristics initially used to identify *An. bancroftii* and *An. pseudobarbirostris* with any of the four genotypes. The distribution of these ITS2 genotypes (putative species) has been further investigated [64], indicating distinct distribution for genotypes A, B, and D. Genotype C is sympatric with B and D without evidence of hybridization, suggesting these genotypes are reproductively isolated and likely biological species. Confirmation of this hypothesis using other nuclear genetic markers is needed. Thus genotype C is sympatric with B and D without evidence of hybridization, suggesting these genotypes are reproductively isolated and likely biological species. Confirmation of this hypothesis using other nuclear genetic markers is needed.

3. Species distribution, biology and vectorial status

3.1. Primary vectors

Three species – *An. farauti, An. koliensis,* and *An. punctulatus* – are considered the primary vectors of malaria in the region. All are widely distributed and can occur in high densities (Fig. 9). They readily feed on humans, and all have been found infected with human malaria parasites.

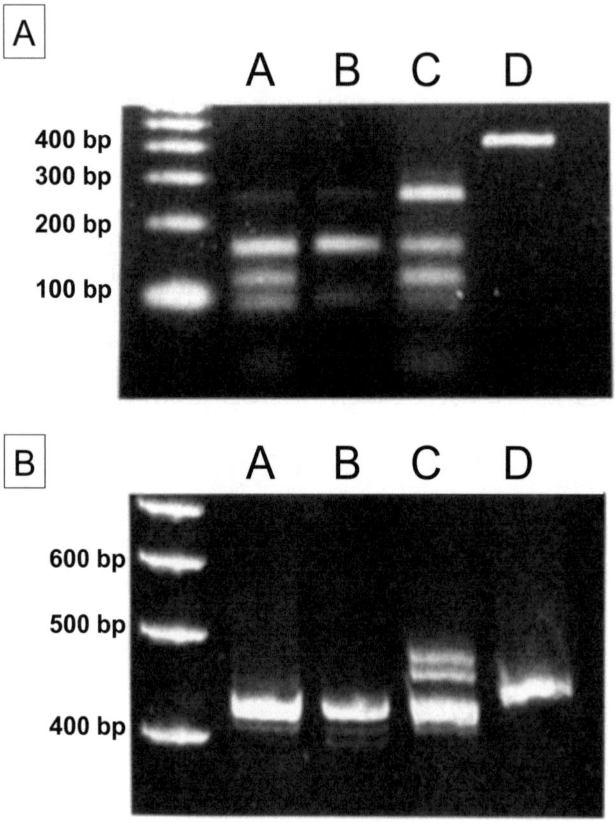

Figure 8. Molecular diagnostic for the cryptic species in the *An. bancroftii* group. **Panel A** are *Msp* I cut ITS2 PCR-RFLP profiles of *An. bancroftii* electrophoresis run through a 3.0% agarose gel. First lane on the left is a 100bp marker. Lanes 2-5 are the RFLP of genotypes A-D with genotype D revealing no *Msp* I restriction sites and the full length of the PCR product (all genotypes produce a 400bp PCR product). **Panel B** are the same PCR products electrophoresed through a 7.0% acrylamide gel that is sensitive to double stranded secondary structure. Lanes A, B and D show a single band for the amplified ITS2 (homogenized single sequence or homoduplex). Lane 4 is genotype C showing both a homoduplex (bottom band) and two heteroduplex products (misspairing in double-stranded duplex alters secondary structure retarding migration). Lane 5 is genotype D that migrates slower due to differences in the secondary structure duplex and not sequence length.

Anopheles farauti has the widest distribution of all the anopheline fauna of the region, occurring in the Moluccas, on New Guinea and its associated islands and archipelagos, in northern Australia, throughout the Solomon Islands and Vanuatu. *Anopheles farauti* has been incriminated as a vector of malaria throughout this range [59, 65-68]. It is a coastal species, whose larvae tolerate brackish water [28, 69], with preferred breeding sites ranging from small ground pools to large coastal swamps and lagoons formed where runoff to the sea is blocked by sand bars (Fig. 10 E). These large sites are ubiquitous along the coastline throughout the region [58, 62] and are often associated with human habitation. Due to their size, they can support high population numbers [62, 70]. *Anopheles farauti*'s ability to breed in brackish water has facilitated its dispersal across the myriad tiny islands throughout the region [20, 71].

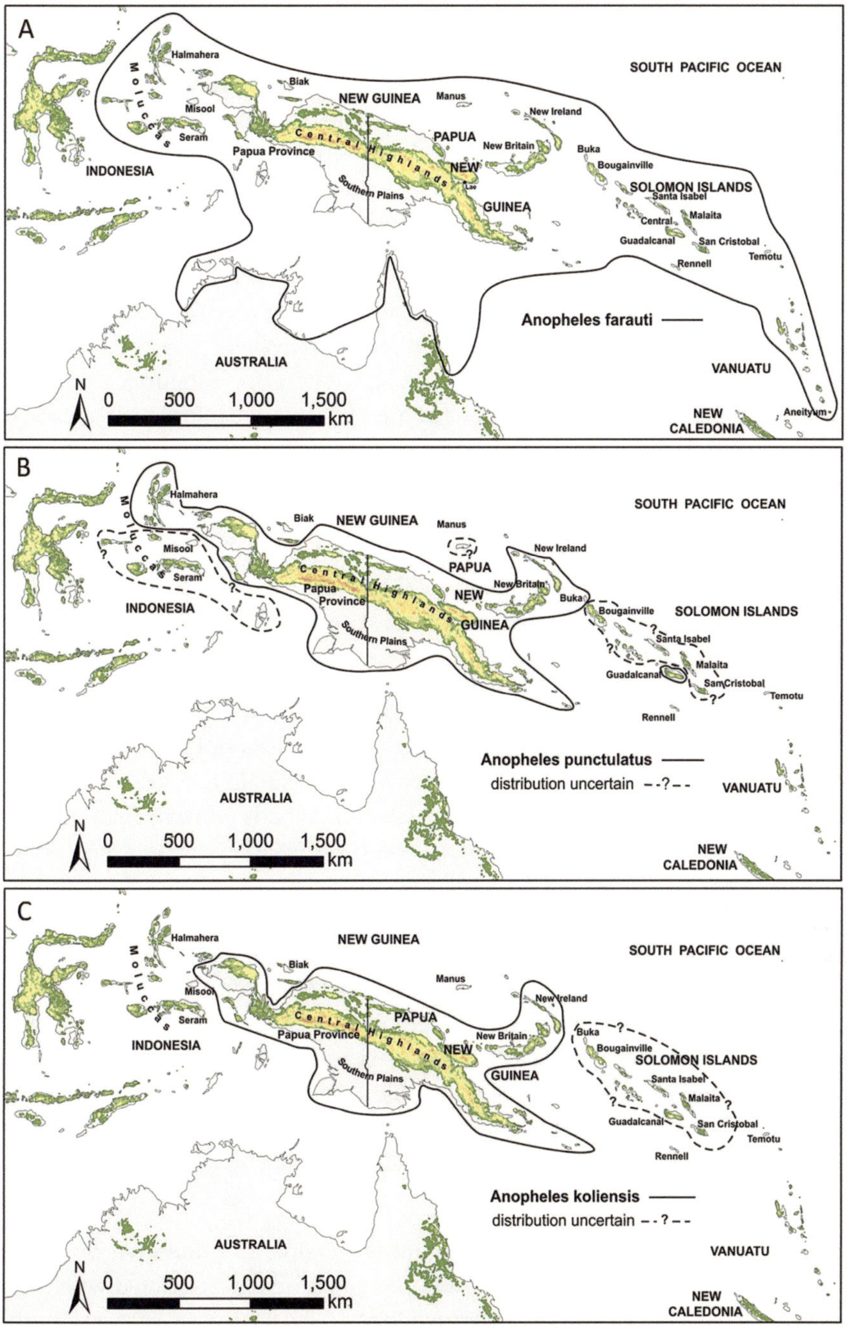

Figure 9. Known distributions of the three main species of the *An. punctulatus* group. **Panel A** is *An. farauti* which throughout its distribution is a coastally restricted species rarely found more that 5 km inland. **Panel B** is *An. punctulatus* which is a fresh water species that exists both coastal, inland and at elevation >1500m. **Panel C**. *An. koliensis* is a lowland inland and coastal species.

In PNG, the Solomon Islands, and Vanuatu, where extensive sampling has occurred and the mosquitoes' distribution is well understood, *An. farauti* is known to exist as several genotypes [53]. These genetically distinct populations are separated by overt barriers: climate disjunction between the northern continuous wet and southern monsoonal region in the Southern Plains of New Guinea (see Fig.1), the central highlands in New Guinea; and sea gaps between New Guinea and Manus Island, the Solomon Islands and Vanuatu [58]. All genotypes appear to have similar behaviours and are malaria vectors wherever they occur.

Given that *An. farauti* remains the dominant species collected in coastal villages, past reference to their biology and behaviour prior to identification using molecular techniques is probably still valid. *Anopheles farauti,* while readily feeding on humans, will also feed on other animals, and anthropophilic indices can be quite low in villages where domestic animals, primarily pigs and dogs, are abundant [27, 67]. Populations of this species were found well outside the flight range of human habitation, indicating that this species will readily feed on native birds and animals [31]. The longevity of this species appears quite variable; in the Solomon Islands province of Temotu the proportion of the population that was parous was 0.42 [70] while in Central Province it was 0.76 (T. Russell, unpublished data). In New Guinea, values ranged from 0.58 in Jayapura [65] to 0.49 in Madang, [27] and 0.73 in the D'Entrecasteaux Islands [66]. It will readily enter houses to feed but is primarily exophilic, leaving the house on the night of feeding to rest outdoors [65, 66].

Anophelespunctulatus has been recorded from the Moluccas, New Guinea, and the larger islands of Manus, New Britain, New Ireland and Buka – but it does not appear to be present on Bougainville Island [48, 72]. During faunal surveys conducted in the early 1970's, *An. punctulatus* was found on all the main islands in the Solomon Islands except Temotu Province [73]. It was found on Malaita in 1987 [74] and on the north coast of Guadalcanal in 1998 [51]. However, recent surveys of Santa Isabel and Central Provinces failed to find this species (62, T. Russell, unpublished data). In New Guinea, it is mainly found in inland lowland regions but is also common in the foothills of central ranges and in the intermountain highland valleys [8, 31, 75]. Its natural larval habitats are rock pools, pools in rivers and streambeds, and pools along the margins of these waterways. It is a highly invasive species and will readily invade sites created by human activity such as wheel ruts in roads, pools in walking tracks, hoof and foot prints, pig wallows and shallow drains around village houses (Table 3, Fig. 10 A) [31, 76]. These sites all have a clay or gravel substrate; are small or transient and are maintained only by regular rainfall; they lack established aquatic fauna and flora; and they have little or no debris.

Given that many rural communities throughout the region are connected by unsealed dirt roads, these thoroughfares – along with roads and construction associated with logging and mining activities – have created both extensive larval sites for this species and the corridors along which it can move. *Anopheles punctulatus* has adapted to these small transient sites with eggs that can survive desiccation for several days, a short larval stage (relative to other species) and highly synchronized larval development [76, 77]. A preference for transient sites binds *An. punctulatus* to areas where the soil contains clay and the rainfall is perennial. Where these conditions exist it can occur in high densities [65]. It is considered the most anthropophilic of all the members of the *An. punctulatus* group [67, 78], and is a late night feeder with a feeding peak between midnight and 2am [79].

Of the three primary malaria vectors in the southwest Pacific, *An. punctulatus* is the most long lived [80]. It is a dangerous vector responsible for maintaining holoendemic transmission rates in a number of areas [78]. It has been incriminated as a malaria vector throughout its range [8, 59, 65, 67, 68, 75].

Anopheleskoliensis has a more complex distribution. It is found throughout New Guinea but not in the Moluccas; it occurs on New Britain and Buka Islands, but not on Bougainville; it was found on all the main islands in the Solomon Islands except those of Temotu Province [31, 72, 73, 81]. However, it can no longer be found in the islands of Santa Isabel, Guadalcanal, and Buka [48, 51, 62]. It was possibly eliminated from most islands in the Solomon Islands by IRS with DDT, with the last occurrence reported on the island of Malaita in 1983 [74]. Predominantly an inland species of the lowlands and river valley flood plains below 300m, its main larval habitats are wheel tracks, drains, natural ground pools, and swamps (Table 3, Fig. 10) [31]. Molecular investigations suggest there may be as many as three independently evolving rDNA genotypes (putative species) within this taxon in the Madang/Maprik areas alone [82], and possibly also elsewhere in PNG (N. Beebe, unpublished data). While *An. koliensis* will feed on pigs and dogs, it prefers humans where available and human blood indices of 0.85 and 0.95 have been recorded [27, 67]. It tends to feed late in the night with a peak biting time similar to *An. punctulatus* [65, 79]. In the village of Entrop, Papua Province, peak biting was at 7pm in DDT sprayed villages most likely due to the selection pressure to avoid the DTT, where in Arso (~50km away), which was not sprayed, peak biting was around midnight [65].

It is a moderately long-lived mosquito with parity rates ranging between 0.52 and 0.75 [65, 83]. It has been incriminated as a vector throughout its range [8, 59, 65, 67, 68]. Along with *An. punctulatus*, it is responsible for maintaining holoendemic transmission in a numbers of areas in New Guinea [65, 78].

3.2. Secondary vectors

A number of species have been found infected with human malaria sporozoites throughout the southwest Pacific, but because they have limited distributions or are relatively uncommon, they are considered secondary vectors.

Anopheleshinesorum (formally *An. farauti* 2) is almost as widespread as *An. farauti*, being found from the Moluccas throughout New Guinea, and on Buka and Bougainville Islands; it is also thought to occur in New Britain, New Ireland, and Manus [31, 48]. In the Solomon Islands, it was found on the islands of Santa Isabel, Central Province and the north coast of Guadalcanal, but does not occur in Vanuatu [51, 62, 70]. Any understanding of its distribution is limited by the paucity of faunal surveys in this region, and it is likely that it will be found on all the main islands in the Solomon Islands except Temotu. In Papua New Guinea this species is most frequently found in lowland inland river valleys and flood plains – however it also occurs on the coast and on small offshore islands [31].

Several genetically structured populations were found within *An. hinesorum* [54], with the genotypes found in Buka and Bougainville in PNG and in the Solomon Islands provinces of Santa Isabel, Central, and Guadalcanal being highly zoophilic and rarely biting humans [35, 48, 51, 62]. On mainland PNG, *An. hinesorum* readily bites humans; it was the most common anopheline found throughout the Southern Plains where it can occur in high densities [59]. It has also been found in the highlands of the central highlands (up to 1740m), though it is less common in this region. This is also the case north of the central highlands, possibly due to competition from other species such as *An. farauti* 4 and *An. koliensis*, which also occur in this region and share similar larval habitats. *Anopheles hinesorum* has been incriminated as a vector in this northern New Guinea region [59].

Anopheles hinesorum oviposits in a range of water bodies, both natural – ground pools, swamps and the edges of streams; and rivers – and human-made drains and ditches, wheel ruts and pig wallows (Table 3, Fig. 10) [31]. On Santa Isabel larvae were found in small, shallow, wheel ruts. These transient sites – turbid, with a clay substrate, and devoid of any vegetation – are, at least in Papua New Guinea, normally the exclusive habitat of *An. punctulatus*, but *An. hinesorum* now appears to occupy this niche in the Solomon Islands [62].

Species	Larval Habitat[1] - incidence (%)								
	Transient pools (A)	Ground pools (B)	Pig wallows (C)	Wheel tracks (D)	Swamp brackish (E)	Swamp fresh (F)	Edge of streams (G)	Drains earthen (H)	Totals
An. punctulatus	115 (49.7)	41 (17.7)	15 (6.5)	34 (14.7)	0	2 (0.8)	3 (1.3)	21 (9.0)	231
An. farauti	7 (4.5)	48 (30.7)	1 (0.6)	22 (14.10	43 (27.5)	2 (1.2)	12 (7.7)	21 (13.40	156
An. koliensis	5 (7.9)	17 (27.0)	4 (6.3)	15 (23.8)	0	2 (3.1)	2 (3.1)	18 (28.5)	63
An. hinesorum	70 (18.7)	141 (37.7)	7 (1.8)	41 (10.9)	12 (3.2)	18 (4.8)	23 (6.1)	52 (13.9)	374
An. farauti 4	0	2 (25.0)	2 (25.0)	1 (12.5)	0	0	0	3 (37.5)	8
An. farauti 6	0	2 (33.3)	0	0	0	1 (16.7)	0	3 (50.0)	6
An. bancroftii	0	0	0	0	0	7 (70.0)	2 (20.0)	1 (10.0)	10

letters after habitat type correspond to illustrations in Fig. 10

Table 3. Larval habitats of some primary and secondary vectors of malaria in the Australian Region.

Little is known about this vector's behaviour with regards to malaria transmission although in northern PNG it appears that human feeding activity peaks early in the evening and then declines through the rest of the night [82].

Anophelesfarauti 4 has been found throughout the inland lowland river valleys and flood plains north of the central highlands in PNG [31, 82]. In some locations it is very abundant, and in villages inland from Lae it can comprise up to 90% of the night-biting catch [31]. It readily utilizes larval sites created by human activity – pig wallows, drains, and wheel ruts (Table 3, Fig. 10) where it was commonly found in association with *An. punctulatus* and *An. koliensis*. It is a vector throughout its range [59, 82]. Little is known of its behaviour mainly due to the fact that there are no reliable morphological characters that separate it from *An. hinesorum* and *An. koliensis*, the two species with which it is commonly sympatric.

Anopheles farauti 6 is restricted in its distribution to the intermontane plains and upland valleys of the highland regions (>1000m, ranging to the highest points of 2000m) of New Guinea. It has adapted to the cool moist climate that prevails at these altitudes and in this habitat it is quite common. It is noticeably larger than any other members of the *An. farauti* complex [31, 84]. In 1960, Peters and Christian [7] found this large *An. farauti* to be the most common anopheline biting humans in the Waghi Valley in the highlands of PNG and recorded sporozoites in 2.2%. It was the most abundant anopheline in human biting catches in the Baliem Valley (Wamena, at 1,500m) in the central highlands of Papua Province [31]. *An. farauti* 6 likely plays an important role in malaria transmission within this restricted range.

Anophelesfarauti 8, the most recent member of the *An. farauti* complex to be recognized, has to date only been found in the inland lowland areas on the east side of the Gulf of Papua in PNG [37]. However, given that this species has an ITS2 RFLP identical to *An. farauti*, it may have been confused with this species in past faunal surveys and its distribution may be more extensive than is currently known. Very little is currently known about this species other than that specimens infected with human malaria parasites have been found [31].

Anopheleslongirostris s.l., now known to be a complex of nine species, [61] is found only on the island of New Guinea. It has a wide distribution below 1000m [31, 81], but has been recorded in large numbers only in a few areas. Its generally low abundance may be due to its preference for jungle pools associated with dense vegetation for oviposition. Behavioural studies have found it to be zoophilic in some areas [27] and anthropophilic in others [64] and these differences in behaviour may possibly be explained by the presence of cryptic species, each exhibiting different host-feeding preferences [61]. Little is known about the biology of these species and the individual role that each species might play in malaria transmission. It has been incriminated as a vector of malaria in the Southern Plains and north of the central highlands in PNG [59, 75].

Anophelesbancroftii s.l. has a wide distribution throughout New Guinea [64, 81]. It is now known to be a species complex containing four independently evolving genotypes [39], although its status with respect to *An. barbiventris* is unknown. *Anopheles bancroftii* A is found throughout northern Australia and the Southern Plains of PNG where it is common, occurring in large numbers and readily biting humans. Genotype B occurs in Papua south of the central highlands and genotype D occurs in the inland river valleys north of the central highlands. The range of *An. bancroftii* C overlaps with genotypes B and D. genotypes B, C, and D are rarely collected near the coast and appear to prefer inland, lowland, river flood plains below 150m. In PNG the members of the *An. bancroftii* complex are rarely found anywhere in large numbers, except for the Southern Plains. Members of the complex have been incriminated as vectors of malaria at only a few locations [59, 75]. Larval habitats are mainly large permanent water bodies such as fresh water swamps and lagoons (Table 3, Fig.10 F). Nothing is yet known about the biology or behaviour of any of these putative species.

3.3. Possible vectors

There are several *Anopheles* species found throughout the southwest Pacific that feed on humans but are not very abundant and have limited distributions – in most cases, little is yet known about their biology or behaviour. These include *An. meraukensis, An. novaguinensis, An. torresiensis,* and *An. hilli* – all of which are found only on the Southern Plains of New Guinea (Fig. 1). All four species are common in northern Australia where a similar climate type also prevails [31, 85, 86]. In Australia these four species will readily bite humans, but in PNG nothing is known about the biology of these species except that *An. hilli* can occur in large numbers, will feed on humans, and will enter houses to do so [87]. *Anopheles hilli* was incriminated as a vector of malaria in Australia during a *Plasmodium vivax* epidemic in Cairns in 1942 [88]. These four species may be involved in malaria transmission but only as minor local vectors at best.

The members of the *Anopheles lungae* complex – *An. lungae, An. solomonis,* and *An. nataliae* – are endemic to the Solomon Islands where they are found on all major islands except Temotu, with *An. lungae* also being recorded from Bougainville [70, 89]. All three species have been recorded to bite humans and there is some circumstantial evidence incriminating *An. lungae* as a malaria vector [18]. On Santa Isabel, *An. solomonis* was found to be the dominant human biting anopheline in inland villages although they were also recorded biting pigs. This species fed outdoors, early in the evening (6pm-9pm) but was short-lived. In a sample of 221 mosquitoes collected via human landing catches, the proportion of parous was 0.33 [62]. No member of the *An. lungae* complex has been found infected with human malaria parasites although their human biting behaviour would make them possible vectors.

3.4. Non-vectors

Several *Anopheles* species present in the southwest Pacific are known not to feed on humans and this zoophilic behaviour precludes them from being vectors of malaria. These species include *An. annulipes* L and *An. annulipes* M, which are part of the *An. annulipes* complex – the members of which are widespread throughout Australia [90]. *Anopheles annulipes* L is found in a small enclave of monsoonal climate, which exists along the southern coast of Papua around Port Moresby, and within this limited distribution, it is quite common (Fig. 1). *Anopheles annulipes* M is a highland species common in intermontane valleys above

1000m [64]. Both species are readily found as larvae but are rarely collected feeding on humans [7, 64].

Anophelesirenicus (formally *An. farauti* 7) is endemic to the Solomon Islands, being recorded only on Guadalcanal. Larvae are commonly collected but the adults have never been recorded as biting humans [35, 51].

Anopheles sp. near *punctulatus* is an uncommon species with a patchy distribution restricted to the upland valleys of the central highlands in Papua New Guinea [31]. Nothing is yet known of its biology though it appears to have little association with humans.

Several species that occur in the region have limited distributions and are too uncommon to play any significant role in malaria transmission. These species include *An. papuensis* and *An. farauti* 5, two rarely recorded species from the highlands of PNG; *Anopheles clowi*, found on only two occasions since 1946 [19, 91]; and *An. rennellensis*, found only on the malaria-free island of Rennell in the Solomon Islands [25].

3.5. Oriental species

Five anopheline species – *An. annulatus, An. kochi, An. indefinitus, An. vanus*, and *An. vagus* – are Oriental species found as far east as the Moluccas Islands, which borders the Australian Region [18]. Two others – *An. karwari* and *An. subpictus* – have made substantial dispersals into New Guinea. While *An. tessellatus* has also been recorded in Papua Province and more recently in the Jayapura area (N. Lobo, unpublished data), it is not considered a vector in the Australian Region.

Anopheleskarwari was first reported in Jayapura in the 1930s where it was believed to be relatively common [92]. In PNG, the first record was from Maprik in 1960 [78], with subsequent confirmation by Hii and colleagues in 1997 [93] who also recorded it from the Maprik area where it made up 14% of the anophelines collected. Its distribution appears to be restricted to inland lowlands, and to foothills (up to 1000m) on the north side of the central highlands in PNG [31]. Nothing is known of its larval habits in PNG, but in Papua Province it was recorded from the edges of slow-moving watercourses, seepages, grassy pools, wheel ruts and hoof prints. *An. karwari* was first incriminated as a vector in 1955 in Papua Province [94]; in PNG it was positive for sporozoites in the Watut Valley inland from Lae [64], and in Maprik [75]. *Anopheles karwari* can be abundant but given its limited distribution, it is considered a secondary vector.

Anophelessubpictus occurs in the Moluccas, in Papua Province, and has been found on the islands of Biak and Misool. It has been found in several isolated populations in Papua New Guinea but only appears to be well established and common along the south coast of PNG from the Gulf of Papua to the D'Entrecasteaux Islands [64, 95]. It is a brackish water breeder and so is restricted to the coast. There are records of it biting humans and being infected with malaria at Bereina west of Port Moresby [95-97]. Apart from the population along the southern coastline of PNG, *An. subpictus* is uncommon with a limited distribution, and so is considered only a secondary vector.

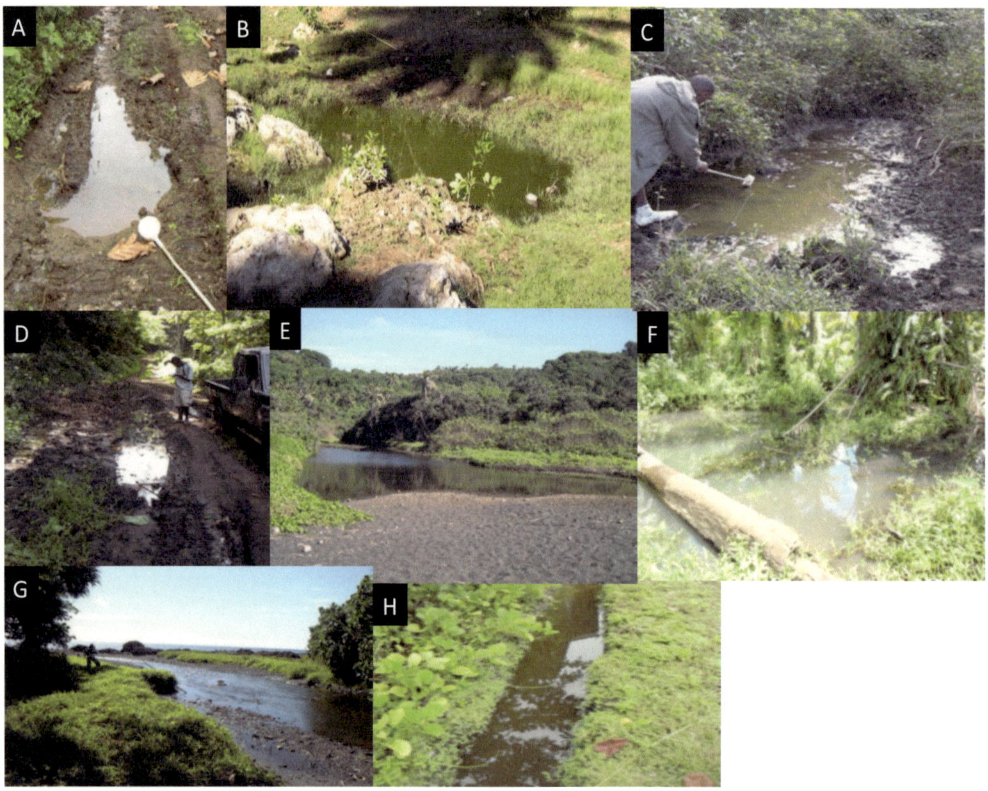

Figure 10. *Anopheles* larval sites as described in Table 3. **Panel A**, transient pool; **Panel B**, ground Pool; **Panel C**, pig wallow; **Panel D**, tyre track; **Panel E**, brackish swamp; **Panel F**, fresh water swamp; **Panel G**, edge of stream; **Panel H**, Drain.

4. Vector control

The strategy behind the use of indoor residual spraying (IRS) and insecticidal treated bed nets (ITNs) is to deliver insecticide to vectors which have entered the house to obtain a blood meal. Given that a female mosquito feeds every second or third night, it will seek a blood meal at least 3 to 5 times during the duration of the extrinsic incubation period, allowing 3 to 5 opportunities to contact the insecticide associated with IRS and ITNs before it develops sporozoites in the salivary glands. Ideally, for IRS and ITNs to successfully control malaria,

http://dx.doi.org/10.5772/55999

the vector should exhibit the following behaviours: a) be highly anthropophilic, b) feed indoors late at night when the humans are indoors, and c) rest on the insecticide treated surfaces of ITNs or IRS either before or after feeding.

The primary vectors in the southwest Pacific initially were reported to exhibit this type of behaviour to varying degrees. *Anopheles punctulatus* is the most anthropophilic of the three vectors [78, 98] and has a peak night-biting time around midnight [79]. *An. koliensis* is the next most anthropophilic and also feeds late at night [78, 79, 98]. On the other hand, *Anopheles farauti* is the least anthropophilic or most opportunistic species, and while it also had a peak feeding time around midnight, it starts feeding earlier in the evening at dusk [99] – when hosts are less likely to be inside or under nets. A pattern of early evening blood feeding was reported in the 1960's [65], 1970's [100] and 1980's [101]. While all species will readily enter houses to obtain a blood meal, none remain inside houses after sunrise [65, 99]. Thus while ITNs and IRS control may well be efficacious against late night biting *An. punctulatus* and *An. koliensis*, adaptation of *An. farauti* to feed primarily early in the evening [100] may minimize the opportunities to contract insecticides and thereby circumvent control efforts with IRS and ITNs.

With the implementation of the eradication program and subsequent control programs using DDT with IRS, populations of *An. punctulatus* were reduced to the point where adults and larvae of this species were virtually impossible to find. This was not an isolated occurrence but was found across all areas where these programs were implemented and the behaviours of the vectors were studied: Arso and Entrop in Papua Province; Maprik and Wewak in PNG; Rabaul in the islands of PNG; and in the Solomon Islands [100-103]. *Anopheles koliensis* populations were also suppressed by IRS though the extent of this suppression varied: in Arso, the reduction was short lived, while in PNG it appeared to be more sustained and in the Solomon Islands this species may have been eliminated [65, 72, 100].

Where *An. farauti*, populations were suppressed by IRS, they returned to pre-spray levels after only a few years [100, 101]. In Wewak, on the coast from Maprik, this happened after the first spray round, and in the Carteret Islands IRS had little effect on the population density of *An. farauti* [72].

Slooff [65] studied the house-visiting behaviour of *An. farauti* and observed that fewer mosquitoes entered DDT sprayed houses compared to the unsprayed houses and that their feeding success was less in sprayed houses. Thevasagayam [104] found that >45% of indoor-feeding *An. farauti* in the Solomon Islands left the house before picking up a lethal dose of insecticide. Slooff [65] suggested that this behaviour was due to an irritant effect of the DDT, a phenomenon that has been understood for some time [105] and which appeared to be pronounced in *An. farauti*.

Studies into the failure of IRS to adequately control populations of *An. farauti* revealed a major shift in the biting time of this species (and to some extent in *An. koliensis* as well) following IRS [65]. Before IRS *An. farauti* commenced feeding at dusk and built up to a peak at midnight [66, 79]. However following IRS, the majority of feeding occurred between 6pm and 8pm [66, 100]. A typical example was New Britain in 1963 where *An. farauti* before IRS with DDT fed throughout the night with a peak at midnight, but after five spray cycles (across two years) there was a distinct peak of feeding between 6pm-7pm, with 76% of feeding occurring before 9pm. [101]. It is common for the human populations in this region to spend the first hours of the night outdoors and so by feeding early in the night, *An. farauti* can obtain a blood meal without entering houses and being exposed to the insecticides used in IRS or ITNs. In the Solomon Islands this change in behaviour was believed responsible, in part, for the inability to interrupt transmission and the eventual failure of the eradication program [106].

This shift in biting time to early in the night appears fixed in some populations: when spraying was withdrawn, the early night-feeding pattern was maintained. In Temotu and Santa Isabel in the Solomon Islands, where DDT IRS was intensively applied during the eradication program of the early 1970s but only intermittently during the subsequent 35 years, *An. farauti* still displays the early night-biting pattern [62, 70]. In Temotu, with the resumption of a malaria elimination program in 2009 (based on the use of pyrethroids in IRS and distribution of ITNs), the early night-biting activity was further enforced with an increase in outdoor biting from 43% to 60% without any significant reduction in biting density post-intervention [70].

On Buka Island, in 1961 prior to spraying with DDT, *An. farauti*, *An. punctulatus*, and *An. koliensis* were all present. A post-spray survey conducted one year later found only *An. farauti* (see Spencer, unpublished report to the Department of Health, Malaria Control Program, Papua and New Guinea, 1961). DDT IRS on Buka continued for the next 20 years (40 spray rounds). Entomological surveys in 2000 failed to find *An. koliensis*; however at this time both *An. farauti* and *An. punctulatus* were abundant, indicating the reintroduction or recovery of the latter species. The night-biting pattern of *An. farauti* at this time showed the classical pre-spray pattern, that is, a rapid build-up in numbers from 6pm to a peak at midnight [48].

There were only a limited number of vector control strategies evaluated in the southwest Pacific in the decades following the cessation of the IRS-based elimination campaigns. While the DDT campaigns did not succeed in eliminating malaria, the campaigns were credited with the elimination of filariasis from the Solomon Islands where that disease was transmitted by the members of the *An. punctulatus* group [107]. Most of the subsequent vector control evaluations were trials of bed nets, either untreated or treated with pyrethroids. Trials evaluated entomological as well as parasitological impacts for malaria and/or filariasis as anophelines vector both of these parasitic diseases. A single-village longitudinal study of untreated bed nets in Madang Province of PNG showed that nets significantly reduced the human blood index of *An. punctulatus*, as well as the infection rates for the *Plasmodium falciparum* CS antigen and *Wuchereria bancrofti* for both early and late stage larvae [108]. On Bagabag Island of Madang, PNG, where *An. farauti* is the vector, one study [109] reported that users of untreated nets had significantly lower microfilariae and filarial antigen positivity rates than individuals not sleeping under bed nets, suggesting that nets were effective in limiting filariasis transmission by *An. farauti.*

The first study of permethrin treated nets in PNG reported significant reductions in the sporozoite rates in the *An. punctulatus* group in two villages as well as a significant reduction in *P. falciparum* incidence in children under the age of four years [10]. At the same time, Charlwood and Dagoro [110], working in a different part of PNG, found that permethrin-treated nets deterred members of the *An. punctulatus* group from entering houses. Prolonged

ITN use in PNG was associated with reduced sporozoite rates, a result hypothesized to be due to a reduction in mosquito survival [111]. Bockarie and Dagoro [112] reported that ITNs were more effective in protecting against *P. falciparum* in PNG and postulated that this was due to vivax-infected members of the *An. punctulatus* group feeding earlier than falciparum-infected mosquitoes.

In the Solomon Islands, ITNs had significantly greater impacts than IRS on vector infectivity and inoculation rates of *An. farauti* and *An. punctulatus*, however the reductions in the entomological inoculation rates were insufficient to effectively control malaria without additional interventions [68]. Later, Hii and colleagues [113] reported that ITNs in villages extended the length of the oviposition cycle by one day compared to DDT or untreated villages, and in 1993, Kere and colleagues reported a 71% reduction in biting rates of *An. farauti* on Guadalcanal, Solomon Islands following the introduction of ITNs but questioned the effectiveness of the nets given that people spend considerable time outside [114]. An analysis of facility-based data showed that both IRS with DDT and permethrin-treated ITNs are associated with reductions in malaria incidence and fever, while larviciding with temephos was not [115]. Recently, Bugoro and colleagues [70] found "little, if any, reduction in biting densities and no reduction in the longevity of the vector population" in Temotu Province of the Solomon Islands following the introduction of LLINs and IRS.

In Vanuatu, malaria was successfully eliminated from the island of Aneityum using a strategy of mass drug administration with pyrimethamine/sulfadoxine (Fansidar), and primaquine, ITNs and larvivorous fish. Falciparum malaria disappeared soon after the start of mass drug administrations [13]. The successful elimination was a function, most likely, of a small island population and the seasonality of transmission together with a high participation of the community in the mass drug administration. The impact of larvivorous fish was believed to be "probably marginal" due to the failure to find all breeding sites and the "incompleteness of predation".

Interpretation of the impact of these interventions must consider the period when the studies were conducted as reports of changes in behaviours of the vectors (discussed earlier) are known to have occurred; the effectiveness of an intervention is not static but is also dependent on the vectors' behaviours (e.g., shifts toward early feeding and outdoor biting may reduce the effectiveness of ITNs and IRS, as was demonstrated by Slooff [65], Taylor [100] and Sweeney [101]). Resistance to pyrethroids (and the existence of knock-down resistance genes) has not yet been found in the few studies thus far conducted in the southwest Pacific [116]; however, 30% of *An. koliensis* in Papua Province, Indonesia, were found to be resistant to DDT [117].

There is now a renewed interest in malaria control with IRS and ITNs in the Solomon Islands and Vanuatu with elimination programs in some areas and intensified control in all other areas. At the most fundamental level, the intervention measures of IRS and ITNS both rely on the vector feeding late at night when people are indoors. As such, these tools have the potential to provide effective control of late night biting *An. punctulatus* and *An. koliensis.* However it is important to emphasize that this behaviour pattern is no longer universally demonstrated by *An. farauti,* the primary coastal vector in the southwest Pacific.

The early biting pattern of the widely distributed *An. farauti* will prevent mosquito control and malaria elimination where this species bites early and outdoors and thereby avoids insecticides in IRS and ITNs. Therefore, additional control measures that target the vectors outside houses are now urgently needed for these programs to achieve effective reductions in malaria transmission. Effective larval control may be feasible with species such as *An. farauti*. Unlike *An. koliensis* and *An. punctulatus*, whose larvae are found in small ground pools that will be difficult to locate and treat where the annual rainfall is >2000mm, the most productive larval sites of *An. farauti* are large permanent coastal swamps and lagoons (Fig. 10 E) [62, 70, 118]. Such sites are easy to locate, few in number and permanent, and thus more easily treated.

5. Conclusion

In 2007, the Bill and Melinda Gates Foundation challenged the malaria community to once again attempt to achieve malaria eradication. The failure of the previous campaigns was due, in part, to attempting to control many vector species with a single intervention that targeted vectors inside houses. Enhancing our chances of eliminating malaria in the southwest Pacific will require the implementation of novel interventions that target vectors based on our knowledge of their behaviours. However, basic knowledge about the biology and behaviours of some vectors and potential vector species in this region is limited. This knowledge gap must be filled before control strategies can be optimized to exploit the vectors' biological vulnerabilities to control measures. The basic parameters essential to understanding transmission such as feeding habits, host preference, longevity, frequency of feeding and seasonal abundance – which are essential for the selection of effective control strategies –, await discovery for many species. Additionally, we remain uncertain of the complete distribution of species, or the importance of the various genotypes that have been recognized to date in a number of taxon.

Significant advances in DNA technologies have enhanced our ability to both discover and identify cryptic species in the southwest Pacific. These technologies, coupled with immunological and molecular assays to detect malaria parasites in mosquitoes, have led to the resurgence in investigations to incriminate vectors and to characterize their behaviors. We now know that there are 13 species in the *An. punctulatus* group (not three); that *An. longirostris* is not one zoophilic mosquito but a complex that includes human-biting malaria vectors; and that *An. bancroftii* is a complex of at least four species (not one as previously thought), two of which are malaria vectors. New studies on species-specific bionomic trails are enabling us to understand the biological basis for how they might be affected by interventions. Because of recent technological advances and their application to field studies, our knowledge on the major vectors in southwest Pacific is much better understood and as a consequence we are now better positioned than ever to study the species in this region and to design and evaluate novel and effective interventions.

Author details

Nigel W. Beebe[1*], Tanya L. Russell[2], Thomas R. Burkot[2], Neil F. Lobo[3] and Robert D. Cooper[4]

*Address all correspondence to: n.beebe@uq.edu.au

1 University of Queensland, St Lucia, Brisbane, Australia and CSIRO Ecosystem Sciences, Brisbane, Australia

2 James Cook University, Cairns, Australia

3 Eck Institute for Global Health, University of Notre Dame, Notre Dame, IN, USA

4 Australian Army Malaria Institute, Brisbane, Australia

References

[1] Black RH. Malaria in Australia. Canberra: Australian Government Publishing Service; 1972.

[2] Hanna JN, Ritchie SA, Eisen DP, Cooper RD, Brookes DL, Montgomery BL. An outbreak of *Plasmodium vivax* malaria in Far North Queensland, 2002. Med J Aust. 2004;180(1):24-8.

[3] Hay SI, Guerra CA, Gething PW, Patil AP, Tatem AJ, Noor AM, et al. A world malaria map: *Plasmodium falciparum* endemicity in 2007. PLoS Med. 2009;6(3):e1000048. Epub 2009/03/28.

[4] Peters W. Ecological factors limiting the extension of malaria in the Southwest Pacific - the bearing on malaria control or eradication programmes. Acta Trop. 1965;22:62-9.

[5] WHO. World malaria report : 2011. World Health Organisation, 2011.

[6] Spencer TET, Spencer M, Jemesen MT, Tommerup JWJ. Special Patrol Report: Malaria in the Mount Hagen area. PNG Med J. 1956;17:61-7.

[7] Peters W, Christian SH. Part V. Unstable highland malaria--the entomological picture. Trans R Soc Trop Med Hyg. 1960;54(6):537-42.

[8] Bangs MJ, Rusmiarto S, Anthony RL, Wirtz RA, Subianto DB. Malaria transmission by *Anopheles punctulatus* in the highlands of Irian Jaya, Indonesia. Ann Trop Med Parasitol. 1996;90(1):29-38. Epub 1996/02/01.

[9] Spencer M. The history of malaria control in the Southwest Pacific region, with particular reference to Papua-New-Guinea and the Solomon-Islands. P N G Med J. 1992;35(1):33-66.

[10] Graves PM, Brabin BJ, Charlwood JD, Burkot TR, Cattani JA, Ginny M, et al. Reduction in incidence and prevalence of *Plasmodium falciparum* in under 5-year-old children by permethrin impregnation of mosquito nets. Bull World Health Organ. 1987;65(6):869-77.

[11] Avery J. A review of the malaria eradication programme in the British Solomon Islands 1970-1972. PNG Med J. 1974;17:50-60.

[12] Kere JF, Kere NK. Bed-nets or spraying? Cost analyses of malaria control in the Solomon Islands. Health Policy and Planning. 1992;7(4):382-6.

[13] Kaneko A, Taleo G, Kalkoa M, Yamar S, Kobayakawa T, Bjorkman A. Malaria eradication on islands. Lancet. 2000;356(9241):1560-4. Epub 2000/11/15.

[14] The Ministries of Health of Vanuatu and Solomon Islands, The Pacific Malaria Initiative Survey Group, Shanks D. Malaria on isolated Melanesian islands prior to the initiation of malaria elimination activities. Malar J. 2010;9(1):218.

[15] McAlpine JR, Keig G, Fall F. Climate of Papua New Guinea. Canberra: 1983.

[16] Döntiz W. Nachrichten aus dem Berliner Entomologischen Verein. Inskten Börse. 1901;18:36-8.

[17] Laveran NA. Sur les Culicides des Nouvelles-Hebrides. C R Soc Biol Paris. 1902;54:908-10.

[18] Lee DJ, Hicks MM, Griffiths M, Debenham ML, Bryan JH, Russell RC, et al. The Culicidae of the Australasian region, Volume 5, Genus Anopheles. Debenham ML, editor. Canberra, Australia: Aust. Gov. Publ Serv.; 1987.

[19] Rozeboom LE, Knight KL. The *punctulatus* complex of *Anopheles* (Diptera: Culicidae). J Parasitol. 1946;32:95-131.

[20] Belkin JN. The mosquitoes of the South Pacific (Diptera: Culicidae): University of California Press, Berkeley; 1962.

[21] Bryan JH, Coluzzi M. Cytogenetic observations on *Anopheles farauti* Laveran. Bull World Health Organ. 1971;45(2):266-7.

[22] Bryan JH. *Anopheles farauti* Laveran from the New Hebrides. Trans R Soc Trop Med Hyg. 1981;75(2):331.

[23] Mahon RJ, Miethke PM. *Anopheles farauti* 3, a hitherto unrecognised biological species of mosquito within the taxon *A. farauti* (Diptera: Culicidae). Trans R Soc Trop Med Hyg. 1982;67:70-84.

[24] Bryan JH. Studies on the *Anopheles punctulatus* complex. I. Identification by proboscis morphological criteria and by cross-mating experiments. Trans R Soc Trop Med Hyg. 1973;67:64-9.

[25] Maffi M. Morphological observations on a population of the *punctulatus* Complex of *Anopheles* (Diptera, Culicidae) from Rennell Island (Solomon Group). Copenhagen: 1973.

[26] Taylor B, Maffi M. *Anopheles* (*Cellia*) *rennellensis*, A new species within the *punctulatus* complex of *Anopheles* (Diptera: Culicidae) from Rennell Island. The natural history of the Rennell Islands, British Solomon Islands. 1991;7.

[27] Charlwood JD, Dagoro H, Paru R. Blood-feeding and resting behaviour in the *Anopheles punctulatus* Dönitz complex (Diptera: Culicidae) from coastal Papua New Guinea. Bull Entomol Res. 1985;75(03):463-76.

[28] Sweeney AW. Larval salinity tolerances of the sibling species of *Anopheles farauti*. J Am Mosq Control Assoc. 1987;3(4):589-92.

[29] Woodhill AR. Observations on the morphology and biology of the subspecies of *Anopheles punctulatus* Döntiz. Proc Linn Soc NSW. 1946;70 276-87.

[30] Foley DH, Paru R, Dagoro H, Bryan JH. Allozyme analysis reveals six species within the *Anopheles punctulatus* complex of mosquitoes in Papua New Guinea. Med Vet Entomol. 1993;7(1):37-48.

[31] Cooper RD, Waterson DGE, Frances SP, Beebe NW, Sweeney AW. Speciation and distribution of the members of the *Anopheles punctulatus* (Diptera : Culicidae) group in Papua New Guinea. J Med Entomol. 2002;39(1):16-27.

[32] Schmidt ER, Foley DH, Bugoro H, Bryan JH. A morphological study of the *Anopheles punctulatus* group (Diptera: Culicidae) in the Solomon Islands, with a description of *Anopheles* (*Cellia*) *irenicus* Schmidt, sp.n. Bull Entomol Res. 2003;93(6):515-26.

[33] Schmidt ER, Foley DH, Hartel GF, Williams GM, Bryan JH. Descriptions of the *Anopheles* (*Cellia*) *farauti* complex of sibling species (Diptera: Culicidae) in Australia. Bull Entomol Res. 2001;91(5):389-411.

[34] Foley DH, Cooper RD, Bryan JH. A new species within the *Anopheles punctulatus* complex in Western Province, Papua New Guinea. J Am Mosq Control Assoc. 1995;11(1):122-7.

[35] Foley DH, Meek SR, Bryan JH. The *Anopheles punctulatus* group of mosquitoes in the Solomon Islands and Vanuatu surveyed by allozyme electrophoresis. Med Vet Entomol. 1994;8(4):340-50.

[36] Beebe NW, Cooper RD, Morrison DA, Ellis JT. A phylogenetic study of the *Anopheles punctulatus* group of malaria vectors comparing rDNA sequence alignments derived from the mitochondrial and nuclear small ribosomal subunits. Mol Phylogenet Evol. 2000;17(3):430-6.

[37] Bower JE, Cooper RD, Beebe NW. Internal repetition and intraindividual variation in the rDNA ITS1 of the *Anopheles punctulatus* group (Diptera: Culicidae): multiple units and rates of turnover. J Mol Evol. 2009;68(1):66-79.

[38] Beebe NW, Foley DH, Saul A, Cooper L, Bryan JH, Burkot TR. DNA probes for identifying the members of the *Anopheles punctulatus* complex in Papua New Guinea. Am J Trop Med Hyg. 1994;50(2):229-34.

[39] Beebe NW, Maung J, van den Hurk AF, Ellis JT, Cooper RD. Ribosomal DNA spacer genotypes of the *Anopheles bancroftii* group (Diptera: Culicidae) from Australia and Papua New Guinea. Insect Mol Biol. 2001;10(5):407-13.

[40] Henry-Halldin CN, Reimer L, Thomsen E, Koimbu G, Zimmerman A, Keven JB, et al. High throughput multiplex assay for species identification of Papua New Guinea malaria vectors: members of the *Anopheles punctulatus* (Diptera: Culicidae) species group. Am J Trop Med Hyg. 2011;84(1):166-73. Epub 2011/01/08.

[41] Mahon RJ. Identification of the three sibling species of *Anopheles farauti* Laveran by the banding pattern of their polytene chromosomes. J Aust Entomol Soc. 1983;22.

[42] Mahon RJ. The status and means of identifying the members of the *Anopheles farauti* Laveran complex of sibling species. In: Bryan JH, Moodie PM, editors. Malaria, Proceedings of a conference to honor Robert H Black. Canberra: Government Publishing Service; 1984. p. 152-6.

[43] Sweeney AW, Cooper RD, Frances SP. Distribution of the sibling species of *Anopheles farauti* in the Cape York Peninsula, northern Queensland, Australia. J Am Mosq Control Assoc. 1990;6(3):425-9.

[44] Cooper RD, Frances SP, Sweeney AW. Distribution of members of the *Anopheles farauti* complex in the Northern Territory of Australia. J Am Mosq Control Assoc. 1995;11(1):66-71.

[45] Foley DH, Bryan JH. Electrophoretic keys to identify members of the *Anopheles punctulatus* complex of vector mosquitoes in Papua New Guinea. Med Vet Entomol. 1993;7(1):49-53.

[46] Cooper L, Cooper RD, Burkot TR. The *Anopheles punctulatus* complex - DNA probes for identifying the Australian species using isotopic, chromogenic, and chemiluminescence detection systems. Exp Parasitol. 1991;73(1):27-35.

[47] Beebe NW, Foley DH, Cooper RD, Bryan JH, Saul A. DNA probes for the *Anopheles punctulatus* complex. Am J Trop Med Hyg. 1996;54(4):395-8.

[48] Cooper RD, Frances SP. Malaria vectors on Buka and Bougainville Islands, Papua New Guinea. J Am Mosq Control Assoc. 2002;18(2):100-6.

[49] Cooper RD. Preservation of anopheline mosquitoes for DNA probe analysis. J Am Mosq Control Assoc. 1998;14(1):58-60.

[50] Beebe NW, Saul A. Discrimination of all members of the *Anopheles punctulatus* complex by polymerase chain reaction--restriction fragment length polymorphism analysis. Am J Trop Med Hyg. 1995;53(5):478-81.

[51] Beebe NW, Bakote'e B, Ellis JT, Cooper RD. Differential ecology of *Anopheles punctulatus* and three members of the *Anopheles farauti* complex of mosquitoes on Guadalcanal, Solomon Islands, identified by PCR-RFLP analysis. Med Vet Entomol. 2000;14(3): 308-12.

[52] Bower JE, Dowton M, Cooper RD, Beebe NW. Intraspecific concerted evolution of the rDNA ITS1 in *Anopheles farauti* sensu stricto (Diptera: Culicidae) reveals recent patterns of population structure. J Mol Evol. 2008;67(4):397-411.

[53] Beebe NW, Cooper RD, Foley D, H., Ellis J, T. Populations of the south-west Pacific malaria vector *Anopheles farauti s.s.* revealed by ribosomal DNA transcribed spacer polymorphisms. Heredity. 2000;84(2):244-53.

[54] Ambrose L, Riginos C, Cooper RD, Leow KS, Ong W, Beebe NW. Population structure, mitochondrial polyphyly and the repeated loss of human biting ability in anopheline mosquitoes from the southwest Pacific. Mol Ecol. 2012. Epub 2012/07/04.

[55] Beebe NW, Ellis JT, Cooper RD, Saul A. DNA sequence analysis of the ribosomal DNA ITS2 region for the *Anopheles punctulatus* group of mosquitoes. Insect Mol Biol. 1999;8(3):381-90.

[56] Beebe NW, Cooper RD, Morrison DA, Ellis JT. Subset partitioning of the ribosomal DNA small subunit and its effects on the phylogeny of the *Anopheles punctulatus* group. Insect Mol Biol. 2000;9(5):515-20.

[57] Foley DH, Bryan JH, Yeates D, Saul A. Evolution and systematics of *Anopheles*: insights from a molecular phylogeny of Australasian mosquitoes. Mol Phylogenet Evol. 1998;9(2):262-75.

[58] Beebe NW, Cooper RD. Distribution and evolution of the *Anopheles punctulatus* group (Diptera: Culicidae) in Australia and Papua New Guinea. Int J Parasitol. 2002;32(5):563-74.

[59] Cooper RD, Waterson DG, Frances SP, Beebe NW, Pluess B, Sweeney AW. Malaria vectors of Papua New Guinea. Int J Parasitol. 2009;39:1495-501.

[60] Collins FH, Kamau L, Ranson HA, Vulule JM. Molecular entomology and prospects for malaria control. Bull World Health Organ. 2000;78(12):1412-23.

[61] Alquezar DE, Hemmerter S, Cooper RD, Beebe NW. Incomplete concerted evolution and reproductive isolation at the rDNA locus uncovers nine cryptic species within *Anopheles longirostris* from Papua New Guinea. BMC Evol Biol. 2010;10:392. Epub 2010/12/28.

[62] Bugoro H, Iro'ofa C, Mackenzie DO, Apairamo A, Hevalao W, Corcoran S, et al. Changes in vector species composition and current vector biology and behaviour

will favour malaria elimination in Santa Isabel Province, Solomon Islands. Malar J. 2011;10:287. Epub 2011/10/04.

[63] Reid JA, Knight KL. Classification within the subgenus *Anopheles* (Diptera: Culicidae). Ann Trop Med Parasitol Res. 1969;33:474–88.

[64] Cooper RD, Waterson DG, Frances SP, Beebe NW, Sweeney AW. The anopheline fauna of Papua New Guinea. J Am Mosq Control Assoc. 2006;22(2):213-21.

[65] Slooff R. Observations on the effect of residual DDT house spraying on behaviour and mortality in species of the *Anopheles punctulatus* group. Final report on a research project in West New Guinea [PhD Thesis]. Leyden, Netherlands: University of Leyden; 1964.

[66] Spencer M. Malaria in the D'Entrecasteaux Islands, Papua, with particular reference to *Anopheles farauti* Laveran. Proceedings of the Linnean Society of New South Wales. 1965;91(1):115-28.

[67] Burkot TR, Graves PM, Paru R, Wirtz RA, Heywood PF. Human malaria transmission studies in the *Anopheles punctulatus* complex in Papua New Guinea: sporozoite rates, inoculation rates, and sporozoite densities. Am J Trop Med Hyg. 1988;39(2): 135-44.

[68] Hii JL, Kanai L, Foligela A, Kan SK, Burkot TR, Wirtz RA. Impact of permethrin-impregnated mosquito nets compared with DDT house-spraying against malaria transmission by *Anopheles farauti* and *An. punctulatus* in the Solomon Islands. Med Vet Entomol. 1993;7(4):333-8. Epub 1993/10/01.

[69] Daggy RH. The biology and seasonal cycle of *Anopheles farauti* on Espirtu Santo, New Hebrides. Ann Entomol Soc Am. 1945;38(1):3-13.

[70] Bugoro H, Cooper RD, Butafa C, Iro'ofa C, Mackenzie DO, Chen CC, et al. Bionomics of the malaria vector *Anopheles farauti* in Temotu Province, Solomon Islands: issues for malaria elimination. Malar J. 2011;10:133. Epub 2011/05/20.

[71] Sweeney AW. Variations in density of *Anopheles farauti* Laveran in the Carteret Islands. P N G Med J. 1968;11(1):11-8.

[72] Spencer T, Spencer M, Venters D. Malaria vectors in Papua New Guinea. P N G Med J. 1974;17(1):22.

[73] Taylor B. Observations on malaria vectors of the *Anopheles punctulatus* complex in the British Solomon Islands Protectorate. J Med Entomol. 1975;11(6):677-87.

[74] Samarawickrema WA, Parkinson AD, Kere N, Galo O. Seasonal abundance and biting behaviour of *Anopheles punctulatus* and *An. koliensis* in Malaita Province, Solomon Islands and a trial of permethrin-impregnated bednets against malaria transmission. Med Vet Entomol. 1992;6:371-8.

[75] Hii JL, Smith T, Mai A, Ibam E, Alpers MP. Comparison between anopheline mosquitoes (Diptera: Culicidae) caught using different methods in a malaria endemic area of Papua New Guinea. Bull Entomol Res. 2000;90(3):211-9.

[76] Charlwood JD, Graves PM, Alpers MP. The ecology of the *Anopheles punctulatus* group of mosqutioes from Papua New Guinea: A review of recent work. P N G Med J. 1986;29:19–26.

[77] Horsfall WR, Porter DA. Biologies of two malaria mosquitoes in New Guinea. Ann Entomol Soc Am. 1946;39:549-60.

[78] Peters W, Standfast HA. Part II. Holoendemic malaria--the entomological picture. Trans R Soc Trop Med Hyg. 1960;54(3):249-54.

[79] Standfast HA. Biting times of nine species of New Guinea Culicidae (Diptera). J Med Entomol. 1967;4(2):192-6.

[80] Graves PM, Burkot TR, Saul A, Hayes RJ, Carter R. Estimation of Anopheline survival rate, vectoral capacity and mosquito infection probability from malaria vector infection rates in villages near Madang, Papua New Guinea. J App Ecol. 1990;27:124-47.

[81] Van Den Assem J, Van Dijk WJ. Distribution of anopheline mosquitoes in Netherlands New-Guinea. Trop Geogr Med. 1958;10(3):249-55. Epub 1958/09/01.

[82] Benet A, Mai A, Bockarie F, Lagog M, Zimmerman P, Alpers MP, et al. Polymerase chain reaction diagnosis and the changing pattern of vector ecology and malaria transmission dynamics in Papua New Guinea. Am J Trop Med Hyg. 2004;71(3): 277-84. Epub 2004/09/24.

[83] Burkot TR, Graves PM. The value of vector-based estimates of malaria transmission. Ann Trop Med Parasitol. 1995;89(2):125-34. Epub 1995/04/01.

[84] Lee DJ. Records of *Anopheles* (Diptera: Culicidae) from high altitudes in New Guinea. Aust J Sci. 1946;8:165.

[85] Cooper RD, Frances SP, Waterson DG, Piper RG, Sweeney AW. Distribution of anopheline mosquitoes in northern Australia. J Am Mosq Control Assoc. 1996;12(4): 656-63. Epub 1996/12/01.

[86] Cooper RD, Waterson DG, Kupo M, Foley DH, Beebe NW, Sweeney AW. Anopheline mosquitoes of the Western Province of Papua New Guinea. J Am Mosq Control Assoc. 1997;13(1):5-12.

[87] Van Den Assem J. A window-trap hut experiment to test the effects of dieldrin under local conditions in the Merauke area (Netherlands New Guinea). Trop Geogr Med. 1959;11(1):32-43. Epub 1959/03/01.

[88] Roberts FHS, O'Sullivan PJ. Studies on the behaviour of adult Australiasian anophelines. Bull Entomol Res. 1948;39:159-78.

[89] Taylor B, Maffi M. A review of the mosquito fauna of the Solomon Islands (Diptera: Culicidae). Pacific Insects. 1978;19(3-4):165-248.

[90] Foley DH, Wilkerson RC, Cooper RD, Volovsek ME, Bryan JH. A molecular phylogeny of *Anopheles annulipes* (Diptera: Culicidae) sensu lato: the most species-rich anopheline complex. Mol Phylogenet Evol. 2007;43(1):283-97.

[91] Cooper RD, Waterson DG, Bangs MJ, Beebe NW. Rediscovery of *Anopheles* (*Cellia*) *clowi* (Diptera: Culicidae), a rarely recorded member of the *Anopheles punctulatus* group. J Med Entomol. 2000;37(6):840-5. Epub 2000/12/29.

[92] Bonne-Wepster J, Swellengrebel NH. The anopheline mosquitoes of the Indo-Australian Region. In: de Bussy JH, editor. Amsterdam1953. p. 473-92.

[93] Hii JLK, Mai A, Mellor S, Lewis D, Alexander N, Alpers M. Spatial and temporal variation in abundance of *Anopheles* (Diptera: Culicidae) in a malaria endemic area in Papua New Guinea. J Med Entomol. 1997;34(2):193-205.

[94] Metselaar D. Some observations on *A. karwari* James. Doc Med Geog et Trop. 1955;7:193-6.

[95] Spencer M. A note on the distribution and prevalence of *Anopheles subpictus* grassi. P N G Med J. 1975;18(2):126-7. Epub 1975/06/01.

[96] Bang FB, Hairston NG, Maier J, Roberts FHS. DDT spraying inside houses as a means of malaria control in New Guinea. Trans R Soc Trop Med Hyg. 1947;40(6): 809-22.

[97] Afifi SE, Spencer M, Hudson PB, Tavil NW. Biting prevalence and malaria transmission patterns in the *Anopheles punctulatus* complex (Diptera: Culicidae) in Papua New Guinea. Aust J Exp Biol Med Sci. 1980;58(1):1-17. Epub 1980/02/01.

[98] Burkot TR, Dye C, Graves PM. An analysis of some factors determining the sporozoite rates, human blood indicies, and biting rates of members of the *Anopheles punctulatus* complex in Papua New Guinea. Am J Trop Med Hyg. 1989;40(3):229-34.

[99] Spencer M. Age-grouping of Anopheline female populations with particular reference to *Anopheles farauti* no. 1 Laveran 1906 revised by Bryan 1973 (Diptera: Culicidae) in Papua New Guinea. Geneva: World Health Organisation. WHO/MAL/76.865, 1976.

[100] Taylor B. Changes in the feeding behaviour of a malaria vector, *Anopheles farauti* Lav., following the use of DDT as a residual spray in houses in the British Solomon Islands Protectorate. Trans R Entomol Soc London. 1975;127:227-92.

[101] Sweeney AW. A review of chemical control of malaria vectors in the south west Pacific region. In: Laird M, Miles JW, editors. Integrated Mosquito Control Methodologies. London: Academic Press London; 1983. p. 143–58.

[102] Metselaar D. A pilot project of residual insecticide spraying in Netherlands New Guinea, contribution to the knowledge of holoendemic malaria. Acta Leiden. 1957;27:1-128. Epub 1957/01/01.

[103] Peters W. A critical survey of the results of malaria-eradication and control programmes in the South-West Pacific. Ann Trop Med Parasitol. 1962;56:20-32. Epub 1962/04/01.

[104] Thevasagayam ES. Malaria control strategies in the Southwest Pacific countries - reappraisal. Proceedings of the Ninth South-West Pacific Malaria Meeting Sydney, Australia. 1983.

[105] Kennedy JS. The excitant and repellent effects on mosquitoes of sublethal contacts with DDT. Bull Entomol Res. 1947;37:593-607.

[106] Paik Y-H, Avery JG. Problem areas in the malaria eradication programme in the British Solomon Islands. P N G Med J. 1973;17(1):61-7.

[107] Webber RH. Eradication of *Wuchereria bancrofti* infection through vector control. Trans R Soc Trop Med Hyg. 1979;73:722-4.

[108] Burkot TR, Garner P, Paru R, Dagoro H, Barnes H, Barnes A, et al. Effects of untreated bed nets on the transmission of *Plasmodium falciparum, P. vivax* and *Wuchereria bancrofti* in Papua New Guinea. Trans R Soc Trop Med Hyg. 1990;84:773-9.

[109] Bockarie MJ, Tavul L, Kastens W, Michael E, Kazura JW. Impact of untreated bednets on prevalence of *Wuchereria bancrofti* transmitted by *Anopheles farauti* in Papua New Guinea. Med Vet Entomol. 2002;16(1):116-9.

[110] Charlwood JD, Dagoro H. Impregnated bed nets for the control of filariasis transmitted by *Anopheles puntulatus* in rural Papua New Guinea. P N G Med J. 1987;30:199-202.

[111] Hii JLK, Smith T, Vounatsou P, Alexander N, Mai A, Ibam E, et al. Area effects of bednet use in a malaria-endemic area in Papua New Guinea. Trans R Soc Trop Med Hyg. 2001;95(1):7-13.

[112] Bockarie MJ, Dagoro H. Are insecticide-treated bednets more protective against *Plasmodium falciparum* than *Plasmodium vivax*-infected mosquitoes? Malar J. 2006;5:15.

[113] Hii JL, Birley MH, Kanai L, Foligeli A, Wagner J. Comparative effects of permethrin-impregnated bednets and DDT house spraying on survival rates and oviposition interval of *Anopheles farauti* No. 1 (Diptera:Culicidae) in Solomon Islands. Ann Trop Med Parasitol. 1995;89(5):521-9. Epub 1995/10/01.

[114] Kere NK, Parkinson AD, Samrawickerema WA. The effect of permethrin impregnated bednets on the incidence of *Plasmodium falciparum*, in children of north Guadalcanal, Solomon Islands. Southeast Asian J Trop Med Public Health. 1993;24(1):130-7. Epub 1993/03/01.

[115] Over M, Bakote'e B, Velayudhan R, Wilikai P, Graves PM. Impregnated nets or DDT residual spraying? Field effectiveness of malaria prevention techniques in Solomon Islands, 1993-1999. Am J Trop Med Hyg. 2004;71(2 Suppl):214-23. Epub 2004/08/28.

[116] Keven JB, Henry-Halldin CN, Thomsen EK, Mueller I, Siba PM, Zimmerman PA, et al. Pyrethroid susceptibility in natural populations of the *Anopheles punctulatus* Group (Diptera: Culicidae) in Papua New Guinea. Am J Trop Med Hyg. 2010;83(6): 1259-61.

[117] Bangs MJ, Annis BA, Bahang ZH, Hamzah N, Arbani PR. Insecticide susceptibility status of *Anopheles koliensis* (Diptera: Culicidae) in northeastern Irian Jaya, Indonesia. Southeast Asian J Trop Med Public Health. 1993;24(2):357-62. Epub 1993/06/01.

[118] Bugoro H, Hii J, Russell TL, Cooper RD, Chan BK, Iro'ofa C, et al. Influence of environmental factors on the abundance of *Anopheles farauti* larvae in large brackish water streams in Northern Guadalcanal, Solomon Islands. Malar J. 2011;10:262. Epub 2011/09/14.

Section 3

Ecology and Spatial Surveillance

Chapter 13

Ecology of Larval Habitats

Eliška Rejmánková, John Grieco, Nicole Achee and Donald R. Roberts

Additional information is available at the end of the chapter

http://dx.doi.org/10.5772/55229

1. Introduction

Mosquito-borne diseases, including malaria are undergoing a global resurgence [1-7]. The factors responsible for the re-emergence are very complex, and management requires integrated cooperation at many levels, however, a need to better understand the ecology of disease vectors remains critical for any control program to succeed. In the case of malaria, the spatial and temporal changes in anopheline mosquito abundance, quantification of transmission potential of vector populations, characterizations of climatic conditions, and description of distributions of host (human) populations are necessary prerequisites for predicting high-risk malaria areas and implementing an effective disease control program [5, 8]. Tools such as remote sensing and geographic information systems (GIS), which are increasingly being used in studies of disease transmission and vector ecology have greatly enhanced our abilities to analyze landscape level relationships of vectors and diseases. Yet these tools can be successfully used only in combination with a thorough understanding of ecologic and epidemiologic processes of disease transmission.

Among the most important determinants of adult mosquito abundance and distribution is the presence and quality of larval habitats.[1] An understanding of the dynamics and productivity of larval habitats in the changing environment is required if efforts to model and predict adult abundance and ultimately limit the disease spread are to succeed [8-12]. While biology of adult mosquitoes has been reviewed from multiple perspectives [13-15], there has been no recent comprehensive review of mosquito larval habitats.[2]

1 terms larval habitat, breeding site, breeding habitat have been used interchangeably for descriptions of places where mosquito females oviposit eggs, larvae hatch, grow and pupate [16]. We will be using the term larval habitat throughout the paper.

2*Anopheles* species included in Sinka's et al [17] list of dominant vector species plus *An. vestitipennis* have been included in this review.

A vast amount of literature on malaria vectors is available. More than 60 years ago, Marston Bates wrote in the Introduction to his The Natural History of Mosquitoes: "Mosquitoes in general, and the malaria carriers in particular, have been the subject of a tremendous amount of study, whose results have been reported in the voluminous literature. Much of this literature is an uncritical accumulation of facts that were easy to record, or of facts that were related to some momentarily fashionable subject of study, or of facts that were needed for the attainment of some immediately practical objective. This accumulation awaits to be converted into an orderly and useful structure of knowledge" [18]. It is hard not to feel the same today, with the Web of Science responding with > 600 references to an inquiry for *Anopheles* larval habitats. We won't be able to provide "an orderly and useful structure of knowledge" in this short chapter, but we will attempt to cover a few important topics:

–History of description of larval habitats

–Determinants of larval habitats

–Habitat selection

–Landscape context

–Human impact and adjustment to new habitats

–Implications for vector control

–Future priorities

Research and reporting efforts and resulting available information are disproportionately distributed and heavily skewed towards the most important malaria vector, *An. gambiae* with over 5440 references in the Web of Science, followed by *An. stephensi, An. arabiensis* and *An. funestus* with 1557, 744 and 537 references respectively. The majority of remaining species from Sinka's [17] list are referenced < 200 times with the exception of *An. albimanus, An. quadrimaculatus, An. darlingi* and *An. dirus* referenced 592, 456, 264 and 255 times, respectively. However, in most cases these species are primary vector species. In considering potential vector replacement following the environmental change (see examples further in the text) it will be important to keep in mind that secondary, little studied and less efficient, vector species might be found replacing primary malaria vector species.

2. History of description of larval habitats

Much of what we know about the detailed behavior of individual insect vectors resulted from observations made during the pre-DDT era of the 1920's and 1930's [8, 19], when programs for malaria control through environmental management and regular larvicidal treatment of larval habitats were developed across Europe, Middle East, Asia, and the Americas [20, 21]. Examples of successful treatment schemes [21] show that they were all accomplished based on a good knowledge of larval ecology. The concept that the prevalence of malaria can more effectively be reduced by destroying vector mosquitoes in their adult stage than in their aquatic, larval stages became central to antimalarial efforts practiced throughout the world's tropical regions beginning first with pyrethrum and later with DDT spraying. Success of those efforts led start-up of the Global Malaria Eradication Strategy, GMES [20, 22]. One of the unfortunate consequences of GMES was a substantial reduction in funding for research related to larval ecology, it was even credited with "exterminating more medical entomologists than mosquitoes" [20]. However, as early as 1983, Service [23] pointed out that "the general disillusionment with chemical control methods has led to the resurrection of biological control from the pre-DDT era" and although funding has not been easy to come by, the 1990's saw an exponential increase in studies on larval ecology and larval habitats. Laird's The Natural History of Laval Mosquito Habitats [24] provided an important source of information.

Although earlier papers are not often cited in the contemporary literature, there are several reasons why older papers are important and should not be ignored:

They provide records of species distributions: The older papers often describing simple surveys or even just few locations where a particular species was found provide historical evidence of species distribution prior to human interference [25, 26]. *Example:* Positive records of the presence of *An. darlin*gi in southern Belize (then British Honduras) published by Komp [25] and Kumm and Ram [26] and a report of absence of this species 30 years later by Bertram [27], made one of the authors of this chapter (DR) suspects that disappearance of *An. darlingi* was most probably a response to DDT house-spraying [28]. The species was eventually recorded again from Belize (a consequence of the interruption of DDT-spraying?). The whole story points to the need to continuously study changing roles of malaria vectors in different geographical areas.

They contain important ecological and ecophysiological observations: Already in the 1940's mosquito entomologists realized what many recent papers present as a new discovery, i.e., that human interference can lead to a vector change. As described by Muirhead-Thomson [29] from the coastal zones of Sierra Leone, draining and dyking of mangroves, which used to be very productive habitats for *An. melas*, and changing land use to rice cultivation, resulted in very productive habitat for *An. gambiae* and eventual replacement of *An. melas* by *An. gambiae*. Goma [30, 31] discarded a long time belief that high incidence of malaria in Uganda is related to the extensive papyrus swamps hypothesizing [30, 31] and eventually experimentally proving [32] that interior of a papyrus swamp is unsuitable for anophelines and only the swamps altered by human activities are significant providers of larval habitats. Numerous interesting observations and results of simple experiments on oviposition and larval development as influenced by environmental factors were published [18, 33] and are well summarized in Bates's Natural History of Mosquitoes [34].

There can be a good information on well executed larval control: A series of detailed studies on larval habitats originated from the US Tennessee Valley Authority, TVA (TVA is a federally owned corporation in the US created in 1933 to provide navigation and flood control, electricity generation, fertilizer manufacturing and economic development in the Tennessee Valley, a region strongly affected by the Great Depression; http://www.tva.com/abouttva/history.htm).

This watershed area of the fifth largest river system in the United States was transformed into a series of reservoirs encompassing more than 11,000 miles of shoreline. Because the impoundment of the river provided enhanced breeding opportunities for *An. quadrimaculatus* in (then) malaria-endemic region, antimalarial measures were required as integral parts of all TVA projects. The general philosophy was to control mosquito breeding through natural measures and limit larvicidal and other temporary controls to an absolute minimum [35]. Papers by Hinman et al [36], Penfound [37], Hess and Hall [38], Hall [39] focused on the importance of aquatic vegetation in anopheline larval habitats (see section on Vegetation).

Older correlative studies can provide a good starting point for hypotheses testing through experimental studies: Starting in early 1990's there is a progression of studies that include habitat characteristics and attempts to relate the presence of larvae to these characteristics [17, 40-51]. An important change compared to the majority of older papers was that in these correlative studies, environmental characteristics of both, larvae positive and negative habitats were recorded. As more information became available on the relationships between larval presence and habitat characteristics, attempts to classify anopheline larval habitats appeared. As an example Rejmankova et al. [44] classified larval habitats of *An. albimanus* on the coastal plain of Chiapas into 16 habitat-types based on the dominant aquatic vegetation. The goal was a hierarchical system of habitat classification that could be universally used for larval habitat description in the study area and it became a basis for many future studies on larval ecology by the Tapachula-based Center for Malaria Studies [52-54]. The analytical methods and hierarchical system described in Rejmankova et al [44] article are applicable to a wide range of studies on phytoecological relationships of vectors to aquatic habitats.

The need for regional classification of larval habitats into higher units became more urgent with the increasing use of remote sensing technology in malaria vector studies [55-57]. The step-wise approach (paradigm) advocated by Roberts and Rodriguez [58] became widely applied [59, 60]. These steps included the following: 1) developing an understanding of vector ecology and defining the environmental determinants for its presence and abundance (this step is based on field studies); 2) constructing a database that characterizes the landscape elements associated with the important aspects of vector biology and human habitation (RS and GIS are suitable tools for this step); and 3) formulating and verifying predictions of vector abundance.

Recently, studies describing larval habitats of anophelines were included in the global database on 41 dominant vector species, DVS, of human malaria. The contemporary distribution of each of the DVS, alongside a comprehensive description of the ecology and behavior of each species, has been published in a series of papers by Sinka and coauthors [17, 61-63]. The authors stated that simple, universal species-specific statements regarding the biology of these vectors are nearly impossible due to the behavioral plasticity of most species, in some cases sympatric distributions of sibling species, changing taxonomic categorization and the influence of environmental disturbance, all contributing to a high level of complexity.

While the descriptive and correlative studies of larval habitats have mushroomed in the 1990's and 2000's, good experimental studies explaining the hypothetical relationships between larvae and the habitat characteristics are still relatively lacking. They are increasingly called for [11, 22], e.g., by proposing development and application of enclosed, pathogen-free, semi-field mesocosms in which vector populations can be experimentally manipulated. There are a few exceptions such as Goma's [31] study from the papyrus swamps in Uganda. Based on his observations on the absence of *An. gambiae* larvae from the swamp interior, Goma hypothesized that the larvae are not found there because the conditions are unfavorable for their development. He conducted a series of experiments in which known amounts of larvae of different instars were placed in floating cages in different locations throughout a swamp and confirmed that larvae in the swamp interior suffered significantly higher mortality and those surviving took longer to develop into adults than larvae in cages placed at the swamp periphery. The high mortality has been later explained as a result of inhibition of larval breathing due to the surface layer of oil produced by papyrus [64]. For other examples of hypotheses driven experimental studies see, e.g., [10, 65-76] and other examples provided in further text.

2.1. Dichotomy between medical entomologists and ecologists in larval studies

There has been quite a deep divide between medical entomologists and ecologist in their approach to studying mosquito larval habitats [22, 77]. Medical entomologists generally study larval habitats with the focus on design of efficient control interventions and often don't realize that it is the ecological approach to studying larval habitats in the context of other ecosystem components that can eventually lead to a thorough understanding of the larvae – habitat relationships. A relatively small number of researchers realize that filling the gap between ecologically based and epidemiologically based information is a necessity [77]. As Chase and Knight [78] put it: because larval mosquitoes are components of a much larger metacommunity of interacting species, the interplay between biotic interactions (competitors and predators) and abiotic constraints (temperature, habitat drying) is essential for understanding the controls on mosquito abundance. By placing mosquitoes into a broader community context, a much better predictive framework can be developed for understanding and predicting year-to-year variation in mosquito abundances [79, 80]. Ecology should—like other basic disciplines such as molecular biology and bioinformatics—be considered an enabling science essential for defining the target product profiles of completely new control technologies and delivery systems [22].

3. Environmental determinants of larval habitats

Larval habitats or breeding sites - places where eggs are laid, larvae hatch, change instars, pupate, and adults emerge - are primary drivers of adult distribution, abundance and fitness [5, 9, 10, 81]. They are always composed of water bodies, natural or man-made, permanent or temporary, large or small, freshwater or saline. The mosquito reproduction is successful only if larval habitats remain stable for a duration equivalent to the development of immature stages [82]. The great diversity of habitats, often combined with inaccessibility, makes studies of the ecology of larval anopheline mosquitoes methodologically quite difficult [9].

Larval densities are controlled by interactions between abiotic (hydrology, temperature, light/shade, pH, salinity, nutrient availability) and biotic (predation, competition) factors [78, 83-85]. For comprehensive analyses of patterns in the productivity of larval habitats the studies should incorporate a landscape context, because presence and abundance of mosquito larvae in aquatic habitats and consequently the number of adults capable of malaria transmission are regulated by a variety of ecosystem processes operating and interacting at several organizational levels and spatial/temporal scales [86]. The conceptual scheme in Figure 1 summarizes the main factors and processes important for good understanding of interactions between larvae and their habitat characteristics in the larger ecosystem context. Humans can affect habitat availability and quality through ecosystem and landscape changes such deforestation/reforestation, desertification, irrigation and other hydrological changes, and agricultural practices (see further). In the following text we will focus on the main determinants of larval development.

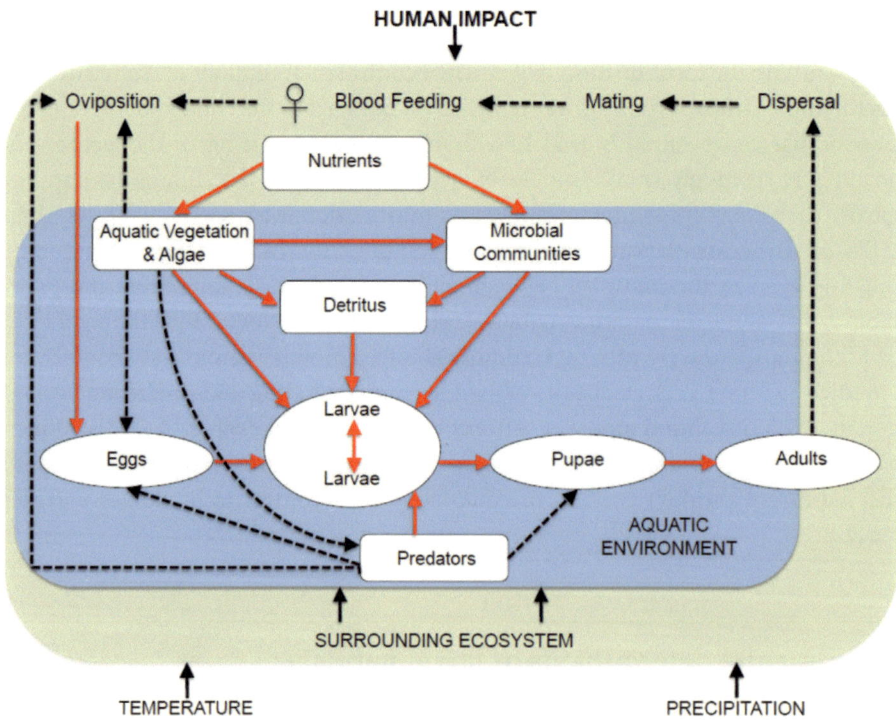

Figure 1. Relationships between larval development and environmental factors on both habitat and ecosystem level. The relationships reviewed in the chapter are indicated in red.

3.1. Temperature

Temperature affects all the important processes such as the rate of larval development and survivorship, pupation rates, larval-to-adult survivorship and larval-to adult development time [81, 87-89]. Water temperature is influenced by various parameters, such as local climate, water depth and movement, habitat size and geometry, land cover type or canopy overgrowth, presence of vegetation and/or algae, soil properties and turbidity [81]. Despite its importance, there are not many detailed outdoor studies on the temperature of larval habitats and the available data are hard to compare due to different methods of temperature measurement (air temperature vs. water temperature; data loggers vs. hand-held thermometers). Available data on *An. gambiae* point to a consensus that one of the main reasons for higher productivity of *An. gambiae* and *An. funestus* in habitats associated with agricultural crops or swamp margins is higher temperature as compared to shaded dense papyrus swamps [72, 90, 91]. Additional proof comes from Wamae et al [88] who compared *An. gambiae* densities in shaded (by napier grass, *Pennisetum purpureum*) and unshaded water channels in reclaimed sites in Western Kenya highlands. In these studies, the shading reduced anopheline larvae by >75%, apparently due to ~3 degrees C reduced water temperature. High water temperature pools (30-33 degrees C) were reported as the most productive habitats for *An. gambiae* in Gambia [92]. In South America, Marten et al [93] found the majority of *An. albimanus* larvae on the coastal plain of Colombia associated with sun-exposed sites with a mid-day temperature range of 27.5 - 30.0° C. Pinault and Hunter [94] report minimum water temperatures that might limit the upper altitudinal distribution of *An. albimanus* (18.7° C) and *An. pseudopunctipennis* (16.0° C). Larvae are not generally able to survive temperatures over 40 degrees C as documented by Muirhead-Thomson [29] for *An. minimus*, (but see *An. bwambae* in hot springs, [95]). Recent detailed study on the longevity and mortality of *An. gambiae* under a wide range of temperatures [87] concluded that under extremely cold (10–12°C) or hot (38–40°C) temperatures all larvae died within a few days. While the low temperature range is rarely experienced in larval habitats of *An. gambiae*, the higher temperatures are frequently encountered in most tropical regions. In nature, however, such high temperatures occur for no more than a few hours and larvae may survive these short periods.

Paaijmans et al [81, 96] stressed the importance of temperature fluctuations for larval development. The authors provided a conceptual model of radiation and energy fluxes at the air–water and soil–water interfaces of small, shallow and clear water pools and did filed measurements comparing smaller and larger water bodies [81]. In general, the small-sized water pool reacted more dynamically to suddenly changing meteorological variables and experienced larger fluctuations. Several important conclusions follow from these experiments: The top layer (upper 2 mm) of each water pool differed in temperature from the layers underneath, which has important consequences for larval dynamics as anopheline larvae generally live horizontally near the air–water interface of aquatic habitats [66]. There can be large differences (> 10 degrees C) between air and water temperature. Larger pools had larger buffering capacity. Mosquito immatures can be exposed to a wide temperature range under natural conditions and they are apparently evolutionarily adapted to their direct environment. The observed differences between air and water temperature have important consequences and should be carefully employed for ecological models that use the air temperature as an input parameter for larval development.

3.2. Light

There are species occurring mostly in sun-exposed environments such as *An. gambiae* s.s., *An. albimanus, An. pseudopunctipennis*, members of the *An. sundaicus* complex, *An. sinensis, An. aconitus* etc., while others seem to prefer shaded water bodies (*An. funestus, An. vestitipennis*). The question of whether sun or shade has a direct effect on the development of larvae or impacts them indirectly through the effect of temperature on food source development has not been answered, although some laboratory experiments seem to show that light is not an important direct factor [83, 97]. It is possible that in some instances, larvae are positively correlated with shaded environment only because shade of trees reduces drying speed of the pools [98]. Little is known about the effects of darkness on larval development in *Anopheles* species. It has been shown, however, that light deprivation causes a significant reduction in the development of adult *An. stephensi* when larvae were bred in the absence of light [33]. In the dark treatment group, only about 60% of pupae transformed into adults.

3.3. Salinity

There are large differences in the tolerance of anopheline larvae to water salinity. While the majority of anopheline larvae are found in fresh waters, there are several species that show high salinity tolerance and are associated with coastal malaria transmission. *Anopheles melas* and *An. merus* within the *An. gambiae* complex are examples from Africa [61]. *Anopheles farauti* s.s. and *An. irenicus* (formerly designated *An. farauti* No. 7) in the Farauti Complex are reported to be salinity-tolerant in Australasia [63, 99]. Malaria vectors of the *An. sundaicus* complex in Southeast Asia are well known brackish water breeders [100, 101]. On the American continent an example of salt tolerant species is *An. aquasalis* [48, 102].

A major challenge faced by all mosquito larvae is the tendency for larval habitats to fluctuate widely in salinity due to changes in rainfall and evaporation [13]. Organisms living in brackish and saline environments have evolved various mechanisms of coping with increased salinity, and in order to survive in these conditions, they have to be able to regulate their osmotic potential. Larvae of salinity tolerant mosquito possess cuticles that are less permeable to water than freshwater forms, and their pupae have thickened and sclerotized cuticles that are impermeable to water and ions. Larval survival depends upon the ability to regulate hemolymph osmolarity by absorbing and excreting ions [103]. Osmoregulatory mechanisms vary among various mosquito genera, for example *An. albimanus* larvae osmoregulate through rectal ion excretion and the larvae undergo a dramatic shift in rectal $Na+/K+$-ATPase (an enzyme important for ion regulation) localization when reared in freshwater *vs.* saline water [103].

Saltwater tolerance is a trait that involves ionic regulation at the aquatic larval stage, and it appears to have been a factor in the adaptive radiation of the *A. gambiae* complex into diverse larval habitats. A mechanistic understanding of the physiology and genetics of ion regulation is important because it can open up new classes of larvicide [104]. Additionally, increasing amounts of saltwater pools and puddles associated with natural disasters (tsunami), land subsidence, or sea level rise would facilitate increased breeding of brackish water malaria vectors (e.g., *An. sundaicus*) and may increase the risk of malaria outbreaks [105, 106].

3.4. Hydrology and geomorphology

Hydrology of a region, i.e., distribution and seasonal dynamics of lotic and lentic water bodies is determined by the geomorphology and precipitation patterns [107, 108]. Water quality in these different water bodies is influenced by rock and soil chemistry, vegetation of the surrounding landscape, and human activities. Both hydrology and water chemistry determine the type of aquatic vegetation present in lakes, pools, and streams [42]. Geomorphological parameters such as elevation, slope, aspect, and ruggedness play an important role in malaria transmission as exemplified, e.g., by Atieli [108] who found broad flat-bottomed valleys in Kenya Highlands to have a significantly higher number of *Anopheles* larvae/dip in their habitats than the narrow valleys. Heavy rains in the tropics can be detrimental to larval survival. In particular, rainstorms are known to flush mosquito larvae from their breeding sites [109, 110] – but see Manguin et al. [47] who reported survival of 3rd and 4th instar larvae in clumps of detritus that was stranded in trees and shrubs in the wake of the flood.

3.5. Vegetation

Many shallow water bodies are dominated by aquatic plants – both microphytes (algae and cyanobacteria) and macrophytes.

Aquatic macrophytes, often also called hydrophytes, are key components of aquatic and wetland ecosystems. As primary producers, they are at the base of herbivorous and detritivorous food chains, providing food to invertebrates, fish and birds, and organic carbon for bacteria. Their stems, roots and leaves serve as a substrate for periphyton, and a shelter for numerous invertebrates and different stages of fish, amphibians and reptiles [66, 111]. Biogeochemical processes in the water column and sediments are to a large extent influenced by the presence/absence and type of macrophyte, and macrophytes can also have a profound impact on water movement and sediment dynamics in water bodies [112].

Phytoecological relationships of many species are strong enough to indicate presence or absence of mosquitoes according to presence or absence of associated plants [44]. The effect of aquatic plants on mosquito oviposition and larval survival and development, particularly among the anophelines, has been recognized since the early 1930's [38, 39, 66, 113-115]. Many aquatic plants provide food and protection for mosquito larvae and create favorable conditions for oviposition. Of special importance is the interface of air-plant-water, which has been termed the intersection line [38]. The intersection line is important to anopheline larvae because it is where the larvae find food and shelter and adults find the water surface broken up into numerous quiet cells favorable for ovipositing [19, 66]. A number of studies have documented a positive correlation between larval density and amount of plant cover or intersection line, e.g., [38, 115-118]. Plants provide favorable conditions for anopheline production if they continuously intersect the water surface during the mosquito breeding season. Collins and Resh [118] present a table showing the evaluation of common wetland plants for habitat suitability including the intersection line value.

Aquatic macrophytes are extremely diverse taxonomically, morphologically and functionally. Thus it is not surprising that different groups of macrophytes provide suitable habitats for different mosquito species (Figure 2). Of the four major macrophyte categories, i.e., freely floating, emergent, submerged, and floating-leaved [112], emergents generally provide the largest number of intersection lines. The positive benefits associated with aquatic macrophyte cover, and dense patches of emergent plants in particular, should result in a strong selective advantage (i.e., increased fitness) to individuals that choose high density macrophyte patches as habitat [66]. Selective pressure for such habitat preferences should operate on both larval and adult stages of *Anopheles* and the strong preferences of larvae and ovipositing adults for higher density patches of *Myriophyllum* were indeed observed by Orr and Resh [66].

While the majority of anopheline species are rather generalists and not very selective for a particular type of vegetation, there are others with tighter phytoecological associations. *Anopheles gambiae* is an example of a generalist whose larval habitats are shallow temporary water bodies with algae or short grasses but also devoid of any vegetation [61], see Figure 2H and papers of Mutuku et al. [119] and Ndenga et al. [89] for illustrations. Among examples of an extremely close association are the larval habitats of *An. pseudopunctipennis,* which are typically sun-exposed streams with abundant filamentous algae [42, 94, 120-124], see Figure 2E. The selection of filamentous algae by *An. pseudopunctipennis* has been confirmed by oviposition experiments [125, 126]. Similarly, the presence and abundance of *An. farauti* larvae was positively associated with filamentous algae in Solomon Islands [99]. Another species whose habitat can be clearly defined by vegetation presence is *An. vestitipennis.* Numerous reports confirm its association with tall dense macrophytes and/or flooded swamp forest [127-130] see Figure 2A. It is perhaps the preference of *An. vestitipennis* for a shaded environment generally that results in it being associated with these two types of habitats [129]. Preferred habitats for *An. darlingi* are patches of detritus often accumulated behind a fallen stump, or vegetation at the shady edges in slowly running streams and rivers [26, 42, 47, 73, 82] see Figure 2F. Barros et al [82] call these habitats "microdams" and they found the presence of microdams to be the most important parameter determining spatial distribution of *An. darlingi* larvae in northern Brazilian Amazon. Achee et al [73] experimentally evaluated the importance of floating detritus patches and overhanging bamboo for *An. darlingi* habitat selection using floating screened enclosures placed in a river at a location with documented presence of both larval and adult *An. darlingi* populations. The detritus treatment had a significantly higher average count of *An. darlingi* larvae documenting that females preferentially oviposited in this habitat.

Even with these tight associations, there are often exceptions, e.g., *An. pseudopunctipennis* found in tall dense macrophytes (*Schoenoplectus californicus*) in the coastal zones of Peru (DR, ER unpublished data), or even without vegetation [124], but these snapshot observations on larval presence don't really provide information about survival and adult fitness.

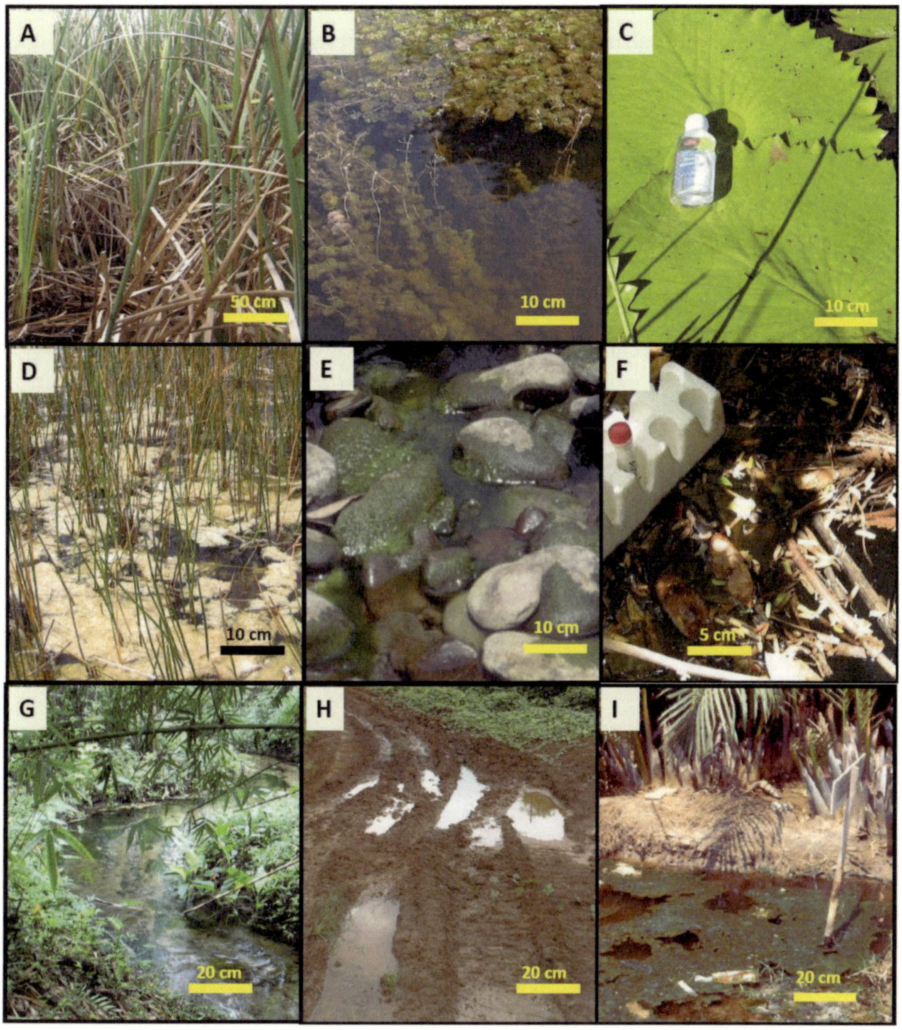

Figure 2. Examples of various larval habitat types as defined by vegetation. A: Freshwater marsh with tall dense macrophyte, *Typha domingensis*, a typical habitat for *Anopheles vestitipennis*; B: River edge vegetation dominated by a dense submersed macrophyte *Cabomba aquatica*, a potential habitat of *An. darlingi*; C: Marsh dominated by floating-leaved macrophyte, *Nymphaea ampla*, an example of an environment where larvae are typically not found; D: Marsh with sparse emergent macrophyte, *Eleocharis cellulosa*, interspersed with floating mats of cyanobacteria, a typical habitat of *An. albimanus*; E: A stream with filamentous green algae, a typical habitat for *An. pseudopunctipennis*; F: Detritus in a protected riverine environment, a typical habitat of *An. darlingi*.G: Small, partially shaded stream with vegetated margins, a tyical habitat for *An. minimus*; H: *An. gambiae* habitat from Equatorial Guinea (Malabo region); I: Stagnant pool of water with floating mats of algae, a habitat of *An. epiroticus* (Sundaicus complex) from southern Vietnam. Note the different scale bars.(Photo G & I courtesy of Sylvie Manguin; photo H courtesy of Pierre Carnevale).

3.6. Rice fields

Considering the large extent of rice fields in the areas with endemic malaria, they deserve their own subchapter. The changing crop practices, such as the shift to irrigated wetland rice affect

Anopheles vector populations, increasing the extent of larval habitats and transmission of malaria [131]. Irrigated rice cultivation extends the time in which vectors breed and in countries with two crops of rice per year, anopheline breeding and biting rates extend well beyond their usual seasons [131, 132].

The aquatic community in rice fields is a dynamic system related closely to rice plant growth, rice cultivation practices, and seasonal climatic changes [133-135]. Each mosquito species often has a preference for a particular phase in rice field development, which may result in an orderly succession of species as the rice plants develop and mature [136]. The pioneer colonizers are typically sun-preferring species, such as *An. gambiae* (Africa) *An. albimanus* (Central America), and *An. fluviatilis* and *An. culicifacies* (Oriental region); but when the rice grows taller it shades the water and shade-preferring species, such as *An. funestus* (Africa), *An. umbrosus* (India), *An. hyrcanus* group (Asia), *An. leucosphyrus* complex (Malaysia), *An. freeborni* (North America), *An. punctimacula* (South America) usually become more abundant [131, 136]. The abundance of aquatic macroinvertebrates, including predators, also changes during the growth of a single rice crop [76, 135, 137]. Compared to Asia and Africa there is less documentation of linkages between rice cultivation and disease in Latin America, although in parts of Mexico and Venezuela rice appears to be associated with seasonal increases in malaria incidence [138].

3.7. Food sources

Aquatic plants (both micro- and macrophytes) provide protection from predators and, together with trees and shrubs, contribute detritus that supports the bacterial community, which, in turn, serves as food for larvae [139]. An understanding of the spatial and temporal distribution of the dietary resources available to larval mosquitoes in their natural habitats could clarify the relationships among food availability, vector competence, and mosquito fitness [19, 140, 141]. Yet, the quantity and quality of food sources available to larvae is often ignored in the study of larval growth and development [9]. Natural food assemblages of larval mosquitoes are extremely diverse biochemically [142]. Generally, bacteria have been considered the most important of the microorganisms that comprise the food of mosquito larvae [19, 24], and mosquito growth can occur on cultures of bacteria alone [19]. In the water column of aquatic ecosystems, bacteria are the major decomposers of organic matter and the presence of particulate heterotrophic bacterial biomass represents an important link between detritus, dissolved organic matter, and higher trophic levels [143]. This bacterial production is controlled by or directly related to the supply of decomposable organic material. Thus, larval habitats with ample supplies of autochthonous and/or allochthonous detritus are capable of providing sufficient supplies of larval food resources. Experiments with diets also demonstrated that mosquito larvae can develop solely by drinking dissolved nutrients [19]. Larval food sources are not distributed homogeneously throughout the water column. The surface microlayer contains relatively high amounts of nutrients, organic material both particulate and dissolved, and various microorganisms as compared to subsurface water [144]. Anopheline larvae are well suited to utilize food sources from the enriched surface layer as they typically feed at the surface of the water where they engage in interfacial feeding behavior [13, 144].

Microalgae and/or small cyanobacteria can also serve as an important food source [19, 53, 93, 145]. Gimnig's et al [10] study demonstrated that larval grazing reduced algal abundances and biomass by an order of magnitude, and changed microeukaryote community structure. Changes in this algal food resource due to larval consumption almost certainly led to the observed density-dependent responses in larval development. Kaufman et al [145] conducted experiments to investigate the importance of algal food resources for larval growth and adult emergence of *An. gambiae* in simulated larval habitats in Kenya. Their results confirmed the importance of algal biomass in the surface microlayers of larval habitats to larval development and production of *An. gambiae* adults. They also showed that soil quality in these ephemeral larval habitats is important as the growth of algae depends on nutrient availability, particularly phosphorus (P). Thus soils releasing more P after flooding would support more algae that can feed more larvae.

While some microalgae are an important food source, other algae can be harmful to anopheline larvae. Marten's [146] review concludes that many species of green algae in the order Chlorococcales are resistant to digestion by mosquito larvae. Larvae are unable to complete their development if indigestible algae are numerous enough in the aquatic habitat to prevent the larvae ingesting enough other food to satisfy their nutritional needs. In addition, cyanobacteria (blue-green algae) can potentially kill larvae by toxins they produce [53].

3.8. Essential fatty acids

Lipids are an important food component for mosquito larvae because they provide a concentrated form of energy storage and a source of essential biochemical nutrients. Fatty acid (FA) constituents of lipids are present in a great structural variety, and are increasingly being used as chemical markers of biogeochemical processes and trophic relationships [147]. While the saturated palmitic acid (16:0) is often one of the most abundant fatty acids in lipid extracts, the interest of nutritional studies has concentrated on polyunsaturated fatty acids (PUFA) with two or more double bonds [148]. Some of these PUFAs are essential to the normal function of cells and they or their corresponding precursors have to be obtained in animal diets. In most animals, the 18-carbon chain, 18C, PUFAs can be converted to the longer-chain essential PUFAs, specifically arachidonic acid, ARA, eicosapentaenoic acid, EPA, and docosahexaenoic acid, DHA. Mosquitoes seem to be an exception because their dietary FA requirements cannot be satisfied by the C-18 PUFAs [149, 150]. They require some 20- and 22-C polyunsaturated fatty acids, EPA, ARA and DHA and without an adequate supply of these PUFAs they are not able to fly [149, 150]. Adult females may get these from a blood meal [151] but these PUFAs are believed essential in the larval stage for flight muscle development. The understanding of the spatial and temporal distribution of dietary resources available to mosquito larvae is needed in order to clarify the relationship among food availability, vector competence, and mosquito fitness. Not only does the nutrient availability within the habitat have to meet a minimum dietary requirement for proper larval development, but the food consumed in the larval stage is critical for a number of physiological processes that impact adult performance [152].

Kominkova et al. [153], in order to reveal the importance of feeding habitats for the nutrition of anopheline larvae, analyzed the FA composition of larvae of three malaria transmitting mosquito species *An. albimanus, An. vestitipennis* and *An. darlingi* and their corresponding habitats. They found that habitats were generally low in essential PUFAs and there were no significant differences among the FA composition of habitat samples. However, there were significant differences in FA composition of larvae. *Anopheles darlingi* contained significantly higher amounts of FA, specifically the linoleic acid. Large differences in PUFA content were found between field collected and laboratory-reared *An. vestitipennis* larvae, however, there were no differences in the total dry weight of the 4th stage larvae between the wild vs. laboratory-reared populations. Total FA in both larvae and samples of habitats of *An. albimanus* and *An. darlingi* were positively correlated with the concentration of particulate organic carbon and nitrogen (POC, PON) in their respective habitats, but no such correlation was found for *An. vestitipennis*. This study revealed that PUFA are a good indicator of nutritional quality although factors controlling the success of anopheline development in larval habitats are likely to be more complex and include, among others, the presence of predators, pathogens and toxins.

3.9. Species interactions (predation and competition)

Understanding species interactions such as competition and predation, across environmental gradients provides insight into how assemblages of mosquitoes are structured. This information is then critical for proper application of biological control [154]. The topic of competition and predation is a good example of the dichotomy in the approach to studying larval stages of mosquitoes. Many papers focus on use of predators for larval control [155-157]. There is a lack of studies focusing on larval competition and predation in the ecological context such as habitat size and temporal stability. But it is what influences the prevalence, pattern, and effects of species interactions across freshwater communities [158-160]. Spatial variation in biotic interactions can explain spatial variation in larval mosquito densities and ultimately the abundance of adult mosquitoes [78, 158]. Studies on predators of mosquito larvae go way back into history. Hinman [161] in his summary of predators on mosquito larvae lists over 100 references. Competition on the other hand is less studied even though interspecific competition for limited resources can be quite important and has been shown to have large effects on mosquito larvae. Mosquitoes compete with tadpoles [162, 163], other species of mosquitoes [164] and cladocerans [165].

Relative impacts of competition and predation change across a gradient of habitat size and permanence [159]. Bodies of water that may serve as larval habitats form a gradient from small and highly ephemeral to large and permanent. At the small, ephemeral end of this gradient, large long-lived predatory organisms (namely fish) are often absent, and aquatic organisms need to develop quickly. These conditions favor rapid growth and development, active foraging, movement, and competitive ability. As water bodies become larger and temporally more stable they can support more diverse community of larger, longer-lived predators. This increase of diversity, number, and voracity of predators favors refuge use, inconspicuousness, predator deterrence, and slow growth and development [159]. Organization of mosquito communities can be viewed in the same way. Interspecific competition among mosquitoes can be more important as a determinant of community structure in small ephemeral habitats, whereas predation can be more important in large permanent habitats [159]. Limited evidence suggests interspecific competition and cannibalism among mosquitoes is common in small pools [70], but comprehensive review of the ecology of competitive interactions of mosquitoes is lacking.

Natural predators of mosquito larvae are quite diverse and include the tadpole stages of amphibians [166], planktivorous fishes [165] and aquatic insects (Coleoptera, adult Heteroptera and larval Odonata). There is a range of papers reviewing predators on mosquito larvae and their potential use in biological control. Kumar and Hwang [167] provided an excellent review of larvicidal efficiency of amphibian tadpoles, larvivorous fish, cyclopoid copepods and aquatic insects. Mogi [168] reviewed insects and invertebrate predation on different life stages of mosquito. Quiroz-Martinez and Rodriguez-Castro [169] summarized the information on arthropods (insects, mites and spiders) that prey on mosquito larvae and discussed the potential of these predators in mosquitoes' biological control programs. Shaalan and Canyon's [156] review covered the predation of different insect species on mosquito larvae, predator prey-habitat relationships, co-habitation developmental issues, survival and abundance, oviposition avoidance, predatorial capacity and integrated vector control. Rozendaal [170] and Chandra et al [171] reviewed information on different larvivorous fish species and the present status of their use in mosquito control.

Despite thorough reviews and much information on different types of predators, there is a paucity of well-designed experimental studies verifying the long term effect of predators on mosquito populations. Although predation has been suggested as one of the important regulation mechanisms for malaria vectors in long lasting aquatic habitats, the predatory efficiency of potential predators is largely unknown [22, 157]. Research on predation of mosquito larvae has relied partly on the identification of larvae in the predators' gut – serological methods [172, 173], partly on correlative field observations evaluating the abundance of larvae and predators in the habitats [52, 174], and partly on laboratory feeding studies [157]. However, many predators that have been shown to be highly successful in eliminating target prey in the laboratory do not show a similar response in their natural habitats [75, 155]. The most basic question is whether predators have an important impact on mosquito populations in the field in the presence of alternative prey. Collins and Resh [118] listed the ecological factors affecting predation that should be considered when designing predation experiments: 1) dietary preference for mosquitoes, 2) abundance of alternative pray; 3) degree of congruity between habitats of the predator and target mosquito; 4) density of predators within habitat; 5) density of mosquito population; 6) quality of habitat as a refuge from predator. Among examples of well-designed experimental studies on multiple predator impacts we can cite Kumar et al [155] who compared the control potential of three larvivorous predators commonly co-occurring in the wetlands of tropical and subtropical regions, the mosquito fish *Gambusia affinis,* the cyclopoid copepod *Mesocyclops aspericornis*, and naiads of the dragonfly *Zyxomma petiolatum,* against the larvae of *An. stephensi* in the presence of alternative cladoceran prey. The presence of the alternative prey significantly reduced larval consumption by all three predators. Kumar et al [155] also discuss the issues related to using non-native mosquito fish considering its potential negative impacts on native assemblages and its lower selectivity for mosquito larvae.

Mosquito control using fish has focused on a limited number of species, primarily *Gambusia affinis* and *Poecilia reticulata* that have traditionally been used for controlling mosquito larvae [175, 176]. One of the most important concerns when introducing exotic fish for mosquito control is their impact on native species [177] and thus information on the predation role of native species is desirable. Louca et al [175] evaluated the role of larval predation by native fishes in Gambia River and they pointed out that the major impact on larvae was actually exerted by a detritivorous *Tilapia*, which is a prevailing species in the system that feeds on larvae only opportunistically in small aquatic habitats.

Blaustein [134] documented an unefficient control of anopheline larvae in the rice fields in California. He pointed out that contrary to what a good system should be composed of, i.e., a relatively permanent habitat, a specialist control agent and a relatively abundant pest species, the fish-mosquito-rice field system does not have any of these attributes. In addition, mosquito fish may have indirect positive effects on mosquito abundance; they also feed on invertebrates which are either natural predators (see [178]) or potential competitors of mosquito immatures [165]. Thus, this strategy attempts to control a relatively rare prey species with a generalist predator. The underlying mechanisms of predator-prey relationships need to be more clearly defined in order to use this biological control agent more effectively. There is a general need for field experiments on competition, predation, and mutualism, and on their context dependence across species and habitats [159].

Predation at larval stages can have important evolutionary consequences for mosquitoes [179]. For example, the predation of aquatic immature stages has been identified as a major evolutionary force driving habitat segregation and niche partitioning in the malaria mosquito *An. gambiae* in humid savannahs of West Africa [160, 180]. These studies explored behavioral responses to the presence of a predator in wild populations of the M and S molecular forms that typically breed in permanent (e.g., rice field paddies) and temporary (e.g., road ruts) water collections. The experiments showed that the M and S forms modify their behavior in the presence of a natural predator by becoming less active and positioning themselves at the wall of the container. These behavioral modifications suggest that mosquitoes are able to detect a predator's presence, through as yet unknown mechanisms which deserve further investigation.

4. Habitat selection

Habitat selection, defined as a process in which individuals preferentially choose and occupy a nonrandom set of available habitats, is of major importance for interpretation of spatial and temporal distributions of populations [139, 181]. The choice for suitable places for female mosquitoes to lay eggs is a key-factor for the survival of immature stages (eggs and larvae). Oviposition site selection has been recognized as critical both for the survival and population dynamics of mosquitoes. It is influenced by several environmental factors [182], including the salinity and turbidity of the water, the size and degree of permanence of the water body, the amount of sunlight, the presence of emergent/floating vegetation and shade, presence of predators, and distance to human habitation [8, 66]. In general, larvae of anopheline mosquitoes prefer clean rather than polluted water [8, 183], although in urban areas in parts of Africa *An. gambiae* appears to be adapting to new habitats such as rubbish-filled pools, sometimes containing sewage [182, 184]. Larvae of several Asian species (*An. dirus, An. punctulatus, An. subpictus*) have been reported from muddy and/or polluted waters [63].

In choosing sites for oviposition, females have to consider multiple—and possibly conflicting—factors to arrive at a site selection strategy that will optimize their reproductive success [185]. As many other oviparous species, mosquitoes also avoid oviposition in habitats with high risk of predation to their larvae [154, 186]. Females perceive these different characteristics of their habitats through a set of various cues both positive and negative. Among positive cues, volatile substances released from larval habitats have been implicated as potential olfactory cues mediating oviposition [54, 126, 139]. Experimental verification of dose response confirmed that low concentrations of volatile materials extracted from species-specific larval habitat materials increased oviposition, while there was a shift to reduced oviposition at high volatile concentrations. Rejmankova et al [139] also confirmed through reciprocal treatment tests that volatile effect was strongly habitat/species-specific.

Different mosquito species may rely on distinct chemical cues to avoid predators [187]. Mosquitoes that can detect aquatic predators often do so by sensing predator-released kairomones [187], see also review in Vonesh and Blaustein [188]. This was confirmed by preferential oviposition of *An. gambiae* in containers with clean water rather than water conditioned with predators (backswimmers, *Notonecta* sp. and tadpoles, *Xenopus* sp.) [72]. The experiment with Notonecta was later successfully repeated on other strains of *An. gambiae* by Warburg et al [187].

After oviposition, the main factors determining larval survival are food availability and refuge from predators. Orr and Resh [66] documented microhabitat selection by larvae of *An. freeborni*. They found that larval distribution throughout the habitat (an emergent macrophyte, *Myriophyllum aquaticum*) was not random, but that the larvae tended to congregate in denser patches of macrophytes. Observational data confirmed an active mechanism of selection, i.e., larvae actively choose patches with higher plant densities.

Larval habitats of the main malaria vectors in Belize are associated with three distinctly different aquatic environments: marshes with sparse macrophytes and cyanobacterial mats (*An. albimanus*), tall dense macrophyte marshes (*An. vestitipennis*), and floating detritus assemblages within freshwater rivers (*An. darlingi*). To assess species specific habitat suitability, we conducted mosquito transplant experiments [74]. First instar larvae of *An. albimanus, An. vestitipenis* and *An. darlingi* were placed in floating containers in the respective habitats of each species. Response of mosquito species to environmental conditions of its own and transplanted habitats clearly showed that each species was performing best in its own habitat. Survivorship of *An. vestitipenis* and *An. darlingi* in the *An. albimanus* habitat was extremely low or none.

5. Landscape context, remote sensing, GIS

Larval habitats are not located in a vacuum, they are an integral part of a broader landscape and their environmental requirements should be studied in this context. The landscape level approach gained momentum when technologies such as remote sensing (RS) and GIS became widely used in 1990's [55, 57, 59, 60, 189-191] and it has continued improving with the progress in RS technology (see review in Machault and coauthors [192, 193]. Direct measurements of the Earth's hydrological and biophysical characteristics, its geological features and its climate from space have provided new data layers with spatial and temporal resolutions relevant to landscape-scale habitat characteristics and ecological processes [194, 195]. The landscape, vegetation, and ecosystem attributes derived from the applied remote sensing data contribute significantly to defining habitat characteristics and help discern patterns and gradients that may exist even within seemingly homogeneous environments.

The use of RS may involve various degree of complexity. The simplest case is when larval habitats are large enough to be directly identified within spatial resolution of remote sensors as, e.g., in Wood et al [55] study from irrigated rice in northern and central California. This study [55] provided a model of rice field mosquito population dynamics using spectral and spatial information. Analysis of field data revealed that rice fields with rapid early season vegetation canopy development, located near livestock pastures (i.e. bloodmeal sources), had greater mosquito larval populations than fields with more slowly developing vegetation canopies located further from pastures. Remote sensing reflectance measurements of early season rice canopy development and GIS measurements of distance to livestock pasture were combined to distinguish between high and low mosquito-producing rice fields. These distinctions were made with 90% accuracy nearly two months before anopheline larval populations peaked.

A more complex approach is needed in situations where larval habitats are spatially below the detection limit of RS data. As an example, a hierarchical approach was used to link larval habitat-types with larger land cover units in an integrated RS, GIS and field study in the Pacific coastal plain of Chiapas, Mexico [57]. Using this approach, villages with high *vs*. low risk for malaria transmission were identified and it was demonstrated that remote sensing-based models generated for one area can be used successfully in another, comparable area [59, 60]. Similarly, RS generated maps of larval habitats in Madagascar rice fields and urban areas were used for predictions of adult densities and definitions of areas that may require indoor insecticide spraying [196, 197]. The landscape determinants of anopheline mosquito larval habitats in Kenya highlands and lowlands and their temporal changes were assessed by Mushinzimana et al. [198], Jacob et al [199], Munga et al [200], Mutuku et al [201], from elsewhere in Central and west Africa by Dambach [193] and Clennon et al [202], and from Malaysia by Ahmad et al [203]. The use of RS as a predictive tool to locate larval habitats has not always been successful as demonstrated by Achee et al [204]. Their results indicated that remotely sensed land cover is not a valuable indicator of the location in which *An. darlingi* larval habitats will form. High-resolution satellite imagery could be used to detect homes along river systems and potentially predict general areas at risk for *An. darlingi* breeding habitat formation based on distances from houses to waterways (Figure 3). The basic idea behind the remotely sensed assessment of larval habitats is to define environmental parameters that can be used to identify areas with increased risk of malaria transmission [193]. Yet, as already stated by

Roberts et al [205], the successful use of RS and GIS technologies to predict potential or actual malaria trouble spots is dependent on clear understandings of environmental factors that determine the presence of malaria vectors.

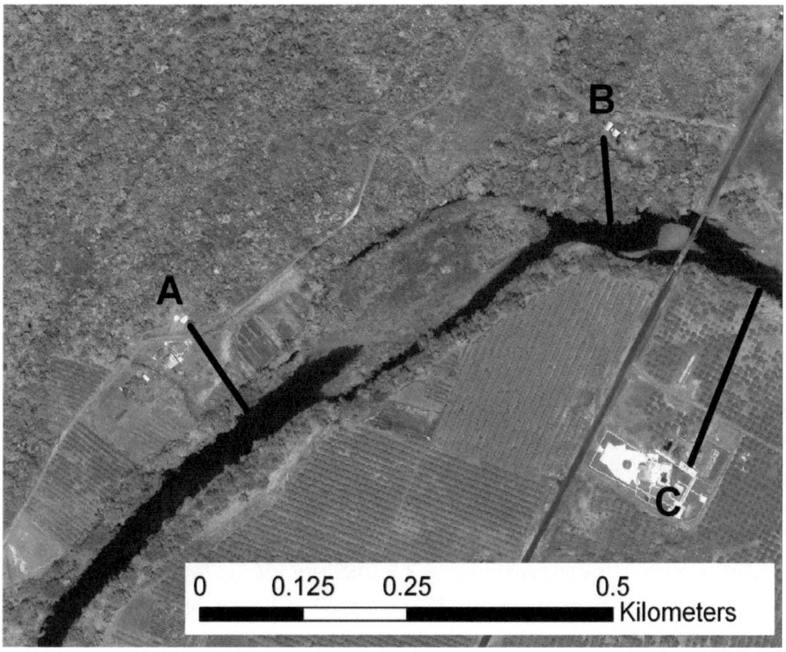

Figure 3. IKONOS 1m-resolution panchromatic image showing three houses (A-C) along a section of the Sibun River. Distance from the river to houses (black lines) was predictive for presence and abundance of *An. darlingi*, the primary malaria vector in Belize.

5.1. Ecological niche models

Populations of mosquito larvae are ideally suited to GIS and remote sensing applications due to their close association with their microenvironment. Specifically, larval mosquitoes have three distinct ecological characteristics that are directly related to predictive risk-modeling: 1) specific habitat preferences, 2) microclimate requirements and 3) vegetation-dependent associations to include plant height and density. Spatial-temporal interactions of mosquito larvae with their natural environment are critical to understanding the risk of contact between the vectors and their human hosts. Due to the fact that mosquitoes spend a substantial portion of their life cycle in the larval stage, population structure and vector survival is greatly influenced by the environmental surroundings. One area that is increasingly being applied to disease ecology which takes advantage of these environmental associations is the use ecological niche models [206]. An ecological niche model is an estimate of the distribution of a species and requires two input data sets: the known locations of a species and environmental data in an image format (such as larval habitats, climate data, elevation data, land cover, etc.). The ecological niche modeling program examines the environmental data at the locations where the species occurs to infer the environmental requirements of the species across a much larger area. The requirements of the species are then used to create a map of the predicted distribution of the species. Any species affected by environmental conditions such as climate can be modeled including disease vectors, disease hosts and pathogens. Models of monthly predictions of dengue fever in Mexico have been created based on mosquito activity [207]. Niche models of malaria vectors in the *An. gambiae* complex have been developed for under-sampled regions of Africa [208]. The benefit of niche modeling is the development of maps showing predicted distribution of an organism based on current and projected vector ecology and environmental data.

6. Human impact land use/global change

Natural ecosystems throughout the world are being severely altered by human intervention. Population pressure results in transformation of natural ecosystems to agriculture, construction of roads and hydroelectric dams, irrigation projects, open pit mines, and uncontrolled human colonization [209, 210]. Anthropogenic modification of the ecosystems also contributes to global climate change represented by an increase in temperature and accompanied by extremes of the hydrologic cycle (e.g., floods and droughts) [211, 212]. The global rate of tropical deforestation continues with nearly 2% to 3% of global forests lost each year and land use change for agriculture represents the largest driver of land cover change across the earth [85, 209, 213]. Arthropod vectors in general, and insect vectors in particular are very sensitive to their environment, which determines their presence, development and behavior. As a consequence, climatic, as well as landscape and land cover factors greatly influence the spatial distribution of vectors and the diseases they transmit [214].

Mosquitoes are among the most sensitive insects to environmental change; their survival, density, and distribution are dramatically influenced by small changes in environmental conditions, such as temperature, humidity, and the availability of suitable larval habitats [48, 88, 215-219]. All these changes can alter the incidence, seasonality and intensity of transmission, and geographic range of diseases such as malaria. Changes in the distribution of malaria cases and intensities of malaria transmission have been documented by many historical examples. As described by Hackett [220], malaria increased in Malaya as jungle was cleared for rubber plantations. Where forest was removed the sun penetrated and populations of *Anopheles maculatus* mosquitoes proliferated, greatly increasing the incidence of human malaria. The better we are able to assess and explain the distribution and dynamics of vector species in relation to fluctuations in their environments, the more accurate prediction can be made of malaria in the context of ongoing environmental change [221, 222]. This will allow us to evaluate the risks associated with current practices, better explain the patterns of increasing and decreasing disease, better identify measures to mitigate the likelihood and impact of disease emergence, and eventually improve its control [213]. Below are specific examples of changes related to important human activities.

6.1. Deforestation

Deforestation is one of the most important factors driving emerging and re-emerging infectious diseases. Through the process of clearing forests and subsequent agricultural development, deforestation changes almost every attribute of local ecosystems such as microclimate, soil, and aquatic conditions, and most significantly, the ecology of local flora and fauna, including human disease vectors. Numerous country and area studies have described the influence of deforestation and subsequent land use on the density of local mosquito vectors [223]. One of the most thorough evaluations of the impact of deforestation combined with the prediction of future changes has been presented by Yasuoka and Levins [224] who conducted a meta-analysis of 60 published studies of changes in ecology of 31 anopheline species and malaria incidence as a consequence of deforestation. In comprehensive tables they summarized density changes by land cover, and for larval habitats the niche-width and sun-preference indices of each species. The conclusion was that mechanisms linking deforestation and agricultural development with mosquito ecology and malaria epidemiology are extremely complex. The impacts of deforestation on mosquito density and malaria incidence are influenced by both the nature of the agricultural development and the ecological characteristics of the local vector mosquitoes. Some species were directly affected by deforestation, some favored or could adapt to the different environmental conditions, and some invaded and/or replaced other species in the process of development and cultivation. The results of the statistical analyses showed that deforestation and agricultural development are favorable for sun-loving species, allowing them to increase in or invade deforested areas where water bodies become exposed to sunlight.

As a specific example of the complexity of a malaria vector to deforestation we present the case of *An. darlingi* in the Amazon region. Vittor et al [225] examined the larval breeding habitat of a major South American malaria vector, *An. darlingi,* in areas with varying degrees of ecologic alteration in the Peruvian Amazon and concluded that deforestation and associated ecologic alterations are conducive to *An. darlingi* larval presence, and thereby increase malaria risk. According to Barros et al [82], deforestation and human presence creates a new habitat, a forest fringe ecosystem, by promoting three changes in *An. darlingi* bionomics: (i) increasing contact with humans; (ii) increasing the number of microdams (small river obstruction causing the accumulation of debris), which increases the number of potential larval habitats as well as the breeding season; and (iii) reducing the number of shaded breeding sites in a given geographical area, which results in a concentration of larvae in remaining shaded areas. The ideal breeding site occurs in the forest fringe, where the three factors, shade, microdams and human blood meals, are located close to each other.

Environmental changes caused by deforestation often lead to vector replacement (for examples referenced in older papers see Service [136]). Conn et al. [226] conducted entomological surveys in malaria areas of Macapá, northeastern Amazonia, and found *An. marajoara* replacing *An. darlingi* as the primary vector. It is hypothesized that the observed change in mosquito population densities was caused by deforestation for agriculture that resulted in newly created ground pools favoring *An. marajoara* larvae. For many regions in the Amazon Basin, populations of *An. darlingi* have increased because road construction in the forest has considerably expanded the breeding sites—large areas of neutral, partially shaded and unpolluted water.

These characteristics also attract human inhabitants. Subsequently, clearing of forests and water pollution reduce the suitability of these for *An. darlingi* breeding. However, these sites, and newly created ponds for agricultural use, attract other mosquito species such as *An. marajoara*. In addition, humans have colonized land near extensive marshy areas, another preferred breeding habitat of *An. marajoara*.

6.2. Dam construction

Water reservoirs have long been recognized to be a risk factor for malaria transmission [227-231]. Hydroelectric or irrigation dam construction increases the habitat availability by the formation of lakes. Shallow parts of these lakes are typically overgrown with macrophytes that provide excellent breeding sites for anopheline mosquitoes [227]. However, compared to the number of studies on land use change due to deforestation and agricultural expansion, research related to the entomological and ecological determinants of the rising malaria burden in the vicinity of large dams is rather limited [232]. There are historical examples, such as that of Tennessee Valley Authority ([35], see also p. 3) of well executed environmental management measures to control malaria vectors [21, 35]. These successfully executed environmental measures can be adapted to control malaria associated with dam construction in sub-Saharan Africa and elsewhere in malaria endemic regions. Construction of new reservoirs under the tropical, sub-humid climatic conditions should therefore be accompanied by entomologic studies to predict the risk of malaria epidemics [233]. Keiser et al [231] calls for institutionalization of health impact assessments for future water development projects analogous to environmental impact assessments as well as the employment of monitoring and surveillance systems that would facilitate systematic evaluation of the impact of these ecosystem interventions over time. The reality is that more dams will be built and thus mitigation strategies to alleviate potential negative health effects are mandatory to reduce the current burden of malaria in settings near irrigation or dam projects.

6.3. Wetland destruction

Draining wetlands has been extensively practiced and promoted as the easiest solution to localized public health threats posed by malaria vectors [21, 234]. Unfortunately, this practice has not always worked. Among many cases of increasing malaria transmission after destruction of natural wetlands are the examples from African papyrus swamps [64]. As stated already by Goma [32, 235] and confirmed recently by others [72, 88, 236], the interior of a papyrus swamp is unsuitable for anophelines, while the swamp periphery and cultivation of natural swamps provides productive larval habitats for *An. gambiae* and consequently, increase the risks of malaria transmission to the human population. Many natural wetlands have been destroyed and changed to brick-making pits – the most abundant habitat type containing *An. gambiae* larvae in Africa [237].

What has not been taken into account when manipulating wetlands for health benefits is the loss of valuable ecosystem services provided by these wetlands, such as water purification, flood control, or provision of food and fiber, and their contributions to human health. This aspect was emphasized by the 2008 Conference of the Contracting Parties to the Ramsar

http://dx.doi.org/10.5772/55229

Convention on Wetlands, whose resolution stated among others: "Those concerned with wetland conservation and management should encourage new and ongoing research regarding the links between wetlands and human health and to bring information on the scientifically proven contributions that functioning wetland ecosystems make to good health to the attention of national ministries and agencies responsible for health, sanitation, and water supply. The human health sector, and all relevant stakeholders should collaborate in assessing the consequences of wetland management linked with human health, and vice versa the consequences for the ecological character of wetlands of current practices which seek to maintain or improve human health, including the identification of appropriate trade-offs in decision-making."

6.4. Wetland creation and restoration

In addition to rice fields, which are the most extensive human made wetlands and their significance as larval habitat has been already described previously, the use of constructed wetlands for wastewater treatment is expanding [236, 238, 239]. Constructed wetland technology has broad applications for the treatment of many types of wastewaters and provides an ecological approach to mitigate the release of nutrients and toxic materials into the environment [240]. However, design features, maintenance activities and the characteristics of the wastewater undergoing treatment contribute differentially to potential levels of mosquito production and, consequently, to threats to human and animal health from mosquito-borne pathogens. Nutrients (nitrogen and phosphorus), and the configuration and maintenance of emergent vegetation can have strong effects on mosquito production. As loading rates of organic matter and nutrients decline, the diversity of mosquitoes produced by treatment wetlands tends to increase and the relative abundance of *Anopheles* species increases in temperate man-made wetlands [239, 241]. A proper design, e.g. subsurface rather than surface flow or flow-through rather than pond-type wetland [242] can help local mosquito problems. Surface-flow wetlands can also be designed to minimize mosquito breeding by increasing macro-invertebrate predators [243]. Greenway [243] concluded that a marsh with a diversity of macrophytes appears optimal for macro-invertebrate biodiversity and the control of mosquito larvae by predation. The key to mosquito management is to ensure a well-balanced ecosystem supporting a diversity of aquatic organisms [240]. A general conclusion from those areas that contain both treatment wetlands and unimpacted natural wetlands is that adequately designed and appropriately managed treatment wetlands do not pose any greater mosquito threat than the existing natural wetlands [244].

To compensate for a large loss of wetlands in the past, we are now witnessing many projects attempting to restore, rehabilitate, or create various types of wetland habitats. The resulting restored wetland areas provide flood control, improve water quality, and provide habitat for wildlife, especially bird species. However, they create great mosquito habitat and only a few restoration project address this issue properly [234] and there is a need for a better coordination between wetland restoration design and management and mosquito larval management.

6.5. Eutrophication

Freshwaters are among the most extensively and rapidly altered ecosystems on the planet [213]. Increased use of fertilizers in agriculture and destruction of natural buffer zones leads to runoff of excessive nutrients, specifically nitrogen and phosphorus to lakes, rivers and reservoirs [245-250]. Nutrient increase is generally responsible for plant production resulting in potential changes in other trophic levels. Several studies have shown positive correlations between concentrations of inorganic nutrients in surface waters and larval abundance for *Anopheles* [43, 251]. Nutrient enriched waters are easily invaded by aggressive aquatic weeds such as water hyacinth (*Eichhornia crassipes*), which are known to be very productive anopheline habitats [37, 44, 252].

The authors' research in Belize [56, 86] provided data in support of the hypothesis that eutrophication causes changes in freshwater communities. The Central American country of Belize contains large wetland areas that used to be dominated by phosphorus limited sparse macrophyte communities interspersed with floating mats of cyanobacteria – a typical *An. albimanus* habitat (Figure 4).

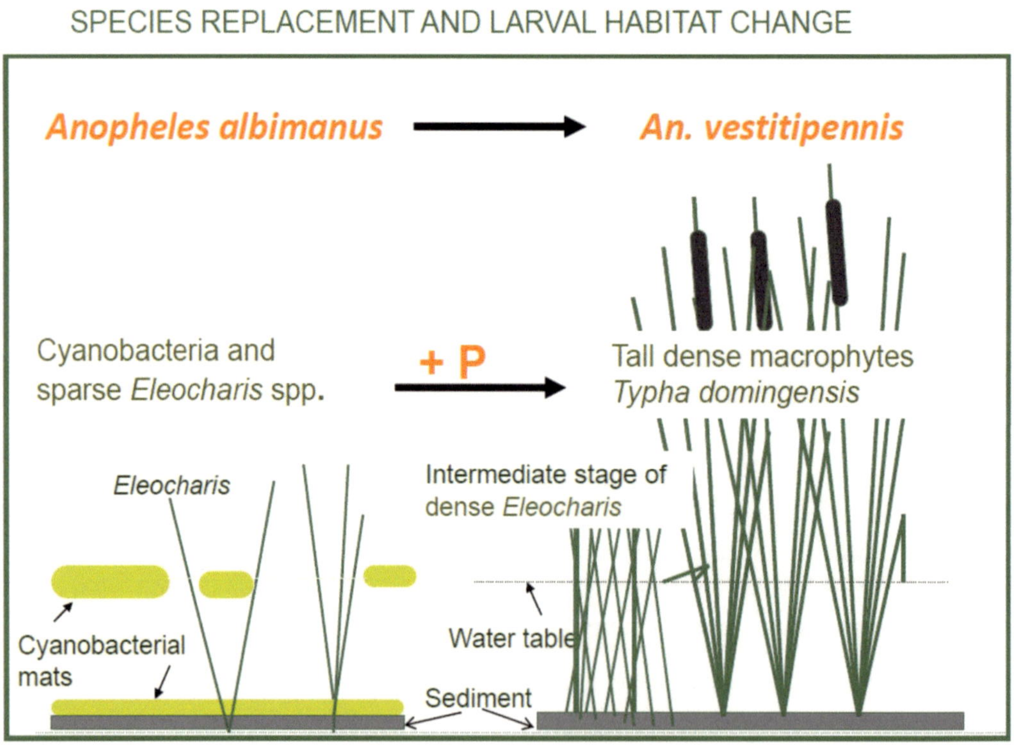

Figure 4. Schematic representation of the change of plant communities in marshes of Belize caused by increased eutrophication by phosphorus. This change is accompanied by the replacement of *An. albimanus* habitat with *An. vestitipennis* habitat.

Anthropogenically mediated P enrichment of wetland plant communities through introduction of fertilizer runoff from expanding sugar cane fields is causing a switch from sparse macrophytes to tall dense macrophytes represented mostly by *Typha domingensis*. Tall dense macrophytes provide favorable habitat for *An. vestitipennis,* which appears to be a more efficient vector of malaria. Thus human-caused nutrient enrichment of marshes may lead to increased risk of malaria transmission in human settlements in proximity to the impacted marshes.

6.6. Temperature and precipitation changes

Malaria transmission is very sensitive to both temperature and precipitation, which makes the issue of change in risk due to past and projected warming trends one of the most important climate change-health questions to follow [253, 254]. Large malaria epidemics in the East African highlands during the mid and late 1990s initiated research on the role that global warming might have on malaria transmission. Historically, these highlands have been used as a shelter against malaria because malaria has been naturally absent due to conditions that limit the biology of the parasite [255]. Several authors proposed that spread of malaria into areas that rarely saw malaria transmission could be related to the impacts of small increases in temperature [253, 256]. The issue became hotly debated [255]. Recently, Chaves et al [257] assessed conclusions from both sides of the argument and found that evidence for the role of climate is robust but they also found a large heterogeneity in malaria trends. They argued that over-emphasizing the importance of climate is misleading for setting a research agenda to understand climate change impacts on emerging malaria patterns. The global change is expected to influence rainfall patterns both seasonal rainfall totals and inter-annual variability in malaria endemic regions, and these events will impact larval habitats availability and thus mosquito population dynamics [258].

6.7. Sea level rise

Along with warming temperatures, any increase in sea levels will affect the extent of saline (>30 ppt) or brackish (0.5-30 ppt) water bodies in coastal areas. These include coastal estuaries, lagoons, marshes and mangroves [106]. An expansion of brackish and saline water bodies in coastal areas, associated with rising sea levels, can increase densities of salinity-tolerant vector mosquitoes and lead to the adaptation of freshwater vectors to breed in brackish and saline waters. Higher vector densities can increase transmission of vector-borne infectious diseases in coastal localities, which can then spread to other areas [106].

The consequences of human-induced ecological changes provide another set of examples. Large-scale shrimp farming in the Mekong delta of Vietnam locally increased the density of *An. sundaicus* [259]. The greater availability of brackish water bodies can also lead to freshwater breeding mosquitoes such as *An. stephensi* and *An. culicifacies* getting adapted to breed in brackish waters as was observed immediately after the 2004 tsunami in India [260] and some years later in eastern Sri Lanka [261].

6.8. Replacability and adaptability

As already indicated by a few examples in the above text, a change in ecology of a region whether due natural factors or human impact can lead to changes in the quality and quantity of larval habitats. This often leads to changes in mosquito population dynamics and species composition [262]. The original anopheline species can be replaced by species better adapted to new conditions or they can adapt themselves. Mosquito species distributed over broad geographic ranges are more likely to have greater habitat diversity than species distributed over a small range [263] and thus their adaptability can be higher. Except for a few examples, our knowledge on the species adaptability is quite limited. But since at least some species are able to adapt to different environmental conditions, an effort needs to be made to obtain data on anopheline population dynamics before, during, and after ecologic alterations. Furthermore, the long-term effectiveness of any control strategy will depend on whether vectors respond to the evolutionary selection pressure created by intervention [22]. For example, mosquitoes may respond by phenotypic plasticity, or by evolving traits such as insecticide resistance or behavioral avoidance.

7. Implication for vector control

Malaria vector control targeting the larval stages of mosquitoes was applied successfully against many species of *Anopheles* in malarious countries until the mid-20th Century [3, 8, 264-266]. Since the introduction of DDT in the 1940s and the associated development of indoor residual spraying (IRS), which usually has a more powerful impact on vectorial capacity than larval control, the focus of malaria prevention programs shifted to the control of adult vectors [8, 267]. However, when it became clear that this strategy is not working (Service 1983), an integrated disease management approach including control of larval stages of malaria vectors, i.e., Integrated Vector Management (IVM) began to be reconsidered [21, 268]. A great step in that direction was made by Keiser et al [264] who provided a systematic review and a meta-analysis of malaria control programs, emphasizing environmental management as their main feature. Most of the 40 studies (85%) were implemented before the Global Malaria Eradication Campaign (1955–69). The authors concluded that malaria control programs that emphasize environmental management are highly effective in reducing malaria. Lessons learned from these past successful programs can guide sound and sustainable malaria control approaches and strategies. The conclusions of Keiser's et al [231] meta-analysis of past control strategies are in agreement with recently developed malaria transmission models showing that substantial reductions of the entomological inoculation rate are possible when an integrated malaria control program with multiple interventions (e.g., environmental management tools) implemented simultaneously is used [269, 270].

The larval source management (LSM) also termed Environmental management that has been successfully used to control mosquitoes in many developed countries (US, Brazil, Canada) is recently becoming an integral component of malaria control methods in Africa [271]. LSM includes: (1) habitat (or environmental) modification, (2) habitat (environmental) manipulation, (3) biological control and (4) larviciding [236, 264, 271]. **Habitat modification** is designed to prevent, eliminate, or reduce vector habitat and it involves a permanent change of land and water, including landscaping, drainage of surface water, land reclamation and filling but also coverage of large water storage containers, wells and other potential breeding sites. **Habitat manipulation** refers to activities that reduce larval habitats of the vector mosquito through temporary changes to the aquatic environment in which larvae develop. It is a recurrent activity, such as water-level manipulation, which includes measures such as flushing, drain clearance, shading or exposing habitats to the sun depending on the ecology of the local vector. It may include planting water-intensive tree species such as *Eucalyptus robusta* to reduce standing water in marshy areas. The best strategies are those that are adapted to local vector ecology, epidemiology and resources, guided by operational research and subject to routine monitoring and evaluation [22, 272]. Bond's et al [122, 123] studies can serve as an example of habitat manipulation. They report on how manual algal removal from breeding pools along a river in southern Mexico significantly reduced both larval and adult densities of *An. pseudopunctipennis*. In a follow up study, the abundance of *An. pseudopunctipennis* larvae + pupae was dramatically reduced by this treatment and remained depressed for two to three months. Algal extraction did not reduce the overall abundance of aquatic insects in river pools. **Biological control** of mosquitoes refers to the introduction of natural enemies into aquatic habitats; these are predatory fish or invertebrates, parasites or disease organisms (see the predator section). *Bacillus thuringiensis israelensis* (Bti) and *Bacillus sphaericus* (Bs) are bacterial species reported to be effective against mosquitoes, and have been widely studied and used as biolarvicides [266, 273, 274]. Recently, researchers have focused on the resident microbiota of insect vectors that can potentially impede transmission of human pathogens. These microbes may prove effective agents for manipulating the vector competence of malaria and other important human pathogens [275-278]. Biological control agents should be evaluated with respect to their climatic compatibility and their capability to maintain very close interactions with target populations [155].

8. What next?

Almost every paper that we reviewed for this chapter ends up with the call for more information on larval stages of malaria vectors, in order to enable a better vector control and more accurate predictions of vector response to changing environment. It is (finally!) becoming clear that understanding the ecology and evolution of mosquito vectors needs to complement epidemiology, genetics and molecular biology in solving malaria problems. Several review papers provide good suggestions for future directions in vector ecology research (see, e.g., Table 2 in Chaves and Koenraadt [255] and Box 3 in Ferguson et al [22]). As stated in the preceding text, almost any factor defining a larval habitat can change as a result of direct human modification (deforestation, agricultural practices, eutrophication) and/or indirectly caused environmental change (temperature, precipitation). In addition, new habitats can be created. All these changes can and will impact the basic environmental determinants of larval habitats – food availability, refuge, predator presence. There are indications that some species will be able to adapt, some will be replaced by other species, and some anophelines that have not traditionally been regarded as vectors may become important ones.

In the context of ecosystem change whether due to nutrient, temperature, precipitation, salinity or vegetation changes, there is a strong need for studies on adaptability of different anopheline species to new conditions. The majority of these studies would be best executed as manipulative field or semi-field experiments focused not only on changing characteristics of species performance but also on interactions with other species (both competition and predation). To be able to accomplish these types of experiments, systems of enclosed, pathogen-free, semi-field mesocosms in which vector populations can be experimentally manipulated will have to be established within environmentally realistic, contained semi-field settings. See, e.g., Ng'habi et al [11] semi-field system of large, netting-enclosed mesocosms, in which vectors can fly freely, feed on natural plant and vertebrate host sources, and access realistic resting and oviposition sites. Ideally, systems of these experimental mesocosms should be established along environmental (temperature, precipitation) gradients or with the capability to experimentally manipulate these variables so that we can conduct the experiments focused on species response to changing environments.

In addition, there is an ongoing need for regular monitoring and good quality long-term dataset on species distributions. High resolution satellite data enable more detailed observations on vegetation changes and regional distribution of precipitations and temperature, which all can results and result in better risk prediction maps [193]. In order to include a temporal component to the risk models, a network of longitudinal population monitoring sites for vector development needs to be established. The ecological niche models [206, 279] mentioned above will undoubtedly play increasingly important role in predictions of disease outbreaks.

Acknowledgements

We thank Stephanie Castle for technical help. Parts of the research referred to in the chapter was supported by the NIH-NSF Ecology of Infectious Diseases program, Grant # R01 AI49726, "Environmental Determinants of Malaria in Belize".

Author details

Eliška Rejmánková[1*], John Grieco[2], Nicole Achee[2] and Donald R. Roberts[2,3]

*Address all correspondence to: erejmankova@ucdavis.edu

1 Department of Environmental Science and Policy, University of California, Davis, USA

2 Department of Preventive Medicine & Biometrics, Uniformed Services University of the Health Sciences, Bethesda, USA

3 Retired, Professor Emeritus, present address: Clifton Forge, VA, USA

References

[1] Zimmerman RH. Ecology of malaria vectors in the America and future direction. Memorias Do Instituto Oswaldo Cruz. 1992; 87 371-83.

[2] Gubler DJ. Resurgent vector-borne diseases as a global health problem. Emerging Infectious Diseases. 1998; 4(3) 442-50.

[3] Townson H, Nathan MB, Zaim M, Guillet P, Manga L, Bos R, et al. Exploiting the potential of vector control for disease prevention. Bulletin of the World Health Organization. 2005; 83(12) 942-7.

[4] Zanetti AR, Zappa A. Emerging and re-emerging infections at the turn of the millennium. Haemophilia. 2010; 16 7-12.

[5] Eckhoff PA. A malaria transmission-directed model of mosquito life cycle and ecology. Malaria Journal. 2011; 10, 303.

[6] Rubbo MJ, Lanterman JL, Falco RC, Daniels TJ. The influence of amphibians on mosquitoes in seasonal pools: can wetlands protection help to minimize disease risk? Wetlands. 2011; 31(4) 799-804.

[7] da Silva-Nunes M, Moreno M, Conn JE, Gamboa D, Abeles S, Vinetz JM, et al. Amazonian malaria: Asymptomatic human reservoirs, diagnostic challenges, environmentally driven changes in mosquito vector populations, and the mandate for sustainable control strategies. Acta Tropica. 2012; 121(3) 281-91.

[8] Walker K, Lynch M. Contributions of *Anopheles* larval control to malaria suppression in tropical Africa: review of achievements and potential. Medical and Veterinary Entomology. 2007; 21(1) 2-21.

[9] Gimnig JE, Ombok M, Kamau L, Hawley WA. Characteristics of larval anopheline (Diptera : Culicidae) habitats in western Kenya. Journal of Medical Entomology. 2001; 38(2) 282-8.

[10] Gimnig JE, Ombok M, Otieno S, Kaufman MG, Vulule JM, Walker ED. Density-dependent development of *Anopheles gambiae* (Diptera : Culicidae) larvae in artificial habitats. Journal of Medical Entomology. 2002; 39(1) 162-72.

[11] Ng'habi KR, Mwasheshi D, Knols BGJ, Ferguson HM. Establishment of a self-propagating population of the African malaria vector *Anopheles arabiensis* under semi-field conditions. Malaria Journal. 2010; 9, 356.

[12] Hiwat H, Bretas G. Ecology of *Anopheles darlingi* Root with respect to vector importance: a review. Parasites & Vectors. 2011; 4, 177.

[13] Clements A. The Biology of Mosquitoes. Volume 1. Development, nutrition and reproduction. London: Chapman & Hall; 1992.

[14] Clements A. The Biology of Mosquitoes. Volume 2. Sensory reception and behavior. Wallingford: Cabi Publishing; 1999.

[15] Clements A. The Biology of Mosquitoes. Volume 3. Transmission of viruses and interactions with bacteria. Wallingford: Cabi Publishing; 2012.

[16] Fournet F, Cussac M, Ouari A, Meyer PE, Toe HK, Gouagna LC, et al. Diversity in anopheline larval habitats and adult composition during the dry and wet seasons in Ouagadougou (Burkina Faso). Malaria Journal. 2010; 9 78.

[17] Sinka ME, Bangs MJ, Manguin S, Rubio-Palis Y, Chareonviriyaphap T, Coetzee M, et al. A global map of dominant malaria vectors. Parasites & Vectors. 2012; 5 69.

[18] Bates M. Oviposition experiments with Anopheline mosquitoes. American Journal of Tropical Medicine and Hygiene. 1940; 20(4) 569-83.

[19] Merritt RW, Dadd RH, Walker ED. Feeding-behavior, natural food, and nutritional relationships of larval mosquitos. Annual Review of Entomology. 1992; 37 349-76.

[20] Killeen GF, Fillinger U, Kiche I, Gouagna LC, Knols BGJ. Eradication of *Anopheles gambiae* from Brazil: lessons for malaria control in Africa? Lancet Infectious Diseases. 2002; 2(10) 618-27.

[21] Kitron U, Spielman A. Suppression of transmission of malaria through source reduction - Antianopheline measures applied in Israel, the United-States, and Italy. Reviews of Infectious Diseases. 1989; 11(3) 391-406.

[22] Ferguson HM, Dornhaus A, Beeche A, Borgemeister C, Gottlieb M, Mulla MS, et al. Ecology: A prerequisite for malaria elimination and eradication. Plos Medicine. 2010; 7(8) e1000303.

[23] Service MW. Biological control of mosquitos - has it a future. Mosquito News. 1983; 43(2) 113-20.

[24] Laird M. The Natural History of Larval Mosquito Habitats. London: Academic; 1988. p. 555.

[25] Komp WHW. The occurrence of *Anopheles darlingi*. Root in British Honduras and Guatemala. Public Health Reports. 1940; 55(16) 693-4.

[26] Kumm HV, Ram LM. Observations on the *Anopheles* of the British Honduras. American Journal of Tropical Medicine and Hygiene. 1941; 21 559-66.

[27] Bertram DS. Mosquitoes of British Honduras, with some comments on malaria, and on arbovirus antibodies in man and equines. Transactions of the Royal Society of Tropical Medicine and Hygiene. 1971; 65(6) 742-62.

[28] Roberts DR, Chan O, Pecor J, Rejmankova E, Manguin S, Polanco J, et al. Preliminary observations on the changing roles of malaria vectors in southern Belize. Journal of the American Mosquito Control Association. 1993; 9(4) 456-9.

[29] Muirhead-Thomson RC. Studies on the behaviour of *Anopheles minimus*. Part III. The influence of water temperature on the choice and suitability of the breeding place. Journal of the Malaria Institute of India. 1940; 3 323-48.

[30] Goma LKH. The productivity of various mosquito breeding places in the swamps of Uganda. Bulletin of Entomological Research. 1958; 49 437-48.

[31] Goma LKH. The swamp-breeding mosquitoes of Uganda: Records of larvae and their habitats. Bulletin of Entomological Research. 1960; 51 77-94.

[32] Goma LKH. Experimental breeding of *Anopheles gambiae* Giles in papyrus swamps. Nature. 1960; 187(4743) 1137-8.

[33] Howland LJ. Bionomical investigation of English mosquito larvae with special reference to their algal food. Journal of Ecology. 1930; 18 81-125.

[34] Bates M. The Natural History of Mosquitoes. New York: MacMillan; 1949.

[35] Authority TV. Malaria Control on Impounded Water. Washington DC: US Government Printing Office; 1947.

[36] Hinman EH. The role of bacteria in the nutrition of mosquito larvae - The growth-stimulating factor. American Journal of Hygiene. 1933; 18(1) 224-36.

[37] Penfound WT, Earle TT. The biology of the water hyacinth. Ecological Monographs. 1948; 18(4) 447-72.

[38] Hess A, Hall T. The intersection line as a factor in anopheline ecology. The Journal of National Malaria Society. 1943; 2(2) 93-8.

[39] Hall TF. Influence of plants on anopheline breeding. American Journal of Tropical Medicine and Hygiene. 1972; 21(5) 787-94.

[40] Orr BK, Resh VH. Experimental test of the influence of aquatic macrophyte cover on the survival of *Anopheles* larvae. Journal of the American Mosquito Control Association. 1989; 5(4) 579-85.

[41] Savage HM, Rejmankova E, Arredondo-Jimenez JI, Roberts DR, Rodriguez MH. Limnological and botanical characterization of larval habitats for 2 primary malarial vectors, *Anopheles albimanus* and *Anopheles pseudopunctipennis*, in coastal areas of Chiapas State, Mexico. Journal of the American Mosquito Control Association. 1990; 6(4) 612-20.

[42] Rejmankova E, Roberts DR, Harbach RE, Pecor J, Peyton EL, Manguin S, et al. Environmental and regional determinants of *Anopheles* (Diptera, Culicidae) larval distribution in Belize, Central-America. Environmental Entomology. 1993; 22(5) 978-92.

[43] Rejmankova E, Savage HM, Rejmanek M, Arredondo-Jimenez JI, Roberts DR. Multivariate-analysis of relationships between habitats, environmental-factors and occur-

rence of anopheline mosquito larvae *Anopheles albimanus* and *A. pseudopunctipennis* in southern Chiapas, Mexico. Journal of Applied Ecology. 1991; 28(3) 827-41.

[44] Rejmankova E, Savage HM, Rodriguez MH, Roberts DR, Rejmanek M. Aquatic vegetation as a basis for classification of *Anopheles albimanus* Weideman (Diptera, Culicidae) larval habitats. Environmental Entomology. 1992; 21(3) 598-603.

[45] Rozendaal JA. Observations on the distribution of anophelines in Surinam with particular reference to the malaria vector *Anopheles darlingi*. Memorias Do Instituto Oswaldo Cruz. 1990; 85(2) 221-34.

[46] Rozendaal JA. Relations between *Anopheles darlingi* breeding habitats, rainfall, river level and malaria transmission rates in the rain-forest of Surinam. Medical and Veterinary Entomology. 1992; 6(1) 16-22.

[47] Manguin S, Roberts DR, Andre RG, Rejmankova E, Hakre S. Characterization of *Anopheles darlingi* (Diptera: Culicidae) larval habitats in Belize, Central America. Journal of Medical Entomology. 1996; 33(2) 205-11.

[48] Grillet ME. Factors associated with distribution of *Anopheles aquasalis* and *Anopheles oswaldoi* (Diptera : Culicidae) in a malarious area, northeastern Venezuela. Journal of Medical Entomology. 2000; 37(2) 231-8.

[49] Rejmankova E, Rubio-Palis Y, Villegas L. Larval habitats of anopheline mosquitoes in the upper Orinoco, Venezuela. Journal of Vector Ecology. 1999; 24(2) 130-7.

[50] Rodriguez AD, Rodriguez MH, Meza RA, Hernandez JE, Rejmankova E, Savage HM, et al. Dynamics of population-densities and vegetation associations of *Anopheles-albimanus* larvae in a coastal area of southern Chiapas, Mexico. Journal of the American Mosquito Control Association. 1993; 9(1) 46-58.

[51] Rojas W, Penaranda F, Echavarria M. Strategies for malaria control in Colombia. Parasitology Today. 1992; 8(4) 141-4.

[52] Danis-Lozano R, Rodriguez MH, Arredondo-Jimenez JI, Hernandez Avila M, Mallorca C. Aquatic insects associated with *Anopheles albimanus* (Diptera: Culicidae) breeding sites in southern Mexico. Environmental Entomology. 1997; 26(4) 828-38.

[53] Vazquez-Martinez MG, Rodriguez MH, Arredondo-Jimenez JI, Mendez-Sanchez JD, Bond-Compean JG, Gold-Morgan M. Cyanobacteria associated with *Anopheles albimanus* (Diptera : Culicidae) larval habitats in southern Mexico. Journal of Medical Entomology. 2002; 39(6) 825-32.

[54] Torres-Estrada JJ, Meza-Alvarez RA, Cibrian-Tovar J, Rodriguez-Lopez MH, Arredondo-Jimenez JI, Cruz-Lopez L, et al. Vegetation-derived cues for the selection of oviposition substrates by *Anopheles albimanus* under laboratory conditions. Journal of the American Mosquito Control Association. 2005; 21(4) 344-9.

[55] Wood B, Washino R, Beck L, Hibbard K, Pitcairn M, Roberts D, et al. Distinguishing high and low anopheline-producing rice fields using remote-sensing and GIS technologies. Preventive Veterinary Medicine. 1991; 11(3-4) 277-88.

[56] Pope K, Masuoka P, Rejmankova E, Grieco J, Johnson S, Roberts D. Mosquito habitats, land use, and malaria risk in Belize from satellite imagery. Ecological Applications. 2005; 15(4) 1223-32.

[57] Pope KO, Rejmankova E, Savage HM, Arredondo-Jimenez JI, Rodriguez MH, Roberts DR. Remote-sensing of tropical wetlands for malaria control in Chiapas, Mexico. Ecological Applications. 1994; 4(1) 81-90.

[58] Roberts DR, Rodriguez MH. The environment, remote-sensing, and malaria control. Disease in Evolution: Global Changes and Emergence of Infectious Diseases. 1994; 740 396-402.

[59] Beck LR, Rodriguez MH, Dister SW, Rodriguez AD, Rejmankova E, Ulloa A, et al. Remote-sensing as a landscape epidemiologic tool to identify villages at high-risk for malaria transmission. American Journal of Tropical Medicine and Hygiene. 1994; 51(3) 271-80.

[60] Beck LR, Rodriguez MH, Dister SW, Rodriguez AD, Washino RK, Roberts DR, et al. Assessment of a remote sensing-based model for predicting malaria transmission risk in villages of Chiapas, Mexico. American Journal of Tropical Medicine and Hygiene. 1997; 56(1) 99-106.

[61] Sinka ME, Bangs MJ, Manguin S, Coetzee M, Mbogo CM, Hemingway J, et al. The dominant *Anopheles* vectors of human malaria in Africa, Europe and the Middle East: occurrence data, distribution maps and bionomic precis. Parasites & Vectors. 2010; 3 117.

[62] Sinka ME, Rubio-Palis Y, Manguin S, Patil AP, Temperley WH, Gething PW, et al. The dominant *Anopheles* vectors of human malaria in the Americas: occurrence data, distribution maps and bionomic precis. Parasites & Vectors. 2010; 3 72.

[63] Sinka ME, Bangs MJ, Manguin S, Chareonviriyaphap T, Patil AP, Temperley WH, et al. The dominant *Anopheles* vectors of human malaria in the Asia-Pacific region: occurrence data, distribution maps and bionomic precis. Parasites & Vectors. 2011; 4 89.

[64] Mouchet J, Manguin S, Sircoulon J, Laventure S, Faye O, Onapa AW, et al. Evolution of malaria in Africa for the past 40 years: Impact of climatic and human factors. Journal of the American Mosquito Control Association. 1998; 14(2) 121-30.

[65] Haddow AJ. Measurements of temperature and light in artificial pools with reference to the larval habitat of *Anopheles (Myzomyia) gambiae* Giles and *A. (M.) funestus* Giles. Bulletin of Entomological Research. 1943; 34 89.

[66] Orr BK, Resh VH. Influence of *Myriophyllum aquaticum* cover on *Anopheles* mosquito abundance, oviposition, and larval microhabitat. Oecologia. 1992; 90(4) 474-82.

[67] Rejmankova E, Roberts DR, Manguin S, Pope KO, Komarek J, Post RA. *Anopheles albimanus* (Diptera: Culicidae) and cyanobacteria: An example of larval habitat selection. Environmental Entomology. 1996; 25(5) 1058-67.

[68] Wallace JR, Merritt RW. Influence of microclimate, food, and predation on *Anopheles quadrimaculatus* (Diptera : Culicidae) growth and development rates, survivorship, and adult size in a Michigan pond. Environmental Entomology. 1999; 28(2) 233-9.

[69] Mutero CM, Blank H, Konradsen F, van der Hoek W. Water management for controlling the breeding of *Anopheles* mosquitoes in rice irrigation schemes in Kenya. Acta Tropica. 2000; 76(3) 253-63.

[70] Koenraadt CJM, Majambere S, Hemerik L, Takken W. The effects of food and space on the occurrence of cannibalism and predation among larvae of *Anopheles gambiae* s.l. Entomologia Experimentalis Et Applicata. 2004; 112(2) 125-34.

[71] Koenraadt CJM, Paaijmans KP, Githeko AK, Knols BGJ, Takken W. Egg hatching, larval movement and larval survival of the malaria vector *Anopheles gambiae* in desiccating habitats. Malaria Journal. 2003; 2 20.

[72] Munga S, Minakawa N, Zhou GF, Barrack OAJ, Githeko AK, Yan GY. Effects of larval competitors and predators on oviposition site selection of *Anopheles gambiae* sensu stricto. Journal of Medical Entomology. 2006; 43(2) 221-4.

[73] Achee NL, Grieco JP, Andre RG, Roberts DR, Rejmankova E. Experimental evaluation of overhanging bamboo in *Anopheles darlingi* larval habitat selection in Belize, Central America. Journal of Vector Ecology. 2006; 31(1) 145-51.

[74] Grieco JP, Rejmankova E, Achee NL, Klein CN, Andre R, Roberts D. Habitat suitability for three species of *Anopheles* mosquitoes: Larval growth and survival in reciprocal placement experiments. Journal of Vector Ecology. 2007; 32(2) 176-87.

[75] Carlson JC, Dyer LA, Omlin FX, Beier JC. Diversity cascades and malaria vectors. Journal of Medical Entomology. 2009; 46(3) 460-4.

[76] Jarju LBS, Fillinger U, Green C, Louca V, Majambere S, Lindsay SW. Agriculture and the promotion of insect pests: rice cultivation in river floodplains and malaria vectors in The Gambia. Malaria Journal. 2009; 8 170.

[77] Montoya-Lerma J, Solarte YA, Giraldo-Calderon GI, Quinones ML, Ruiz-Lopez F, Wilkerson RC, et al. Malaria vector species in Colombia - A review. Memorias Do Instituto Oswaldo Cruz. 2011; 106 223-38.

[78] Chase JM, Knight TM. Drought-induced mosquito outbreaks in wetlands. Ecology Letters. 2003; 6(11) 1017-24.

[79] Chase JM, Shulman RS. Wetland isolation facilitates larval mosquito density through the reduction of predators. Ecological Entomology. 2009; 34(6) 741-7.

[80] Blaustein L, Ostfeld RS, Holt RD. A community-ecology framework for understanding vector and vector-borne disease dynamics. Israel Journal of Ecology & Evolution. 2010; 56(3-4) 251-62.

[81] Paaijmans KP, Jacobs AFG, Takken W, Heusinkveld BG, Githeko AK, Dicke M, et al. Observations and model estimates of diurnal water temperature dynamics in mosquito breeding sites in western Kenya. Hydrological Processes. 2008; 22(24) 4789-801.

[82] Barros FSM, Arruda ME, Gurgel HC, Honorio NA. Spatial clustering and longitudinal variation of *Anopheles darlingi* (Diptera: Culicidae) larvae in a river of the Amazon: The importance of the forest fringe and of obstructions to flow in frontier malaria. Bulletin of Entomological Research. 2011; 101(6) 643-58.

[83] Bates M, De Zulueta J. The seasonal cycle of Anopheline mosquitoes in a pond in eastern Colombia. American Journal of Tropical Medicine. 1949; 29(1) 129-50.

[84] Washburn JO. Regulatory factors affecting larval mosquito populations in container and pool habitats - Implications for biological-control. Journal of the American Mosquito Control Association. 1995; 11(2) 279-83.

[85] Stresman GH. Beyond temperature and precipitation: Ecological risk factors that modify malaria transmission. Acta Tropica. 2010; 116(3) 167-72.

[86] Rejmankova E, Grieco J, Achee N, Masouka P, Pope K, Roberts D, et al. Freshwater community interactions and malaria. In: Collinge SK, Ray C, editors. Disease Ecology. Oxford: Oxford University Press; 2006.

[87] Bayoh MN, Lindsay SW. Temperature-related duration of aquatic stages of the Afrotropical malaria vector mosquito *Anopheles gambiae* in the laboratory. Medical and Veterinary Entomology. 2004; 18(2) 174-9.

[88] Wamae PM, Githeko AK, Menya DM, Takken W. Shading by napier grass reduces malaria vector larvae in natural habitats in Western Kenya highlands. Ecohealth. 2010; 7(4) 485-97.

[89] Ndenga BA, Simbauni JA, Mbugi JP, Githeko AK, Fillinger U. Productivity of malaria vectors from different habitat types in the western Kenya highlands. Plos One. 2011; 6(4) e19473.

[90] Lindblade KA, Walker ED, Onapa AW, Katungu J, Wilson ML. Land use change alters malaria transmission parameters by modifying temperature in a highland area of Uganda. Tropical Medicine & International Health. 2000; 5(4) 263-74.

[91] Imbahale SS, Mweresa CK, Takken W, Mukabana WR. Development of environmental tools for anopheline larval control. Parasites & Vectors. 2011; 4 130.

[92] Fillinger U, Sombroek H, Majambere S, van Loon E, Takken W, Lindsay SW. Identifying the most productive breeding sites for malaria mosquitoes in The Gambia. Malaria Journal. 2009; 8 62.

[93] Marten GG, Suarez MF, Astaeza R. An ecological survey of *Anopheles albimanus* larval habitats in Colombia. Journal of Vector Ecology. 1996; 21(2) 122-31.

[94] Pinault LL, Hunter FF. Characterization of larval habitats of *Anopheles albimanus, Anopheles pseudopunctipennis, Anopheles punctimacula,* and *Anopheles oswaldoi* s.l. populations in lowland and highland Ecuador. Journal of Vector Ecology. 2012; 37(1) 124-36.

[95] White GB. *Anopheles bwambae* sp-n, a malaria vector in the Semliki Valley, Uganda, and its relationships with other sibling species of the *An. gambiae* complex (Diptera, Culicidae). Systematic Entomology. 1985; 10(4) 501-22.

[96] Paaijmans KP, Blanford S, Bell AS, Blanford JI, Read AF, Thomas MB. Influence of climate on malaria transmission depends on daily temperature variation. Proceedings of the National Academy of Sciences of the United States of America. 2010; 107(34) 15135-9.

[97] Chahad-Ehlers S, Lozovei AL, Marques MD. Reproductive and post-embryonic daily rhythm patterns of the malaria vector *Anopheles (Kerteszia) cruzii*: Aspects of the life cycle. Chronobiology International. 2007; 24(2) 289-304.

[98] Obsomer V, Defourny P, Coosemans M. The *Anopheles dirus* complex: spatial distribution and environmental drivers. Malaria Journal. 2007; 6 26.

[99] Bugoro H, Hii J, Russell TL, Cooper RD, Chan BKK, Iro'ofa C, et al. Influence of environmental factors on the abundance of *Anopheles farauti* larvae in large brackish water streams in Northern Guadalcanal, Solomon Islands. Malaria Journal. 2011; 10 262.

[100] Surendran SN, Jude PJ, Ramasamy R. Variations in salinity tolerance of malaria vectors of the *Anopheles subpictus* complex in Sri Lanka and the implications for malaria transmission. Parasites & Vectors. 2011; 4 117.

[101] Dusfour I, Harbach RE, Manguin S. Bionomics and systematics of the oriental *Anopheles sundaicus* complex in relation to malaria transmission and vector control. American Journal of Tropical Medicine and Hygiene. 2004; 71(4) 518-24.

[102] Berti J, Navarro-Bueno E, Zoppi E, Gordon E, Delgado L. Estacionalidad de la densidad larval del mosquito *Anopheles aquasalis* (Diptera: Culicidae) y otros insectos asociados a su habitat en Sucre, Venezuela. Revista de Biologia Tropical. 2010; 58(2) 777-87.

[103] Smith KE, VanEkeris LA, Okech BA, Harvey WR, Linser PJ. Larval anopheline mosquito recta exhibit a dramatic change in localization patterns of ion transport proteins in response to shifting salinity: a comparison between anopheline and culicine larvae. Journal of Experimental Biology. 2008; 211(19) 3067-76.

[104] White BJ, Collins FH, Besansky NJ. Evolution of *Anopheles gambiae* in relation to humans and malaria. Annual Review of Ecology, Evolution, and Systematics, Vol 42. 2011; 42 111-32.

[105] Krishnamoorthy K, Jambulingam P, Natarajan R, Shriram AN, Das PK, Sehgal SC. Altered environment and risk of malaria outbreak in South Andaman, Andaman & Nicobar Islands, India affected by tsunami disaster. Malaria Journal. 2005; 4 32.

[106] Ramasamy R, Surendran SN. Possible impact of rising sea levels on vector-borne infectious diseases. BMC Infectious Diseases. 2011; 11 18.

[107] Mitsch WJ, Gosselnk JG. Wetlands. 4th edition ed. Hoboken, New Jersey: John Wiley & Sons, Inc.; 2007.

[108] Atieli HE, Zhou GF, Lee MC, Kweka EJ, Afrane Y, Mwanzo I, et al. Topography as a modifier of breeding habitats and concurrent vulnerability to malaria risk in the western Kenya highlands. Parasites & Vectors. 2011; 4 241.

[109] Paaijmans KP, Wandago MO, Githeko AK, Takken W. Unexpected high losses of *Anopheles gambiae* larvae due to rainfall. Plos One. 2007; 2(11) e1146.

[110] Charlwood JD, Braganca M. The effect of rainstorms on adult *Anopheles funestus* behavior and survival. Journal of Vector Ecology. 2012; 37(1) 252-6.

[111] Timms RM, Moss B. Prevention of growth of potentially dense phytoplankton populations by zooplankton grazing, in the presence of zooplanktivorous fish, in a shallow wetland ecosystem. Limnology and Oceanography. 1984; 29 472-86.

[112] Rejmankova E, Sirova D, Carlson E. Patterns of activities of root phosphomonoesterase and phosphodiesterase in wetland plants as a function of macrophyte species and ambient phosphorus regime. New Phytologist. [Article]. 2011; 190(4) 968-76.

[113] Ancona AH. Las Lemnaces y las larvas de los mosquitos. Anales del Instituto de Biología de México. 1930; 1(3) 3-37.

[114] Matheson R. The utilization of aquatic plants as aids in mosquito control. American Naturalist. 1930; 64 56-86.

[115] Balling SS, Resh VH. Seasonal pattern of pondweed standing crop and *Anopheles occidentalis* densities in Coyote Hills marsh. Proceedings of the California Mosquito Vector Control Association. 1985; 52 122-5.

[116] Rozeboom LE, Hess AD. The relation of the intersection line to the production of *Anopheles quadrimaculatus*. Journal of the National Malaria Society. 1944; 3 169-79.

[117] Walker ED, Merritt RW, Wotton RS. Analysis of the distribution and abundance of *Anopheles-quadrimaculatus* (Diptera, Culicidae) larvae in a marsh. Environmental Entomology. 1988; 17(6) 992-9.

[118] Collins JN, Resh VH. Measurements of temperature and light in artificial pools with reference to the larval habitat of *Anopheles (Myzomyia) gambiae* Giles and *A. (M.) funestus* Giles: California MVCA and University of California Mosquito Research Program1989.

[119] Mutuku FM, Alaii JA, Bayoh MN, Gimnig JE, Vulule JM, Walker ED, et al. Distribution, description, and local knowledge of larval habitats of *Anopheles gambiae* s.l. in a village in western Kenya. American Journal of Tropical Medicine and Hygiene. 2006; 74(1) 44-53.

[120] Fernandez-Salas I, Roberts DR, Rodriguez MH, Marina-Fernandez CF. Bionomics of larval populations of *Anopheles pseudopunctipennis* in the Tapachula foothills area, southern Mexico. Journal of the American Mosquito Control Association. 1994; 10(4) 477-86.

[121] Rueda LM, Peyton EL, Manguin S. *Anopheles (Anopheles) pseudopunctipennis* Theobald (Diptera: Culicidae): Neotype designation and description. Journal of Medical Entomology. 2004; 41(1) 12-22.

[122] Bond JG, Rojas JC, Arredondo-Jimenez JI, Quiroz-Martinez H, Valle J, Williams T. Population control of the malaria vector *Anopheles pseudopunctipennis* by habitat manipulation. Proceedings of the Royal Society of London Series B-Biological Sciences. 2004; 271(1553) 2161-9.

[123] Bond JG, Quiroz-Martinez H, Rojas JC, Valle J, Ulloa A, Williams T. Impact of environmental manipulation for *Anopheles pseudopunctipennis* Theobald control on aquatic insect communities in southern Mexico. Journal of Vector Ecology. 2007; 32(1) 41-53.

[124] Manguin S, Roberts DR, Peyton EL, Rejmankova E, Pecor J. Characterization of *Anopheles pseudopunctipennis* larval habitats. Journal of the American Mosquito Control Association. 1996; 12(4) 619-26.

[125] Bond JG, Arredondo-Jimenez JI, Rodriguez MH, Quiroz-Martinez H, Williams T. Oviposition habitat selection for a predator refuge and food source in a mosquito. Ecological Entomology. 2005; 30(3) 255-63.

[126] Torres-Estrada JL, Meza-Alvarez RA, Cruz-Lopez L, Rodriguez MH, Arredondo-Jimenez JI. Attraction of gravid *Anopheles pseudopunctipennis* females to oviposition substrates by *Spirogyra majuscula* (Zygnematales : Zygnemataceae) algae under laboratory conditions. Journal of the American Mosquito Control Association. 2007; 23(1) 18-23.

[127] Johnson HA. Occurence of *Anopheles vestitipennis* in Porto Rico. The American Journal of Tropical Medicine. 1925; 6(2) 153-5.

[128] Loyola EG, Arredondo-Jimenez I, Rodriguez MH, Brown DN, Vacamarin MA. *Anopheles vestitipennis*, the Probable Vector of *Plasmodium vivax* in the Lacandon Forest of Chiapas, Mexico. Transactions of the Royal Society of Tropical Medicine and Hygiene. 1991; 85(2) 171-4.

[129] Rejmankova E, Pope KO, Roberts DR, Lege MG, Andre R, Grieco J, et al. Characterization and detection of *Anopheles vestitipennis* and *Anopheles punctimacula* (Diptera :

Culicidae) larval habitats in Belize with field survey and SPOT satellite imagery. Journal of Vector Ecology. 1998; 23(1) 74-88.

[130] Ulloa A, Rodriguez MH, Arredondo-Jimenez JI, Fernandez-Salas I. Biological variation in two *Anopheles vestitipennis* populations with different feeding preferences in southern Mexico. Journal of the American Mosquito Control Association. 2005; 21(4) 350-4.

[131] Gratz NG. Emerging and resurging vector-borne diseases. Annual Review of Entomology. 1999; 44 51-75.

[132] Forattini OP, Kakitani I, Massad E, Marucci D. Studies on mosquitos (Diptera, Culicidae) and anthropic environment - 3-survey of adult stages at the rice irrigation system and the emergence of *Anopheles albitarsis* in South-Eastern, Brazil. Revista De Saude Publica. 1993; 27(5) 313-25.

[133] Mogi M, Okazawa T, Miyagi I, Sucharit S, Tumrasvin W, Deesin T, et al. Development and survival of anopheline immatures (Diptera, Culicidae) in rice fields in northern Thailand. Journal of Medical Entomology. 1986; 23(3) 244-50.

[134] Blaustein L. Larvivorous fishes fail to control mosquitos in experimental rice plots. Hydrobiologia. 1992; 232(3) 219-32.

[135] Mogi M, Miyagi I. Colonization of rice fields by mosquitoes (Diptera, Culicidae) and larvivorous predators in asynchronous rice cultivation areas in the Philippines. Journal of Medical Entomology. 1990; 27(4) 530-6.

[136] Service MW. Agricultural-development and arthropod-borne diseases - A review. Revista De Saude Publica. 1991; 25(3) 165-78.

[137] Ohba SY, Huynh TTT, Le LL, Ngoc HT, Hoang SL, Takagi M. Mosquitoes and their potential predators in rice agroecosystems of the Mekong Delta, southern Vietnam. Journal of the American Mosquito Control Association. 2011; 27(4) 384-92.

[138] Lacey LA, Lacey CM. The medical importance of riceland mosquitos and their control using alternatives to chemical insecticides. Journal of the American Mosquito Control Association. 1990; 1-93.

[139] Rejmankova E, Higashi R, Grieco J, Achee N, Roberts D. Volatile substances from larval habitats mediate species-specific oviposition in *Anopheles* mosquitoes. Journal of Medical Entomology. 2005; 42(2) 95-103.

[140] Lyimo EO, Takken W, Koella JC. Effect of rearing temperature and larval density on larval survival, age at pupation and adult size of *Anopheles-gambiae*. Entomologia Experimentalis Et Applicata. 1992; 63(3) 265-71.

[141] Koella JC, Lyimo EO. Variability in the relationship between weight and wing length of *Anopheles gambiae* (Diptera: Culicidae). Journal of Medical Entomology. 1996; 33(2) 261-4.

[142] Peck GW, Walton WE. Effect of bacterial quality and density on growth and whole body stoichiometry of *Culex quinquefasciatus* and *Culex tarsalis* (Diptera: Culicidae). Journal of Medical Entomology. 2006; 43(1) 25-33.

[143] Cole JJ, Findlay S, Pace ML. Bacterial production in fresh and saltwater ecosystems - a cross-system overview. Marine Ecology-Progress Series. 1988; 43(1-2) 1-10.

[144] Walker ED, Merritt RW. Bacterial enrichment in the surface microlayer of an *Anopheles quadrimaculatus* (Diptera, Culicidae) larval habitat. Journal of Medical Entomology. 1993; 30(6) 1050-2.

[145] Kaufman MG, Wanja E, Maknojia S, Bayoh MN, Vulule JM, Walker ED. Importance of algal biomass to growth and development of *Anopheles gambiae* larvae. Journal of Medical Entomology. 2006; 43(4) 669-76.

[146] Marten GG. Larvicidal algae. Journal of the American Mosquito Control Association. 2007; 23(2) 177-83.

[147] Napolitano GE. Fatty acids as trophic and chemical markers in freshwater ecosystems. In: Arts MT, Wainman BC, editors. Lipids in Freshwater Ecosystems. Verlag: Springer; 1999. p. 21-44.

[148] Parish CC. Determination of total lipid, lipid classes and fatty acids in aquatic samples In: Arts MT, Wainman BC, editors. Lipids in Freshwater Ecosystems. Verlag: Springer; 1999. p. 4-20.

[149] Dadd RH, Kleinjan JE, Stanley-Samuelson DW. Polyunsaturated fatty acids of mosquitoes reared with single dietary polyunsaturates. Insect Biochemistry. 1987; 17 7-16.

[150] Dadd RH, Kleinjan JE. Prostaglandin sparing of dietary arachidonic-acid in the mosquito *Culex pipiens*. Journal of Insect Physiology. 1988; 34(8) 779-85.

[151] Nor Aliza AR, Stanley DW. A digestive phospholipase A2 in larval mosquitoes, *Aedes aegypti*. Insect Biochemistry and Molecular Biology. 1998; 28 561-9.

[152] Timmermann SE, Briegel H. Effect of plant, fungal and animal diets on mosquito development. Entomologia Experimentalis Et Applicata. 1996; 80(1) 173-6.

[153] Kominkova D, Rejmankova E, Grieco J, Achee N. Fatty acids in anopheline mosquito and their habitats. Journal of Vector Ecology. 2012; 37(2) 382-395.

[154] Blaustein L, Kiflawi M, Eitam A, Mangel M, Cohen JE. Oviposition habitat selection in response to risk of predation in temporary pools: mode of detection and consistency across experimental venue. Oecologia. 2004; 138(2) 300-5.

[155] Kumar R, Muhid P, Dahms HU, Tseng LC, Hwang JS. Potential of three aquatic predators to control mosquitoes in the presence of alternative prey: a comparative experimental assessment. Marine and Freshwater Research. 2008; 59(9) 817-35.

[156] Shaalan EAS, Canyon DV. Aquatic insect predators and mosquito control. Tropical Biomedicine. 2009; 26(3) 223-61.

[157] Kweka EJ. Predation efficiency of *Anopheles gambiae* larvae by aquatic predators in western Kenya highlands. Tropical Medicine & International Health. 2012; 17 53.

[158] Knight TM, Chase JM, Goss CW, Knight JJ. Effects of interspecific competition, predation, and their interaction on survival and development time of immature *Anopheles quadrimaculatus*. Journal of Vector Ecology. 2004; 29(2) 277-84.

[159] Juliano SA. Species interactions among larval mosquitoes: context dependence across habitat gradients. Annual Review of Entomology. 2009; 54 37-56.

[160] Gimonneau G, Pombi M, Dabire RK, Diabate A, Morand S, Simard F. Behavioural responses of *Anopheles gambiae* sensu stricto M and S molecular form larvae to an aquatic predator in Burkina Faso. Parasites & Vectors. 2012; 5 56.

[161] Hinman EH. Predators of the Culicidae (mosquitoes). I. The predators of larvae and pupae, exclusive of fish. Journal of Tropical Medicine and Hygiene. 1934; 37 129-34.

[162] Blaustein L, Margalit J. Mosquito larvae (*Culiseta-longiareolata*) prey upon and compete with toad tadpoles (*Bufo-viridis*). Journal of Animal Ecology. 1994; 63(4) 841-50.

[163] Mokany A, Shine R. Biological warfare in the garden pond: tadpoles suppress the growth of mosquito larvae. Ecological Entomology. 2003; 28(1) 102-8.

[164] Grill CP, Juliano SA. Predicting species interactions based on behaviour: Predation and competition in container-dwelling mosquitoes. Journal of Animal Ecology. 1996; 65(1) 63-76.

[165] Blaustein L, Karban R. Indirect effects of the mosquitofish *Gambusia-affinis* on the mosquito *Culex-tarsalis*. Limnology and Oceanography. 1990; 35(3) 767-71.

[166] Mokany A. Impact of tadpoles and mosquito larvae on ephemeral pond structure and processes. Marine and Freshwater Research. 2007; 58(5) 436-44.

[167] Kumar R, Hwang JS. Larvicidal efficiency of aquatic predators: A perspective for mosquito biocontrol. Zoological Studies. 2006; 45(4) 447-66.

[168] Mogi M. Insects and other invertebrate predators. Journal of the American Mosquito Control Association. 2007; 23(2) 93-109.

[169] Quiroz-Martinez H, Rodriguez-Castro A. Aquatic insects as predators of mosquito larvae. Journal of the American Mosquito Control Association. 2007; 23(2) 110-7.

[170] Rozendaal JA. Vector Control: Methods for Use by Individuals and Communities. Geneva: World Health Organization; 1997.

[171] Chandra G, Bhattacharjee I, Chatterjee SN, Ghosh A. Mosquito control by larvivorous fish. Indian Journal of Medical Research. 2008; 127(1) 13-27.

[172] Service MW. Identification of predators of *Anopheles gambiae* resting in huts, by precipitin test. Transactions of the Royal Society of Tropical Medicine and Hygiene. 1973; 67(1) 33-4.

[173] Service MW. Mortalities of immature stages of species-b of *Anopheles gambiae* complex in kenya - comparison between rice fields and temporary pools, identification of predators, and effects of insecticidal spraying. Journal of Medical Entomology. 1977; 13(4-5) 535-45.

[174] Caillouet KA, Keating J, Eisele TP. Characterization of aquatic mosquito habitat, natural enemies, and immature mosquitoes in the Artibonite Valley, Haiti. Journal of Vector Ecology. 2008; 33(1) 191-7.

[175] Louca V, Lucas MC, Green C, Majambere S, Fillinger U, Lindsay SW. Role of fish as predators of mosquito larvae on the floodplain of the Gambia River. Journal of Medical Entomology. 2009; 46(3) 546-56.

[176] Walton WE. Larvivorous fish including Gambusia. Journal of the American Mosquito Control Association. 2007; 23(2) 184-220.

[177] Preston DL, Henderson JS, Johnson PTJ. Community ecology of invasions: direct and indirect effects of multiple invasive species on aquatic communities. Ecology. 2012; 93(6) 1254-61.

[178] Bence JR. Indirect effects and biological-control of mosquitos by mosquitofish. Journal of Applied Ecology. 1988; 25(2) 505-21.

[179] Diabate A, Dabire RK, Heidenberger K, Crawford J, Lamp WO, Culler LE, et al. Evidence for divergent selection between the molecular forms of *Anopheles gambiae*: role of predation. BMC Evolutionary Biology. 2008; 8 5.

[180] Gimonneau G, Bouyer J, Morand S, Besansky NJ, Diabate A, Simard F. A behavioral mechanism underlying ecological divergence in the malaria mosquito *Anopheles gambiae*. Behavioral Ecology. 2010; 21(5) 1087-92.

[181] Morris DW. Toward an ecological synthesis: a case for habitat selection. Oecologia. 2003; 136(1) 1-13.

[182] Impoinvil DE, Keating J, Mbogo CM, Potts MD, Chowdhury RR, Beier JC. Abundance of immature *Anopheles* and Culicines (Diptera : Culicidae) in different water body types in the urban environment of Malindi, Kenya. Journal of Vector Ecology. 2008; 33(1) 107-16.

[183] Munga S, Minakawa N, Zhou GF, Barrack OOJ, Githeko AK, Yan GY. Oviposition site preference and egg hatchability of *Anopheles gambiae*: Effects of land cover types. Journal of Medical Entomology. 2005; 42(6) 993-7.

[184] Keating J, MacIntyre K, Mbogo C, Githeko A, Regens JL, Swalm C, et al. A geographic sampling strategy for studying relationships between human activity and malaria

http://dx.doi.org/10.5772/55229

vectors in urban Africa. American Journal of Tropical Medicine and Hygiene. 2003; 68(3) 357-65.

[185] Blaustein L. Oviposition site selection in response to risk of predation: evidence from aquatic habitats and consequences for population dynamics and community structure. In: Wasser SP, editor. Evolutionary theory and processes: modern perspectives. Dordrecht: Kluwer Academic Publishers; 1999. p. 441-56.

[186] Kershenbaum A, Spencer M, Blaustein L, Cohen JE. Modelling evolutionarily stable strategies in oviposition site selection, with varying risks of predation and intraspecific competition. Evolutionary Ecology. 2012; 26(4) 955-74.

[187] Warburg A, Faiman R, Shtern A, Silberbush A, Markman S, Cohen JE, et al. Oviposition habitat selection by *Anopheles gambiae* in response to chemical cues by *Notonecta maculata*. Journal of Vector Ecology. 2011; 36(2) 421-5.

[188] Vonesh JR, Blaustein L. Predator-induced shifts in mosquito oviposition site selection: A meta-analysis and implications for vector control. Israel Journal of Ecology & Evolution. 2010; 56(3-4) 263-79.

[189] Beck LR, Lobitz BM, Wood BL. Remote sensing and human health: New sensors and new opportunities. Emerging Infectious Diseases. 2000; 6(3) 217-27.

[190] Stoops CA, Gionar YR, Shinta, Sismadi P, Rachmat A, Elyazar IF, et al. Remotely-sensed land use patterns and the presence of *Anopheles* larvae (Diptera : Culicidae) in Sukabumi, West Java, Indonesia. Journal of Vector Ecology. 2008; 33(1) 30-9.

[191] Lourenco PM, Sousa CA, Seixas J, Lopes P, Novo MT, Almeida APG. *Anopheles atroparvus* density modeling using MODIS NDVI in a former malarious area in Portugal. Journal of Vector Ecology. 2011; 36(2) 279-91.

[192] Machault V, Vignolles C, Borchi F, Vounatsou P, Pages F, Briolant S, et al. The use of remotely sensed environmental data in the study of malaria. Geospatial Health. 2011; 5(2) 151-68.

[193] Dambach P, Machault V, Lacaux JP, Vignolles C, Sie A, Sauerborn R. Utilization of combined remote sensing techniques to detect environmental variables influencing malaria vector densities in rural West Africa. International Journal of Health Geographics. 2012; 11, 8.

[194] Turner W, Spector S, Gardiner N, Fladeland M, Sterling E, Steininger M. Remote sensing for biodiversity science and conservation. Trends in Ecology & Evolution. 2003; 18(6) 306-14.

[195] Buermann W, Saatchi S, Smith TB, Zutta BR, Chaves JA, Mila B, et al. Predicting species distributions across the Amazonian and Andean regions using remote sensing data. Journal of Biogeography. 2008; 35(7) 1160-76.

[196] Rakotomanana F, Randremanana RV, Rabarijaona LP, Duchemin JB, Ratovonjato J, Ariey F, et al. Determining areas that require indoor insecticide spraying using Multi

Criteria Evaluation, a decision-support tool for malaria vector control programmes in the Central Highlands of Madagascar. International Journal of Health Geographics. 2007; 6, 2.

[197] Rakotomanana F, Ratovonjato J, Randremanana RV, Randrianasolo L, Raherinjafy R, Rudant JP, et al. Geographical and environmental approaches to urban malaria in Antananarivo (Madagascar). BMC Infectious Diseases. 2010; 10, 173.

[198] Mushinzimana E, Munga S, Minakawa N, Li L, Feng CC, Bian L, et al. Landscape determinants and remote sensing of anopheline mosquito larval habitats in the western Kenya highlands. Malaria Journal. 2006; 5, 13.

[199] Jacob BG, Muturi EJ, Mwangangi JM, Funes J, Caamano EX, Muriu S, et al. Remote and field level quantification of vegetation covariates for malaria mapping in three rice agro-village complexes in Central Kenya. International Journal of Health Geographics. 2007; 6 21.

[200] Munga S, Yakob L, Mushinzimana E, Zhou GF, Ouna T, Minakawa N, et al. Land use and land cover changes and spatiotemporal dynamics of anopheline larval habitats during a four-year period in a highland community of Africa. American Journal of Tropical Medicine and Hygiene. 2009; 81(6) 1079-84.

[201] Mutuku FM, Bayoh MN, Hightower AW, Vulule JM, Gimnig JE, Mueke JM, et al. A supervised land cover classification of a western Kenya lowland endemic for human malaria: associations of land cover with larval *Anopheles* habitats. International Journal of Health Geographics. 2009; 8, 19.

[202] Clennon JA, Kamanga A, Musapa M, Shiff C, Glass GE. Identifying malaria vector breeding habitats with remote sensing data and terrain-based landscape indices in Zambia. International Journal of Health Geographics. 2010; 9, 58.

[203] Ahmad R, Ali WN, Nor ZM, Ismail Z, Hadi AA, Ibrahim MN, et al. Mapping of mosquito breeding sites in malaria endemic areas in Pos Lenjang, Kuala Lipis, Pahang, Malaysia. Malaria Journal. 2011; 10, 361.

[204] Achee NL, Grieco JP, Masuoka P, Andre RG, Roberts DR, Thomas J, et al. Use of remote sensing and geographic information systems to predict locations of *Anopheles darlingi*-positive breeding sites within the Sibun River in Belize, central America. Journal of Medical Entomology. 2006; 43(2) 382-92.

[205] Roberts DR, Paris JF, Manguin S, Harbach RE, Woodruff R, Rejmankova E, et al. Predictions of malaria vector distribution in Belize based on multispectral satellite data. American Journal of Tropical Medicine and Hygiene. 1996; 54(3) 304-8.

[206] Peterson AT. Biogeography of diseases: a framework for analysis. Naturwissenschaften. 2008; 95(6) 483-91.

[207] Peterson AT, Martinez-Campos C, Nakazawa Y, Martinez-Meyer E. Time-specific ecological niche modeling predicts spatial dynamics of vector insects and human

dengue cases. Transactions of the Royal Society of Tropical Medicine and Hygiene. 2005; 99(9) 647-55.

[208] Levine RS, Peterson AT, Benedict MQ. Geographic and ecologic distributions of the *Anopheles gambiae* complex predicted using a genetic algorithm. American Journal of Tropical Medicine and Hygiene. 2004; 70(2) 105-9.

[209] Patz JA, Olson SH, Uejio CK, Gibbs HK. Disease emergence from global climate and land use change. Medical Clinics of North America. 2008; 92(6) 1473-91.

[210] Myers SS, Patz JA. Emerging threats to human health from global environmental change. Annual Review of Environment and Resources. 2009; 34 223-52.

[211] IPCC. Climate Change 2007: The Physical Science Basis. Contribution of Working Group I to the Fourth Assessment Report of the Intergovernmental Panel on Climate Change. Cambridge and New York 2007.

[212] McMichael AJ, Friel S, Nyong A, Corvalan C. Global environmental change and health: impacts, inequalities, and the health sector. British Medical Journal. 2008; 336(7637) 191-4.

[213] Carpenter SR, Stanley EH, Vander Zanden MJ. State of the world's freshwater ecosystems: Physical, chemical, and biological changes. Annual Review of Environment and Resources, Vol 36. 2011; 36 75-99.

[214] Tran A, Poncon N, Toty C, Linard C, Guis H, Ferre JB, et al. Using remote sensing to map larval and adult populations of *Anopheles hyrcanus* (Diptera: Culicidae) a potential malaria vector in Southern France. International Journal of Health Geographics. 2008; 7, 9.

[215] Martens P, Kovats RS, Nijhof S, de Vries P, Livermore MTJ, Bradley DJ, et al. Climate change and future populations at risk of malaria. Global Environmental Change-Human and Policy Dimensions. 1999; 9 S89-S107.

[216] Molyneux DH. Vectorborne parasitic diseases - an overview of recent changes. International Journal for Parasitology. 1998; 28(6) 927-34.

[217] Molyneux DH. Common themes in changing vector-borne disease scenarios. Transactions of the Royal Society of Tropical Medicine and Hygiene. 2003; 97(2) 129-32.

[218] Afrane YA, Githeko AK, Yan GY. The ecology of *Anopheles* mosquitoes under climate change: Case studies from the effects of deforestation in East African highlands. Year in Ecology and Conservation Biology. 2012; 1249 204-10.

[219] Berger F, Flamand C, Musset L, Djossou F, Rosine J, Sanquer MA, et al. Investigation of a sudden malaria outbreak in the isolated Amazonian village of Saul, French Guiana, January-April 2009. American Journal of Tropical Medicine and Hygiene. 2012; 86(4) 591-7.

[220] Hackett LW. Distribution of Malaria. In: Boyd MF, editor. Malariology. Philadelphia: Saunders; 1949. p. 722-35.

[221] Fontenille D, Simard F. Unravelling complexities in human malaria transmission dynamics in Africa through a comprehensive knowledge of vector populations. Comparative Immunology Microbiology and Infectious Diseases. 2004; 27(5) 357-75.

[222] Gimonneau G, Pombi M, Choisy M, Morand S, Dabire RK, Simard F. Larval habitat segregation between the molecular forms of the mosquito *Anopheles gambiae* in a rice field area of Burkina Faso, West Africa. Medical and Veterinary Entomology. 2012; 26(1) 9-17.

[223] Laporta GZ, Ramos DG, Ribeiro MC, Sallum MAM. Habitat suitability of *Anopheles* vector species and association with human malaria in the Atlantic Forest in southeastern Brazil. Memorias Do Instituto Oswaldo Cruz. 2011; 106 239-49.

[224] Yasuoka J, Levins R. Impact of deforestation and agricultural development on anopheline ecology and malaria epidemiology. American Journal of Tropical Medicine and Hygiene. 2007; 76(3) 450-60.

[225] Vittor AY, Pan W, Gilman RH, Tielsch J, Glass G, Shields T, et al. Linking deforestation to malaria in the Amazon: Characterization of the breeding habitat of the principal malaria vector, *Anopheles darlingi*. American Journal of Tropical Medicine and Hygiene. 2009; 81(1) 5-12.

[226] Conn JE, Wilkerson RC, Segura MNO, De Souza RTL, Schlichting CD, Wirtz RA, et al. Emergence of a new neotropical malaria vector facilitated by human migration and changes in land use. American Journal of Tropical Medicine and Hygiene. 2002; 66(1) 18-22.

[227] Tadei WP, Thatcher BD, Santos JMH, Scarpassa VM, Rodrigues IB, Rafael MS. Ecologic observations on anopheline vectors of malaria in the Brazilian Amazon. American Journal of Tropical Medicine and Hygiene. 1998; 59(2) 325-35.

[228] Lerer LB, Scudder T. Health impacts of large dams. Environmental Impact Assessment Review. 1999; 19(2) 113-23.

[229] Jobin WR. Dams and Disease: Ecological Design and Health Impacts of Large Dams, Canals and Irrigation Systems. London: Routledge; 1999.

[230] Hunter JM. Inherited burden of disease: agricultural dams and the persistence of bloody urine (*Schistosomiasis hematobium*) in the Upper East Region of Ghana, 1959-1997. Social Science & Medicine. 2003; 56(2) 219-34.

[231] Keiser J, De Castro MC, Maltese MF, Bos R, Tanner M, Singer BH, et al. Effect of irrigation and large dams on the burden of malaria on a global and regional scale. American Journal of Tropical Medicine and Hygiene. 2005; 72(4) 392-406.

[232] Kibret S, Lautze J, Boelee E, McCartney M. How does an Ethiopian dam increase malaria? Entomological determinants around the Koka reservoir. Tropical Medicine & International Health. 2012; 17(11), 1320-8.

[233] Zeilhofer P, dos Santos ES, Ribeiro ALM, Miyazaki RD, dos Santos MA. Habitat suitability mapping of *Anopheles darlingi* in the surroundings of the Manso hydropower plant reservoir, Mato Grosso, Central Brazil. International Journal of Health Geographics. 2007; 6, 7.

[234] Willott E. Restoring nature, without mosquitoes? Restoration Ecology. 2004; 12(2) 147-53.

[235] Goma LKH. The influence of man's activities on swamp-mosquito breeding in Uganda (Diptera: Culicidae). Journal of the Entomological Society of South Africa. 1961; 24 231-47.

[236] Malan HL, Appleton CC, Day JA, Dini J. Wetlands and invertebrate disease hosts: Are we asking for trouble? Water Sa. 2009; 35(5) 753-67.

[237] Carlson JC, Byrd BD, Omlin FX. Field assessments in western Kenya link malaria vectors to environmentally disturbed habitats during the dry season. BMC Public Health. 2004; 4, 33.

[238] Thullen JS, Sartoris JJ, Walton WE. Effects of vegetation management in constructed wetland treatment cells on water quality and mosquito production. Ecological Engineering. 2002; 18(4) 441-57.

[239] Walton WE, Popko DA, Van Dam AR, Merrill A, Lythgoe J, Hess B. Width of planting beds for emergent vegetation influences mosquito production from a constructed wetland in California (USA). Ecological Engineering. 2012; 42 150-9.

[240] Knight RL, Walton WE, O'Meara GF, Reisen WK, Wass R. Strategies for effective mosquito control in constructed treatment wetlands. Ecological Engineering. 2003; 21(4-5) 211-32.

[241] Sanford MR, Chan K, Walton WE. Effects of inorganic nitrogen enrichment on mosquitoes (Diptera : Culicidae) and the associated aquatic community in constructed treatment wetlands. Journal of Medical Entomology. 2005; 42(5) 766-76.

[242] Yadav P, Foster WA, Mitsch WJ, Grewal PS. Factors affecting mosquito populations in created wetlands in urban landscapes. Urban Ecosystems. 2012; 15(2) 499-511.

[243] Greenway M. The role of constructed wetlands in secondary effluent treatment and water reuse in subtropical and arid Australia. Ecological Engineering. 2005; 25(5) 501-9.

[244] Carlson DB, Knight RL. Mosquito production and hydrological capacity of southeast Florida impoundments used for waste-water retention. Journal of the American Mosquito Control Association. 1987; 3(1) 74-83.

[245] Vitousek PM, Aber JD, Howarth RW, Likens GE, Matson PA, Schindler DW, et al. Human alteration of the global nitrogen cycle: Sources and consequences. Ecological Applications. 1997; 7(3) 737-50.

[246] Carpenter SR, Caraco NF, Correll DL, Howarth RW, Sharpley AN, Smith VH. Non-point pollution of surface waters with phosphorus and nitrogen. Ecological Applications. 1998; 8(3) 559-68.

[247] Howarth RW, Anderson D, Cloern J, Elfring C, Hopkinson C, Lapointe B, et al. Nutrient pollution of coastal rivers, bays, and seas. Issues in Ecology. 2000; 7 1-15.

[248] Galloway JN, Cowling EB. Reactive nitrogen and the world: 200 years of change. Ambio. 2002; 31(2) 64-71.

[249] Camargo JA, Alonso A. Ecological and toxicological effects of inorganic nitrogen pollution in aquatic ecosystems: A global assessment. Environment International. 2006; 32(6) 831-49.

[250] Townsend AR, Howarth RW, Bazzaz FA, Booth MS, Cleveland CC, Collinge SK, et al. Human health effects of a changing global nitrogen cycle. Frontiers in Ecology and the Environment. 2003; 1(5) 240-6.

[251] Teng HJ, Wu YL, Wang SJ, Lin C. Effects of environmental factors on abundance of *Anopheles minimus* (Diptera : Culicidae) larvae and their seasonal fluctuation in Taiwan. Environmental Entomology. 1998; 27(2) 324-8.

[252] Minakawa N, Dida GO, Sonye GO, Futami K, Njenga SM. Malaria vectors in Lake Victoria and adjacent habitats in western Kenya. Plos One. 2012; 7(3) e32725.

[253] Patz JA, Olson SH. Malaria risk and temperature: Influences from global climate change and local land use practices. Proceedings of the National Academy of Sciences of the United States of America. 2006; 103(15) 5635-6.

[254] Reiter P, Thomas CJ, Atkinson PM, Hay SI, Randolph SE, Rogers DJ, et al. Global warming and malaria: a call for accuracy. Lancet Infectious Diseases. 2004; 4(6) 323-4.

[255] Chaves LF, Koenraadt CJM. Climate change and highland malaria: Fresh air for a hot debate. Quarterly Review of Biology. 2010; 85(1) 27-55.

[256] Pascual M, Ahumada JA, Chaves LF, Rodo X, Bouma M. Malaria resurgence in the East African highlands: Temperature trends revisited. Proceedings of the National Academy of Sciences of the United States of America. 2006; 103(15) 5829-34.

[257] Chaves LF, Hashizume M, Satake A, Minakawa N. Regime shifts and heterogeneous trends in malaria time series from Western Kenya Highlands. Parasitology. 2012; 139(1) 14-25.

[258] Bomblies A. Modeling the role of rainfall patterns in seasonal malaria transmission. Climatic Change. 2012; 112(3-4) 673-85.

[259] Trung HD, Van Bortel W, Sochantha T, Keokenchanh K, Quang NT, Cong LD, et al. Malaria transmission and major malaria vectors in different geographical areas of Southeast Asia. Tropical Medicine & International Health. 2004; 9(2) 230-7.

[260] Gunasekaran K, Jambulingam P, Srinivasan R, Sadanandane C, Doss PSB, Sabesan S, et al. Malaria receptivity in the tsunami-hit coastal villages of southern India. Lancet Infectious Diseases. 2005; 5(9) 531-2.

[261] Jude PJ, Dharshini S, Vinobaba M, Surendran SN, Ramasamy R. *Anopheles culicifacies* breeding in brackish waters in Sri Lanka and implications for malaria control. Malaria Journal. 2010; 9, 106.

[262] Reinbold-Wasson DD, Sardelis MR, Jones JW, Watts DM, Fernandez R, Carbajal F, et al. Determinants of *Anopheles* seasonal distribution patterns across a forest to periurban gradient near Iquitos, Peru. American Journal of Tropical Medicine and Hygiene. 2012; 86(3) 459-63.

[263] Charlwood JD. Biological variation in *Anopheles darlingi* root. Memorias Do Instituto Oswaldo Cruz. 1996; 91(4) 391-8.

[264] Keiser J, Singer BH, Utzinger J. Reducing the burden of malaria in different eco-epidemiological settings with environmental management: a systematic review. Lancet Infectious Diseases. 2005; 5(11) 695-708.

[265] Lambrechts L, Knox TB, Wong J, Liebman KA, Albright RG, Stoddard ST. Shifting priorities in vector biology to improve control of vector-borne disease. Tropical Medicine & International Health. 2009; 14(12) 1505-14.

[266] Raghavendra K, Barik TK, Reddy BPN, Sharma P, Dash AP. Malaria vector control: from past to future. Parasitology Research. 2011; 108(4) 757-79.

[267] Najera JA, Gonzalez-Silva M, Alonso PL. Some lessons for the future from the Global Malaria Eradication Programme (1955-1969). Plos Medicine. 2011; 8(1) e1000412.

[268] Worrall E, Fillinger U. Large-scale use of mosquito larval source management for malaria control in Africa: A cost analysis. Malaria Journal. 2011; 10 338.

[269] McKenzie FE, Baird JK, Beier JC, Lal AA, Bossert WH. A biologic basis for integrated malaria control. American Journal of Tropical Medicine and Hygiene. 2002; 67(6) 571-7.

[270] Gu WD, Novak RJ. Habitat-based modeling of impacts of mosquito larval interventions on entomological inoculation rates, incidence, and prevalence of malaria. American Journal of Tropical Medicine and Hygiene. 2005; 73(3) 546-52.

[271] Fillinger U, Lindsay SW. Larval source management for malaria control in Africa: myths and reality. Malaria Journal. 2011; 10 353.

[272] Minakawa N, Mutero CM, Githure JI, Beier JC, Yan GY. Spatial distribution and habitat characterization of anopheline mosquito larvae in western Kenya. American Journal of Tropical Medicine and Hygiene. 1999; 61(6) 1010-6.

[273] Abdul-Ghani R, Al-Mekhlafi AM, Alabsi MS. Microbial control of malaria: Biological warfare against the parasite and its vector. Acta Tropica. 2012; 121(2) 71-84.

[274] Mittal PK. Biolarvicides in vector control: challenges and prospects. Journal of Vector Borne Diseases. 2003; 40 20-32.

[275] Favia G, Ricci I, Damiani C, Raddadi N, Crotti E, Marzorati M, et al. Bacteria of the genus Asaia stably associate with *Anopheles stephensi*, an Asian malarial mosquito vector. Proceedings of the National Academy of Sciences of the United States of America. 2007; 104(21) 9047-51.

[276] Cirimotich CM, Ramirez JL, Dimopoulos G. Native microbiota shape insect vector competence for human pathogens. Cell Host & Microbe. 2011; 10(4) 307-10.

[277] Chouaia B, Rossi P, Epis S, Mosca M, Ricci I, Damiani C, et al. Delayed larval development in *Anopheles* mosquitoes deprived of *Asaia* bacterial symbionts. BMC Microbiology. 2012; 12, suppl. 1, S2.

[278] Rani A, Sharma A, Rajagopal R, Adak T, Bhatnagar RK. Bacterial diversity analysis of larvae and adult midgut microflora using culture-dependent and culture-independent methods in lab-reared and field-collected *Anopheles stephensi*-an Asian malarial vector. BMC Microbiology. 2009; 9, 96.

[279] Peterson AT. Shifting suitability for malaria vectors across Africa with warming climates. BMC Infectious Diseases. 2009; 9, 59.

Chapter 14

From *Anopheles* to Spatial Surveillance: A Roadmap Through a Multidisciplinary Challenge

Valérie Obsomer, Nicolas Titeux,
Christelle Vancustem, Grégory Duveiller,
Jean-François Pekel, Steve Connor,
Pietro Ceccato and Marc Coosemans

Additional information is available at the end of the chapter

http://dx.doi.org/10.5772/55622

1. Introduction

Anopheles mosquito species are diverse and vector of many pathogens. A review of the genus *Anopheles* [1] recently updated [2] listed more than 520 species, some of which including subspecies and cryptic species. Each of them presents ecologic requirements and behaviours that can influence their status as vector for specific pathogens. Pathogen transmission dynamics vary greatly from one region to another such as documented for the biodiversity of malaria in the world [3]. Acknowledging these variations at local scale within a country through detailed mapping can lead to better targeted measures and improved monitoring. Interactions between vectors, pathogens and humans in a given area can be better comprehended using a spatial framework leading to what we call here a spatial surveillance.

Part of spatial variation is explained by differences in pathogen species or by successful control in some areas. Nevertheless, *Anopheles* species play a major part in the occurrence, seasonality and spatial variation of *Anopheles*-borne diseases. The environment in a given region provides or not support for a given species to breed, thrive and live long enough to be an efficient vector. Because of these variations a species might be an efficient vector in one settlement and then only a secondary vector in another. The need to clarify *Anopheles* distribution is recognised as a crucial step towards malaria eradication [4]. A recent effort to provide detailed maps of malaria and vectors has been carried out [5–8] including a description of ecological requirements. While these distribution maps are essential for an overview, some issues [9] (described further) linked to the data and modelling impede usage in an operational world. Modelling and surveillance are key activities for successful control but integration of all components for effective operational surveillance is not straightforward.

In this chapter we review the challenges posed by spatial surveillance of *Anopheles*-borne diseases with particular attention for malaria surveillance. This challenge will mainly reside in the difficulty of getting the appropriate raw data and the large spectrum of multidisciplinary expertise. We propose here a roadmap from *Anopheles* sampling to a spatial surveillance.

2. Problem statement and application area

When working on vector-borne-diseases, decision makers and researchers often face a lack of specific quality data required for optimal targeting the intervention and surveillance. However, the results/decisions are critical as they impact on the lives of many people. Numerous studies use suboptimal vector dataset, and proxies for environmental drivers to map vector distribution or provide basis for vector surveillance. However, the uncertainties linked to the original dataset are not always well documented, in particular regarding proxies for environmental drivers derived from satellite imagery. Analysis methods also do not always take into account the specificity of species ecological distribution and inaccuracies linked to the vector dataset.

3. Research course and method used

Spatial surveillance of vector-borne diseases should integrate specialised knowledge in entomology, ecology, parasitology, epidemiology, human health, ecological modelling and social sciences. The authors of this chapter are specialized in those different fields and teamed up to offer an overview of the challenges posed by spatial surveillance. As vector-borne-diseases are linked to the environment, a spatial analysis using geographical information or remote sensing related technologies seems then appropriate.

4. Following the road map

Reliable outputs to go from *Anopheles* to spatial surveillance first depend on the data entering any analysis or decision process, being the data on *Anopheles* or on environmental factors. Environmental factors provided by remote sensing techniques that could be used to predict distribution or occurrence of malaria and *Anopheles* have already been reviewed [10]. Based on this inventory, we analyse pros and cons of *Anopheles* sampling strategies, various types of data and modelling techniques. Finally, useful initiatives to make research efforts available and operational in the field are discussed. The general scheme is provided in figure 1.

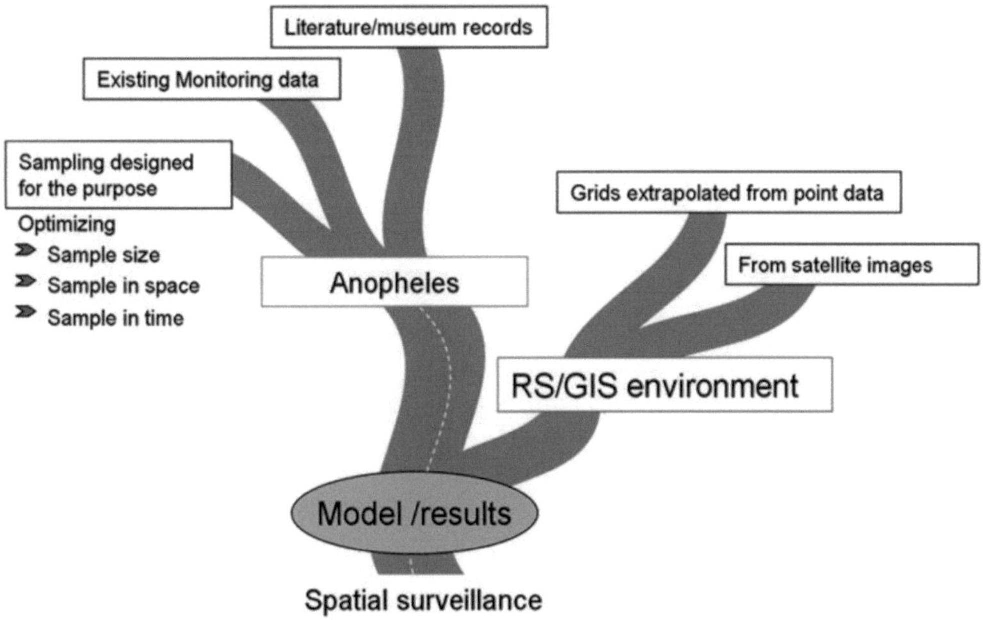

Figure 1. General scheme of the roadmap for *Anopheles* spatial surveillance

4.1. *Anopheles* and sampling strategies

Many useful attributes can be collected on *Anopheles* such as the list of species and their vector status in a given area, resistance to insecticides, behaviour influencing human vector contact, control effort avoidance (early biting, outdoor resting). Research and monitoring programmes might be based on existing entomological data whose particularities should be dealt with at the modelling step. However the most direct way is to design the collection protocol in relation to the objective, i.e. mapping the *Anopheles* species. In this last case, the quality of the dataset could be high if some rules are followed. Monitoring data are typically collected in a network of sampling locations according to a variety of standardized procedures [11] and used for mapping species distributions [12]. However, records are generally collected only in a restricted number of locations often loosely distributed across the region of interest, which is inconvenient for documenting species distribution.

Species distribution modelling techniques [13,14] provide assistance to achieve mapping based on monitoring data [15] such as detailed further in the road map. When coupling *Anopheles* monitoring and mapping efforts, defining an optimal sampling strategy becomes of highest interest. Indeed, well-designed monitoring projects have the potential to produce appropriate data to estimate changes in species attributes [16] but also document the distribution in space and time [12]. An appropriate sampling design should address key issues: what constitutes a sampling location? How many are needed? Where do they have to be located? How often to survey? When monitoring data are used to generate species distribution models, designing the sampling strategy is a challenge because these issues are to be addressed relatively to the monitoring and the modelling objectives.

4.1.1. Optimizing sample size

Sampling locations may be sites, squares, transects or any spatial unit from which the measurements are made in the field to document attributes (e.g. presence, population density, infected/infective mosquitoes, reproductive status, insecticide resistance) that describe the *Anopheles* species. A sample is a set of sampling locations where attributes of the species are measured to estimate its characteristics over the entire study area. Hence, a sample must be representative of the whole study area and more than one sampling location is needed to account for the variation in the measurements made in the field. For instance, the population density or even the presence of a species depend on environmental conditions and this is to be taken into account to estimate the mean population density or the infection rate of the species in the study area or to document its spatial distribution with sufficient accuracy. Precision (typically measured by standard error) reflects how similar to each other are the different measurements made in the sampling locations, thereby providing a measure of sampling uncertainty. When sample measurements are similar to each other, the sample mean is likely to be estimated with an acceptable level of precision from a few sampling locations. In contrast, when the between-location variation in the measurements is high, a larger number of sampling locations is needed [11]. Achieving a sufficient level of precision is of critical importance: the higher the precision of the estimates, the better the chances to detect temporal changes using statistical hypothesis testing procedures. Sample size is also known to impact on the performance of species distribution models [17–19]: predictions based on few records are likely to be less accurate than predictions based on larger sample sizes [18]. A sufficient number of sampling locations is needed to capture in the statistical models the response of the species to the environmental conditions. A balance is, therefore, to be achieved between ensuring statistical robustness (i.e. increasing the sample size) and reducing sampling effort (i.e. decreasing the sample size) because sampling is time- and/or budget-consuming.

For monitoring purpose, a power analysis may be performed to evaluate the number of sampling locations required to detect a given level of change over time in the attributes of the species with a predetermined level of statistical certainty. First, decisions are to be made by the users on (1) the minimum level of change that is to be detected in the analysis (for instance, 10% of change between time t and t+1) and (2) the acceptable chances of making type-1 (i.e. concluding that change is taking place when it is not) and type-2 (i.e. concluding that no change is taking place when it is) errors in hypothesis testing procedures [15]. Such decisions are often based on the precautionary principle and the relative importance of type-1 and type-2 errors also depends on the objective. Then, the analysis integrates information on the precision of the estimates to calculate the optimal sample size needed to detect the desired level of change. A pilot survey is, however, required to obtain an initial approximation of the precision of the estimates linked to the variation in the field measurements. For modelling applications, modelling performance increases with sample size and impact of sample size on modelling performance may strongly depend on the modelling technique used [20]. A series of studies have also recently shown that the performance may be sensitive to particularly small sample sizes and may reach an asymptote level beyond a sufficiently large sample size [18,19]. In order to examine how large the sample size should be to obtain sufficiently well-performing models, different alternative options are available: (1) using readily available datasets in the study area [12] or (2) creating virtual species in real landscapes [19,21]. With such data, it becomes possible to manipulate the number of sampling locations to represent a range of sample size and to examine the impact of restricted sample size on modelling performance.

4.1.2. Optimizing sampling strategy in space

An appropriate sampling design also involves positioning the sampling locations so that the full range of environmental conditions across the study area may be covered to ensure the representativeness of the sample. Several approaches are available to position the sampling locations (only some are presented below) [21] with different advantages and disadvantages (details in [11]): Those include:

Expert-based sampling – Sampling units are located based on a priori knowledge of the study area and the status of the species. This subjective strategy is to be avoided because the sample is most likely not representative of the study area and may thus not be used for statistical inference.

Random sampling – Random selection of sampling locations among a list is an easy-to-use procedure that is recommended when the aim of the sampling is to provide a picture of the situation across the study area. However, the precision of the estimates may be much lower than when using a stratified sampling (see below), especially in heterogeneous environments.

Systematic (or regular) sampling – A regular distribution of the sampling locations may prove to be appealing because the whole study area is covered with the same sampling effort. However, the sample may provide a biased picture when the fixed distance between sampling locations coincides with a particular structure in the spatial arrangement of the environmental conditions.

Stratified sampling – The study area is first divided in strata assumed to influence differently the attributes of the species measured in the field. A random sampling procedure is applied to select a number of sampling locations within the strata in ratio to their relative geographical extent. The main advantage of stratification is that the precision of the estimates based on the sample may be considerably improved compared to a simple random sampling. Stratification requires preliminary survey to be conducted to minimize the within-strata variation in the measurements. In practice, however, stratification is often applied according to environmental layers representing heterogeneity of the environment conditions that are assumed to exert an influence on the attributes of the species.

4.1.3. Optimizing sampling strategy in time

Presence-only techniques can deal with the issue of false absences in species distribution modelling studies [14,22], and failure to consider the detectability of a species (i.e. the probability of detecting it when present at a site) when designing a monitoring programme might lead to misleading conclusions [23,24]. In order to account for detection probabilities and to provide an unbiased estimate of *Anopheles* species occupancy or infection rate, it becomes necessary to carry out repeated survey at least in some sampling locations over a single season of data collection. If the emphasis of the programme is on estimating changes in the species occupancy or infection rate over time, it is also required to repeat the surveys from one season to the other. Site occupancy modelling is a statistical framework specifically designed to jointly estimate detectability and occupancy of the species as well as changes in those parameters over time [24]. Designing effective sampling schemes to estimate *Anopheles* species dynamics in space and time requires decisions to be made about how to allocate sampling effort among spatial and temporal replicates. Power analyses may be implemented to optimize the sampling design in space and time, i.e. to achieve a compromise between the number of sampling locations and the number of repeated surveys within sampling locations in relation to (1) the acceptable level of imprecision associated with the estimates of species occupancy, (2) the occupancy and detectability of the species, (3) the available manpower and possible sampling effort.

4.2. Environmental factors

Once environmental factors of interest are identified, their importance according to the type of climate (e.g. semi-arid or humid), type of species, and altitude must be further discussed. Any place where surface water is available for breeding and emergence might lead to *Anopheles* occurrence. Vector status requires above plus (1) presence of human/animal host and their disease parasites. Then (2) suitable temperature and humidity which have then an effect on (3) vector dynamics and parasite development. A review [10] of the current state of the art in the context of remote sensing applications for malaria underlines that, temperature, humidity, surface water, climate seasonality, vegetation type and growth stage influence vector abundance irrespective of their association with rainfall. The vegetation around breeding sites may also determine abundance associated with the breeding site by providing resting sites, sugar feeding supplies for adult mosquitoes and protection from climatic conditions [25]. Furthermore, vegetation type or land use may influence mosquito abundance by affecting the presence of animal or human hosts and thus availability of blood meals [10]. Factors are of two kinds [9]: (1) abiotic slow changing factors such as long term climatic variables, soils, topography, (2) fast changing biotic factors such as vegetation, presence of predator, hosts, interactions with other *Anopheles*, seasonal temperature/ rainfall, water bodies,....

Remote sensing products provide environmental characteristics on large surfaces even in areas of limited accessibility and can provide recent information on an area compared to commonly available maps. The quality of the information provided is however dependent of the original remote sensing data quality and suitabilility. The processing required to mosaic images in order to cover a large area, to make various types of image correction, cloud screening operations and image interpretation are not straightforward for non-specialists. Derived products, such as land cover maps or composited time series of simple vegetation indices, are therefore often more adapted to the need of the users. However, the process behind the final product must be understood to a certain extent by the users, in order for them to be aware of the assumptions and simplifications done in the processing. Furthermore, different methods are typically available to reach a given goal, and the choice of the method can strongly influence on the quality of the results.

4.2.1. Long term abiotic variables

Abiotic slow changing factors might be used to delineate a species distribution area or maximum potential extend for a species. Those factors include topography, soil types, long term climate and ecoregions (Table 1). Available source are not many but cover the world. Consistent topography is available from the USGS GTOPO 30 suite [26] including derived variables such as digital elevation model, flow accumulation, slope or aspect or from the NASA Shuttle Radar Topographic Mission (SRTM) dataset reprocessed by the CGIAR [27]. The digital soils map of the world compiled by the FAO [28] is still a reference. Long term climatic datasets of monthly temperature and rainfall are available from Worldclim [29] which provided also bioclimatic variables. A second dataset CRU CL2.0 [30] provided also monthly temperature and rainfall but also number of monthly rainy days, rainfall monthly variation and relative humidity. The datasets are based on meteorological stations data from 1950 to 1990 or 2000. The quality of the data is high in some areas and less in others due to availability of meteorological station which can be quite low, particularly in Africa. The ecoregions [31] are a useful dataset to delineate sample stratification at regional level. Those dataset are mostly not derived from remote sensing (RS) images but grids developed from point data.

Variables	Sensor/ source	Resolution	Date
Topography	USGS (not RS) (http://www1.gsi.go.jp/geowww/ globalmap-gsi/gtopo30/gtopo30.html)	1km	1996
Topography	SRTM (http://srtm.csi.cgiar.org)	100 m	February 2000
Soils	FAO (not RS) (http://www.fao.org/nr/land/soils/ digital-soil-map-of-the-world/en/	17km	1990
Climate	Worldclim (not RS) (http://www.worldclim.org/)	1km	Published 2005, (1960 to 2000)
Climate	CRU. 10 (http://www.cru.uea.ac.uk/cru/data/ hrg/)	15km	Published 2005, (1961 to 1990)
Ecoregions	OLSON		1998

Table 1. Relevant long term abiotic variables

4.2.2. Monitoring air temperature

Air temperature *Ta*, is commonly obtained from measurements in weather stations, which depend on the regional infrastructure. Data are collected as point samples whose distribution is rarely designed to capture the range of climate variability within a region especially in developing countries. The data is also not readily available for real time applications and need to be interpolated to obtain information everywhere in a given region. On the other hand satellite images can provide land surface temperature *Ts* which is different from the air temperature and corresponds to the temperature of the top of the features present on the land surface (i.e. snow, ice, grass of a lawn, roof of a building, leaves of the canopy in a forest). Specific methods (split-windows techniques) can derive daily *Ts* at 1 km resolution [32,33] from two types of sensors, namely the Advanced Very High Resolution Radiometer (AVHRR) and the Moderate Resolution Imaging Spectroradiometer (MODIS) [33,34] (see description table of MODIS Ts: https://lpdaac.usgs.gov/products/modis_products_table). On the contrary, the derivation of air temperature (*Ta*) is far from straightforward. Recent research showed that minimum *Ts* retrieved from MODIS night images provide estimates of minimum *Ta* in different ecosystems in Africa [35]. Information on maximum *Ta* is also needed to study heat waves and can influence the transmission of vector-borne diseases in regions where temperature is a limiting factor. During daytime the retrieval of maximum *Ta* from *Ts* is more complex due to factors which influence (*Ts-Ta*): i.e. solar radiation, soil moisture and surface brightness. Methods based on Temperature Vegetation index, Normalized Difference Vegetation Index and Solar Zenith Angle to correct (*Ts-Ta*) are not sufficiently accurate to retrieve maximum Ta in different ecosystems [35]. Therefore, a new approach has been recently proposed [36] to estimate maximum *Ta* based on night AQUA-MODIS *Ts* data in combination with Worldclim [29] which provides long term monthly average of maximum and minimum air temperature. These inputs allow to characterize the diurnal cycle (amplitude and phase) and determine maximum *Ta* by extrapolating in time minimum *Ta* according to the determined diurnal cycle. The method is used to produce maximum *Ta* maps at 1km every 8 days over Africa available in real time from the International Research Institute for Climate and Society (IRI). Unfortunately *Ta* does represent temperature outside but no proxies are available to monitor indoor temperature or other stable microenvironment which can explain transmission in Finland when temperature in -20°c outside and is important in highlands malaria in Africa.

4.2.3. Monitoring rainfall

In some regions, the spatial distribution of weather stations is limited and the dissemination of rainfall data is variable, therefore limiting their use for real-time applications. If satellite-based data can partly compensate and help to monitor rainfall, unfortunately, no satellite yet exists which can reliably identify rainfall and accurately estimate the rainfall rate in all circumstances. Some sensors can make indirect estimates of rainfall by measuring parameters such as the thickness of clouds or the temperature of the cloud tops. Advantages and drawbacks of existing methods are summarized in [37]. Various satellite rainfall products exist at continental or global scales. The most relevant are:

- The Tropical Rainfall Measuring Mission **(TRMM)** products [38] provide better spatial (25 km) and temporal estimation (3 hours) of rainfall in Africa [39] than most products but are available only between 35° North and South latitudes.

- Products from the CPC MORPHing technique **(CMORPH)** [40] cover the world at 8 km resolution every 30 min. This technique uses precipitation estimates derived from low orbite satellite microwave observations obtained entirely from various geostationary satellite infrared (IR) data. The estimation method developed for these products is extremely flexible such that any precipitation estimates from any microwave satellite source can be incorporated.

http://dx.doi.org/10.5772/55622

- African Rainfall Estimation **(RFE)** products cover Africa. The current version (RFE2) uses microwave estimates in addition to the use of cloud top temperature and station rainfall data to provide daily rainfall estimation at 10 km resolution. Comparison between CMORPH and RFE over complex terrain in Africa [39] and over the Desert Locust recession regions [41] shows that no single product stands out as having the best or the worst overall performance [42,43].
- The TAMSAT African Rainfall Climatology And Time-series data version 2 **(TARCAT2)** product [44] covers Africa at 4 km resolution and is derived from the MeteoSat thermal infra-red (TIR) satellite imagery. It consists of rainfall information every 10 days.
- The Multi-sensor Precipitation Estimate **(GRIB MPE)** [45] derives instantaneous rain rate from the infrared (IR) data of the geo-stationary EUMETSAT satellites over Europe and Africa by continuous re-calibration of the algorithm with rain-rate data from polar orbiting microwave sensors. The algorithm is only suitable in convective weather. Frontal precipitation, especially at warm fronts is very often wrongly located and overestimated. Two quality indicators distributed together with the MPE product give indications where the product should be used and where it may be problematic. Temporal resolution is high (15 min) and the product available in real time.

4.2.4. Remote sensing indicators of vegetation status

Monitoring the status of green biomass from space is made possible thanks to the particular spectral properties of green vegetation. In order to drive the exothermic reaction of photosynthesis, plant pigments absorb electromagnetic radiation over different parts of the visible spectrum (400-700 nm). This is known as photosynthetically active radiation (PAR). Additionally, much of the near-infrared light (740-1100 nm) is scattered by green plant tissues to avoid overheating, and this scatter results in strong spectral reflectance at these wavelengths. These unusual spectral properties, which are directly linked to photosynthesis, stomatal resistance and evapotranspiration, facilitate the retrieval of information on plant canopies from the electromagnetic signal measured by satellite remote sensing instruments [46]. Satellites dedicated to vegetation monitoring have been equipped with sensors capable of measuring reflected electromagnetic radiations in various wavebands, with a particular emphasis on the red (Red) and near-infrared (NIR), to assess the green biomass in a canopy.

A common and simple way to resume the information content within these bands is the use of spectral vegetation indices, which is an algebraic combination of the spectral bands designed to be as sensitive to the desired factor (green biomass) and as insensitive as possible to perturbing factors affecting spectral reflectance (such as atmospheric and illumination conditions, soil properties and the viewing geometry of the imaging instrument). Indices based on red and near-infrared reflectance have been shown to be a measure of chlorophyll abundance and energy absorption [47]. Variations of across one year can help spotting vegetation types, and the quantification of the water content can help identifying areas in a similar vegetation class which retain more humidity and might thus be more favourable to mosquito breeding or survival in dry season. Dozens of vegetation indices assess the state of the vegetation qualitatively and quantitatively on the basis of reflectance values:

- The Normalized Difference Vegetation Index **(NDVI)** (NDVI = (NIR - Red) / (NIR + Red)) [48] is the most popular of such vegetation indices. NDVI is easily available because it is based only on Red and NIR bands, which are present in most satellite sensors dedicated to land surface observation. The GIMMS (Global Inventory Modelling and Mapping Studies) NDVI dataset based on NOAA-AVHRR offer the longest coherent dataset from July 1981 to December 2011 which can be useful for long term studies [49]. However the spatial resolution of 8 km limits some applications. SPOT-VEGETATION provides a regular product since 1998 at a better spatial resolution of 1 km and geo-location. Similarly, the MODIS sensor provides NDVI at 250 m resolution. NDVI can also be calculated from images with a higher spatial resolution, such as those from the Landsat or SPOT series. The NDVI is used extensively but has several disadvantages such as its sensibility to atmospheric aerosols and to soil background (particularly in sparsely vegetated areas) [50]. Additionally, NDVI also tends to saturate in forested areas and is therefore not responsive to variations in the full range of canopy vegetation content [51].
- The Enhanced Vegetation Index **(EVI)** remains sensitive to variations in dense forests where NDVI saturates [52]. EVI calculated from MODIS imagery is provided, alongside NDVI, as standard freely available product. A disadvantage of EVI is that it requires an additional blue band, which is not available in NOAA-AVHRR, thereby blocking the possibility to exploit the long term dataset. To remediate that, a simplified 2-band EVI has also been proposed [53].
- The Normalized Difference Water Index (**NDWI** = (NIR - SWIR) / (NIR + SWIR)) [54], where SWIR is the Short wave infrared, is sensitive to vegetation water content and to the spongy mesophyll structure in vegetation canopies. Regarding vegetation water content, [55] summarized the limitations of using the NDVI: a decrease in chlorophyll content does not imply a decrease in vegetation water content and inversely. It might also help target vegetation retaining humidity in the dry season. Few studies have attempted to retrieve directly vegetation water content using operational satellite data such as provided by SPOT-VEGETATION [55], MODIS [56] and Landsat [51]. A disadvantage of NDWI is that several instruments are not equipped with detectors in the SWIR domain, and when they do they are often at lower spatial resolution than other bands.
- The **Hue index** is a qualitative index proposed recently by [57] for the monitoring of the Locust habitat. This exploits simultaneously three wavelengths (the SWIR, the NIR, and red) and has two main advantages: (i) avoiding confusions between bare soils and vegetation, and (ii) allowing the identification of green vegetation independently from the observation conditions, i.e., atmosphere and acquisition geometry, and from its intrinsic variations, i.e., the phenological stage. Potential for monitoring crops, forests and other applications still need to be assessed.

Albeit their widespread use, the use of vegetation indices over large geographic extents has its limits for describing canopy status in a fine and robust way, since both the desired information and the perturbing factors vary spatially, temporally and spectrally. Another type of information on canopy status that can be retrieved from remote sensing data is biophysical variables. The most common are the fraction of Absorbed Photosynthetically Active Radiation

(fAPAR) and the Leaf Area Index **(LAI)**, defined as half the total developed area of green leaves per unit of ground horizontal area [58]. Unlike vegetation indices, which are a convenient way to resume spectral information related to vegetation behaviour, biophysical variables such as fAPAR and LAI have a real physiological meaning. These variables govern the process of photosynthesis and the exchange of energy, water and carbon between the canopy and the atmosphere. To retrieve LAI and fAPAR from satellite remote sensing observations, the radiative transfer of photons within the canopy and through the atmosphere must be modelled. A thorough description of the physical problem, alongside caveats on its application to satellite remote sensing of vegetation, is presented in [59]. Dorigo et al. [60] provide a review of the various methods that exist to use such radiative transfer models to relate satellite observations to LAI and fAPAR. Up to recently, the two main datasets of global fAPAR and LAI are products from MODIS and CYCLOPES with different methodologies described in [61] and [62]. These datasets have been inter-compared and evaluated against ground measurements over different land cover types [63–65]. A combined product has recently been made available, GEOV1, in the framework of the Geoland2 project, in view of providing it as an operational land product service of the Global Monitoring for Environment and Security (GMES) programme [66]. This product is currently based on SPOT-Vegetation, but a compatible long term data record from 1981 to 2000 has been also constructed based on NOAA-AVHRR data (with a spatial resolution of 0.05°) [67], and in the future it is expected to be produced based on the future operational Sentinel3-OLCI mission. Such biophysical products are increasingly used but seldom in epidemiological studies.

4.2.5. Land cover

Detailed information from land cover maps is generally available in national geographical institutes but this information is often out of date due to the long process implied in developing such dataset for a whole country. Moreover, the diverse origin and scale of these datasets when considering more than one country impeded proper comparison between sites. One could thus consider producing national or regional land cover maps using satellite high-resolution data. This exercise includes the pre-processing, the interpretation of the images, and the validation through field surveys. For instance, Landsat images were used in the framework of the Food and Agriculture Organization of the United Nations (FAO) Africover program [68] to map land cover types at 30 m resolution for 11 countries in Africa. Such land cover maps present a great level of detail, but may suffer for some inconsistencies because of heterogeneity in acquisition dates, images and interpretation from one scene to another. Moreover this approach hardly takes into account the seasonal variation and phenological behaviour of different vegetation types. These datasets are also limited in their spatial coverage and cannot be regularly updated following the methodology commonly used (i.e. visual interpretation). Finally, if the whole Landsat images archive was made freely available in 2009, images from Landsat 7 present gaps since May 2003 and Landsat 5 back to activity in 2003 is now failing since November 2011.

Medium to coarse resolution imagery (250 to 1 km) can improve some major issues: the information is acquired consistently over the whole area and frequent images (every 1 or 3 days) of a same area can be combined to eliminate cloud contamination and angular effects, and characterize the vegetation phenology. These time series can be used to produce global maps such as (i) the Global Land Cover 2000 **(GLC2000)** map that is based on SPOT-VEGETATION data (1 km) thanks to an international partnership of research groups coordinated by the European Commission's Joint Research Centre (JRC) [69], (ii) the 500 m **MODIS global land cover** derived from collection 5 Nadir BRDF-Adjusted Reflectance (NBAR) and Land Surface Temperature (LST) products [70], (iv) the **GlobCover** map [71] at 300 m derived from a Medium Resolution Imaging Spectrometer (MERIS) time series for year 2005. These types of time series were also used to produce land cover and vegetation maps at national and regional scales such as for example [72]. These types of products have the advantage that the data preprocessing and the methodology used are adapted to the local constraints and application needs but are limited in their spatial coverage. The possibility to regularly update global land cover information has been proved recently with the second run of the GlobCover processing system [73], thus offering the potential to use such product in a monitoring program. The delineation of the vector habitat underlines the essential role of these land cover datasets which makes the necessary link between the technical remote sensing world and application requirements. Land cover dataset are one of the essential variables for the Group on Earth Observations (GEO). A major effort is to be continuously invested in the development and improvement of such dataset. The quality of this dataset can only be really tested if used for applications. Close interactions with final users remain the guarantee for the relevancy of the Earth observation product.

4.2.6. Monitoring water bodies

In order to identify the presence of water, it is also possible to use satellite-derived products that detect water bodies instead of approximate water availability using rainfall estimates. In the last 10 years, only a few operational methods applied to datasets with a spatial resolution equal or higher than 1 km, were proposed to monitor surface water at continental or global scale. Among these, two most recent offer dynamic detections in near real-time through an operational monitoring system:

- First, the Small Water Bodies **(SWB)** product based on SPOT-VEGETATION [74] available via the DevCoCast project website makes use of 10 day NDVI, the NDWI and syntheses of the SWIR band data. It is based on a contextual algorithm [75] exploiting the local contrast of the water surface with respect to the surrounding area. The product performs well in sub-humid and semi-arid regions, but limitations have been observed over dense vegetation areas. The 1 km spatial resolution is an intrinsic limitation. Nevertheless, the combination of eight years of small water body monitoring data demonstrated the value of multi-annual approaches to capture water bodies that do not replenish every year in relation with seasonal rainfall patterns [74][97].

- **The HSV WATER** product [76] based on Hue Saturation Value (HSV) transformation of SPOT-VEGETATION and MODIS time series allows consistent detection at continental scale. This pixel based approach uses SWIR, NIR and red bands and transform the RGB color space into HSV that decouples chromaticity and luminance. It presents the advantage to have a robust and reliable image-independent discrimination between water and other land cover types. An automatic processing chain based on SPOT-VEGETATION was designed to provide a dekadal water surface product at the continental scale. The product can be ordered freely through the geoland2 web portal following the link http://www.geoland2.eu/core-mapping-services/biopar.html.

The analysis of eight years of small water body data demonstrated the capacity of such methods to capture inter-annual water bodies variability and the relation with seasonal rainfall patterns [98]. Nevertheless, the 1 km spatial resolution of products derived from SPOT-VEGETATION is still a strong intrinsic limitation. The operational production of a MODIS based product at 250 m using the second method is in progress and should be available soon.

4.2.7. *Caveats on remote sensing data*

Various issues have to be highlighted when looking from the application angle:

- The spatial resolution for all environmental factors necessary for a study is often not similar (table 2) and transformation to similar resolution might lead to increase geolocation imprecision when pixels limits do not correspond. The pixel size selected for the analysis is dependent of the available datasets and not the best cell size to describe the phenomena under study. Datasets not available at high resolution thus limit spatial details of results.
- Some useful dataset are not covering the world or not available at the appropriate date.
- Too detailed datasets such as rainfall products with data every 3 hours (TRMM) would require long summarizing process for non-specialists to get information per week or month.
- At high spatial resolution, geo-location accuracy can be jeopardized by the viewing angle, particularly in accidented terrain. Image distorsion needs to be corrected using a topographic information not always available at high resolution.

Spatial resolution: Remote sensing is typically characterized by a trade-off between the different types of resolutions: spatial, temporal, spectral and to a certain extent also radiometric and angular. High spatial resolution is desired to characterise the land in a detailed way. However, cloud occurrence limits its availability. Basis for land cover map might be a puzzle of images from different seasons or even years thus creating artifacts of land cover differences at the limits between the images. As it is discussed further, coarse spatial resolution imagery, with its frequent revisit and through the use of compositing can partially remediate the problem, but this can be a problem with high resolution imagery where images are costly and revisit not frequent. Having regular observations at fine spatial resolution typically limit the geographic extend that can be monitored. Even over a limited coverage, satellites providing such services are typically commercial ones for which the cost is currently high and for which there is competition for their observation capacity between different geographic sites. Such images are thus often used in studies of limited spatial extend from which the results are difficult to extrapolate to a country level needed for spatial surveillance. It is however just a matter of time before high spatial resolution (5 – 20 m) becomes available for the entire globe

Type of variable	Sensor/ source	Spatial	Timing	Area	Date
Minimum air temperature	Terra/Aqua MODIS http:// iridl.ldeo.columbia.edu/ maproom/.Health/.Regional/. Africa/.Malaria/.TMR/)	1 km		World	
Maximum air temperature	MODIS/ Worldclim	1 km		World	
Rainfall	TRMM	25 km	3 hours	35° N & 35° S	Since 1998
Rainfall	CMORPH : Mixt IR data, NOAA-CPC	8 km	30 min	World	Since December 2002
African Rainfall Estimation (RFE)	produced by NOAA-CPC	10 km	daily	Africa	Since January 2001
Rainfall	TARCAT http:// www.met.reading.ac.uk/ ~tamsat/data	4 km		Africa	Since 1983
Rainfall	EUMETSAT/ GRIB MPE				From January 2007
NDVI	GIMMS products from NOAA-AVHRR	8 km		World	Since 1981
NDVI	Spot VEGETATION	1 km	daily	World	
NDVI MODIS	Terra/Aqua MODIS	250 m		World	
EVI	Terra/Aqua MODIS	500 m		World	
NDWI	Spot VEGETATION	1 km	daily	World	
Hue Index	Spot-VEGETATION	1 km	daily	World	
fAPAR + LAI	Terra/Aqua MODIS	1 km	8 days	World	Since 2000
fAPAR+LAI	CYCLOPES products fSpot-VEGETATION	1 km	10 days	World	Since 2000
faPAR+LAI	GEOV1 products Spot-VEGETATION	1km	10 days	World	Since 2000
fAPAR+LAI	GEOV1 products from NOAA-AVHRR	5 km	10 days	World	1981 - 2000

Table 2. Some important remote sensing related products

and the European Space Agency is currently preparing its Sentinel-2 constellation (with an expected launch of its first satellite in 2014), which aims at operationally providing multispectral imagery, at spatial resolutions of 10 to 60 m for different bands, and with a 5-day revisit period. However, the challenge of collecting, processing and delivering this data may still limit its practical use for years.

Clouds and compositing: The quality of the spatial and temporal spectral consistency of coarse resolution optical time series may be limited by processing steps of cloud-screening and compositing. The efficiency of the cloud-screening, i.e. its ability to remove clouds while keeping a maximum of useful information, depends on three factors: (i) the methodology used to identify cloud-free pixels, (ii) the type of clouds (thick clouds are easier to overcome than veils of clouds which change surreptitiously radiation values), and (iii) the sensor characteristics. The detection of clouds is often based on specific bands, i.e. the blue, the middle infrared and the thermic infrared, and the choice of the wavelengths may vary according to the sensor. Depending on these factors, residuals clouds and haze may still remain after the cloud-screening step. Quality of time series may strongly vary according to the compositing strategy used. The most common method used for producing temporal syntheses consists of selecting the Maximum Value Composite (MVC) NDVI [77] (Figure 2) that minimizes the effect of undetected clouds since these would typically have a lower NDVI value. However, the composited reflectance bands may exhibit substantial radiometric variations, since composite radiances are generally recorded under varying atmospheric and geometric conditions. This may cause serious spatial inconsistencies in the composites and in the subsequent processing.

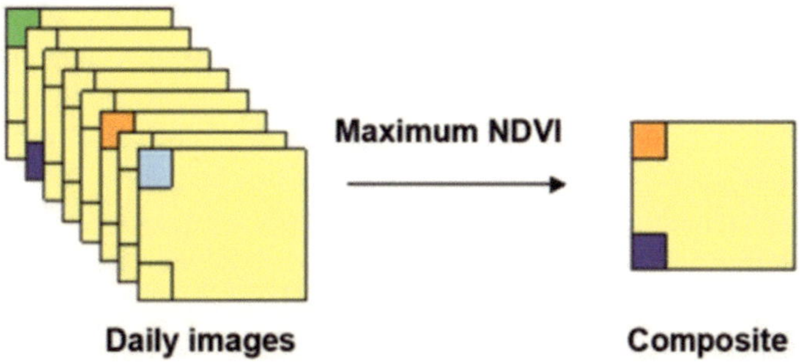

Figure 2. Maximum NDVI standard compositing

A more advanced approach consists of normalizing the bidirectional reflectance by fitting a bi-directional reflectance distribution function (BRDF) model to the available cloud free observations [78] which considerable improve the result. But operational implementation requires a large number of cloud-free observations, the BRDF retrieval has a high sensitivity to residual clouds [79] (Figure 3), the algorithm is complex and requires ancillary data. A more flexible and "user-friendly" compositing approach was recently proposed [80] where cloud free reflectance values are averaged after a quality control.

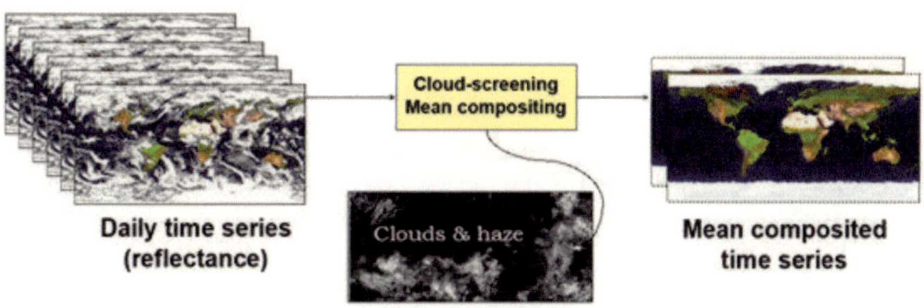

Figure 3. Mean composting method

It presents the advantages to reduce both the anisotropy effects and the possible remaining perturbation after atmospheric correction and cloud removal. Despite the benefits of compositing, for some applications it may be more interesting to avoid it altogether. Indeed, to follow vegetation changes at a finer time scale it may be better to exploit all available observations within a period (typically 10 days or more) instead of combining them together. In agriculture monitoring, considerable changes in biomass or phenology can occur within a week and exploiting all available observations should thus be preferred. Such approach has been used, to provide crop specific biophysical variable time series at regional scale by fitting a simplified model of the canopy dynamics over daily data [81] and might be of use to identify processing occurring in potential *Anopheles* habitat such as rice paddies.

What is in a pixel? Coarse spatial resolution satellite imagery has several advantages. Frequent observations enable timely detection of environmental changes that may indicate potential changes in the presence of *Anopheles*. Second, the higher frequency of available observations allows to better address the problem of lack of data due to cloud contamination and anisotropy through compositing or temporal smoothing. Third, their (relatively) long archives enable to have a picture of the past with which the actual conditions can be compared to. In the short coming future, coarse datasets may also serve as a benchmark in order to calibrate products to their signal, which could be more stable thanks to their higher revisit frequency. Finally, coarse spatial resolution data are also often the only data available and there is thus a tendency to use them at the limit of their spatial resolution by looking at individual pixels. A common misconception is that the observational footprint is the geometric projection of a rectangular pixel onto the Earth's surface [82]. The footprint rather depends on some properties of the instrument, resumed under the concept of spatial response [83], and which results in an observation footprint generally larger than the pixel delivered to the user (Figure 4).

This problem is compounded for sensors such as AVHRR, MODIS and VIIRS (the successor of MODIS), which scan the Earth with large angles, leading to an expansion of the observation footprint along the scanline (while the grid in which the data is provided keeps the same size). Furthermore, the pre-processing step of gridding, i.e. assigning an observation to a predefined system of grid, introduces a ``pixel-shift'' [84], which means that the centre of the pixel does not correspond with the centre of the observation. Such gridding artefacts have serious consequences on the quality of the MODIS signal, and more specifically on composites and band-to-band registration across various spatial resolutions [85]. Recent work [86] has further demonstrated the impact of gridding artefacts and the scan angle on the spatial purity of an observation, i.e. on the percentage of the target land cover within an observation footprint that effectively contributes to the signal encoded in the pixel.

Mosquito Land cover: Land cover provides the more understandable information to non-specialist in terms of vegetation and habitat but the classes are not always adapted to the user needs. Instead of choosing between vegetation indices which represent continuous values and land cover of more or less 20 classes, it might be useful to give access to intermediary products of land cover classification. Indeed, processing chains of a land cover such as GlobCover include a correction process, cloud screening and image compositing to improve overall quality of the data [71]. Then vegetation indices and reflectance bands linked to vegetation

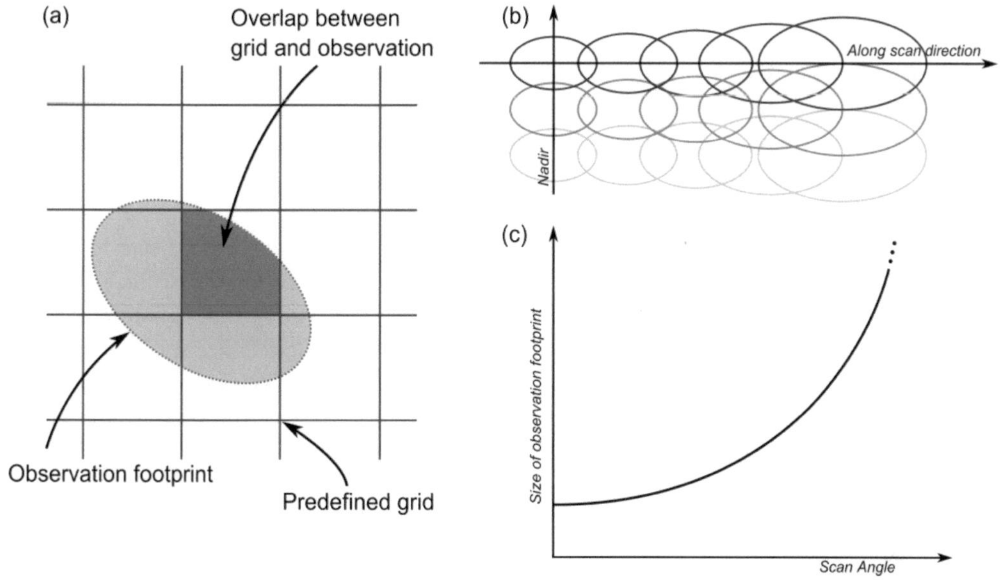

Figure 4. Some effects influencing what is really in a pixel of a satellite remote sensing image. (a) Schematic mis-alignment between the observation footprint and the arbitrary grid remote sensing observations are encoded into (i.e. the pixel). (b) Illustration of the expansion and overlap of the observation footprint along the scanline for whiskbroom sensors such as AVHRR and MODIS; and (c) representation of how this size increase as the sensor scans with larger viewing angles. Figure adapted from [87] with permission from Elsevier.

status are used to group similar adjacent pixels and assign to those a same class label through clustering method which creates a chosen number of classes. In the next step, each class is compared to classes of a reference existing dataset or other existing data. According to a set of decision rules, the classes are interpreted and grouped in definitive classes. This last step raises several issues. The transformation of continuous dataset and the separation of the continuous landscape into a set of discrete classes are bound to a loss of information and inaccuracy particularly at the border of the classes. For example, the transition from a forest to a meadow might not always present a clear cut border. Other land cover initiatives work with continuous fields to avoid this issue [88]. Moreover, at the end of the process, up to 30% of the pixels are integrated into mosaic classes used when it is impossible to attribute the group of pixels to a single class, the pixel itself being a mixture for example of forest and meadow and thus providing a signal which is neither corresponding to forest, neither corresponding to meadow. Using mosaic classes in models and analysis can create confusion, particularly if several mosaic classes are grouped together. In this context, access to intermediate products such as classes based on cluster of similar pixels produced by remote sensing specialist might allow to integrate those into ecological models integrating ecological information relevant to *Anopheles* into the building of the final land cover would allow to define a better suited product for the purpose. Integrating several sensors to build a Landover might also improve the results. Indeed, GlobCover is based on MERIS satellite images which do not contain the Short Wavelength Infrared (SWIR) useful for discrimination of the forest vegetation. A combination with spot VEGETATION could result into better discrimination power for a similar resolution.

4.3. Model development

Sampling strategies, detailed field studies and casual observations can provide data which constitute the baseline information for model development. While remote sensing products are still too coarse resolution or maybe not adapted to define microhabitats, they can however provide proxies for environmental factors influencing general habitat and might be used in two ways. (1) Environmental values can be extracted at the sampling sites or in a buffer around the sites and then related to *Anopheles* data in descriptive models. Buffer size is often a compromise between some meaningful ecological feature such as flying range and the spatial resolution of the environmental factors [89]. (2) For question regarding habitat, spatial variation in vector capacity and spatial surveillance, spatial models are needed. In these models, environmental factors are related to the species records collected in the sampling locations and this relation is then used to predict the distribution of the species beyond the sampling locations [90–93].

When working with existing data, sampling protocol cannot be influenced a posteriori but an adapted methodology can be used to take into account potential peculiarity of each dataset. Field data may be obtained as a by-product of existing operational projects. However, depending on the finality which determined sampling design, the data might not be used straightforwardly for spatial surveillance. The dataset might include non standardized data collected during different years, according to a variety of sampling strategies but might be the only data available covering many countries. Existing datasets can consist of a collection of literature records covering wide regions. However, the collection sites are seldom well geo-referenced, large areas are not covered by the studies which might use different collection techniques at different seasons. With such datasets lack of records might be linked to inefficient sampling method, wrong timing for the survey or absence of survey and according to the source of data, abundance and absence need to be treated with caution. Even certified presence might not reflect current situation if recorded years ago. These issues may partly be addressed by methods similar to the previously mentioned subsampling procedures to reduce the potential biases in readily available datasets or using adapted modelling techniques.

4.3.1. Species distribution modelling

Early development in the field of remote sensing and vector-borne diseases risk mapping used the following methodological steps: collecting human cases (or mosquito presence/absence), collecting relevant environmental gridded data (pixel), extracting data at sampling sites to build a logistic regression model explaining cases of occurrence according to the environmental conditions, then mapping the probabilities by calculation of the model output for each gridded cell of the original environmental maps [94]. Numerous methods have now been used to model vector-borne diseases spatially [95] and suggestions to improve frequent drawbacks include (1) using several models and select the best suited for prediction and (2) make a summary model from the best-fitting models. On the other hand innovative methods are constantly improved in spatial ecology. Quantifying the link between species and their environment is a central research area in quantitative ecology. When absence data are available / reliable, numerous methods now do exist, ranging from logistic regression, ordinary multiple regressions and its generalized form (GLM), ordination, classification method, distance metrics such as Mahalonobis distances, neural networks, boosted regression tree, random forest and even more sophisticated support vector machines are some examples among the plethora of recently developed methods [14]. Multi-species community modelling methods have also been developed. One advantage of this kind of techniques is that it becomes possible to build species assemblage models that take into account the relationships between the different species in the community and so their relative location in the "environmental hyperspace", instead of modelling single species distribution independently from each other [96].

However, mapping elusive species such as mosquitoes is often a challenge mainly because of the impossible collection of reliable absence data such as described earlier. Discriminant approaches such as logistic regression analysis developed for specific diseases are thus not suited anymore because they compare environmental conditions in sites where the species is present and absent (not recorded). When only occurrence data are available, some niche-based modelling approaches offer adapted solution as they can use presence-only record information to build the statistical models. The concept of ecological niche has been defined [97] as follows: considering the n variables corresponding to all of the ecological factors relevant for the species, an n-dimensional hyper-volume can be defined in the environmental hyperspace between the limiting values permitting a species to survive and reproduce. This volume is called the fundamental niche of the species. This niche can be related to the two-dimensional geographical area of distribution considering that any point of the niche may represent a combination of environmental values that corresponds to some locations in the geographical space. Mechanistic approaches to ecological niche modelling [90] use direct measurements or physical modelling of response of individuals to parameters and infer from them individuals fitness values of different combinations of physical variables. On the contrary, correlative approaches to ecological niche models such as developed for species distribution models intend in a first step to define niches using the environmental variables at sampling point of occurrence, then assess for each spatial location in a study area probability to belong to the niche. Many large-scale species modelling techniques inspired by the principle of environmental envelopes were developed including BIOCLIM [98] based on a very simple classification tree, DOMAIN [99] based on a measure of multivariate distance, ENFA [100] based on the same principle of distance measure in an environmental hyperspace. Elith *et al.* [14] provide a good overview of most currently used methods including the Maxent method [22] based on presence data which seems to perform particularly well.

In this context classical presence-only modeling can also be integrated [9] into a hierarchical framework [101]. The first step is to model entomological data using environmental data relevant for the same time period. Indeed, mapping *Anopheles* information from literature records dating back several decades should be based on long term environmental factors such as climatic factors and not on factors such as land cover, or NDVI which are changing fast in some regions. The mapping of a first potential distribution based on long term slows changing information and literature records is then refined using a mask of fast changing updatable information such as land cover or current meteorological prediction. This allows producing a risk map or distribution map relevant for a specific date corresponding to the date of environmental factors used to refine the map. The resulting map is thus ecologically meaningful and relevant for a precise date. Recent other improvements in the field of presence only models include selection of pseudo-absence with a spatial bias similar to the potential bias of presence data [102], selection of the environmental factors to enter the model based on ecological requirements, adapted method for species with low number of occurrence [103].

Some issues still need to be tackled however. Ecological model should be based on source populations. Those are sustainable populations in suitable habitat. To the contrary, sink populations are surviving in habitat not suitable for population persistence but persist thanks to immigration from nearby source population. Typical museum records include both sink and source populations [104]. Moreover, current vector-borne disease distribution may be limited by a number of factors both environmental and socio-economic. For example, during the past 100 years, malaria risk zone has reduced from around a half down to a quarter of the Earth's land surface. However malaria remains prevalent in 106 countries of the tropical and semitropical world, with 35 countries in central Africa bearing the highest burden of cases and deaths [105,106]. The latitudinal limits apparent today are in effect 'control frontiers' reflecting the interplay of control interventions combined with changes in environmental management and socio-economic developments that reduce community vulnerability to the disease [107]. Altitudinal limits to malaria transmission have been the subject of much discussion regarding shifting of malaria risk into highland regions, such as East Africa. If documented climate change [108] might have add a small impact, major factors for extension to new areas seem to be changes in land use and landscape leading to changes in local ecology for human and vector [109].

4.3.2. Time or space prediction — Evolution in time — Forecast

While delineation of potential habitat for a species is a first step in risk mapping for *Anopheles*-borne species, forecasting seasonal events and variation in (micro-) habitat suitability and mosquito population is essential. Remote sensing and Geographical Information Systems (GIS) contributed to the development of environmental systems to support vector control or more sophisticated early warning systems. Those systems usually target situations of epidemic malaria which occurs in regions where malaria is not present continuously but associated to climatic events such as a particularly wet season in near desert areas [110] or a hot season in African highlands [111]. Epidemic situation are predicted to increase preparedness in public health [112]. These first experiences are reviewed in [10]. Several trends are observed in current research, but a major effort is targeted towards the prediction of malaria epidemic season based on climatic/meteorological variables, particularly in the context of climate changes and availability of new meteorological data sources [35]. The disease risk is forecasted using seasonal climate prediction and in particular rainfall and sea-surface temperature [110], and influence of climate change analysed [113]. Following the development of the European ENSEMBLE System for seasonal to inter - annual prediction [114], challenging researches are now proposing to integrate the seasonal climate forecasts from climate model into malaria early warnings systems [115]. Regional specificity still needs to be integrated in such models as for example the fact that low rainfall may trigger epidemics in the highlands [116].

4.3.3. *Anopheles vector capacity*

When trying to assess disease occurrence risk, not only vector presence is necessary but the capacity and eagerness to transmit the diseases is essential. This capacity is well summarized in the vectorial capacity (VC) concept [117] derived from the Basic reproduction rate of MacDonald [118]. Vectorial capacity is a series of biological features that determine the ability of mosquitoes to transmit *Plasmodium*. It is defined as the daily rate at which future inoculations could arise from a currently infected case [119] and it is generally used as a convenient way to express malaria transmission risk. Interestingly, a spatial version of the VC called VCAP has been developed to propose a spatial version of the formula, allowing assessment of vectorial capacity for each pixel in a given area [120]. To be able to do so, the VCAP is VC only driven by minimum *Ta* and rainfall. Rainfall and temperature are used as inputs to the model because they have an impact on vectorial capacity. Temperature has an effect on both the vector and the parasite. For the vector, it affects the juvenile development rates, the length of the gonotrophic cycle and survivorship of larvae and adults with an optimal temperature and upper and lower lethal boundaries. For the parasite, it effects the extrinsic incubation period [121]. *Plasmodium falciparum* (the dominant parasite in Africa) requires warmer minimum temperature than *Plasmodium vivax*. This can account for the geographic limits of malaria transmission for this species in Africa [122]. At 26ºC the extrinsic incubation period of this species is about 9-10 days whereas at 20-22ºC it may take as long as 15-20 days. In highlands, where cold temperatures preclude vector and/or parasite development during part/or all of the year, increased prevalence rates may be associated with higher than average minimum temperatures [123] which might be led by period of low rainfall [116]. It is possible to use minimum *Ta* derived from MODIS for monitoring risks of malaria transmission in highlands regions including Eritrea and Ethiopia where a high proportion of the population lives at risk of epidemic malaria. Currently, the USGS EROS Center uses this temperature derived from MODIS night *Ts* on an 8-day basis jointly with rainfall data derived from the Tropical Rainfall Measuring Mission (TRMM) downscaled to 1 km spatial resolution to produce a 1 km VCAP map every 8-days specifically for the epidemic regions of sub-Saharan Africa [118]. In Eq. 1, the two raster images MODIS night time (T_s) and rainfall (TRMM) are integrated as follows:

$$VCAP = \frac{-\left(m\,a^2\right)\,p^n}{\ln\left(p\right)} \tag{1}$$

Where:

m = 10.0 * TRMM

a = 0.7/gonotrophic

gonotrophic =[36.5/(T_s+2.0-9.9)]+0.5

$p=0.5^{(1.0/\text{gonotrophic}))}$

n=111.0/{[2.0*(36.5/ T_s+2.0-9.9)/gonotrophic]+T_s-18.0}

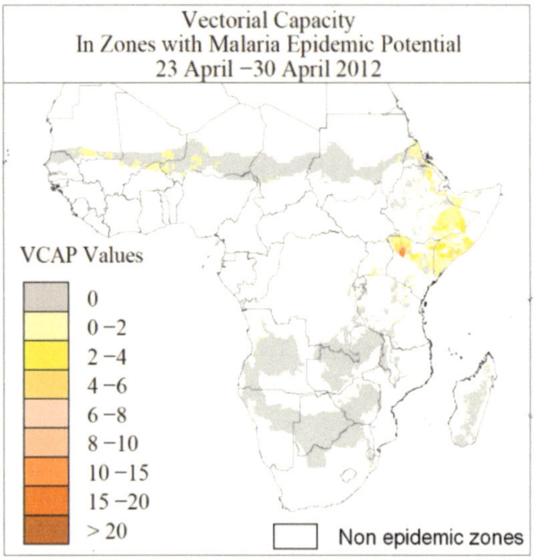

Figure 5. Vectorial capacity map VCAP provided for the epidemic zones of Africa at 1 km spatial resolution.

Parameter, m is the density of vectors (per human), a is the frequency of daily vector-man contact, p is the probability of a mosquito surviving through one whole day, and n is the extrinsic incubation period of malaria parasites or 'the time taken for completion of the extrinsic cycle'. Here the density m is estimated as a function of rainfall while the duration of the gonotrophic cycle and the extrinsic incubation period n are function of the temperature. The coefficients used in the VCAP equation are at this stage not optimized to specific regions. The variability in VCAP is only driven by the T_s and rainfall. This is a first attempt to spatially map risk of malaria transmission based on a vectorial capacity model. The product (Figure 5) is made available on a regular basis for the period Jan 2004 to present on the FEWS NET Africa Data Portal: http://earlywarning.usgs.gov/fews/africa/web and IRI data library: (http://iridl.ldeo.columbia.edu/maproom/.Health/.Regional/.Africa/.Malaria/.VCAP/)

The analysis of VCAP in relation to rainfall, temperature, and malaria incidence data in Eritrea and Madagascar shows that the VCAP correctly tracks the risk of malaria both in regions where rainfall is the limiting factor and in regions where temperature is the limiting factor [118]. However, in Burundi highlands, low rainfall triggered higher temperature and increased the risk of epidemics [116] and thus lower rainfall might be the trigger particularly because houses provide microenvironment with stable temperature 5°c higher than outside temperature and reduce influence of temperature on epidemic risk. The VCAP could also be further detailed by carrying analysis per vector species.

4.4. Transferring spatial information to health professionals

Roberts *et al.* [124] demonstrated many potential uses of remotely sensed data in managing and targeting vector and disease control measures. Just mapping the existing *Anopheles* species attributes can already bring information. Recently a map of all existing records for the *Anopheles dirus* complex was proposed [125] to document ecological settings, but also to demonstrate that detailed mapping could bring much more information and could lead to more sophisticated models [9] from those datasets such as developed [6] for *Anopheles* vectors. In this context, major effort were made in the past to provide mapping expertise through customized GIS application to malaria control staff and help them to map their entomological and diseases cases records. Simply overlaying this information with existing environmental information can lead to new working hypotheses better defined by people with experience in the field. Current availability of easy to use packages such as Google earth and Google map offer new opportunities particularly in areas covered by detailed imagery. Studies carried out by scientist devoted to research provide outputs in scientific publications, in pdf format or might target small study areas not representative of the whole country. While this type of output is useful for advances in sciences it is often of little use to the health worker in the field. Two types of approaches are more adapted to the field and complementary. One is to provide ready-to-use product to integrate into operating systems, updated regularly to feed into early warning systems, or informative enough to provide the necessary clues for control and forecast. Those include vector capacity maps. The other approach is to bring the most expertise possible into the hands of the health worker.

However, to be fully operational the development of new products and early warning systems presented above must be integrated into a decision/action framework. There is currently a good deal of policy congruence through international, regional and local levels to support this effort (e.g. the Global Framework for Climate Services whose aims are to develop more effective services to meet the increasing demand coming from climate sensitive sectors including health). The remaining challenge is to get the knowledge into practice and sustaining it where it is needed. It is crucial that appropriate policies are developed and implemented to improve health system performance [126]. This may be helped by enhancing the workforces' ability to detect and treat diseases, monitor and predict spatio-temporal patterns and implement intervention and control strategies in a timely and cost-effective manner through the use of tools and analysis informed by climate data.

In order to get research outcomes into policy and practice it is important to understand the context in which policies are adopted and supported in a practical manner. Below is an example of how policies developed at the district and national level connect to the larger political agenda of international policy makers. At the global scale improved early warning, prevention and control of epidemics is one of the key technical elements of the current Global Strategy for Malaria Control [127] the RBM Partnership referenced earlier in this section. In Africa, Heads-of-State declared their support for the Roll Back Malaria initiative in April 2000 with the Abuja Targets [128]. In these targets, national malaria control services are expected to detect sixty per cent of malaria epidemics within two weeks of onset, and respond to sixty per cent of epidemics within two weeks of their detection. With the support of the WHO Regional Office for Africa, the WHO Inter-Country Programme Teams engage in the development of recommendations, guidelines and technical support to improve prevention and control of epidemics and transboundary/cross border within their various sub-regions (e.g. Regional Economic Communities (RECS) ECOWAS, IGAD and SADC) including collaborative activities with the

African Development Bank. As a consequence of these policy developments, nations epidemic prone have enhanced capabilities for delimiting epidemic/endemic prone areas; established epidemic malaria surveillance systems; and strengthening their epidemic response capacities with the help of the Global Fund to Fight AIDS, Tuberculosis and Malaria (GFATM) and other donor support.

In many national malaria control policy documents, countries now recognize that to achieve the Roll Back Malaria (RBM) and Millennium Development Goals (MDG) targets they need better information on where epidemics are most likely to occur, and some indication of when they are likely to happen. As a consequence, they have begun to explore the use of climate information in the development of integrated early warning systems. Thus, there is increasing congruence in policy initiatives from multilateral, bilateral, national and non-governmental agencies in relation to epidemic disease control and a growing demand for climate information and robust early warning systems to support these efforts. This is reflected in the newly emerging Global Framework for Climate Services. This policy congruence extends to the current discussions on adaptation to climate change. Strengthened health systems are also seen as vital to improving the management of climate-sensitive disease in the context of climate change. The IPCC identified building public health infrastructure as: *The most important, cost effective and urgently needed adaptation strategy.* Other measures endorsed by the IPCC include public health training programs, more effective surveillance and emergency response systems, and sustainable prevention and control programs. These measures are familiar to the public health community and are needed regardless of climate change and constitute what is the basis of a *no regrets* adaptation strategy [129,130].

5. Further research

In terms of data, interactions between *Anopheles* species should be investigated, those being sympatric on the same habitat or even breeding site or one dominant species deterring another species. Adapted methodology based on asymmetrical similarity coefficients, indirect clustering and the search of indicative species [131] have been proposed [132] to identify species association to help assess the risk of presence of elusive species, if another often associated species is present. Caveats and potential improvements to environmental factors have already been discussed. Remote sensing offers already a wide range of useful products but improvements could target easier delivery of products such as proposed by the IRI data library (http://iridl.ldeo.columbia.edu/) in similar standardised format and resolution and availability of all useful derived products over the world.

In terms of modelling, various issues have also already been discussed such as the necessity to better integrate ecological issues such as sink and source population [104]. Regarding the outputs, quality assessment could be attached to the resulting maps. Bayesian inference can be used [133] to quantify the uncertainty in the predictions. Rather than mapping the prevalence, what is mapped is the probability, given the data, that a particular location exceeded the predetermined high-risk prevalence threshold for which a change in strategy for control or the delivery of the drug is required. A level of uncertainty attached to each location help the decision maker choose which areas are at risk or not.

There is a necessity to document in details the data entered in models and choices of the modellers particularly when dealing with results which might trigger decision in public health [134]. Indeed, the final results do not only depend on input data but on pre-processing of those data, selection of useful variables, selection of a best model between various potential models, a whole process of model building which leads to one final result dependant on choices of the modeller. More details on dates of satellite images used to derived RS product, or even detailing quality spatially could also improve the final results and potential interpretation. Providing maps of the dataset entered in the model could help spot good spatial consistency or mismatch between adjacent raw images.

While disease occurrence prediction is generally the objective of forecasting, targeting the vector instead of the disease cases might provide several advantages. Indeed, some diseases might be present in a high number of asymptomatic carriers (lymphatic filariasis), or might not be accurately reported because the disease is not notifiable or misdiagnosis is frequent such as confusion between malaria and *Borrelia duttoni* in parts of Senegal and Togo [135]. Targeting the vector can help identify areas where asymptomatic cases might occur, target several diseases at once and predict epidemics or seasonal occurrence of diseases in advance based on fluctuations in mosquito populations.

6. Conclusions

In conclusion, providing relevant information to help disease spatial surveillance is not straighforwards and resemble more to a multidisciplinary challenge. In order to improve the current situation, increased sharing of existing data and increase transparency and documentation in the building of models could help target low quality areas such as places with low information or part of modelling process which could be improved. The quality of the entomological and environmental dataset as well as documentation of the relevant dates of each parameter such as original satellite images included in land cover maps and potential issues such as source-sink population sample could help identify new questions. Meanwhile, the information is still needed for the support of essential activities such as malaria control or for scientific research. A better interaction between research and operational work also seems to be necessary. Research product and results can only be useful if validated in the field and the best research questions are defined by people working in the field. Constant interactions can improve quality of research products and finally improve surveillance. Reinforcing the research capabilities in the region and in the malaria centres is of up-most importance. Indeed malaria workers in-countries have an extended experience of the field. They are in a better position to analyze the situation, identify their needs and find the answers. This would help bringing the data and the expertise where it is mostly needed: in the malaria centres.

Abbreviations

AVHRR Advanced Very High Resolution Radiometer

BRDF bi-directional reflectance distribution function

CGIAR Consultative Group on International Agricultural Research

CMORPH Products from the CPC MORPHing technique

CRU Climate Research Unit, University of East Anglia, UK

ECOWAS Economic Community Of West African States

EUMETSAT European Organisation for the Exploitation of Meteorological Satellites

EVI The Enhanced Vegetation Index

FAO Food and Agriculture Organization of the United Nations

fAPAR fraction of Absorbed Photosynthetically Active Radiation

FEWS NET Famines Early Warning Systems Network

GFATM Global Fund to Fight AIDS, Tuberculosis and Malaria

GIMMS Global Inventory Modelling and Mapping Studies

GIS Geographical Information Systems

GMES Global Monitoring for Environment and Security

GRIB MPE The Multi-sensor Precipitation Estimate

HSV Hue saturation value

IGAD The Intergovernmental Authority on Development, East Africa

IPCC Intergovernmental Panel on Climate Change

IR Infrared

IRI International Research Institute for Climate and Society

LAI Leaf Area Index

LST Land Surface Temperature

MDG Millennium Development Goals

MERIS Medium Resolution Imaging Spectrometer

MODIS Moderate Resolution Imaging Spectroradiometer

MPE Multisensor Precipitation Estimator

MVC Maximum Value Composite

NASA National Aeronautic and Space Administration

NBAR Nadir BRDF-Adjusted Reflectance

NDVI The Normalized Difference Vegetation Index

NDWI The Normalized Difference Water Index

http://dx.doi.org/10.5772/55622

NIR Near-Infrared

NOAA-CPC National Oceanic and Atmospheric Administration – Climate Prediction Centre

RBM Roll Back Malaria

RECS Regional Economic Communities

RFE African Rainfall Estimation

SADC Southern African Development Community

SRTM Shuttle Radar Topographic Mission

SWIR Short Wavelength Infrared

TARCAT The TAMSAT African Rainfall Climatology And Time-series

TIR Thermal infra-red

TRMM The Tropical Rainfall Measuring Mission

USGS United states Geological Survey Agency

VC (VCAP) Vectorial Capacity (spatial version)

WHO World Health Organisation

Author details

Valérie Obsomer[1*], Nicolas Titeux[2], Christelle Vancustem[3], Grégory Duveiller[3], Jean-François Pekel[3], Steve Connor[4], Pietro Ceccato[5] and Marc Coosemans[6]

*Address all correspondence to: valerie.obsomer@uclouvain.be

1 Earth and Life Institute, Université Catholique de Louvain, Louvain-la-Neuve, Belgium

2 Department Environment & Agro-biotechnologies, Public Research Centre - Gabriel Lippmann, Belvaux, Luxembourg

3 Joint Research Centre of the European Commission (JRC), Ispra, Italy

4 School of Environmental Sciences, University of Liverpool, Liverpool, United Kingdom

5 International Research Institute for Climate and Society, The Earth Institute, Columbia University, New York, USA

6 Institute for Tropical Medicine, Antwerp, Belgium

References

[1] Harbach RE. The classification of genus *Anopheles* (Diptera: Culicidae): a working hypothesis of phylogenetic relationships. Bulletin of Entomological Research 2004; 94(6) 537-553.

[2] Harbach R. Mosquito Taxonomic Inventory. 2012. http://mosquito-taxonomic-inventory.info /sites/mosquito-taxonomic-inventory.info/files/Anopheles%20classification_25.pdf

[3] Manguin S, Carnevale P, Mouchet J, Coosemans M, Julvez J, Richard-Lenoble D, Sircoulon J. Biodiversity of malaria in the world. John Libbey; 2008.

[4] The malERA Consultative Group on Vector Control. A research agenda for malaria eradication: Vector control. PLoS Medicine 2011; 8(1):e1000401.

[5] Hay SI, Guerra CA, Gething PW, Patil AP, Tatem AJ, Noor AM, et al. A World malaria map: *Plasmodium falciparum* endemicity in 2007. PLoS Medicine 2009; 6(3):e1000048.

[6] Sinka ME, Bangs MJ, Manguin S, Chareonviriyaphap T, Patil AP, Temperley WH, Gething PW, Elyazar IRF, Kabaria CW, Harbach RE, Hay SI. The dominant *Anopheles* vectors of human malaria in the Asia-Pacific region: occurrence data, distribution maps and bionomic précis. Parasites & Vectors 2011; 4:89.

[7] Sinka M, Bangs M, Manguin S, Coetzee M, Mbogo C, Hemingway J, Patil AP, Temperley WH, Gething PW, Kabaria CW, Okara RM, Van Boeckel T, Godfray HCJ, Harbach RE, I Hay S. The dominant *Anopheles* vectors of human malaria in Africa, Europe and the Middle East: occurrence data, distribution maps and bionomic précis. Parasites & Vectors 2010; 3 (1) 117.

[8] Sinka M, Rubio-Palis Y, Manguin S, Patil A, Temperley W, Gething P, Van Boeckel T, Kabaria CW, Harbach RE, Hay SI. The dominant *Anopheles* vectors of human malaria in the Americas: occurrence data, distribution maps and bionomic précis. Parasites & Vectors 2010; 3 (1) 72.

[9] Obsomer V, Defourny P, Coosemans M. Predicted distribution of major malaria vectors belonging to the *Anopheles dirus* Complex in Asia: ecological niche and environmental influences. PLoS ONE 2012; 7(11):e50475.

[10] Ceccato P, Connor SJ, Jeanne I, Thomson MC. Application of geographical information systems and remote sensing technologies for assessing and monitoring malaria risk. Parassitologia 2005;47 (1) 81-96.

[11] Hill D, Fasham M, Tucker G, Shewry M, Shaw P. Handbook of Biodiversity Methods: Survey, Evaluation and Monitoring. Cambridge University Press 2005.

[12] Brotons L, Herrando S, Pla M. Updating bird species distribution at large spatial scales: applications of habitat modelling to data from long-term monitoring programs. Diversity and Distributions 2007; 13 (3) 276-88.

[13] Guisan A, Thuiller W. Predicting species distribution: offering more than simple habitat models. Ecology Letters 2005; 8 (9) 993-1009.

[14] Elith J, Graham C, Anderson R, Dudík M, Ferrier S, Guisan A, Hijmans RJ, Huettmann F, Leathwick JR, Lehmann A, Li J, Lohmann LG, Loiselle BA, Manion G, Moritz C, Nakamura M, Nakazawa Y, Overton JMM, Peterson AT, Phillips SJ, Richardson K, Scachetti-Pereira R, Schapire RE, Soberón J, Williams S, Wisz MS, Zimmermann NE. Novel methods improve prediction of species' distributions from occurrence data. Ecography 2006; 29 (2) 129-151.

[15] Brotons L, Sierdsemama H, Newson S, Jiguet F, Gregory R. Spatial modeling of large-scale bird monitoring data: Towards pan-European quantitative distribution maps. Journal of Ornithology. 2006; 147:29.

[16] Kéry M, Dorazio RM, Soldaat L, Van Strien A, Zuiderwijk A, Royle JA. Trend estimation in populations with imperfect detection. Journal of Applied Ecology 2009; 46 (6) 1163-72.

[17] Pearce J, Ferrier S. An evaluation of alternative algorithms for fitting species distribution models using logistic regression. Ecological Modelling 2000; 128 (2–3) 127-147.

[18] Wisz MS, Hijmans RJ, Li J, Peterson AT, Graham CH, Guisan A, et al. Effects of sample size on the performance of species distribution models. Diversity and Distributions 2008; 14 (5) 763-773.

[19] iménez-Valverde A, Lobo JM, Hortal J. The effect of prevalence and its interaction with sample size on the reliability of species distribution models. Community Ecology 2009; 10(2) 196-205.

[20] Feeley KJ, Silman MR. Keep collecting: accurate species distribution modelling requires more collections than previously thought. Diversity and Distributions 2011; 17(6) 1132-1140.

[21] Hirzel A, Guisan A. Which is the optimal sampling strategy for habitat suitability modelling. Ecological Modelling 2002; 157 (2–3) 331-341.

[22] Phillips SJ, Anderson RP, Schapire RE. Maximum entropy modeling of species geographic distributions. Ecological Modelling 2006; 190 (3–4) 231-259.

[23] Mackenzie DI, Royle JA. Designing occupancy studies: general advice and allocating survey effort. Journal of Applied Ecology 2005; 42 (6) 1105-1114.

[24] MacKenzie DI, Nichols JD, Royle JA, Pollock KH, Bailey LL, Hines JE. Occupancy Estimation and Modeling: Inferring Patterns and Dynamics of Species Occurrence. 1er éd. Academic Press 2005.

[25] Beck LR, Rodriguez MH, Dister SW, Rodriguez AD, Rejmankova E, Ulloa A, et al. Remote sensing as a landscape epidemiologic tool to identify villages at high risk for malaria transmission. American Journal of Tropical Medicine and Hygiene 1994; 51 (3) 271-280.

[26] USGS United States Geological Survey. Hydro 1km, elevation derivative database. Sioux Falls, South Dakota, USA. 2001

[27] CGIAR CIAT International Center for Tropical Agriculture. Void-filled seamless SRTM data VI. 2004.

[28] FAO United Nation Food and Agriculture Organisation. Digital soil map of the world 1990.

[29] Hijmans RJ, Cameron SE, Parra JL, Jones PG, Jarvis A. Very high resolution interpolated climate surfaces for global land areas. International Journal of Climatology 2005; 25 (15) 1965-1978.

[30] New M, Lister D, Hulme M, Makin I. A high-resolution dataset of surface climate over global land areas. Climate research 2002; 21:1-25.

[31] Olson DM, Dinerstein E, Wikramanayake ED, Burgess ND, Powell GVN, Underwood EC, et al. Terrestrial Ecoregions of the World: A New Map of Life on Earth. BioScience 2001; 51(11) 933-938.

[32] Price JC. Land surface temperature measurements from the split window channels of the NOAA 7 Advanced Very High Resolution Radiometer. Journal of Geophysical Research 1984; 89 (D5): 7231-7237.

[33] Wan Z, Zhang Y, Zhang Q, Li Z. Validation of the land-surface temperature products retrieved from Terra Moderate Resolution Imaging Spectroradiometer data. Remote Sensing of Environment 2002; 83 (1–2) 163-80.

[34] Pinheiro ACT, Mahoney R, Privette JL, Tucker CJ. Development of a daily long term record of NOAA-14 AVHRR land surface temperature over Africa. Remote Sensing of Environment 2006; 103 (2) 153-164.

[35] Vancutsem C, Ceccato P, Dinku T, Connor SJ. Evaluation of MODIS land surface temperature data to estimate air temperature in different ecosystems over Africa. Remote Sensing of Environment 2010; 114 (2) 449-465.

[36] Ceccato P, Vancutsem C, Temimi M. Monitoring air and Land Surface Temperatures from remotely sensed data for climate-human health applications. Geoscience and Remote Sensing Symposium (IGARSS), 2010 IEEE International. 2010. page 178 -180.

[37] Ceccato P, Dinku T. Introduction to remote sensing for monitoring rainfall, temperature, vegetation and water bodies. Palisades, New York: International Research Institute for Climate and Society; 2010 page 15 pp. Report No.: 10-04.

[38] Huffman GJ, Bolvin DT, Nelkin EJ, Wolff DB, Adler RF, Gu G, Hong Y, Bowman KP, Stocker EF. The TRMM Multisatellite Precipitation Analysis (TMPA): Quasi-Global,

Multiyear, Combined-Sensor Precipitation Estimates at Fine Scales. Journal of Hydrometeorology 2007; 8 (1) 38-55.

[39] Dinku T, Chidzambwa S, Ceccato P, Connor SJ, Ropelewski CF. Validation of high-resolution satellite rainfall products over complex terrain. International Journal of Remote Sensing 2008; 29(14) 4097-4110.

[40] Joyce RJ, Janowiak JE, Arkin PA, Xie P. CMORPH: A Method that Produces Global Precipitation Estimates from Passive Microwave and Infrared Data at High Spatial and Temporal Resolution. Journal of Hydrometeorology 2004; 5:487.

[41] Dinku T, Ceccato P, Cressman K, Connor SJ. Evaluating Detection Skills of Satellite Rainfall Estimates over Desert Locust Recession Regions. Journal of Applied Meteorology and Climatology 2010; 49 (6) 1322-1332.

[42] Dinku T, Ceccato P, Connor SJ. Challenges of satellite rainfall estimation over mountainous and arid parts of east Africa. International Journal of Remote Sensing 2011; 32 (21) 5965-5979.

[43] Dinku T, Connor S, Ceccato P. Evaluation of Satellite Rainfall Estimates and Gridded Gauge products over the Upper Blue Nile Region. In: Melesse AM, (ed.) Nile River Basin. Part II.; 2011. p109-127.

[44] Maidment RI, Grimes DIF, Allan RP, Greatrex H, Rojas O, Leo O. Evaluation of satellite-based and model re-analysis rainfall estimates for Uganda. Meteorological Applications 2012; ISSN 1469-8080 (in press)

[45] Heinemann T, Kenényi J. The Eumestsat multi sensor precipitation estimate (MPE): concept et validation. Proceedings of the EUMETSAT users conference. Weimar, Germany; 2003.

[46] Tucker CJ, Sellers PJ. Satellite remote sensing of primary production. International Journal of Remote Sensing 1986; 7 (11) 1395-1416.

[47] Myneni RB, Hall FG, Sellers PJ, Marshak AL. The interpretation of spectral vegetation indexes. IEEE Transactions on Geoscience and Remote Sensing 1995; 33 (2)481 -486.

[48] Rouse JW, Haas RH, Schell JA, Deering DW. Monitoring Vegetation Systems in the Great Plains with Erts. NASA Special Publication 1974; 351:309.

[49] Tucker CJ, Pinzon JE, Brown ME, Slayback DA, Pak EW, Mahoney R, Vermote, EF, El Saleous, N. An extended AVHRR 8-km NDVI dataset compatible with MODIS and SPOT vegetation NDVI data. International Journal of Remote Sensing 2005; 26(20) 4485-4498

[50] Huete R. Soil influence in remote sensed vegetation-canopy spectra. Introduction to the physics and techniques of remote sensing. Wiley-interscience. New York; 1987. page 107-41.

[51] Jackson TJ, Chen D, Cosh M, Li F, Anderson M, Walthall C, Doriaswamy P, Hunt ER. Vegetation water content mapping using Landsat data derived normalized difference water index for corn and soybeans. Remote Sensing of Environment 2004; 92(4) 475-82.

[52] Huete A, Didan K, Miura T, Rodriguez E., Gao X, Ferreira L. Overview of the radiometric and biophysical performance of the MODIS vegetation indices. Remote Sensing of Environment 2002; 83(1–2) 195-213.

[53] Jiang Z, Huete AR, Didan K, Miura T. Development of a two-band enhanced vegetation index without a blue band. Remote Sensing of Environment 2008; 112(10) 3833-3845.

[54] Gao B. NDWI: A normalized difference water index for remote sensing of vegetation liquid water from space. Remote Sensing of Environment 1996; 58 (3) 257-266.

[55] Ceccato P, Gobron N, Flasse S, Pinty B, Tarantola S. Designing a spectral index to estimate vegetation water content from remote sensing data: Part 1: Theoretical approach. Remote Sensing of Environment. 2002; 82 (2–3) 188-97.

[56] Zarco-Tejada P., Rueda C., Ustin S. Water content estimation in vegetation with MODIS reflectance data and model inversion methods. Remote Sensing of Environment 2003; 85 (1) 109-24.

[57] Pekel J-F, Ceccato P, Vancutsem C, Cressman K, Vanbogaert E, Defourny P. Development and Application of Multi-Temporal Colorimetric Transformation to Monitor Vegetation in the Desert Locust Habitat. IEEE Journal of Selected Topics in Applied Earth Observations and Remote Sensing 2011; 4(2) 318 -326.

[58] Chen JM, Black TA. Defining leaf area index for non-flat leaves. Plant, Cell & Environment 1992; 15(4): 421-429.

[59] Myneni RB, Maggion S, Iaquinta J, Privette JL, Gobron N, Pinty B, Kimes DS, Verstraete MM, Williams DL. Optical remote sensing of vegetation: Modeling, caveats, and algorithms. Remote Sensing of Environment 1995; 51(1) 169-188.

[60] Dorigo WA, Zurita-Milla R, de Wit AJW, Brazile J, Singh R, Schaepman ME. A review on reflective remote sensing and data assimilation techniques for enhanced agroecosystem modeling. International Journal of Applied Earth Observation and Geoinformation 2007; 9(2) 165-193.

[61] Myneni R., Hoffman S, Knyazikhin Y, Privette J., Glassy J, Tian Y, Wang Y, Song X, Zhang Y, Smith GR, Lotsch A, Friedl M, Morisette JT, Votava P, Nemani RR, Running SW. Global products of vegetation leaf area and fraction absorbed PAR from year one of MODIS data. Remote Sensing of Environment 2002; 83 (1–2) 214-31.

[62] Baret F, Hagolle O, Geiger B, Bicheron P, Miras B, Huc M, Berthelot B, Niño F, Weiss M, Samain O, Roujean J-L, Leroy M. LAI, fAPAR and fCover CYCLOPES global

products derived from VEGETATION: Part 1: Principles of the algorithm. Remote Sensing of Environment 2007; 110 (3) 275-86.

[63] Weiss M, Baret F, Garrigues S, Lacaze R. LAI and fAPAR CYCLOPES global products derived from VEGETATION. Part 2: validation and comparison with MODIS collection 4 products. Remote Sensing of Environment 2007; 110 (3) 317-331.

[64] Garrigues S, Lacaze R, Baret F, Morisette JT, Weiss M, Nickeson JE, Fernandes R, Plummer S, Shabanov NV, Myneni RB, Knyazikhin Y, Yang W. Validation and intercomparison of global Leaf Area Index products derived from remote sensing data. Journal of Geophysical Research 2008; 113(G2):G02028.

[65] Fang H, Wei S, Liang S. Validation of MODIS and CYCLOPES LAI products using global field measurement data. Remote Sensing of Environment 2012; 119(0) 43-54.

[66] Baret F, Weiss M. Biopar Methods Compendium LAI, FAPAR, FCOVER, NDVI. Geoland2 rep. BP-RP038. 2010. 50pp.

[67] Baret F, Pacholczyk P, Lacaze R. BioPar Product User Manual: LAI, FAPAR, FCover from AVHRR-LTDR data. Geoland 2 rep BR-RP053.2012. Geoland 2 rep BR-RP053.2012; 2012.

[68] Latham J. Africover eastern Africa. LUUC NewsLetter 2001; (7) 15-6.

[69] Bartholomé E, Belward AS. GLC2000: a new approach to global land cover mapping from Earth observation data. International Journal of Remote Sensing 2005; 26 (9)1959-1977.

[70] Friedl MA, Sulla-Menashe D, Tan B, Schneider A, Ramankutty N, Sibley A, et al. MODIS Collection 5 global land cover: Algorithm refinements and characterization of new datasets. Remote Sensing of Environment 2010; 114 (1) 168-182.

[71] Defourny P, Vancutsem C, Pekel J-F, Bicheron P, Brockmann C, Nino F, Schouten L, Leroy M. Towards a 300 m global land cover product - the Globcover initiative. Snd workshop of the EARSeL Special Interest Group on land use and land cover: application & development. Bonn (Germany): Braun M; 2008.

[72] Giri C, Jenkins C. Land cover mapping of Greater Mesoamerica using MODIS data. Canadian Journal of Remote Sensing 2005; 31(4) 274-282.

[73] Bontemps S, Arino O, Bicheron P, Carsten B, Leroy M, Vancutsem C, Defourny P. Operational service demonstration for global land cover mapping: the GlobCover and GlobCorine expertience for 2005 and 2009. Remote sensing of land use and land cover: principle and applications. 2012.

[74] Haas EM, Bartholomé E, Combal B. Time series analysis of optical remote sensing data for the mapping of temporary surface water bodies in sub-Saharan western Africa. Journal of Hydrology 2009; 370(1–4) 52-63.

[75] Gond V, Bartholomé E, Ouattara F, Nonguierma A, Bado L. Surveillance et cartographie des plans d'eau et des zones humides et inondables en régions arides avec l'in-

strument VEGETATION embarqué sur SPOT-4. International Journal of Remote Sensing 2004; 25(5) 987-1004.

[76] Pekel J-F, Vancutsem C, Bastin L, Clerici M, Vanbogaert E, Bartholomé E, et al. A water surface detection method based on hSV transformation of MODIS multi-spetral time series suitable for near real-time monitoring in Africa. Remote Sensing of Environment (submitted). 2013

[77] Holben BN. Characteristics of maximum-value composite images from temporal AVHRR data. International Journal of Remote Sensing 1986; 7(11) 1417-1434.

[78] Schaaf CB, Gao F, Strahler AH, Lucht W, Li X, Tsang T, Strugnella NC, Zhanga X, Jina Y, Mullerc J-P, Lewis P, Barnsley M, Hobson P, Disney M, Roberts G, Dunderdale M, Doll C, d'Entremont RP, Hug B, Liangh S, Privettei JL, Royh D. First operational BRDF, albedo nadir reflectance products from MODIS. Remote Sensing of Environment 2002; 83 (1-2) 135-148.

[79] Hagolle O, Lobo A, Maisongrande P, Cabot F, Duchemin B, De Pereyra A. Quality assessment and improvement of temporally composited products of remotely sensed imagery by combination of VEGETATION 1 and 2 images. Remote Sensing of Environment 2005; 94 (2) 172-86.

[80] Vancutsem C, Pekel J -F., Bogaert P, Defourny P. Mean Compositing, an alternative strategy for producing temporal syntheses. Concepts and performance assessment for SPOT VEGETATION time series. International Journal of Remote Sensing 2007; 28(22) 5123-5141.

[81] Duveiller G, Baret F, Defourny P. Remotely sensed green area index for winter wheat crop monitoring: 10-Year assessment at regional scale over a fragmented landscape. Agricultural and Forest Meteorology 2012; 166–167 (0) 156-168.

[82] Cracknell AP. Review article Synergy in remote sensing-what's in a pixel? International Journal of Remote Sensing 1998; 19(11) 2025-47.

[83] Schowengerdt. Remote sensing models and methods for image processing. San Diego, USA: San Diego Academic Press; 2007.

[84] Wolfe RE, Roy DP, Vermote E. MODIS land data storage, gridding, and compositing methodology: Level 2 grid. IEEE Transactions on Geoscience and Remote Sensing 1998; 36(4) 1324 -1338.

[85] Tan B, Woodcock CE, Hu J, Zhang P, Ozdogan M, Huang D, Yang W, Knyazikhin Y, Myneni RB. The impact of gridding artifacts on the local spatial properties of MODIS data: Implications for validation, compositing, and band-to-band registration across resolutions. Remote Sensing of Environment 2006; 105(2) 98-114.

[86] Duveiller G. Caveats in calculating crop specific pixel purity for agricultural monitoring using MODIS time series. Proc. SPIE 8531, Remote Sensing for Agriculture, Ecosystems, and Hydrology XIV, 85310J (October 19, 2012).

[87] Duveiller G, Baret F, Defourny P. Crop specific green area index retrieval from MODIS data at regional scale by controlling pixel-target adequacy. Remote Sensing of Environment 2011; 115 (10) 2686-2701.

[88] Hansen MC, DeFries RS, Townshend JRG, Carroll M, Dimiceli C, Sohlberg RA. Global Percent Tree Cover at a Spatial Resolution of 500 Meters: First Results of the MODIS Vegetation Continuous Fields Algorithm. Earth Interactions 2003; 7 (10) 1-15.

[89] Overgaard HJ, Ekbom B, Suwonkerd W, Takagi M. Effect of landscape structure on anopheline mosquito density and diversity in northern Thailand: Implications for malaria transmission and control. Landscape ecology 2003; 18 (6) 605-619.

[90] Guisan A, Zimmermann NE. Predictive habitat distribution models in ecology. Ecological Modelling 2000; 135 (2–3) 147-186.

[91] Brotons L, Thuiller W, Araújo MB, Hirzel AH. Presence-absence versus presence-only modelling methods for predicting bird habitat suitability. Ecography 2004; 27(4) 437-448.

[92] Araújo MB, Guisan A. Five (or so) challenges for species distribution modelling. Journal of Biogeography 2006; 33 (10) 1677-1688.

[93] Franklin J. Mapping Species Distributions: Spatial Inference and Prediction. Cambridge University Press; 2010.

[94] Thomson M, Obsomer V, Dunne M, Connor S, Molyneux D. Satellite mapping of *Loa loa* prevalence in relation to ivermectin use in west and central Africa. The Lancet 2000; 356 (9235) 1077-1078.

[95] Rogers DJ. Models for vectors and vector-borne diseases. Advances in Parasitology 2006; 62: 1-35.

[96] Titeux N, Dufrêne M, Jacob J-P, Paquay M, Defourny P. Multivariate analysis of a fine-scale breeding bird atlas using a geographical information system and partial canonical correspondence analysis: environmental and spatial effects. Journal of Biogeography 2004; 31 (11) 1841-1856.

[97] Hutchinson G. Concluding remarks 1957. Cold Spring Harbor Symposia on Quantitative Biology. p415-427.

[98] Busby J. BIOCLIM - A bioclimate analysis and prediction system. In: Margules C, Austin M,. Nature conservation: cost effective biological surveys and data analysis. Melbourne: CSIRO; 1991.

[99] Carpenter G, Gillison AN, Winter J. DOMAIN: a flexible modelling procedure for mapping potential distributions of plants and animals. Biodiversity and Conservation 1993; 2 (6) 667-80.

[100] Hirzel AH, Hausser J, Chessel D, Perrin N. Ecological-niche factor analysis: how to compute habitat-suitability maps without absence data? Ecology 2002; 83(7) 2027-2036.

[101] Soberón J. Grinnellian and Eltonian niches and geographic distributions of species. Ecology Letters 2007; 10 (12) 1115-1123.

[102] Phillips SJ, Dudík M, Elith J, Graham CH, Lehmann A, Leathwick J, Ferrier S. Sample selection bias and presence-only distribution models: implications for background and pseudo-absence data. Ecological Applications 2009; 19(1) 181-197.

[103] Pearson RG, Raxworthy CJ, Nakamura M, Townsend Peterson A. Predicting species distributions from small numbers of occurrence records: a test case using cryptic geckos in Madagascar. Journal of Biogeography 2007; 34(1) 102-117.

[104] Rascalou G, Pontier D, Menu F, Gourbière S. Emergence and Prevalence of Human Vector-Borne Diseases in Sink Vector Populations. PLoS ONE. 2012; 7(5):e36858.

[105] Mouchet J, Manguin S, Sircoulon J, Laventure S, Faye O, Onapa AW, Carnevale P, Julvez J, Fontenille D. Evolution of malaria in Africa for the past 40 years: impact of climatic and human factors. Journal of the American Mosquito Control Association 1998; 14 (2) 121-130.

[106] Bouma MJ. Methodological problems and amendments to demonstrate effects of temperature on the epidemiology of malaria. A new perspective on the highland epidemics in Madagascar, 1972–1989. Transactions of the Royal Society of Tropical Medicine and Hygiene 2003; 97 (2) 133-139.

[107] WHO/UNICEF. The World Malaria Report 2010. 2011.

[108] Omumbo JA, Lyon B, Waweru SM, Connor SJ, Thomson MC. Raised temperatures over the Kericho tea estates: revisiting the climate in the East African highlands malaria debate. Malaria Journal. 2011; 10(1)12.

[109] Reiter P. Global warming and malaria: knowing the horse before hitching the cart. Malaria Journal 2008; 7(Suppl 1): S3

[110] Thomson MC, Mason SJ, Phindela T, Connor SJ. Use of rainfall and sea surface temperature monitoring for malaria early warning in Botswana. The American journal of tropical medicine and hygiene 2005; 73(1): 214-221.

[111] Abeku TA, Hay SI, Ochola S, Langi P, Beard B, de Vlas SJ, Cox J. Malaria epidemic early warning and detection in African highlands. Trends in Parasitology 2004; 20 (9):400-405.

[112] Hay SI, Were EC, Renshaw M, Noor AM, Ochola SA, Olusanmi I, Alipui N, Snow RW. Forecasting, warning, and detection of malaria epidemics: a case study. The Lancet 2003; 361(9370):1705-1706.

[113] Hay SI, Shanks GD, Stern DI, Snow RW, Randolph SE, Rogers DJ. Climate variability and malaria epidemics in the highlands of East Africa. Trends in Parasitology 2005; 21(2):52-53.

[114] Palmer TN, Doblas-Reyes FJ, Hagedorn R, Alessandri A, Gualdi S, Andersen U, Feddersen H, Cantelaube P, Terres J-M, Davey M, Graham R, Délécluse P, Lazar A, Déqué M, Guérémy J-F, Díez E, Orfila B, Hoshen M, Morse AP, Keenlyside N, Latif M, Maisonnave E, Rogel P, Marletto V, Thomson MC. Development of an European multimodel ensemble system for seasonal-to-interannual prediction (DEMETER). Bulletin of the American Meteorological Society 2004; 85 (6) 853-72.

[115] Thomson MC, Doblas-Reyes FJ, Mason SJ, Hagedorn R, Connor SJ, Phindela T, Morse AP, Palmer TN. Malaria early warnings based on seasonal climate forecasts from multi-model ensembles. Nature 2006; 439(7076) 576-9.

[116] Protopopoff N, Van Bortel W, Speybroeck N, Van Geertruyden J-P, Baza D, D'Alessandro U, Coosemans M. Ranking Malaria Risk Factors to Guide Malaria Control Efforts in African Highlands. PLoS ONE 2009; 4:e8022.

[117] Garret-Jones C. Prognosis for interruption of malaria transmission through assessment of the mosquito's vectorial capacity. Nature 1964; 204: 1173–1175.

[118] Macdonald G. Theory of the eradication of malaria. Bulletin of the World Health Organisation 1956; 15: 369–387.

[119] Dye C. The Analysis of parasite transmission by bloodsucking insects. Annual Review of Entomology 1992; 37 (1) 1-19.

[120] Ceccato P, Vancutsem C, Klaver R, Rowland J, Connor SJ. A Vectorial Capacity product to monitor changing malaria transmission potential in epidemic regions of Africa. Journal of Tropical Medicine 2012; 2012 (595948) 1-6.

[121] Lactin DJ, Holliday NJ, Johnson DL, Craigen R. Improved rate model of temperature-dependent development by arthropods. Environmental entomology 1995; 24(1) 68-75.

[122] Bruce-Chwatt L. Essential malariology. London, UK: Heinemann medical books; 1991.

[123] Bouma M, Sondorp H, van der Kaay H. Health and climate change. The Lancet 1994; 343 (8892) 302-304.

[124] Roberts DR, Rodriguez MH. The environment, remote sensing, and malaria control. Annals of the New York Academy of Sciences 1994; 15 (740) 396-402.

[125] Obsomer V, Defourny P, Coosemans M. The *Anopheles dirus* complex: spatial distribution and environmental drivers. Malaria Journal 2007; 6(1):26.

[126] Travis P, Bennett S, Haines A, Pang T, Bhutta Z, Hyder AA, et al. Overcoming health-systems constraints to achieve the Millennium Development Goals. The Lancet 2004; 364 (9437) 900-906.

[127] WHO. A global strategy for malaria control. Geneva: World Health Organisation; 1993.

[128] WHO. The Abuja declaration on Roll Back Malaria. Geneva: World Health Organisation; 2000.

[129] Grambsch A, Menne B. Adaptation and adaptive capacity in the public health context. Climate change and human health. Geneva: World Health organisation; 2003. p220-236.

[130] Ceccato P, Connor S. Early Warning Systems. In: Morain S, Budge A. (ed.) Environmental tracking for public health surveillance. International society for photogrammetry and remote sensing (ISPRS) Commission VIII/WG-2; 2012.

[131] Dufrene M, Legendre P. Species assemblages and indicator species: the need for a flexible asymmetrical approach. Ecological Monographs 1997; 1(67)3: 345-66.

[132] Obsomer V, Dufrene M, Defourny P, Coosemans M. *Anopheles* species associations in Southeast Asia: indicator species and environmental influences. Parasites & vectors (submitted).

[133] Diggle P, Thomson M, Christensen O, Rowlingson B, Obsomer V, Gardon J, et al. Spatial modeling and prediction of *Loa loa* risk: decision making under uncertainty. Annals of Tropical Medicine and Parasitology 2007; 101(6) 499-509.

[134] Pineros Garcet J. Quality assessment of environmental simulation scenarios: Scientific, expertise, interpretive and participatory methods based on mathematical, epistemological and socio-anthropological approaches. PhD thesis. Université catholique de Louvain, Louvain-la-Neuve; 2012.

[135] Nordstrand A, Bunikis I, Larsson C, Tsogbe K, Schwan TG, Nilsson M, et al. Tickborne relapsing fever diagnosis obscured by malaria, Togo. Emerging Infectious Diseases 2007; 13(1) 117-23.

Section 4

Pathogen Transmission and Influencing Factors

Chapter 15

Simian Malaria Parasites: Special Emphasis on *Plasmodium knowlesi* and Their *Anopheles* Vectors in Southeast Asia

Indra Vythilingam and Jeffery Hii

Additional information is available at the end of the chapter

http://dx.doi.org/10.5772/54491

1. Introduction

Simian malaria parasites were first reported in Malayan monkeys by Daniels in 1908 [1]. It had been assumed for a long time that transmission of simian malaria to humans would not be possible. However, an accidental infection of scientists in Atlanta, USA by mosquito bites in the laboratory proved that a simian malaria species– *Plasmodium cynomolgi* can be transmitted to humans [2, 3]. In 1965 the first natural infection in human was reported in an American surveyor who was infected in the jungles of Pahang, Malaysia [4]. Fortunately he returned to USA and was detected first as *Plasmodium falciparum* and later revised to *Plasmodium malariae* due to the band form of the parasite. Further examination proved that it was actually *Plasmodium knowlesi* [4].

Plasmodium knowlesi was first found in *Macaca fascicularis* monkeys that were brought to India from Singapore. Drs Knowles and Das Gupta knew that they were dealing with a new malaria parasite but did not provide a binomial nomenclature. It was Sinton and Muligan who formally named the new species as *P. knowlesi* [5] after Dr. Knowles. Studies that were carried out before the first human case was reported unveiled many new simian malaria parasites but no human cases. After the first human case was reported in 1965, blood samples were collected from about 1000 people from surrounding villages in West Malaysia where the case of *P. knowlesi* was found but none were positive for simian malaria [6]. However, a presumptive case was reported from Johore, a southern state in peninsular Malaysia [7].

Mosquito surveys carried out in the area where the first case occurred did not reveal any sporozoite infections in the mosquitoes. However, studies in the coastal areas of Selangor in peninsular Malaysia found *Anopheles hackeri* to be a vector of *P. knowlesi* [8] and this mosquito was attracted only to non-human primates and would not come to bite humans. Thus, at that time it was concluded that simian malaria parasites would not easily affect humans and if it did human malaria cases would occur at very low levels [9]. In 2004 a large focus of knowlesi malaria among humans in Sarawak, Malaysian Borneo was reported [10]. This significant finding stimulated many scientists who were interested in the field of simian malaria in humans and their vectors and hosts. Southeast Asia has now become a focal point for the distribution of *P. knowlesi* in humans. This chapter will describe the simian malaria parasites in non-human primates, the bionomics of vectors involved in transmission, human cases of knowlesi malaria and the challenges in relation to elimination of malaria.

2. Simian malaria parasites and their hosts

In Southeast Asia, there are 13 species of *Plasmodium* affecting non-human primates [11]. Of these *Plasmodium coatneyi, P. cynomolgi, P. fieldi, P. fragile, P. inui, P. knowlesi* and *P. simiovale* are known to occur in macaques and leaf monkeys [12]. However, of the seven species, *P. fragile* has been reported in both India and Sri Lanka while *P. simiovale* is restricted only to Sri Lanka [12]. *Plasmodium eylesi, P. jefferyi, P. youngi* and *P. hylobati* are found in gibbons while *P. pitheci* and *P. silvaticum* are found in orangutans in Borneo. These malaria parasites are found throughout mainland Southeast Asia and associated islands within the Wallace's line [13].

Information is currently available on the non-human primate malaria especially in Malaysia. Thus, so far five species of simian malaria parasites in non-human primates (macaques) have been reported from Malaysia [12, 14]. The simian malaria parasite *P. cynomolgi* is a species that had been experimentally transmitted to humans [3, 15]. *Plasmodium cynomolgi* in monkeys has many of the characteristics seen during infection of humans with *P. vivax* [16]. It was always believed that monkey malaria was specific for monkeys and human malaria was specific for humans. However, in 1960 accidental infections in the laboratory of simian malaria to humans by mosquito bites led to investigative studies to be carried out in Malaysia and this resulted in the description of many new simian malaria parasites [17-20].

Simian malaria parasites have been detected in three main species of non-human primates. They are *Macaca fascicularis, Macaca nemestrina* and *Presbytis melalophos* [19, 20]. In the 1960's studies on malaria parasites of *M. nemestrina* revealed that this non-human primate can harbour the following simian malaria species: *P. cynomolgi, P. inui, P. knowlesi* and *P. fieldi* [19] Of these *P. fieldi* was a new species found in this macaque [17]. Currently, *P. fieldi* has been found as mixed infection in longtailed macaques but less frequently compared to the other simian malaria parasites [14]. Only 4% of the macaques had *P.fieldi* mono-infection in a study in Sarawak, Malaysian Borneo [14]. In Malaysian Borneo the predominant species found in the longtailed macaques was *P. inui* (82%) followed by *P. knowlesi* (78%), *P. coatneyi* (66%) and *P. cynomolgi* (56%) [14]. However, in Singapore *P. knowlesi* was the predominant species among long-tailed macaques (68.2%), followed by *P. cynomolgi* (66.6%), *P. fieldi* (16.7 %), *P. coatneyi* (3%) and *P. inui* (1.5%) [21]. In Selangor, out of the 107 samples of macaque blood tested for malaria, 64.5% were positive for *Plasmodium* of which 23.3 % were positive for *P. knowlesi* [22].

Plasmodium coatneyi was successfully established when sporozoites from *An. hacker* collected from Rantau Panjang Selangor, were inoculated into an uninfected rhesus monkey. The monkey exhibited infection after a prepatent period of 14 days. The young trophozoites were not easily distinguishable from those of *P. falciparum* and demonstrated a tertian cycle thus leading to a new species [23]. This is the first instance of finding a new species of malaria in the vector before it was known from the primate host. Subsequently *P. coatneyi* was also isolated from *M. fascicularis* from the same area and also from the Philippines [24].

The pig-tailed macaque – *Macaca nemestrina* occurs in various sub-species from easternmost India and Bangladesh, through Myanmar and Thailand, Malaysia, Sumatra and Kalimantan [19]. This animal is trained to harvest coconuts from tall trees and is kept as a pet by their owners. They coexist with long-tailed macaques-*M. fascicularis* but are ecologically less diverse in their choice of habitats [19].They are also less commonly seen compared to *M. fascicularis*. The parasites found in the pig-tailed macaques were *P. cynomolgi, P. inui, P. knowlesi, P. fieldi* and Hepatocystis [19].

3. History of natural infection of *P. knowlesi* in human host

Scientists have always been curious as to the possibility of humans being infected with non-human primate malaria. This interest was intensified when two scientists working in the Memphis laboratory were infected with *P. cynomolgi*. They were conducting infection studies in the laboratory and they were dissecting a large number of mosquitoes heavily infected with malaria parasites two weeks prior to coming down with the illness [2]. Following these infections, scientists decided to survey areas in peninsular Malaysia and search for natural transmission of simian malaria in humans. There were also attempts by scientists to probe into the natural transmission of monkey malaria to humans in the northernmost state of peninsular Malaysia [25]. In the first survey they did not come across any human cases but described new species of monkey malaria parasites in macaques [6].

In 1965, an American surveyor working in Bukit Kertau in Pahang, Malaysia came down with malaria. Fortunately he returned to USA where he was diagnosed as *P. knowlesi* [4]. This was the first natural infection reported in humans. The surveyor was apparently working in the forested area at night. American scientists along with the scientists from the Institute for Medical Research carried out extensive surveys in that area where the surveyor was infected. Blood from 1117 persons from 17 villages were examined for malaria parasites by microscopy using Giemsa stained slides. Blood was also inoculated into rhesus monkeys to determine if there were natural infections of simian malaria in humans. Of these only 28 had malaria infection, 11 were *P. falciparum*, 13 *P.vivax* and four were not identifiable. None of the rhesus monkeys developed malaria parasites [6]. Thus it was concluded that simian malaria would not easily infect humans. In 1970's a presumptive case of *P. knowlesi* was reported from Johore, peninsular Malaysia [7].

4. Cases of knowlesi malaria in Southeast Asia

In 2004, a large focus of human knowlesi malaria cases were reported from Sarawak, Malaysian Borneo [10]. In that study it was found that 58% of the patients, admitted at the Sarawak hospital, were found to be infected with knowlesi malaria using molecular tools. These were misidentified by microscopy as *P. malariae*. Early trophozoites of *P. knowlesi* in the erythrocyte resemble that of *P. falciparum* such as double chromatin dots, multiple-infected erythrocytes and appliqué forms [26]. Besides the late and mature trophozoites, schizonts and gametocytes of *P. knowlesi* in human infections were generally indistinguishable from those of *P. malariae*. Moreover, 'band form' trophozoites, which are a characteristic feature for *P. malariae* parasites [27, 28] were observed in more than half of the blood films examined by Lee *et al* [26]. 'Sinton and Mulligan's stippling' in erythrocytes infected with *P. knowlesi* was noted previously in infections in rhesus monkeys [27] and humans [7]. However, in present knowlesi cases only faint stippling was evident in some of the infected erythrocytes with mature trophozoite and schizont stages [10, 26]. Thus, human infections with *P. knowlesi* have been mistaken for *P. falciparum* malaria when the infecting parasites were predominantly at the early trophozoite or ring form developmental stage and as *P. malariae* when in the late trophozoite or band form. Figure 1 shows the different stages of development of *P. knowlesi*.

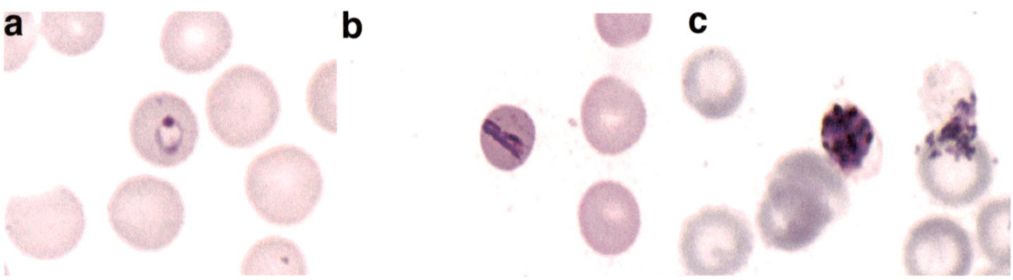

Figure 1. Giemsa stained thin blood film of *P. knowlesi* as seen with 100 x objective. a). trophozoite b) band form of trophozoite, c) schizont

After the publication in 2004 [10], more cases were reported in Malaysia [29-32] and also from other countries in Southeast Asia with the exception of Lao PDR. To date cases have been reported from Thailand [33-35], Philippines [36],Vietnam [37], Indonesia [38], Cambodia [39], Myanmar [40] and Singapore [41]. Malaysia has reported the highest number of cases in the region. *Plasmodium knowlesi* is now considered as the fifth malaria parasite affecting humans [42] and is detected by molecular methods. However, some still believe that it is a simian malaria since human to human transmission has not been proven [13].

A study has shown that *M. fascicularis* experimentally infected with *P. knowlesi* erythrocytic parasites from humans developed pre patent infection on day seven and demonstrated diurnal sub-periodic pattern [43]. It is the only primate malaria with a 24-hour erythrocytic cycle [44] while *P. falciparum* has a 48 hour cycle and *P. malariae* a 72 hour cycle.

Knowlesi malaria has shown to be life threatening and mortality has been reported [29, 31]. From December 2007 to November 2009 six (27%) out of 22 patients with severe knowlesi malaria died in Sabah [31]. Cases of knowlesi malaria are also occurring in areas where human malaria cases have been reduced or in malaria free areas [45]. People can contract malaria either outside their houses in rural settings, in farms where they work or in the forest while hunting or working.

5. Knowlesi malaria associated with travellers to Southeast Asia

Naturally acquired cases of *P. knowlesi* have been reported from travellers visiting this region. A New Zealand pilot working in Sabah and Sarawak north of Bintulu Malaysian Borneo was diagnosed as *P. knowlesi* in New Zealand when he fell ill. The sequence of the parasite had a 100% homology to the Vietnam strain [46]. A lady born in the Philippines and residing in USA for more than 25 years came down with knowlesi malaria after visiting Palawan in the Philippines where she stayed in a log cabin close to the forest edge. She fell ill and on her return to USA was diagnosed as *P. knowlesi* [47]. A Finish traveller spent about 5 days in the jungle on the north-western coast of peninsular Malaysia and fell ill after he returned to Finland. He was diagnosed with *P. knowlesi* parasitaemia by PCR and sequencing showed 100% homology with *P. knowlesi* sequence from Malaysian Borneo and a *Macaca mullata* from Colombia [48]. A Swede who travelled to the Bario Highlands in Malaysian Borneo came down ill on his return to Sweden and was diagnosed as suffering from knowlesi malaria [49]. A Spanish traveller who spent six months travelling around Southeast Asia – in forested areas was diagnosed as knowlesi malaria when he returned to Spain [50]. A French tourist returning from Thailand was diagnosed as *P. knowlesi* [51]. This shows that the knowlesi malaria is currently a serious public health problem and not just single occasional episodes.

6. Bionomics of simian malaria vectors and trapping techniques

6.1. Distribution

The distribution of *P. knowlesi* in the natural monkey hosts and transmission to humans are restricted to mosquito vectors of the *Anopheles* Leucosphyrus Group confined to Southeast Asia [52]. It is currently recognized that under natural forest conditions, most if not all members of the Leucosphyrus Group apparently feed primarily on monkeys in the canopy, transmitting various plasmodia [53]. In Harbach's review [54], the Leucosphyrus Group in the Neomyzomyia Series contains 20 named species [55, 56], one unnamed species (aff. *takasagoensis*) and two geographical forms (Con Son form from island off South Vietnam and Negros form from Negros island in Philippines) [55] divided between the Hackeri, Leucosphyrus and Riparis Subgroups. According to Manguin *et al.* [57] and Sallum *et al.* [56], the Leucosphyrus Subgroup consists of the Dirus and Leucosphyrus complexes, which includes seven and five sibling species, respectively. Species belonging to the Leucosphyrus complex are also important vectors of human malaria and lymphatic filariasis and are distributed in the South and Southeast Asia regions. The current vectorial status and geographical distribution of the Leucosphyrus Group are listed in Table 1 and Figure 2.

Complex	Vector species	Species of *Plasmodium*	Vertebrate hosts	Distribution
Leucosphyrus	*An. leucosphyrus Donitz (hv)*[1]	*Pf, Pv, Pm*[2]	Human	Indonesia, Sumatra
	An. latens Sallum & Peyton (hv, sv, fv)	Pf, Pv, Pm *P. inui* [78] *P. knowlesi, P. inui, P. coatneyi, P. fieldi*[79]	Human *M. fascicularis, M. nemestrina* *P. melalophos* [19-22]	Indonesia, East Malaysia, West Malaysia, Thailand Sarawak: East Malaysia: Sarawak[45,75] West Malaysia [56]
	An. introlatus Colless (sv)	*P. cynomolgi, P. fieldi* [78]	*M. fascicularis, M. nemestrina* *P. melalophos* [19-22]	Indonesia West Malaysia, Thailand [56]
	An. balabacensis Colless (hv, sv, fv)	*P. knowlesi* [45]; possibly *P. coatneyi* & *P. inui*[73]	*M. fascicularis* [73]	Brunei, Indonesia, East Malaysia, Philippines [56]
	An. baisasi Colless	Information inadequate		Luzon, Philippines
Dirus	*An. dirus* Peyton & Harrison (hv, sv fv)	*P. knowlesi* [76-77]	Human *M. fascicularis*, [35]	Cambodia, China, Vietnam, Laos, Thailand
	An. cracens Sallum & Peyton (hv, sv, fv)	Probable vector of human malaria [56] *P. knowlesi* [30,72] *P. cynomolgi, P. inui* [80]	*M. fascicularis* [30]	Indonesia, West Malaysia, Thailand
	An. baimaii Sallum & Peyton (hv, fv)	Pf, Pv Pm	Human	Bangladesh, India, Thailand, Myanmar, China
Hackeri	*An. mirans* Sallum & Peyton (sv)	*P. cynomolgi, P. inui* [56] *P. inui shortii; P. fragile* [56]		India, Sri Lanka
	An. hackeri Edwards (sv)	*P. cynomolgi, P. inui, P. fieldi, P. coatneyi, P. knowlesi* [52]	*M. fascicularis*	East and West Malaysia, Philippines, Thailand
	An. pujutensis Colless (sv)?	Probable vector of simian malaria parasites [52]		Indonesia, East and West Malaysia, Thailand

[1] hv,sv and fv indicate human malarial, simian malarial and human lymphatic filarial vectors; sv? Vectorial status awaiting confirmation

Table 1. Simian malaria parasites of Southeast Asia: their Leucosphyrus Group natural vectors, hosts and geographical distribution (modified from Sallum et al [56]

http://dx.doi.org/10.5772/54491

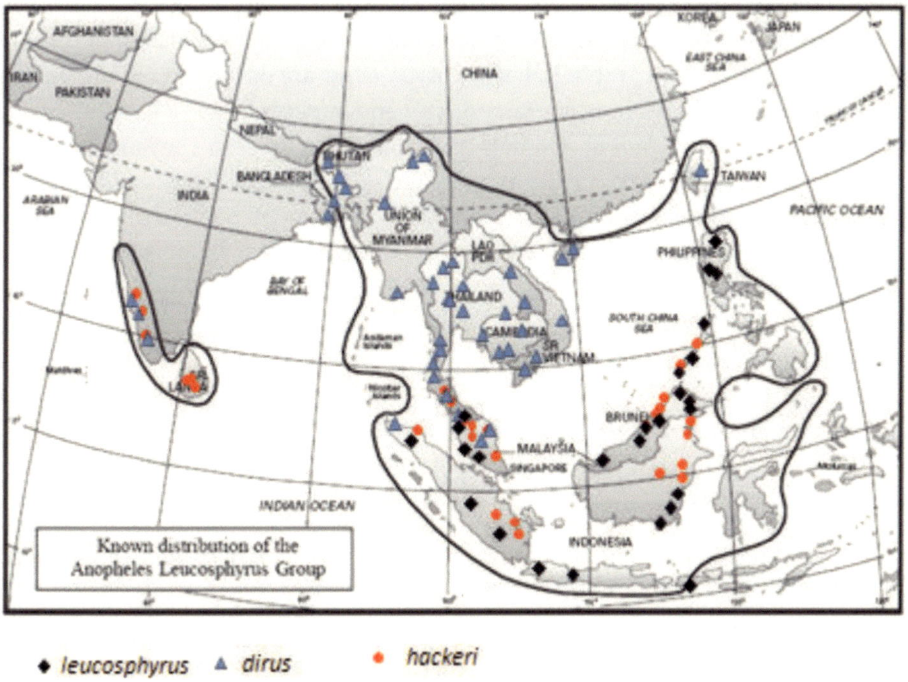

Figure 2. Known limit of the distribution of the *An. leucosphyrus* Group (*An. hackeri* Subgroup, *An, dirus* complex and *An. leucosphyrus* complex) of mosquitoes in South and Southeast Asia adopted from Sallum et al 2005. Only the distribution of those species mentioned in Table 1 are shown

As a member of the Leucosphyrus complex, *An. latens* is widely distributed in Borneo (Kalimantan, Sarawak, Sabah) together with *An. balabacensis* in the forested areas of eastern Borneo (Figure 2). *Anopheles latens* and *An. introlatus* are sympatric with members of the closely related Dirus complex in the Malay Peninsula, including southern Thailand [58, 59] (Figure 2).

The Dirus complex is well known because its species are widespread in forest and forest foothills throughout the Oriental Region from southwestern India eastwards and from 30° north parallel to the Malaysian peninsula [60-62] (Figure2), whereas the Leucosphyrus complex has been investigated to a much lesser degree in Malaysia Borneo and Kalimantan Borneo. *Anopheles cracens* (Dirus complex) was the predominant mosquito species in a recent study and was never reported previously from Pahang, Malaysia [30]. Earlier reports indicate that *An. cracens* was found in Perlis (Northern most state of Peninsular, Malaysia) and in Terengganu (east Coast State of Peninsular Malaysia [56]. Its geographic distribution within peninsular Malaysia is unknown [63].

6.2. Larval biology

Table 2 shows a summary of *Anopheles* larval habitat characteristics adapted from Sinka et al [64]. As forest-dwelling species, the immature stages share an affinity for humid, shaded environments where they make use of transient or temporary larval habitats such as pools and puddles. Like other members of the Leucosphyrus complex, larval habitats of *An. lateens* and *An. balabacensis* are mostly shaded temporary pools and natural containers of clear or turbid water on the ground in forest areas (Table 2). Larvae of *An. latens* are usually found in clear seepage pools in forest swamps in peninsular Malaysia [65] and in pools beside a forest stream and in swampy patches in hilly areas [66]. Habitats occupied by *An. latens* in Thailand include stump ground holes, sand pools, stream margins, seepage-springs, wheel tracks and elephant foot prints [53, 59]. Typical breeding places of *An. balabacensis* are small pools in clay soil containing fairly clean seepage or rainwater, still or slow moving, and under some shade, with the upper altitudinal limit of 4000 ft in Borneo (1220 meters) [66]. Other adventitious and rare breeding sites include swamp edges or in rock pools, bamboo stumps, split bamboos, tins and other artificial containers [66] and wells in Sandakan, Sabah (unpublished report by Dr David Muir, WHO consultant). In inland forest *An. hackeri* was found breeding in split bamboo while in the coastal area it was found breeding in the cavities of leaf bases of nipah palm [8].

Species	Light intensity	Turbidity	Water movement	Small natural water collections	Small man-made water collections
An. latens & leucosphyrus	Heliophobic	Clear, turbid, fresh water Muddy pool (W Malaysia [56])	Still or stagnant	Small streams, seepage streams, pools	Wheel ruts, hoof prints
An. balabacensis	Typical heliophobic	Fresh water	Still or stagnant	Pools; dips in the ground	Wheel ruts, hoof prints
An. dirus	Heliophobic	Clear, turbid, fresh water	Still or stagnant	Small streams, pools, wells, dips in the ground	Borrow pits, wheel ruts, hoof prints
An. hackeri	Heliophobic	Clean non saline water, but found in water containing up to 4% sea-water	Still or stagnant	In split bamboo and cavities at the leaf base of nipa palm	In Thailand, in elephant footprints [56]

Table 2. Larval habitat characteristics of monkey malaria vectors (adapted from Sinka et al [64]) including individual studies reported in the literature.

6.3. Biological characteristics

The important biological charactersitics of the known vectors of simian malaria are shown in Table 3 which has been modified from Meek [67]. Of the known vectors, *An. hackeri* is known to bite only monkeys and rarely comes to bite humans [8]. Although *An. latens* is a vector of human malaria in East Malaysia [68-70], the current studies have shown that the species is more attracted to monkeys compared to humans [71], whilst *An. cracens* is attracted to both monkeys and humans [72]. In Palawan Island, Philippines, *An. balabacensis* was more attracted to a monkey bait trap compared to carabao (water buffalo) and human bait traps [73, 74]. It was also found positive for oocysts and sporozoites but could not be confirmed if it was of monkey origin [73]. However, infection studies carried out by the same authors proved that *An. balabacensis* was the vector of simian malaria in Palawan [73]. So far only the *An.* Leucosphyrus Group (*An. latens, An. cracens, An. balabacensis, An. hackeri* and *An. dirus*) of mosquitoes have been found positive for simian malaria parasites in nature [30, 45, 71, 72, 75-80]. However, *An. dirus* is also a main vector of both human malaria, with sporozoite rates as high as 14% in Myanmar and as low as 2.5% in Lao PDR [61, 81], and *Wuchereria bancrofti* [82].

Species	Peak biting time	Host preference or MBT:HBT	Survivorship	Sporozoite rate/EIR
An. latens	Sarawak: Around midnight in forested areas and soon after dusk in village settlements [68] Forest: 1900-2000 h; farm: 0100-0200 h [69] Monkey biting rate at 6, 3 m above ground and at ground: 6.8:3.2:1.0. HBR highest at forest fringe (6.74%), within the forest (1.85%) and at long house (0.28%) [71]	Similar host preference 1.0 : 1.3 [71]	Sarawak: parous rate 65.8% (farm), 53.7% (forest), 65.8% (longhouse) [71] VC: 2.86 (farm), 0.60 (forest), 0.85 (longhouse) [71]	Sarawak: 1.18% (pooled from forest fringe, forest & longhouse) , 0.7% (farm), 1.4% (forest), all confirmed Pk by PCR; EIR 11.98 (farm), 14.1 (forest) [71]
An. balabacensis	Palawan: In and out; 20.00-03.00 h [73] Sabah: 22:00-02:00 h [85- 86];after midnight [87] Out (76%): 19:00-20:00 h, in(24%): 22:00-23:00 h;[83] Lombok: 19:00-21:00h) [84]	Attracted to humans, monkey & water buffalo; more frequently caught in monkey traps [74]	Sabah: highest in Nov, lowest in July [83]	Kalimantan: 1.3% [88] Palawan: 12.5% sporozoite rate; 29% attracted to monkeys were positive for oocysts [74]
An. dirus	Late or early biting, usually around 22:00 h [60-62]	Highly anthropophilic,	Higher parous rate (76%) & life expectancy during dry season	Human sporozoite rates vary with season and location: from

Species	Peak biting time	Host preference or MBT:HBT	Survivorship	Sporozoite rate/EIR
	9 of 13 *Plasmodium* positive bites occur before 21:00 h (Vietnam) [91]	exophagic as well as endophagic and exophilic [61-62]	compared to wet season (62.4%) in Lao [81]	7.8% in Assam (India) to 14% in Myanmar [61] and 2.5% in Laos [81] 43% of 72 salivary glands were PCR-positive for Pk CSP and Pk 18s rRNA. Mixed infections of Pk with Pv and Pf were common in Vietnam [77]
An. cracens	Thailand: 1900-2100 h [60] West Malaysia: 2000-2100 h; 74% biting before 2100 h; predominantly exophagic (1.11 bites/ man-night) in both forest (1.24 bites/man-night) and fruit orchard (4.15 bites/man-night); 60% biting at ground level to 3 m high before 00:00 h; more biting at canopy level (6 m) compared to earlier collections at the same level [72].	West Malaysia: 1: 2.6 [7.2]	West Malaysia: parous rate 65.7% (fruit orchard), 71.5% (forest) VC: 2.46 (fruit orchard), 1.09 (forest) [72]	West Malaysia: 0.60% (fruit orchard), 2.9% (forest) EIR: 0.08 [72]
An. hackeri	Not known since most bite monkeys and rarely found in human bait traps [78]	Most attracted to monkeys at canopy level in mangrove forest does not come to bite humans [78]	No data available	In coastal area of Rantau Panjang West Malaysia 0.7% [78]

[1]VC - vectorial capacity; EIR - entomological inoculation rate; PCR - polymerase chain reaction; HBR - human biting rate; MBT- Monkey bait trap; HBT- human bait trap; CSP - circumsporozoite

Table 3. Biological variations among adults of simian malaria vectors in Southeast Asia (modified from Meek 1995 [67].

http://dx.doi.org/10.5772/54491

The peak biting times of *An. balabacensis* vary from place to place as shown in Table 3. It seems to bite as early as 19:00 h in recent years compared to being late night biters in the previous decades [83-89]. *An. dirus s.s.* tends to bite between 20:00 and 23:00 h [53, 56, 60] and and there is significant biological variability within the Dirus complex, depending on the local circumstances [90]. In Vietnam, sporozoite positive bites from *An. dirus* occur before 21:00 h [91] and co-infections of *P. knowlesi, P. falciparum* and *P. vivax* [76, 77] in mosquitoes are indicative of simultaneous transmission. *Plasmodium knowlesi*-sporozoite infective *An. latens* and *An. cracens* were detected from human landing and monkey bait collections in Sarawak and Pahang, Malaysia, respectively [71, 72] suggesting that *P. knowlesi* is being transmitted to both humans and macaques by these two vector species. Generally the parous rates of the Leucosphyrus Group of mosquitoes where relatively high as shown in Table 3. Overall parous rate of *An. latens* was 59% and those caught in the forest was significantly lower than those caught at the farm or long house (where native people of Sarawak live) [71], while for *An. cracens* the parous rate in the forest was higher than in the farm (Table 3), and on average was above 60% [72]. Heterogeneity in biting rates and parous rates indicates that the vectorial capacities are relatively higher in farms or orchards compared to forests (Table 3), and has significant implications for vector control. Understanding the importance of natural heterogenity in *P. knowlesi* transmission is necessary to elucidate the key variation undermining existing control efforts and to target the vector species for focused interventions [92].

6.4. Laboratory susceptibility studies

In laboratory experiments with *P. knowlesi, An. balabacensis* was found to be a successful vector [93]. However, *An. maculatus* only developed few oocysts and sporozoite infection in salivary glands was of low intensity. Laboratory feeding experiments, *An. maculatus* was susceptible to *P. inui* and was able to transmit the parasite to the non-human primate host after a prepatent period of 11 days [94]. In a series of experiments infectivity conducted in the Institute for Medical Research, with the Gombak strain of *P. cynomolgi,* the following mosquitoes were found with salivary gland infections: *An. maculatus, An. kochi, An. sundaicus* (=*An. epiroticus*), *An. vagus* and *An. introlatus* [16]. However, in field situation it was observed that *An. maculatus* was not attracted to macaques, with only three female mosquitoes entering the monkey bait trap [72]. While *An. kochi* was the second predominant mosquito entering monkey baited trap, none were positive for oocyst or sporozoites [72]. Thus, although species other than the Leucosphyrus Group were able to develop the simian malaria parasites to sporozoites, none were incriminated in nature except the Leucosphyrus Group.

6.5. Trapping techniques

Various trapping methods were tested for the collection of *Anopheles* mosquitoes attracted to non-human primates. Earlier observations indicated that these mosquitoes prefer to feed well above ground level and especially about 6-8 m above ground level. Thus, platforms were built among foliage in the forest or plantations to house the non-human primates for mosquito collections. The following traps that were tested [95] are described hereunder.

Net Traps

This is similar to the human–bait-net trap introduced by Gater [96]. This method provided the best results when tested [95]. The platforms were constructed among the branches of trees to a height of 6 meters. Special metal cages measuring 90 cm x 90 cm x 90 cm and covered by wire mesh were used to house the monkeys on the platform measuring 300 cm X 200 cm. The meshed cages provided a physical barrier to prevent the monkeys from grabbing the collectors and also to prevent the entry of snakes. It is ideal to have two monkeys sharing a cage to increase vector attraction. A mosquito net measuring 190 cm x 180 cm x 150 cm with an opening of about 40 cm lifted on either ends was used to cover the cages with monkeys on each platform. The traps were operated from 18:00 to 06:00 hours and were searched at regular intervals [71, 72]. A collector, upon entering the net, closed the openings and collected all resting mosquitoes with the use of aspirators. Mosquitoes in the aspirator were then transferred to paper cups and were brought to the laboratory for identification and dissection. Platforms were built at various heights, ground level, 3 and 6 meters above ground. Figure 3 shows two different platforms in operation.

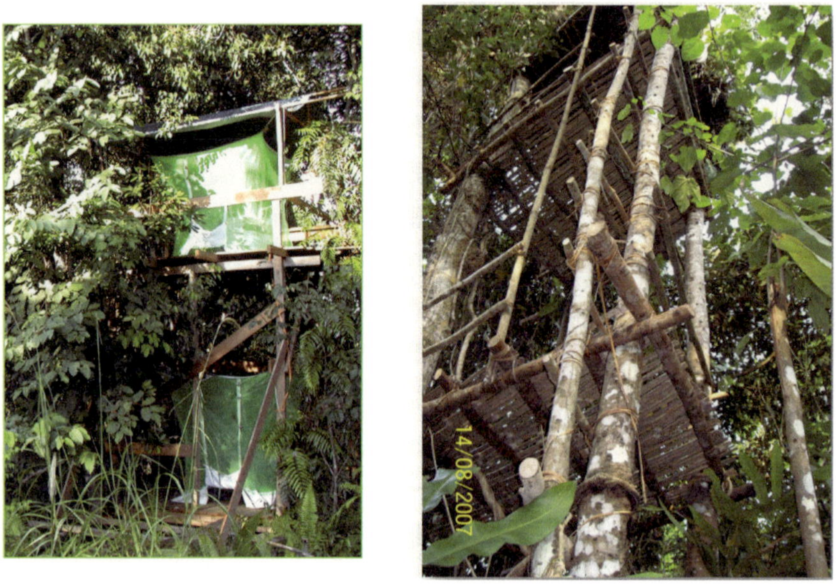

Figure 3. Monkey Baited Net Traps at different levels on platform.

The other traps used were Shannon net trap, drum funnel-trap, Lumsden suction trap and light traps. Detailed descriptions can be found in Wharton [95]. Of all the traps tested, it was found that the monkey- baited traps were superior compared to other types of traps. Although it is a difficult task to collect mosquitoes from the platforms at regular intervals, it is no doubt important to study the behaviour of the mosquitoes. Studies by Wharton [95] demonstrated that 83% of the *An. hackeri* were collected in catches made before midnight, compared to only 62% and 65.8% of *An. latens* and *An. cracens* caught before midnight respectively [71, 72]. Thus, it seems that all night collection is still important despite logistical difficulties, costliness, tediousness and human fatigue.

7. Implications for control

Currently insecticide treated bednets (ITN) and indoor residual spraying (IRS) are the two most important tools for the control of malaria vectors. Scaling up ITN, IRS, artemisinin-based combination therapies and intermittent preventive treatment for infants and pregnant women have contributed to the reported reductions in malaria on a global scale [97]. As part of the Global Malaria Action Plan, the RBM Partnership and World Health Organization has recommended "malaria eradication worldwide by reducing the global incidence to zero through progressive malaria elimination in countries" [98]. However, if human malaria could be eliminated, forests in Southeast Asia provide favourable environments for zoonotic transmission of *P. knowlesi* thus, thwarting efforts to eliminate malaria.

The vectors of *P. knowlesi* malaria have been incriminated only from certain districts or locations in Malaysia [71, 72, 75]. Given that the vectors of monkey malaria show anthropophagic, exophagic and exophilic tendencies, it is obvious that the existing front-line vector control tools (IRS, ITN) will not be sufficient to reduce vector density and break the transmission cycle of *P. knowlesi* in the most intensively endemic parts of Southeast Asia. Innovative interventions are needed to control simio-anthropophagic and acrodendrophilic vectors that do not rest and feed indoors. There are two major problems that need to be addressed before considering malaria elimination. It is known that *P. knowlesi* can be life threatening [99] and mortality due to it is increasing [31, 100]. Thus it is important to determine the vectors throughout the country; study the behavior and ecology of the species of mosquitoes and apply the most effective strategy(ies) for control of these vector. To achieve these outcomes, several key areas for strategic investment relevant for malaria elimination have been proposed [101]. Second, there will always be a problem of human population movement (HPM) and thus people moving into the jungle may introduce the parasite which could give rise to new infections if suitable vectors are present and readily establish local transmission. HPM is common among migrants in the Greater Mekong Subregion [102] and in Southeast Asia [103].

In Vietnam, forest malaria caused by *An. dirus* was controlled because workers going into the forest used long lasting insecticide hammocks (LLIH) [104]. The use of LLIH can be encouraged in ecotourism areas where people stay overnight in the community managed guest houses or camps in the forest. However, other types of personal protection methods need to be evaluated for forest workers. A study has demonstrated that military personnel who used permethrin treated uniforms were protected against mosquito bites, thereby reducing malaria transmission [105].

The use of repellents as personal protection measures have been advocated for malaria control. However, this needs to be evaluated in forest settings and large scale implementation will be a public health challenge. Among US Military troops, malaria cases have been reported due to non-compliance of personal protective measures and failure of chemoprophylaxis [106].

Currently in Malaysia people are getting infected when they visit plantations or forests for work or recreational activities as some important vectors do not enter houses [72].

8. Challenges

There is no reason to doubt the possibility and biological capacity of other simian malaria species to infect humans [13, 107]. *An. latens* can develop all the five species of simian malaria [79] and has a biting preference for both humans and macaques, the possibility of humans being infected with *P. cynomologi* or *P. inui* needs to be addressed. As stated by Baird [108], in areas where macaques and vectors are in close proximity to humans and when malaria occurs other species should also be considered and not just the human malarias and *P. knowlesi.*

Currently only three species of mosquitoes have been incriminated as simian malaria vectors in Malaysia (*An. balabacensis, An. cracens* and *An. latens*) [45, 71, 72, 75] and one in Vietnam (*An. dirus*) [76, 77]. However, it is beyond doubt that there would be several more species involved that would feed on both humans and monkeys and establish natural transmission. Before the inception of the malaria eradication program there were many more *Anopheles* species that were vectors [109], but some species were successfully brought down to very low levels due to their endophilic/endophagic behaviours and susceptibility to residual insecticides. Thus the aggressive national control programme has resulted controlling in only three to four important vectors occurring in Malaysia (*An. balabacensis, An. flavirostris, An. latens, An. maculatus*), [110-113].

In Thailand, the main vectors for human malaria are *An. dirus, An. minimus* and *An. maculatus,* mosquitoes [114]. Although *An. dirus* mosquitoes which belong to the Leucosphyrus Group and have been identified as potential vectors for *P. knowlesi* in Vietnam [76, 77], its distribution and abundance have significantly decreased in all major malaria-endemic areas of Thailand during the past decade [34]. Human cases of *P. knowlesi* have been reported from Thailand at a low prevalence (0.57% in 2006-2007), however the vector remains unknown [34].

According to Obsomer et al [61] the mean temperature below 20° C seems to limit the northern distribution of the Dirus complex to just beyond the border of India with Nepal and Bhutan. Rainfall is probably the limiting factor to the west with annual rainfall per year under 800 mm. Thus the lack of information on the distribution and occurrence of *P. knowlesi* cases in large non-forested areas of Thailand, southern Vietnam and central India is probably linked with the lack of suitable habitats [61]. The absence of the complex (besides the newly described species aff. *takasagoensis*) in north of Vietnam is puzzling as this area is still forested and members of the complex occur at the same latitude in neighbouring countries. Laos PDR is the only country in the Greater Mekong Subregion that has not reported the occurrence of *P. knowlesi* malaria. This may be due to the fact that so far investigations have not been carried out for *P. knowlesi.*

Thus it is timely to determine all the vectors of simian malaria throughout the Southeast Asian region. Although old records stating the distribution of the various *Anopheles* species are available, it may not depict the current situation since landscape ecology and vegetation cover have significantly changed over time. The distribution of vectors, in relation to forest areas and human settlements using modern technology such as the GPS, GIS and the behavioral ecology of the vectors, needs to be addressed. These and other key areas identified for specific strategic investment in ecological research [101] should assist to define the target product profiles of completely new control technologies and delivery systems.

9. Conclusion

Since many malaria control programmes in Southeast Asia are moving towards elimination of malaria [115], it is important to determine the prevalence of knowlesi malaria in these countries. In the Greater Mekong Subregion including Bangladesh and India *An. dirus* is one of the primary vector of human malaria and thus it is important to determine if other vectors are involved in knowlesi transmission. Among habitats shared by macaques and vector mosquitoes, it is possible for humans who encroach these areas to be infected. Thus, important issues that need to be determined are as follows: Are other simian malaria parasites affecting humans? Is human to human transmission occurring? What are the other vectors transmitting simian malaria to humans (apart from *An. cracens*, *An. latens*, *An.dirus* and *An. balabacensis*) in the region and what roles do they play in host switching? What innovative technologies or biting prevention are appropriate for the control of these vectors? Thus, knowlesi malaria remains a great challenge for the future.

Acknowledgements

The authors thank Pollie Rueda for his constructive comments. The first author was supported by a grant from University of Malaya UM.C/625/1/HIR/099.J-20011-73822

Author details

Indra Vythilingam[1,3*] and Jeffery Hii[2,3]

*Address all correspondence to: indra.vythilingam@gmail.com

1 Parasitology Department, Faculty of Medicine, University of Malaya, Kuala Lumpur, Malaysia

2 Taman Damai, Jalan Fung Yei Ting, Kota Kinabalu, Sabah, Malaysia

3 Formerly WHO Malaria Scientist, World Health Organization, Philippines

References

[1] Daniels CW. Animal parasites in man and some of the lower animals in Malaya. Studies Instite for Medical Research FMS 1908;3:1-13.

[2] Coatney GR. Simian malaria: Its importance to world wide eradication of malaria. Journal of American Medical Association 1963;184:876-7.

[3] Contacos PG, Elder HA, Coatney GR. Man to man transfer of two strains of *Plasmodium cynomolgi* by mosquito bites. American Journal of Tropical Medicine and Hygiene 1962;11:186-93.

[4] Chin W, Contacos PG, Coatney GR, Kimball HR. A naturally acquired quotidian-type malaria in man transferable to monkeys. Science 1965;149:865.

[5] Sinton JA MH. A critical review of the literature relating to the identification of the malaria parasites recorded from monkeys of the families Cercopithecidae and Colobidae. Rec Malaria Surv India 1932-1933;III:357–443.

[6] Warren MW, Cheong WH, Fredericks HK, Coatney GR. Cycles of jungle malaria in West Malaysia. American Journal of Tropical Medicine and Hygiene 1970;19:383.

[7] Fong YL, Cadigan FC, Coatney GR. A presumptive case of naturally occurring *Plasmodium knowlesi* malaria in man in Malaysia. Transactions of Royal Society of Tropical Medicine and Hygiene 1971;65:839.

[8] Wharton RH, Eyles DE. *Anopheles hackeri*, a vector of *Plasmodium knowlesi* in Malaya. Science 1961;134:279.

[9] Chin W, Contacos PG, Collins WE, Jeter MH, Alpert E. Experimental mosquito-transmission of *Plasmodium knowlesi* to man and monkey. American Journal of Tropical Medicine and Hygiene 1968;17:355-8.

[10] Singh B, Sung LK, Matusop A, Radhakrishnan A, Shamsul SSG, Cox-Singh J, et al. A large focus of naturally acquired *Plasmodium knowlesi* infections in human beings. Lancet 2004;363:1017-24.

[11] Collins WE. Major animal models in malaria research: Simian. In: Wernsdofer WH and McGregor editors. Malaria: Principles and Practice of Malariology. Edinburgh: Churchill Livingstone; 1988. p. 1473-501.

[12] Fodden J. Malaria in Macaques. International Journal of Primatology 1994;15:573-96.

[13] Galinski MR, Barnwell JW. Monkey malaria kills four humans. Trends in Parasitology 2009;25:200-4.

[14] Lee KS, Divis PCS, Zakaria SK, Matusop A, Julin RA, Conway DJ, et al. *Plasmodium knowlesi:* reservoir hosts and tracking the emergence in humans and macaques. PLoS Pathogens 2011;7:e1002015.

[15] Coatney GR, Elder HA, Contacos PG, Getz ME, Greenland R, Rossan RN, et al. Transmission of the M strain of *Plasmodium cynomolgi* to man. The American Journal of Tropical Medicine and Hygiene 1961;10:673-8.

[16] Collins WE, Warren MW, Sullivan JAS, Galland GG, Nace D, Williams A, et al. Studies on two strains of *Plasmodium cynomolgi* in New World and Old World monkeys and mosquitoes. Journal of Parasitology 2005;91:280-3.

[17] Eyles DE, Laing ABG, Fong YL. *Plasmodium fieldi* sp nov, a new species of malaria parasite from the pig-tailed macaque in Malaya. Annals of Tropical Medicine and Parasitology 1962;56:242-7.

[18] Eyles DE. The species of simian malaria: Taxonomy, morphology, life cycle, and geographical distribution of the monkey species. Journal of Parasitology 1963:866-87.

[19] Eyles DE, Laing ABG, Dobrovolny CG. The malaria parasites of the pig-tailed macaque, *Macaca nemestrina* (Linnaeus). Indian Journal of Malariology 1962;16:285-98.

[20] Eyles DE, Laing ABG, Warren M, Sandosham AA. Malaria parasites of the Malayan leaf monkeys of the genus *Presbytis*. Medical Journal of Malay 1962;17:85-6.

[21] Li M. Identification and molecular characterization of simian malaria parasites in wild monkeys of Singapore. Singapore: National University of Singapore; 2011.

[22] Ho G, Lee C, Abie M, Zainuddin Z, Japnin J, Topani R, et al. Prevalance of *Plasmodium* in the Long-tailored Macaque (*Macaca fasicularis*) from Selangor, Malaysia. Proceedings 13th Association of Institutions for Tropical Veterinary Medicine (AITVM) Conference 2010:49.

[23] Eyles DE, Fong, Y.l.,Warren, Mc,W., Guinn,E.,Sabdosham,AA.,Wharton,R.H. *Plasmodium coatneyi,* a new species of primate malaria from Malaya. American Journal of Tropical Medicine and Hygiene 1962;11:597-604.

[24] Eyles DE, Dunn F, Warren McW, Guinn E. *Plasmodium coatneyi* from the Philippines. Journal of Parasitology 1963;49:1038.

[25] Sandosham A. Recent researchers on malaria at the Institute for Medical Research, Kuala Lumpur. Medical Journal of Malaysia 1967;22:145-60.

[26] Lee KS, Cox-Singh J, Singh B. Morphological features and differential counts of *Plasmodium knowlesi* parasites in naturally acquired human infections. Malaria Journal 2009;8:73.

[27] Coatney RG, Collins WE, Warren M, Contacos PG. The Primate Malarias. Washington: U.S. Government Printing Office; 1971.

[28] Sandosham AA. Malariology with special reference to Malaya Singapore. Kuala Lumpur: University of Malaya Press; 1959.

[29] Cox Singh J, Davis TME, Lee KS, Shamsul SSG, Matusop A, Ratnam S, et al. *Plasmodium knowlesi* malaria in humans is widely distributed and potentially life threatening. Clinical Infectious Diseases 2008;46:165-71.

[30] Vythilingam I, NoorAzian YM, Huat TC, Jiram AI, Yusri YM, Azahari AH, et al. *Plasmodium knowlesi* in humans, macaques and mosquitoes in peninsular Malaysia. Parasite Vectors 2008;1:26.

[31] William T, Menon J, Rajahram G, Chan L, Ma G, Donaldson S, et al. Severe *Plasmodium knowlesi* malaria in a tertiary care hospital, Sabah, Malaysia. Emerging Infectious Diseases 2011;17:1248-54.

[32] Barber BE, William T, Jikal M, Jilip J, Dhararaj P, Menon J, et al. *Plasmodium knowlesi* malaria in children. Emerging Infectious Diseases 2011;17:20.

[33] Jongwutiwes S, Putaporntip C, Iwasaki T, Sata T, Kanbara H. Naturally acquired *Plasmodium knowlesi* malaria in human, Thailand. Emerging Infectious Diseases 2004;10:2211-3.

[34] Jongwutiwes S, Buppan P, Kosuvin R, Seethamchai S, Pattanawong U, Sirichaisinthop J, et al. *Plasmodium knowlesi* Malaria in humans and macaques, Thailand. Emerging Infectious Diseases 2011;17:1799-806.

[35] Putaporntip C, Hongsrimuang T, Seethamchai S, Kobasa T, Limkittikul K, Cui L, et al. Differential prevalence of *Plasmodium* infections and cryptic *Plasmodium knowlesi* malaria in humans in Thailand. Journal of Infectious Diseases 2009;199:1143.

[36] Luchavez J, Espino F, Curameng P, Espina R, Bell D, Chiodini P, et al. Human infections with *Plasmodium knowlesi*, the Philippines. Emerging Infectious Diseases 2008;14:811-3.

[37] Eede P, Van H, Van Overmeir C, Vythilingam I, Duc T, Hung L, et al. Human *Plasmodium knowlesi* infections in young children in central Vietnam. Malaria Journal 2009;8:249.

[38] Sulistyaningsih E, Fitri LE, Löscher T, Berens-Riha N. Diagnostic difficulties with *Plasmodium knowlesi* infection in humans. Emerging Infectious Diseases 2010;16:1033.

[39] Khim N, Siv S, Kim S, Mueller T, Fleischmann E, Singh B, et al. *Plasmodium knowlesi* infection in humans, Cambodia, 2007-2010. Emerging Infectious Diseases 2011;17:1900.

[40] Zhu H, Li J, Zheng H. Human natural infection of *Plasmodium knowlesi*. Zhongguo ji sheng chong xue yu ji sheng chong bing za zhi= Chinese Journal Parasitology Parasite Diseases 2006;24:70.

[41] Ng OT, Ooi EE, Lee CC, Lee PJ, Ng LC, Pei SW, et al. Naturally acquired human *Plasmodium knowlesi* infection, Singapore. Emerging Infectious Diseases 2008;14:814.

[42] White N. *Plasmodium knowlesi*: the fifth human malaria parasite. Clinical Infectious Diseases 2008;46:172.

[43] Anderios F, NoorRain A, Vythilingam I. In vivo study of human *Plasmodium knowlesi* in *Macaca fascicularis*. Experimental Parasitology 2010;124:181-9.

[44] Garnham P. Malaria parasites and other haemosporidia. Oxford: Blackwell Scientific Publications; 1966.

[45] Vythilingam I. Review Paper *Plasmodium knowlesi* in humans: a review on the role of its vectors in Malaysia. Tropical Biomedicine 2010;27:1-12.

[46] Hoosen A, Shaw M. *Plasmodium knowlesi* in a traveller returning to New Zealand. Travel Medicine and Infectious Disease 2011;9:144-8.

[47] Mali S, Steele S, Slutsker L, Arguin PM. Malaria surveillance–United states, 2006. MMWR Surveill Summ 2008;57:24-39.

[48] Kantele A, Marti H, Felger I, Muller D, Jokiranta TS. Monkey Malaria in a European Traveler Returning from Malaysia. Emerging Infectious Diseases 2008;14:1434-6.

[49] Bronner U, Divis PCS, Farnert A, Singh B. Swedish traveller with *Plasmodium knowlesi* malaria after visiting Malaysian Borneo: a case report. Malaria Journal 2009;8:15.

[50] Tang TH, Salas A, Ali-Tammam M, Martínez M, Lanza M, Arroyo E, et al. First case of detection of *Plasmodium knowlesi* in Spain by Real Time PCR in a traveller from Southeast Asia. Malaria Journal 2010;9:219.

[51] Berry A, Iriart X, Wilhelm N, Valentin A, Cassaing S, Witkowski B, et al. Imported *Plasmodium knowlesi* malaria in a French tourist returning from Thailand. American Journal of Tropical Medicine and Hygiene 2011;84:535-8.

[52] Warren MW, Wharton RH. The vectors of simian malaria: identity, biology, and geographical distribution. Journal of Parasitology 1963:892-904.

[53] Sallum MAM, Peyton EL, Wilkerson RC. Six new species of the *Anopheles leucosphyrus* group, reinterpretation of *An. elegans* and vector implications. Medical and Veterinary Entomology 2005;19:158-99.

[54] Harbach RE. The classification of genus *Anopheles* (Diptera: Culicidae): a working hypothesis of phylogenetic relationships. Bulletin of Entomological Research 2004;94:537-54.

[55] Peyton E. A new classification for the Leucosphyrus Group of *Anopheles* (*Cellia*). Mosquito Systematics 1989;21:197-205.

[56] Sallum MAM, Peyton EL, Harrison BA, Wilkerson RC. Revision of the Leucosphyrus group of *Anopheles* (*Cellia*)(Diptera, Culicidae). Revista Brasileira de Entomolo 2005;49:01-152.

[57] Manguin S, Garros C, Dusfour I, Harbach RE, Coosemans M. Bionomics, taxonomy, and distribution of the major malaria vector taxa of *Anopheles* subgenus *Cellia* in

Southeast Asia: An updated review. Infection, Genetics and Evolution 2008;8:489-503.

[58] Rattanarithikul R, Harrison BA. An illustrated key to the *Anopheles* larvae of Thailand. United State Army Medical Component, South East Asia Treaty Organization, Bangkok 1973.

[59] Rattanarithikul R, Harrison BA, Harbach RE, Panthusiri P, Coleman RE. Illustrated keys to the mosquitoes of Thailand. IV. *Anopheles*. Southeast Asian Journal of Tropical Medicine Public Health 2006;37 1-128.

[60] Baimai V, Kijchalao U, Sawadwongporn P, Green CA. Geographic distribution and biting behaviour of four species of the *Anopheles dirus* complex (Diptera: Culicidae) in Thailand. Southeast Asian Journal of Tropical Medicine Public Health 1988;19:151-61.

[61] Obsomer V, Defourny P, Coosemans M. The *Anopheles dirus* complex: spatial distribution and environmental drivers. Malaria Journal 2007;6:26.

[62] Trung HD, Bortel WV, Sochantha T, Keokenchanh K, Briët OJT, Coosemans M. Behavioural heterogeneity of *Anopheles* species in ecologically different localities in Southeast Asia: a challenge for vector control. Tropical Medicine & International Health 2005;10:251-62.

[63] Vythilingam I. *Plasmodium knowlesi* and *Wuchereria bancrofti*: their vectors and challenges for the future. Frontiers in Systems Biology 2012;3.

[64] Sinka ME, Bangs MJ, Manguin S, Chareonviriyaphap T, Patil AP, Temperley WH, et al. The dominant *Anopheles* vectors of human malaria in the Asia-Pacific region: occurrence data, distribution maps and bionomic précis. Parasite Vectors 2011;4:1-46.

[65] Reid JA. Anopheline Mosquitoes of Malaya and Borneo. Malaysia: Institute for Medical Research Malaysia; 1968.

[66] Colless D. The *Anopheles leucosphyrus* group. Transactions of Royal Entomological Society London 1956;108:37-116.

[67] Meek S. Vector control in some countries of Southeast Asia: comparing the vectors and the strategies. Annals of Tropical Medicine and Parasitology 1995;89:135-47.

[68] Chang MS, Doraisingam P, Hardin S, Nagum N. Malaria and filariasis transmission in a village/forest setting in Baram District, Sarawak, Malaysia. Journal of Tropical Medicine and Hygiene 1995;98:192.

[69] Colless DH. Observations on Anopheline mosquitoes of the Akah river, 4th Division, Sarawak. Bulletin of Entomological Research 1956;47:115-23.

[70] Zulueta J. Malaria in Sarawak. Bulletin World Health Organisation 1956;15:651-71.

[71] Tan CH, Vythilingam I, Matusop A, Chan ST, Singh B. Bionomics of *Anopheles latens* in Kapit, Sarawak, Malaysian Borneo in relation to the transmission of zoonotic simian malaria parasite *Plasmodium knowlesi*. Malaria Journal 2008;7:52.

[72] Jiram AI, Vythilingam I, NoorAzian YM, Yusof YM, Azahari AH, Fong MY. Entomologic investigation of *Plasmodium knowlesi* vectors in Kuala Lipis, Pahang, Malaysia. Malaria Journal 2012;11:213.

[73] Tsukamoto M, Miyata A, Miyagi I. Surveys on simian malaria parasites and their vector in Palawan Island, the Philippines. Tropical Medicine 1978;20:39-50.

[74] Miyagi I. Studies on malaria vectors in Philippines especially on *Anopheles balabacensis balabacensis* and monkey malaria in Palawan. The Journal of Tropical Medicine 1973;2:163.

[75] Vythilingam I, Tan CH, Asmad M, Chan ST, Lee KS, Singh B. Natural transmission of *Plasmodium knowlesi* to humans by *Anopheles latens* in Sarawak, Malaysia. Transactions Royal Society Tropical Medicine Hygiene 2006;100:1087-8.

[76] Nakazawa S, Marchand RP, Quang NT, Culleton R, Manh ND, Maeno Y. *Anopheles dirus* co-infection with human and monkey malaria parasites in Vietnam. International Journal of Parasitology 2009;39:1533-7.

[77] Marchand RP, Culleton R, Maeno Y, Quang NT, Nakazawa S. Co-infections of *Plasmodium knowlesi, P. falciparum, and P. vivax* among humans and *Anopheles dirus* mosquitoes, southern Vietnam. Emerging Infectious Diseases 2011;17:1232-9.

[78] Wharton RH, Eyles DE, Warren M, Cheong WH. Studies to determine the vectors of monkey malaria in Malaya. Annals of Tropical Medicine and Parasitology 1964;58:56.

[79] Tan CH. Identification of vectors of *Plasmodium knowlesi* and other malaria parasites, and studies on their bionomics in Kapit, Sarawak, Malaysia. MSc Thesis University Malaysia, Sarawak (UNIMAS) 2008.

[80] Cheong WH, Warren MW, Omar AH, Mahadevan S. A*nopheles balabacensis balabacensis* identified as vector of simian malaria in Malaysia. Science 1965;150:1314.

[81] Vythilingam I, Phetsouvanh R, Keokenchanh K, Yengmala V, Vanisaveth V, Phompida S, et al. The prevalence of *Anopheles* (Diptera: Culicidae) mosquitoes in Sekong Province, Lao PDR in relation to malaria transmission. Tropical Medicine International Health 2003;8:525-35.

[82] Pothikasikorn J, Bangs MJ, Boonplueang R, Chareonviriyaphap T. Susceptibility of various mosquitoes of Thailand to nocturnal subperiodic *Wuchereria bancrofti*. Journal of Vector Ecology 2008;33:313-20.

[83] Vythilingam I, Chan ST, Shanmugratnam C, Tanrang H, Chooi KH. The impact of development and malaria control activities on its vectors in the Kinabatangan area of Sabah, East Malaysia. Acta Tropica 2005;96:24-30.

[84] Maekawa Y, Tsuda Y, Dachlan YP, Yotopranoto S, Gerudug IK, Yoshinaga K, et al. Anopheline fauna and incriminatory malaria vectors in malaria endemic areas on Lombok Island, Indonesia. Medical Entomology and Zoology 2009;60:1-11.

[85] Hii J. Evidence for the existence of genetic variability in the tendency of *Anopheles balabacensis* to rest in houses and to bite man. The Southeast Asian Journal of Tropical Medicine and Public Health 1985;16:173.

[86] Rohani A, Lokman Hakim S, Hassan AR, Chan ST, Ong YF, Abdullah AG, Lee HL Bionomics of *Anopheles balabacensis* Baisas, the Principal Malaria Vector in Ranau, Sabah. Tropical Biomedicine 1999;16:31-8.

[87] Chiang G, Cheong W, Samarawickrema W, Mak J, Kan S. Filariasis in Bengkoka Peninsula, Sabah, Malaysia: vector studies in relation to the transmission of filariasis. The Southeast Asian Journal of Tropical Medicine and Public Health 1984;15:179.

[88] Schultz G. Biting activity of mosquitoes (Diptera: Culicidae) at a malarious site in Palawan, Republic of The Philippines. Southeast Asian Journal Tropical Medicine and Public Health 1992;23:464-9.

[89] Harbach RE, Baimai V, Sukowati S. Some observations on sympatric populations of the malaria vectors *Anopheles leucoshpyrus* and *Anopheles balabacensis* in a village forest setting in South Kalimantan. Southeast Asian Journal of Tropical Medicine and Public Health 1987;18:241-7.

[90] Sungvornyothin S, Kongmee M, Muenvorn V, Polsomboon S, Bangs MJ, Prabaripai A, et al. Seasonal abundance and bloodfeeding activity of *Anopheles dirus* sensu lato in western Thailand. Journal of the American Mosquito Control Association 2009;25:425-30.

[91] Van Bortel W, Trung HD, Hoi le X, Van Ham N, Van Chut N, Luu ND, Roelants P, et al. Malaria transmission and vector behaviour in a forested malaria focus in central Vietnam and the implications for vector control. Malaria Journal 2010;9:373.

[92] Lambrechts L, Knox TB, Wong J, Liebman KA, Albright RG, Stoddard ST. Shifting priorities in vector biology to improve control of vector borne disease. Tropical Medicine & International Health 2009;14:1505-14.

[93] Collins WE, Contacos PG, Guinn EG. Studies on the transmission of simian malarias II. Transmission of the H strain of *Plasmodium knowlesi* by *Anopheles balabacensis balabacensis*. Journal of Parasitology 1967:841-4.

[94] Collins WE, Contacos PG, Guinn EG, Held JR. Studies on the transmission of simian malarias, I. Transmission of two strains of *Plasmodium inui* by *Anopheles maculatus* and *A. stephensi*. Journal of Parasitology 1966:664-8.

[95] Wharton RH, Eyles DE, Warren McW. The development of methods for trapping the vectors of monkey malaria. Annals of Tropical Medicine and Parasitology 1963;57:32-46.

[96] Gater BAR. Aids to the identification of anopheline imagines in Malaya. Singapore: Government Printer; 1935.

[97] Takken W, Knols BGJ. Malaria vector control: current and future strategies. Trends in Parasitology 2009;25:101-4.

[98] WHO. The global malaria action plan for a malaria free world. http://wwwrollbackmalariaorg/gmap accessed 18Sept 2012. Geneva 2008.

[99] Cox-Singh J, Singh B. Knowlesi malaria: newly emergent and of public health importance? Trends in Parasitology 2008;24:406-10.

[100] Rajahram GS, Barber BE, William T, Menon J, Anstey NM, Yeo TW. Deaths due to *Plasmodium knowlesi* malaria in Sabah, Malaysia: association with reporting as *Plasmodium malariae* and delayed parenteral artesunate. Malaria Journal 2012;11:284.

[101] Ferguson HM DA, Beeche A, Borgemeister C, Gottlieb M, et al. Ecology: A Prerequisite for Malaria Elimination and Eradication. PLoS Medicine 2012;7(8):e1000303. doi: 10.1371/journal.pmed.

[102] Delacollette C, D'Souza C, Christophel E, Thimasarn K, Abdur R, Bell D, et al. Malaria trends and challenges in the Greater Mekong Subregion. Southeast Asian Journal of Tropical Medicine and Public Health 2009;40:674.

[103] Organisation Internationale pour les Migration. Situation report on international migration in East and Southeast Asia. 2008.

[104] Thang ND, Erhart A, Speybroeck N, Xa NX, Thanh NN, Van Ky P, et al. Long-lasting insecticidal hammocks for controlling forest malaria: a community-based trial in a rural area of central Vietnam. PloS One 2009;4:e7369.

[105] Deparis X, Frere B, Lamizana M, N'Guessan R, Leroux F, Lefevre P, et al. Efficacy of permethrin-treated uniforms in combination with DEET topical repellent for protection of French military troops in Cote d'Ivoire. Journal of Medical Entomology 2004;41:914-21.

[106] Wallace MR, Sharp TW, Smoak B, Iriye C, Rozmajzl P, Thornton SA, et al. Malaria among United States troops in Somalia. The American Journal of Medicine 1996;100:49-55.

[107] Collins WE. *Plasmodium knowlesi*: A Malaria Parasite of Monkeys and Humans. Annual Review of Entomology 2012;57.

[108] Baird JK. Malaria zoonoses. Travel Med and Infect Dis 2009;7:269-77.

[109] Sandosham AA, Thomas V. Malariology: with special reference to Malaya: Coronet Books; 1983.

[110] Rahman WA, Che'Rus A, Ahmad AH. Malaria and *Anopheles* mosquitos in Malaysia. Southeast Asian Journal of Tropical Medicine and Public Health 1997;28:599.

[111] Vythilingam I, Foo LC, Chiang GL, Chan ST, Eng KL, Mahadevan S, et al. The impact of permethrin impregnated bednets on the malaria vector *Anopheles maculatus* (Diptera: Culicidae) in aboriginal villages of Pos Betau Pahang, Malaysia. Southeast Asian Journal of Tropical Medicine and Public Health 1995;26:354-8.

[112] Chang MS, Hii J, Buttner P, Mansoor F. Changes in abundance and behaviour of vector mosquitoes induced by land use during the development of an oil palm plantation in Sarawak. Trans Roy Soc Trop Med Hyg 1997;91:382-6.

[113] Hii JLK, Kan S, Vun YS, Chin KF, Lye MS, Mak JW, et al. *Anopheles flavirostris* incriminated as a vector of malaria and Bancroftian filariasis in Banggi Island, Sabah, Malaysia. Transactions of the Royal Society of Tropical Medicine and Hygiene 1985;79:677-80.

[114] Chareonviriyaphap T, Bangs MJ, Ratanatham S. Status of malaria in Thailand. Southeast Asian Journal of Tropical Medicine and Public Health 2000;31:225-37.

[115] APMEN. Vietnam joins Asia Pacific Malaria Elimination Network (APMEN). http://apmenorg/storage/newsmedia/Vietnam assessed 18 Sept 2012.

Chapter 16

Thermal Stress and Thermoregulation During Feeding in Mosquitoes

Chloé Lahondère and Claudio R. Lazzari

Additional information is available at the end of the chapter

http://dx.doi.org/10.5772/56288

1. Introduction

Many arthropods have acquired the ability to use the blood of endothermic vertebrates as their main or even unique food. Among insects, haematophagy has evolved independently in different groups [1], which have converged to this way of life under strong selective pressures that modelled many morphological, physiological and behavioural traits.

Blood is a rich source of nutrients and, except for the possible presence of parasites, otherwise sterile. However, being haematophagous is a risky task, as the food circulates inside vessels hidden beneath the skin of mobile hosts, able to defend themselves from biting or even predate on blood-sucking species. Thus, in order to minimize the contact with the host, blood-sucking insects need to pierce the host-skin without being noticed and gather blood in relatively high amounts and as quick as possible. Large blood-meals produce a strong osmotic misbalance at its ingestion and toxic metabolites as by products of its digestion. In addition, the rapid ingestion of a fluid which temperature can exceed that of the insects by 20°C or more and account for many times the insect's own body weight also implies a rapid transfer of heat into the insect's body. Thus, the inner temperature of the insect could exceed the physiological limits of certain functions, causing deleterious effects [2]. Numerous studies report the impact of temperature on different behavioural [3] and physiological processes such as development [4-6], metabolism [7, 8], blood-feeding and reproduction [9] of mosquitoes and insects in general.

Thermal stress may not only affect the insect itself but also its symbiotic flora [10-12] and the parasites that it transmits with an important impact on vector infectivity [13-15]. Finally, heat constitutes a main cue to find a food source (*i.e.* a warm-blooded vertebrate). Consequently, a recently fed insect could be exposed to cannibalism if its body temperature is higher than that of the surrounding environment, facilitating the horizontal transmission of parasites between vectors [16-17].

Provided their ectothermic nature, as well as their ability to colonize all kind of habitats, insects must cope with highly variable temperatures. Therefore, many insect species have developed particular physiological and behavioural mechanisms and strategies to avoid the risk to be submitted to thermal stress [18, 19]. To avoid the effect of environmental heat, insects can seek for fresher environments or adjust their water loss to increase evaporation. In the case of haematophagous insects such as mosquitoes, they must in addition confront the exposition to thermal stress at each feeding event.

The problem of heat transfer between hosts and blood-sucking insects during blood feeding remained largely overlooked until recently, when unexpected physiological mechanisms against thermal stress were unravelled in mosquitoes. We present in this chapter a brief account of these findings and the perspectives that they open in both, fundamental and applied research.

2. Thermal stress and protective strategies in *Anopheles*

The first evidences of thermal stress during feeding in haematophagous insects were obtained only recently [20]. The variation of the temperature of the body during the feeding process was measured in different species of blood-sucking insects, including two mosquitoes, *Aedes aegypti* and *Anopheles gambiae* using thermocouples. As soon as feeding begins, a steady increase of the body temperature occurs, reaching peak values of up to +10°C a few minutes later. After feeding, the temperature decreases gradually to come back similar to the environmental one. Depending on the values of environmental temperature, which is the initial temperature of the insect, and that of the blood, the amplitude and dynamics of heating and cooling vary.

Physiological responses of insects to heat include molecular changes, as is a rapid increase in the level of heat shock proteins (Hsps), which have a role as molecular chaperones that preserve the function of enzymes and other critical proteins [20]. More than a dozen Hsps are synthetized after exposure to high temperature, being the Hsp70 the most widely recognised as associated to thermal and other stresses. As in many other organisms, mosquito Hsp70s have been shown to increase during environmental stress [21, 22].

Benoit and co-workers [20] showed that, correlated with feeding and the associated elevation of the body temperature, a synthesis of heat-shock proteins occurs in *Aedes aegypti* in the few hours following a blood meal, in particular of Hsp70. In this species, the Hsp70 synthesis peaks 1 hour after feeding, reaching maximal expression in the mosquito midgut, where the relative amount of Hsp70 increases about 7 times after feeding. Similar increases in Hsp70 were showed immediately after blood feeding in *Culex pipiens* and in *Anopheles gambiae*, as well as in the bed bug *Cimex lectularius*. Nevertheless this increase, measured as the relative increase of mRNA by Northern blot, is not identical in the three mosquito species. Whereas in *Aedes aegypti* and

http://dx.doi.org/10.5772/56288

Culex pipiens the relative level increases between nine and ten times, in *Anopheles gambiae* only three times. This last result is particularly interesting, since it is probable that the last named species would be less submitted to thermal stress, as we will discuss in the following sections.

3. Heterothermy during feeding in *Anopheles*

To better understand to what extent mosquitoes are exposed to thermal stress during feeding, we recently conducted a real-time infrared thermographic analysis of the evolution of the body temperature of *Anopheles stephensi* during feeding on live hosts at different skin temperatures and using an artificial feeder [23].

Thermal imaging analysis has first revealed that during feeding, the different regions of the mosquito's body exhibited different temperatures. When *Anopheles stephensi* fed on mice or human volunteers, their head temperature remained close to that of the ingested blood while the abdomen temperature stayed closer to that of the ambient temperature (Figure 1). The thermal profile along a mosquito's body during feeding, notwithstanding the exact temperature of the host skin, can be summarized as in this: $T°_{head} > T°_{thorax} > T°_{abdomen}$. The fact of maintaining different temperatures in different regions of the body by an animal is named "regional heterothermy" and it is common in vertebrates living in cold aquatic or terrestrial environments. When the body temperature changes with time, this condition is called "temporal heterothermy". A combination of both types of heterothemy is frequently found in insects that perform pre-heating of flight muscles before taking off. By means of simultaneous isometric contractions of antagonist muscles, insects like bumble-bees and moths heat their thorax up to reach the optimal temperature for muscular work [18].

In the case of *Anopheles stephensi*, an average difference of 3.3° C between $T°_{head}$ and $T°_{abdomen}$ was measured when the $T°_{host}$ was 34° C and 2.2° C when T_{host} was 28° C. At the end of feeding, when mouthparts are retracted from the skin, the mosquito temperature returns rapidly to environmental temperature (ectothermy).

Infrared thermography revealed a quite different pattern of body temperature in *Aedes aegypti*. In this species, the abdominal temperature during feeding remains close to that of the host, rather than to that of the environment as in *Anopheles stephensi* [23]. On the other hand, when the two species fed on sugar solution, despite the muscular activity of the ingestion pump, no heterothermy occurs: the temperature of the whole body remained that of the environment. As a consequence males, which don't feed on blood, exhibit a typically ectothermic thermal profile even when resting on a warm host, demonstrating that heating is only due to blood ingestion and not to the proximity of the host [23].

4. Prediuresis and drop-keeping

During blood feeding, most haematophagous species excrete drops of fluid, a process referred in mosquitoes as "prediuresis". The physiological function of prediuresis has been related to

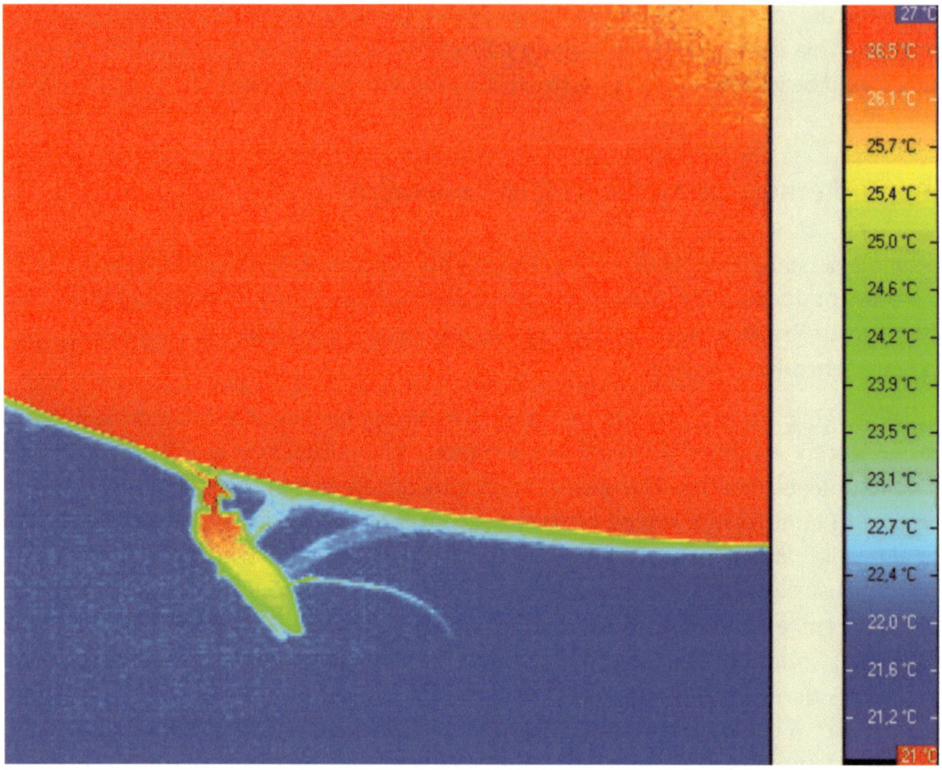

Figure 1. Thermographic image of an *Anopheles stephensi* female at the beginning of feeding on an anesthetized mouse ($T°_{host}$ = 28° C, $T°_{environment}$ = 22° C). The temperature of the head is very close to the mouse one and a temperature gradient along the mosquito body can be observed (i.e., heterothermy).

erythrocytes concentration and elimination of water excess. The eliminated fluid is in most insects composed of urine, but in some blood-sucking species, such as mosquitoes and sandflies, it also contains fresh ingested blood that gives to the drop a bright red appearance. In mosquitoes, which feed not only on vertebrate blood, but also on nectar, prediuresis occurs during blood-feeding but it is rare or absent when they take a sugar meal.

In *Anopheles stephensi*, notwithstanding the nature of the host, blood-feeding almost always proceeds in a similar way: drops of fluid start being excreted during the first or second minute after the insect begins to feed. Frequently, a drop remains attached to the end of the abdomen for several minutes, increasing its size during feeding. Eventually the drop felt, and a new one is emitted and retained at the abdomen's end. The number of drops produced until complete gorging may vary.

Real-time thermography revealed that when *Anopheles stephensi* performs prediuresis and keeps a drop attached to its anus, a transient fall of 2° C or more of the abdominal temperature occurs and the characteristic heterothermy along its body becomes even more pronounced (Figure 2). The same phenomenon was observed in females of this species feeding in mice, human volunteers or using an artificial feeder [23]. Besides, when ingesting blood at the same temperature, the abdominal temperature of drop-keepers is significantly lower than that of mosquitoes that just perform prediuresis but that do not keep drops. These results demonstrate the existence of a physical cooling process in *Anopheles stephensi*. Conversely, drop-keeping was never observed to occur in *Aedes aegypti* among the individuals producing pre-urine while feeding, even if the frequency of prediuresis is the same in both mosquito species [23].

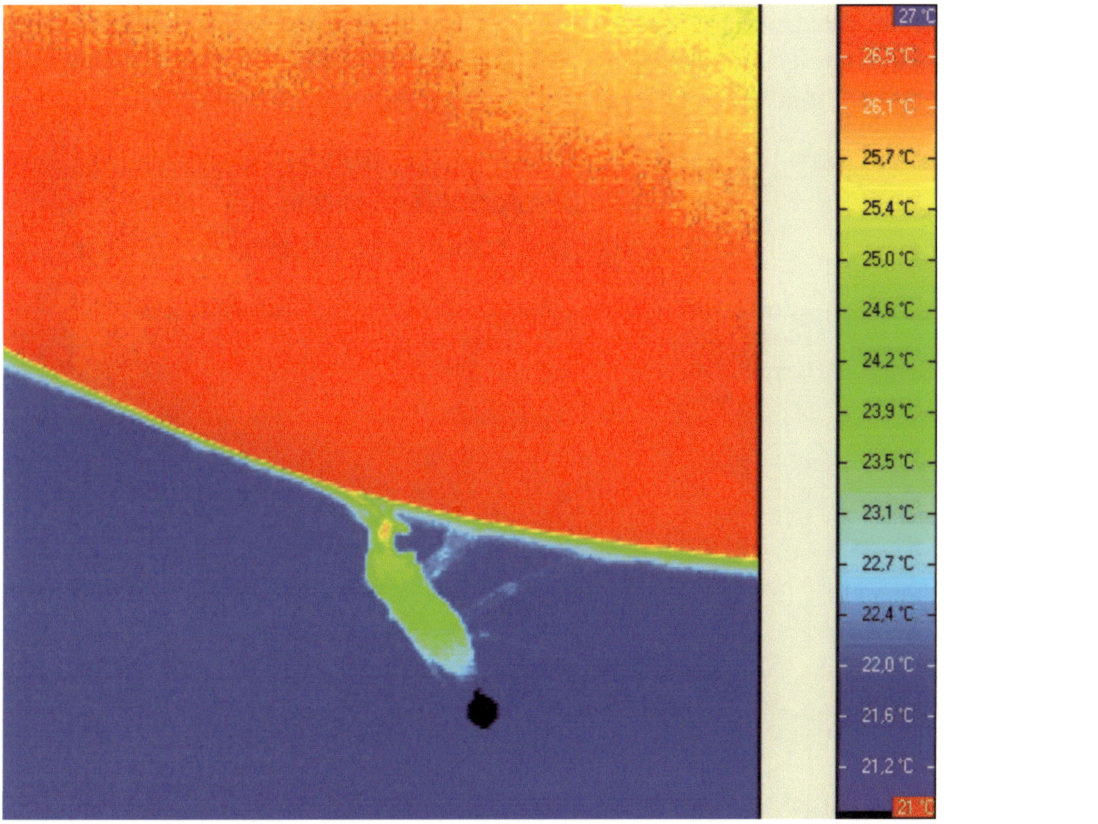

Figure 2. Thermographic image of the same *Anopheles stephensi* female as Figure 1, but during prediuresis. The mosquito performs evaporative cooling. The retention of the fluid drop attached to the abdomen end leads to a fall of the abdomen temperature causing a clear temperature gradient along the mosquito body. The colour of the droplet does not reflect the real temperature, because of the difference in the emissivity between the cuticle of the mosquito and the drop surface.

5. Thermoregulation in *Anopheles*

Many insects, in particular those having easy access to water, produce and retain drops of fluid, such as nectar, honey-dew, water or urine, depending on species, which evaporates in contact with the air, causing heat loss by evaporative cooling and the consequent decrease of the temperature of the insect body. Evaporative cooling constitutes an adaptive and effective response to risks associated to high temperature and has been observed in different groups of insects [24, 25].

This decrease of temperature helps them to avoid the deleterious physiological consequences of thermal stress. Some insects such as honeybees and bumblebees produce heat with their thoracic muscles while flying (endothermy) and regurgitate a droplet of nectar through their mouthparts to cool down their head, thus keeping the brain safe from overheating [26, 27]. Moths emit fluid, which is retained on the proboscis to refresh their head whereas others, like aphids, excrete honey-dew through their anus that consequently refresh their abdomen. The recorded loss of temperature is between 2 and 8° C depending on species [28].

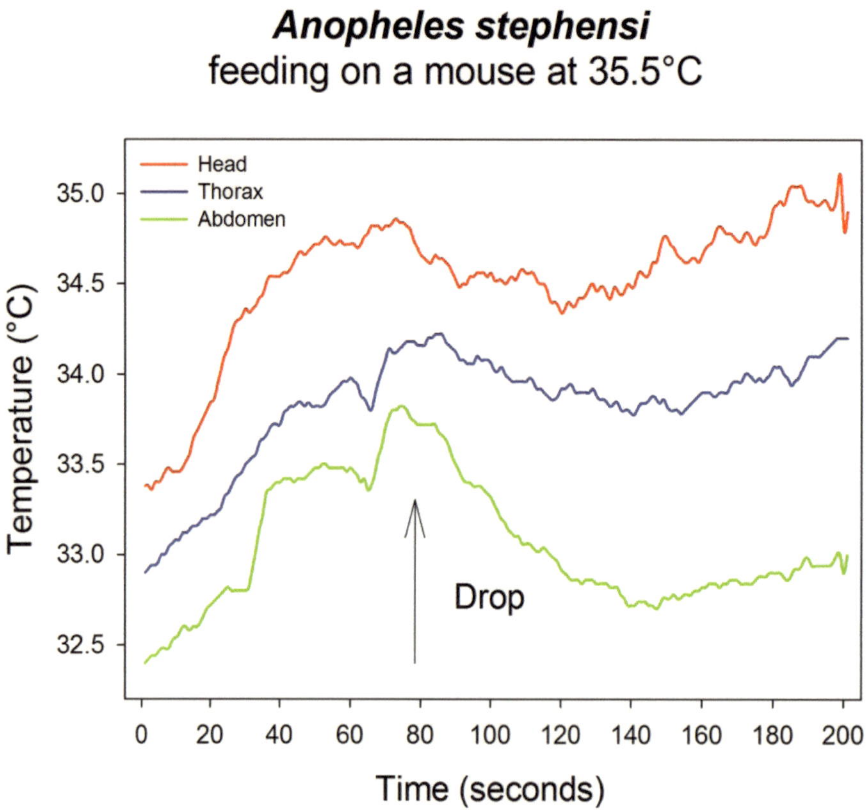

Figure 3. Evolution of the body temperatures of *Anopheles stephensi* during feeding on an anesthetized mouse. The arrow indicates the excretion of a droplet. ($T°_{host}$ = 35.5° C, $T°_{environment}$ = 28° C)

In *Anopheles* mosquitoes, the abdominal temperature of drop-keepers decreases of about 2° C during drop retention. For mosquitoes and in general for all haematophagous insects that need to manage an excess of water into their body during feeding and keep a well-adjusted water balance, evaporative cooling represents an efficient protective mechanism against overheating.

To what extent prediuresis and drop-keeping occurs is variable and it is known that the rate of production and the size of the droplets excreted in mosquitoes during prediuresis differ not only between species but also within the same species, as also differs the amount of erythrocytes from the ingested blood [29].

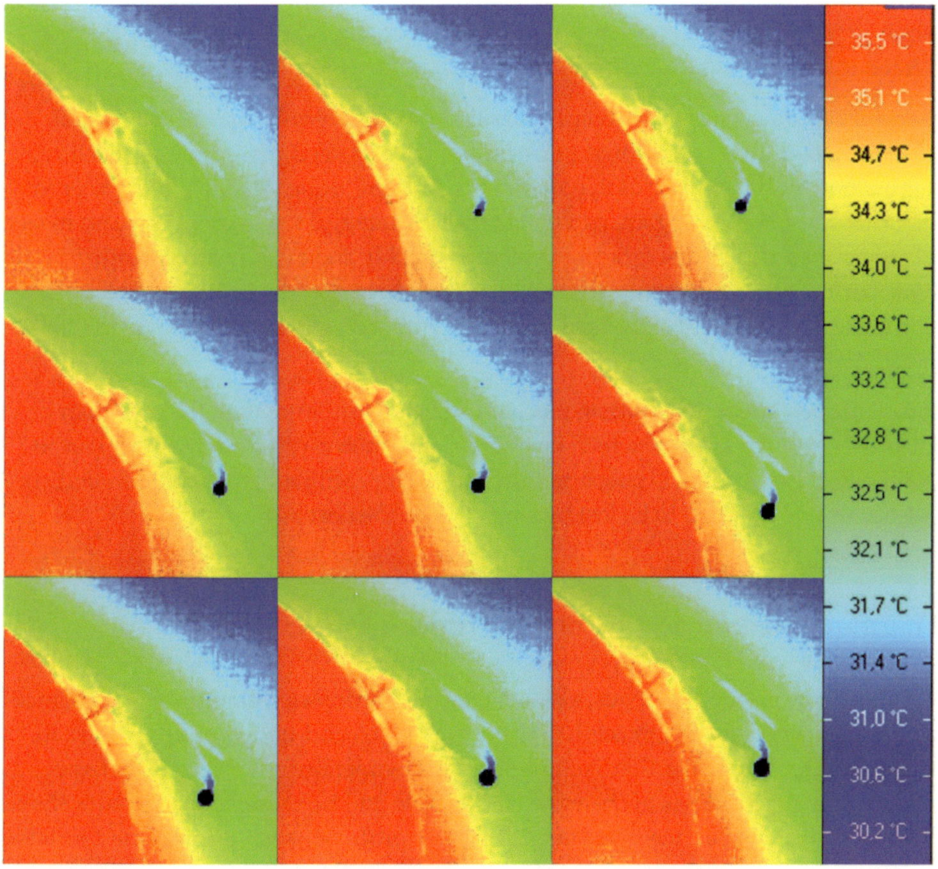

Figure 4. Sequence of thermographic images showing the production of a drop during feeding and the subsequent cooling of the abdomen in an *Anopheles stephensi* female. The insect fed on a human host ($T°_{host}$ = 36° C, $T°_{environment}$ = 23° C). Images were taken every 5 seconds.

6. A novel significance of prediuresis

Even though the occurrence of prediuresis and the elimination of fresh blood have been largely reported, it has been always considered just a way of concentrating erythrocytes and reducing the insect weight for take-off [30]. Nevertheless, two puzzling aspects of prediuresis in mosquitoes remained unsolved. The first one is the elimination during feeding of some of the just ingested blood containing erythrocytes [29]. It is widely accepted that strong selective pressures made blood-sucking insects minimize their contact time with a host in order to reduce the risk of being predated [1]. Thus, throwing away some of the food they ingest appears, at first glance, as a maladaptive strategy. From a point of view of thermoregulation, however, this "waste" makes sense, since it allows a quick increase in the volume (and evaporative surface) of the droplet and perhaps the surface properties of the drop, influencing its retention. Thus, the excretion of fresh blood during feeding in mosquitoes can be explained in terms of an adaptive response of evaporative cooling when exposed to thermal stress associated to feeding.

The second puzzling aspect of prediuresis is that not all mosquito species perform it. In fact, it has been shown that species that perform prediuresis need more time to reach repletion during a blood meal than species that do not produce pre-urine [31, 32]. Thus, the production of pre-urine could be seen, again, as a maladaptive strategy. However, an increase in feeding time could represent a trade-off between feeding quickly and avoiding overheating in species that are particularly sensitive to thermal stress. Others may be less sensitive or, as *Aedes* minimize the consequences of thermal stress by synthetizing more heat-shock proteins as, for example, *Anopheles* mosquitos.

Drop-keeping as evaporative cooling mechanism is in accordance with the particular position adopted by *Anopheles* species, which keep their abdomen away from the host surface. This causes the drop to be more exposed to the ambient air facilitating evaporation and cooling, and also avoiding the drop to be lost by contact with the host skin.

7. Thermoregulation and pathogens transmission

When anopheline mosquitoes ingest a blood meal from an infected host, mature and functional *Plasmodium* gametocytes are present in the erythrocytes and undergo differentiation in the mosquito midgut, a process that is influenced by temperature. Indeed, high temperatures negatively affect early stages of the parasite life cycle and no exflagellation occurs above 30° C, holding parasites in an inactive state [14]. Later processes such as ookinete formation or migration of sporozoites towards the salivary glands are also influenced by temperature [15, 33, 34]. Furthermore, it has been well demonstrated that different species of *Plasmodium* are thermo-sensitive and that temperature has a direct impact on the incubation period of parasites in the mosquito [13]. On the other hand, the proliferation and dispersion of flaviviruses in *Aedes* mosquitoes is also under the influence of temperature but contrary to *Plasmodium*, this latter constitutes one of the most important factor positively influencing the extrinsic incubation period (*EIP*). It has been shown that high temperatures are important for flaviviruses, acting on the rate of viral multiplication and consequently on the vector competence [35, 36, 37].

Moreover, *Plasmodium* parasites have to cope with the formation of the peritrophic matrix that follows each blood meal, which restrain their penetration through the gut wall [38, 39]. During the process of differentiation, *Plasmodium* ookinetes have to cross the peritrophic matrix and the midgut epithelium, before they turn into oocysts [40]. The time needed for the formation of the peritrophic matrix positively correlates with the vectorial capacity of mosquitoes, taking a longer time in *Anopheles* species than in species of *Aedes* or *Culex* [1, 41]. Thus, for *Plasmodium* parasites, insect's heterothermy could represent an important advantage, since when they enter into the mosquito's body, they are exposed to a rapid fall in temperature, which could immediately trigger exflagellation. Parasites could therefore penetrate the gut wall before the peritrophic matrix is fully formed.

From an evolutionary point of view, it makes sense that *Plasmodium* parasites take an advantage to be associated with species that undergo evaporative cooling, protecting them from lethal temperatures. On the other hand, flaviviruses associated with non drop-keeper species would benefit from a necessary warmer environment.

Evaporative cooling could also protect from heat stress the symbiotic microorganisms associated to mosquitoes and that can play an important role in haematophagous insects [10]. *Asaia* bacteria have been found in high density in the gut of *Anopheles stephensi* females as well as in ovaries [11]. Recently many genera have been identified in the midgut of natural populations of *Anopheles gambiae* [42]. In particular, the abundance of *Enterobacteriaceae* in the mosquito midgut has been found to correlate significantly with the *Plasmodium* infection status [42].

8. Thermoregulation and thermotolerance in mosquitoes

Finally, it is possible to speculate on two further implications of our interpretation of the functionality of prediuresis as thermoregulatory mechanisms. The first one concerns how environmental temperature may affect the survival of less thermotolerant mosquitoes. If we consider that the species that perform evaporative cooling could be more sensitive to heat, any change in the environmental temperature, due to local or global warming, would have a higher impact on them than on species that do not perform it, as for example *Culex spp.* that feed quickly and do not perform prediuresis while feeding [43]. It can be predicted that such species have been selected to reduce the contact time with their host and consequently to be more thermotolerant to temperature increases. Indeed, *Aedes aegypti* and its ability to produce Hsps represent an example of this [20].

The second implication of our finding is related to the control of mosquito populations. Prediuresis has deeper physiological consequences than just diuresis. In addition to excretion, it implies blood concentration and thermoregulation. The exploitation of the knowledge about excretion physiology to control disease vector insects by interfering with the function of Malpighian tubules has been already proposed for other haematophagous insects [44], and the same can be expected for mosquitoes. In this case, blocking or delaying the production of urine would have a double impact on disease transmission by affecting microorganisms transmitted by prediuresis [45, 46] and/or affecting the survival of mosquitoes exposed to overheating.

9. Conclusion

Anopheles mosquitoes are capable to perform thermoregulation by evaporative cooling during blood intake. This mechanism protects the insect itself, as well as the associated microorganisms (both symbionts and parasites) from thermal stress. Thus, prediuresis which plays such different roles in the mosquito physiology, appears one more time as an interesting possible target for the control of disease vectors.

Acknowledgements

We are very grateful to Catherine Bourgouin and the CEPIA staff (Institut Pasteur, France) for providing us anopheline mosquitoes and rearing advices as well as Rogerio Amino (Institut Pasteur, France) for his valuable comments on the manuscript and helpful discussions. We also thank Fabrice Chandre and Marie-Noelle Lacroix (IRD Montpellier, France) for providing us *Aedes aegypti* eggs. This work received financial support from ANR (EcoEpi), CNRS and the University of Tours (France).

Author details

Chloé Lahondère and Claudio R. Lazzari*

*Address all correspondence to: claudio.lazzari@univ-tours.fr

Institut de Recherche sur la Biologie de l'Insecte, UMR CNRS - Université François Rabelais, Tours, France

References

[1] Lehane MJ. The biology of blood-sucking in insects Cambridge University Press, New York. 2nd ed.; 2005.

[2] Kirby MJ, Lindsay SW. Responses of adult mosquitoes of two sibling species, *Anopheles arabiensis* and *Anopheles gambiae s.s.* (Diptera: Culicidae), to high temperatures. Bulletin of Entomological Research 2004; 94 441-448.

[3] Muirhead Thomson CR. The reactions of mosquitoes to temperature and humidity. Bulletin of Entomological Research 1938; 125-140.

[4] Lanciani CA, Le TM. Effect of temperature on the wing length body-weight relationship in *Anopheles quadrimaculatus*. Journal of the American Mosquito Control Assocation 1995; 11 241-243.

[5] Lyimo EO, Takken W, Koella JC. Effect of rearing temperature and larval density on larval survival, age at pupation and adult size of *Anopheles gambiae*. Entomoligia Experimentalis et Applicata 1992; 63 265-271.

[6] Rueda LM, Patel KJ, Axtell RC, Stinner RE. Temperature-dependent development and survival rates of *Culex quinquefasciatus* and *Aedes aegypti* (Diptera: Culicidae). Journal of Medical Entomology 1980; 27 892-898.

[7] Clements AN. The biology of mosquitoes. Chapman & Hall, London, UK, Vol. 1; 1992.

[8] Mellanby K. The influence of athmospheric humidity on the thermal death point of a number of insects. Journal of Experimental Biology 1932; 9 222-231.

[9] Eldridge BF. Effect of temperature and photoperiod on blood-feeding and ovarian development in mosquitoes of *Culex pipiens* complex. American Journal of Tropical Medicine and Hygiene 1968; 17 133-140.

[10] Brooks MA. Symbiotes and nutrition of medically important insects. Bulletin of the World Health Organisation 1964; 31 555-559.

[11] Favia G, Ricci I, Damiani C, Raddadi N, Crotti E, Marzorati M, Rizzi A, Urso R, Brusetti L, Borin S, et al. Bacteria of the genus *Asaia* stably associate with *Anopheles stephensi,* an Asian malarial mosquito vector. Proceeding of the National Academy of Science of the United States of America 2007; 104 9047-9051.

[12] Gusmão DS, Santos AV, Marini DC, Russo ES, Peixoto AMD, Bacci MJr, Berbert-Molina MA, Lemos, FJA. First isolation of microorganisms from the gut diverticulum of *Aedes aegypti* (Diptera: Culicidae): new perspectives for an insect-bacteria association. Memorias do Instituto Oswaldo Cruz 2007; 102 919-924.

[13] Boyd MF. Epidemiology: factors related to the definitive host. In Malariology. ed Boyd MF, W.B. Saunders & Co, Philadelphia, Vol 1; 1949.

[14] Ogwan'g RA, Mwangi JK, Githure J, Were JBO, Roberts CR, Martin SK. Factors affecting exflagellation of in-vitro cultivated *Plasmodium falciparum* gametocytes. American Journal of Tropical Medicine and Hygiene 1993; 49 25-29.

[15] Vanderberg JP, Yoeli M. Effects of temperature on sporogonic development of *Plasmodium berghei*. Journal of Parasitology 1966; 52 559-564.

[16] Jones JC, Pilitt DR. Blood-feeding behavior of adult *Aedes aegypti* mosquitoes. Biological Bulletin 1973; 145 127-139.

[17] Weathersby AB, Ah HS, Mccall JW. Mosquitoes feeding on engorged mosquitoes. Mosquito News 1971; 31 110-111.

[18] Heinrich, B. The hot-blooded insects : strategies and mechanisms of thermoregulation Harvard University Press, Cambridge, Massachusetts; 1993.

[19] May ML. Insect thermoregulation. Annual Review of Entomology 1979; 24 313-349.

[20] Benoit JB, Lopez-Martinez G, Patrick KR, Phillips ZP, Krause TB, Denlinger, DL. Drinking a hot blood meal elicits a protective heat shock response in mosquitoes. Proceeding of the National Academy of Science of the United States of America 2011; 108 8026-8029.

[21] Gross TL, Myles KM, Adelman ZN. Identification and characterization of heat shock 70 genes in *Aedes aegypti* (Diptera: Culicidae). Journal of Medical Entomology 2009; 46 496–504.

[22] Benoit JB, Lopez-Martinez G, Phillips ZP, Patrick KR, Denlinger DL. Heat shock proteins contribute to mosquito dehydration tolerance. Journal of Insect Physiology 2010; 56 151–156.

[23] Lahondère C, Lazzari CR. Mosquitoes cool down during blood feeding to avoid overheating. Current Biology 2012; 22, 40–45.

[24] Adams PA, Heath JE. An evaporative cooling mechanism in *Pholus achemon*. Journal of Research on the Lepidoptera 1964; 3 69-72.

[25] Mittler TE. The excretion of honey-dew by *Tuberolachnus salignus* (Gmelin) (Homoptera: Aphididae). Proceeding of the Royal Entomological Society, Series A General Entomology 1958; 33 49-55.

[26] Heinrich B. Heat-exchange in relation to blood-flow between thorax and abdomen in bumblebees. Journal of Experimental Biology 1976; 64 561-585.

[27] Heinrich B. Keeping a cool head - honeybee thermoregulation. Science 1979; 205 1269-1271.

[28] Prange HD. Evaporative cooling in insects. Journal of Insect Physiology 1996; 42 493-499.

[29] Chege GMM, Beier JC Blood acquisition and processing by three *Anopheles* (Diptera: Culicidae) species with different innate susceptibilities to *Plasmodium falciparum*. Journal of Medical Entomology 1998; 35(3) 319-323.

[30] Briegel H, Rezzonico L. Concentration of host blood protein during feeding by Anopheline mosquitoes (Diptera, Culicidae). Journal of Medical Entomology 1985; 22 612-618.

[31] Vaughan JA, Noden BH, Beier JC. Concentration of human erythrocytes by Anopheline mosquitoes (Diptera, Culicidae) during feeding. Journal of Medical Entomology 1991; 28 780-786.

[32] Chadee DD, Beier JC, Mohammed RT. Fast and slow blood-feeding durations of *Aedes aegypti* mosquitoes in Trinidad. Journal of Vector Ecology 2002; 27 172-177.

[33] Ball GH, Chao J. Temperature stresses on mosquito phase of *Plasmodium relictum*. Journal of Parasitology 1964; 50 748-752.

[34] Noden BH, Kent MD, Beier JC. The impact of variations in temperature on early *Plasmodium falciparum* development in *Anopheles stephensi*. Parasitology 1995; 111 539-545.

[35] Davis NC. The effect of various temperatures in modifying the extrinsic incubation period of the yellow fever virus in *Aedes aegypti*. American Journal of Epidemiology 1932; 16 163-176.

[36] Hardy JL, Houk EJ, Kramer LD, Reeves WC. Intrinsic factors affecting vector competence of mosquitoes for arboviruses. Annual Review of Entomology 1983; 28 229-262.

[37] Kramer LD, Ebel GD. Dynamics of flavivirus infection in mosquitoes. Advances in Virus Research 2003; 60 187-232.

[38] Baton LA, Ranford-Cartwright LC. How do malaria ookinetes cross the mosquito midgut wall? Trends in Parasitology 2005; 21 22-28.

[39] Freyvogel TA, Staeubli W. The formation of the peritrophic membrane in Culicidae. Acta Tropica 1965; 22 118-147.

[40] Sinden RE. *Plasmodium* differentiation in the mosquito. Parassitologia 1999; 41 139-148.

[41] Devenport M, Jacobs-Lorena M. The peritrophic matrix of hematophagous insects. In Biology of Disease Vectors, ed. W.C. Marquardt Elsevier Academic Press, Amsterdam; 2005.

[42] Boissière A, Tchioffo MT, Bachar D, Abate L, Marie A, Nsango SE, Shahbazkia HR, Awono-Ambene PH, Levashina EA, Christen R, Morlais I. Midgut microbiota of the malaria mosquito vector *Anopheles gambiae* and interactions with *Plasmodium falciparum* infection. Public Library of Science Pathogens 2012; 8(5): e1002742. doi: 10.1371/journal.ppat.1002742

[43] Vaughan JA, Azad AF Passage of host immunoglobulin-G from blood meal into hemolymph of selected mosquito species (Diptera, Culicidae). Journal of Medical Entomology 1988; 25 472-474.

[44] Santini MS, Ronderos JR. Allatotropin-like peptide released by Malpighian tubules induces hindgut activity associated with diuresis in the Chagas disease vector *Triatoma infestans* (Klug). Journal of Experimental Biology 2007; 210 1986-1991.

[45] Sadlova J, Reishig J, Volf P. Prediuresis in female *Phlebotomus* sandflies (Diptera: Psychodidae). European Journal of Entomology 1998; 95 643-647.

[46] Blow JA, Turell MJ, Walker ED, Silverman AL. Post-bloodmeal diuretic shedding of hepatitis B virus by mosquitoes (Diptera: Culicidae). Journal of Medical Entomology 2002; 39 605-612.

Chapter 17

The *Anopheles* Mosquito Microbiota and Their Impact on Pathogen Transmission

Mathilde Gendrin and George K. Christophides

Additional information is available at the end of the chapter

http://dx.doi.org/10.5772/55107

1. Introduction

An ecosystem is composed of a biological community and its physical environment. A unique ecosystem is the metazoan digestive tract, which contains and interacts with many microorganisms, e.g. a single human gut contains 10^{13}-10^{14} bacteria belonging to hundreds of species [4, 5]. These microorganisms are important for the host physiology, particularly in shaping the mucosal immune system [6] and protecting the host against infections by colonization resistance [7].

The term microbiota defines the microbial communities that live in contact with the body epithelia. They are composed of bacteria, viruses, yeasts and protists. To date, the bacterial component of the microbiota is the most studied and best characterized. Studies from *Drosophila* to mice have revealed that the microbial flora is tightly regulated by the immune system and that failures in this can have detrimental effects on the host [8, 9]. The microbiota composition and numbers undergo significant changes during a host's lifetime, in particular upon changes of the environment and feeding habits.

Anopheles mosquitoes are of great importance to human health. They transmit pathogens including malaria parasites, filarial worms and arboviruses (arthropod-borne viruses). These pathogens infect the mosquito gut when ingested with a bloodmeal, disseminate through the hemolymph (insect blood) to other tissues and are transmitted to a new human host upon another mosquito bite some days later. The time pathogens spend in mosquitoes is known as extrinsic incubation period. The malaria parasite, *Plasmodium*, undergoes sexual reproduction in the midgut lumen and develops into a motile form that, approximately 24h after infection, traverses the gut epithelium establishing an infection on the basal side that is bathed in the hemolymph [10]. A week to 10 days later, parasites travel to the salivary glands where they become infectious to man. Similarly, after shedding their protective sheath in the mosquito midgut lumen, the elephantiasis nematodes *Wuchereria* and *Brugia* microfilariae migrate through the midgut epithelium to the thoracic muscles where they embark on larval development [11]. Some 10-14 days later, infectious larvae emerge from the mosquito cuticle or the proboscis and infect the human host via a skin wound, such as that caused by the mosquito bite. The O'Nyong Nyong virus (ONNV), the only arbovirus known to be transmitted exclusively by *Anopheles*, mosquitoes infects the muscle bands of the midgut and other visceral tissues after dissemination from infected gut cells [12, 13]. The next steps of the virus migration through the mosquito are not well characterized but it is thought that, as shown for its cousin Chikungunya virus, it infects the salivary glands from where it can be transmitted to the human host. Thus, for all three types of pathogens, the *Anopheles* mosquito midgut is an obligatory gateway to infection and transmission.

The mosquito gut microbiota has recently emerged as an important factor of resistance against pathogens. In particular, midgut bacteria have been shown to have a substantial negative impact on malaria parasite burden through colonization mechanisms involving either direct *Plasmodium*-microbiota interactions or bacteria-mediated induction of the mosquito immune response [1, 2, 14]. Equivalent effects of the microbiota on infection with the Dengue virus and *Brugia* microfilariae are shown in the mosquito *Aedes aegypti* [15-17]. Therefore, the research field of mosquito microbiota has received great attention in the last years and new concepts of microbiota-mediated transmission blocking are currently investigated. These studies face an important challenge: the microbiota of a female mosquito changes considerably as the mosquito shift environments during metamorphosis, from the aqueous developing larva to an air-living adult, and yet during adulthood as its feeding behaviour alternates between flower-nectar feeding and blood feeding [18, 19]. The diversity of the bacterial community is shown to decrease during mosquito development and after the first bloodmeal, whereas bacteria massively proliferate, with a 10 to 900-fold increase registered 24h to 30h after a bloodmeal [18, 20, 21].

In this chapter, we provide an overview on the current knowledge of the composition of the *Anopheles* mosquito microbiota, including important findings from recent high-throughput sequencing studies. We then review studies about the impact of the microbiota on mosquito physiology and infection, focusing in particular on resistance to infection by human pathogens. Finally, we discuss the potential use of this knowledge toward reducing the mosquito vectorial capacity and transmission blocking.

2. The diversity of the *Anopheles* microbiota

The microbiota composition has been studied in several anophelines mainly by culturing or sequencing of the 16S rRNA [14, 18, 20, 22-41]. Together, studies on field-collected or laboratory-reared mosquitoes identified as many as 98 bacterial genera excluding genera of low abundance identified by high-throughput sequencing analyses (Table 1). Of these, 41 genera were found in more than one *Anopheles* species while 9 were reported in at least 7 of these 23 studies and thus appear to be frequently associated with *Anopheles*. *Pseudomonas* was the most frequent of those genera, detected in 16 studies, followed by *Aeromonas, Asaia, Comamonas, Elizabethkingia, Enterobacter, Klebsiella, Pantoea* and *Serratia*, detected in 7-10 studies. No single bacterial genus was found in all the studies, even if culture-dependent studies are not considered – as culturing techniques might be an issue. Thus, there is presumably no obligate symbiont in the *Anopheles* genus, as is the case of some other blood-sucking insects such as the Tsetse fly that hosts *Wigglesworthia spp.*, an obligatory bacterial symbiont important for fly fecundity [42] or the head louse that hosts *Riesia pediculicola* [43]. As the most frequent genera are present in both laboratory and field-collected mosquitoes, it is suggestive that laboratory colonies retain bacterial communities established prior to laboratory colonisation (Table 1 and [18]). There are, however, substantial differences between field-collected and laboratory-reared mosquitoes, as reflected by the loss of microbiota species richness in laboratory-reared mosquitoes [18, 22].

Genus	Family	Class	Example	Condi-tions	stag	*Anopheles* species	Deep seq	Culture	Non-culture
Actinobacteria									
Agromyces	*Microbacteriaceae*	*Actinobacteria*	JX186590	F*	L	*gambiae*	[17]		
Brevibacterium	*Brevibacteriaceae*	*Actinobacteria*	FJ608062	F	L	*stephensi*			[38]
Corynebacterium	*Corynebacteria-ceae*	*Actinobacteria*	GQ109703	F, F*	A	*funestus, gambiae*	[17, 36]		
Janibacter	*Intrasporangiaceae*	*Actinobacteria*	NR_043218	F	A	*arabiensis*		[22]	
Kocuria	*Micrococcaceae*	*Actinobacteria*	HQ591424	F	L	*stephensi*		[23]	
Microbacterium	*Microbacteriaceae*	*Actinobacteria*	HQ591431	F, L	L	*gambiae, stephensi*		[11, 23]	
Micrococcus	*Micrococcaceae*	*Actinobacteria*	FJ608230	F, L	A	*gambiae, stephensi*		[38, 37]	
Propionibacterium	*Propionibacteria-ceae*	*Actinobacteria*	GQ003306	F, F*	A	*funestus, gambiae*	[17, 36]		
Rhodococcus	*Nocardiaceae*	*Actinobacteria*	AY837749	F	L, A	*arabiensis, stephensi*		[22, 23]	
Bacteroidetes									
Chryseobacterium	*Flavobacteriaceae*	*Flavobacteriia*	HQ591432	F, F*, L	L, P, A	*coustani, funestus, gambiae, stephensi*	[17, 36]	[11, 38, 23]	[38]
Dysgonomonas	*Porphyromonada-ceae*	*Bacteroidia*	FJ608061	F	L	*stephensi*			[38]
Elizabethkingia	*Flavobacteriaceae*	*Flavobacteriia*	EF426434	F*, L	A	*gambiae, stephensi*	[17, 21]	[22, 37]	[38, 27, 32]
Flavobacterium	*Flavobacteriaceae*	*Flavobacteriia*		F, L	A	*albimanus, funestus, gambiae, stephensi*		[19]	[30]
Flexibacteraceae		*Cytophagia*	FJ608195	F	A	*stephensi*			[38]
Myroides	*Flavobacteriaceae*	*Flavobacteriia*	HQ832872	F	L, A	*stephensi*		[23]	
Prevotella	*Prevotellaceae*	*Bacteroidia*	JN867317	F*	A	*gambiae*	[21]		
Sediminibacterium	*Chitinophagaceae*	*Sphingo-bacteriia*	FJ915158	F*	A	*gambiae*	[21]		
Sphingobacterium	*Sphingobacteria-ceae*	*Sphingo-bacteriia*	EF426436	L	P, A	*gambiae*		[35]	
Firmicutes									
Bacillus	*Bacillaceae*	*Bacilli*	AY837746	F, L	L, A	*arabiensis, funestus, gambiae (ss, sl), stephensi*		[11, 38, 22, 24]	[38, 27, 30]
Clostridium	*Clostridiaceae*	*Clostridia*	JN391577	F*	L	*gambiae*	[17]		
Enterococcus	*Enterococcaceae*	*Bacilli*	HQ591441	F	L, A	*funestus, gambiae, stephensi*	[36]	[23]	
Exiguobacterium	*Bacillales Family XII. Incertae Sedis*	*Bacilli*	HQ591439	F	L	*stephensi*		[38, 23]	

Lactobacillus	*Lactobacillaceae*	*Bacilli*	FJ608053	F, F*	L, A	*gambiae, stephensi*	[17]		[38]
Lysinibacillus	*Bacillaceae*	*Bacilli*	GU204964	F	L	*maculipennis, stephensi*		[24]	
Paenibacillus	*Paenibacillaceae*	*Bacilli*	EF426449	F	A	*arabiensis, stephensi*			[38, 22]
Staphylococcus	*Staphylococcaceae*	*Bacilli*	FJ608067	F, F*, L	L, A	*funestus, gambiae, maculipennis, quadrimaculatus, stephensi*	[21, 36]	[25, 38, 40]	[38, 26]
Streptococcus	*Streptococcaceae*	*Bacilli*	FJ608047	F, F*	L, A	*funestus, gambiae, stephensi*	[21, 36]		[38]

Proteobacteria

Acetobacter	*Acetobacteraceae*	*Alpha-proteobacteria*		L	A	*stephensi*			[26]
Achromobacter	*Alcaligenaceae*	*Beta-proteobacteria*	FJ608301	F	A	*stephensi*			[38]
Acidovorax	*Comamonadaceae*	*Beta-proteobacteria*	AY837725	F	A	*arabiensis*			[22]
Acinetobacter	*Moraxellaceae*	*Gamma-proteobacteria*	FJ608267	F, F*, L	L, A	*albimanus, funestus, gambiae, stephensi*	[17, 21, 36]	[19, 38]	[38, 26]
Aeromonas	*Aeromonadaceae*	*Gamma-proteobacteria*	FJ608130	F, F*, L	L, A	*coustani, darlingi, funestus, gambiae, maculipennis, stephensi*	[17, 36]	[19, 38, 23, 24]	[22, 33]
Agrobacterium	*Comamonadaceae*	*Beta-proteobacteria*	FJ607997	L	A	*stephensi*		[38]	[38]
Alcaligenes	*Alcaligenaceae*	*Beta-proteobacteria*	HQ832875	F	A	*funestus, stephensi*		[23]	[30]
Anaplasma	*Anaplasmataceae*	*Alpha-proteobacteria*	AY837739	F	A	*arabiensis*			[22]
Aquabacterium	*Burkholderiales Genera incertae sedis*	*Beta-proteobacteria*		F	A	*gambiae*			[26]
Asaia	*Acetobacteraceae*	*Alpha-proteobacteria*	FN821398	F, F*, L	L, A	*coustani, funestus, gambiae, maculipennis, stephensi*	[21, 36]	[11, 26-28, 37]	[26, 28]
Azoarcus	*Rhodocyclaceae*	*Beta-proteobacteria*	FJ608071	F	L	*stephensi*			[38]
Bordetella	*Alcaligenaceae*	*Beta-proteobacteria*	HQ832874	F	A	*stephensi*		[23]	
Bradyrhizobium	*Bradyrhizobiaceae*	*Alpha-proteobacteria*	AB740924	F*	A	*gambiae*	[21]		
Brevundimonas	*Caulobacteraceae*	*Alpha-proteobacteria*	GU204962	F	L, A	*funestus, stephensi*		[24]	[30]
Burkholderia	*Burkholderiaceae*	*Beta-proteobacteria*	AY391283	F, F*, L	A	*gambiae, stephensi*	[21]		[26, 27]
Buttiauxella	*Enterobacteriaceae*	*Gamma-proteobacteria*		F	A	*darlingi*			[33]
Cedecea	*Enterobacteriaceae*	*Gamma-proteobacteria*	DQ068869	F, F*, L	A	*funestus, gambiae (ss, sl), stephensi*	[21]	[19, 29]	[30]
Citrobacter	*Enterobacteriaceae*	*Gamma-proteobacteria*	FJ608234	F	A	*darlingi, stephensi*		[38]	[33]
Comamonas	*Comamonadaceae*	*Beta-proteobacteria*	EF426440	F, F*	P, A	*dureni, funestus, gambiae, quadrimaculatus, stephensi*	[17, 21]	[38, 35, 39, 40]	[30]

Delftia	*Comamonadaceae*	*Beta-proteobacteria*	EF426438	L	P	*gambiae*		[35]	
Ehrlichia	*Anaplasmataceae*	*Alpha-proteobacteria*		F	A	*arabiensis*			[22]
Enterobacter	*Enterobacteriaceae*	*Gamma-proteobacteria*	HQ832863	F, F*, L	L, A	*albimanus, darlingi, funestus, gambiae (ss, sl), stephensi*	[17]	[11, 38, 23, 30, 31]	[38, 23, 26]
Erwinia	*Enterobacteriaceae*	*Gamma-proteobacteria*	FJ816023	F, L	A	*darlingi, funestus, gambiae*		[37]	[30, 33]
Escherichia-Shigella	*Enterobacteriaceae*	*Gamma-proteobacteria*	FJ608223	F, F*, L	A	*arabiensis, darlingi, funestus, gambiae (ss, sl), stephensi*	[21, 36]	[11, 38, 30]	[30, 33]
Ewingella	*Enterobacteriaceae*	*Gamma-proteobacteria*		L	A	*stephensi*		[25]	
Gluconacetobacter	*Acetobacteraceae*	*Alpha-proteobacteria*	FN814298	F*, L	A	*gambiae*	[21]	[27]	
Gluconobacter	*Acetobacteraceae*	*Alpha-proteobacteria*		F, L	A	*funestus, stephensi*			[26, 30]
Herbaspirillum	*Oxalobacteraceae*	*Beta-proteobacteria*	FJ608162	F, L	A	*gambiae, stephensi*		[11]	[38]
Hydrogenophaga	*Comamonadaceae*	*Beta-proteobacteria*	FJ608063	F, F*	L	*gambiae (ss, sl), stephensi*	[17]		[38, 30]
Ignatzschineria	*Xanthomonada-ceae*	*Gamma-proteobacteria*	FJ608103	F	L	*stephensi*			[38]
Klebsiella	*Enterobacteriaceae*	*Gamma-proteobacteria*	HQ591433	F, F*, L	L, A	*darlingi, funestus, gambiae (ss, sl), stephensi*	[17]	[23, 30, 37, 39]	[38, 30, 33]
Kluyvera	*Enterobacteriaceae*	*Gamma-proteobacteria*		F		*funestus, gambiae*		[19]	[30]
Leminorella	*Enterobacteriaceae*	*Gamma-proteobacteria*	FJ608283	F	A	*stephensi*			[38]
Leptothrix	*Burkholderiales Genera incertae sedis*	*Beta-proteobacteria*	FJ608083	F	L	*stephensi*			[38]
Morganella	*Enterobacteriaceae*	*Gamma-proteobacteria*		F	A	*gambiae sl*			[30]
Methylobacterium	*Methylobacteria-ceae*	*Alpha-proteobacteria*	AB673246	F, F*	A	*funestus, gambiae*	[21, 36]		
Methylophilus	*Methylophilaceae*	*Beta-proteobacteria*	FJ517736	F*	P	*gambiae*	[17]		
Neisseria	*Neisseriaceae*	*Beta-proteobacteria*	JX010905	F*	A	*gambiae*	[21]		
Novosphingobium	*Sphingomonada-ceae*	*Alpha-proteobacteria*	JX222980	F*	A	*gambiae*	[17]		
Pantoea	*Enterobacteriaceae*	*Gamma-proteobacteria*	JF690934	F, L	L, A	*albimanus*, darlingi, funes-tus, gambiae (*) (ss, sl), stephensi (*)*		[11, 19, 24, 35]	[38, 30, 33]
Pelagibacter	*SAR11 cluster* (no family)	*Alpha-proteobacteria*	GQ340243	F*	A	*gambiae*	[17]		
Phenylobacterium	*Caulobacteraceae*	*Alpha-proteobacteria*		F	A	*gambiae*			[26]
Phytobacter	*Enterobacteriaceae*	*Gamma-proteobacteria*		L	A	*gambiae*		[11]	
Porphyrobacter	*Erythrobacteraceae*	*Alpha-proteobacteria*	JQ923889	F*	L	*gambiae*	[17]		

Pseudomonas	*Pseudomonada-ceae*	*Gamma-proteobacteria*	EF426444	F, F*, L	L, P, A	*albimanus, darlingi, dure-ni, funestus, gambiae (ss, sl), maculi-pennis, qua-drimaculatus stephensi*	[17, 21, 36]	[11, 19, 22-24, 29, 35, 38, 39, 40]	[38, 26, 30, 33]
Rahnella	*Enterobacteriaceae*	*Gamma-proteobacteria*	GU204974	F	L	*stephensi*		[24]	
Ralstonia	*Burkholderiaceae*	*Beta-proteobacteria*	AY191852	F*	A	*gambiae*	[21]		
Raoultella	*Enterobacteriaceae*	*Gamma-proteobacteria*	HQ811336	F*	A	*gambiae*	[17]		
Rhizobium	*Rhizobiaceae*	*Alpha-proteobacteria*	DQ814410	F*	L	*gambiae*	[17]		
Salmonella	*Enterobacteriaceae*	*Gamma-proteobacteria*		F		*funestus, gambiae sl*			[30]
Schlegelella	*Comamonadaceae*	*Beta-proteobacteria*	FR774570	F*	A	*gambiae*	[21]		
Serratia	*Enterobacteriaceae*	*Gamma-proteobacteria*	FJ608101	F, F*, L	L, A	*albimanus, dureni, gambiae, maculipennis,q uadrimacula-tus, stephensi*	[17, 21]	[11, 19, 25, 31, 37-40]	[38]
Shewanella	*Shewanellaceae*	*Gamma-proteobacteria*	HQ591421	F	L	*stephensi*		[23]	
Sphingobium	*Sphingomonada-ceae*	*Alpha-proteobacteria*	GU940735	F*	A	*gambiae*	[17]		
Sphingomonas	*Sphingomonada-ceae*	*Alpha-proteobacteria*	GU204960	F, F*, L	L, A	*funestus, gambiae, stephensi*	[21, 36]	[11, 24]	[26]
Stenotrophomonas	*Xanthomonada-ceae*	*Gamma-proteobacteria*	EF426435	F, F*	A	*arabiensis, funestus, gambiae*	[17, 21]	[35]	[22, 30]
Thorsellia	*Enterobacteriaceae*	*Gamma-proteobacteria*	NR_043217	F, F*	L, A	*gambiae, stephensi*	[17]	[38, 22]	[38, 34]
Vibrio	*Vibrio*	*Gamma-proteobacteria*	FJ608116	F	L, A	*arabiensis*		[38, 22]	
Xenorhabdus	*Enterobacteriaceae*	*Gamma-proteobacteria*	FJ608329	F	A	*stephensi*			[38]
Yersinia	*Enterobacteriaceae*	*Gamma-proteobacteria*		F	A	*darlingi*			[33]
Zymobacter	*Halomonadaceae*	*Gamma-proteobacteria*	FR851711	F	A	*funestus, gambiae*	[36]		
Others									
Bacillariophyta (Eukaryota: Diatom)			JQ727029	F*	L	*gambiae*	[17]		
Chlorophyta (green algae)			EF114678	F*	L	*gambiae*	[17]		
Calothrix	*Rivulariaceae*	(no data)	FJ608095	F	L	*stephensi*			[38]
Deinococcus	*Deinococcaceae*	*Deinococci*	FJ608089	F	L	*stephensi*		[38]	[38]
Mycoplasma	*Mycoplasmataceae*	*Mollicutes*	AY837724	F	A	*arabiensis*			[22]
Spiroplasma	*Spiroplasmataceae*	*Mollicutes*	AY837733	F	A	*funestus*			[22]
Cyanobacteria-GpI			HM573452	F*	P	*gambiae*	[17]		
Cyanobacteria-GpIIa			JQ305084	F*	L	*gambiae*	[17]		
Cyanobacteria-GpV			AB245143	F*	L	*gambiae*	[17]		
Fusobacterium	*Fusobacteriaceae*	*Fusobacteriia*	JX548360	F*	A	*gambiae*	[17, 21]		

Table 1. List of bacterial genera associated with *Anopheles* mosquitoes reported in the following studies: [11, 17, 19, and 21-40]. For high-throughput sequencing studies; only genera found to represent at least 1% of the total population in at least one study/condition are listed. Genera are classified by phyla, which are indicated in bold. In column "Conditions", F, F* and L indicate field, semi-natural and laboratory conditions, respectively. In column "Stage", L, P and A indicate larvae, pupae and adults, respectively. Column "Example" shows NCBI accession number of a sequence example for each genus (first hit after BLAST). Columns "Deep seq", "Culture", "Non culture" list studies based on 16S rRNA gene deep sequencing, culture-dependent methods, conventional sequencing (including 16S rRNA gene libraries and DGGE) and gas chromatography, respectively. In the line "*Pantoea*", * refers to what was identified in [19] as *Enterobacter agglomerans*, since then renamed *Pantoea agglomerans*.

Three metagenomics studies were recently carried out using 16S RNA from bacteria found in the *Anopheles* gut [18, 22, 37]. Wang and co-workers examined the microbiota composition throughout the mosquito life cycle, using a laboratory colony of *A. gambiae* mosquitoes (the main vector of malaria in sub-Saharan Africa) reared in semi-natural microcosms in Kenya [18]. The microcosms contained local rainwater and topsoil and were kept outside to allow microbial colonization. Boissière and co-workers investigated the microbiota of adult *A. gambiae* mosquitoes in Cameroon and how these microbiota may be related to *Plasmodium* infection [22]. They collected larvae from the field, reared them to adulthood in the laboratory and monitored the microbiota composition of individual mosquitoes 8 days after infection with *Plasmodium falciparum* sampled directly from gametocytemic patients. Finally, Osei-Poku and co-workers collected adult mosquitoes in Kenya and analysed the microbiota of individual mosquitoes of 8 different species, including 3 species of *Anopheles* (*A. coustani, A. funestus* and *A. gambiae*) [37].

These studies led to 5 main observations. First, the microbiota diversity is high: when defining species as $OTU_{97\%, V1-V3}$[1], Wang et al. detected more than 2,000 species in a pool of 30 adult *A. gambiae* [18]. The highest diversity was registered in larvae and pupae, with an estimate of 4,000-8,000 species in a pool of 30 individuals of each stage. Diversity decreased during adulthood to 2,000-4,000 species upon emergence and dropped further to 600-900 species after a bloodmeal. As all of these high-throughput sequencing studies used bacterial DNA, which is a very stable molecule, an important question is whether these results genuinely reflect the *Anopheles* gut communities or include environmental contaminants. By direct sampling of the larval aquatic environment, Wang et al. indeed showed that the microbial communities differed from those in the larvae, suggesting that – at least in this study – bacteria were able to persist in, if not colonise, the mosquito host (Figure 1A).

Second, this diversity is partially explained by significant diversity within a single mosquito [22, 37], varying from 5 to 71 $OTUs_{97\%, V3}$ per individual (median: 42 $OTUs_{97\%, V3}$) [37]. Diversity is higher than what observed by metagenomics studies in other insects such as the honeybee which hosts 8 dominant species ($OTU_{97\%, V6-V8}$), the estimated species richness within a colony being 9-10 [44], and *Drosophila* where 31 $OTUs_{97\%,V2}$ were observed in a pool of 50 females [45]. Nevertheless, a single $OTU_{97\%, V3}$ represents on average 67% of a mosquito bacterial community and the median mosquito gut species richness is only 17% to that of humans, where an individual hosts 150-300 $OTUs_{99\%, whole\ 16S}$ [4, 37].

Third, another component of the observed biodiversity lies within the high variability in microbial communities between individuals. This is quantified by calculating the UniFrac distance between mosquitoes. UniFrac varies from 0 when two mosquitoes have exactly the same microbiota to 1 when there is no phylogenetic overlap between the microbiota of two mosquitoes. The mean UniFrac distance between individuals is high, 0.72 and 0.74 in *A. funestus* and *A. gambiae*, respectively [37]. This variability is almost as high between *Anopheles* individuals of the same species as between mosquitoes of different species and/or genera [37].

1 As not all the studies were based on the same region of 16S or the same threshold of differences, we refer here to OTU97%, V1-V3 as the operational taxonomic unit with more than 97% identity in the V1-V3 regions of 16S rRNA gene sequences.

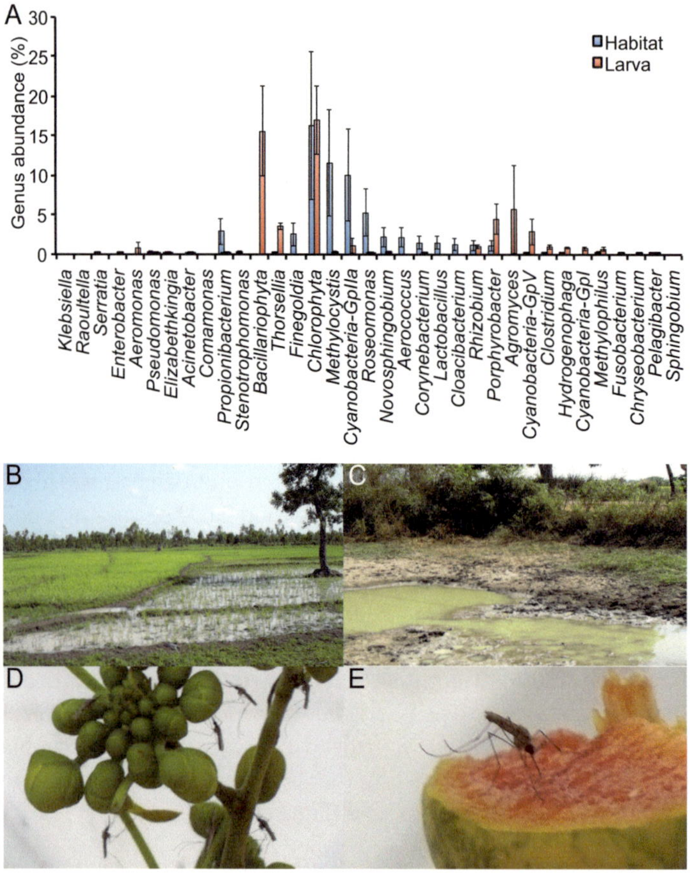

Figure 1. Anopheles microbiota and environment. A: Abundance of bacterial genera in larval habitat and in larvae found in [17]. B, C: Natural habitat of *A. gambiae*. Permanent habitats such as rice fields (B) are colonized with M molecular form of *A. gambiae* and temporary water ponds (C) with S plus M forms (mostly S). D, E: Mosquitoes feeding on *Senna siamea* flowers (D) and papaya fruit-*Carica papaya* (E).

Fourth, the microbiota composition partly reflects the larval origin but bacteria acquired during adulthood may affect the microbiota composition to the extent that the geographic origin cannot be traced. Osei-Poku and co-workers did not observe any correlation between geographic location and microbiota composition in their Kenyan adult collections [37]. This is in sharp contrast to the Boissière et al. observations that microbiota were more similar between adults derived from larvae breading in the same pond than between adults derived from larvae of different geographic origins [22]. These results are, however, not contradictory if we consider differences in experimental designs of these studies. The latter study focused almost exclusively on bacteria transmitted from larvae to adults since larvae from the field were sampled and adults where fed with sterile sugar upon emergence, while the former study additionally sampled bacteria acquired during adulthood, and related to presumably diverse adult life histories. Together, these studies suggest that the acquisition of new strains of bacteria during adulthood can potentially increase the inter-individual diversity and mask similarities linked to the larval origin. However, this hypothesis requires further investigation, as mosquitoes from the two geographical origins reported in the Boissière et al. study belonged to the M and S molecular forms of *A. gambiae*, respectively, which are thought to be emerging species breading in different types of aquatic environments, i.e. permanent and temporary (rain-dependent) water pools, respectively (see Figures 1B, C) [22]. These environments are likely to contain different microbiota that largely determine the mosquito enterotype. Additionally, genetic differences between the two molecular forms may also partly account for the observed differences in microbiota composition.

Fifth, when considering the *Plasmodium* infection status, Boissière and co-workers found that the abundance of bacteria of the *Enterobacteriaceae* family was higher in *P. falciparum*-infected mosquitoes than in non-infected mosquitoes fed with the same infectious bloodmeal. This observation may indicate that *Enterobacteriaceae* favour *P. falciparum* infection or, conversely, that *P. falciparum* infection influences the composition of microbiota to the benefit of *Enterobacteriaceae* [22].

3. Bacterial colonization of mosquitoes

In addition to metagenomics studies, factors determining the composition of the adult mosquito microbiota were also investigated by conventional methods. Evidence that mosquitoes are colonized by bacteria both found in the environment and transmitted between individuals or developmental stages was revealed, but the relative contribution of these transmission routes to the microbiota diversity remains largely unknown. Laboratory studies investigated the vertical (from parent to progeny), transstadial (between developmental stages) and horizontal (between individuals of the same stage) transmission of specific bacterial strains. In particular, horizontal transfer of *Asaia sp.* is found to occur both by feeding and by mating (from male to female), but it is yet unclear whether vertical transmission occurs via egg spreading or by contamination of the environment during egg-laying [27]. Transstadial transmission of *Pantoea stewartii* is shown to occur from larvae to pupae but not from pupae to adults [36]. This is likely due to gut sterilization during metamorphosis; bacterial counts are high in the gut of fourth instar larvae, decrease after final larval defecation, increase again during pupal development and are very low or null in newly emerged adults [46].

Two mechanisms are thought to be involved in gut sterilization during adult emergence [46]. Firstly, bacteria are enclosed in the degenerated larval midgut, the meconium, enveloped by 2 meconial peritrophic matrixes and egested during molting. Secondly, during emergence, adults ingest exuvial liquid that has bactericidal properties. Nevertheless, sterilisation is thought to be incomplete, thus allowing some direct transmission from pupae to adults [46] and being responsible for the contribution of the larval/pupal breading sites to the adult microbiota, as mentioned earlier [22]. Moreover, emerging adults have been reported to ingest water and uptake bacteria during or shortly after emergence, with colonization efficiencies depending on the bacterial strains, e.g. *Elizabethkingia anophelis* (previously thought to be *E.*

meningoseptica) is more successful than *Pantoea stewartii* [33, 36]. During adulthood, mosquitoes take sugar-meals of floral and extra-floral nectar, sap, ripe fruit and honeydew (Figure 1D, E) [47-49]. These meals potentially provide new bacterial species and are likely to affect the relative growth of existing species or strains depending on their properties, such as the concentration of each sugar type, typically glucose, fructose or gulose [50]. This might well be the case for *Asaia* and *Gluconacetobacter*, two genera usually found in flowers, and which have been identified as part of the adult *Anopheles* microbiota [22, 27].

The *Anopheles* tissue specificity of *Asaia sp.* was studied using a bacterial strain expressing GFP (green fluorescent protein) [27]. *Asaia* was found in the female gut and salivary glands, two tissues of particular interest to vector biology, but also in the male reproductive tract and the larval gut, which are potentially important tissues for the bacterial spread [27]. The microbiome of *Anopheles* other tissues than the gut has not yet been characterized. Interestingly, *Wolbachia sp.*, a maternally transmitted intracellular bacterium able to colonize multiple tissues in other insects, has not yet been found in any *Anopheles* species. This is of particular interest, as this endosymbiont colonizes around half of the insect species including several *Culex* and *Aedes* mosquito species [51]. Reasons for the apparent incompatibility between *Anopheles* and *Wolbachia* are unknown, but the generation of *Wolbachia*-infected *Anopheles* colonies is currently being pursued. Laboratory infection has been achieved for *Ae. aegypti* [52, 53], where *Wolbachia* is a promising candidate for reducing the vector competence (see below). To our knowledge, no endosymbiont has been described in *Anopheles* to date.

Non-bacterial members of the *Anopheles* microbiota are poorly understood. Such studies are of special interest, as these microorganisms can potentially interact directly with the bacterial microbiota as well as the human pathogens and are likely to affect the mosquito physiology. An initial study, based on sequencing a 18S-library, identified 6 fungal clones related to *Candida sp., Hanseniaspora uvarum, Pichia sp., Wallemia sebi, Wickerhamomyces anomalus* and uncultured fungi in laboratory-reared *A. stephensi* [54]. *W. anomalus* is also found in wild and laboratory-reared *A. gambiae* [55]. TEM observation of mosquito tissues revealed the presence of yeasts in the female midgut and of actively dividing yeasts in the male gonoduct of *A. stephensi* [54, 55].

4. Impact of microbiota on *Anopheles* physiology and pathogen transmission

The studies reviewed above suggest that *Anopheles* mosquitoes do not host any particular obligate symbiont. However, bacteria as a whole appear to be essential for mosquito physiology. In particular, it has not been possible to date to maintain *Anopheles* colonies on conventional laboratory diet in axenic conditions. In addition, *A. stephensi* larval development is slowed down in the presence of antibiotics and putatively blocked at the 3rd or 4th instar, but an antibiotic-resistant strain of *Asaia* is sufficient to revert this effect [56]. Although the mechanism involved in this dependence is unknown, several lines of experimental evidence point to the important nutritional role of gut commensals. First, the development of aseptic

A. stephensi mosquitoes was achieved from sterilized eggs to adults in a custom aseptic medium [57], although no mention is made about adult fertility under these conditions. Second, a delay in the development was also observed in *Drosophila melanogaster* raised in axenic conditions under protein deprivation, which was rescued by the addition of live *Lactobacillus plantarum* in the fly medium [58]. *L. plantarum* was shown to promote larval growth under poor dietary conditions by enhancing nutrient sensing in a TOR-dependent manner, thus acting on ecdysone and insulin-like-peptide pathways [58]. Third, larval mortality was reported in the clothing louse deprived of its bacterial symbionts and can be avoided by supplementing the blood with B-vitamins (ß-biotin, pantothenate and nicotinic acid) [59]. The *Anopheles* microbiota may also participate in metabolism, as adult mosquitoes fed with radiolabelled-Glycine *Pseudomonas* displayed radioactive signal throughout their body [40]. Interestingly, *Plasmodium* oocysts and sporozoites developing in these mosquitoes also contained radioactive compounds, suggesting that bacteria also participate in parasite nutrition [40].

Anopheles females appear to also sense bacterial presence in the water, which influences oviposition in a bacterial strain dependent manner [60]. The underlying stimuli are not known but they are likely semiochemicals, i.e. messenger molecules produced by bacteria [60]. A principal component analysis of volatiles emitted by 17 bacterial strains, including 6 oviposition-inducing strains, failed to identify compounds shared between all oviposition-inducing bacterial strains, suggesting that such semiochemicals are acting as cocktails [60].

An aspect of the *Anopheles* microbiota that received great interest recently is the colonisation resistance effect towards *Plasmodium* infection, as depicted in Figure 2. First, bacterial growth after a bloodmeal is reported to trigger an immune response via the Immune-deficiency (Imd) pathway, which causes synthesis of antimicrobial peptides and other immune effectors [2]. These effectors target bacterial populations in the mosquito midgut and exert antiparasitic effects. Second, an *Enterobacter* strain (*EspZ*) isolated from wild *A. arabiensis* mosquitoes is shown to directly affect *Plasmodium* development in the mosquito gut via elevated synthesis of ROS (reactive oxygen species) [1]. Third, microbiota-dependent immune priming is reported upon *Plasmodium* infection. This effect protects mosquitoes from subsequent *Plasmodium* infections and is likely to be mediated by hemocyte differentiation [3].

As mentioned above, *Anopheles* mosquitoes are also vectors of filarial worms and ONNV (anophelines are also secondary vectors of West Nile virus). The effect of gut microbiota on infection with these pathogens has not been thoroughly investigated to date, but feeding *A. quadriannulatus* with an antibiotic/antimycotic mixture is shown to increase *Brugia malayi* infection [61]. In *Ae. aegypti*, antibiotic treatment increases the susceptibility of mosquitoes to Dengue virus via a decrease in antimicrobial gene transcription [53]. This can be reverted by addition of bacterial strains such as *Proteus sp.* and *Paenibacillus sp.* [62]. The role of *Anopheles* microbiota upon viral infections is still unclear, but our unpublished observations suggest that antibiotic treatment of *A. gambiae* increases significantly the prevalence of infection with ONNV.

Vertically-transmitted *Wolbachia* endosymbionts are under special focus as promising candidates to stop pathogen transmission. Research in this field has advanced in *Ae. aegypti*, where stable infections of *Wolbachia* strains have been established in laboratory colonies [52, 53]. The

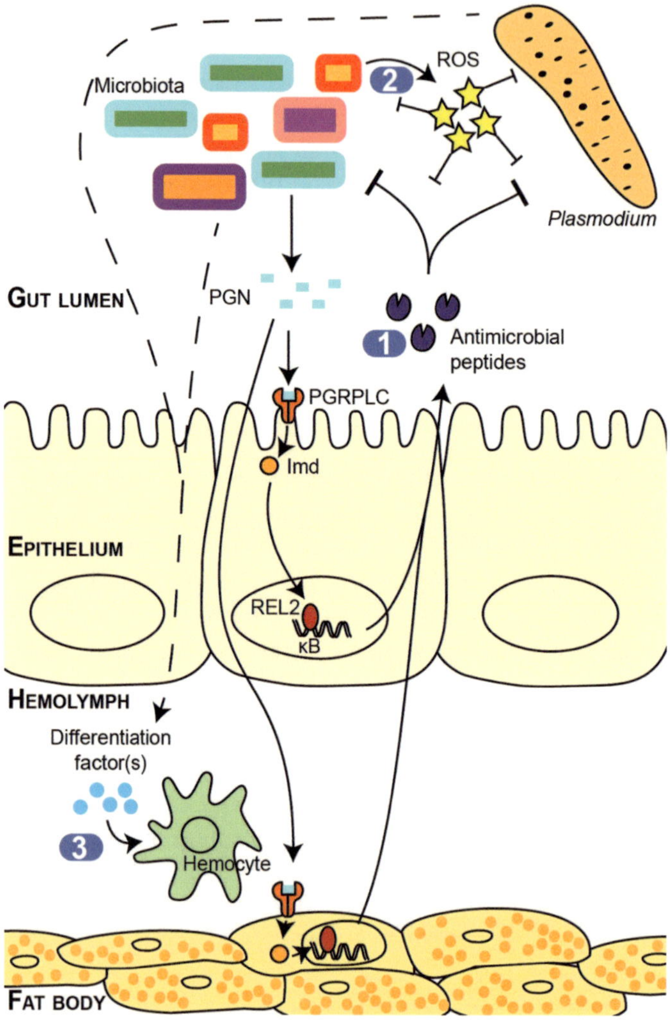

Figure 2. Mechanisms of colonization resistance conferred by *Anopheles* microbiota against *Plasmodium* infection. 1 — Direct effect via synthesis of ROS by the *Enterobacter EspZ* strain [1]. 2 — Indirect effect via induction of NF-κB antibacterial responses that have antiparasitic effects [2]. This is likely to be the most general mechanism. 3 — Induction of hemocyte differentiation by unknown soluble hemolymph factors during *Plasmodium* infection, which has a priming effect against asubsequent *Plasmodium* infection [3].

fast growing wMelPop strain of *Wolbachia* halves the mosquito lifespan, thus potentially affecting the capacity of mosquitoes to transmit pathogens with long extrinsic incubation periods [52]. It also induces a constitutively elevated immune response that negatively impacts on the infection prevalence and intensity of *Brugia pahangi* microfilariae, Chikungunya and Dengue viruses and the avian parasite *Plasmodium gallinaceum* [15, 17]. wAlbB and wMel, which naturally infect the Asian tiger mosquito *Aedes albopictus* and *D. melanogaster*, respectively, also render *Aedes* mosquitoes resistant to Dengue virus when introduced into laboratory populations [16, 63, 64]. Moreover, wMel is shown to successfully spread into wild *Ae. aegypti* populations in North-Eastern Australia [65] and is a strong candidate for Dengue biocontrol. When injected into *Anopheles* mosquitoes, *Wolbachia* seems to positively or negatively impact on *Plasmodium* infection depending on the *Wolbachia/Plasmodium* strain/species combination [66-68].

The immune system of *Anopheles* is known to control the microbiota population, by both resistance and tolerance mechanisms. On the one hand, the Imd pathway is shown to control the midgut bacterial numbers, especially after a bloodmeal [2], together with the production of ROS [21]. The melanization reaction might also contribute to limiting the bacterial numbers, as shown in the hindgut of the silkworm *Bombyx mori* [69]. On the other hand, induction of the Duox-IMPer (Dual oxidase - Immunomodulatory peroxidase) pathway after a bloodmeal leads to the formation of a dityrosine-linked mucus layer in the space between the peritrophic membrane and the midgut epithelium that reduces the permeability to immune elicitors. This tolerance mechanism leads to increased bacterial and *Plasmodium* loads [21]. Interestingly, such protection from oxidative stress is also identified in *Ae. aegypti*, where blood heme induces a protein kinase C-dependent mechanism leading to decreased ROS production and bacterial proliferation [70]. In *Drosophila*, several negative regulators of the Imd pathway are involved in tolerance to gut bacteria, but equivalent tolerance mechanisms have not yet been described in *Anopheles*. In particular, PGRP-LB and PGRP-SC1A/B degrade peptidoglycan into non-immunogenic fragments and Pirk downregulates the activity of the PGRP-LC and PGRP-LE receptors [71-76]. Orthologs of these regulators PGRPs, but not of Pirk, are present in *Anopheles* [77, 78].

In several insect species, microbiota are shown to also impact on host behavior. Notably, *Drosophila* mating preference is influenced by the microbiota composition [79]. *Klebsiella oxytoca* is proposed as a probiotic able to rescue the loss of copulatory performance that follows male sterilization by irradiation in medfly (*Ceratitis capitata*), by restoring the *Klebsiella/Pseudomonas* ratio to its normal levels [80]. In termites, a Rifampicin treatment is shown to reduce the queen oviposition rate and to decrease longevity and fecundity of termite reproductives [81]. As *Anopheles* mosquitoes are able to sense the presence of bacteria in water as well as on human skin and modulate their oviposition rate and feeding behavior accordingly [60, 82], the microbiota composition could also influence the mosquito social and/or reproductive behavior and feeding preference. This may prove to be of particular importance to vector control.

5. Potential exploitations to reduce *Anopheles* vector competence

Reduction of the *Anopheles* competence to transmit human pathogens, especially malaria, will have great implications on public health. Any perspective of reducing vector competence should affect at least one of the parameters of the Ross-McDonald model of disease transmission [83]. These parameters include the mosquito-to-man ratio, the mosquito biting rate, the probability of successful man-to-mosquito and mosquito-to-man transmission, the mosquito daily survival probability, the days needed for the parasite in the mosquito to become infective and the daily rate at which humans become non-infectious to mosquitoes. From studies carried out to date and reviewed in preceding sections, it is evident that the mosquito microbiota can potentially affect most of these parameters except those referring only to disease progression in the vertebrate host. The most important of these parameters are mosquito longevity, feeding behavior and capacity to support pathogen development and/or replication.

A direct way to reduce vector competence using our current knowledge of the *Anopheles* microbiota would be to use bacterial strains that are naturally incompatible with pathogen development and/or replication. Potential candidates are either natural microbiota such as the EspZ strain of *Enterobacter* that causes resistance to *Plasmodium* [1] or artificially introduced bacteria such as *Wolbachia,* which apparently induce a wide spectrum of resistance to human pathogens [15]. The great advantage of the latter is its ability to spread into populations by manipulating insect reproduction in several ways. In particular, *Wolbachia* induces death of young embryos laid by *Wolbachia*-free females mated with infected males; *Wolbachia*-infected females are always fertile independently of the male infection status [84]. This so-called cytoplasmic incompatibility confers a reproductive benefit to *Wolbachia*-infected females and leads to propagation of *Wolbachia* even if it bears small fitness cost to the host, including reduced fecundity (discussed in [85, 86]). The challenge of this approach is the fact that *Wolbachia* and *Anopheles* seem to be incompatible in nature and introduction of the endosymbiont in laboratory colonies of *Anopheles* has not yet been achieved. Screening of *Wolbachia* strains able to infect the *Anopheles* reproductive tissues, when cultured *ex vivo,* has been reported [87]. Alternatively, preadaptation of *Wolbachia* strains by long-term culturing in mosquito cell lines has been suggested as a strategy to infect new hosts, as shown successfully for *Aedes* [52, 88]. As previously reported in *Aedes* [15-17], *Wolbachia* might impact both on mosquito longevity and successful development and/or replication of all three taxa of *Anopheles*-borne pathogens, i.e. *Plasmodium,* viruses and nematodes.

An alternative approach is paratransgenesis, the introduction of genetically modified bacteria into the vector, which would confer resistance to pathogens. *Pantoea agglomerans,* a natural *Anopheles* symbiont, is a candidate for this approach and has been successfully engineered to express and secrete proteins that either inhibit midgut invasion by *Plasmodium,* such as $[EPIP]_4$ (*Plasmodium* enolase-plasminogen interaction peptide) that competes with *Plasmodium* EPIP for plasminogen binding, or by directly targeting the parasite, such as the scorpion-derived antiplasmodial scorpine [89, 90]. Green fluorescent protein (GFP)-tagged *P. agglomerans* persists and grows in the *Anopheles* gut, while transgenic *P. agglomerans* confers resistance against *P. falciparum* infection in both *A. stephensi* and *A. gambiae* without affecting the mosquito lifespan [90]. Applicability to more than one mosquito species is particularly advantageous for a transmission blocking approach. *Asaia* has also been proposed as a candidate for paratransgenesis, as it is quite frequent in *Anopheles* microbiota and can be successfully transformed [27]. Interestingly, this genus has been found in all of the 30 individuals assessed in the metagenomics study of Boissière et al. suggesting that it can easily spread into field populations [22]. *Asaia* can be transmitted both horizontally and vertically presenting an additional advantage for the spread of a transgenic strain into mosquito populations [27]. The introduction of such microbiota into mosquito populations could be achieved by using baiting stations, i.e. clay jars containing cotton balls soaked with sugar and bacteria, around malaria endemic villages, but this approach requires further investigation [90].

Finally, transmission-blocking interventions could involve drugs or other interventions that would impact on the microbiota, thus affecting mosquito homeostasis and efficiency of pathogen development. For example, the effects of antibiotics in the human blood could significantly impact the mosquito microbiota upon blood feeding, indirectly influencing mosquito physiology and infection with pathogens. Depending on its spectrum, an antibiotic could influence the microbiota composition and thus have a positive or negative impact on pathogen development and/or replication.

6. Conclusion

Recent high-throughput sequencing studies of the *Anopheles* microbiota have revealed the extent of the microbiota diversity, mostly in field or semi-natural conditions. A diverse range of bacteria is able to colonize the *Anopheles* gut, and there is a vast diversity of microbiota between mosquitoes. To some extent, this diversity needs to be considered at the bacterial strain level, as different strains of one species may have diverse effects on the mosquito physiology and other microbes of the gut ecosystem. Although bacteria may be the most abundant and important members of the gut microbiota, characterization of the viral, fungal and protist communities could prove insightful into the understanding of the homeostasis of this complex biological system (e.g. phage predation is thought to regulate bacterial populations [91]) and its effects on pathogen transmission. An important question that may arise from further studies is whether variability and/or discrepancies in experimental findings about the interactions between mosquitoes and pathogens could be attributed to differences in the microbiota between laboratories. Toward exploiting the knowledge on *Anopheles* microbiota to reduce vector competence, research is currently at its infancy, but some bacteria such as *Pantoea* and *Asaia* already emerge as promising candidates of paratransgenesis. The use of *Wolbachia* to reduce *Aedes* vectorial capacity and fitness may be of particular importance, if this technology can be effectively transferred to *Anopheles*. Finally, the possibility to use drugs such as antibiotics to target specific mosquito microbiota and affect vector competence or fitness is a new concept that merits further investigation.

Acknowledgements

We thank Jiannong Xu, Jewelna Osei-Poku, Anne Boissière and Isabelle Morlais for providing example sequences of some of the bacterial genera shown in Table 1 and Thierry Lefèvre for helping with mosquito pictures presented in Figure 1.

Author details

Mathilde Gendrin and George K. Christophides*

*Address all correspondence to: g.christophides@imperial.ac.uk

Department of Life Sciences, Imperial College London, UK

References

[1] Cirimotich CM, Dong Y, Clayton AM, Sandiford SL, Souza-Neto JA, Mulenga M, et al. Natural microbe-mediated refractoriness to *Plasmodium* infection in *Anopheles gambiae*. Science. 2011 May 13;332(6031):855-8.

[2] Meister S, Agianian B, Turlure F, Relogio A, Morlais I, Kafatos FC, et al. *Anopheles gambiae* PGRPLC-mediated defense against bacteria modulates infections with malaria parasites. PLoS pathogens. 2009 Aug;5(8):e1000542. DOI: 10.1371/journal.ppat.1000542.g006

[3] Rodrigues J, Brayner FA, Alves LC, Dixit R, Barillas-Mury C. Hemocyte differentiation mediates innate immune memory in *Anopheles gambiae* mosquitoes. Science. 2010 Sep 10;329(5997):1353-5.

[4] Eckburg PB, Bik EM, Bernstein CN, Purdom E, Dethlefsen L, Sargent M, et al. Diversity of the human intestinal microbial flora. Science. 2005 Jun 10;308(5728):1635-8.

[5] Dethlefsen L, McFall-Ngai M, Relman DA. An ecological and evolutionary perspective on human-microbe mutualism and disease. Nature. 2007 Oct 18;449(7164):811-8.

[6] Bouskra D, Brezillon C, Berard M, Werts C, Varona R, Boneca IG, et al. Lymphoid tissue genesis induced by commensals through NOD1 regulates intestinal homeostasis. Nature. 2008 Nov 27;456(7221):507-10.

[7] Stecher B, Hardt WD. Mechanisms controlling pathogen colonization of the gut. Current opinion in microbiology. 2011 Feb;14(1):82-91.

[8] Ryu JH, Kim SH, Lee HY, Bai JY, Nam YD, Bae JW, et al. Innate immune homeostasis by the homeobox gene caudal and commensal-gut mutualism in *Drosophila*. Science. 2008 Feb 8;319(5864):777-82.

[9] Saha S, Jing X, Park SY, Wang S, Li X, Gupta D, et al. Peptidoglycan recognition proteins protect mice from experimental colitis by promoting normal gut flora and preventing induction of interferon-gamma. Cell host & microbe. 2010 Aug 19;8(2): 147-62.

[10] Yassine H, Osta MA. *Anopheles gambiae* innate immunity. Cell Microbiol. 2010 Jan; 12(1):1-9.

[11] Manguin S, Bangs MJ, Pothikasikorn J, Chareonviriyaphap T. Review on global co-transmission of human *Plasmodium* species and *Wuchereria bancrofti* by *Anopheles* mosquitoes. Infection, genetics and evolution : journal of molecular epidemiology and evolutionary genetics in infectious diseases. 2010 Mar;10(2):159-77.

[12] Brault AC, Foy BD, Myles KM, Kelly CL, Higgs S, Weaver SC, et al. Infection patterns of O'nyong nyong virus in the malaria-transmitting mosquito, *Anopheles gambiae*. Insect Mol Biol. 2004 Dec;13(6):625-35.

[13] Waldock J, Olson KE, Christophides GK. *Anopheles gambiae* antiviral immune response to systemic O'nyong-nyong infection. PLoS neglected tropical diseases. 2012;6(3):e1565. DOI: 10.1371/journal.pntd.0001565.

[14] Dong Y, Manfredini F, Dimopoulos G. Implication of the mosquito midgut microbiota in the defense against malaria parasites. PLoS pathogens. 2009 May;5(5):e1000423. DOI: 10.1371/journal.ppat.1000423.

[15] Moreira LA, Iturbe-Ormaetxe I, Jeffery JA, Lu G, Pyke AT, Hedges LM, et al. A *Wolbachia* symbiont in *Aedes aegypti* limits infection with dengue, Chikungunya, and *Plasmodium*. Cell. 2009 Dec 24;139(7):1268-78.

[16] Bian G, Xu Y, Lu P, Xie Y, Xi Z. The endosymbiotic bacterium *Wolbachia* induces resistance to dengue virus in *Aedes aegypti*. PLoS pathogens. 2010;6(4):e1000833. DOI: 10.1371/journal.ppat.1000833.g006.

[17] Kambris Z, Cook PE, Phuc HK, Sinkins SP. Immune activation by life-shortening *Wolbachia* and reduced filarial competence in mosquitoes. Science. 2009 Oct 2;326(5949):134-6.

[18] Wang Y, Gilbreath TM, 3rd, Kukutla P, Yan G, Xu J. Dynamic gut microbiome across life history of the malaria mosquito *Anopheles gambiae* in Kenya. PloS one. 2011;6(9):e24767. DOI: 10.1371/journal.pone.0024767.

[19] Muller GC, Beier JC, Traore SF, Toure MB, Traore MM, Bah S, et al. Field experiments of *Anopheles gambiae* attraction to local fruits/seedpods and flowering plants in Mali to optimize strategies for malaria vector control in Africa using attractive toxic sugar bait methods. Malaria journal. 2010;9:262.

[20] Pumpuni CB, Demaio J, Kent M, Davis JR, Beier JC. Bacterial population dynamics in three anopheline species: the impact on *Plasmodium* sporogonic development. The American journal of tropical medicine and hygiene. 1996 Feb;54(2):214-8.

[21] Kumar S, Molina-Cruz A, Gupta L, Rodrigues J, Barillas-Mury C. A peroxidase/dual oxidase system modulates midgut epithelial immunity in *Anopheles gambiae*. Science. 2010 Mar 26;327(5973):1644-8.

[22] Boissiere A, Tchioffo MT, Bachar D, Abate L, Marie A, Nsango SE, et al. Midgut microbiota of the malaria mosquito vector *Anopheles gambiae* and interactions with *Plasmodium falciparum* infection. PLoS pathogens. 2012 May;8(5):e1002742. DOI: 10.1371/journal.ppat.1002742.

[23] Lindh JM, Terenius O, Faye I. 16S rRNA gene-based identification of midgut bacteria from field-caught *Anopheles gambiae sensu lato* and *A. funestus* mosquitoes reveals new species related to known insect symbionts. Applied and environmental microbiology. 2005 Nov;71(11):7217-23.

[24] Chavshin AR, Oshaghi MA, Vatandoost H, Pourmand MR, Raeisi A, Enayati AA, et al. Identification of bacterial microflora in the midgut of the larvae and adult of wild caught *Anopheles stephensi*: a step toward finding suitable paratransgenesis candidates. Acta tropica. 2012 Feb;121(2):129-34.

[25] Dinparast Djadid N, Jazayeri H, Raz A, Favia G, Ricci I, Zakeri S. Identification of the midgut microbiota of *An. stephensi* and *An. maculipennis* for their application as a paratransgenic tool against malaria. PloS one. 2011;6(12):e28484. DOI: 10.1371/journal.pone.0028484.

[26] Pumpuni CB, Beier MS, Nataro JP, Guers LD, Davis JR. *Plasmodium falciparum*: inhibition of sporogonic development in *Anopheles stephensi* by gram-negative bacteria. Experimental parasitology. 1993 Sep;77(2):195-9.

[27] Favia G, Ricci I, Damiani C, Raddadi N, Crotti E, Marzorati M, et al. Bacteria of the genus *Asaia* stably associate with *Anopheles stephensi*, an Asian malarial mosquito vector. Proceedings of the National Academy of Sciences of the United States of America. 2007 May 22;104(21):9047-51.

[28] Chouaia B, Rossi P, Montagna M, Ricci I, Crotti E, Damiani C, et al. Molecular evidence for multiple infections as revealed by typing of *Asaia* bacterial symbionts of four mosquito species. Applied and environmental microbiology. 2010 Nov;76(22):7444-50.

[29] Damiani C, Ricci I, Crotti E, Rossi P, Rizzi A, Scuppa P, et al. Mosquito-bacteria symbiosis: the case of *Anopheles gambiae* and *Asaia*. Microbial ecology. 2010 Oct;60(3):644-54.

[30] Noden BH, Vaughan JA, Pumpuni CB, Beier JC. Mosquito ingestion of antibodies against mosquito midgut microbiota improves conversion of ookinetes to oocysts for *Plasmodium falciparum*, but not *P. yoelii*. Parasitology international. 2011 Dec;60(4):440-6.

[31] Straif SC, Mbogo CN, Toure AM, Walker ED, Kaufman M, Toure YT, et al. Midgut bacteria in *Anopheles gambiae* and *An. funestus* (*Diptera*: *Culicidae*) from Kenya and Mali. Journal of medical entomology. 1998 May;35(3):222-6.

[32] Gonzalez-Ceron L, Santillan F, Rodriguez MH, Mendez D, Hernandez-Avila JE. Bacteria in midguts of field-collected *Anopheles albimanus* block *Plasmodium vivax* sporogonic development. Journal of medical entomology. 2003 May;40(3):371-4.

[33] Kampfer P, Matthews H, Glaeser SP, Martin K, Lodders N, Faye I. *Elizabethkingia anophelis sp. nov.*, isolated from the midgut of the mosquito *Anopheles gambiae*. Int J Syst Evol Microbiol. 2011 Nov;61(Pt 11):2670-5.

[34] Terenius O, de Oliveira CD, Pinheiro WD, Tadei WP, James AA, Marinotti O. 16S rRNA gene sequences from bacteria associated with adult *Anopheles darlingi* (*Diptera: Culicidae*) mosquitoes. Journal of medical entomology. 2008 Jan;45(1):172-5.

[35] Briones AM, Shililu J, Githure J, Novak R, Raskin L. *Thorsellia anophelis* is the dominant bacterium in a Kenyan population of adult *Anopheles gambiae* mosquitoes. The ISME journal. 2008 Jan;2(1):74-82.

[36] Lindh JM, Borg-Karlson AK, Faye I. Transstadial and horizontal transfer of bacteria within a colony of *Anopheles gambiae* (Diptera: Culicidae) and oviposition response to bacteria-containing water. Acta tropica. 008 Sep;107(3):242-50.

[37] Osei-Poku J, Mbogo CM, Palmer WJ, Jiggins FM. Deep sequencing reveals extensive variation in the gut microbiota of wild mosquitoes from Kenya. Molecular ecology. 2012 Sep 18. DOI: 10.1111/j.1365-294X.2012.05759.x.

[38] Kajla MK, Andreeva O, Gilbreath TM, 3rd, Paskewitz SM. Characterization of expression, activity and role in antibacterial immunity of *Anopheles gambiae* lysozyme c-1. Comparative biochemistry and physiology Part B, Biochemistry & molecular biology. 2010 Feb;155(2):201-9.

[39] Rani A, Sharma A, Rajagopal R, Adak T, Bhatnagar RK. Bacterial diversity analysis of larvae and adult midgut microflora using culture-dependent and culture-independent methods in lab-reared and field-collected *Anopheles stephensi*-an Asian malarial vector. BMC Microbiol. 2009;9:96.

[40] Jadin J. [Role of bacteria in the digestive tube of insects, vectors of plasmodidae and trypanosomidae]. Annales des sociétés belges de médecine tropicale, de parasitologie, et de mycologie. 1967;47(4):331-42.

[41] Jadin J, Vincke IH, Dunjic A, Delville JP, Wery M, Bafort J, et al. [Role of *Pseudomonas* in the sporogenesis of the hematozoon of malaria in the mosquito]. Bulletin de la Société de pathologie exotique et de ses filiales. 1966 Jul-Aug;59(4):514-25.

[42] Aksoy S. *Wigglesworthia gen. nov.* and *Wigglesworthia glossinidia sp. nov.*, taxa consisting of the mycetocyte-associated, primary endosymbionts of tsetse flies. International journal of systematic bacteriology. 1995 Oct;45(4):848-51.

[43] Kirkness EF, Haas BJ, Sun W, Braig HR, Perotti MA, Clark JM, et al. Genome sequences of the human body louse and its primary endosymbiont provide insights into the

permanent parasitic lifestyle. Proceedings of the National Academy of Sciences of the United States of America. 2010 Jul 6;107(27):12168-73.

[44] Moran NA, Hansen AK, Powell JE, Sabree ZL. Distinctive gut microbiota of honey bees assessed using deep sampling from individual worker bees. PloS one. 2012;7(4):e36393. DOI: 10.1371/journal.pone.0036393.

[45] Wong CN, Ng P, Douglas AE. Low-diversity bacterial community in the gut of the fruitfly *Drosophila melanogaster*. Environmental microbiology. 2011 Jul;13(7):1889-900.

[46] Moll RM, Romoser WS, Modrzakowski MC, Moncayo AC, Lerdthusnee K. Meconial peritrophic membranes and the fate of midgut bacteria during mosquito (Diptera: Culicidae) metamorphosis. Journal of medical entomology. 2001 Jan;38(1):29-32.

[47] Gary RE, Jr., Foster WA. *Anopheles gambiae* feeding and survival on honeydew and extra-floral nectar of peridomestic plants. Medical and veterinary entomology. 2004 Jun;18(2):102-7.

[48] Muller G, Schlein Y. Plant tissues: the frugal diet of mosquitoes in adverse conditions. Medical and veterinary entomology. 2005 Dec;19(4):413-22.

[49] Gouagna LC, Poueme RS, Dabire KR, Ouedraogo JB, Fontenille D, Simard F. Patterns of sugar feeding and host plant preferences in adult males of *An. gambiae* (Diptera: Culicidae). Journal of vector ecology : journal of the Society for Vector Ecology. 2010 Dec;35(2):267-76.

[50] Manda H, Gouagna LC, Foster WA, Jackson RR, Beier JC, Githure JI, et al. Effect of discriminative plant-sugar feeding on the survival and fecundity of *Anopheles gambiae*. Malaria journal. 2007;6:113.

[51] Wiwatanaratanabutr I. Geographic distribution of *Wolbachia* infection in mosquitoes from Thailand. Journal of invertebrate pathology. 2012 May 23. DOI: 10.1016/j.jip.2012.04.010.

[52] McMeniman CJ, Lane RV, Cass BN, Fong AW, Sidhu M, Wang YF, et al. Stable introduction of a life-shortening *Wolbachia* infection into the mosquito *Aedes aegypti*. Science. 2009 Jan 2;323(5910):141-4.

[53] Xi Z, Ramirez JL, Dimopoulos G. The *Aedes aegypti* toll pathway controls dengue virus infection. PLoS pathogens. 2008 Jul;4(7):e1000098. http://www.ncbi.nlm.nih.gov/entrez/query.fcgi?cmd=Retrieve&db=PubMed&dopt=Citation&list_uids=18604274.

[54] Ricci I, Damiani C, Scuppa P, Mosca M, Crotti E, Rossi P, et al. The yeast *Wickerhamomyces anomalus* (*Pichia anomala*) inhabits the midgut and reproductive system of the Asian malaria vector *Anopheles stephensi*. Environmental microbiology. 2011 Apr;13(4):911-21.

[55] Ricci I, Mosca M, Valzano M, Damiani C, Scuppa P, Rossi P, et al. Different mosquito species host *Wickerhamomyces anomalus* (*Pichia anomala*): perspectives on vector-borne diseases symbiotic control. Antonie van Leeuwenhoek. 2011 Jan;99(1):43-50.

[56] Chouaia B, Rossi P, Epis S, Mosca M, Ricci I, Damiani C, et al. Delayed larval development in *Anopheles* mosquitoes deprived of *Asaia* bacterial symbionts. BMC Microbiol. 2012 Jan 18;12 Suppl 1:S2.

[57] Lyke KE, Laurens M, Adams M, Billingsley PF, Richman A, Loyevsky M, et al. *Plasmodium falciparum* malaria challenge by the bite of aseptic *Anopheles stephensi* mosquitoes: results of a randomized infectivity trial. PloS one. 2010;5(10):e13490. DOI: 10.1371/journal.pone.0013490.

[58] Storelli G, Defaye A, Erkosar B, Hols P, Royet J, Leulier F. *Lactobacillus plantarum* promotes *Drosophila* systemic growth by modulating hormonal signals through TOR-dependent nutrient sensing. Cell metabolism. 2011 Sep 7;14(3):403-14.

[59] Puchta O. Experimentelle Untersuchungen ueber die Symbiose der Kleiderlaus *Pediculus vestimenti* Burm. Die Naturwissenschaften. 1954 1954;41(3):71-2.

[60] Lindh JM, Kannaste A, Knols BG, Faye I, Borg-Karlson AK. Oviposition responses of *Anopheles gambiae s.s.* (Diptera: Culicidae) and identification of volatiles from bacteria-containing solutions. Journal of medical entomology. 2008 Nov;45(6):1039-49.

[61] Nayar JK, Knight JW. Nutritional factors and antimicrobials on development of infective larvae of subperiodic *Brugia malayi* (Nematoda: Filarioidea) in *Anopheles quadrimaculatus* and *Aedes aegypti* (Diptera: Culicidae). Journal of medical entomology. 1991 Mar;28(2):275-9.

[62] Ramirez JL, Souza-Neto J, Torres Cosme R, Rovira J, Ortiz A, Pascale JM, et al. Reciprocal tripartite interactions between the *Aedes aegypti* midgut microbiota, innate immune system and dengue virus influences vector competence. PLoS neglected tropical diseases. 2012;6(3):e1561. DOI: 10.1371/journal.pntd.0001561.

[63] Blagrove MS, Arias-Goeta C, Failloux AB, Sinkins SP. *Wolbachia* strain *wMel* induces cytoplasmic incompatibility and blocks dengue transmission in *Aedes albopictus*. Proceedings of the National Academy of Sciences of the United States of America. 2012 Jan 3;109(1):255-60.

[64] Walker T, Johnson PH, Moreira LA, Iturbe-Ormaetxe I, Frentiu FD, McMeniman CJ, et al. The *wMel Wolbachia* strain blocks dengue and invades caged *Aedes aegypti* populations. Nature. 2011 Aug 25;476(7361):450-3.

[65] Hoffmann AA, Montgomery BL, Popovici J, Iturbe-Ormaetxe I, Johnson PH, Muzzi F, et al. Successful establishment of *Wolbachia* in *Aedes* populations to suppress dengue transmission. Nature. 2011 Aug 25;476(7361):454-7.

[66] Hughes GL, Koga R, Xue P, Fukatsu T, Rasgon JL. *Wolbachia* infections are virulent and inhibit the human malaria parasite *Plasmodium falciparum* in *Anopheles gambiae*. PLoS pathogens. 2011 May;7(5):e1002043. DOI: 10.1371/journal.ppat.1002043.

[67] Hughes GL, Vega-Rodriguez J, Xue P, Rasgon JL. *Wolbachia* strain *wAlbB* enhances infection by the rodent malaria parasite *Plasmodium berghei* in *Anopheles gambiae* mosquitoes. Applied and environmental microbiology. 2012 Mar;78(5):1491-5.

[68] Kambris Z, Blagborough AM, Pinto SB, Blagrove MS, Godfray HC, Sinden RE, et al. *Wolbachia* stimulates immune gene expression and inhibits *Plasmodium* development in *Anopheles gambiae*. PLoS pathogens. 2010;6(10):e1001143. DOI: 10.1371/journal.ppat.1001143.

[69] Shao Q, Yang B, Xu Q, Li X, Lu Z, Wang C, et al. Hindgut innate immunity and regulation of fecal microbiota through melanization in insects. The Journal of biological chemistry. 2012 Apr 20;287(17):14270-9.

[70] Oliveira JH, Goncalves RL, Lara FA, Dias FA, Gandara AC, Menna-Barreto RF, et al. Blood meal-derived heme decreases ROS levels in the midgut of *Aedes aegypti* and allows proliferation of intestinal microbiota. PLoS pathogens. 2011 Mar;7(3):e1001320. DOI: 10.1371/journal.ppat.1001320.

[71] Bischoff V, Vignal C, Duvic B, Boneca IG, Hoffmann JA, Royet J. Downregulation of the *Drosophila* Immune Response by Peptidoglycan-Recognition Proteins SC1 and SC2. PLoS pathogens. 2006 Feb;2(2):e14. DOI: 10.1371/journal.ppat.0020014.sg002.

[72] Zaidman-Remy A, Herve M, Poidevin M, Pili-Floury S, Kim MS, Blanot D, et al. The *Drosophila* amidase PGRP-LB modulates the immune response to bacterial infection. Immunity. 2006 Apr;24(4):463-73.

[73] Paredes JC, Welchman DP, Poidevin M, Lemaitre B. Negative regulation by amidase PGRPs shapes the *Drosophila* antibacterial response and protects the fly from innocuous infection. Immunity. 2011 Nov 23;35(5):770-9.

[74] Aggarwal K, Rus F, Vriesema-Magnuson C, Erturk-Hasdemir D, Paquette N, Silverman N. Rudra interrupts receptor signaling complexes to negatively regulate the IMD pathway. PLoS pathogens. 2008;4(8):e1000120. DOI: 10.1371/journal.ppat.1000120.t001.

[75] Kleino A, Myllymaki H, Kallio J, Vanha-aho LM, Oksanen K, Ulvila J, et al. Pirk is a negative regulator of the *Drosophila* Imd pathway. J Immunol. 2008 Apr 15;180(8):5413-22.

[76] Lhocine N, Ribeiro PS, Buchon N, Wepf A, Wilson R, Tenev T, et al. PIMS modulates immune tolerance by negatively regulating *Drosophila* innate immune signaling. Cell host & microbe. 2008 Aug 14;4(2):147-58.

[77] Waterhouse RM, Kriventseva EV, Meister S, Xi Z, Alvarez KS, Bartholomay LC, et al. Evolutionary dynamics of immune-related genes and pathways in disease-vector mosquitoes. Science. 2007 Jun 22;316(5832):1738-43.

[78] Waterhouse RM, Zdobnov EM, Tegenfeldt F, Li J, Kriventseva EV. OrthoDB: the hierarchical catalog of eukaryotic orthologs in 2011. Nucleic acids research. 2011 Jan; 39(Database issue):D283-8.

[79] Sharon G, Segal D, Ringo JM, Hefetz A, Zilber-Rosenberg I, Rosenberg E. Commensal bacteria play a role in mating preference of *Drosophila melanogaster*. Proceedings of the National Academy of Sciences of the United States of America. 2010 Nov 16;107(46):20051-6.

[80] Ben Ami E, Yuval B, Jurkevitch E. Manipulation of the microbiota of mass-reared Mediterranean fruit flies *Ceratitis capitata* (Diptera: Tephritidae) improves sterile male sexual performance. The ISME journal. 2010 Jan;4(1):28-37.

[81] Rosengaus RB, Zecher CN, Schultheis KF, Brucker RM, Bordenstein SR. Disruption of the termite gut microbiota and its prolonged consequences for fitness. Applied and environmental microbiology. 2011 Jul;77(13):4303-12.

[82] Verhulst NO, Beijleveld H, Knols BG, Takken W, Schraa G, Bouwmeester HJ, et al. Cultured skin microbiota attracts malaria mosquitoes. Malaria journal. 2009;8:302.

[83] Smith DL, Battle KE, Hay SI, Barker CM, Scott TW, McKenzie FE. Ross, macdonald, and a theory for the dynamics and control of mosquito-transmitted pathogens. PLoS pathogens. 2012;8(4):e1002588. DOI: 10.1371/journal.ppat.1002588.

[84] Engelstadter J, Telschow A. Cytoplasmic incompatibility and host population structure. Heredity. 2009 Sep;103(3):196-207.

[85] Douglas AE. The microbial dimension in insect nutritional ecology. Funct Ecol. 2009 Feb;23(1):38-47.

[86] Walker T, Moreira LA. Can *Wolbachia* be used to control malaria? Mem I Oswaldo Cruz. 2011 Aug;106:212-7.

[87] Hughes GL, Pike AD, Xue P, Rasgon JL. Invasion of *Wolbachia* into *Anopheles* and other insect germlines in an ex vivo organ culture system. PloS one. 2012;7(4):e36277. DOI: 10.1371/journal.pone.0036277.

[88] McMeniman CJ, Lane AM, Fong AW, Voronin DA, Iturbe-Ormaetxe I, Yamada R, et al. Host adaptation of a *Wolbachia* strain after long-term serial passage in mosquito cell lines. Applied and environmental microbiology. 2008 Nov;74(22):6963-9.

[89] Bisi DC, Lampe DJ. Secretion of anti-*Plasmodium* effector proteins from a natural *Pantoea agglomerans* isolate by using PelB and HlyA secretion signals. Applied and environmental microbiology. 2011 Jul;77(13):4669-75.

[90] Wang S, Ghosh AK, Bongio N, Stebbings KA, Lampe DJ, Jacobs-Lorena M. Fighting malaria with engineered symbiotic bacteria from vector mosquitoes. Proceedings of the National Academy of Sciences of the United States of America. 2012 Jul 31;109(31):12734-9.

[91] Rohwer F, Prangishvili D, Lindell D. Roles of viruses in the environment. Environmental microbiology. 2009 Nov;11(11):2771-4.

Chapter 18

Bacterial Biodiversity in Midguts of *Anopheles* Mosquitoes, Malaria Vectors in Southeast Asia

Sylvie Manguin, Chung Thuy Ngo,
Krajana Tainchum, Waraporn Juntarajumnong,
Theeraphap Chareonviriyaphap,
Anne-Laure Michon and Estelle Jumas-Bilak

Additional information is available at the end of the chapter

http://dx.doi.org/10.5772/55610

1. Introduction

Factors allowing the development of a pathogen to reach the infecting stage in a mosquito are poorly known. On the 528 species of mosquitoes recorded within the *Anopheles* genus [1], only 70 to 60 are able to transmit parasites responsible for malaria and filariasis [2, 3]. In vector-parasite interactions, the mosquito gut represents the first point of contact between parasites ingested and the vector epithelial surfaces. In the midgut, the parasites will have the opportunity to undergo their life cycle, but of the tens of thousands of *Plasmodium* gametocytes ingested by mosquitoes, less than five oocysts might be produced [4]. The factors responsible for this drastic reduction are still poorly understood. Recent studies showed that one of these factors concerns the primordial role played by the bacteria naturally present in mosquito midgut. Then, there is a growing interest on bacterial biodiversity in *Anopheles* mosquitoes and particularly those based on the identification of bacteria to be used for malaria transmission blocking based on bacterial genetic changes to deliver antiparasite molecules or paratransgenic approach [5-13]. Recent studies reported the presence of symbiotic bacteria, such as *Pantoea agglomerans* or *Asaia* in midgut lumen with anti-*Plasmodium* effector proteins that render host mosquitoes refractory to malaria infection [6, 10, 13]. Engineered *P. agglomerans* strains were able to inhibit *Plasmodium falciparum* development by 98% [13]. Other studies showed that insects with an important microbiota seem more resistant to infections and certain bacteria, such as *Enterobacter* sp. (Esp Z) inhibit partially or totally ookinete, oocyst and sporozoite formation [14-16]. In *Anopheles albimanus*, co-infections with the bacteria, *Serratia marcescens*, and *Plasmodium vivax* resulted in only 1% of mosquitoes being infected with oocysts, compared with 71% infection for control mosquitoes without bacteria [17]. A recent meta-taxogenomic study provides an in-depth description of the microbial communities in the midgut of *Anopheles gambiae* exposed to *P. falciparum* infection and the links between microbiota and parasitic status by comparing midgut microbiota in *P. falciparum*-positive and *P. falciparum*-negative individuals. Authors found significant correlation between the high enterobacterial content and malaria infection. Despite conflicting results on the role of enterobacteria, it has now clearly been established that bacteria present in *Anopheles* populations have a great influence on parasite transmission [18].

In Thailand and Vietnam, malaria is a public health priority with a strong prevalence of this disease in forested regions, in particular along the international borders with Myanmar and Cambodia respectively. In these malaria endemic areas, another parasitic disease occurs, Bancroftian lymphatic filariasis (BLF) for which only limited data are available [2]. Malaria and BLF are mosquito-borne diseases with *Plasmodium* species, especially *P. falciparum, P. vivax*, and rural strains of *Wuchereria bancrofti* sharing the same *Anopheles* vector species. In Southeast Asia, *Anopheles* vectors belong to species complexes with different involvement in the transmission of pathogens [19]. Few sibling species of the Dirus and Minimus Complexes and the Maculatus Group are involved in malaria and BLF, but specific role of each sibling species and factors influencing this role have never been studied due to the lack of reliable methods for species identification, now available [20-22]. As mosquito microbiota is one of the factors influencing pathogen transmission, this chapter is presenting the biodiversity of bacteria in the midgut of field-collected adults of 10 *Anopheles* species, topic less studied compared to the large number of studies presenting bacteria in the defense against parasites in laboratory conditions.

1.1. Midgut microbiome of mosquitoes

Many insects contain large communities of diverse microorganisms that probably exceed the number of cells in the insect itself [23]. More specifically, complex microbiotae have been described in mosquito midgut reporting the presence of numerous Gram-negative rods, including *Serratia marcescens, Klebsiella ozaenae, Pseudomonas aeruginosa, Escherichia coli, Enterobacter* spp. [14]. Recently, three metagenomic studies provided a more comprehensive picture of the diversity of midgut microbiota in *Anopheles gambiae*, the main malaria vector in Africa [18, 24, 25]. In wild caught adults of *Anopheles* species, the microbiota showed the common presence of *Pseudomonas* and *Aeromonas* species reported from at least five species among which malaria vectors (Table 1). The following five genera, *Asaia, Bacillus, Chryseobacterium, Klebsiella,* and *Pantoea* have been reported from four field collected *Anopheles* species, while *Serratia* and *Stenotrophomonas* were identified in three species (Table 1). At least three mosquito-specific bacterial species, isolated from the midgut of main malaria vectors of the Gambiae Complex, have been described, such as *Thorsellia anophelis* [26], *Janibacter anophelis* [27] and *Elizabethkingia anophelis* [28]. The first of the three species represents a new genus and species found predominant in the midgut of *Anopheles arabiensis* [29], the same *Anopheles* species in which *J. anophelis* was isolated. The third newly described species is closely related to *Elizabethkingia meningoseptica* as they share 98.6% similarity, and both species have been found in the midgut of *Anopheles gambiae* [11, 28]. The latter species, *E. meningoseptica,* was also isolated from diseased birds, frogs, turtles, cats, being most likely an agent of zoonotic infections, as well as a human meningitis especially in newborn infants [30]. Bacteria of the genus *Asaia* have also been associated with *Anopheles* species, in particular field-collected *An. gambiae, An. funestus, An. coustani* and *An. maculipennis* (Table 1), as well as a colony of *An. stephensi* in which *Asaia* bacteria was dominant and stably associated [9]. The presence of *Asaia* species in *Anopheles* could serve as candidate for malaria control based on the production of antiparasite molecules in mosquitoes for use in paratransgenic control of malaria [6, 9, 31]. Other bacterial species have been defined as antimalarial agents, especially those producing prodigiosin, a pigment produced by various bacteria, including *S. marcescens* [14].

The number of bacteria not only varied between individuals but also changed markedly during development, depending on both the stage of development and the blood-feeding status of the mosquitoes [31]. The normal midgut microbiota of *Anopheles* mosquitoes need to be further identified [5] as only few studies have reported the microbiota of wild caught malaria vectors (Table 1) [5-7, 9, 11, 12, 17, 24, 26-29, 31-35]. Further investigations of gut microbiota, especially of wild-caught insect vectors, might contribute to understanding the annual and regional variations recorded for vector transmitted diseases [17] and yield novel vector-control strategies [14].

1.2. Exploring bacterial communities by 16S PCR-TTGE

Bacterial communities are classically assessed through culture-dependent methods based on colony isolation on solid medium, sometimes after enrichment by growth in liquid medium. But, it is now obvious that the microbial diversity is poorly represented by the cultured fraction, and culture have been shown to explore less than 1% of the whole bacterial diversity in environment samples [36]. Thanks to sophisticated biotechnological and computational tools of the metagenomics, molecular ecology offers the potential of determining microbial diversity in an ecosystem by assessing the genetic diversity. The complete metagenomic approach will give the total gene content of a community, thus providing data about biodiversity but also function and interactions [37]. For the purpose of biodiversity studies, metagenomics can focus on one common gene shared by all members of the community. The most commonly used culture-independent method relies on amplification and analysis of the 16S rRNA genes in a microbiota [38].

The 16S rRNA genes are widely used for documentation of the evolutionary history and taxon assignment of individual organisms because they have highly conserved regions for construction of universal primers and highly variable regions for identification of individual species [39]. The notion developed by Woese that rRNA genes could identify living organisms by reconstructing phylogenies resulted in the adoption of 16S rRNA gene in microbiology [39]. Its universality and the huge number of sequences stored in databases have established 16S rRNA gene as the "gold standard" not only in microbial phylogeny, systematics, and identification but also microbial ecology [40].

	Anopheles									Total
Bacteria genera (species)	***albimanus***	***arabiensis***	***coustani***	***darlingi***	***dureni***	***funestus***	***gambiae***	***maculipennis***	***stephensi***	***Anopheles* species**
Achromobacter (A. xylosoxidans)							[31]		[5, 34]	2
Acidovorax (A. temperans)		[12]								1
Acinetobacter sp. (A. hemolyticus, A. radioresistens)						[24]			[34]	2
Aeromonas sp. (A. hydrophila)			[24]*	[35]		[24]	[12, 24]		[5]	5
Anaplasma (A. ovis)		[12]								1
Asaia spp. (A. bogorensis, A. siamensis)			[24]			[24]	[9, 24]	[9]		4
Bacillus spp. (B. cereus, B. coagulans, B. megaterium, B. mucoides, B. silvestris, B. simplex, B. thuringensis)		[12]				[31]	[31]		[34]	4
Bordetella									[5]	1
Brevundiumonas (B. diminuta)						[31]				1
Cedecea (C. davisae)						[31]	[31]			2
Chryseobacterium (C. indologenes)			[24]			[24]	[24]		[34]	4
Citrobacter (C. freundii)									[34]	1
Enterobacter spp. (E. amnigenus, E. cloacae, E. sakazaki)	[17]								[34]	2
Ehrlichia		[12]								1
Erwinia (E. ananas, E. chrysanthenum)						[31]	[31]			2
Escherichia (E. coli, E. senegalensis)		[12]				[31]				2
Elizabethkingia (E. anophelis, E. meningoseptica)							[11, 28]			1
Flavobacterium (F. resinovorum)						[31]				1
Gluconobacter (G. cerinus)						[31]				1
Janibacter (J. anophelis, J. limosus)		[12, 27]								1
Klebsiella spp. (K. pneumoniae)					[33]	[31]	[31]		[32]	4
Kluyvera (K. cryocrescens)						[31]				1
Leuconostoc (L. citreum)									[34]	1
Leminorella (L. grimontii)									[34]	1
Morganella (M. morgani)							[31]			1
Mycoplasma (M. wenyonii)		[12]								1
Myroides									[5]	1
Nocardia (N. corynebacterioides)		[12]								1
Paenibacillus sp.		[12]								1
Pantoea (P. agglomerans, P. stewartii)				[35]		[31]	[11, 31]		[7]	4

http://dx.doi.org/10.5772/55610

					Anopheles					Total *Anopheles* species
Bacteria genera (species)	***albimanus***	***arabiensis***	***coustani***	***darlingi***	***dureni***	***funestus***	***gambiae***	***maculipennis***	***stephensi***	
Pseudomonas spp. (P. aeruginosa, P. mendosina, P. pseudoflava, P. putida, P. stutzeri, P. synxantha, P. testosteroni)				[35]	[33]	[29, 31]	[12, 31]		[5, 34]	5
Salmonella spp. (S. choleraesuis, S. enteritidis)						[31]	[31]			2
Serratia (S. marcescens, S. nematodiphila, S. odorifera, S. proteamaculans)	[17]	[12]							[32, 34]	3
Sphingobacterium (S. multivorum)							[11]			1
Spiroplasma sp.						[12]				1
Stenotrophomonas (S. maltophilia)		[12]				[31]	[11, 12]			3
Thorsellia (T. anophelis)		[26, 29]								1
Vibrio (V. metschnikovii)		[12]								1
Xenorhabdus (X. nematophila)									[34]	1
Zymobacter							[24]			1

°, *An. gambiae* s.l. or s.s.; *, For Osei-Poku et al (2012) [24], genera with low frequency were not considered in this table.

Table 1. Bacterial genera isolated from the midgut of wild-caught adults of 9 *Anopheles* species linked to the associated reference numbers.

The complete 16S rRNA gene (1500 bp) gives the accurate affiliation to a species in most cases. In metagenomics, the amplified fragments are shorter, ranging from 200 to 400 bp, but contain nine hypervariable regions (V1-V9) [41], which compensate the lack of information due to the small sequence size by a high rate of mutation. In most studies, the V3 region located in the 5′ part of the gene is chosen [42]. However, the phylogenetic information is sometimes insufficient to achieve species identification. Depending on the bacterium, sequences provide identification to the genus or family level only. Consequently, the diversity of the community is not described by a list of bacterial species but by a list of operational taxonomic units (OTUs) corresponding to the lower taxonomic level being accurately identified. The 16S rRNA gene, in spite of some recognized pitfalls [43], remains today the most popular marker for studying the specific diversity in a bacterial community. Alternative markers can also be proposed such as *rpoB* [40] but universal *rpoB* PCR primers allowing the exploration of the whole bacterial diversity cannot be designed (Jumas-Bilak E, personal data) and the databases remain poor in *rpo* sequences.

Molecular approaches for assessing biodiversity avoid the bias of cultivability but displayed several pitfalls that should be evaluated and considered for a sound interpretation of the data. Particularly, DNA should be recovered and amplified from all the genotypes in the community, i.e. extraction and PCR should be as universal as possible. Special attention should be given to *Firmicutes* and *Actinobacteria* because they display thick and resistant cell wall. The extraction efficiency should be tested on a wide panel of bacteria to scan a large range of bacterial types. Extraction is generally improved by the use of large-spectrum lytic enzymes and/or by a mechanical grinding [44, 45]. The PCR itself is another cause of limitations in the molecular approaches. It often praises for its detection sensitivity but this sensitivity can fail when complex samples are analyzed. For example, detection thresholds of 10^3-10^4 CFU (colony forming units)/mL are currently described for universal PCR and migration in denaturing gels [44-46]. The detection limit cannot be easily assessed as it depends on both CFU/g count of each OTU and the relative representation of OTUs in the community. Minor populations of less than 1% of total population are generally undetectable for denaturing-gel-based methods used in microbial ecology [45, 47, 48].

In biodiversity studies, the different 16S rRNA genes representative of the community are amplified by PCR and then separated and identified either by cloning and Sanger sequencing or by direct pyro-sequencing [38]. Tools for sequence-specific separation after bulk PCR amplification, such as T-RFLP (Terminal-Restriction Fragment Length Polymorphism) [49], D-HPLC (Denaturing High Performance Liquid Chromatography) [50], CDCE (Constant Denaturing Capillary Electrophoresis) [51], SSCP (Single Stranded Conformation Polymorphism) [52], DGGE (Denaturing Gradient Gel Electrophoresis) [53], TGGE (Temperature Gradient Gel Electrophoresis), [48] and TTGE (Temporal Temperature Gradient Gel Electrophoresis) [47], can also be used. Methods based upon separation in denaturing electrophoresis allow the comparison of microbiotae with low or medium diversity [54]. They easily provide a "fingerprint" of the community diversity and therefore they are suitable for the follow-up of large collection of samples.

PCR-TTGE is a PCR-denaturing gradient gel electrophoresis that allows separation of DNA fragments in a temporal gradient of temperature [47, 55]. PCR amplicons of the same size but with different sequences are separated in the gel. In a denaturing acrylamide gel, DNA denatures in discrete regions called melting domains, each of them displaying a sequence specific melting temperature. When the melting temperature (*Tm*) of the whole amplicon is reached, the DNA is denatured creating branched molecules. This branching reduces DNA mobility in the gel. Therefore, amplicons of the same size but with different nucleotide compositions can be separated based on differences in the behavior of their melting domains. When DNA is extracted and amplified from a complex community, TTGE leads to the separation of the different amplicons and produces a banding pattern characteristic of the community. Counting bands on the TTGE profile provides a diversity score that roughly corresponds to the number of molecular species in the sample. The banding profile can be further analyzed by measuring distance migration of bands and comparing with patterns from known species. This comparison allows the affiliation of band to some representative species. Affiliation of all bands can be achieved by cutting bands from the gel, extracting DNA from bands and sequencing. A method associating migration distances measurement and sequencing of selected bands has shown its efficiency in describing bacterial communities of low complexity such as the gut microbiota of neonates [45]. Such an approach is simple enough and cost-effective to survey bacterial communities on a wide range of samples [56].

This chapter presents the bacterial biodiversity in the midguts of malaria vectors from Thailand and Vietnam based on the amplification of the V3 region of the 16S rRNA gene, separation of amplicon by TTGE and sequencing. The bacterial biodiversity among specimens and species in relation to the collection site are discussed.

2. Material and methods

2.1. Mosquito collections and species identification

In Thailand, populations of *Anopheles* mosquitoes were collected from three different sites located in malaria endemic area along the Thai-Myanmar border (Figure 1). One study site is in Pu Teuy, a village located in Sai Yok District, Kanchanaburi Province, western Thailand (14° 17′N, 99° 01′E). The rural site is located in mountainous terrain mostly surrounded by forest. The main water body near the collection site is a narrow, slow running stream, bordered with native vegetation [57]. This stream represents the main larval habitat for *An. minimus* s.l. [58]. A total of 1,330 malaria cases were reported in 2011 in the Sai Yok District with a prevalence of 389 cases of *P. falciparum* (44.7%) and 481 cases of *P. vivax* (55.3%) with a mortality rate per 100,000 inhabitants of 0.71 [59]. The second site located in Mae Sod District, Tak Province, is in the northern part of Thailand (16° 67′N, 98° 68′E). This is a forested area associated to agricultural fields and small streams. In 2011, 1,876 malaria cases were reported in this district with 187 cases of *P. falciparum* (28.3%) and 473 cases of *P. vivax* (71.7%). The mortality rate per 100,000 was of 0.56 [59]. The third site in Sop Moei District is the most southern district of Mae Hong Son Province (17° 86′N, 97° 96′E). This mountainous province is located north of Tak Province with a high malaria transmission occurring from June to August, during the rainy season [60]. In 2011, 1,643 malaria cases were found in this district due to *P. falciparum* with 419 cases (45.0%) and *P. vivax* with 511 cases (55.0%) and a mortality rate per 100,000 of 0.41 [59].

The specimens from Vietnam were collected from six sites located in Dak Ngo Commune, Tuy Duc District, Dak Nong Province (11°59′N, 107°42′E - central Highlands) where 848 malaria cases were reported in 2011, of which, 322 cases (54.9%) were caused by *P. falciparum*, 209 cases (35.6%) by *P. vivax* and 56 cases (9.5%) were mixed infections [61]. This province was named in 2004 after integrating parts from northern area of Binh Phuoc Province and southern area of Dak Lak Province. The average temperature in this province is around 24° C with the rainy season ranging from May to October and the dry season from November to April. The climate is favorable for agriculture, especially coffee, pepper and rubber plantations. Crops of coffee, pepper or cashew nuts were normally cultivated around houses. Villages were surrounded by cassava, corn and rice fields and located in the fringe forest. Every year, during harvest period, workers from neighbourhood come to work in the field, which generate high population movements in this area.

Anopheles mosquitoes were morphologically sorted by taxon before using specific AS-PCR assays for species identification within the complex or the group [20-22]. Each individual was split in two pieces, head-thorax for species identification and abdomen for midgut bacteria analysis.

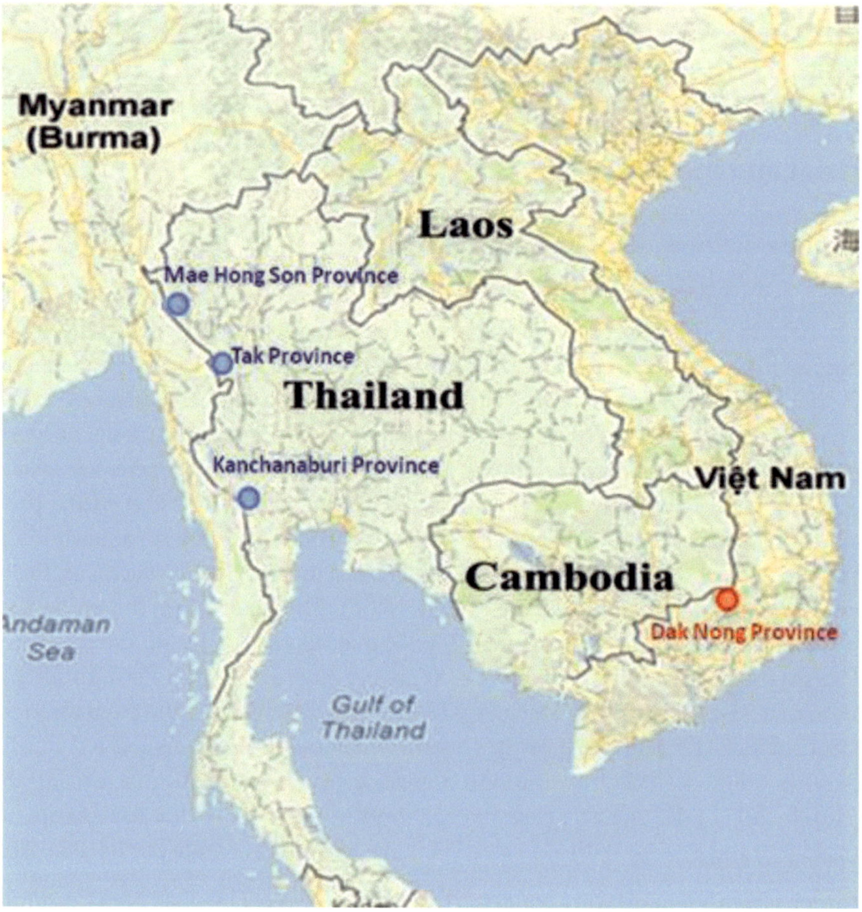

Figure 1. Map of Southeast Asia showing the locations of three provinces in Thailand (blue dots) and the province in Vietnam (red dot) where the mosquito collections were implemented.

2.2. DNA extraction

Mosquitoes stored at -20°C were surface rinsed twice in purified water prepared for injectable solution, and abdomen was thoroughly disrupted using a tissue crusher device in 150 µl of TE buffer. DNA was extracted using the Master Pure Gram Positive DNA purification kit as recommended by the supplier (Epicentre Biotechnologics, Madison, USA).

2.3. PCR

The V2–V3 region of the 16S rRNA gene of bacteria in the samples was amplified using the primers HDA1/HDA2 [45]; HDA1: 5′-ACTC CTA CGG GAG GCA GCA GT-3′, HDA2: 5′-GTA TTA CCG CGG CTG CTG GCA-3′. A 40-bp clamp, named GC (5′-CGC CCG GGG CGC GCC

CCG GGC GGG GCG GGG GCA CGG GGG G-3') flanked the 5' extremity of HDA1 [47] in order to form HDA1-GC. PCR was performed using an Eppendorf thermal cycler® (Eppendorf, Le Pecq, France) and 0.5 ml tubes. The reaction mixture (50 µl) contained 2.5 units of Taq DNA Polymerase (FastStart High fidelity PCR system, Roche, Meylan, France), 0.2 mM of each primer and 1 µl of DNA in the appropriate reaction buffer. Amplification was 95°C for 2 min, 35 cycles of 95°C for 1 min, 62°C for 30 s, 72°C for 1 min and 7 min at 72°C for final extension. To avoid contamination, solutions were prepared with sterile DNA-free water and preparation of the mastermix, addition of template DNA and gel electrophoresis of PCR products were carried out in separate rooms. PCR amplification was checked by DNA electrophoresis in 1.5% agarose gels containing ethidium bromide and visualized under ultraviolet light.

2.4. TTGE migration

TTGE was performed using the DCode universal mutation detection system (Bio-Rad Laboratories, Marne-la-Coquette, France) in gels that were 16 cm × 16 cm by 1 mm. The gels (40 ml) were composed of 8% (wt/vol) bisacrylamide (37.5:1), 7 M urea, 40 µl of N,N,N',N'-tetramethylethylenediamine (TEMED), and 40 mg ammonium persulfate (APS). Gels were run with 1X Tris–acetate–EDTA buffer at pH 8.4. The 5 µl of DNA was loaded on gel with 5 µl of in-house dye marker (saccharose 50%, Bromophenol Blue 0.1%) using capillary tips. Denaturing electrophoresis was performed at 46 V with a temperature ramp from 63°C to 70°C during 16 h (0.4°C/h) after a pre-migration of 15 min at 20 V and 63°C. Gels were stained with ethidium bromide solution (5 µg/ml) for 20 minutes, washed with de-ionized water, viewed using a UV transillumination system (Vilbert-Lourmat, France) and photographed.

2.5. TTGE band sequencing and OTU affiliation

TTGE bands were excised and the DNA was eluted with 50 µl of elution buffer (EB) of the Qiaquick PCR purification kit (Qiagen, Courtabeuf, France) overnight at 37°C before PCR amplification with HDA1/HDA2 used without GC clamp. The reaction conditions were identical to those described above. PCR products were sequenced on an ABI 3730xl sequencer (Cogenics, Meylan, France). Each sequencing chromatograph was visually inspected and corrected. The sequences were analyzed by comparison with Genbank (http://www.ncbi.nlm.nih.gov/) and RDPII databases (http://rdp.cme.msu.edu/) using Basic Local Alignment Search Tool (BLAST) and Seqmatch programs, respectively. The reference sequence with the highest percentage was used for OTU affiliation. A sequence was affiliated to a species-level OTU when the percent of sequence similarity was above 99.0%, as previously proposed [62]. This value is over the recognized cut-off value for the delineation of species [63], but warrants high stringency for species-level OTU affiliation. Below 99.0%, the sequence is affiliated to the genus of the reference sequence with the highest percentage. When several species reference sequences match equally, affiliation was done to the genus level. For example, sequence with 99.5% in similarity to the species *Aeromonas caviae* and *Aeromonas hydrophila* was only assigned to the genus *Aeromonas*. Low cut-off is not defined for the genus delineation since affiliation to a higher taxonomic rank such as family or order will be done considering the taxonomic frame of the clade using Greengenes database [64]. On each TTGE gel, about

50% of the bands were sequenced, the others being affiliated to an OTU by comparison of their migration distance with that of sequenced bands.

2.6. Phylogeny

The sequences for phylogenetic analysis were selected in the GenBank database using BLAST program and taxonomy browser (http://www.ncbi.nlm.nih.gov). The sequences were then quality checked using SEQMATCH program in the 16S rDNA-specialized database, RDPII (http://rdp.cme.msu.edu). Sequences were aligned using the ClustalX program [65], and the alignment was manually corrected to exclude gaps and ambiguously aligned regions. Maximum-likelihood (ML) phylogenetic analysis was performed using PhyML v2.4.6 [66], the model being General Time Reversible plus gamma distribution plus invariable site. ML bootstrap support was computed on 100 reiterations using PhyML.

3. Results

3.1. *Anopheles* species

Among the 175 specimens of *Anopheles* collected in Thailand and Vietnam, a total of 10 species were identified including six species per country of which two, *An. maculatus* and *An. dirus*, were common to both countries (Table 2). Eight species out of 10 belong to a group or a complex of which the sibling species were identified using the appropriate PCR assay (see Material and Methods). The Maculatus Group was represented by two species, *An. maculatus* and *An. sawadwongporni*, the latter collected in Thailand only. Within the Dirus Complex, three species were identified, *An. dirus*, *An. baimaii* and *An. scanloni*, the latter two were also collected in Thailand, as well as two species of the Minimus Complex, *An. minimus* and *An. harrisoni*. Three additional species were collected in Vietnam, *An. gigas* belonging to the Gigas Complex, *An. barbumbrosus*, and *An. crawfordi*. Among the 10 collected species, the former seven species of the Maculatus Group, Dirus and Minimus Complexes are defined as important malaria vectors and the latter three species have not been reported as being involved in malaria transmission [19, 67].

3.2. PCR-TTGE profiles and diversity index in midgut bacterial communities of *Anopheles*

The midgut microbiota of 175 specimens of *Anopheles* mosquitoes was investigated by 16S rRNA gene PCR-TTGE anchored in the V3 hypervariable region. A representative gel is given in Figure 2. TTGE profiles were obtained for 144 samples, 31 samples (17.7%) giving no amplification in PCR or a faint PCR signals leading to non-detectable TTGE profiles. Negative results suggested a low bacterial inoculum rather than a total absence of bacteria in the corresponding samples. Most negative samples came from Vietnam mosquitoes (n=26), compared to Thailand (n=5), and seemed to be unrelated to the *Anopheles* species. Finally, V3 16S PCR-TTGE approach led to the description of a microbial community for about 80% of the specimens analyzed and therefore appeared as an efficient tool to investigate midgut bacterial diversity in a large population of mosquitoes.

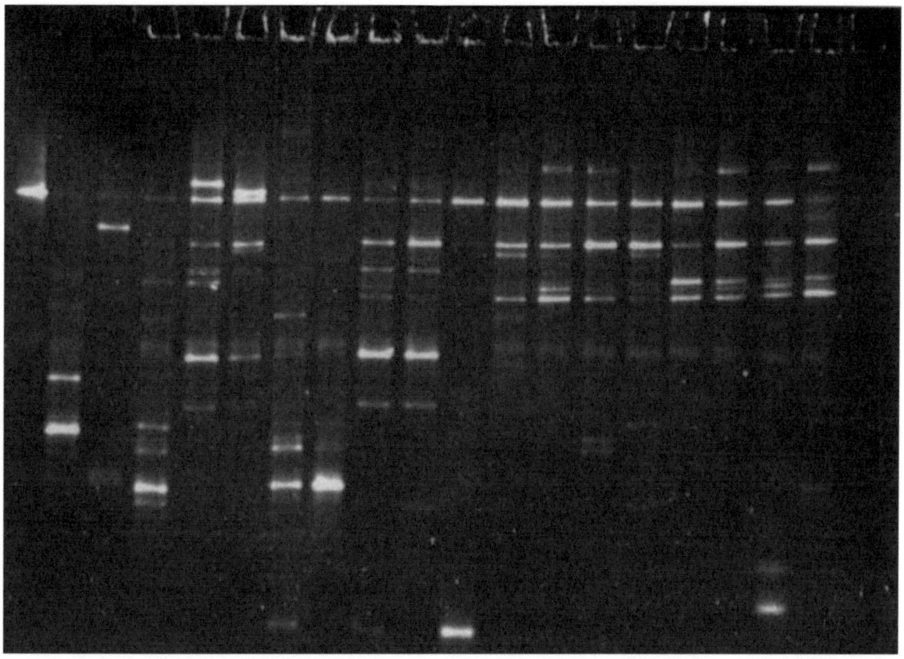

Figure 2. Representative TTGE analysis of V3 16S rRNA gene PCR products amplified from midgut samples of *Anopheles* mosquitoes from Thailand. Each lane corresponded to a specimen microbiota.

A raw diversity index that globally reflects the bacterial diversity in a sample is classically evaluated by counting the bands in TTGE profiles. At a first glance, the number of bands on TTGE profiles (Figure 2) ranged from 1 to 10 suggesting that the bacterial diversity per specimen ranged from 1 to 10 OTUs. However, sequencing showed that bands with different distance of migration could belong to the same OTU. This atypical phenomenon was observed for bacteria displaying sequence heterogeneity among their 16S rRNA gene copies. For instance, members of the genus *Acinetobacter* as well as most members of the genera affiliated to the family *Enterobacteriaceae* displayed a high level of 16S rRNA gene heterogeneity leading to complex banding patterns in V3 16S PCR-TTGE. Considering that *Acinetobacter* and *Enterobacteriaceae* were prevalent in our samples, the raw diversity index drastically overestimated the bacterial diversity. Therefore, a refined diversity index was calculated after affiliation of each band to an OTU by sequencing or by comparative approach (see Material and Methods).

The refined diversity index showed a low bacterial diversity per specimen with an average of 1.5 OTU per specimen. Most positive samples displayed a diversity index of 1 or 2 (Figure 3). Five OTUs is the maximal biodiversity per specimen observed in our population of *Anopheles* mosquitoes. Figure 3 showed that the number of OTUs per specimen differed slightly between populations from different origin, with an average of 1.7 and 1.3 OTU per specimen in Thailand and Vietnam, respectively. Considering mosquito species, the average diversity varied between 0 for *An. sawadwongporni* and 3 for *An. harrisoni* (Table 2).

	COUNTRY		VECTORS									NON VECTORS		
			Maculatus			*Minimus*		*Dirus*						
	Thailand (n=75)	Vietnam (n=100)	*An. maculatus* (n=28)	*An. maculatus* (n=11)	*An. sawadwongporni* (n=1)	*An. minimus* (n= 37)	*An. harrisoni* (n=13)	*An. baimaii* (n=4)	*An. scanloni* (n=3)	*An. dirus* (n=6)	*An. dirus* (n=23)	*An. gigas* (n=24)	*An. barbumbrosus* (n=13)	*An. crawfordi* (n=12)
Acinetobacter	■	■	14			10	10	1	1		11	18	3	5
Aeromonas	■					8								
Asaia	■	■	2				4							
Bacillus	■	■	1					1						1
*Cellvibrio**		■									1			
*Chromobacterium**	■					1								
Chryseobacterium	■	■					1		1				1	
Citrobacter	■					1								
*Corynebacterium**		■												1
*Cronobacter**	■					5								
*Diaphorobacter**	■					1								
*Diplorickettsia**		■									1	1		
Elizabethkingia	■					4				1				
*Enhydrobacter**		■											1	
Enterobacter	■	■		1		11		1		1	2			
Escherichia	■					1								
*Gluconacetobacter**	■						2							
Kluyvera	■						3							
*Microbacterium**		■											1	
*Moraxella**		■	1								1			2
*Nitrincola**		■										3		
Pantoea	■					1								
Pseudomonas	■	■		8		1	8		1	1				2
*Psychrobacter**		■										1		
*Raoultella**	■	■				2	9				2			
*Riemerella**		■											1	
Serratia	■	■		8		6			1	2				3
*Shewanella**	■						1							
*Sphingomonas**		■	20								16	8	1	1
*Staphylococcus**		■										1	1	
Stenotrophomonas		■									2			
Diversity Index	1.7	1.3	1.3	1.8	0	1.5	3	0.6	1.3	1.2	1.7	1.4	0.6	0.3

Table 2. Bacterial genera detected in midgut of *Anopheles* species caught in Thailand (blue) and Vietnam (red) with the number of specimens carrying each genus. Diversity index links to *Anopheles* species and origin is given at the bottom of the table. Genera described for the first time in *Anopheles* are marked with asterisk. Vertical lines delineated, from left to right, both countries with their respective number of *Anopheles* specimens, and groupings of *Anopheles* species, such as the Maculatus Group, the Minimus and Dirus Complexes, and the non-vector species including the Gigas Complex and 2 additional species.

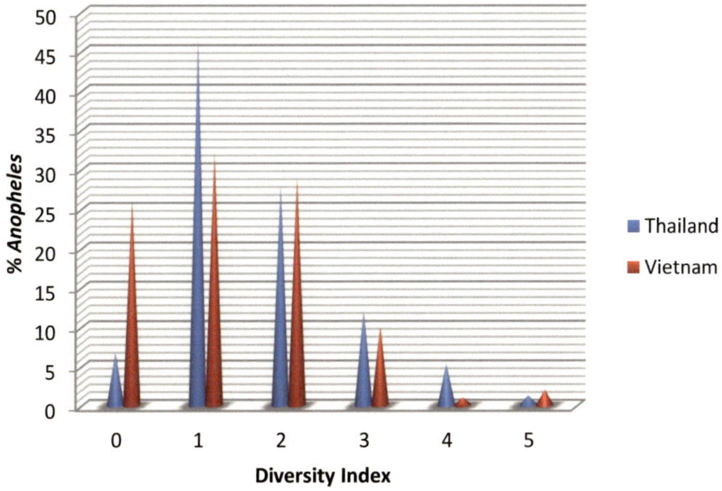

Figure 3. Distribution of the *Anopheles* mosquito populations from Thailand and Vietnam according to their refined diversity index

3.3. Bacterial diversity in the whole population of *Anopheles* mosquitoes

16S rRNA gene PCR-TTGE is focused on hypervariable region V3 produced sequences of about 200 bp, which are generally not informative enough for species affiliation. Consequently, we presented here the bacterial diversity to the genus level. However, probable species affiliation will be proposed for several genera when the phylogenetic signal of the V3 region was significant.

Contrasting with the low diversity per specimen, OTU diversity in the whole population was high with the detection of 31 different bacterial genera (Table 2) distributed in four phyla, *Proteobacteria, Bacteroidetes/Chlorobi, Firmicutes* and *Actinobacteria. Proteobacteria* largely dominated the midgut microbiota of *Anopheles* mosquitoes with 232 OTUs in the population studied. Their diversity encompassed *Alpha, Beta-* and *Gamma* superclasses of *Proteobacteria.*

The gamma-proteobacterial genera *Acinetobacter, Pseudomonas, Enterobacter, Serratia* and *Raoultella* were widely detected in our populations. A total of 40% of specimens and 70% of *Anopheles* species were colonized by members of the genus *Acinetobacter*, which therefore could be considered as a 'core genus' of the midgut microbiota of *Anopheles*. The sequences affiliated to the genus *Acinetobacter* were identified to the species level by a phylogenetic approach (Figure 4). The *Anopheles* midgut microbiota included 6 main species, *Acinetobacter baumannii, Acinetobacter calcoaceticus, Acinetobacter johnsonii, Acinetobacter soli, Acinetobacter guillouiae* and *Acinetobacter junii*, the two latter being more represented. The genus *Acinetobacter* belongs to the order *Pseudomonadales* in gamma-proteobacteria together with *Pseudomonas* (*Pseudomonas fluorescens* and *Pseudomonas alcaligenes*), *Moraxella, Enhydrobacter, Psychrobacter* and *Cellvibrio. Enterobacteriales* was the second main order of gamma-proteobacteria represented in the midgut microbiota of *Anopheles*. In enterobacteria, the species affiliation could not be achieved since genera are very close together in 16S rRNA gene phylogeny, particularly for *Enterobacter* and its relatives *Cronobacter* and *Pantoea*. Members of gamma-proteobacteria of the orders *Legionellales* (*Diplorickettsia*), *Oceanospirillales* (*Nitrincola*), *Alteromonadales* (*Shewanella*), *Xanthomonadales* (*Stenotrophomonas*) and *Aeromonadales* (*Aeromonas*) were also detected showing the very wide diversity of gamma-proteobacteria in the midgut microbiota of *Anopheles*.

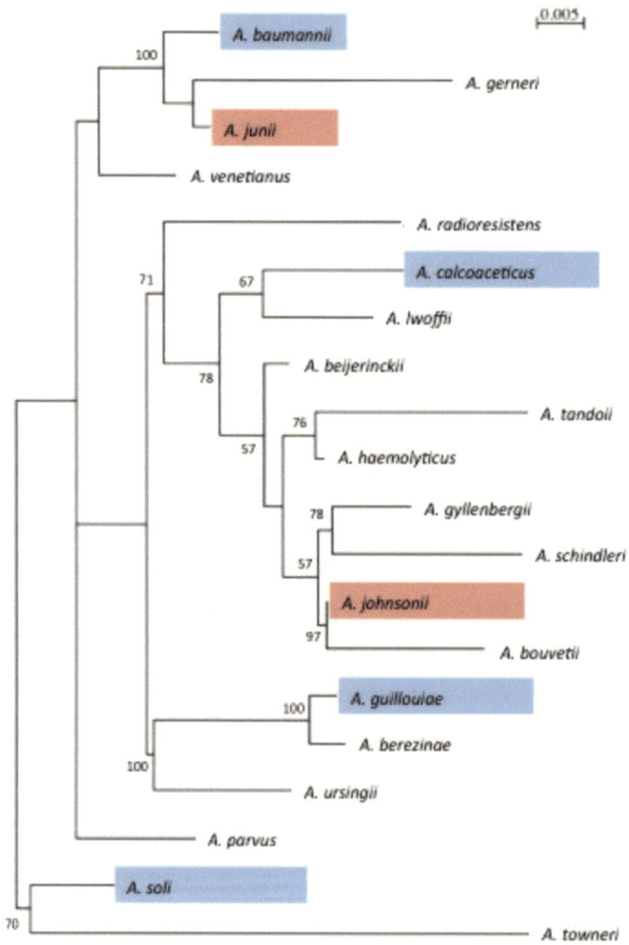

Figure 4. Maximum Likelihood phylogenetic tree of the genus *Acinetobacter.* Lineages of strains detected in the microbiota of *Anopheles* mosquitoes are in color, blue for Thailand, red for Vietnam. Bootstrap percentages (>50 %) after 100 resamplings are shown. Bar: 0.5 % sequence divergence.

The diversity was lower in alpha- and beta-proteobacteria. However, the genus *Sphingomonas* that belonged to *Alphaproteobacteria,* was the second main genus detected in this study (26% of the *Anopheles* species colonized) mostly represented by sequences affiliated or related to the species *Sphingomonas aromaticivorans* and *Sphingomonas glacialis*. Acetic-acid bacteria (*Asaia* and *Gluconacetobacter*) belonged to *Alphaproteobacteria* and were sporadically represented as well as *Chromobacterium* and *Diaphorobacter*, the two members of *Betaproteobacteria*.

Beside *Proteobacteria,* the phyla *Bacteroidetes/Chlorobi, Actinobacteria* and *Firmicutes* were represented by only few genera: 15, 9 and 5 respectively. *Chryseobacterium, Elizabethkingia* and *Riemerella,* which colonized only 8 mosquitoes, belonged to *Bacteroidetes/Chlorobi* and class *Flavobacteriia.* Sequences affiliated to the genus *Elizabethkingia* could not be related with certainty to *Elizabethkingia anophelis,* because the V3 region did not discriminate between this *Anopheles*-specific species and the human pathogen *Elizabethkingia meningoseptica. Bacillus* and *Staphylococcus* (*Firmicutes*), *Corynebacterium* and *Microbacterium* (*Actinobacteria*) were the sole Gram-positive genera found in the population of *Anopheles* mosquitoes. The most related species were *Bacillus cereus, Corynebacterium freiburgense* and *Microbacterium trichothecenolyticum.* The *Staphylococcus* sequences found in two mosquitoes were identical to those of a strain isolated in the midgut of the ladybug *Harmonia axyridis* and were linked to the species *Staphylococcus sciuri.*

3.4. Bacterial associations and relationship

Acinetobacter spp. was present in all mosquito specimens except in *An. maculatus* and *An. dirus* from Thailand. Specimens of these two *Anopheles* species were mainly colonized by *Pseudomonas* and *Serratia* (Table 2). When the microbiota of each specimen is considered (data not shown), the pair *Pseudomonas / Serratia* never co-habited with *Acinetobacter* in the same midgut. *Pseudomonas* strains associated with *Serratia* were related to the species *P. fluorescens* whereas *P. alcaligenes* was never associated with *Serratia* and inhabited midguts colonized with *Acinetobacter.* These results suggested that the association *P. fluorescens / Serratia* might specifically inhibit the colonization of *Anopheles* midgut by *Acinetobacter.*

Negative relationships between *Sphingomonas* and enterobacteria were also suggested in Table 2 for mosquitoes from Vietnam. Considering each specimen, we always observed the absence of enterobacteria when *Sphingomonas* colonized the midgut (data not shown).

3.5. Comparison of bacterial diversity in the midgut of *Anopheles* from Thailand and Vietnam

Table 2 and Figure 5 showed the differential distribution of bacterial genera according to the geographic origin of mosquitoes. Eight genera were shared between specimens from Thailand and Vietnam and corresponded to genera with high prevalence such as *Enterobacter, Serratia, Pseudomonas* and *Acinetobacter.* In Thailand, each of these four genera colonized more than 10% of specimens, each of the genera *Raoultella, Cronobacter, Aeromonas, Elizabethkingia* and *Asaia* colonized 3 to 10% of the specimens, and 10 other genera colonized 2% or less of the specimens (Figure 5A).

Except for the core genus *Acinetobacter,* main genera found in Thailand were not prevalent in specimens from Vietnam, *Enterobacter, Serratia, Pseudomonas, Raoultella,* and *Asaia* colonizing each 2% or less of the Vietnam specimens (Figure 5B). *Cronobacter, Aeromonas* and *Elizabethkingia* were not detected in *Anopheles* mosquitoes from Vietnam. Except for the genus *Acinetobacter* again (40%), the more prevalent genera in specimens from Vietnam appeared origin-specific. Indeed, *Sphingomonas* and *Moraxella* present in *Anopheles* from Vietnam at 36% and 3% respectively, were not detected in mosquitoes from Thailand (Figure 5B). When the species forming the genus *Acinetobacter* were considered, we observed again an origin-specific distribution with *A. junii* and *A. johnsonii* dominating the microbiota of mosquitoes from Vietnam but absent from the Thailand samples. Gut microbiota of mosquitoes from Thailand displayed a wider *Acinetobacter* diversity with four species represented, *A. baumannii, A. calcoaceticus, A. soli* and *A. guillouiae* (Figure 4). In the same phylogenetic clade of *Acinetobacter*, bacterial lineages from Thailand mosquitoes differed from bacterial lineages of Vietnam mosquitoes. For instance, the lineages *A. baumannii* and *A. junii* belonged to the same clade in the 16S rRNA gene tree but inside this clade, each lineage was origin-specific (Figure 4).

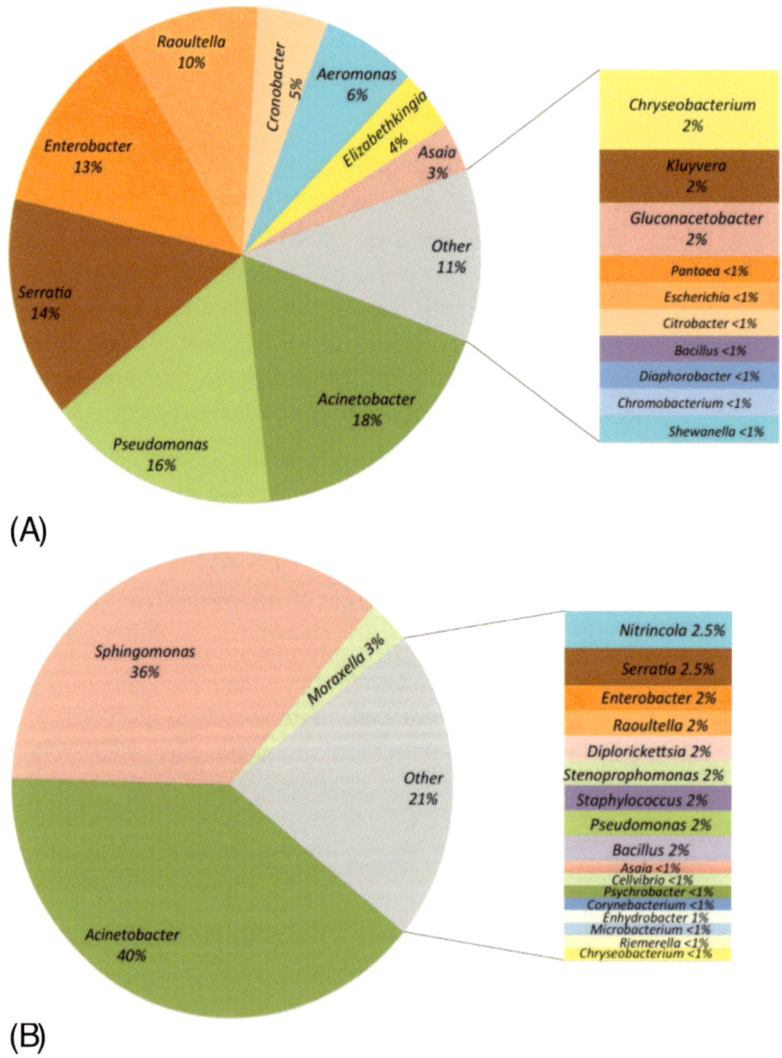

Figure 5. Repartition in genera of OTU assigned bands obtained by PCR-TTGE from 175 specimens of *Anopheles* mosquitoes from Thailand (A) and from Vietnam (B).

http://dx.doi.org/10.5772/55610

Considering bacterial taxa higher than the genus, the microbiotae of *Anopheles* from Thailand and Vietnam were both dominated by *Pseudomonadales* (Figure 6) due to the general high prevalence of *Acinetobacter*. *Enterobacteriaceae* largely dominated the microbiota of *Anopheles* from Thailand but contributed little to bacterial diversity in *Anopheles* from Vietnam.

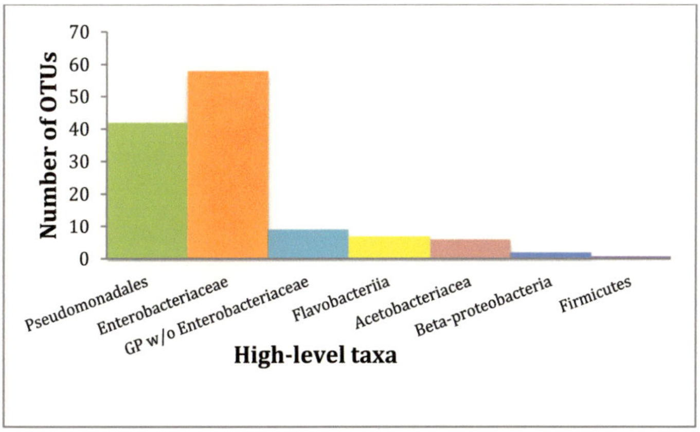

(A)

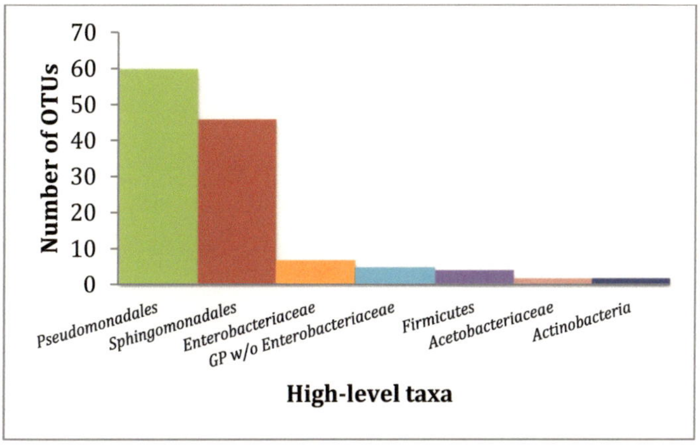

(B)

Figure 6. Repartition in significative high-level bacterial taxa of OTU from 175 specimens of *Anopheles* mosquitoes from Thailand (A) and from Vietnam (B). GP for *Gammaproteobacteria*.

This low prevalence of enterobacteria in the midgut of *Anopheles* from Vietnam was particularly noteworthy (Fig. 6B). In opposite, *Sphingomonadales* was the major high-level taxon in Vietnam specimens but absent from Thailand specimens. Therefore, the ratio *Enterobacteriaceae / Sphingomonadales* appeared as a signature differentiating Thailand and Vietnam *Anopheles* specimens. Other signatures, which should be confirmed with more specimens, were *Betaproteobacteria* and *Actinobacteria* in specimens from Thailand and Vietnam, respectively.

3.6. Links between microbiota composition and *Anopheles* species or species complexes

Table 2 showed the distribution of bacterial genera according to the species of *Anopheles*. To evaluate the link between bacteria and host species, we first compared the microbiotae of the same mosquito species but from different origins. Specimens of *An. maculatus* gave a good model for this comparison because it was enough represented in both geographic sites (Figure 7). The two groups of microbiotae differed clearly, in particular considering the origin-specific signature, i.e. the ratio *Enterobacteriaceae* / *Sphingomonadales* (Figure 7). Therefore, the case of *An. maculatus* indicated that the microbiota composition was influenced by sampling geographic sites rather than *Anopheles* species. Comparison of the microbiotae between *An. dirus* from Thailand and Vietnam resulted in the same conclusion (Table 2).

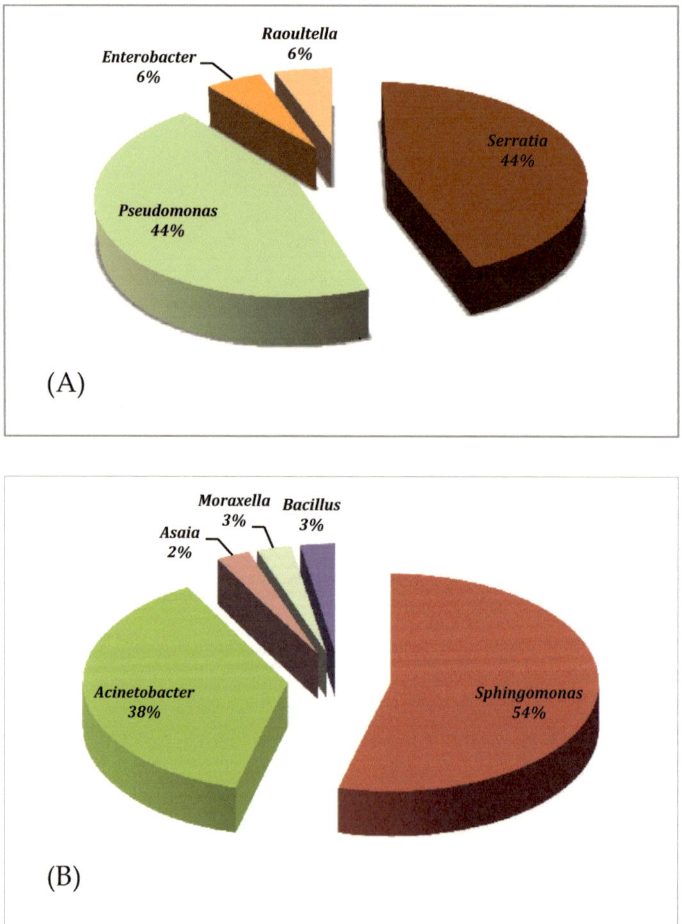

Figure 7. Comparison of the microbiota of *An. maculatus* caught in Thailand (n=11) (A) and in Vietnam (n=28) (B).

Sibling species within a group or a complex have been linked to the microbial content of the midgut. As previously observed for the species *An. maculatus*, the corresponding complex displayed a non-specific microbiota but its bacterial colonization is influenced by the geographic origin. Similar situation was observed in the Dirus Complex for which the shared bacterial genera were *Acinetobacter* and *Enterobacter*, as well as for *An. gigas* of the Gigas Complex with shared bacteria belonging to the dominating genera *Acinetobacter* and *Enterobacter*.

In the Minimus Complex, *An. minimus* and *An. harrisoni* were colonized by 18 different bacterial genera but only three were shared by both species. Two shared genera corresponded to bacteria widely represented in the whole population, *Acinetobacter* and *Pseudomonas*, while the third one, *Raoultella*, seemed to be more specific, represented in two and nine specimens of *An. minimus* and *An. harrisoni* respectively, showing its higher association to the latter species.

4. Discussion

To our knowledge, this study describes the midgut microbiotae of the largest population of field-collected *Anopheles* species with 10 species (Table 2) when the literature shows 9 analyzed species, *An. gambiae* being the most studied species of all (Table 1). Thereby, 16S rRNA gene PCR-TTGE focused on hypervariable region V3 proves its efficiency to study microbiota of *Anopheles* mosquitoes. This method, that presents a relative low resolution, is efficient to follow bacterial communities with low to moderate diversities. This limit is due to the number of bands that can be separated within the length of the gel. Optimization of TTGE conditions allows separation of bands by a minimum of 0.1 mm over all the gel length. Therefore, TTGE would be difficult to interpret if the diversity exceeds 25 to 30 OTUs [45]. Microbiotae of *Anopheles* displays TTGE profiles that do not exceed 10 bands but the profiles have been interpreted with difficulties due to heterogeneities in rRNA genes for most bacteria in the mosquito midgut ecosystem. At the genomic level, rRNA genes are generally organized in multigene families [68] in which sequences show low variability within species, subspecies or genome [69]. However, intra-genomic heterogeneity in the form of nucleotide differences between 16S rRNA gene copies are described in relation to fine-tuning of the ribosome function to optimize bacterial niche fitness [70]. In PCR-TTGE, heterogeneities lead to multiple bands for a single OTU and then to an overestimation of OTU diversity. This pitfall has been avoided here by band sequencing that led to the definition of a refined diversity index drastically lowered in comparison with the raw diversity index. The level of ribosomal heterogeneity in bacteria genome from midgut of mosquitoes suggested adaptation processes in a rather instable niche.

With the development of high-output sequencing, twenty-one century metagenomics consider fingerprint approaches as obsolete. However, these methods remain of great interest to give a snapshot of microbiota in large populations of hosts. Thereby, we described herein the midgut microbiotae of 175 specimens of 10 *Anopheles* species with a sequencing effort of less than 150 reads compared to 5 millions of reads estimated for the same study by pyrosequencing. A pyrosequencing study of the midgut microbiota of *An. gambiae* (30 laboratory breed and two field-collected mosquitoes) has been recently published [18]. Authors described bacteria belonging to 26 phyla, among which, five represented more than 99% of the total microbiota: *Proteobacteria, Bacteroidetes, Actinobacteria, Firmicutes,* and *Fusobacteria*. Except the latter, four phyla corresponded to those described in this study, suggesting that PCR-TTGE explored the majority of bacterial populations in the microbiota. Among 147 OTUs detected by pyrosequencing, only 28 genera had an abundance of >1% in at least one mosquito midgut [18]. This is in accordance with our results describing 31 bacterial genera in the microbiota of field-collected *Anopheles*. Fourteen of the 31 genera have been previously detected in diverse studies on field-collected *Anopheles* (Table 1). Then, we would like to highlight the fact that 17 bacterial genera were described herein for the first time (Table 2), 6 (32%) and 12 (60%) from the populations of Thailand and Vietnam respectively, suggesting that the bacterial diversity associated to midgut of *Anopheles* remains underestimated. It is noteworthy that twice as many new genera were found in specimens from Vietnam compared to Thailand. Newly described genera were scarcely represented in few specimens except for *Sphingomonas* found in 46 specimens belonging to five species from Vietnam and *Raoultella* found in 13 specimens belonging to 3 species from Thailand and Vietnam. Of note the genus *Sphingomonas* has been detected by pyrosequencing in the midgut of a population of *An. gambiae* maintained in standard insectary conditions [18].

The gut microbiota of mosquitoes presented a large inter-specimen variability but was dominated by few genera, *Acinetobacter, Pseudomonas, Enterobacter, Serratia, Raoultella* and *Sphingomonas*. Among them, *Acinetobacter* was considered as a mosquito midgut core genus because it was detected in most specimens. *Acinetobacter, Pseudomonas* and *Sphingomonas* also belong to the *An. gambiae* midgut core microbiota defined by Boissière et al. [18]. *Asaia* was found in all samples by pyrosequencing but its relative abundance showed great variations ranging from 0.04 to 98.95% according the *An. gambiae* specimen [18]. We detected *Asaia* in only 6 specimens of *An. maculatus* and *An. harrisoni*. Again, our result compared to pyrosequencing data suggested that PCR-TTGE failed to detect minority and/or low loaded populations. This low resolution is certainly a limit but we also see it as a benefit because the majority taxa detected by TTGE probably corresponds to true colonizers of the midgut and not to transient or contaminant bacteria.

Anopheles-associated bacterial species recently described were not detected or identified with confidence in this study. Members of the genus *Elizabethkingia* detected in *Anopheles* from Thailand could not be identified as *E. anophelis* owing to its relatedness in 16S rRNA gene sequence with *E. meningosepticum*. Of note, *Thorsellia anophelis* has been detected in mosquitoes used in the optimization step of this study but not in mosquitoes included in the study population.

In spite of the large inter-specimen variability, sub-populations from different geographic origins exhibit drastically different midgut microbiotae. High prevalence of *Enterobacteriacea* and absence of *Sphingomonas* spp. characterize microbiotae of *Anopheles* caught in Thailand whereas *Anopheles* in Vietnam displayed high prevalence of *Sphingomonas* and low rate of enterobacteria. Similar differences in enterobacteria prevalence have been described in *An. gambiae* originating from two sampling sites in Cameroon [18]. Composition of the midgut microbiota seems unrelated to *Anopheles* species, except for *Raoultella* and *An. harrisoni* but their relationship needs to be confirmed on additional specimens. Some positive and negative associations of bacteria suggested complex interactions in the microbiota. The most striking result was the pair *P. fluorescens / Serratia* which never co-habited with *Acinetobacter*. *Pseudomonas fluorescens* is well known as a great anti-microbial and bacteriocin-like substances producer [71] exhibiting negative effect on diverse Gram-negative bacteria and biofilm formation [72]. The bacteriocins are narrow-spectrum toxins that typically kill bacteria related to the producing strain as is the case for *P. fluorescens* and *Acinetobacter,* which both belong to the order *Pseudomonadales*. Moreover, bacteriocins can play an important role in the fitness of a strain by killing or inhibiting bacterial co-inhabitants that compete for the limited resources probably found in the midgut environment [71]. Similar antagonism was observed between *Sphingomonas* and enterobacteria in mosquitoes from Vietnam. *Sphingomonas* is a sparsely known genus but antimicrobial activities against *Candida* have been described recently [73]. Culture of the natural isolates of *P. fluorescens, Serratia, Acinetobacter* and *Sphingomonas* should confirm these potential antagonisms and give insights about their mechanism.

Antagonism against enterobacteria is of particular interest because it has been suggested that mosquitoes harboring *Enterobacteriacae* are more likely to be infected by *P. falciparum* [18]. In our collection, *An. minimus* specimen KAN-27 from Pu Teuy, Kanchanaburi was infected by *P. falciparum* and displayed a microbiota containing exclusively enterobacteria that belonged to four genera, *Pantoea, Enterobacter, Cronobacter* and *Escherichia*. This specimen displayed the highest enterobacterial diversity of the *Anopheles* collection and the core genus *Acinetobacter* was not detected. Identification of the *Enterobacter* species in our samples will be the next step with the search for *Enterobacter* (Esp_Z), which was reported to inhibit *P. falciparum* development in *An. gambiae* [15]. As the microbiota might have an impact on pathogen development in *Anopheles* mosquitoes and disease transmission, more studies need to be done for better understanding the role of some specific bacteria in wild mosquito populations before developing potential method of control.

5. Conclusion

Based on the analysis of the midgut microbiota of 10 field-caught *Anopheles* species from Thailand and Vietnam, we described 17 bacterial genera for the first time in *Anopheles* mosquitoes, suggesting that the bacterial diversity associated to midgut of *Anopheles* remains underestimated. Low bacterial diversity ranging from one to three per specimen was found which contrasted with a high OTU diversity in the whole *Anopheles* population that presented 31 different bacterial genera distributed in four phyla, *Proteobacteria, Bacteroidetes/Chlorobi, Firmicutes,* and *Acinetobacteria*. More specifically, the association of *Pseudomonas* and *Serratia* never co-habited with *Acinetobacter* in the same mosquito midgut. The same presence/absence was observed between *Sphingomonas* and enterobacteria. Midgut microbiota was drastically different for the *Anopheles* from Thailand compared to those from Vietnam showing the importance of the geographic origin. The ratio *Enterobacteriaceae / Sphingomonadales* appeared as a signature differentiating the *Anopheles* specimens from Thailand and Vietnam.

Acknowledgements

We are thankful to Naritsara Malaithong and Wanapa Ritthison, students of the Department of Entomology (Kasetsart University, Bangkok, Thailand) for their involvement in the optimization step of this study. This study was funded by the French Ministry of Foreign Affairs in the framework of the "Partenariat Hubert Curien" - PHC Thai project 20627SD.

Author details

Sylvie Manguin[1*], Chung Thuy Ngo[1,2], Krajana Tainchum[3], Waraporn Juntarajumnong[3], Theeraphap Chareonviriyaphap[3], Anne-Laure Michon[4] and Estelle Jumas-Bilak[4]

*Address all correspondence to: sylvie.manguin@ird.fr

1 Institut de Recherche pour le Développement (IRD), Faculté de Pharmacie, Montpellier, France

2 National Institute of Veterinary Research, Ha Noi, Viet Nam

3 Department of Entomology, Faculty of Agriculture, Kasetsart University, Bangkok, Thailand

4 University Montpellier, Equipe Pathogènes et Environnements, Faculté de Pharmacie, Montpellier, France

References

[1] Harbach RE. *Anopheles* classification. Mosquito Taxonomic Inventory, http://mosquito-taxonomic-inventory.info/, accessed on 8 November 2012.

[2] Manguin S, Bangs MJ, Pothikasikorn J, Chareonviriyaphap T. Review on global co-transmission of human *Plasmodium* species and *Wuchereria bancrofti* by *Anopheles* mosquitoes. Infection, Genetics and Evolution : journal of molecular epidemiology and evolutionary genetics in infectious diseases 2010;10:159-177.

[3] Manguin S, Carnevale P, Mouchet J, Coosemans M, Julvez J, Richard-Lenoble D, et al. Biodiversity of malaria in the world. Paris, France: John Libbey Eurotext; 2008.

[4] Al-Olayan EM, Williams GT, Hurd H. Apoptosis in the malaria protozoan, *Plasmodium berghei*: a possible mechanism for limiting intensity of infection in the mosquito. International Journal for Parasitology 2002;32:1133-1143.

[5] Chavshin AR, Oshaghi MA, Vatandoost H, Pourmand MR, Raeisi A, Enayati AA, et al. Identification of bacterial microflora in the midgut of the larvae and adult of wild caught *Anopheles stephensi*: a step toward finding suitable paratransgenesis candidates. Acta Tropica 2012;121:129-134.

[6] Damiani C, Ricci I, Crotti E, Rossi P, Rizzi A, Scuppa P, et al. Mosquito-bacteria symbiosis: the case of *Anopheles gambiae* and *Asaia*. Microbial Ecology 2010;60:644-654.

[7] Dinparast Djadid N, Jazayeri H, Raz A, Favia G, Ricci I, Zakeri S. Identification of the midgut microbiota of *An. stephensi* and *An. maculipennis* for their application as a paratransgenic tool against malaria. PloS One 2011;6:e28484.

[8] Dong Y, Das S, Cirimotich C, Souza-Neto JA, McLean KJ, Dimopoulos G. Engineered *Anopheles* immunity to *Plasmodium* infection. PLoS Pathogens 2011;7:e1002458.

[9] Favia G, Ricci I, Damiani C, Raddadi N, Crotti E, Marzorati M, et al. Bacteria of the genus *Asaia* stably associate with *Anopheles stephensi*, an Asian malarial mosquito vector. Proceedings of the National Academy of Sciences of the United States of America 2007;104:9047-9051.

[10] Favia G, Ricci I, Marzorati M, Negri I, Alma A, Sacchi L, et al. Bacteria of the genus *Asaia*: a potential paratransgenic weapon against malaria. Advances in Experimental Medicine and Biology 2008;627:49-59.

[11] Lindh JM, Borg-Karlson AK, Faye I. Transstadial and horizontal transfer of bacteria within a colony of *Anopheles gambiae* (Diptera: Culicidae) and oviposition response to bacteria-containing water. Acta Tropica 2008;107:242-250.

[12] Lindh JM, Terenius O, Faye I. 16S rRNA gene-based identification of midgut bacteria from field-caught *Anopheles gambiae* sensu lato and *A. funestus* mosquitoes reveals new species related to known insect symbionts. Applied and Environmental Microbiology 2005;71:7217-7223.

[13] Wang S, Ghosh AK, Bongio N, Stebbings KA, Lampe DJ, Jacobs-Lorena M. Fighting malaria with engineered symbiotic bacteria from vector mosquitoes. Proceedings of the National Academy of Sciences of the United States of America 2012;109:12734-12739.

[14] Azambuja P, Garcia ES, Ratcliffe NA. Gut microbiota and parasite transmission by insect vectors. Trends in Parasitology 2005;21:568-572.

[15] Cirimotich CM, Dong Y, Clayton AM, Sandiford SL, Souza-Neto JA, Mulenga M, et al. Natural microbe-mediated refractoriness to *Plasmodium* infection in *Anopheles gambiae*. Science 2011;332:855-858.

[16] Dong Y, Manfredini F, Dimopoulos G. Implication of the mosquito midgut microbiota in the defense against malaria parasites. PLoS Pathogens 2009;5:e1000423.

[17] Gonzalez-Ceron L, Santillan F, Rodriguez MH, Mendez D, Hernandez-Avila JE. Bacteria in midguts of field-collected *Anopheles albimanus* block *Plasmodium vivax* sporogonic development. Journal of Medical Entomology 2003;40:371-374.

[18] Boissiere A, Tchioffo MT, Bachar D, Abate L, Marie A, Nsango SE, et al. Midgut microbiota of the malaria mosquito vector *Anopheles gambiae* and interactions with *Plasmodium falciparum* infection. PLoS Pathogens 2012;8:e1002742.

[19] Manguin S, Garros C, Dusfour I, Harbach RE, Coosemans M. Bionomics, taxonomy, and distribution of the major malaria vector taxa of *Anopheles* subgenus *Cellia* in Southeast Asia: An updated review. Infection, Genetics and Evolution : journal of molecular epidemiology and evolutionary genetics in infectious diseases 2008;8:489-503.

[20] Garros C, Koekemoer LL, Coetzee M, Coosemans M, Manguin S. A single multiplex assay to identify major malaria vectors within the African *Anopheles funestus* and the Oriental *An. minimus* groups. American Journal of Tropical Medicine & Hygiene 2004;70:583-590.

[21] Walton C, Handley JM, Kuvangkadilok C, Collins FH, Harbach RE, Baimai V, et al. Identification of five species of the *Anopheles dirus* complex from Thailand, using allele-specific polymerase chain reaction. Medical and Veterinary Entomology 1999;13:24-32.

[22] Walton, C, Somboon, P, O'Loughlin, S. M, Zhang, S, Harbach, R. E, Linton, Y. M, et al. Genetic diversity and molecular identification of mosquito species in the *Anopheles maculatus* group using the ITS2 region of rDNA. Infection, Genetics and Evolution: journal of molecular epidemiology and evolutionary genetics in infectious diseases (2007); 7, 93-102.

[23] Dillon RJ, Dillon VM. The gut bacteria of insects: nonpathogenic interactions. Annual Review of Entomology 2004;49:71-92.

[24] Osei-Poku J, Mbogo CM, Palmer WJ, Jiggins FM. Deep sequencing reveals extensive variation in the gut microbiota of wild mosquitoes from Kenya. Molecular Ecology 2012;21:5138-5150.

[25] Wang Y, Gilbreath TM, 3rd, Kukutla P, Yan G, Xu J. Dynamic gut microbiome across life history of the malaria mosquito *Anopheles gambiae* in Kenya. PloS One 2011;6:e24767.

[26] Kampfer P, Lindh JM, Terenius O, Haghdoost S, Falsen E, Busse HJ, et al. *Thorsellia anophelis* gen. nov., sp. nov., a new member of the Gammaproteobacteria. International Journal of Systematic and Evolutionary Microbiology 2006;56:335-338.

[27] Kampfer P, Terenius O, Lindh JM, Faye I. *Janibacter anophelis* sp. nov., isolated from the midgut of *Anopheles arabiensis*. International Journal of Systematic and Evolutionary Microbiology 2006;56:389-392.

[28] Kampfer P, Matthews H, Glaeser SP, Martin K, Lodders N, Faye I. *Elizabethkingia anophelis* sp. nov., isolated from the midgut of the mosquito *Anopheles gambiae*. International Journal of Systematic and Evolutionary Microbiology 2011;61:2670-2675.

[29] Briones AM, Shililu J, Githure J, Novak R, Raskin L. *Thorsellia anophelis* is the dominant bacterium in a Kenyan population of adult *Anopheles gambiae* mosquitoes. The ISME Journal 2008;2:74-82.

[30] Bernardet JF, Vancanneyt M, Matte-Tailliez O, Grisez L, Tailliez P, Bizet C, et al. Polyphasic study of *Chryseobacterium* strains isolated from diseased aquatic animals. Systematic and Applied Microbiology 2005;28:640-660.

[31] Straif SC, Mbogo CN, Toure AM, Walker ED, Kaufman M, Toure YT, et al. Midgut bacteria in *Anopheles gambiae* and *An. funestus* (Diptera: Culicidae) from Kenya and Mali. Journal of Medical Entomology 1998;35:222-226.

[32] Jadin J. [Role of bacteria in the digestive tube of insects, vectors of plasmodidae and trypanosomidae]. Annales des Sociétés Belges de Médecine Tropicale, de Parasitologie, et de Mycologie 1967;47:331-342.

[33] Jadin J, Vincke IH, Dunjic A, Delville JP, Wery M, Bafort J, et al. [Role of *Pseudomonas* in the sporogenesis of the hematozoon of malaria in the mosquito]. Bulletin de la Société de Pathologie Exotique et de ses filiales 1966;59:514-525.

[34] Rani A, Sharma A, Rajagopal R, Adak T, Bhatnagar RK. Bacterial diversity analysis of larvae and adult midgut microflora using culture-dependent and culture-independent methods in lab-reared and field-collected *Anopheles stephensi*-an Asian malarial vector. BMC Microbiology 2009;9:96.

[35] Terenius O, de Oliveira CD, Pinheiro WD, Tadei WP, James AA, Marinotti O. 16S rRNA gene sequences from bacteria associated with adult *Anopheles darlingi* (Diptera: Culicidae) mosquitoes. Journal of Medical Entomology 2008;45:172-175.

[36] Riesenfeld CS, Schloss PD, Handelsman J. Metagenomics: genomic analysis of microbial communities. Annual Review of Genetics 2004;38:525-552.

[37] Tyson GW, Chapman J, Hugenholtz P, Allen EE, Ram RJ, Richardson PM, et al. Community structure and metabolism through reconstruction of microbial genomes from the environment. Nature 2004;428:37-43.

[38] Nossa CW, Oberdorf WE, Yang L, Aas JA, Paster BJ, Desantis TZ, et al. Design of 16S rRNA gene primers for 454 pyrosequencing of the human foregut microbiome. World Journal of Gastroenterology : WJG 2010;16:4135-4144.

[39] Woese CR. Bacterial evolution. Microbiological Reviews 1987;51:221-271.

[40] Case RJ, Boucher Y, Dahllof I, Holmstrom C, Doolittle WF, Kjelleberg S. Use of 16S rRNA and rpoB genes as molecular markers for microbial ecology studies. Applied and Environmental Microbiology 2007;73:278-288.

[41] Van de Peer Y, Chapelle S, De Wachter R. A quantitative map of nucleotide substitution rates in bacterial rRNA. Nucleic Acids Research 1996;24:3381-3391.

[42] Jany JL, Barbier G. Culture-independent methods for identifying microbial communities in cheese. Food Microbiology 2008;25:839-848.

[43] von Wintzingerode F, Gobel UB, Stackebrandt E. Determination of microbial diversity in environmental samples: pitfalls of PCR-based rRNA analysis. FEMS Microbiology Reviews 1997;21:213-229.

[44] Le Bourhis AG, Dore J, Carlier JP, Chamba JF, Popoff MR, Tholozan JL. Contribution of *C. beijerinckii* and *C. sporogenes* in association with *C. tyrobutyricum* to the butyric fermentation in Emmental type cheese. International Journal of Food Microbiology 2007;113:154-163.

[45] Roudiere L, Jacquot A, Marchandin H, Aujoulat F, Devine R, Zorgniotti I, et al. Optimized PCR-Temporal Temperature Gel Electrophoresis compared to cultivation to assess diversity of gut microbiota in neonates. Journal of Microbiological Methods 2009;79:156-165.

[46] Temmerman R, Masco L, Vanhoutte T, Huys G, Swings J. Development and validation of a nested-PCR-denaturing gradient gel electrophoresis method for taxonomic characterization of bifidobacterial communities. Applied and Environmental Microbiology 2003;69:6380-6385.

[47] Ogier JC, Son O, Gruss A, Tailliez P, Delacroix-Buchet A. Identification of the bacterial microflora in dairy products by temporal temperature gradient gel electrophoresis. Applied and Environmental Microbiology 2002;68:3691-3701.

[48] Zoetendal EG, Akkermans AD, De Vos WM. Temperature gradient gel electrophoresis analysis of 16S rRNA from human fecal samples reveals stable and host-specific communities of active bacteria. Applied and Environmental Microbiology 1998;64:3854-3859.

[49] Kitts CL. Terminal restriction fragment patterns: a tool for comparing microbial communities and assessing community dynamics. Current Issues in Intestinal Microbiology 2001;2:17-25.

[50] Penny C, Nadalig T, Alioua M, Gruffaz C, Vuilleumier S, Bringel F. Coupling of denaturing high-performance liquid chromatography and terminal restriction fragment length polymorphism with precise fragment sizing for microbial community profiling and characterization. Applied and Environmental Microbiology 2010;76:648-651.

[51] Thompson JR, Randa MA, Marcelino LA, Tomita-Mitchell A, Lim E, Polz MF. Diversity and dynamics of a north atlantic coastal Vibrio community. Applied and Environmental Microbiology 2004;70:4103-4110.

[52] Ege MJ, Mayer M, Normand AC, Genuneit J, Cookson WO, Braun-Fahrlander C, et al. Exposure to environmental microorganisms and childhood asthma. The New England Journal of Medicine 2011;364:701-709.

[53] Muyzer G, de Waal EC, Uitterlinden AG. Profiling of complex microbial populations by denaturing gradient gel electrophoresis analysis of polymerase chain reaction-amplified genes coding for 16S rRNA. Applied and Environmental Microbiology 1993;59:695-700.

[54] Roudiere L, Lorto S, Tallagrand E, Marchandin H, Jeannot JL, Jumas-Bilak E. [Molecular fingerprint of bacterial communities and 16S rDNA intra-species heterogeneity: a pitfall that should be considered]. Pathologie-Biologie 2007;55:434-440.

[55] Yoshino K, Nishigaki K, Husimi Y. Temperature sweep gel electrophoresis: a simple method to detect point mutations. Nucleic Acids Research 1991;19:3153.

[56] Jacquot A, Neveu D, Aujoulat F, Mercier G, Marchandin H, Jumas-Bilak E, et al. Dynamics and clinical evolution of bacterial gut microflora in extremely premature patients. The Journal of Pediatrics 2011;158:390-396.

[57] Chareonviriyaphap T, Prabaripai A, Bangs MJ, Aum-Aung B. Seasonal abundance and blood feeding activity of *Anopheles minimus* Theobald (Diptera: Culicidae) in Thailand. Journal of Medical Entomology 2003;40:876-881.

[58] Kengluecha A, Singhasivanon P, Tiensuwan M, Jones JW, Sithiprasasna R. Water quality and breeding habitats of anopheline mosquito in northwestern Thailand. Southeast Asian Journal of Tropical Medicine & Public Health 2005;36:46-53.

[59] MoPH. Report of Vector Borne Disease. In: Department DC, editor: Ministry of Public Health, Bangkok, Thailand; 2011.

[60] Thimasarn K, Jatapadma S, Vijaykadga S, Sirichaisinthop J, Wongsrichanalai C. Epidemiology of Malaria in Thailand. Journal of Travel Medicine 1995;2:59-65.

[61] IMPEQN. Malaria cases reported in 2011 - The Central and Highland provinces. Institute of Malaria, Parasite and Entomology sub., Quy Nhon; 2012.

[62] Drancourt M, Bollet C, Carlioz A, Martelin R, Gayral JP, Raoult D. 16S ribosomal DNA sequence analysis of a large collection of environmental and clinical unidentifiable bacterial isolates. Journal of Clinical Microbiology 2000;38:3623-3630.

[63] Stackebrandt E, Goebel BM. Taxonomic note: a place for DNA-DNA reassociation and 16S rRNA sequence analysis in the present species definition in bacteriology. International Journal of Systematic Bacteriolgy 1994;44:846-849.

[64] McDonald D, Price MN, Goodrich J, Nawrocki EP, DeSantis TZ, Probst A, et al. An improved Greengenes taxonomy with explicit ranks for ecological and evolutionary analyses of bacteria and archaea. The ISME Journal 2012;6:610-618.

[65] Thompson JD, Gibson TJ, Higgins DG. Multiple sequence alignment using ClustalW and ClustalX. Current protocols in bioinformatics / editoral board, Andreas D Baxevanis [et al] 2002;Chapter 2:Unit 2 3.

[66] Guindon S, Delsuc F, Dufayard JF, Gascuel O. Estimating maximum likelihood phylogenies with PhyML. Methods of Molecular Biology 2009;537:113-137.

[67] Sinka ME, Bangs MJ, Manguin S, Chareonviriyaphap T, Patil AP, Temperley WH, et al. The dominant *Anopheles* vectors of human malaria in the Asia-Pacific region: occurrence data, distribution maps and bionomic précis. Parasites & Vectors 2011;4:89.

[68] Acinas SG, Marcelino LA, Klepac-Ceraj V, Polz MF. Divergence and redundancy of 16S rRNA sequences in genomes with multiple rrn operons. Journal of Bacteriology 2004;186:2629-2635.

[69] Liao D. Gene conversion drives within genic sequences: concerted evolution of ribosomal RNA genes in bacteria and archaea. Journal of Molecular Evolution 2000;51:305-317.

[70] Roger F, Lamy B, Jumas-Bilak E, Kodjo A, Marchandin H. Ribosomal Multi-Operon Diversity: An Original Perspective on the Genus *Aeromonas*. PloS One 2012;7:e46268.

[71] Loper JE, Hassan KA, Mavrodi DV, Davis EW, 2nd, Lim CK, Shaffer BT, et al. Comparative genomics of plant-associated *Pseudomonas* spp.: insights into diversity and inheritance of traits involved in multitrophic interactions. PLoS Genetics 2012;8:e1002784.

[72] Guerrieri E, Bondi M, Sabia C, de Niederhausern S, Borella P, Messi P. Effect of bacterial interference on biofilm development by *Legionella pneumophila*. Current Microbiology 2008;57:532-536.

[73] Lee LH, Cheah YK, Nurul Syakima AM, Shiran MS, Tang YL, Lin HP, et al. Analysis of Antarctic proteobacteria by PCR fingerprinting and screening for antimicrobial secondary metabolites. Genetics and Molecular Research, 2012;11:1627-1641.

Section 5

Vector Control: Current Situation, New Approaches and Perspectives

Chapter 19

Distribution, Mechanisms, Impact and Management of Insecticide Resistance in Malaria Vectors: A Pragmatic Review

Vincent Corbel and Raphael N'Guessan

Additional information is available at the end of the chapter

http://dx.doi.org/10.5772/56117

1. Introduction

Malaria is still a major burden causing the death of nearly 655,000 people each year, mostly in children under the age of five, and affecting those living in the poorest countries [1]. Currently, the major obstacles to malaria control and elimination are the absence of a protective vaccine, the spread of parasite resistance to anti-malarial drugs and the mosquito resistance to insecticides [2]. Controlling mosquito vectors is fundamental to reduce mosquito-borne diseases by targeting vectorial capacity and hence the transmission. Vector control through the use of chemicals for mosquito bed nets and indoor residual spraying is still the cornerstone of malaria prevention [1]. Unfortunately, the extensive use of insecticides since the 1950s has led to the development of strong resistance worldwide hence representing a major public health problem where insecticidal vector control is implemented. Here, we propose to review the current level, distribution and mechanisms of insecticide résistance in malaria vectors and address their impact on the efficacy of vector control interventions. Strategies to prevent and/or delay the spread of insecticide resistance in natural mosquito populations are also discussed.

2. Definition of resistance

According to the *World Health Organization* (WHO), resistance is defined as the ability of an insect to withstand the effects of an insecticide by becoming resistant to its toxic effects by means of natural selection and mutations [3]. This definition differs from that provided by the *Insecticide Resistance Action committee* (IRAC) (www.irac-online.org) that gathers independent scientists and experts belonging to Agrochemical Companies who define operational (field) resistance as a heritable change in the sensitivity of a pest population that is reflected in the repeated failure of a product to achieve the expected level of control when used according to the label recommendation for that pest species. The IRAC definition, although pragmatic, is less "sensitive" with the scope to implement early *Insecticide Resistance Management* (IRM) strategies in the field. In both cases however, appropriate tools (biological, biochemical and/or molecular) are needed to identify the mechanisms involved and to conduct surveillance at individual and/or population levels [4].

Resistance has been observed in more than 500 insect species worldwide among which more than 50 *Anopheles* species (Diptera: Culicidae) are responsible for the transmission of malaria parasites to humans [5]. Resistance is a heritable character that relies on a genetic basis. Resistance results from the selection of a genetic modification in one or several genes occurring by migration and/or mutation. For example, when a mosquito population is exposed to an insecticide A, the individuals having resistant genes to this insecticide A survive and reproduce until the resistant allele becomes almost fixed. The use of insecticides for agricultural purposes and more recently for public health has played pivotal step in the selection of resistance in malaria vectors [6]. Resistance can involve several physiological and/or behavioural changes. Changes in the insecticide target site that reduce its binding to insecticides (known as target-site resistance) is the best understood type of resistance mechanism and molecular diagnostics to detect this resistance mechanism are now integrated into insecticide resistance monitoring strategies in malaria control programmes [7, 8]. Enhanced insecticide metabolism that lowers the amount of insecticide reaching the target site (known as metabolic resistance) is more complex but recent advances have identified key enzymes responsible for insecticide detoxification, paving the way for the development of molecular markers for this type of resistance mechanism [9, 10]. Other physiological changes (e.g. reduce penetration through cuticular resistance) and/or behavioural changes in the mosquito population were identified but their impact on the efficacy of insecticides is still poorly understood.

It is commonly accepted that the enhanced metabolism and target site modifications are responsible for high level of insecticide resistance in malaria vectors. To date, malaria vectors have developed resistance to the main chemical classes used in public health (i.e. pyrethroids, DDT, carbamates and organophosphates) (table 1) and the occurrence of cross-resistance[1] and multiple resistance[2] represent a serious threat to achieving the Millennium Development Goals for malaria control (i.e 75% reduction of global malaria cases by 2015). Surveillance and routine monitoring campaigns to assess the level and type of resistance are essential to help Malaria Control Programme (MCPs) to design more effective and sustainable malaria vector control strategies at an operational scale [4].

3. History of resistance to public health insecticides

Since the humans used chemicals for crop protection and/or the prevention of vector borne diseases, cases of resistances have been reported [11, 12]. Insecticides used for malaria control

---

1**Cross resistance:** occurs when a resistance mechanism, which allows insects to resist one insecticide, also confers resistance to another insecticide. Cross resistance can occur between insecticides from different chemical classes.

2**Multiple resistance:** occurs when insects develop resistance to several compounds by expressing multiple resistance mechanisms. The different resistance mechanisms can combine to provide resistance to multiple classes of products.

have included organochlorine, organophosphorus, carbamate, and pyrethroid insecticides, with the latter now taking increasing market share for both indoor residual spraying and Long Lasting Insecticidal mosquito Nets (LLINs) programmes [13]. Resistance has naturally tended to follow the use and switches of these insecticides [5].

Insecticides	Molecular target	Resistance mechanisms		References
		target site	enzymatic mechanisms	
Pyrethroids, type I	sodium channel	Kdr and super Kdr mutations	monooxygenases + esterases	[10,61,62]
Pyrethroids, Type II	sodium channel	Kdr mutations	monooxygenases + esterases	[10,61,62]
Organochlorates	sodium channel	Kdr mutations	GS-tranferases + monooxygenases	[10,61,62]
N-alkyl-amides	sodium channel	no resistance reported against insect of public health importance		
Organophosphates	acetylcholinesterase	Ace1 ^{R} mutation	esterases + GS-tranferases + monooxygenases	[10,59,63-67]
Carbamates	acetylcholinesterase	Ace1 ^{R} mutation		[10,59,63-67]
Neonicotinoids	nicotinic acetycholine receptor	not reported	monooxygenases	[68,69]
Spinosad	nicotinic acetycholine receptor	not reported		
Cyclodienes, Lindane, Bicyclic phosphates	GABA receptor	Rdl mutation	GS-transferases	[62,70]
Phenylpyrazoles	GABA receptor	Rdl mutation	GS-transferases	[62,70]
Avermectines	GABA receptor	undiscribed	monooxygenases + esterases	[62,70]
Insect Growth Regulators	Ecdysone agonist/disruptor or inhibitor of ATP synthase, chitin biosynthesis or lipid synthesis	no resistance reported against insect of public health importance		
Bacillus thuringiensis var. israelensis	microbial disruptors of insect midgut membranes	reported against Culex pipiens s.l. but non discribed		[71]

Table 1. Mechanisms of insect resistance to the main insecticide families of public health interest

Historically, DDT was first introduced for mosquito control and malaria eradication programme in 1946. The first case of DDT resistance was reported in *An. sacharovi* in Greece in 1953 and was followed by dieldrin resistance in 1954 [15]. Onset of resistance was marked by deterioration in malaria control that has continued for more than 30 years with sporadic epidemics of disease [16]. Resistance in *An. sacharovi* has been later reported in Bulgaria, Lebanon, Iran, Iraq, and Syria [12]. Pronounced DDT resistance appeared in *An. stephensi* in Iran and Iraq when full scale house spraying operations began in 1957 and dieldrin resistance appeared three years later. In India, house-spraying of DDT and Lindane (HCH) under the public health programme was introduced in the 1950s. Resistance of the main malaria vector *An. culicifacies* to dieldrin developed in 1958 [17] and resistance to DDT in 1959 [18], but the malaria control programme continued until 1965-1966 when both DDT and HCH failed to control outbreaks of malaria [19]. As a result, malathion was introduced in some areas in 1969 with some success but *An. culicifacies* rapidly developed resistance by 1973 [20]. Malathion resistance resulted in colossal epidemics of malaria in 1975 with 4 million cases reported as compared with 125,000 in 1965. The experience in Pakistan was similar with DDT resistance appearing in 1963. The importance of the resistance was not recognized until outbreaks of malaria began in 1969 and neither DDT nor HCH was effective. By 1975, malaria cases were reported in Pakistan to number 100 million as compared to 9,500 in 1961 [12]. DDT resistance in *An. culicifacies* was reported in Sri Lanka in 1968 resulting in a severe epidemic of malaria

[21]. This vector is now resistant to DDT, dieldrin, organophosphates, carbamates and pyrethroids [11].

Similar trend was noted in Central America and the Caribbean. Dieldrin spraying against *An. albimanus* begun in 1956 and widespread resistance appeared in 1958 [12]. A return to DDT spraying produced generalized resistance by 1960 [18]. The carbamate propoxur was employed in El Salvador, Guatemala, Honduras and Nicaragua in 1970 and resistance developed by 1974. *An albimanus* now exhibits multiple resistances to DDT, dieldrin, lindane and other chemical recently used in public health [22].

Much less information is however available for South East Asian malaria vectors, most probably because resistance monitoring was not carried out in routine before the 80s. In Vietnam, DDT resistance was found in 1989 in *An. epiroticus* of the Sundaicus Complex and is still occurring [23]. From 1990 till 2000, pyrethroid resistance was almost absent in all tested species except in some populations of *An. vagus* and *An. minimus s.l.* [24]. In Thailand, no evidence of insecticide resistance in malaria vectors was present before 1985 [25]. In 1986, development of physiological resistance to DDT was detected in *An. aconitus* from the north where DDT was commonly used for malaria control. One year later, DDT resistance was found in field collected mosquitoes of *An. philippinenis, An. nivipes* and *An. aconitus* from the same northern region. Between 1990 and 1997, DDT resistance has been detected in the three primary malaria vectors *An. dirus s.l., An. minimus s.l.* and *An. maculatus s.l.* and permethrin resistance was suggested in a population of *An. minimus s.l.* from northern Thailand, based however on a lower discriminative dosage (0.25%) of permethrin than that used today [25].

In Africa, resistance was initially found in *An. gambiae* in Bobo Dioulasso by 1967 (Burkina Faso), hence less than 7 years after the end of DDT use for malaria control [12]. DDT resistance was found in neighbouring countries including Cote d'Ivoire, Nigeria and Mali [26] and was then reported in most of Central and East African countries [27]. Strong association was observed between the level of DDT resistance in malaria vectors and the amount of DDT use for cotton protection [28]. Regarding BHC/dieldrin, the first cases of resistance were reported in Nigeria in 1954 hence only few months after the introduction of this molecule for malaria control. Initially found in very limited geographical areas, dieldrin resistance has spread in areas free of any insecticide treatments [29]. Few years later, resistance was reported in Bobo-Dioulasso and Cote d'Ivoire [30]. Today, resistance to BHC/dieldrin is still widespread in wild field anopheline populations despite its abandon in public health for many decades [31]. As for DDT, dieldrin resistance in malaria vectors arose and persisted from intensive use of pesticide for agricultural practices and in some specific settings due to public health programmes [32, 33].

After the 80s, DDT has been more or less abandoned worldwide and replaced by organophosphate (OP), pyrethroids and, to lesser extent, carbamates. However, insecticide resistance continued to be a problem, and vector control operations were affected, particularly in India, Africa and Latin America, by extensive use of agricultural pesticides. OP resistance, either in the form of broad-spectrum OP resistance or malathion-specific resistance was found in the major malaria vector species worldwide [12]. Pyrethroids were introduced in late 70s in public health and increasingly used in the 90s; however, cases of resistance were rapidly reported in the main malaria vectors worldwide including *An. albimanus* [34], *An. darlingi* [35], *An. culicifacies* [36], *An. stephensi* [37], *An. gambiae* [38], *An. funestus* [39] and *An minimus* [40]. Despite a sporadic use (compared to DDT and pyrethroids), resistance to carbamates was earlier reported in several mosquito species including *An. albimanus* [41], *An. atroparvus* [42], *An. sacharovi* [5] and *An. gambiae* [43]. Carbamate resistance is now spreading in malaria vectors especially in West Africa where it has been reported in Cote d'Ivoire [44], Burkina Faso [45, 46], Benin [47] and Nigeria [48]. Increased level of carbamate resistance in African mosquito populations is worrying for malaria control because these chemicals are increasingly used in replacement to pyrethroids for Indoor Residual Spraying (IRS) [49].

It is obvious that insecticide resistance in malaria vectors is increasing worldwide due to the increasing selection pressure on mosquito populations caused by the presence of urban, domestic and/or agricultural pollutants in the environment [50]. Transversal and longitudinal monitoring surveys are essential to address the spatio-temporal changes in resistance (dynamic) and to design appropriate strategies for a better control of resistant malaria vector populations worldwide.

4. Resistance mechanisms

The various mechanisms that enable insects to resist the action of insecticides can be grouped into four distinct categories including metabolic resistance, target-site resistance, reduce penetration and behavioral avoidance. These mechanisms that are shown in the figure 1 are briefly described in the following sections.

4.1. Metabolic resistance

Metabolic resistance is the most common resistance mechanism that occurs in insects. This mechanism is based on the enzyme systems which all insects possess to help them to detoxify naturally occurring xenobiotics/insecticides. It is commonly accepted that insect detoxification systems derived from the plant-insect evolutionary arm race and several insect detoxification enzymes have been associated to the detoxification of plant toxins and all types of chemicals, including insecticides [51]. Over-expression of enzymes capable of detoxifying insecticides or amino acid substitutions within these enzymes, which alter the affinity of the enzyme for the insecticide, can result in high levels of insecticide resistance (see [52] for review). Increased expression of the genes encoding the major xenobiotic metabolizing enzymes is the most common cause of insecticide resistance in mosquitoes. Over expression of detoxyfing enzymes can occur as the result of gene amplification (e.g. duplication) or due to changes in either trans-acting regulator elements or in the promoter region of the gene [5, 53, 54]. The consequence is a significant increase of enzyme production in resistant insects that enables them to metabolize or degrade insecticides before they are able to exert a toxic effect. Three categories of enzymes, namely esterases, P450s and glutathione-S-transferases are known to confer resistance to insecticides in insect pest such as malaria vectors. These large enzyme families contain multiple enzymes with broad overlapping substrate specificities, and one member of the family might

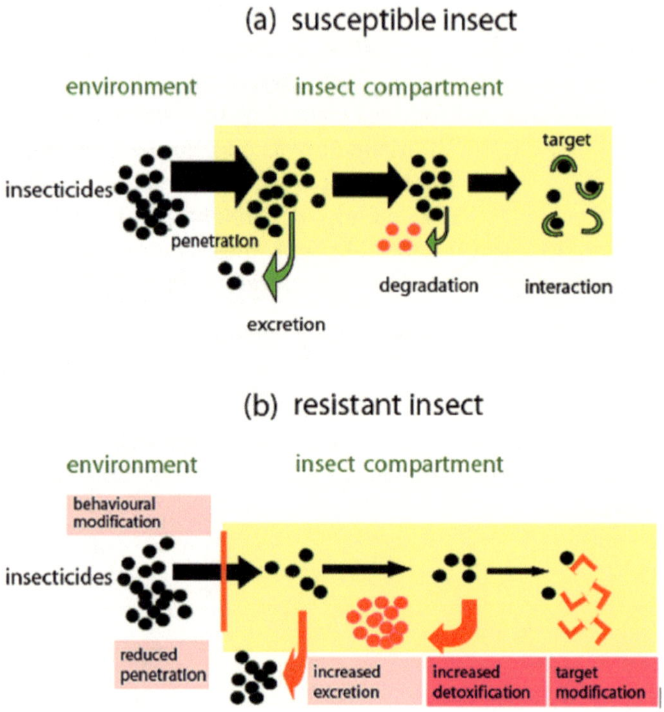

Figure 1. Scheme of potential behavioral and physiological changes associated with insecticide resistance in malaria vectors; (a) susceptible insect; (b) resistant insect *(source ; see [14])*

be capable of metabolizing limited number of insecticides. Similarly, the level of resistance conferred can vary from low to very high and may differ from compound to compound. Metabolic resistance mechanisms have been identified in mosquito populations for all major classes of insecticides currently used for vector control, including organochlorine, organophosphates, carbamates, and pyrethroids.

Esterases. One of the most common metabolic resistance mechanisms is that of elevated levels, or activity, of esterase enzymes which hydrolyze ester bonds or sequester insecticides. A striking example comes from studies on *Culex quinquefasciatus* that resist to a broad range of OP insecticides. In this species, multiple copies of EST-genes was already found hence enabling it to overproduce this type of enzyme [55]. In contrast to the situation in *Culex,* a number of *Anopheles* species (ie *An. culicifacies*, *An. stephensi* and *An. arabiensis*) have a non-elevated esterase mechanism that confers resistance specifically to malathion through increased rates of metabolism. Malathion resistance in *Anopheles* spp was associated with an altered form of esterase that specifically metabolizes the molecule at a much faster rate than that in susceptible counterparts [56, 57]. Although Carboxylesterase (CCEs) have been mostly associated to organophosphate resistance in mosquitoes, their role in pyrethroid resistance is probable. Indeed, the ability of esterases to metabolize pyrethroids has been suggested in mosquitoes [58, 59] even if no specific mosquito CCE has yet been validated as a pyrethroid metabolizer

[50]. Clearly much more information is needed on the esterase-mediated resistance in malaria vectors.

P450s. Cytochrome P450-dependent monooxygenases are an important and diverse family of enzymes involved in the metabolism of numerous endogenous and exogenous compounds. P450 belong to six families and increased transcription of genes belonging to the CYP4, CYP6, and CYP9 has been observed in various insecticide-resistant species from different taxa [60]. There is increasing number of reports demonstrating elevated P450 monooxygenase activities in insecticide-resistant mosquitoes, frequently in conjunction with altered activities of other enzymes. In most cases where a link between insecticide resistance and elevated P450 activity has been shown, the CYP gene belongs to the CYP6 family. Since the publication of the *An. gambiae* genome [61], P450s were extensively studied in the primary malaria vector in Africa. A total of 111 P450 enzymes were identified [62] and, as in other insects, only a small number of these enzymes are capable of detoxifying insecticides. However, higher activity of enzymes and/or expression of detoxification genes in insecticide resistant colonies do not necessarily correlate with insecticide resistance. For example, some authors have shown elevated transcript levels of an adult-specific CYP6 P450 gene, CYP6Z1, in pyrethroid-resistant strain *of An. gambiae* [63, 64] and *An. funestus* [65]. Further validation studies conducted in *An. gambiae* showed that cyp6z1 was however not capable to metabolize pyrethroids but was capable to metabolize DDT [66]. Another study showed that CYP6z2 displays broad substrate specificity, which may be associated with xenobiotics metabolism and detoxification [67]. Despite, CYP6Z2 being able to bind to permethrin and cypermethrin, this gene does not metabolise any of these insecticides. Microarray-based approaches have lately identified three new "candidate" P450 genes that were found to be repeatedly over-produced in pyrethroid resistant populations of *An. gambiae*: CYP6M2, CYP6P3 and CYP6Z2 [68-70]. All of these genes encode for enzymes that are able to bind to type I and type II pyrethroids but only CYP6P3 and CYP6M2 showed to metabolize the insecticides [10, 71]. More recently, some authors demonstrated that CYP6M2 is also capable of metabolizing the organochlorine insecticide DDT in *An. gambiae,* hence demonstrating the first evidence for a metabolic cross-resistance in malaria vectors [9]. Interestingly the putative ortholog of *An. gambiae* CYP6P3, CYP6P9, as being the prime candidate for conferring pyrethroid resistance, have been identified in *An. funestus* [72, 73] but only the CYP6P9 showed to metabolize types I and II pyrethroids [74]. Recent works showed that overproduction of CYP6P9 in *An. funestus* result from gene duplication [72]. In *An. minimus* mosquito, CYP6AA3 and CYP6P7 were up-regulated in pyrethroid-resistance population of Thailand [75] and seem to possess activities toward pyrethroid degradation [76, 77].

Glutathione S-transferases (GSTs). Glutathione transferases (GSTs) are multifunctional enzymes involved in the detoxification of many endogenous and xenobiotic compounds. Conjugation of Glutathione (GSH) to such organic molecules enhances solubility, thus facilitating their eventual elimination [78]. Elevated GST activity has been implicated in resistance to at least four classes of insecticides in insects. Higher enzyme activity is usually due to an increase in the amount of one or more GST enzymes, either as a result of gene amplification or more commonly through increases in transcriptional rate, rather than qualitative changes in individual enzymes [52]. At least six classes of insect GSTs have been identified in *An. gambiae* [79], found in several large clusters on all three chromosomes. The Delta and Epsilon classes found exclusively in insects are the largest classes of insect GSTs. Members of both classes have been implicated in resistance to all the major classes of insecticide. The primary role of GSTs in mosquito insecticide resistance is in the metabolism of DDT to DDE (non toxic products), although they also have a secondary role in organophosphate resistance [80]. GST-based DDT resistance is common in a number of anopheline species including *An. gambiae* [81-83], reflecting the heavy use of this insecticide for malaria control over several decades. Molecular biology and *in vitro* expression studies showed that *aggst3-2* was over expressed in resistant strain of *An. gambiae* and that recombinant *aggst3-2* was very efficient at metabolizing DDT [84]. Most studies of GSTs suggested that regulation occurs at the transcriptional level. Several regulatory elements have been identified in the promoter regions of GSTs that may mediate their induction but the significance of these findings is unclear. Genetic mapping of the major genes controlling GST-based DDT resistance in *An. gambiae* provided however evidence for a trans-acting regulator [84], although in this species, mutations in promoter elements of the Epsilon GST cluster are also associated with resistance [81]. It has been suggested that GSTs may play a role in pyrethroid resistance by detoxifying lipid peroxidation products induced by pyrethroids and/or by protecting from insecticide exposure induced oxidative stress [85]. Furthermore, GST might confer secondary role in pyrethroid resistance by sequestering the insecticide hence reducing the total *in vivo* concentration of insecticide [86].

Despite the great advance obtained recently in the identification of the role of detoxifying enzymes in insecticide resistance, force is to note that the function of >90% of metabolic genes is still unknown. Although only a limited number of resistance mechanisms have been implicated to date, the diversity within enzyme families involved in metabolic resistance is likely to contribute substantially to resistance to many insecticide classes. Further functional genomics and post-genomic technology are needed to reveal the contributions of hitherto unsuspected enzymes in insecticide metabolism and/or sequestration and to identify the causal mutations associated with metabolic resistance in mosquitoes. The contribution that these enzymes make towards various insecticide resistance phenotypes in malaria vectors is yet to be elucidated.

4.2. Target-site resistance

The second most common resistance mechanism encountered in insects is target-site resistance. Insecticides generally act at a specific site within the insect, typically within the nervous system (e.g. OP, carbamate, DDT and pyrethroid insecticides). The site of action can be modified in resistant strains of insects such that the insecticide no longer binds effectively. Reduce sensitivity of the target receptors to insecticide results from non-silent point mutations in the gene encoding the protein. For example, the target site for OP and carbamate insecticides is acetylcholinesterase (AChE) in the nerve cell synapses. Several mutations in the gene encoding for an acetylcholinesterase have been found in insects" [87] which result in reduced sensitivity to inhibition of the enzyme by these insecticides [88, 89]. In malaria vectors, the

G119S mutation (i.e. glycine to serine substitution at position 119) responsible for carbamate and OP resistance has been reported in *An. gambiae* and *An. albimanus,* essentially at the heterozygous state [90]. Recent sequence analysis of some resistant mosquitoes collected in Benin revealed the presence of a duplication of the *ace-1* gene in both A*n*. *A. gambiae* M and S forms [91]. In addition, mutations at a single codon (position 302) in the Rdl (resistance to dieldrin) gene encoding one receptor subunit, from an alanine residue to a serine (or more rarely to a glycine), have been documented in dieldrin-resistant insect species [92] including the malaria vectors *An. stephensi* [93], *An. gambiae s.l.* [94] and *An. funestus* [31]. Similarly, mutations in the amino acid sequence in the voltage-gated sodium channels of nerve cell membranes leads to a reduction in the sensitivity of the channels to the binding of DDT and pyrethroid insecticides [95]. Alterations in the target site that cause resistance to insecticides are often referred to as knockdown resistance (*kdr*) in reference to the ability of insects with these alleles to withstand prolonged exposure to insecticides without being 'knocked-down" [96]. One of the most common amino acid replacements associated with pyrethroid resistance in malaria vectors is a substitution of the leucine residue found at codon 1014 with either phenylalanine (1014F) [97] or serine (1014S) [98] in the Voltage-Gated Sodium Channel (VGSC). Interestingly, residue 1014 does not appear to interact directly with the insecticide but is predicted to alter channel activation kinetics [99]. Note that a *de novo* mutation (N1575Y) recently emerged within domains III-IV of voltage gate sodium channel in pyrethroid resistant populations of *An. gambiae* and seems to occurs only in a single long-range haplotype, also bearing 1014F allele [100]. It has been suggested that the N1575Y mutation may compensates for deleterious fitness effects of 1014F and/or confers additional resistance to pyrethroid insecticides.

4.3. Reduced penetration

Modifications in the insect cuticle or digestive tract linings that prevent or slow the absorption or penetration of insecticides can be found is some resistant insects. This resistance mechanism is not specific and can affect a broad range of insecticides. Reduced uptake of insecticide, often referred to as cuticular resistance, is frequently described as a minor resistance mechanism. Certainly for pests where the major route of insecticide delivery is via ingestion, this is likely to be the case. However, for malaria control, where insecticides are typically delivered on bed nets or on wall surfaces, uptake of insecticides is primarily through the appendages. An increase in the thickness of the tarsal cuticle, or a reduction in its permeability to lipophilic insecticides, could have a major impact on the bioavailability of an insecticide *in vivo*. Examples of reduced-penetration mechanisms are however limited; cuticular resistance was reported for the domestic Fly *Musca domestica* [101] and the lymphatic filariasis vector *Culex quinque-fasciatus* [102]. In *Anopheles*, microarrays studies have recently identified two genes, cplcg3 and cplcg4, encoding cuticular proteins that were upregulated in pyrethroid resistant strains from four populations and two different species (i.e. *An. gambiae* and *An. stephensi*) ([69, 103, 104]. Recently, measures of mean cuticle thickness in a laboratory strain of *An. funestus* using scanning electron microscopy (SEM) showed that the mean cuticle thickness was significantly greater in pyrethroid tolerant mosquitoes than their susceptible counterparts [105]. Clearly much more work is required in order to identify the significance of cuticular resistance in phenotypic resistance.

4.4. Behavioural resistance

Insecticide resistance in mosquitoes is not always based on biochemical mechanisms such as metabolic detoxification or target site mutations, but may also be conferred by behavioural changes in response to prolonged exposure to an insecticide. Behavioural resistance does not have the same "importance" as physiological resistance but may be considered to be a contributing factor, leading to the avoidance of lethal doses of an insecticide [106, 107]. For example, the first study on the irritant effect of DDT residual deposits was conducted using *Anopheles quadrimaculatus* where females were found to be irritated shortly after making contact with the treated surfaces resulting in a rapid escape response from a treated house prior to taking a blood meal [108]. This type of response can be further divided into direct contact excitation (sometimes referred to as 'irritancy') and non-contact spatial repellency that is used when insects move away from the insecticide-treated area before making direct contact [106, 109]. Examples of behavioral resistance or avoidance are few. Change in vector composition (i.e. switch from *An. minimus* to *An. harrisoni*) has been observed following implementation of ITNs in a village form central Vietnam [110]. With regard to *An. funestus*, recent findings showed a shift from indoor to outdoor biting preferences in Tanzania in relation to increasing coverage of pyrethroid-impregnated net [111]. Significant changes in the host-seeking behavior of the *An. funestus* population was confirmed in Benin (West Africa) where scaling up of LLINs at community level induced a change from night biting to early-morning biting behaviour [112]. It is unclear however whether adaptation of malaria vectors species to insecticidal based vector control interventions such as LLIN may result from a phenotypic plasticity or from selected behavioral traits (see Durnez & Coosemans for details).

5. Method to detect insecticide resistance

Currently most resistance monitoring is dependent on bioassays, using fixed insecticide concentrations and exposure times, and the data is reported as percentage mortality and/or Knock Down (KD) effect. The World Health Organisation (WHO) has defined diagnostic doses (i.e. twice the dosage that killed 100% susceptible mosquitoes of a given species) for most insecticides used in malaria control and produces susceptibility test kits consisting of exposure chambers and insecticide treated filter papers [113-115]. Although simple to perform, these diagnostic dose assays provide limited information and several alternative methods for detecting resistance are available (Table 2). These alternative assays generally detect specific resistance mechanisms, and should always be performed as an addition, not a substitute, to bioassays, to avoid the risk that unknown resistance mechanisms go undetected. It should be noted that none of the current methods listed in Table 2 are suitable for detecting cuticular and/or behavioural resistance. Regular monitoring for insecticide resistance is essential in order to react proactively to prevent insecticide resistance from compromising control. If the frequency of resistance alleles is going to build up unchecked, resistance may eventually become 'fixed' in the populations. Once resistance reaches very high levels, strategies to restore susceptibility are unlikely to be effective.

Method	Advantages	Disadvantages
Bioassays using WHO defined diagnostic doses of insecticide	Standardized, simple to perform, detect resistance regardless of mechanism	Lack sensitivity and provide no information about level and type of resistance (except when using with synergists), to be done on live mosquitoes
Dose response bioassays	Provides data on level of resistance in population, regardless of mechanism	Require large numbers of alive mosquitoes, and data from different groups not readily comparable
Biochemical assays to detect activity of enzymes associated with insecticide resistance	Provides information on specific mechanisms responsible for resistance	Requires cold chain. Not available for all resistance mechanisms, sensitivity and specificity issues for some assays (e.g. GST)
Molecular assays to detect resistant alleles	Very sensitive. Can detect recessive alleles and therefore provide an 'early warning' of future resistance.	Requires specialized and costly equipment. Only available for a limited number of resistance mechanisms.

Table 2. Methods for detecting insecticide resistance (source: see [6])

5.1. Bioassays

Guidelines for test procedures and interpretation of results are available from the WHOPES[3] (see http://www.who.int/whopes/resistance/en/). It is important that the mosquitoes used for the bioassays are standardized for age, sex and physiological status as all of these can affect the outcome of the tests. Typically either adults raised from isofemale lines or F1 progeny from field collected blood fed females are used. The limitations and advantages of these two alternatives have recently been discussed [116].

These diagnostic dose assays are simple to perform and provide standardized data sets that, assuming the guidelines are followed, can be readily compared to identify temporal and/or geographical variations in the resistant status of malaria vector populations. However, it is important to recognize some of the limitations of these susceptibility tests. As only a single concentration of insecticide is used, the results do not provide any information about the level of resistance in a population. For example if 50 % of population A and 20 % of population B were killed after exposure to the diagnostic dose of permethrin, it cannot be concluded that population B is more resistant than population A. The results only indicate that both populations are resistant (according to WHO definitions if there is < 80 % mortality, the population is defined as resistant) and that, subject to tests of significance, there is a higher frequency of

3 World Health Organization Pesticide Evaluation Scheme

resistant individuals in population B than in A. Dose response assays would be needed to compare the levels of resistance in two populations (e.g. by measuring the Resistant Ratios and their 95% confidence intervals). For pyrethroids, median knock down time (MKDT) is also a useful quantifiable variable [117]. Similarly, the results of these tests cannot be used to compare the levels of resistance to two different insecticides. If 50 % mortality was observed after exposure to the diagnostic dose of permethrin (0.75 %) whereas mortality was 70% after exposure to the diagnostic dose of deltamethrin (0.05%), it is not correct to state that the population is more resistant to permethrin than deltamethrin. Again, all that can be stated is that the population is resistant to both insecticides.

Partly due to the limitations of the diagnostic dose assays described above and partly due to the difficulties that are sometimes incurred in obtaining a regular supply of the insecticide impregnated papers from WHO, an alternative bioassay methodology has been developed [118] and is being adopted by some monitoring programmes. This method, known as the CDC bottle bioassay, uses glass bottles coated with a known concentration of insecticide. As these test kits are assembled in the users own laboratory, the concentration of insecticide can be readily adjusted enabling dose response curves to be developed to compare two or more strains. A caveat to this is that the flexibility, and the potential variation in the insecticide grade used in the tests, impairs comparison of results between two separate studies.

Both WHO diagnostic doses and CDC bottle bioassays can be modified to incorporate synergists. Synergists such as piperonyl butoxide, that block the activity of two major detoxification enzyme families, can be used to explore the role of different resistance mechanisms. If resistance is due to increased metabolism, exposure to an appropriate synergist prior to insecticide bioassays should increase the level of mortality observed.

5.2. Biochemical tests

Biochemical tests to detect alterations in activities of enzyme families associated with insecticide resistance have been available for over two decades and are sometimes used in combination with insecticide bioassays [119]. These assays employ model substrates to record the overall activity of glutathione transferases, carboxylesterases or cytochrome P450s in individual insects. Biochemical assays are also available to detect target site resistance to organophosphate and carbamate insecticides caused by insensitive acetylcholinesterase (AChE). The enzymatic reaction produces a colour change that is generally visible to the naked eye and hence these assays do not require access to expensive equipment (spectrophotometer is appropriate). However, it is important that the mosquitoes are kept on ice from the point of collection to the performance of the assay and this can often pose logistical challenges. Furthermore, there are sensitivity and specificity issues that limit the utility of some of these assays. For example, with over 100 different cytochrome P450 enzymes in malaria vectors, an assay that measures the total level or activity of this enzyme family may not have the sensitivity to detect over production of the single or small number of P450 enzymes that are thought to be involved in pyrethroid metabolism. This may explain the lack of significant correlation observed in many studies between cytochrome P450 activity and bioassay mortality results [120, 121]. In addition not all members of the enzyme family will have the same affinity for the model substrates used in these assays (e.g. CDNB (1-chloro 2-4, dinitrobenzene) is the substrate typically used to assess glutathione transferase activity but the Epsilon class of GSTs which are responsible for DDT resistance have relatively low activity with this substrate). In order to incorporate data from resistance monitoring into evidence based decisions on appropriate insecticide based interventions for malaria control, it is clearly essential that the data is both reliable and accessible. Although guidelines for conducting the various assays exist, there is little consensus on the number of sites and frequency with which resistance monitoring should occur [122]. It is clear that resistance is a dynamic trait, and wide fluctuations in resistance levels throughout the malaria transmission season have been reported [116, 123, 124]. Resistance can also be very focal, particularly when vector composition differs between sites [125], hence a minimum number of sampling sites should be established, taking into account patterns of vector distribution and insecticide usage. The WHO/AFRO African Network for Vector Resistance was established in 2000 and amongst its objectives was the important goal of improving the dissemination of resistance data. Accordingly a database was established to store the results of resistance monitoring activities by the African Network for Vector Resistance (ANVR) members but until recently, this database was not readily accessible by outside users. The recent establishment of new data base (see section 6), as an online centralized resource for collating data on insecticide resistance in disease vectors and the integration of this with the ANVR database, will hopefully ensure that both published and unpublished data on resistance in malaria vectors are more readily available to all interested parties.

5.3. Molecular tests

A multitude of molecular assays have been developed to detect *kdr* alleles in malaria mosquitoes, several of which were recently compared in a study by Bass et al (see [126]). These are routinely used by research laboratories monitoring for insecticide resistance and are gradually being incorporated into some national malaria control resistance monitoring programmes. Unfortunately, despite the recent identification of the key enzymes responsible for metabolic resistance to pyrethroids in *An gambiae* and *An funestus*, there are currently no simple DNA based assays to detect these resistance mechanisms. Detection of these genes is presently dependent on RNA based approaches using relatively sophisticated equipment (e.g. RT-qPCR). Assays to detect the genetic mutation(s) responsible for the resistance phenotype in individual insects can provide an early warning of the emergence of resistance which may not have been detectable by bioassays that can only record the population response. The presence of a single individual with an allele known to confer resistance should be cause for concern as experience dictates that resistance can spread very rapidly in a population unless the selection pressure is eased and/or the genetic cost associated with the resistant allele is high. Conversely, a negative result from a molecular assay should not lead to complacency. As discussed above, molecular assays are presently only available for target site resistance and the failure to detect *kdr* clearly cannot be interpreted as an absence of resistance in a population. Hence molecular assays should be seen as a complement rather than a substitute for bioassays.

6. Current distribution of insecticide resistance

Insecticide resistance has been reported in the main malaria vectors worldwide. Resistance is however not uniformly distributed among vector species and can greatly differ from one village, province, country, region and continent to another. Unfortunately, the highest levels of insecticide resistance were reported in Africa where malaria burden is still the highest in the world [1]. Resistance to pyrethroids, the gold standard insecticides used for LLIN and IRS will be extensively discussed in the present chapter as it remains a real and ever-present danger to future success of malaria vector control. Note that more information on the distribution of insecticide resistance in malaria vectors can be found in *Anobase,* http://anobase.vector-base.org/ir/; *MARA* http://www.mara.org.za; *Arthropod Pesticide Resistance Database,* http:// www.pesticideresistance.org.; and IR mapper, http://www.irmapper.com.

6.1. Africa

Although the occurrence of insecticide resistance in malaria vectors in Africa is not a "new" event (see section 2.), the speed at which pyrethroid-resistance recently evolved in field populations is worrying as it may jeopardize the current malaria vector control initiatives carried out in the continent. As shown in figure 2, pyrethroid resistance in *Anopheles* sp. is widespread but not uniformly distributed among the different countries. In the 49 African countries that have been investigated (see [6] for details), 15 did not report any data on resistance in the last 10 years i.e. Algeria, Botswana, Democratic Republic of Congo, Djibouti, Sierra Leone, Lesotho, Liberia, Libya, Maurice, Mauritania, Namibia, Rwanda, Somalia, Swaziland, Tunisia. If a lot of data has been generated in West Africa (as far as *An. gambiae s.l.* is concerned), a lack of information is globally observed in Central, Eastern and Austral Africa. It is obvious that the frequent conflicts that has occurred in the last decades in some African countries has rendered difficult the conduct of routine monitoring surveys by NMCP, International Organisation (WHO/ANVR) and/or research institutions.

Globally, pyrethroid resistance is high in *An. gambiae s.l.* in West Africa including Benin [127], Burkina Faso [128], Guinea Konakry ([129], Ghana [130], Mali [131], Niger [132], Nigeria [133] and Cote d'Ivoire [134]). In this region, pyrethroid resistance is predominant in *An. gambiae s.s.*, compared to *An. arabiensis*. Surprisingly, susceptibility to pyrethroids (permethrin and/or deltamethrin) was reported in *An. gambiae* s.l. in Guinea Bissau [135] despite the presence of the L1014F mutation. In Central Africa, pyrethroid resistance/tolerance is widespread in *An. gambiae s.l* in Cameroon [136-138], Chad [116, 139], Gabon [140, 141], Equatorial Guinea [8] and Sudan [142, 143]. In Chad, North Cameroon and Sudan, pyrethroid resistance is present essentially in *An. arabiensis,* which is consistent with the higher prevalence of this mosquito species in more arid areas with higher mean annual temperatures [144]. In East and Austral Africa, *An. gambiae* and *An. arabiensis* populations are mostly susceptible to pyrethroids in Tanzania [145, 146], Mozambique [147] and Madagascar [148], but highly resistant in eastern Uganda [149, 150], Ethiopia [151], Kenya [152, 153], Zambia [154], South Africa [155] and the Gwave Region of Zimbabwe [120]. Regarding *An. funestus,* most of the literature reporting pyrethroid resistance comes from South Africa [39, 156] and Mozambique [157-159], most probably because *An. funestus* is the main malaria vector in these countries. The data available

http://dx.doi.org/10.5772/56117

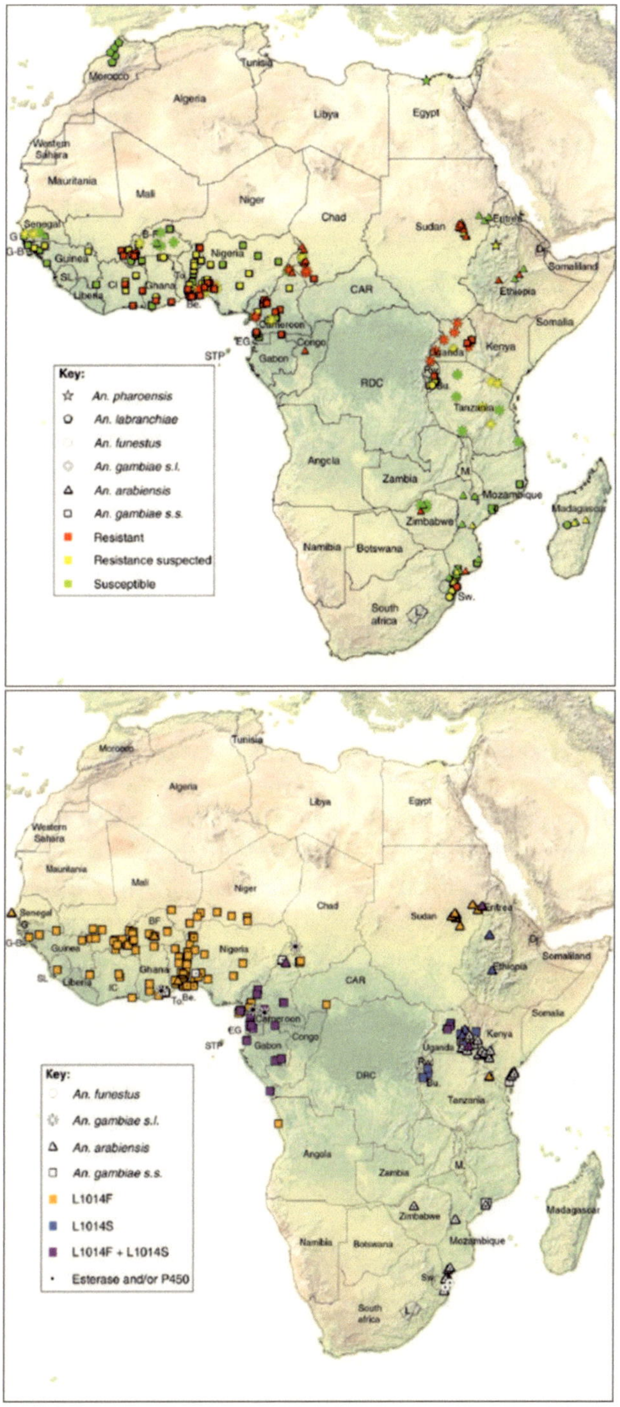

Figure 2. Maps showing the distribution of pyrethroid-resistance in African malaria vectors; A) status of pyrethroid resistance according to WHO criteria ; B) Target site (*kdr*) and metabolic resistance reported for a given mosquito species (Source; see [6]).

in other African countries is very limited in partly due to the difficulty to colonize *An. funestus* species in laboratory. Pyrethroid resistance/tolerance was detected in Malawi [160, 161] and suspected in Obusi and Kassena-Nankana Regions from Ghana [121, 162] and Benin [163] whereas full susceptibility to permethrin and deltamethrin was found in Burkina Faso [164] and Tanzania [145]. There is a lack of information on secondary vectors e.g. *An. moucheti* and *An. nili* which can play important role in malaria transmission in specific settings (e.g. Cameroon, Congo, Côte d'Ivoire). Regarding other vectors species, full susceptibility to pyrethroids has been reported in *An. labranchiae* in Morocco [165] and in *An. pharoensis* in Egypt [166] and Ethiopia [167].

In Africa, the L1014F mutation is widespread (figure 2) and predominant in the molecular S form compared to the M form, except in Benin [168], Guinea Equatorial [8] and Niger [132]. Some authors suggested that the *kdr* alleles may have arisen from at least four independent mutation events in the *An. gambiae* S-form [169]. Regarding the M form, it is not clear whether the *kdr* mutation resulted from an introgression from the S form only [170, 171] and/or from independent mutation events, has recently suggested for Bioko Island [172]. The second mutation, a leucine–serine substitution at the same codon (L1014S), was identified first in a colony of *An. gambiae s.l.* from Kenya [98]. This substitution has been lately reported in Burundi [173], Cameroon [136, 138], Gabon [174], Equatorial Guinea [175], Uganda [176], Republic of Congo [177] and Angola [140], mainly in co-occurrence with the 1014F *kdr* allele. Although some authors have reported that the 1014S allele may confer lower level of pyrethroid resistance than the 1014F allele [178], its spread from eastern to central Africa and more recently to West Africa [124, 179] suggest a survival advantage of mosquitoes sharing this mutation in presence of pyrethroids. So far, the L1014S substitution has always been detected in the S molecular form [180] but recent findings showed the occurrence of the 1014S allele in the M form in Equatorial Guinea [181] and Cameroon [182]. In these two countries, the 1014S allele was present at very low frequencies, alone or associated with the L1014F allele. It is currently impossible to know whether the *kdr* alleles have arisen first in Cameroon or Equatorial Guinea. The higher frequency of the 1014S allele in the S form compared with the M form could either be attributed to an introgression from the S taxon or to a *de novo* mutation. Regarding the sister taxa *An. arabiensis*, both of these mutations were reported in Western [124], Central [183] and Eastern Africa [184]. Interestingly, a new *kdr* mutation (N1575Y) occurring within domains III-IV of voltage gate sodium channel was found in both S and M molecular forms of *An. gambiae* and occurs upon a 1014F haplotypic background only [100]. Additive resistance of *1575Y* was demonstrated for permethrin and DDT in both molecular forms of *An. gambiae*. The prevalence of the 1575Y mutation has increased in West Africa in the last years hence indicating that the 1014F-1575Y haplotype is under strong selection pressure (Djégbé pers. com). It is possible that besides the 1014F/1014S *kdr* mutation, other mutations in the para-type sodium channel gene might be needed for mosquitoes to survive after exposure to a discriminating concentration of an insecticide. Further investigation is needed to better address the distribution and the role of the N1575Y mutation in pyrethroid resistance as well as to assess the fitness benefits conferred by this allele on the L1014F mutation in malaria vectors.

Beyond the spread of *kdr* alleles, metabolic-based resistance due to detoxifying enzymes namely oxidase, the GST (epsilon) and CCE families have expanded in African malaria vectors.

In *An. gambiae s.l.* metabolic resistance involving increased levels of P450 has been reported at least in Kenya [185], Cameroon [186], Benin [69], Nigeria [69], Ghana [70], Mozambique [147], South Africa [187] and Zimbabwe [120]. Up to now, only genes encoding CYP6P3 and CYP6M2 P450 enzymes have been clearly involved in cellular mechanisms known to metabolize deltamethrin and permethrin [10, 71].These genes were found over-expressed in pyrethroid-resistant *An. gambiae* populations from Benin, Nigeria and Ghana [69, 70], mainly in co-association with the *kdr* L1014F allele. In *An. funestus*, pyrethroid resistance involving increased activity of P450 monooxygenase and/or GST was demonstrated in South Africa [157], Mozambique [188] and Malawi [161].

To conclude, the immense challenge in Africa will be not to manage and control *kdr*-resistant mosquitoes only but to deal with the development of "multiple resistant" populations that could resist to different class of insecticides used in public health. One other issue is the occurrence and development of carbamate resistance in some countries (eg Benin, Nigeria) where this chemical class is in use for IRS through the PMI programme [47, 48]. The spread of carbamate resistance in malaria vectors in Africa is worrying for insecticide resistance management and alternative insecticides, and innovative strategies are urgently needed to better reduce the vectorial capacity of mosquitoes and hence effectively reduce the burden of malaria in the region. Resistance management strategy for malaria control is discussed in section 8.

6.2. South-East Asia and India

The South East Asia Region (SEAR) that account for 13% of the total malaria cases worldwide (2nd position after Africa) [1] is not spare of insecticide resistance in the main malaria vector species.

In the Mekong region, cross-country monitoring of insecticide resistance has been conducted through the MALVECASIA network (http://www.itg.be/malvecasia/) to help MCPs in the choice of insecticide to use at regional level. Large differences in insecticide resistance status were observed among species and countries. *Anopheles dirus s.s.*, the main vector in forested malaria foci, was mainly susceptible to permethrin except in central Vietnam where it showed possible resistance to type II pyrethroids [23]. *Anopheles minimus* s.l. populations were found resistant / tolerant in Vietnam and northern Thailand [189] but almost susceptible in Cambodia and Laos. No *kdr* mutation has been observed so far in these species [190] and pyrethroid resistance seems to result from increased detoxification by esterases and/or P450 monooxygenases [191]. Indeed, increased mRNA expression of two P450 genes, *CYP6P7* and *CYP6AA3*, suspected to metabolize some pyrethroids [76] have been reported in a deltamethrin-resistant population of *An. minimus* in Thailand [75, 192].

Anopheles epiroticus of the Sundaicus Complex showed to be highly resistant to all pyrethroids in the Mekong Delta [23] but susceptible to DDT, except near Ho Chi Minh City. DDT and pyrethroid-resistant populations of *An. subpictus* were reported in Vietnam and Cambodia. Biochemical assays suggest an esterase-mediated pyrethroid detoxification in both *An. epiroticus* and *An. subpictus* whereas DDT resistance in *An. subpictus* might be conferred to a higher GST activity. In Vietnam and Cambodia, *An. vagus* and *An sinensis* showed various levels of pyrethroid resistance and sequence-analysis of the DIIS6 region of the VGSC revealed the presence of the 1014S *kdr* allele [193]. Pyrethroid resistant populations of *An. sinensis* were also reported in the Republic of Korea (ROK) [194] and in China [195]. In China, cypermethrin resistance in *An. sinensis* was associated with the presence of both 1014F and L1014C substitutions, whereas only 1014F and 1014S mutations were found in the ROK and Vietnam, respectively. In Indonesia, molecular analysis carried out in field mosquito samples revealed the presence of the 1014F allele in the four main malaria vectors i.e. *An. sundaicus, An. aconitus, An. subpictus* and *An. vagus* [196]. At the present time, it is difficult to speculate on the relative contribution of the *kdr* mutations *versus* metabolic detoxification on pyrethroid and DDT resistance in malaria vectors from the SEA region and more work are needed to establish a clear trend.

Insecticide resistance is known to be widespread in other part of Asia such as India. In this country, resistance has a long history (see section 2) and it represents a big challenge for malaria vector control. Among the *Anopheles* species, *An. culicifacies s.l.*, the major vector of malaria in most parts of the country, has developed strong resistance to pyrethroids [36], DDT [197, 198], dieldrin/HCH [199], and malathion [198]. The 1014F mutation, which generates the *kdr* phenotype was detected in pyrethroid and DDT resistant *An. culicifacies s.l.* populations sometimes in co-occurrence with the 1014S mutation [197]. Note that a novel mutation V1010L (resulting from G-to-T or -C transversions) in the VGSC was recently identified in Indian *An. culicifacies* and was tightly linked to 1014S substitution [197]. Elevated activities of GST seem to play also an important role in DDT-resistance in this mosquito species [82]. Similarly, strong level of pyrethroid resistance due to the presence of both 1014F and 1014S mutations was found in the urban malaria vector *An. stephensi* particularly in the Rajasthan District [200]. Other vectors that are reported to be resistant to pyrethroid, DDT and/or dieldrin/HCH in India are *An. annularis, An. subpictus* and *An. philippinensis* [201]. In contrast, *An. minimus* has still not showed pyrethroid and DDT resistance [202].

The same trend was noted in Sri Lanka where the main malaria vectors species, i.e. *An. culificifacies s.l.* and *An. subpictus* have developed DDT, pyrethroid and malathion resistance in several districts [203, 204]. However, the main mechanisms associated with DDT and malathion resistance in *An. culicifacies s.l.* and *An. subpictus* are primarily metabolic and involve carboxylesterases (malathion) or monooxygenases and GSTs (for DDT) [205, 206]. An altered acetylcholinesterase conferring organophosphate resistance has been suspected in both vector species [205].

In the delta region of Bangladesh, the *An. sundaicus* malaria vector is fully susceptible to DDT but other malaria vectors such as *An. philippinensis, An. maculatus s.l.,* and *An. aconitus* have all developed resistance to DDT [207]. *Anopheles aconitus,* additionally, has been reported to be resistant to dieldrin/HCH. Bhutan records *An. maculatus s.l.* as resistant to DDT, but there is no record of its resistance to any other insecticides [207]. Two vectors of malaria in Nepal, *An. maculatus s.l.* and *An. aconitus,* also have developed resistance to DDT whereas only malathion resistance was reported in *An. stephensi* in Pakistan [208]. Finally, in Iran and Turkey, *An. stephensi* and *An. sacharovi* showed resistance to DDT and dieldrin but both species are mostly susceptible to pyrethroids [209-211].

6.3. Latin America

The countries of the Amazon Basin (Bolivia, Brazil, Colombia, Ecuador, Guyana, Peru, Surinam and Venezuela) carry the greatest burden of malaria in the Americas. The primary vectors of this disease in the Amazon basin are *An. darlingi* and *An. albimanus*. Surprisingly, much less data on insecticide resistance is available for these two mosquito species comparatively to African and/or Asian malaria vector species [212].

In Colombia, DDT resistance was reported in the late 80's in some populations of *An. darlingi* in the districts of Quibdó and close to the Atrato River [213, 214]. Successive insecticide susceptibility evaluations revealed resistance to pyrethroids in both *An. darlingi* and *An. albimanus* mainly in the Chocó State [215]. In *An. darlingi*, increased levels of both Multi function Oxidase (MFO) and Non specific Esterase (NSE) were reported in a deltamethrin and DDT-resistant population, hence suggesting a possible involvement of these detoxifying enzymes in cross resistance to DDT and deltamethrin [35]. Note that various levels of resistance to organophosphate and pyrethroids were also reported in the secondary malaria vector *An. nuneztovari* [216].

In neighboring countries, DDT, permethrin and deltamethrin resistance was found in laboratory colonized populations of *An. albimanus* from Guatemala, whereas full susceptibility was noted in field populations from El Salvador and Belize [217, 218]. The colonies from Guatemala showed significant increase in the specific activity of esterase and/or oxidase as measured by spectrophotometer suggesting their potential involvement in pyrethroid-resistance [34, 217]. In Peru, monitoring campaigns carried out since 2000 showed that *An. albimanus* was the only Anopheline species to exhibit pyrethroid-resistance [219].

In Mexico, high level of DDT resistance and low levels of resistance to organophosphate, carbamate and pyrethroid insecticides were detected in field populations of *An. albimanus* in Chiapas, prior to a large-scale resistance management project [220]. Biochemical assays revealed that the DDT resistance was caused by elevated levels of GST activity leading to increased rates of metabolism of DDT to DDE [22], whereas carbamate resistance was attributed to an altered acetylcholinesterase (AChE). More recent studies conducted in the southern Yucatan Peninsula showed high levels of DDT, deltamethrin and pirimiphos-methyl resistance in the *An. albimanus* populations tested [221]. Biochemical tests revealed elevated levels of GST, P450 and esterases activities that could be involved in DDT and pyrethroid-resistance. As for carbamate, pirimiphos-methyl resistance was strongly correlated with the presence of an insensitive acetylcholinesterase.

To our knowledge, it is the main "published" information available on the distribution, levels and mechanisms of resistance (i.e. accessible through Medline and pub med) in malaria vectors in Latin America. It is then essential to strengthen the capacity of all Latin America countries that suffering from malaria to make insecticide monitoring in routine to obtain much accurate information on the insecticide resistance situation in the malaria vectors. This will provide stake holders with useful information for the implementation of more effective and sustainable malaria control programmes in the region.

7. Impact of pyrethroid-resistance on programmatic malaria control

Few operational reports exist that measure the impact of pyrethroid resistance on epidemiological outcomes of malaria, owing to body of factors that mislead the attributable component of resistance. Where tentative evidence is provided in most cases, the design of the study has been observational and the effect of confounding factors can never be excluded with confidence, making difficult the interpretation of data.

Most probably, the only clearest evidence of control failure being directly linked to pyrethroid resistance was reported from the borders of Mozambique and South Africa. In 1996, the malaria control programme in KwaZulu Natal switched from using DDT to deltamethrin for indoor spraying. Within four years, notified malaria cases had increased about four fold, *An. funestus* had re-appeared and was observable emerging alive from pyrethroid sprayed houses. Bioassays showed that this species was resistant to pyrethroids but susceptible to DDT [39]. A decision was taken to switch back to DDT spraying and, within the two years after this switch was made, *An. funestus* was no longer observed emerging alive from insecticide sprayed houses. The combination of DDT and antimalarial drugs in KwaZulu-Natal has resulted in a 91% decline in the malaria incidence rate [222, 223]. There is no doubt that that the emergence of pyrethroid resistance and the avoidance of its effects by switching to DDT, has been of major operational importance [224].

Additional evidence was brought on the island of Bioko on the West African Coast. A malaria control strategy based on IRS with lambdacyhalothrin was launched by the Bioko Island Malaria Control Project (BIMCP) funded by the Government of Equatorial Guinea and a consortium of private donors led by Marathon Oil Corporation. One round of IRS using the pyrethroid deltamethrin (K-Orthrine WP50, Bayer Crop Sciences, Isando, South Africa) failed to curtail an increase in the population density of *An. gambiae* M form because of evidence in the rise of the knock-down resistance (*kdr*) gene in this species [8]. The programme switched to carbamate insecticide before a substantial decline in the mosquito population, transmission index and malaria prevalence in children was seen. Nevertheless, in an observational study such as this, the possible contribution of other confounding factors to the failure of pyrethroid IRS cannot be overlooked so the direct consequence of the *kdr* frequency is unclear.

Another programmatic study was conducted in the highland provinces of Burundi. Between 2002 and 2005, a well targeted vector control programme (conducted in foot of valleys only) combining IRS with pyrethroids and/or PermaNet 1.0 LLINs was initiated in one of the most affected island provinces, Karuzi [225]. Initially, one round per year of pyrethroid-IRS was carried out in all human dwellings and cattle sheds before the seasonal increase in transmission. LLIN distribution preceded the first IRS round in the same year. The S-form of *An. gambiae* was the predominant vector species in Karuzi District and showed resistance to pyrethroids due to the *kdr* mutation. The entomological data showed that the intervention, overall, effectively reduced *Anopheles* density by 82% and malaria transmission was decreased by 90% despite high frequencies of the L1014S allele in the local *An. gambiae* population [173].

In a more recent observational study conducted in Malawi, the impact of pyrethroid resistance on operational malaria control has been assessed with more controversial evidence of resistance impacting pyrethroid-based vector control [161]. In this trial, pyrethroid-LLINs were distributed to communities in 2007 followed by a pilot campaign of IRS with lambda-cyhalothrin supported by the President's Malaria Initiatives between 2008-2010 within districts. A series of sentinel sites were established during these periods to track the effect of the increase in pyrethroid resistance in the local malaria vectors (*An. gambiae* and *An. funestus*) and assess any impact on malaria transmission and prevalence of infection. Pyrethroid resistance had been selected over the 3 years of the programme in these two major malaria vectors with the resistance in the later vector (i.e; *An. funestus*) being metabolically-mediated and involving the up-regulation of two duplicated P450s. The selection of resistance over 3 years had however not triggered a major increase in parasite prevalence in Malawian children, but it may have reduced the benefit of introducing IRS alone in several districts [161]. The impact of this pyrethroid resistance on the ability of LLIN and IRS to reduce malaria infection in Malawi needs to be further elucidated.

Similarly, in the Dielmo Village of Senegal, a longitudinal study of inhabitants was carried out between January, 2007, and December, 2010 [226]. In July, 2008, deltamethrin-LLINs were provided to all villagers and asymptomatic carriage of malaria parasites was assessed from cross-sectional surveys. Overall, the incidence density of malaria attacks decreased from 5.45 per 100 person-months before LLINs distribution in 2007 to 0.41 by August 2010, but increased sharply back to 4.57 between September and December, 2010, i.e, in less than 3 years after the distribution of LLINs. Within the same time frame, the malaria vector became gradually resistant to pyrethroids and the prevalence of the 1014F *kdr* resistance allele increased from scratch, i.e. 8% in 2007 to 48% in 2010. Once again, these results should be considered with caution as the study was conducted in an unique village and the conclusions drawn could not be extrapolated or extended to Senegal or other areas of Western Africa. Moreover, the link between the slight rise of pyrethroid resistance and the rebound in malaria cases cannot be established with accuracy and such rebound could be due to other sources of factors totally independent of resistance.

Another recent study reports the presence of pyrethroid-resistance in malaria vectors *versus* the gain in current efforts to control malaria in the Zambia [154]. In line with the Global trend to improve malaria control efforts, a country wide campaign of Olyset Nets and PermaNets (LLIN) distribution was initiated in 1999 and indoor residual spraying with DDT or pyrethroids was reintroduced in 2000 in the country by the NMCP. In 2006, these efforts were strengthened by the PMI. Both major malaria vectors, *An. gambiae* and *An. funestus* were controlled effectively with the ITN and IRS programme in Zambia, maintaining a reduced disease transmission and burden, despite the discovery of DDT and pyrethroid resistance in the country.

There have been extensive randomized controlled trials (RCTs) (phase III) in part of Africa aiming at investigating the efficacy of ITNs for malaria prevention [227], but very few have assessed how pyrethroid resistance might affect the effectiveness of such intervention. RCTs entail a set of communities randomly divided into groups, one that receives the novel form of vector control intervention, and comparison arms that often receive the old form of vector control tools or nothing. The key difficulty is that it is impossible to address the question to whether vector control would produce a smaller reduction in malaria if the vector mosquitoes are resistant than it would have done if they were susceptible, using RCT methods. This is simply because resistance is not an easy factor that can be allocated randomly to some communities and not to others. The distribution of resistance is patchy and its severity seems to differ from one location (village) to another. Moreover there may be more resistance or survival trend of mosquitoes in some villages than others because of variations in the quality of vector control operations, or in mosquito behavior [228, 229]. This is important to mention, because many health scientists regard evidence from randomized-controlled studies as the only reliable basis for decision-making in public health.

The first RCT that investigated the impact of pyrethroid-resistance on LLIN efficacy was conducted in the Korhogo area in the north of Côte d'Ivoire. The trial encompassed multiple villages where the 1014F *kdr* allele frequency was >90% [28] and malaria was endemic. The regular use of conventionally lambdacyhalothrin-treated nets had a significant impact on the entomological inoculation rate (55% reduction) and on malaria incidence in children < 5 (56% reduction of clinical attacks) compared to a control group having no nets [230]. This was the first clear-cut evidence of ITNs continuing to provide effective personal protection against malaria in an area with a very high frequency of *kdr* in the vector population. However, as reported in Ranson et al. [6], the absence of a physical barrier in the control group may have overestimated the impact of pyrethroid treated nets against *kdr* mosquitoes in this study.

More recently, another RCT of LLINs and/or IRS was conducted in 28 villages in southern Benin, from 2007 to 2010 [231]. The objective of the study was to examine whether carbamate-IRS applied every 8 months, as practiced by the PMI programme in Benin provided additional benefit over LLINs (ie Permanet 2.0) in term of malaria prevention and management of pyrethroid resistance in malaria vectors. Results showed that combination of LLINs and IRS did not reduce malaria transmission and morbidity compared to LLIN alone in an area of pyrethroid resistance [124]. Significant increase of 1014F *kdr* frequency was observed in the reference and treated arms only 18 months post intervention hence indicating that LLIN and IRS failed to reduce the spread of the 1014F allele in malaria vectors. The authors suggested that the increase in pyrethroid resistance might have accounted for the reduction of LLIN efficacy at a community level. Clearly, further investigation is needed to assess whether pyrethroid-resistance can reduce efficiency of LLINs and IRS for malaria prevention in Africa.

Given the many obstacles for evaluating the epidemiological impact of resistance, other alternative methods to measure operational impact has been to measure proxy entomological outcomes, such as the relative mortality and feeding success of resistant and susceptible vectors in experimental huts [232, 233]. Although such results can be remarkably clear, and definitively linked to resistance, experimental hut methods have their own limitations owing to the controlled hut structures that differ in many ways to normal houses in rural African context.

An early experimental hut trial of ITNs was conducted in the western African country of Benin. In southern Benin (Ladji), pyrethroid resistance has evolved in the M form of *An. gambiae* mosquitoes that appear to combine the knockdown resistance (*kdr*) gene with oxidase mechanisms [127, 234]. In Ladji, carrier mosquitoes of this resistance were not controlled by pyrethroid treatments in experimental hut trials of ITNs or the leading brands of LLINs, PermaNet 2.0 (Vestergaard Frandsen SA, Aarhus, Denmark) and Olyset (Sumitomo Chemi-

http://dx.doi.org/10.5772/56117

cals, Osaka, Japan) [235]), compared to Malanville in the north where the vector was largely susceptible to pyrethroids [127]. Further household randomized trial conducted in northern susceptible and southern resistance areas demonstrated that lambdacyalothrin-ITNs (regardless the physical condition) lose their capacity to confer personal protection against pyrethroid-resistant A*n. gambiae* [236].

One of the problems associated with many of these studies is that, due to the lack of molecular markers for alternative resistance mechanisms (i.e. metabolic or even cuticular and behavioral), the frequency of *kdr* alleles is frequently used as a proxy for resistance. It has been recently demonstrated in Southern Benin that *kdr* by itself in *An. gambiae* does not seem to bear more malaria parasites than in a susceptible [237] but this conception can be misleading when metabolic or other resistance mechanisms are predominant or combine with *kdr* to confer resistance. There is an urgent need for properly controlled large-scale trials to assess the impact of pyrethroid resistance on IRS and ITNs in Africa but also in different regions affected by malaria (e.g. Asia and Latin America). Such studies should use both entomological and epidemiological indices and should be conducted in areas where alternative resistance mechanisms are known to be responsible for pyrethroid resistance. Furthermore, these studies must consider the possibility of behavioural resistance as recently suggested in Benin [238] and Tanzania [111] and monitor for changes in key traits such as location of resting and feeding which may impact on the efficacy of current insecticide based interventions.

8. Resistance management strategies

As a general statement, the use of insecticides does not create resistance by itself but select small proportion of individuals having a genetic mutation that allow them to resist and survive the effects of the insecticide. If this advantage is maintained by constant use of the same insecticide, the resistant insects will reproduce and the genetic changes that confer resistance will be transferred to offspring so that they become more prevalent within the population (figure 3). This selection process will take longer time to occur if the gene conferring resistance is rare or present at a low prevalence. Resistance should not be confused with "induction" that can occur after sub-lethal (or low dose) exposure to any insecticide and/or xenobiotic and is not passed on to offspring [239].

8.1. Main factors influencing resistance development

The evolution of insecticide resistance is complex and depends on several genetic, biological and operational factors [240-242]. The biological factors relate by the life cycle of the insect (e.g. rate of reproduction, number of generation/offspring, rate of migration and isolation, etc), while the genetic factors include the intrinsic characteristics of the resistant genes (e.g. mono *versus* polygenic resistance, dominance, fitness cost and gene interaction). Operational factors concern the treatment itself including the method and frequency of application, dosage and residual activity of the insecticides as well as insecticide coverage.

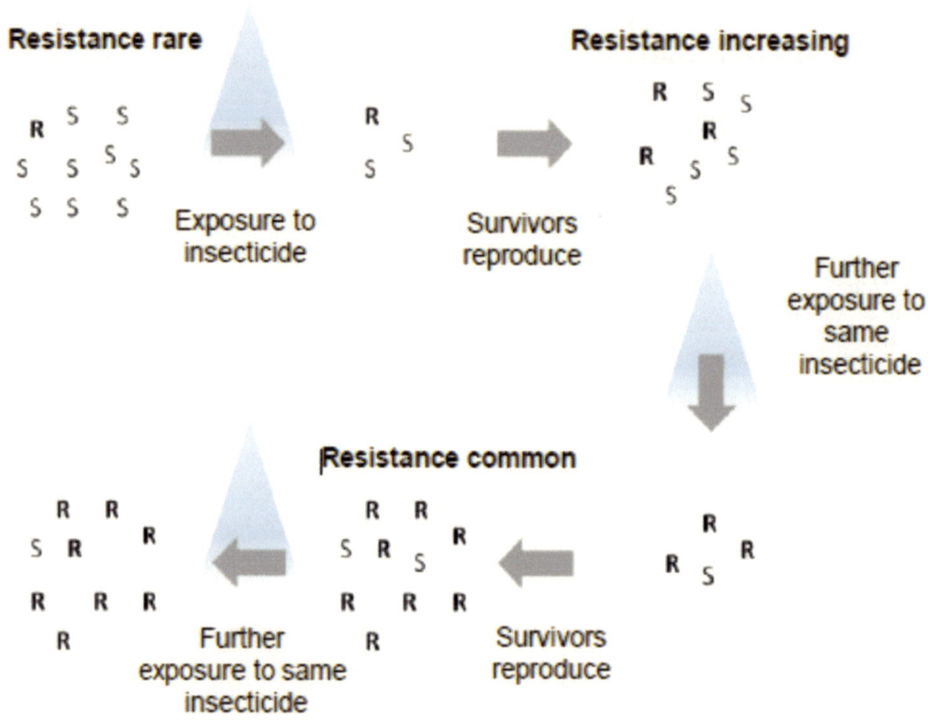

Figure 3. Possible scenario for resistance development in a mosquito population (source; [240])

8.1.1. Biological factors

Rate of reproduction

Insect species that have a short life cycle and high rates of reproduction are likely to develop resistance more rapidly than species that have a lower rate of reproduction, as any resistance genes can rapidly spread throughout the population. Because mosquitoes can produce high number of offspring (i.e. females can lay several hundred eggs during their reproductive life) they are much likely to develop resistance to insecticides than other species.

Population migration / isolation

With mosquitoes, the goal is to eliminate all or the majority of the population, however the greater the selection pressure that is put on a population, the faster susceptibility may be lost. Immigration of individuals possessing susceptible genes from untreated areas can beneficially dilute and compete with the resistance genes in the overall population. An early step in a malaria vector control programme should therefore be to estimate the susceptibility status of vector populations (see section 5 for details) and estimate potential immigration of untreated insects. This can be achieved by using genetic markers to estimate the gene flow (migrants) and genetic structure between populations. For example, an isolated area (e.g. island) where the entire area is treated would have a higher risk of developing resistance as few "susceptible" genotypes would join the treated population. The risk of insecticide resistance developing should be considered when planning a resistance management strategy. Awareness of and coordination with neighboring vector control programmes and agricultural activities should be encouraged, so that the regional and potential "side effect" on the target population is considered.

8.1.2. Genetics factor

Dominance

Resistance genes can range from dominant through semi-dominant to recessive. If dominant or semi-dominant, only one parent needs to possess the characteristic to be fully or partially expressed in the offspring. If recessive, both parents must possess the trait. Fortunately, most resistance mechanisms (e.g. *kdr*) are controlled by recessive or semi-recessive genes, which slows their spread within the population at early stage of resistance development when most individuals are present at heterozygous state. In contrast, when the resistance is genetically dominant, e.g. the *Ace.1*^{R} gene conferring cross-resistance to carbamates and OPs [243], it can rapidly become established within the population and will be difficult to manage. Fortunately, strong genetic cost is often associated with dominant resistant gene that can compensate the effect of the dominance and slow down the increase of resistance gene frequency in natural populations [244].

Gene interactions

Epistasis is the non-additive interaction (synergistic *versus* antagonistic) between different loci which contribute to a phenotype [245]. Epistasis between independent loci conferring insecticide resistance is important to investigate as this phenomenon can shape the rate at which resistance evolves and can dictate the level of resistance in the field. Epistasis can be measured in laboratory studies on susceptible and resistant colonies, but without these data, it is generally impossible to predict whether or not it will occur when two genes are being evaluated. Studies of the interactions between resistance loci have been most commonly conducted in house flies [246-248]. Generally, a greater than additive interaction was observed between two loci that were both homozygous resistant, whereas additively (i.e. lack of epistasis) occurs between two loci that were both heterozygous. In mosquitoes, Harstone and colleagues [249] showed multiplicative interactions between *kdr* and P450 detoxification in *Culex pipiens quinquefasciatus* whether the resistance alleles were homozygous or heterozyges. For example, resistance ratio 50 (i.e. LC50 resistant strain/LC50 susceptible strain) to permethrin in the double homozygote mosquitoes (RR50 of 30,000) was much higher than that expected (RR50 of 1,400) by simple additive effect of the two loci. Overall, interactions between independent resistant genes are complex. It is therefore important to better understand the interactions between resistant loci as well as to address how the fitness costs/benefits of the mechanisms can manipulate the observed interactions.

Fitness cost

Populations of insects that have never been exposed to insecticides are usually fully susceptible, and resistance genes within those populations are very rare. This usually occurs through a "fitness cost", which means that insects sharing the resistance allele lack some other attribute or "quality" such that it gives an advantage to the susceptible insects in an insecticide free environment [250]. For example, resistant insects may have lower mating success, be more susceptible to natural enemies [251], or more prone to mortality during over-wintering [252]. Increased production of metabolic enzymes generally shows lower associated fitness cost than those associated with alterations in the structural genes most probably because the primary function of the enzyme is not disrupted [253]. There is good laboratory and field evidence to suggest that the deficit of insecticide selection pressure, in most cases, selects for susceptible genotypes. For example, the absence of homozygote's resistant genotypes in *An. gambiae* populations in West Africa is most probably due to the strong genetic cost associated with the carbamate-resistance allele *ace.1*^{R} (G119S) [254]. In addition, once resistance in the field has been selected it often rapidly reverts once the insecticide treatment regime is changed. A good example of this occurred in *An. arabiensis* in Sudan, where malathion specific insecticide resistance was selected in the early 1980s through antimalarial house spraying. The development of resistance prompted a switch of insecticide treatment to fenitrothion and the malathion resistance rapidly reverted in the following years. However, reversion rates are variable and may be very slow, particularly when an insecticide has been used for many years. For example, DDT was used extensively for malaria control over a 20 year period up to the 1960s in Sri Lanka to control *An. culicifacies s.l.* and *An. subpictus.* DDT was replaced by malathion in Sri Lanka in the early 1970s when a total and effective ban on DDT use was implemented. Subsequent regular monitoring has shown that DDT resistance has reverted very slowly towards susceptibility; around 80% of the adult mosquito population was resistant in the 1970s compared to about 50% in the 1990s. The same is true with the R*dl* gene that was maintained in field mosquito populations despite the abandon of cyclodiene for mosquito control for more than 30 years [33]. Rate of reversion is an important parameter to consider before implementing any resistance management strategy in the field.

8.1.3. Operational factors

In practice, only operational factors such as the insecticide(s) used, the area of coverage (for example for IRS or LLIN), and the timing, rate, and method of application can be manipulated directly to reduce the selection pressure for resistance. Operational factors influence selection by determining the overall fraction of a population exposed (larvae/adults) to a selecting agent and the degree of contact and pick-up of toxicant by exposed pests at what has been termed the "interface between insects and insecticides" [242]. At both stages, operational and intrinsic factors interact in complex ways to establish the net effect of a control treatment on both genetic composition and total population size. Management of resistance therefore entails resolving these interactions to anticipate with some confidence both the suppressive and selective effects of potential control strategies.

Frequency of application, dosage and persistence of effect

How often an insecticide is used is one of the most important factors that influence resistance development [240]. With each use, an advantage is given to the resistant insects within a population. The rate of increase of resistance on any population will generally be faster in the presence of a lower fitness cost and high reproductive and short life cycles producing several generations per season. The length of time that an insecticide remains effective, also called its persistence, is dependent upon the physical chemistry of the insecticide, the type of formulation, the application rate and the substrate. Products which provide a persistent effect provide continual selection pressure in a similar manner to multiple treatments. For example, a space spray will persist for a very short time and will select only against a single generation of mosquitoes. In contrast, a residual wall application (IRS) or Insecticide Treated nets treatment (especially Long Lasting Nets) will persist for months or years providing a selection pressure against many generations of the same insect. For example, repeated application of DDT for indoor residual spraying has contributed to increase the number of DDT-resistant malaria vector species in various geographical settings [255]. Several studies showed however that the use of insecticides in agriculture play a key role in the selection of resistance in mosquitoes [256, 257]. Indeed, most insecticides used in agriculture are of the same chemical classes and have the same targets and modes of action as those used in public health programme. In practice, VC programmes cannot influence the choice of the pesticide used for crop protection and the only thing that can be done is to appropriately select the most judicious insecticide for mosquito control. However, there is more published evidence that public health insecticides can contribute to select for pyrethroid resistance alleles (see section 7 for details). It is obvious that we can expect enhanced selection pressure on resistance genes through the scaling up of LLIN and/or IRS for malaria elimination.

Choice of the insecticide

The speed at which an insecticide effectively kills an insect can also influence the evolution of resistance. All current insecticides approved for ITNs or IRS kill extremely rapidly after contact. While fast-acting conventional insecticides can produce even more effective initial control, they impose enormous selection for resistance by killing young female adults. The consequence is that spectacular initial mosquito control can last as little as a few years, thus providing very poor medium- to long-term disease control [258]. Some authors recently suggest that Late Acting insecticides (e.g. entomofungus) may be a more tactical strategy to manage resistance if female mosquitoes are killed after 2 or more gonotrophic cycles [259]. Indeed, the less the insecticide impact on mosquito fitness, the less the strength of selection, especially if the resistance allele is associated with a strong genetic cost. In theory, it would be possible to create an insecticide that would provide effective malaria control yet never be undermined by the evolution of resistant mosquitoes. However, further studies are required as "proof of principle" i.e. to demonstrate that this strategy can be effective for vector management and malaria prevention in a real setting.

8.2. Resistance management — Strategies and tactics

Historically, the practice of using an insecticide until resistance becomes a limiting factor has rapidly eroded the number of suitable/available insecticides for vector control. Rotations, mosaics, and mixtures have all been proposed as resistance management tools [260, 261] but there are very few "success stories" in public health. Numerous mathematical models have been produced to estimate how these tools could be optimally used [262-264] but these models have rarely been tested under field conditions due to the practical difficulties in estimating changes in resistance gene frequencies (especially for metabolic resistance) in large samples of insects [220]. With the advent of different molecular techniques for resistance-gene frequency estimation, field trials of resistance management strategies have now become more feasible.

8.2.1. Approaches to resistance management

Ideally insecticide resistance management should be undertaken using insecticide based approaches in conjunction with other non-insecticidal vector control methods, i.e. as part of Integrated Vector Management (IVM[4]) [265]. The insecticides used have to be safe to humans and comply with WHO specifications. In practice, most of IVM programmes work well in experimental trials but become challenging when programmes are scaling up into long-term (operational) control. Operationally, the simplest form of resistance management is likely to be "insecticide" based, and this could take several forms.

Rotations

Rotational strategies are based on the rotation over time of two or preferably more insecticide classes with different modes of action. This approach assumes that if resistance to each insecticide is rare, then multiple resistances will be extremely rare [266]. Rotation allows any resistance developed to the first insecticide to decline over time when the second insecticide class is introduced. As for other strategy, rotations are particularly effective if the resistance gene has an associated fitness cost. The timeframe for rotation needs to be sufficiently short to prevent significant levels of resistance to develop to any one rotation partner. Rotations have been successful in many applications in agriculture and are considered to be effective in slowing the evolution of resistance (see [240] for details*)*. The most striking example of "success story" using this strategy was within the framework of the Onchocerciasis Control Programme (OCP) carried in West Africa 40 years ago. Indeed, weekly application of unrelated larvicides in rivers was successful to kill the larvae of the blackfly vector and mitigate the spread of temephos resistance over the 17 years of its implementation [267]. However, the rotation was introduced at early stage of the OCP, as soon as the operators faced temephos resistance problems in pilot localities. As for all IRM strategies, the status of resistance of the insecticide used in the rotation must be known when implementing rotations and the chemicals used should not present any (known) cross-resistance. For LLIN, it is difficult to implement this method knowing that only pyrethroids are recommended so far by WHO for the impregnation [268]. For IRS, the pragmatic approach would be to rotate insecticides annually. Indeed, changing insecticides more than once a year (which could be the case in areas where two spray rounds are conducted each year) is not recommended, because of procurement and other financial and logistical challenges (see [4]). Despite higher cost of implementing rotation than single spray (as available alternatives to pyrethroids —the carbamates organophosphates, insect growth regulators, pyroles —are currently more expensive), this is probably the price to pay to preserve the arsenal of cost-effective insecticides for malaria vector control.

4*Integrated Vector Management* can be defined as "a rational decision making process for the optimal use of resources for vector control". IRM is therefore an integral part of IVM, as only through the active management of insecticide resistance can the available resources be optimally and sustainably used.

Mosaics

Spatially separated applications of different compounds against the same insect constitute a "mosaic" approach to resistance management [240]. Fine scale mosaics can be achieved in malaria vector control programmes, for example, by using two insecticides in different dwellings within the same village. The aim of this strategy is to preserve susceptibility by spatial restriction of insecticides [4]. If such a fine scale mosaic is to be used, careful records of which insecticide was used in each house are essential. Larger scale mosaics have been shown to be effective for the management of pyrethroid resistance in *An. albimanus* in Mexico [22]. Indeed, pyrethroid resistance rose more rapidly in the areas under pyrethroid treatment alone than in the mosaic areas using OP, Pyrethroid and carbamate [240]. Whilst there are some practical difficulties implementing a mosaic in a vector control programme (eg spray with different insecticides, dosages, apparatus, etc), it may offer the advantages of a mixture strategy with lower insecticide inputs and hence cost. The scale at which a mosaic needs to be applied has not been clearly established. In South Africa for example, different insecticides have been used in different types of houses within the same community and this is considered by some to be a mosaic-like strategy [240]. Similarly, mosquito bed nets from panels treated with different insecticides achieve a similar mosaic effect to treating houses with different compounds but on a much finer scale. Industry has recently developed mosaic LLINs containing a pyrethroid insecticide and a synergist (Piperonyl butoxide or PBO an oxidase inhibitor) on the roof to increase efficacy against pyrethroid-resistant malaria vectors. Small scale field trial [235, 269] and mathematical exercises [270] suggested that mosaic LLIN may provide better insecticidal effect against resistant mosquitoes and enhanced community-level protection against malaria compared to "classical" LLIN in area of pyrethroid resistance. Clearly further operational research is required to establish the applicability and effectiveness of mosaics approaches for malaria control.

Mixtures

A mixture is defined by the simultaneous use of two or more insecticides of unrelated mode of action. If two insecticides A and B, with independent resistance mechanisms, are applied together in a mixture, and if resistance to A and resistance to B are both rare, then we expect doubly resistant insects to be extremely rare, and almost all insects resistant to A will be killed by B, and vice versa [266]. This system of "redundant killing" means that resistance to the two insecticides will evolve much more slowly than if either had been used on its own [271]. This approach may be not successful if resistance to one of the components used is already present at a detectable level and/or if linkage disequilibrium is present in the targeted population [4]. Unlike rotations, the effectiveness of mixtures is not directly related to the degree of fitness cost. Rather the mixture aims to overpower resistance instead of preserving susceptibility. However, for mixtures to work well in practice both insecticides need to be used at their full application rate in order that the efficacy and persistence of the two insecticides would be broadly similar (same decay rate). Further, theoretical models suggest that mixtures might delay resistance longer than rotations or broad mosaics [271, 272]. However, mixtures of products were rarely adopted in malaria vector control programmes on grounds of cost, logistics, and safety issue and because of the limited number of recommended compounds available for both

IRS and LLIN. It is not yet clear however how much the addition of a second active ingredient will add to the total cost of manufacturing since the cost of additional insecticide can greatly vary according to the strategy, ie. cost for LLINs would be much lower than that for IRS. For LLIN, previous laboratory and field trials showed interesting prospects for reducing mosquito survival and biting rates with the use of insecticide mixtures applied on mosquito nets against *kdr*-resistant *An. gambiae* in Africa [273, 274]. Other chemicals, such as insect growth regulators (IGR), represent also promising alternative to be included in mixture formulations as they may impact on mosquito longevity, fertility and fecundity [275, 276]. With the development of next-generation of LLIN, combined use of non-pyrethroids and pyrethroids on bed nets is technically achievable and has the potential to provide better control of malaria and prevent further development of pyrethroid-resistance in malaria vectors. Risk assessment and acceptability of such new tools should be however carefully investigated before any trial being implemented at operational level.

Combinations

In this context, combinations expose the vector population to two vector control tools, such that a mosquito that survives contact with one (e.g. LLIN) is exposed to the other one (e.g. IRS), or vice versa. In practice, exposure to two insecticides is not guaranteed but there is some evidence to indicate that this is likely [277]. The effectiveness of combinations in IRM does not depend on the ability to reduce the level of resistance, but on the ability to kill the vector despite the existence of resistance, through the use of another insecticide or intervention, which compensates for resistance [231]. As for other strategy, the combination should not contain insecticides with same mode of action (e.g. avoid pyrethroids for both IRS and LLINs), as this would increase selection pressure rather than reducing it. As combinations require doubling of interventions, cost would be significantly higher than rotations and mosaics. This might nevertheless be warranted in some circumstances, for example where malaria transmission is very high and/or where targeted IRS can help overcome identified resistance to pyrethroids in areas with high LLIN coverage. In practice, combinations would be more easily implemented in countries having sufficient human and financial resources allocated to public health programmes. So far, a small number of observational studies [278-280] and mathematical modeling exercises [263, 264] suggest that VC combination has an added benefit for reduction of the risk of infection because the people not protected by one of the interventions are protected by the other. A recent cluster randomized controlled trial carried out in Benin showed however that neither clinical malaria in children younger than 6 years nor transmission intensity differ between LLIN and carbamate-IRS or Carbamate Treated Plastic Sheeting and the reference group (LLIN alone) and the insecticide combinations did not slow down the evolution of the *kdr* allele in *An gambiae s.s.* compared with LLIN [231]. It was concluded from this study that IRS should be timely implemented (i.e. using appropriate insecticide, dosage and time interval) to ensure optimum efficacy of the IRS intervention over LLIN. Clearly, cost-effectiveness of combined vector control interventions need to be carefully considered to ensure that increased efforts and cost dedicated to combinations effectively contribute to better control and management of pyrethroid-resistant malaria vectors.

9. Conclusions

Insecticide resistance develops in an insect population when individuals carrying genes that allow them to survive exposure to the insecticide pass these genes on. Thus, any activities that control the individuals with the resistance trait will delay the spread of the resistance genes in the population. IRM should then be seen in the context of IVM and should therefore also include activities such as habitat management, community education, and/or larval source management (e.g. biological control). In order to successfully develop and implement any resistance management strategies based on rotations, mosaics, mixtures or combinations, knowledge of the mode of action, chemical properties, and residual life of the available insecticide products is essential. Although insecticides with novel modes of action have recently been introduced in public health (neonicotinoids, pyroles, oxadiazin, etc) few of them appear to have the optimum biological and/or physical properties required for residual wall spray and/or mosquito net. Unfortunately, the exorbitant costs associated with developing and registering new insecticides (see [281] for details) mean that products appear in the more profitable agricultural markets before consideration is given to their public health potential. We have then no other option than to make an appropriate and judicious use of the current insecticides if we want to avoid any disillusion with pyrethroids as we faced before with DDT or dieldrin. The philosopher George Santayana said *"those who cannot remember the past are condemned to repeat it."* Hope it's not too late for malaria vector control.

Author details

Vincent Corbel[1,2*] and Raphael N'Guessan[3,4]

*Address all correspondence to: vincent.corbel@ird.fr

1 Institut de Recherche pour le Développement, Maladies Infectieuses et Vecteurs, Ecologie, Génétique, Evolution et Contrôle (IRD 224-CNRS 5290 UM1-UM2), Benin

2 Department of Entomology, Kasetsart University, Bangkok, Thailand

3 London School of Hygiene & Tropical Medicine, London, UK

4 Centre de Recherches Entomologiques de Cotonou, Cotonou, Benin

References

[1] World Health Organization: WHO malaria report : 2011. In: *WHO Global Malaria Programme.* Edited by Data WLC-i-P. Geneva: WHO; 2011: 259.

[2] Yassine H, Osta MA: *Anopheles gambiae* innate immunity. *Cell Microbiol,* 12(1):1-9.

[3] Davidson G: Insecticide resistance in *Anopheles sundaicus. Nature* 1957, 180(4598): 1333-1335.

[4] World Health Organization: Global Plan for Insecticide Resistance Management in Malaria Vectors (GPIRM). In: *WHO/HTM/GMP/20125.* Edited by Organization WH. Geneva, Switzerland: World Health Organization; 2012: 130.

[5] Hemingway J, Ranson H: Insecticide resistance in insect vectors of human disease. *Annu Rev Entomol* 2000, 45:371-391.

[6] Ranson H, N'Guessan R, Lines J, Moiroux N, Nkuni Z, Corbel V: Pyrethroid resistance in African anopheline mosquitoes: what are the implications for malaria control? *Trends Parasitol* 2011, 27(2):91-98.

[7] Ridl FC, Bass C, Torrez M, Govender D, Ramdeen V, Yellot L, Edu AE, Schwabe C, Mohloai P, Maharaj R *et al*: A pre-intervention study of malaria vector abundance in Rio Muni, Equatorial Guinea: their role in malaria transmission and the incidence of insecticide resistance alleles. *Malar J* 2008, 7:194.

[8] Sharp BL, Ridl FC, Govender D, Kuklinski J, Kleinschmidt I: Malaria vector control by indoor residual insecticide spraying on the tropical island of Bioko, Equatorial Guinea. *Malar J* 2007, 6:52.

[9] Mitchell SN, Stevenson BJ, Muller P, Wilding CS, Egyir-Yawson A, Field SG, Hemingway J, Paine MJ, Ranson H, Donnelly MJ: Identification and validation of a gene causing cross-resistance between insecticide classes in *Anopheles gambiae* from Ghana. *Proc Natl Acad Sci U S A* 2012, 109(16):6147-6152.

[10] Stevenson BJ, Bibby J, Pignatelli P, Muangnoicharoen S, O'Neill PM, Lian LY, Muller P, Nikou D, Steven A, Hemingway J *et al*: Cytochrome P450 6M2 from the malaria vector *Anopheles gambiae* metabolizes pyrethroids: Sequential metabolism of deltamethrin revealed. *Insect Biochem Mol Biol* 2011, 41(7):492-502.

[11] Brown AWA: Insecticide Resistance Mosquitoes: A Pragmatic Rewiew. *J Am Mosq Control Assoc* 1986, 2(2):123-140.

[12] Metcalf RL: Insect resistance to insecticides. *Pesticide Science* 1989, 26(4):333-358.

[13] WHO: Global Insecticide Use for Vector-Borne Disease Control- 4th edition. *In Edited by World Health Organization Geneva: World Health Organization* 2009, WHO/HTM/NTD/WHOPES/GCDPP/2009.6.

[14] Lapied B, Pennetier C, Apaire-Marchais V, Licznar P, Corbel V: Innovative applications for insect viruses: towards insecticide sensitization. *Trends Biotechnol* 2009, 27(4):190-198.

[15] Livadas GA, Georgopoulos G: Development of resistance to DDT by *Anopheles sacharovi* in Greece. *Bull World Health Organ* 1953, 8(4):497-511.

[16] Brown AWA, Haworth J, Zahar AR: Malaria eradication and control from a global standpoint. *Journal of Medical Entomology* 1976, 13(1):1-25.

[17] Patel TB, Ramachandra Rao T, Halgeri AV, Deobhankar RB: A preliminary note on a probable case of dieldrin kesistance in *Anopheles culicifacies* in Thana District, Bombay State. *Indian J Malariol* 1958, 12:367-370.

[18] Brown AW, Pal R: Insecticide resistance in arthropods. *Public Health Pap* 1971, 38(0): 1-491.

[19] Brown AW, Haworth J, Zahar AR: Malaria eradication and control from a global standpoint. *J Med Entomol* 1976, 13(1):1-25.

[20] Rajagopal R: Malathion resistance in *Anopheles culicifacies* in Gujarat. *Indian J Med Res* 1977, 66(1):27-28.

[21] Rawlings P, Herath PR, Kelly S: *Anopheles culicifacies* (Diptera: Culicidae): DDT resistance in Sri Lanka prior to and after cessation of DDT spraying. *J Med Entomol* 1985, 22(4):361-365.

[22] Penilla RP, Rodriguez AD, Hemingway J, Torres JL, Arredondo Jimenez JI, Rodriguez MH: Resistance management strategies in malaria vector mosquito control. Baseline data for a large-scale field trial against *Anopheles albimanus* in Mexico. *Medical and Veterinary Entomology* 1998, 12(3):217-233.

[23] Van Bortel W, Trung HD, Thuan le K, Sochantha T, Socheat D, Sumrandee C, Baimai V, Keokenchanh K, Samlane P, Roelants P *et al*: The insecticide resistance status of malaria vectors in the Mekong region. *Malar J* 2008, 7:102.

[24] Trung HD, Van Bortel W, Sochantha T, Keokenchanh K, Quang NT, Cong LD, Coosemans M: Malaria transmission and major malaria vectors in different geographical areas of Southeast Asia. *Trop Med Int Health* 2004, 9(2):230-237.

[25] Chareonviriyaphap T, Aum-aung B, Ratanatham S: Current insecticide resistance patterns in mosquito vectors in Thailand. *Southeast Asian J Trop Med Public Health* 1999, 30(1):184-194.

[26] Hamon J, Subra R, Sales S, Coz J: [Presence in the southwestern part of Upper Volta of a population of *Anopheles gambiae* "A" resistant to DDT]. *Med Trop (Mars)* 1968, 28(4):521-528.

[27] Carnevale P, Robert V: *Anopheles*: Biologie, transmission du *Plasmodium* et lutte antivectorielle. Bondy: IRD; 2009.

[28] Chandre F, Darriet F, Manguin S, Brengues C, Carnevale P, Guillet P: Pyrethroid cross resistance spectrum among populations of *Anopheles gambiae* s.s. from Cote d'Ivoire. *J Am Mosq Control Assoc* 1999, 15(1):53-59.

[29] Armstrong JA, Ramsdale CD, Ramakrishna V: Insecticide resistance in *Anopheles gambiae* Giles in Western Sokoto, Northern Nigeria. *Ann Trop Med Parasitol* 1958, 52(3):247-256.

[30] Hamon J, Garrett-Jones C: [Resistance to insecticides in the major malaria vectors and its operational importance]. *Bull World Health Organ* 1963, 28(1):1-24.

[31] Wondji CS, Dabire RK, Tukur Z, Irving H, Djouaka R, Morgan JC: Identification and distribution of a GABA receptor mutation conferring dieldrin resistance in the malaria vector *Anopheles funestus* in Africa. *Insect Biochem Mol Biol* 2011, 41(7):484-491.

[32] Mouchet J: Mini-Review : Agriculture and Vector Resistance. *Insect Sci Applic* 1988, 9(3):291-302.

[33] Mahande AM, Dusfour I, Matias JR, Kweka EJ: Knockdown Resistance, rdl Alleles, and the Annual Entomological Inoculation Rate of Wild Mosquito Populations from Lower Moshi, Northern Tanzania. *J Glob Infect Dis* 2012, 4(2):114-119.

[34] Brogdon WG, McAllister JC, Corwin AM, Cordon Rosales C: Oxidase-based DDT-pyrethroid cross-resistance in Guatemalan *Anopheles albimanus*. *Pesticide Biochemistry and Physiology* 1999, 64(2):101-111.

[35] Fonseca-Gonzalez I, Quinones ML, McAllister J, Brogdon WG: Mixed-function oxidases and esterases associated with cross-resistance between DDT and lambda-cyhalothrin in *Anopheles darlingi* Root 1926 populations from Colombia. *Mem Inst Oswaldo Cruz* 2009, 104(1):18-26.

[36] Raghavendra K, Verma V, Srivastava HC, Gunasekaran K, Sreehari U, Dash AP: Persistence of DDT, malathion & deltamethrin resistance in *Anopheles culicifacies* after their sequential withdrawal from indoor residual spraying in Surat district, India. *Indian J Med Res* 2010, 132:260-264.

[37] Tiwari S, Ghosh SK, Ojha VP, Dash AP, Raghavendra K: Reduced susceptibility to selected synthetic pyrethroids in urban malaria vector *Anopheles stephensi*: a case study in Mangalore city, South India. *Malar J* 2010, 9:179.

[38] Elissa N, Mouchet J, Riviere F, Meunier JY, Yao K: Resistance of *Anopheles gambiae* s.s. to pyrethroids in Cote d'Ivoire. *Ann Soc Belg Med Trop* 1993, 73(4):291-294.

[39] Hargreaves K, Koekemoer LL, Brooke BD, Hunt RH, Mthembu J, Coetzee M: *Anopheles funestus* resistant to pyrethroid insecticides in South Africa. *Medical and Veterinary Entomology* 2000, 14(2):181-189.

[40] Chareonviriyaphap T, Rongnoparut P, Juntarumporn P: Selection for pyrethroid resistance in a colony of *Anopheles minimus* species A, a malaria vector in Thailand. *J Vector Ecol* 2002, 27(2):222-229.

[41] Ayad H, Georghiou GP: Resistance to organophosphates and carbamates in *Anopheles albimanus* based on reduced sensitivity of acetylcholinesterase. *Journal of Economic Entomology* 1975, 68(3):295-297.

[42] Hemingway J: Genetics of organophosphate and carbamate resistance in *Anopheles atroparvus* (Diptera: Culicidae). *J Econ Entomol* 1982, 75(6):1055-1058.

[43] Elissa N, Mouchet J, Riviere F, Meunier JY, Yao K: [Susceptibility of *Anopheles gambiae* to insecticides in the Ivory Coast]. *Sante* 1994, 4(2):95-99.

[44] N'Guessan R, Darriet F, Guillet P, Carnevale P, Traore-Lamizana M, Corbel V, Koffi AA, Chandre F: Resistance to carbosulfan in *Anopheles gambiae* from Ivory Coast, based on reduced sensitivity of acetylcholinesterase. *Med Vet Entomol* 2003, 17(1): 19-25.

[45] Dabire KR, Diabate A, Namontougou M, Djogbenou L, Kengne P, Simard F, Bass C, Baldet T: Distribution of insensitive acetylcholinesterase (ace-1R) in *Anopheles gambiae* s.l. populations from Burkina Faso (West Africa). *Trop Med Int Health* 2009, 14(4): 396-403.

[46] Djogbenou L, Dabire R, Diabate A, Kengne P, Akogbeto M, Hougard JM, Chandre F: Identification and geographic distribution of the ACE-1R mutation in the malaria vector *Anopheles gambiae* in south-western Burkina Faso, West Africa. *Am J Trop Med Hyg* 2008, 78(2):298-302.

[47] Djogbenou L, Pasteur N, Akogbeto M, Weill M, Chandre F: Insecticide resistance in the *Anopheles gambiae* complex in Benin: a nationwide survey. *Med Vet Entomol* 2011, 25(3):256-267.

[48] Oduola AO, Idowu ET, Oyebola MK, Adeogun AO, Olojede JB, Otubanjo OA, Awolola TS: Evidence of carbamate resistance in urban populations of *Anopheles gambiae* s.s. mosquitoes resistant to DDT and deltamethrin insecticides in Lagos, South-Western Nigeria. *Parasit Vectors* 2012, 5:116.

[49] USAID: The President's Malaria Initiative: fourth annual report. In. Washigton: U.S. Agency for International Development; 2010.

[50] Nkya TE, Akhouayri I, Kisinza W, David JP: Impact of environment on mosquito response to pyrethroid insecticides: Facts, evidences and prospects. *Insect Biochem Mol Biol* 2012.

[51] Despres L, David JP, Gallet C: The evolutionary ecology of insect resistance to plant chemicals. *Trends Ecol Evol* 2007, 22(6):298-307.

[52] Hemingway J, Hawkes NJ, McCarroll L, Ranson H: The molecular basis of insecticide resistance in mosquitoes. *Insect Biochem Mol Biol* 2004, 34(7):653-665.

[53] Guillemaud T, Makate N, Raymond M, Hirst B, Callaghan A: Esterase gene amplification in *Culex pipiens*. *Insect Molecular Biology* 1997, 6(4):319-327.

[54] Hawkes NJ, Hemingway J: Analysis of the promoters for the beta-esterase genes associated with insecticide resistance in the mosquito *Culex quinquefasciatus*. *Biochim Biophys Acta* 2002, 1574(1):51-62.

[55] Vaughan A, Hawkes N, Hemingway J: Co-amplification explains linkage disequilibrium of two mosquito esterase genes in insecticide-resistant *Culex quinquefasciatus*. *Biochem J* 1997, 325 (Pt 2):359-365.

[56] Herath PR, Miles SJ, Davidson G: Fenitrothion (OMS 43) resistance in the taxon *Anopheles culicifacies* Giles. *J Trop Med Hyg* 1981, 84(2):87-88.

[57] Hemingway J: The genetics of malathion resistance in *Anopheles stephensi* from Pakistan. *Trans R Soc Trop Med Hyg* 1983, 77(1):106-108.

[58] Vontas J, Blass C, Koutsos AC, David JP, Kafatos FC, Louis C, Hemingway J, Christophides GK, Ranson H: Gene expression in insecticide resistant and susceptible *Anopheles gambiae* strains constitutively or after insecticide exposure. *Insect Mol Biol* 2005, 14(5):509-521.

[59] Somwang P, Yanola J, Suwan W, Walton C, Lumjuan N, Prapanthadara LA, Somboon P: Enzymes-based resistant mechanism in pyrethroid resistant and susceptible *Aedes aegypti* strains from northern Thailand. *Parasitol Res* 2011, 109(3):531-537.

[60] Feyereisen R, Lawrence IG, Kostas I, Sarjeet SG: Insect Cytochrome P450. In: *Comprehensive Molecular Insect Science.* Amsterdam: Elsevier; 2005: 1-77.

[61] Holt RA, Subramanian GM, Halpern A, Sutton GG, Charlab R, Nusskern DR, Wincker P, Clark AG, Ribeiro JM, Wides R *et al*: The genome sequence of the malaria mosquito *Anopheles gambiae*. *Science* 2002, 298(5591):129-149.

[62] Ranson H, Nikou D, Hutchinson M, Wang X, Roth CW, Hemingway J, Collins FH: Molecular analysis of multiple cytochrome P450 genes from the malaria vector, *Anopheles gambiae*. *Insect Mol Biol* 2002, 11(5):409-418.

[63] Nikou D, Ranson H, Hemingway J: An adult-specific CYP6 P450 gene is overexpressed in a pyrethroid-resistant strain of the malaria vector, *Anopheles gambiae*. *Gene* 2003, 318:91-102.

[64] David JP, Strode C, Vontas J, Nikou D, Vaughan A, Pignatelli PM, Louis C, Hemingway J, Ranson H: The *Anopheles gambiae* detoxification chip: a highly specific microarray to study metabolic-based insecticide resistance in malaria vectors. *Proc Natl Acad Sci U S A* 2005, 102(11):4080-4084.

[65] Irving H, Riveron JM, Ibrahim SS, Lobo NF, Wondji CS: Positional cloning of rp2 QTL associates the P450 genes CYP6Z1, CYP6Z3 and CYP6M7 with pyrethroid resistance in the malaria vector *Anopheles funestus*. *Heredity (Edinb)* 2012, 109(6):383-392.

http://dx.doi.org/10.5772/56117

[66] Chiu TL, Wen Z, Rupasinghe SG, Schuler MA: Comparative molecular modeling of *Anopheles gambiae* CYP6Z1, a mosquito P450 capable of metabolizing DDT. *Proc Natl Acad Sci U S A* 2008, 105(26):8855-8860.

[67] McLaughlin LA, Niazi U, Bibby J, David JP, Vontas J, Hemingway J, Ranson H, Sutcliffe MJ, Paine MJ: Characterization of inhibitors and substrates of *Anopheles gambiae* CYP6Z2. *Insect Mol Biol* 2008, 17(2):125-135.

[68] Muller P, Chouaibou M, Pignatelli P, Etang J, Walker ED, Donnelly MJ, Simard F, Ranson H: Pyrethroid tolerance is associated with elevated expression of antioxidants and agricultural practice in *Anopheles arabiensis* sampled from an area of cotton fields in Northern Cameroon. *Mol Ecol* 2008, 17(4):1145-1155.

[69] Djouaka RF, Bakare AA, Coulibaly ON, Akogbeto MC, Ranson H, Hemingway J, Strode C: Expression of the cytochrome P450s, CYP6P3 and CYP6M2 are significantly elevated in multiple pyrethroid resistant populations of *Anopheles gambiae* s.s. from Southern Benin and Nigeria. *BMC Genomics* 2008, 9:538.

[70] Muller P, Donnelly MJ, Ranson H: Transcription profiling of a recently colonised pyrethroid resistant *Anopheles gambiae* strain from Ghana. *BMC Genomics* 2007, 8:36.

[71] Muller P, Warr E, Stevenson BJ, Pignatelli PM, Morgan JC, Steven A, Yawson AE, Mitchell SN, Ranson H, Hemingway J *et al*: Field-caught permethrin-resistant *Anopheles gambiae* overexpress CYP6P3, a P450 that metabolises pyrethroids. *PLoS Genet* 2008, 4(11):e1000286.

[72] Wondji CS, Irving H, Morgan J, Lobo NF, Collins FH, Hunt RH, Coetzee M, Hemingway J, Ranson H: Two duplicated P450 genes are associated with pyrethroid resistance in *Anopheles funestus*, a major malaria vector. *Genome Res* 2009, 19(3):452-459.

[73] Wondji CS, Morgan J, Coetzee M, Hunt RH, Steen K, Black WCt, Hemingway J, Ranson H: Mapping a quantitative trait locus (QTL) conferring pyrethroid resistance in the African malaria vector *Anopheles funestus*. *BMC Genomics* 2007, 8:34.

[74] Riveron JM, Irving H, Ndula M, Barnes KG, Ibrahim SS, Paine MJ, Wondji CS: Directionally selected cytochrome P450 alleles are driving the spread of pyrethroid resistance in the major malaria vector *Anopheles funestus*. *Proc Natl Acad Sci U S A* 2012, 110(1):252-257.

[75] Rongnoparut P, Boonsuepsakul S, Chareonviriyaphap T, Thanomsing N: Cloning of cytochrome P450, CYP6P5, and CYP6AA2 from *Anopheles minimus* resistant to deltamethrin. *J Vector Ecol* 2003, 28(2):150-158.

[76] Duangkaew P, Kaewpa D, Rongnoparut P: Protective efficacy of *Anopheles minimus* CYP6P7 and CYP6AA3 against cytotoxicity of pyrethroid insecticides in *Spodoptera frugiperda* (Sf9) insect cells. *Trop Biomed* 2011, 28(2):293-301.

[77] Duangkaew P, Pethuan S, Kaewpa D, Boonsuepsakul S, Sarapusit S, Rongnoparut P: Characterization of mosquito CYP6P7 and CYP6AA3: differences in substrate preference and kinetic properties. *Arch Insect Biochem Physiol* 2011, 76(4):236-248.

[78] Ranson H, Cornel AJ, Fournier D, Vaughan A, Collins FH, Hemingway J: Cloning and Localization of a Glutathione S-transferase Class I Gene from *Anopheles gambiae*. *J Biol Chem* 1997, 272(9):5464-5967.

[79] Ranson H, Hemingway J: Mosquito glutathione transferases. *Methods Enzymol* 2005, 401:226-241.

[80] Fournier D, Bride JM, Poirie M, Berge JB, Plapp FW, Jr.: Insect glutathione S-transferases. Biochemical characteristics of the major forms from houseflies susceptible and resistant to insecticides. *Journal of Biological Chemistry* 1992, 267(3):1840-1845.

[81] Ranson H, Rossiter L, Ortelli F, Jensen B, Wang XL, Roth CW, Collins FH, Hemingway J: Identification of a novel class of insect glutathione S-transferases involved in resistance to DDT in the malaria vector *Anopheles gambiae*. *Biochemical Journal* 2001, 359 Part 2:295-304.

[82] Gunasekaran K, Muthukumaravel S, Sahu SS, Vijayakumar T, Jambulingam P: Glutathione S transferase activity in Indian vectors of malaria: A defense mechanism against DDT. *J Med Entomol* 2011, 48(3):561-569.

[83] Prapanthadara LA, Ketterman AJ: Qualitative and quantitative changes in glutathione S-transferases in the mosquito *Anopheles gambiae* confer DDT-resistance. *Biochem Soc Trans* 1993, 21 (Pt 3)(3):304S.

[84] Ranson H, Jensen B, Wang X, Prapanthadara L, Hemingway J, Collins FH: Genetic mapping of two loci affecting DDT resistance in the malaria vector *Anopheles gambiae*. *Insect Mol Biol* 2000, 9(5):499-507.

[85] Vontas JG, Small GJ, Hemingway J: Glutathione S-transferases as antioxidant defence agents confer pyrethroid resistance in *Nilaparvata lugens*. *Biochem J* 2001, 357(Pt 1): 65-72.

[86] Kostaropoulos I, Papadopoulos AI, Metaxakis A, Boukouvala E, Papadopoulou-Mourkidou E: Glutathione S-transferase in the defence against pyrethroids in insects. *Insect Biochem Mol Biol* 2001, 31(4-5):313-319.

[87] Fournier D: Mutations of acetylcholinesterase which confer insecticide resistance in insect populations. *Chem Biol Interact* 2005.

[88] Weill M, Lutfalla G, Mogensen K, Chandre F, Berthomieu A, Berticat C, Pasteur N, Philips A, Fort P, Raymond M: Comparative genomics: Insecticide resistance in mosquito vectors. *Nature* 2003, 423(6936):136-137.

[89] Alout H, Labbe P, Berthomieu A, Pasteur N, Weill M: Multiple duplications of the rare ace-1 mutation F290V in *Culex pipiens* natural populations. *Insect Biochem Mol Biol* 2009.

[90] Weill M, Malcolm C, Chandre F, Mogensen K, Berthomieu A, Marquine M, Raymond M: The unique mutation in ace-1 giving high insecticide resistance is easily detectable in mosquito vectors. *Insect Mol Biol* 2004, 13(1):1-7.

[91] Djogbenou L, Chandre F, Berthomieu A, Dabire R, Koffi A, Alout H, Weill M: Evidence of introgression of the ace-1(R) mutation and of the ace-1 duplication in West African *Anopheles gambiae* s. s. *PLoS ONE* 2008, 3(5):e2172.

[92] Ffrench-Constant RH: The molecular and population genetics of cyclodiene insecticide resistance. *Insect Biochem Mol Biol* 1994, 24(4):335-345.

[93] Andreasen MH, Ffrench-Constant RH: In situ hybridization to the Rdl locus on polytene chromosome 3L of *Anopheles stephensi*. *Med Vet Entomol* 2002, 16(4):452-455.

[94] Du W, Awolola TS, Howell P, Koekemoer LL, Brooke BD, Benedict MQ, Coetzee M, Zheng L: Independent mutations in the Rdl locus confer dieldrin resistance to *Anopheles gambiae* and *An. arabiensis*. *Insect Mol Biol* 2005, 14(2):179-183.

[95] Davies TG, Field LM, Usherwood PN, Williamson MS: DDT, pyrethrins, pyrethroids and insect sodium channels. *IUBMB Life* 2007, 59(3):151-162.

[96] Donnelly MJ, Corbel V, Weetman D, Wilding CS, Williamson MS, Black WCt: Does *kdr* genotype predict insecticide-resistance phenotype in mosquitoes? *Trends Parasitol* 2009, 25(5):213-219.

[97] Martinez Torres D, Chandre F, Williamson MS, Darriet F, Berge JB, Devonshire AL, Guillet P, Pasteur N, Pauron D: Molecular characterization of pyrethroid knockdown resistance (*kdr*) in the major malaria vector *Anopheles gambiae* s.s. *Insect Molecular Biology* 1998, 7(2):179-184.

[98] Ranson H, Jensen B, Vulule JM, Wang X, Hemingway J, Collins FH: Identification of a point mutation in the voltage-gated sodium channel gene of Kenyan *Anopheles gambiae* associated with resistance to DDT and pyrethroids. *Insect Molecular Biology* 2000, 9(5):491-497.

[99] O'Reilly AO, Khambay BP, Williamson MS, Field LM, Wallace BA, Davies TG: Modelling insecticide-binding sites in the voltage-gated sodium channel. *Biochem J* 2006, 396(2):255-263.

[100] Jones CM, Liyanapathirana M, Agossa FR, Weetman D, Ranson H, Donnelly MJ, Wilding CS: Footprints of positive selection associated with a mutation (N1575Y) in the voltage-gated sodium channel of *Anopheles gambiae*. *Proc Natl Acad Sci U S A* 2012, 109(17):6614-6619.

[101] Plapp FW, Jr.: The genetic basis of insecticide resistance in the house fly: evidence that a single locus plays a major role in metabolic resistance to insecticides. *Pesticide Biochemistry and Physiology* 1984, 22(2):194-201.

[102] Georghiou GP, Ariaratnam V, Pasternak ME, Lin CS: Organophosphorus multiresistance in *Culex pipiens quinquefasciatus* in California. *Journal of Economic Entomology* 1975, 68(4):461-467.

[103] Vontas J, David JP, Nikou D, Hemingway J, Christophides GK, Louis C, Ranson H: Transcriptional analysis of insecticide resistance in *Anopheles stephensi* using cross-species microarray hybridization. *Insect Mol Biol* 2007, 16(3):315-324.

[104] Awolola TS, Oduola OA, Strode C, Koekemoer LL, Brooke B, Ranson H: Evidence of multiple pyrethroid resistance mechanisms in the malaria vector *Anopheles gambiae* sensu stricto from Nigeria. *Trans R Soc Trop Med Hyg* 2009, 103(11):1139-1145.

[105] Wood O, Hanrahan S, Coetzee M, Koekemoer L, Brooke B: Cuticle thickening associated with pyrethroid resistance in the major malaria vector *Anopheles funestus*. *Parasit Vectors* 2010, 3:67.

[106] Roberts DR, Chareonviriyaphap T, Harlan HH, Hshieh P: Methods of testing and analyzing excito-repellency responses of malaria vectors to insecticides. *J Am Mosq Control Assoc* 1997, 13(1):13-17.

[107] Chandre F, Darriet F, Duchon S, Finot L, Manguin S, Carnevale P, Guillet P: Modifications of pyrethroid effects associated with *kdr* mutation in *Anopheles gambiae*. *Medical and Veterinary Entomology* 2000, 14(1):81-88.

[108] Gahan JB, Lindquist AW: DDT residual sprays applied in buildings to control *Anopheles quadrimaculatus*. *Journal of Economic Entomology* 1945, 38 (2):223-230.

[109] Chareonviriyaphap T, Roberts DR, Andre RG, Harlan HJ, Manguin S, Bangs MJ: Pesticide avoidance behavior in *Anopheles albimanus*, a malaria vector in the Americas. *J Am Mosq Control Assoc* 1997, 13(2):171-183.

[110] Garros C, Marchand RP, Quang NT, Hai NS, Manguin S: First record of *Anopheles minimus* C and significant decrease of *An. minimus* A in central Vietnam. *J Am Mosq Control Assoc* 2005, 21(2):139-143.

[111] Russell TL, Govella NJ, Azizi S, Drakeley CJ, Kachur SP, Killeen GF: Increased proportions of outdoor feeding among residual malaria vector populations following increased use of insecticide-treated nets in rural Tanzania. *Malar J* 2011, 10:80.

[112] Moiroux N, Gomez MB, Pennetier C, Elanga E, Djenontin A, Chandre F, Djegbe I, Guis H, Corbel V: Changes in *Anopheles funestus* Biting Behavior Following Universal Coverage of Long-Lasting Insecticidal Nets in Benin. *J Infect Dis* 2012, 206(10): 1622-1629.

[113] WHO: Guidelines for testing mosquito adulticides intended for Indoor Residual Spraying (IRS) and Insecticide Treated Nets (ITNs). 2006, WHO/CDS/NTD/WHOPES/GCDDP/2006.3.

[114] WHO: Report of the WHO Informal Consultation Tests procedures for insecticide resistance monitoring in malaria vectors, bio-efficacy and persistence of insecticides on treated surfaces. In. Geneva: World Health Organization: Parasitic Diseases and Vector Control (PVC)/Communicable Disease Control, Prevention and Eradication (CPE); 1998: 43.

[115] Williams J, Pinto J: Training Manual on Malaria Entomology; For Entomology and Vector Control Technicians (Basic Level) In. Edited by USAID. Washington, D.C.; 2012: 78.

[116] Ranson H, Abdallah H, Badolo A, Guelbeogo WM, Kerah-Hinzoumbe C, Yangalbe-Kalnone E, Sagnon N, Simard F, Coetzee M: Insecticide resistance in *Anopheles gambiae*: data from the first year of a multi-country study highlight the extent of the problem. *Malar J* 2009, 8(1):299.

[117] Skovmand O, Bonnet J, Pigeon O, Corbel V: Median knock-down time as a new method for evaluating insecticide-treated textiles for mosquito control. *Malar J* 2008, 7:114.

[118] Brogdon WG, McAllister JC: Simplification of adult mosquito bioassays through use of time-mortality determinations in glass bottles. *J Am Mosq Control Assoc* 1998, 14(2): 159-164.

[119] World Health Organization: Techniques to detect insecticide resistance mechanisms (field and laboratory manual). In. Edited by WHO/CDS/CPC/MAL/98.6 WHO. Geneva: World Health Organization; 1998.

[120] Munhenga G, Masendu HT, Brooke BD, Hunt RH, Koekemoer LK: Pyrethroid resistance in the major malaria vector *Anopheles arabiensis* from Gwave, a malaria-endemic area in Zimbabwe. *Malar J* 2008, 7:247.

[121] Okoye PN, Brooke BD, Koekemoer LL, Hunt RH, Coetzee M: Characterisation of DDT, pyrethroid and carbamate resistance in *Anopheles funestus* from Obuasi, Ghana. *Trans R Soc Trop Med Hyg* 2008, 102(6):591-598.

[122] Kelly-Hope L, Ranson H, Hemingway J: Lessons from the past: managing insecticide resistance in malaria control and eradication programmes. *Lancet Infect Dis* 2008.

[123] Chouaibou M, Etang J, Brevault T, Nwane P, Hinzoumbe CK, Mimpfoundi R, Simard F: Dynamics of insecticide resistance in the malaria vector *Anopheles gambiae* s.l. from an area of extensive cotton cultivation in Northern Cameroon. *Trop Med Int Health* 2008, 13(4):476-486.

[124] Djegbe I, Boussari O, Sidick A, Martin T, Ranson H, Chandre F, Akogbeto M, Corbel V: Dynamics of insecticide resistance in malaria vectors in Benin: first evidence of the

presence of L1014S *kdr* mutation in *Anopheles gambiae* from West Africa. *Malaria Journal* 2011, 10(1):261.

[125] Dabire KR, Diabate A, Pare-Toe L, Rouamba J, Ouari A, Fontenille D, Baldet T: Year to year and seasonal variations in vector bionomics and malaria transmission in a humid savannah village in west Burkina Faso. *J Vector Ecol* 2008, 33(1):70-75.

[126] Bass C, Nikou D, Donnelly MJ, Williamson MS, Ranson H, Ball A, Vontas J, Field LM: Detection of knockdown resistance (*kdr*) mutations in *Anopheles gambiae*: a comparison of two new high-throughput assays with existing methods. *Malar J* 2007, 6:111.

[127] Corbel V, N'Guessan R, Brengues C, Chandre F, Djogbenou L, Martin T, Akogbeto M, Hougard JM, Rowland M: Multiple insecticide resistance mechanisms in *Anopheles gambiae* and *Culex quinquefasciatus* from Benin, West Africa. *Acta Trop* 2007, 101(3): 207-216.

[128] Diabate A: The Role of Agricultural Uses of Insecticides in Resistance to Pyrethroids in *Anopheles gambiae* S.L. in Burkina Faso. *Am J Trop Med Hyg* 2002, 67(6):617-622.

[129] Carnevale P, Toto JC, Guibert P, Keita M, Manguin S: Entomological survey and report of a knockdown resistance mutation in the malaria vector *Anopheles gambiae* from the Republic of Guinea. *Trans R Soc Trop Med Hyg*, 104(7):484-489.

[130] Yawson AE, McCall PJ, Wilson MD, Donnelly MJ: Species abundance and insecticide resistance of *Anopheles gambiae* in selected areas of Ghana and Burkina Faso. *Med Vet Entomol* 2004, 18(4):372-377.

[131] C. Fanello VP, A. della Torre, F. Santolamazza, G. Dolo, M. Coulibaly, A. Alloueche, C. F. Curtis, Y. T. Touré and M. Coluzzi: The pyrethroid knock-down resistance gene in the *Anopheles gambiae* complex in Mali and further indication of incipient speciation within *An. gambiae* s.s. *Insect Molecular Biology* 2003, 12(3):241-245.

[132] Czeher C, Labbo R, Arzika I, Duchemin J-B: Evidence of increasing Leu-Phe knockdown resistance mutation in *Anopheles gambiae* from Niger following a nationwide long-lasting insecticide-treated nets implementation. *Malaria Journal* 2008, 7(1):189.

[133] Awolola TS, Brooke BD, Hunt RH, Coetze M: Resistance of the malaria vector *Anopheles gambiae* s.s. to pyrethroid insecticides, in south-western Nigeria. *Annals of Tropical Medicine and Parasitology* 2002, 96(8):849-852.

[134] Koffi AA, Alou LP, Adja MA, Kone M, Chandre F, N'Guessan R: Update on resistance status of *Anopheles gambiae* s.s. to conventional insecticides at a previous WHOPES field site, "Yaokoffikro", 6 years after the political crisis in Cote d'Ivoire. *Parasit Vectors* 2012, 5:68.

[135] Dabire KR, Diabate A, Agostinho F, Alves F, Manga L, Faye O, Baldet T: Distribution of the members of *Anopheles gambiae* and pyrethroid knock-down resistance gene (*kdr*) in Guinea-Bissau, West Africa. *Bull Soc Pathol Exot* 2008, 101(2):119-123.

[136] Etang J, Fondjo E, Chandre F, Morlais I, Brengues C, Nwane P, Chouaibou M, Ndjemai H, Simard F: First report of knockdown mutations in the malaria vector *Anopheles gambiae* from Cameroon. *Am J Trop Med Hyg* 2006, 74(5):795-797.

[137] Ndjemai HN, Patchoke S, Atangana J, Etang J, Simard F, Bilong CF, Reimer L, Cornel A, Lanzaro GC, Fondjo E: The distribution of insecticide resistance in *Anopheles gambiae* s.l. populations from Cameroon: an update. *Trans R Soc Trop Med Hyg* 2009.

[138] Nwane P, Etang J, Chouaibou M, Toto JC, Kerah-Hinzoumbe C, Mimpfoundi R, Awono-Ambene HP, Simard F: Trends in DDT and pyrethroid resistance in *Anopheles gambiae* s.s. populations from urban and agro-industrial settings in southern Cameroon. *BMC Infect Dis* 2009, 9:163.

[139] Kerah-Hinzoumbe C, Peka M, Nwane P, Donan-Gouni I, Etang J, Same-Ekobo A, Simard F: Insecticide resistance in *Anopheles gambiae* from south-western Chad, Central Africa. *Malar J* 2008, 7:192.

[140] Janeira F, Vicente JL, Kanganje Y, Moreno M, Do Rosario VE, Cravo P, Pinto J: A primer-introduced restriction analysis-polymerase chain reaction method to detect knockdown resistance mutations in *Anopheles gambiae*. *J Med Entomol* 2008, 45(2): 237-241.

[141] Mourou JR, Coffinet T, Jarjaval F, Pradines B, Amalvict R, Rogier C, Kombila M, Pages F: Malaria transmission and insecticide resistance of *Anopheles gambiae* in Libreville and Port-Gentil, Gabon. *Malar J* 2010, 9:321.

[142] Himeidan YE, Chen H, Chandre F, Donnelly MJ, Yan G: Short report: permethrin and DDT resistance in the malaria vector *Anopheles arabiensis* from eastern Sudan. *Am J Trop Med Hyg* 2007, 77(6):1066-1068.

[143] Abdalla H, Matambo TS, Koekemoer LL, Mnzava AP, Hunt RH, Coetzee M: Insecticide susceptibility and vector status of natural populations of *Anopheles arabiensis* from Sudan. *Transactions of the Royal Society of Tropical Medicine and Hygiene* 2008, 102(3):263-271.

[144] Costantini C, Ayala D, Guelbeogo WM, Pombi M, Some CY, Bassole IH, Ose K, Fotsing JM, Sagnon N, Fontenille D *et al*: Living at the edge: biogeographic patterns of habitat segregation conform to speciation by niche expansion in *Anopheles gambiae*. *BMC Ecol* 2009, 9(1):16.

[145] Kulkarni MA, Malima R, Mosha FW, Msangi S, Mrema E, Kabula B, Lawrence B, Kinung'hi S, Swilla J, Kisinza W *et al*: Efficacy of pyrethroid-treated nets against malaria vectors and nuisance-biting mosquitoes in Tanzania in areas with long-term insecticide-treated net use. *Trop Med Int Health* 2007, 12(9):1061-1073.

[146] Kabula B, Tungu P, Matowo J, Kitau J, Mweya C, Emidi B, Masue D, Sindato C, Malima R, Minja J *et al*: Susceptibility status of malaria vectors to insecticides commonly used for malaria control in Tanzania. *Trop Med Int Health* 2012, 17(6):742-750.

[147] Coleman M, Casimiro S, Hemingway J, Sharp B: Operational impact of DDT reintroduction for malaria control on *Anopheles arabiensis* in Mozambique. *J Med Entomol* 2008, 45(5):885-890.

[148] Ratovonjato J, Le Goff G, Rajaonarivelo E, Rakotondraibe EM, Robert V: [Recent observations on the sensitivity to pyrethroids and DDT of *Anopheles arabiensis* and *Anopheles funestus* in the central Highlands of Madagascar; preliminary results on the absence of the *kdr* mutation in *An. arabiensis*]. *Arch Inst Pasteur Madagascar* 2003, 69(1-2):63-69.

[149] Ramphul U, Boase T, Bass C, Okedi LM, Donnelly MJ, Muller P: Insecticide resistance and its association with target-site mutations in natural populations of *Anopheles gambiae* from eastern Uganda. *Trans R Soc Trop Med Hyg* 2009.

[150] Verhaeghen K, Bortel WV, Roelants P, Okello PE, Talisuna A, Coosemans M: Spatio-temporal patterns in *kdr* frequency in permethrin and DDT resistant *Anopheles gambiae* s.s. from Uganda. *Am J Trop Med Hyg* 2010, 82(4):566-573.

[151] Abate A, Hadis M: Susceptibility of *Anopheles gambiae* s.l. to DDT, malathion, permethrin and deltamethrin in Ethiopia. *Trop Med Int Health* 2011, 16(4):486-491.

[152] Ochomo E, Bayoh MN, Brogdon WG, Gimnig JE, Ouma C, Vulule JM, Walker ED: Pyrethroid resistance in *Anopheles gambiae* s.s. and *Anopheles arabiensis* in western Kenya: phenotypic, metabolic and target site characterizations of three populations. *Med Vet Entomol* 2012.

[153] Mathias DK, Ochomo E, Atieli F, Ombok M, Bayoh MN, Olang G, Muhia D, Kamau L, Vulule JM, Hamel MJ *et al*: Spatial and temporal variation in the *kdr* allele L1014S in *Anopheles gambiae* s.s. and phenotypic variability in susceptibility to insecticides in Western Kenya. *Malar J* 2011, 10:10.

[154] Chanda E, Hemingway J, Kleinschmidt I, Rehman AM, Ramdeen V, Phiri FN, Coetzer S, Mthembu D, Shinondo CJ, Chizema-Kawesha E *et al*: Insecticide resistance and the future of malaria control in Zambia. *PLoS ONE* 2011, 6(9):e24336.

[155] Mouatcho JC, Munhenga G, Hargreaves K, Brooke BD, Coetzee M, Koekemoer LL: Pyrethroid resistance in a major African malaria vector *Anopheles arabiensis* from Mamfene, northern KwaZulu-Natal, South Africa. *South African Journal of Science* 2009, 105(3-4):127-131.

[156] Mouatcho JC, Hargreaves K, Koekemoer LL, Brooke BD, Oliver SV, Hunt RH, Coetzee M: Indoor collections of the *Anopheles funestus* group (Diptera: Culicidae) in sprayed houses in northern KwaZulu-Natal, South Africa. *Malar J* 2007, 6:30.

[157] Brooke BD, Kloke G, Hunt RH, Koekemoer LL, Temu EA, Taylor ME, Small G, Hemingway J, Coetzee M: Bioassay and biochemical analyses of insecticide resistance in southern African *Anopheles funestus* (Diptera: Culicidae). *Bulletin of Entomological Research* 2001, 91(4):265-272.

[158] Cuamba N, Morgan JC, Irving H, Steven A, Wondji CS: High level of pyrethroid resistance in an *Anopheles funestus* population of the Chokwe District in Mozambique. *PLoS ONE* 2010, 5(6):e11010.

[159] Kloke RG, Nhamahanga E, Hunt RH, Coetzee M: Vectorial status and insecticide resistance of *Anopheles funestus* from a sugar estate in southern Mozambique. *Parasit Vectors* 2011, 4:16.

[160] Hunt R, Edwardes M, Coetzee M: Pyrethroid resistance in southern African *Anopheles funestus* extends to Likoma Island in Lake Malawi. *Parasit Vectors* 2010, 3:122.

[161] Wondji CS, Coleman M, Kleinschmidt I, Mzilahowa T, Irving H, Ndula M, Rehman A, Morgan J, Barnes KG, Hemingway J: Impact of pyrethroid resistance on operational malaria control in Malawi. *Proc Natl Acad Sci U S A* 2012, 109(47):19063-19070.

[162] Anto F, Asoala V, Anyorigiya T, Oduro A, Adjuik M, Owusu-Agyei S, Dery D, Bimi L, Hodgson A: Insecticide resistance profiles for malaria vectors in the Kassena-Nankana district of Ghana. *Malaria Journal* 2009, 8(1):81.

[163] Djouaka R, Irving H, Tukur Z, Wondji CS: Exploring mechanisms of multiple insecticide resistance in a population of the malaria vector *Anopheles funestus* in Benin. *PLoS ONE* 2011, 6(11):e27760.

[164] Dabire KR, Baldet T, Diabate A, Dia I, Costantini C, Cohuet A, Guiguemde TR, Fontenille D: *Anopheles funestus* (Diptera: Culicidae) in a humid savannah area of western Burkina Faso: bionomics, insecticide resistance status, and role in malaria transmission. *J Med Entomol* 2007, 44(6):990-997.

[165] Faraj C, Adlaoui E, Brengues C, Fontenille D, Lyagoubi M: [Resistance of *Anopheles labranchiae* to DDT in Morocco: identification of the mechanisms and choice of replacement insecticide]. *Eastern Mediterranean health journal = La revue de sante de la Mediterranee orientale = al-Majallah al-sihhiyah li-sharq al-mutawassit* 2008, 14(4):776-783.

[166] Mostafa AA, Allam KA: Studies on the present status of insecticides resistance on mosquitoes using the diagnostic dosages in El-Fayium Governorate, a spot area of malaria in Egypt. *J Egypt Soc Parasitol* 2001, 31(1):177-186.

[167] Balkew M, Elhassan I, Ibrahim M, GebreMichael T, Engers H: Very high DDT-resistant population of *Anopheles pharoensis* Theobald (Diptera: Culicidae) from Gorgora, northern Ethiopia. *Parasite* 2006, 13(4):327-239.

[168] Yadouleton AW, Padonou G, Asidi A, Moiroux N, Bio-Banganna S, Corbel V, N'Guessan R, Gbenou D, Yacoubou I, Gazard K *et al*: Insecticide resistance status in *Anopheles gambiae* in southern Benin. *Malar J* 2010, 9:83.

[169] Pinto J, Lynd A, Vicente JL, Santolamazza F, Randle NP, Gentile G, Moreno M, Simard F, Charlwood JD, do Rosario VE *et al*: Multiple Origins of Knockdown Resistance Mutations in the Afrotropical Mosquito Vector *Anopheles gambiae*. *PLoS ONE* 2007, 2(11):e1243.

[170] della Torre A, Fanello C, Akogbeto M, Dossou-yovo J, Favia G, Petrarca V, Coluzzi M: Molecular evidence of incipient speciation within *Anopheles gambiae* s.s. in West Africa. *Insect Mol Biol* 2001, 10(1):9-18.

[171] Weill M, Chandre F, Brengues C, Manguin S, Akogbeto M, Pasteur N, Guillet P, Raymond M: The *kdr* mutation occurs in the Mopti form of *Anopheles gambiae* s.s. through introgression. *Insect Molecular Biology* 2000, 9(5):451-455.

[172] Reimer LJ, Tripet F, Slotman M, Spielman A, Fondjo E, Lanzaro GC: An unusual distribution of the *kdr* gene among populations of *Anopheles gambiae* on the island of Bioko, Equatorial Guinea. *Insect Mol Biol* 2005, 14(6):683-688.

[173] Protopopoff N, Verhaeghen K, Van Bortel W, Roelants P, Marcotty T, Baza D, D'Alessandro U, Coosemans M: A significant increase in *kdr* in *Anopheles gambiae* is associated with an intensive vector control intervention in Burundi highlands. *Trop Med Int Health* 2008, 13(12):1479-1487.

[174] Pinto J, Lynd A, Elissa N, Donnelly MJ, Costa C, Gentile G, Caccone A, do Rosario VE: Co-occurrence of East and West African *kdr* mutations suggests high levels of resistance to pyrethroid insecticides in *Anopheles gambiae* from Libreville, Gabon. *Med Vet Entomol* 2006, 20(1):27-32.

[175] Moreno M, Vicente JL, Cano J, Berzosa PJ, de Lucio A, Nzambo S, Bobuakasi L, Buatiche JN, Ondo M, Micha F *et al*: Knockdown resistance mutations (*kdr*) and insecticide susceptibility to DDT and pyrethroids in *Anopheles gambiae* from Equatorial Guinea. *Trop Med Int Health* 2008, 13(3):430-433.

[176] Verhaeghen K, Van Bortel W, Roelants P, Backeljau T, Coosemans M: Detection of the East and West African *kdr* mutation in *Anopheles gambiae* and *Anopheles arabiensis* from Uganda using a new assay based on FRET/Melt Curve analysis. *Malaria Journal* 2006, 5(1):16.

[177] Koekemoer LL, Spillings BL, Christian RN, Lo TC, Kaiser ML, Norton RA, Oliver SV, Choi KS, Brooke BD, Hunt RH *et al*: Multiple insecticide resistance in *Anopheles gambiae* (Diptera: Culicidae) from Pointe Noire, Republic of the Congo. *Vector Borne Zoonotic Dis* 2011, 11(8):1193-1200.

[178] Reimer L, Fondjo E, Patchoke S, Diallo B, Lee Y, Ng A, Ndjemai HM, Atangana J, Traore SF, Lanzaro G *et al*: Relationship between *kdr* mutation and resistance to pyrethroid and DDT insecticides in natural populations of *Anopheles gambiae*. *J Med Entomol* 2008, 45(2):260-266.

[179] Badolo A, Traore A, Jones CM, Sanou A, Flood L, Guelbeogo WM, Ranson H, Sagnon N: Three years of insecticide resistance monitoring in *Anopheles gambiae* in Burkina Faso: resistance on the rise? *Malar J* 2012, 11:232.

[180] Santolamazza F, Calzetta M, Etang J, Barrese E, Dia I, Caccone A, Donnelly MJ, Petrarca V, Simard F, Pinto J *et al*: Distribution of knock-down resistance mutations in

Anopheles gambiae molecular forms in west and west-central Africa. *Malar J* 2008, 7(1): 74.

[181] Ridl F, Bass C, Torrez M, Govender D, Ramdeen V, Yellot L, Edu A, Schwabe C, Mohloai P, Maharaj R *et al*: A pre-intervention study of malaria vector abundance in Rio Muni, Equatorial Guinea: Their role in malaria transmission and the incidence of insecticide resistance alleles. *Malaria Journal* 2008, 7(1):194.

[182] Reimer L, Fondjo E, Patchok, Salomon, Diallo B, Lee Y, Ng A, Ndjemai HM, Atangana J, Traore SF *et al*: Relationship Between *kdr* Mutation and Resistance to Pyrethroid and DDT Insecticides in Natural Populations of *Anopheles gambiae*. *Journal of Medical Entomology* 2008, 45:260-266.

[183] Matambo TS, Abdalla H, Brooke BD, Koekemoer LL, Mnzava A, Hunt RH, Coetzee M: Insecticide resistance in the malarial mosquito *Anopheles arabiensis* and association with the *kdr* mutation. *Medical and Veterinary Entomology* 2007, 21(1):97-102.

[184] Kulkarni M, Rowland M, Alifrangis M, Mosha F, Matowo J, Malima R, Peter J, Kweka E, Lyimo I, Magesa S *et al*: Occurrence of the leucine-to-phenylalanine knockdown resistance (*kdr*) mutation in *Anopheles arabiensis* populations in Tanzania, detected by a simplified high-throughput SSOP-ELISA method. *Malaria Journal* 2006, 5(1):56.

[185] Chen H, Githeko AK, Githure JI, Mutunga J, Zhou G, Yan G: Monooxygenase Levels and Knockdown Resistance (*kdr*) Allele Frequencies in *Anopheles gambiae* and *Anopheles arabiensis* in Kenya. *Journal of Medical Entomology* 2008, 45:242-250.

[186] Etang J, Manga L, Toto JC, Guillet P, Fondjo E, Chandre F: Spectrum of metabolic-based resistance to DDT and pyrethroids in *Anopheles gambiae* s.l. populations from Cameroon. *J Vector Ecol* 2007, 32(1):123-133.

[187] Hargreaves K, Hunt RH, Brooke BD, Mthembu J, Weeto MM, Awolola TS, Coetzee M: *Anopheles arabiensis* and *An. quadriannulatus* resistance to DDT in South Africa. *Med Vet Entomol* 2003, 17(4):417-422.

[188] Amenya DA, Naguran R, Lo TC, Ranson H, Spillings BL, Wood OR, Brooke BD, Coetzee M, Koekemoer LL: Over expression of a cytochrome P450 (CYP6P9) in a major African malaria vector, *Anopheles funestus*, resistant to pyrethroids. *Insect Mol Biol* 2008, 17(1):19-25.

[189] Somboon P, Prapanthadara LA, Suwonkerd W: Insecticide susceptibility tests of *Anopheles minimus* s.l., *Aedes aegypti*, *Aedes albopictus*, and *Culex quinquefasciatus* in northern Thailand. *Southeast Asian J Trop Med Public Health* 2003, 34(1):87-93.

[190] Verhaeghen K, Van Bortel W, Trung HD, Sochantha T, Coosemans M: Absence of knockdown resistance suggests metabolic resistance in the main malaria vectors of the Mekong region. *Malar J* 2009, 8:84.

[191] Chareonviriyaphap T, Rongnoparut P, Chantarumporn P, Bangs MJ: Biochemical detection of pyrethroid resistance mechanisms in *Anopheles minimus* in Thailand. *J Vector Ecol* 2003, 28(1):108-116.

[192] Rodpradit P, Boonsuepsakul S, Chareonviriyaphap T, Bangs MJ, Rongnoparut P: Cytochrome P450 genes: molecular cloning and overexpression in a pyrethroid-resistant strain of *Anopheles minimus* mosquito. *J Am Mosq Control Assoc* 2005, 21(1):71-79.

[193] Verhaeghen K, Van Bortel W, Trung HD, Sochantha T, Keokenchanh K, Coosemans M: Knockdown resistance in *Anopheles vagus, An. sinensis, An. paraliae* and *An. peditaeniatus* populations of the Mekong region. *Parasit Vectors* 2011, 3(1):59.

[194] Kang S, Jung J, Lee S, Hwang H, Kim W: The polymorphism and the geographical distribution of the knockdown resistance (*kdr*) of *Anopheles sinensis* in the Republic of Korea. *Malar J* 2012, 11:151.

[195] Tan WL, Wang ZM, Li CX, Chu HL, Xu Y, Dong YD, Wang ZC, Chen DY, Liu H, Liu DP *et al*: First report on co-occurrence knockdown resistance mutations and susceptibility to beta-cypermethrin in *Anopheles sinensis* from Jiangsu Province, China. *PLoS ONE* 2012, 7(1):e29242.

[196] Syafruddin D, Hidayati AP, Asih PB, Hawley WA, Sukowati S, Lobo NF: Detection of 1014F *kdr* mutation in four major Anopheline malaria vectors in Indonesia. *Malar J* 2010, 9:315.

[197] Singh OP, Dykes CL, Das MK, Pradhan S, Bhatt RM, Agrawal OP, Adak T: Presence of two alternative *kdr*-like mutations, L1014F and L1014S, and a novel mutation, V1010L, in the voltage gated Na+ channel of *Anopheles culicifacies* from Orissa, India. *Malar J* 2010, 9:146.

[198] Mishra AK, Chand SK, Barik TK, Dua VK, Raghavendra K: Insecticide resistance status in *Anopheles culicifacies* in Madhya Pradesh, central India. *J Vector Borne Dis* 2012, 49(1):39-41.

[199] Sharma SN, Shukla RP, Raghavendra K: Susceptibility status of *An. fluviatilis* and *An. culicifacies* to DDT, deltamethrin and lambdacyhalothrin in District Nainital, Uttar Pradesh. *Indian J Malariol* 1999, 36(3-4):90-93.

[200] Singh OP, Dykes CL, Lather M, Agrawal OP, Adak T: Knockdown resistance (*kdr*)-like mutations in the voltage-gated sodium channel of a malaria vector *Anopheles stephensi* and PCR assays for their detection. *Malar J* 2011, 10:59.

[201] Tikar SN, Mendki MJ, Sharma AK, Sukumaran D, Veer V, Prakash S, Parashar BD: Resistance status of the malaria vector mosquitoes, *Anopheles stephensi* and *Anopheles subpictus* towards adulticides and larvicides in arid and semi-arid areas of India. *J Insect Sci* 2011, 11:85.

[202] Baruah K, Lal S: A report on the susceptibility status of *Anopheles minimus* (Theobald) against DDT and deltamethrin in three districts of Assam. *J Vector Borne Dis* 2004, 41(1-2):42-44.

[203] Karunaratne SH, Hemingway J: Malathion resistance and prevalence of the malathion carboxylesterase mechanism in populations of mosquito vectors of disease in Sri Lanka. *Bull World Health Organ* 2001, 79(11):1060-1064.

[204] Kelly-Hope LA, Yapabandara AM, Wickramasinghe MB, Perera MD, Karunaratne SH, Fernando WP, Abeyasinghe RR, Siyambalagoda RR, Herath PR, Galappaththy GN *et al*: Spatiotemporal distribution of insecticide resistance in *Anopheles culicifacies* and *Anopheles subpictus* in Sri Lanka. *Trans R Soc Trop Med Hyg* 2005, 99(10):751-761.

[205] Perera MD, Hemingway J, Karunaratne SP: Multiple insecticide resistance mechanisms involving metabolic changes and insensitive target sites selected in anopheline vectors of malaria in Sri Lanka. *Malar J* 2008, 7:168.

[206] Surendran SN, Jude PJ, Weerarathne TC, Parakrama Karunaratne SH, Ramasamy R: Variations in susceptibility to common insecticides and resistance mechanisms among morphologically identified sibling species of the malaria vector *Anopheles subpictus* in Sri Lanka. *Parasit Vectors* 2012, 5:34.

[207] Mittal PK, Wijeyaratne P, Pandey S: Status of Insecticide Resistance of Malaria, Kala-azar and Japanese Encephalitis Vectors in Bangladesh, Bhutan, India and Nepal (BBIN). In. Edited by Project EH. Washington 2004.

[208] Rowland M: Location of the gene for malathion resistance in *Anopheles stephensi* (Diptera: Culicidae) from Pakistan. *J Med Entomol* 1985, 22(4):373-380.

[209] Abai MR, Mehravaran A, Vatandoost H, Oshaghi MA, Javadian E, Mashayekhi M, Mosleminia A, Piyazak N, Edallat H, Mohtarami F *et al*: Comparative performance of imagicides on *Anopheles stephensi*, main malaria vector in a malarious area, southern Iran. *J Vector Borne Dis* 2008, 45(4):307-312.

[210] Lak SH, vatandoost H, Entezarmahdi MR, Ashraf H, Abai MR, Nazari M: Monitoring of Insecticide Resistance in *Anopheles sacharovi* (Favre, 1903) in Borderline of Iran, Armenia, Naxcivan and Turkey, 2001. *Iranian J Publ Health* 2002, 31(3-4):96-99.

[211] Vatandoost H, Mashayekhi M, Abaie MR, Aflatoonian MR, Hanafi-Bojd AA, Sharifi I: Monitoring of insecticides resistance in main malaria vectors in a malarious area of Kahnooj district, Kerman province, southeastern Iran. *J Vector Borne Dis* 2005, 42(3): 100-108.

[212] Malcolm CA: Current status of pyrethroid resistance in anophelines. *Parasitol Today* 1988, 4(7):S13-15.

[213] Quinones ML, Suarez MF: Irritability to DDT of natural populations of the primary malaria vectors in Colombia. *J Am Mosq Control Assoc* 1989, 5(1):56-59.

[214] Suarez MF, Quinones ML, Palacios JD, Carrillo A: First record of DDT resistance in *Anopheles darlingi*. *J Am Mosq Control Assoc* 1990, 6(1):72-74.

[215] Fonseca-Gonzalez I: Estatus de la resistencia a insecticidas de los vectores primarios de malaria y dengue en Antioquia, Chocó, Norte de Santander y Putumayo, Colombia. Universidad de Antioquia, Colombia; 2008.

[216] Fonseca-Gonzalez I, Cardenas R, Quinones ML, McAllister J, Brogdon WG: Pyrethroid and organophosphates resistance in *Anopheles (N.) nuneztovari* Gabaldon populations from malaria endemic areas in Colombia. *Parasitol Res* 2009, 105(5):1399-1409.

[217] Chareonviriyaphap T, Golenda CF, Roberts DR, Andre RG: Identification of Elevated Esterase Activity in a Pyrethroid-Resistant Population of *Anopheles albimanus* Wiedemann. *ScienceAsia* 1999, 25 153-156.

[218] Brogdon WG, McAllister JC, Corwin AM, Cordon Rosales C: Independent selection of multiple mechanisms for pyrethroid resistance in Guatemalan *Anopheles albimanus* (Diptera: Culicidae). *Journal of Economic Entomology* 1999, 92(2):298-302.

[219] Zamora Perea E, Balta Leon R, Palomino Salcedo M, Brogdon WG, Devine GJ: Adaptation and evaluation of the bottle assay for monitoring insecticide resistance in disease vector mosquitoes in the Peruvian Amazon. *Malar J* 2009, 8:208.

[220] Hemingway J, Penilla RP, Rodriguez AD, James BM, Edge W, Rogers H, Rodriguez MH: Resistance management strategies in malaria vector mosquito control. A large-scale field trial in Southern Mexico. *Pesticide Science* 1997, 51(3):375-382.

[221] Dzul FA, Patricia Penilla R, Rodriguez AD: [Susceptibility and insecticide resistance mechanisms in *Anopheles albimanus* from the southern Yucatan Peninsula, Mexico]. *Salud Publica Mex* 2007, 49(4):302-311.

[222] South Africa Department of Health: Malaria Updates. In. Pretoria, S.A: S.A.D.H.; 2003.

[223] Maharaj R, Mthembu DJ, Sharp BL: Impact of DDT re-introduction on malaria transmission in KwaZulu-Natal. *S Afr Med J* 2005, 95(11):871-874.

[224] Roberts DR, Manguin S, Mouchet J: DDT house spraying and re-emerging malaria. *Lancet* 2000, 356(9226):330-332.

[225] Protopopoff N, Van Bortel W, Marcotty T, Van Herp M, Maes P, Baza D, D'Alessandro U, Coosemans M: Spatial targeted vector control in the highlands of Burundi and its impact on malaria transmission. *Malar J* 2007, 6:158.

[226] Trape J-F, Tall A, Diagne N, Ndiath O, Ly AB, Faye J, Dieye-Ba F, Roucher C, Bouganali C, Badiane A *et al*: Malaria morbidity and pyrethroid resistance after the introduction of insecticide-treated bednets and artemisinin-based combination therapies: a longitudinal study. *The Lancet Infectious Diseases* 2011.

[227] Lengeler C: Insecticide-treated bed nets and curtains for preventing malaria. *Cochrane Database of Systematic reviews* 2009(2):1-58.

[228] Kitau J, Oxborough RM, Tungu PK, Matowo J, Malima RC, Magesa SM, Bruce J, Mosha FW, Rowland MW: Species shifts in the *Anopheles gambiae* complex: do LLINs successfully control *Anopheles arabiensis*? *PLoS ONE* 2012, 7(3):e31481.

[229] Bradley J, Matias A, Schwabe C, Vargas D, Monti F, Nseng G, Kleinschmidt I: Increased risks of malaria due to limited residual life of insecticide and outdoor biting versus protection by combined use of nets and indoor residual spraying on Bioko Island, Equatorial Guinea. *Malar J* 2012, 11:242.

[230] Henry MC, Assi SB, Rogier C, Dossou-Yovo J, Chandre F, Guillet P, Carnevale P: Protective efficacy of lambda-cyhalothrin treated nets in *Anopheles gambiae* pyrethroid resistance areas of Cote d'Ivoire. *Am J Trop Med Hyg* 2005, 73(5):859-864.

[231] Corbel V, Akogbeto M, Damien GB, Djenontin A, Chandre F, Rogier C, Moiroux N, Chabi J, Banganna B, Padonou GG *et al*: Combination of malaria vector control interventions in pyrethroid resistance area in Benin: a cluster randomised controlled trial. *Lancet Infect Dis* 2012, 12(8):617-626.

[232] Darriet F, N' Guessan R, Koffi AA, Konan L, Doannio JMC, Chandre F, Carnevale P: Impact of the resistance to pyrethroids on the efficacy of impregnated bednets used as a means of prevention against malaria: results of the evaluation carried out with deltamethrin SC in experimental huts. *Bulletin de la Société de Pathologie Exotique* 2000, 93(2):131-134.

[233] Corbel V, Chandre F, Brengues C, Akogbeto M, Lardeux F, Hougard JM, Guillet P: Dosage-dependent effects of permethrin-treated nets on the behaviour of *Anopheles gambiae* and the selection of pyrethroid resistance. *Malar J* 2004, 3(1):22.

[234] N'Guessan R, Corbel V, Akogbeto M, Rowland M: Reduced efficacy of insecticide-treated nets and indoor residual spraying for malaria control in pyrethroid resistance area, Benin. *Emerg Infect Dis* 2007, 13(2):199-206.

[235] N'Guessan R, Asidi A, Boko P, Odjo A, Akogbeto M, Pigeon O, Rowland M: An experimental hut evaluation of PermaNet(R) 3.0, a deltamethrin-piperonyl butoxide combination net, against pyrethroid-resistant *Anopheles gambiae* and *Culex quinquefasciatus* mosquitoes in southern Benin. *Trans R Soc Trop Med Hyg* 2010, 104(12):758-765.

[236] Asidi A, N'Guessan R, Akogbeto M, Curtis C, Rowland M: Loss of household protection from use of insecticide-treated nets against pyrethroid-resistant mosquitoes, Benin. *Emerg Infect Dis* 2012, 18(7):1101-1106.

[237] Osse R, Gnanguenon V, Sezonlin M, Aikpon R, Padonou G, Yadouleton A, Akogbeto M: Relationship between the presence of *kdr* and Ace-1 mutations and the infection with *Plasmodium falciparum* in *Anopheles gambiae* s.s. in Benin. *Journal of Parassitology & Vector Biology* 2012, 4(3):31-39.

[238] Moiroux N, Boussari O, Djenontin A, Damien G, Cottrell G, Henry MC, Guis H, Corbel V: Dry season determinants of malaria disease and net use in Benin, West Africa. *PLoS ONE* 2012, 7(1):e30558.

[239] Poupardin R, Reynaud S, Strode C, Ranson H, Vontas J, David JP: Cross-induction of detoxification genes by environmental xenobiotics and insecticides in the mosquito *Aedes aegypti*: impact on larval tolerance to chemical insecticides. *Insect Biochem Mol Biol* 2008, 38(5):540-551.

[240] IRAC: Prevention and Management of Insecticide Resistance in Vectors of Public Health Importance In: *Resistance Management for Sustainable Agriculture and Improved Public Health : Second Edition 2010* Insecticide Resistance Action Commitee; 2010: 72pp.

[241] Georghiou GP, Taylor CE: Genetic and biological influences in the evolution of insecticide resistance. *Journal of Economic Entomology* 1977, 70(3):319-323.

[242] Denholm I, Rowland MW: Tactics for managing pesticide resistance in arthropods: theory and practice. *Annu Rev Entomol* 1992, 37:91-112.

[243] Djogbenou L, Weill M, Hougard JM, Raymond M, Akogbeto M, Chandre F: Characterization of insensitive acetylcholinesterase (ace-1R) in *Anopheles gambiae* (Diptera: Culicidae): resistance levels and dominance. *J Med Entomol* 2007, 44(5):805-810.

[244] Berticat C, Bonnet J, Duchon S, Agnew P, Weill M, Corbel V: Costs and benefits of multiple resistance to insecticides for *Culex quinquefasciatus* mosquitoes. *BMC Evol Biol* 2008, 8:104.

[245] Moore JH, Williams SM: Traversing the conceptual divide between biological and statistical epistasis: systems biology and a more modern synthesis. *Bioessays* 2005, 27(6):637-646.

[246] Shono T, Zhang L, Scott JG: Indoxacarb resistance in the house fly, *Musca domestica*. *Pesticide Biochemistry and Physiology* 2004, 80(2):106-112.

[247] Shono T, Kasai S, Kamiya E, Kono Y, Scott JG: Genetics and mechanisms of permethrin resistance in the YPER strain of house fly. *Pesticide Biochemistry and Physiology* 2002, 73(1):27-36.

[248] Scott JG, Shono T, Georghiou GP: Genetic analysis of permethrin resistance in the house fly, *Musca domestica* L. *Experientia* 1984, 40(12):1416-1418.

[249] Hardstone MC, Leichter CA, Scott JG: Multiplicative interaction between the two major mechanisms of permethrin resistance, *kdr* and cytochrome P450-monooxygenase detoxification, in mosquitoes. *J Evol Biol* 2009, 22(2):416-423.

[250] Berticat C, Boquien G, Raymond M, Chevillon C: Insecticide resistance genes induce a mating competition cost in *Culex pipiens* mosquitoes. *Genet Res* 2002, 79(1):41-47.

[251] Agnew P, Berticat C, Bedhomme S, Sidobre C, Michalakis Y: Parasitism increases and decreases the costs of insecticide resistance in mosquitoes. *Evolution Int J Org Evolution* 2004, 58(3):579-586.

[252] Foster SP, Harrington R, Devonshire AL, Denholm I, Devine GJ, Kenward MG: Comparative survival of insecticide-susceptible and resistant peach-potato aphids, *Myzus persicae* (Sulzer) (Hemiptera: Aphididae), in low temperature field trials. *Bull Ent Res* 1996, 86:17-27.

[253] Shi MA, Lougarre A, Alies C, Fremaux I, Tang ZH, Stojan J, Fournier D: Acetylcholinesterase alterations reveal the fitness cost of mutations conferring insecticide resistance. *BMC Evol Biol* 2004, 4:5.

[254] Djogbenou L, Noel V, Agnew P: Costs of insensitive acetylcholinesterase insecticide resistance for the malaria vector *Anopheles gambiae* homozygous for the G119S mutation. *Malar J* 2010, 9(1):12.

[255] Brogdon WG, McAllister JC: Insecticide resistance and vector control. *Emerg Infect Dis* 1998, 4(4):605-613.

[256] Diabate A, Baldet T, Chandre F, Akoobeto M, Guiguemde TR, Darriet F, Brengues C, Guillet P, Hemingway J, Small GJ *et al*: The role of agricultural use of insecticides in resistance to pyrethroids in *Anopheles gambiae* s.l. in Burkina Faso. *Am J Trop Med Hyg* 2002, 67(6):617-622.

[257] Yadouleton A, Martin T, Padonou G, Chandre F, Asidi A, Djogbenou L, Dabire R, Aikpon R, Boko M, Glitho I *et al*: Cotton pest management practices and the selection of pyrethroid resistance in *Anopheles gambiae* population in northern Benin. *Parasit Vectors* 2011, 4:60.

[258] Harrison G: Mosquitoes, malaria and man: A history of hostilities since 1880.; 1978.

[259] Read AF, Lynch PA, Thomas MB: How to make evolution-proof insecticides for malaria control. *PLoS Biol* 2009, 7(4):e1000058.

[260] Roush RT, Hoy CW, Ferro DN, Tingey WM: Insecticide resistance in the Colorado potato beetle (Coleoptera: Chrysomelidae): influence of crop rotation and insecticide use. *Journal of Economic Entomology* 1990, 83(2):315-319.

[261] Georghiou GP: Insecticide resistance and prospects for its management. *Residue Reviews* 1980, 76:131-145.

[262] Tabashnik BE: Managing resistance with multiple pesticide tactics: theory, evidence, and recommendations. *J Econ Entomol* 1989, 82(5):1263-1269.

[263] Chitnis N, Schapira A, Smith T, Steketee R: Comparing the effectiveness of malaria vector-control interventions through a mathematical model. *Am J Trop Med Hyg* 2010, 83(2):230-240.

[264] Yakob L, Dunning R, Yan G: Indoor residual spray and insecticide-treated bednets for malaria control: theoretical synergisms and antagonisms. *J R Soc Interface* 2011, 8(59):799-806.

[265] World Health Organization: Global strategic framework for integrated vector management. Geneva; 2004.

[266] Curtis CF: Theoretical models of the use of insecticide mixtures for management of resistance. *Bull Ent Res* 1985, 75: 259-265.

[267] Hougard JM, Poudiougo P, Guillet P, Back C, Akpoboua LK, Quillevere D: Criteria for the selection of larvicides by the Onchocerciasis Control Programme in west Africa. *Ann Trop Med Parasitol* 1993, 87(5):435-442.

[268] WHO: Pesticides and their application for the control of vectors and pests of public health importance; Sixth edition. In. Edited by WHO/CDS/NTD/WHOPES/GCDPP/2006.1 WHO, Geneva; 2006: 1-125.

[269] Corbel V, Chabi J, Dabire RK, Etang J, Nwane P, Pigeon O, Akogbeto M, Hougard JM: Field efficacy of a new mosaic long-lasting mosquito net (PermaNet 3.0) against pyrethroid-resistant malaria vectors: a multi centre study in Western and Central Africa. *Malar J* 2010, 9:113.

[270] Killeen GF, Okumu FO, N'Guessan R, Coosemans M, Adeogun A, Awolola S, Etang J, Dabire RK, Corbel V: The importance of considering community-level effects when selecting insecticidal malaria vector products. *Parasit Vectors* 2011, 4:160.

[271] Mani GS: Evolution of resistance in the presence of two insecticides. *Genetics* 1985, 109(4):761-783.

[272] Roush RT: Designing resistance management programs: how can you choose? *Pesticide Science* 1989, 26(4):423-441.

[273] Hougard JM, Corbel V, N'Guessan R, Darriet F, Chandre F, Akogbeto M, Baldet T, Guillet P, Carnevale P, Traore-Lamizana M: Efficacy of mosquito nets treated with insecticide mixtures or mosaics against insecticide resistant *Anopheles gambiae* and *Culex quinquefasciatus* (Diptera: Culicidae) in Cote d'Ivoire. *Bull Entomol Res* 2003, 93(6):491-498.

[274] Asidi AN, N'Guessan R, Koffi AA, Curtis CF, Hougard JM, Chandre F, Corbel V, Darriet F, Zaim M, Rowland MW: Experimental hut evaluation of bednets treated with an organophosphate (chlorpyrifos-methyl) or a pyrethroid (lambdacyhalothrin) alone and in combination against insecticide-resistant *Anopheles gambiae* and *Culex quinquefasciatus* mosquitoes. *Malar J* 2005, 4(1):25.

[275] Ohashi K, Nakada K, Ishiwatari T, Miyaguchi J, Shono Y, Lucas JR, Mito N: Efficacy of pyriproxyfen-treated nets in sterilizing and shortening the longevity of *Anopheles gambiae* (Diptera: Culicidae). *J Med Entomol* 2012, 49(5):1052-1058.

[276] Mosqueira B, Duchon S, Chandre F, Hougard JM, Carnevale P, Mas-Coma S: Efficacy of an insecticide paint against insecticide-susceptible and resistant mosquitoes - part 1: laboratory evaluation. *Malar J* 2010, 9:340.

[277] Ngufor C, N'Guessan R, Boko P, Odjo A, Vigninou E, Asidi A, Akogbeto M, Rowland M: Combining indoor residual spraying with chlorfenapyr and long-lasting insecticidal bed nets for improved control of pyrethroid-resistant *Anopheles gambiae*: an experimental hut trial in Benin. *Malar J* 2011, 10:343.

[278] Kleinschmidt I, Schwabe C, Shiva M, Segura JL, Sima V, Mabunda SJ, Coleman M: Combining indoor residual spraying and insecticide-treated net interventions. *Am J Trop Med Hyg* 2009, 81(3):519-524.

[279] Okumu FO, Moore SJ: Combining indoor residual spraying and insecticide-treated nets for malaria control in Africa: a review of possible outcomes and an outline of suggestions for the future. *Malar J* 2011, 10:208.

[280] Brosseau L, Drame PM, Besnard P, Toto JC, Foumane V, Le Mire J, Mouchet F, Remoue F, Allan R, Fortes F *et al*: Human antibody response to *Anopheles saliva* for comparing the efficacy of three malaria vector control methods in Balombo, Angola. *PLoS ONE* 2012, 7(9):e44189.

[281] Bill_&_Melinda_Gates_Fondation, Boston_Consulting_Group: Market Assessment for Public Health Pesticide Products. In.; 2007.

Chapter 20

Perspectives on Barriers to Control of *Anopheles* Mosquitoes and Malaria

Donald R. Roberts, Richard Tren and Kimberly Hess

Additional information is available at the end of the chapter

http://dx.doi.org/10.5772/55466

1. Introduction

Though mankind has struggled against malaria for countless generations, it remains a major global health problem. The malaria parasite and the *Anopheles* mosquito have evolved and developed with mankind since earliest recorded history, but there is nothing inevitable about the disease. Although thousands of children die from malaria every year, the disease is preventable and entirely curable, and the history of malaria control in the 20th century demonstrates that with the right tools and funding, malaria can be controlled, or even eradicated. The key, of course, is the cost-effective use of the right tools.

2. Statement of the problem

This chapter will examine arguably the most important tool for malaria control – public health insecticides (PHIs). Insecticide opponents often mischaracterize the public health use of insecticides, to include how they are used and consequences of their use in public health programs. Common inferences are that public health use of insecticides results in broad-scale environmental contamination and harm to wildlife. It is important for the reader to understand that there are internationally accepted guidelines for public health use of insecticides and that public health use is very different from how insecticides are used for agriculture. Optimum public health use of PHIs is to spray small quantities on inside walls of houses. In the case of DDT, it is approved only for use in public health programs. Applying it to inside walls leverages DDT's powerful repellent actions, giving continual protection from malaria-infected mosquitoes, for months on end, to those living inside the sprayed house. It should be obvious that a small amount of an insecticide on house walls is a far cry from spraying insecticides on vast acreages of cropland, as one might envisage for insecticides used in agriculture. Thus we emphasize that the subject of this chapter is public health use of insecticides, with no connotations whatsoever for the use of insecticides in agriculture.

We will summarize, with specific examples, the way that modern PHIs, and DDT in particular, have saved millions of lives since the 1940s. Despite this remarkable achievement, popular campaigns by activists, some scientists and even United Nations (UN) agencies, have stigmatized and often demonized PHIs. Instead of regarding insecticides in the same light as medicines and diagnostics, essential elements of a malaria control program, insecticide opponents have mounted vocal campaigns to halt their use. Frequently these campaigns avoid or ignore the scientific process and rely on the flimsiest of evidence to make great claims about human health or ecological effects of PHIs. We will characterize examples of studies and claims against PHIs used by the activist communities and we will describe the major failings of each as they relate to the use of PHIs.

The claims by those who oppose PHIs, as we will explain and demonstrate with specific examples, do not comply with even the most basic epidemiologic criteria to prove a cause and effect relationship – yet those claims drive public opinion and policy. We will also document how UN bureaucrats have made outrageous claims that malaria can be controlled without PHIs. At the same time, the UN has set grand goals of achieving near-zero deaths from malaria by 2015. There is a valid debate to be had about whether or not this goal can be met, or even properly defined and measured; however, what is clear, is that progress against malaria cannot be achieved and sustained without access to PHIs. For access to be secured, the malaria community, including program managers, researchers, advocates and others, must defend PHIs rigorously and emphatically. The overarching goal of this chapter is to help with that defense. Without it, the lives of men, women and children living at risk of malaria will be greatly imperiled. However, for proper defense of PHIs, there must be a clear understanding about how insecticide opponents have succeeded in past anti-insecticide campaigns, and that influential groups and UN organizations actively oppose the use of PHIs. As anti-insecticide campaigners employ distinct strategies and tactics, it is important to know what they are and how they are used.

3. Malaria control today versus the early years of PHI use

Today there is great enthusiasm and substantial funding to advance global efforts to control and, in some regions, eradicate malaria. Indeed, and as suggested by recent outcomes of control programs, we are beginning to see promising results [1,2]. The necessary change for refocusing efforts to control malaria started in 1998, when, faced with mounting evidence that the global burden of malaria was increasing, and had been for some time, the World Health Organization (WHO) formed a new malaria control partnership, Roll Back Malaria (RBM). The RBM Partnership is made up of WHO and several UN agencies, such as UNICEF and UNDP, and development agencies, such as the World Bank and the US Agency for International Development (USAID), along with the private sector and NGOs. RBM's stated goal in 1998 was to halve the burden of malaria by 2010 [3].

RBM began with limited funding and an apparent disdain for scientific evidence. The early efforts were disappointing. Far from achieving any reduction in malaria cases, by 2004 there was evidence that malaria cases were in fact increasing. RBM was described in a stinging editorial in the *British Medical Journal* as a 'failing public health campaign [4].' One of the main reasons for this was the Partnership's dogged support for the use of insecticide treated bednets (ITNs) over other vector control interventions, e.g., indoor residual spraying (IRS) with insecticides such as DDT. The limited and controlled spraying of insecticides inside houses has long been known to rapidly reduce malaria cases and deaths, yet in the early years of the RBM Partnership was roundly ignored. In addition RBM's Partners failed to support any change in treatment policy away from failing drug therapies to the new artemisinin-based combination therapies (ACTs).

It was not until 2006 that progress against malaria finally started to be made. To its credit RBM acknowledged some of the problems it faced and set about restructuring and reforming. Much of impetus for these reforms came from a newly appointed head of the WHO's Global Malaria Program, Dr. Arata Kochi. Dr. Kochi had little history in malaria control and perhaps because of this had no need to defend any misguided previous policy decisions. One of Kochi's first acts was to re-issue WHO's treatment guidelines, recommending ACTs.

Shortly thereafter Kochi re-addressed WHO's policy on both DDT and IRS, and in a public and, for WHO, aggressive gesture issued a statement strongly endorsing the use of DDT. At the same time the US global malaria control program run by USAID underwent a major reform, creating the President's Malaria Initiative (PMI). A distinguishing feature of the PMI, which sets it apart from other major bi-lateral donor funded malaria control programs, is its support for IRS and its willingness to pay for use of DDT [5].

Together these reforms marked a change in global malaria control and as a result, malaria cases began to decline. As described below, malaria funding increased by more than 20 fold in a decade and malaria deaths, according to WHO modeling data, have fallen.

Malaria funding for the PMI and the Global Fund to Fight AIDS, TB and Malaria (Global Fund) through 2011 is estimated at $1,858,370,500 for the PMI [6], and $6,156,000,000 in malaria grants through 2011 for the Global Fund (based on $22.8b value of grant portfolio as of December 31, 2011, of which 27% is for malaria) [7].

International funding for malaria control has gone from less than $100 million in 2000 to $2 billion in 2011 [8]. Likewise, the estimated changes in global malaria burden since 2000 are compliant with improved funding of control efforts after 2005. For example, estimated numbers of malaria cases and malaria deaths in 2000 were 223 million and 755,000 respectively. In 2005 the values were 237 million cases and 801,000 deaths, whereas in 2011, the values were 216 million cases and 655,000 deaths [8].

Clearly progress is being made in the renewed focus on malaria. The positive changes with regard to funding IRS and DDT's place in malaria control are obviously welcomed. However these advances can be reversed at any time and as we explain in this chapter, the forces opposing the careful and effective use of PHIs are well-funded, organized, and aggressive. The malaria control community should remember, and learn from history, that we have been at this stage before. We can get a sense of this by looking back to what was happening in 1959. At this time DDT was used widely in agriculture and for pest management around the world. Aerial spraying of DDT was common as farmers sought to protect their crops, but in malaria control DDT use was entirely different. Most malaria vectors enter houses in search of blood meals, and so protecting people while they are at home, often asleep, is crucial. Soon after the Allied forces first used DDT during World War II, scientists discovered that DDT acts primarily as a spatial repellent. In other words, if the interior of a house is sprayed with DDT, mosquitoes are driven away and are unlikely to enter. DDT will also act as a contact irritant, so if a mosquito lands on a sprayed surface, it is likely to exit the house rapidly, often before feeding. Of course DDT will also act as a toxicant, killing the mosquito. However it is a relatively weak toxicant and its spatial repellency is the insecticide's most important mode of action by far. Widespread area spraying of DDT would have been pointless for malaria control.

In 1959 malaria was in rapid retreat in many endemic countries as a consequence of effective DDT use. The global malaria eradication program was just barely underway. By that time, the malaria control community had already used DDT to free 300 million people from the burdens of endemic disease. By the program's end in 1969, the lives of almost one billion people would be equally improved. In 1959 there was a wealth of malaria control expertise, substantial funding, and programmatic emphasis on malaria prevention; there were powerful and successful national programs, goal-oriented malaria control policies, and great enthusiasm for the goals of the global program. We suggest that few, if any workers of that time could, in their wildest imaginings, have predicted what was to come. In just 20 years from that auspicious beginning most highly effective national control programs would begin grinding to a halt. Their malaria control expertise would be frittered away, their funding would be gone, the price of DDT would be up and its availability down, and the international policies for malaria control would be changed from disease prevention to case detection and treatment. The declining population of malaria control workers would begin seeing the disease they had worked so hard to control expanding back into malaria-free areas. Malaria would once again be inflicting ever-greater harm on the people they had tried to help. We should pause and consider how that happened, how our community failed to recognize the threat, and why it failed to respond.

The answers to these questions are perhaps more simple than one might think. During the 1960s, and into the 1970s, our community was committed, and had its nose to the grindstone, so to speak. From the initial use of DDT in the mid-1940s, our community had been in a position to observe any adverse effects from insecticides, if they were to occur. The community had close and continuous contact with the populations living in sprayed houses, and they saw no meaningful adverse effects. In brief, it had no evidence of any problems that appeared suddenly or gradually with the public health use of insecticides. Simultaneously the community saw great improvements in health when DDT was used to prevent the diseases it sought to eliminate. It was, perhaps, beyond the community's ability to think that anyone would work against a worthy and effective public health program; but the community was wrong. Additionally, the community had not focused on diverging malaria control interests of developed and developing countries. Divergences occurred because the developed countries had used DDT to eliminate malaria and no longer needed it. Meanwhile the developing

http://dx.doi.org/10.5772/55466

countries still needed DDT to help with their disease control problems. Last but not least, the community had no prior experience with the ruthless and scientifically indefensible fear tactics that were being unleashed against its disease control programs.

Threats to the old malaria eradication effort evolved from two ideologies within the environmental movement. One was that there are too many people on planet earth and malaria elimination allowed excessive population growth of poor people in developing countries. The second theme was that man-made chemicals endangered wildlife and human health. In 1970, George Woodwell, a prominent and entrenched anti-insecticide campaigner, captured the two ideologies in a paper he published in *Science* magazine. He concluded that the answer to the problem of environmental pollution was "Fewer people, unpopular but increasing restrictions on technology (making it more and more expensive) [9]." His concluding comment captured the thinking of major stakeholders within the environmental movement at that time. Through the careful use of fear tactics, global campaigns grew up around each ideology. Eventually the ideologies became established at the highest levels of the UN and national governments of developed countries. Those campaigns eventually destroyed effective disease control programs. The campaigns against PHIs achieved success through misrepresentations of science, by dragging companies and public organizations into courts in order to grab headlines for their fear-invoking claims, by using smear tactics against those who spoke in defense of insecticides, and, lastly, through extremely well-funded anti-insecticide advocacy. Through it all, anti-insecticide campaigners were supported by a popular press that fed off the fear invoked by the movement's predictions of insecticides causing catastrophic harm to wildlife and human health.

Naysayers will claim this is an exaggeration and that the old disease eradication programs were eliminated for a slew of reasons not mentioned here. Indeed there were other factors; but the overwhelming factors, as documented in annual proceedings of the WHO's Executive Board, discussions of the World Health Assembly (WHA), internal documents of UNICEF, and other published and unpublished reports, were those delineated above. Those who choose to believe current programs are not at risk of a similar fate may venture the opinion that regardless of past events, circumstances are entirely different now. They might even conclude movements that brought down the old programs are no longer active. For certain, the people, the claims, and the organizations have changed; but the themes and the scare tactics are the same. Nevertheless we will concede one point. The circumstances facing disease control programs today are entirely different from those that confronted the old disease eradication programs. Chief among the differences are that the old programs were not confronted by:

- Global networks of well-funded anti-insecticide advocacy,
- A WHO that, aside from its support for DDT under Dr. Kochi's brief leadership of the Global Malaria Program, frequently prioritizes the agenda of environmentalist groups over public health interests,
- Educational systems seeded with anti-insecticide propaganda,
- A Conference of the Parties to the Stockholm Convention on persistent organic pollutants that has independent authority to select insecticides for global elimination,

- Large national and international bureaucracies for regulatory control of insecticides,
- A vast, and largely anti-insecticide, research establishment functioning in universities and research institutes around the world,
- Billions of dollars for regulatory control and research against insecticides,
- A declining arsenal of insecticides for malaria control, and
- Regulatory controls that are major impediments to the research and development of new PHIs.

4. Environmentalism over public health policies

With an annual caseload estimated at 216 million and 655,000 deaths, malaria continues as one of the most important insect-borne diseases [10]. Yet, it is just one of many insect-borne diseases that collectively claim millions of lives and stifle economic growth and development in disease endemic countries. PHIs and other public health chemicals are vital to the global struggle to control these diseases. Where PHIs are removed or their use restricted, disease rates increase. For example, two large eradication programs that were based almost entirely on public health use of DDT, freed Bolivia of malaria, dengue fever, and risk of urban yellow fever from the 1950s to the mid-1970s. The WHO acknowledges the importance of one program as follows: "Historically, mosquito control campaigns [that employed DDT] successfully eliminated *Aedes aegypti*, the urban yellow fever vector, from most mainland countries of central and South America. However, this mosquito species has re-colonized urban areas [with cessation of the *Aedes aegypti* eradication program] in the region and poses a renewed risk of urban yellow fever [11]." In spite of marvelous improvements in human health that were achieved by use of PHIs, international anti-insecticide pressures were brought to bear on those programs.

Bolivia abandoned *Aedes aegypti* eradication in the 1970s. This occurred because Bolivia, as with many countries of the Americas, ramped down eradication efforts once the US buckled to anti-DDT pressures in 1969 and ended use of DDT for *Aedes aegypti* eradication. Almost all countries of the Americas followed the US example in the 1970s. Years later Bolivia abandoned use of DDT for malaria control. As a consequence, malaria and threats of urban yellow fever are once again commonplace in Bolivia [12], and in 2009 Bolivia was savaged by a major dengue epidemic.

India is another case study. In the early 1950s, India had an estimated 75 million malaria infections, with roughly 800,000 deaths each year. Spraying DDT brought numbers of cases down to 49,151 by 1961. Today, the number of malaria cases each year is in doubt. What seems certain however is that the number of cases is huge and the number of deaths is on an order of hundreds of thousands. Estimates for cases vary from a few million to tens of millions of cases per year [13].

Despite the considerable human and economic toll caused by past increases in diseases like malaria and dengue, the current arsenal of PHIs for spraying on house walls is limited to just

12 compounds from four chemical classes, namely pyrethroids, organophosphates, carbamates and organochlorines. Most PHIs are pyrethroids. DDT, the only organochlorine permitted for use, is one of the 12 approved compounds.

Even though production and use of DDT has declined continuously during the last four decades, DDT has grown as a convenient target of environmental science research. A recent PubMed search (in early 2011) for research papers on insecticides uncovered almost 60,000 papers, and about one sixth (9,459) were on DDT. These are remarkable statistics considering that DDT is hardly in use anymore. The decline in usage was sudden and corresponds to precipitous drops in human body burdens of DDT residues. Today, for example, the amount of DDT in human breast milk, based on serial surveys in many countries, is an infinitesimal fraction of what it was in the 1960s—and even those exceedingly low levels are declining [14]. Along with precipitous reductions in DDT use, one could reasonably expect that research on DDT would decline. However, as revealed in Figure 1, the numbers of published papers on DDT have actually increased, and more so in recent years than in the past. Furthermore, papers on DDT and malaria account for only a minor proportion (2.6 to 14.8% per year) of those published papers. So, why is the research effort on DDT increasing even as the use of DDT fades to inconsequential levels? To answer this question we will delve more into the modern themes of environmental research and anti-insecticide advocacy.

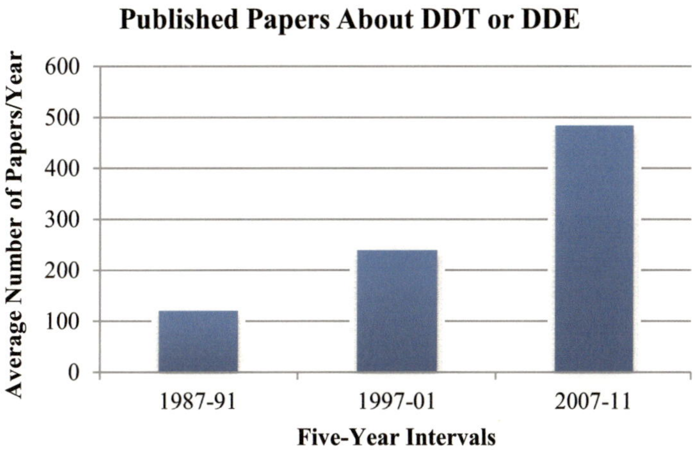

Figure 1. Average number of papers published per year on DDT or DDE. Data based on PubMed searches on key words--DDT and/or DDE. Counts summed for five-year intervals of 1987-1991, 1997-2001, and 2007-2011.

5. Why increased research on insecticides?

A 2005 paper by Dr. Stephen Safe, a Distinguished Professor and recipient of the Distinguished Lifetime Toxicology Scholar Award from the Society of Toxicology, explains much about the modern trend of increased funding and research on DDT [15]. Professor Safe is a professor at

Texas A&M and is a specialist in toxicology and molecular biology of estrogenic and anti-estrogenic compounds. To summarize introductory comments in his 2005 paper, modern emphasis on DDT is linked to a series of 1990 papers and the concept of the precautionary principle. The papers proposed that endocrine disrupting chemicals (EDCs), which include both man-made (synthetic) and naturally occurring chemicals, were contributing to diverse health problems worldwide. The diverse harms include decreased male sperm counts, increased birth defects, decreased fertility, increased incidence of breast and testicular cancers, etc. As Dr. Safe states, the role of synthetic EDCs as a cause of diverse health problems has been subjected to multiple challenges, to include a lack of biological plausibility for some responses and failure to consider that people are more heavily exposed to natural or dietary EDCs compared to relatively low exposures to the synthetic EDCs. Additionally, the natural compounds are often far more potent endocrine disruptors than synthetic EDCs.

The 1990s papers and the concept of the precautionary principle resulted in new funding and renewed interests in insecticides. As described by Dr. Safe, "Regulatory and research funding agencies have taken the endocrine disruptor hypothesis seriously [15]." Funds for research grew and, as a result, "... numerous laboratory animal and clinical studies have been initiated to test the validity of the hypothesis and to determine the association between health problems and exposure to EDCs [15]." This, in large part, seems to explain the huge growth in research and numbers of publications about potential harms from DDT and other insecticides. It is worth noting that extremely sensitive assays are available for DDT and other synthetic EDCs; but assays are often not available for more abundant and more diverse populations of natural EDCs. Thus it seems that the selection of DDT as a research topic is more closely related to availability and familiarity with quantitative assays opposed to some understanding of what the real threats are from synthetic versus natural EDCs.

In his 2005 paper Dr. Safe reviews many recent studies, and we refer the reader to his paper for more in-depth analyses. He comments on the synthetic EDCs as casual agents in breast cancer and male reproductive track anomalies. For the former, he reviews several studies, to include a meta-analysis, and concludes that the evidence does not support the hypothesis that DDE causes breast cancer. He concludes further that "If organochlorines do not significantly impact on this disease [breast cancer], it is now time to generate new hypotheses and focus on identifying other etiological factors that are linked to the high incidence of sporadic breast cancer in women [15]."

Dr. Safe reviewed numerous studies on DDT and other synthetic organochlorines (OCs) reportedly causing diseases of the male reproductive tract. The claim that sperm counts are declining is central to the thesis of many alarmists who propose that synthetic OCs are causing declining male sexual function. Dr. Safe reviews past reports and concludes, "results from various clinics are not sufficient to support a global decrease or increase [15]" in sperm counts. He also concludes "the hypothesized role of *in utero* exposure to estrogens as a factor in regulating sperm count in adult males is also questionable [15]." Dr. Safe goes on to review studies on possible associations between levels of synthetic EDCs with urogenital birth defects and increasing trends of testicular cancer. For the former, he found that both the evidence of increasing rate of birth defects and the hypothetical associations between those rates and exposures to synthetic EDCs were not persuasive. Additionally, evidence of multiple studies did not support the hypothesis that synthetic EDCs were a cause of testicular cancer.

In this brief section we have described the major themes of research that will be the source of future claims against PHIs. Dr. Safe sounded a warning in his comments about EDCs and breast cancer. He pointed out that our abilities to detect EDCs and a wealth of other variables (for example, biomarkers, genotypes, and a wealth of other biological, biochemical, environmental, and sociological variables) "increases the probability of 'chance' correlations, and there are several examples of these associations that are not consistent across all studies [15]." So, it seems clear that we should expect a greater frequency of claims against PHIs in the future. That said, anti-insecticide advocacy more so than research poses the greatest threat to the future of effective disease control programs. As we observed in the negotiations for the Stockholm Convention on Persistent Organic Pollutants (POPs) described below, well-funded anti-insecticide advocacy is the operational arm of the environmental movement. But unlike the careful deliberations of most environmental scientists, anti-insecticide groups are not constrained by subtle considerations of consistent and meaningful evidence and other criteria for cause-effect relationships, or by considerations of harm versus benefits of insecticide use.

6. Renewed malaria control programs beset by opposition to PHIs

As stated in an earlier section, today there is great enthusiasm and considerable funding to advance the goals of global control of malaria. We arrive at this period of enthusiasm only because we lived through many years of almost no hope at all.

The steady increase in malaria cases that led to RBM's formation had several underlying causes. Among them was the spread of drug resistance around the world. Since the 1940s chloroquine had been a mainstay of malaria treatment programs, but resistance by the *Plasmodium falciparum* parasite to the drug first appeared in the 1950s and slowly spread worldwide. Chloroquine was duly replaced by sulphadoxine-pyrimethamine (SP) in the 1980s, but resistance soon emerged to this drug as well.

Another cause of the growing burden of malaria was the lack of interest in malaria control by major donor agencies and malarial country governments. Enthusiasm for malaria dissipated when the great push against malaria - the global malaria eradication campaign of the 1950s and 60s – was called off. Malaria control is expensive, requiring the employment of trained personnel, logistics specialists, scientists and large quantities of drugs and vector control products. Continuing to pay for malaria control year in and year out when it was clear that global eradication was not feasible was a tough sell. Concurrently the focus for many development agencies was away from disease control and towards population control, as we touch on in this chapter and explain in more detail in *The Excellent Powder, DDT's Political and Scientific History* [16]. Few newly independent and highly malarial African countries sustained malaria control programs that had been run by colonial rulers. In Zambia, for instance, malaria control programs that had been set up when the country was ruled by Great Britain as Northern Rhodesia collapsed along with the Zambian economy in the 1980s.

However, as illustrated in the examples of disease control history in Bolivia and India, arguably one of the greatest obstacles to sustained malaria control was the growing campaign against PHIs, and DDT in particular. DDT had been used in malaria control since World War II. The effectiveness of this insecticide in controlling malaria was unprecedented. As we explain above, DDT, when sprayed on the inside walls of houses, acts to repel mosquitoes, but it will also irritate mosquitoes so they exit houses sooner than they otherwise would and will kill mosquitoes that rest on a sprayed surface long enough.

Through these multiple modes of action, and thanks to the dedicated work of thousands of hard working malaria control program officers, DDT saved around one billion people from malaria during the eradication era. But what some people heralded as a great savior, others decried as a harbinger of doom. Chief among the anti-DDT crusaders was Rachel Carson whose 1962 book, *Silent Spring*, is a florid and grossly exaggerated attack on the chemical for its supposed impact on wildlife and human health [17]. There were, and are, no shortages of Carson acolytes who have joined in with their own attacks on DDT, as we explain later in this chapter.

Following the banning of DDT for most uses in the US and Western Europe in the 1970s, production fell dramatically. Although DDT was still permitted for use in disease control, supplies dwindled and predictably the cost began to rise. It mattered little that the WHO's malaria control advisers still supported the use of DDT, when the reality was that fewer countries could obtain it. In 1969, Scandinavian countries, Canada and the US started to place 'severe' restrictions on the use of DDT [18]. Thus, it was no coincidence that global malaria eradication and the United State's *Aedes aegypti* eradication programs were both stopped in 1969—just as it was no coincidence that both relied on use of DDT [16]. Unsurprisingly, within just a few years, malarial countries were complaining to the WHO of their inability to obtain the chemical and use it to save lives [19]. Along with the growing campaigns against DDT, donor agencies like USAID, under pressure of legal actions, began to withdraw funding for DDT and malaria control in the 1970s.

In the following section we will detail, with a specific example, how the bio-politics of environmental activism against DDT and other PHIs translated into real world harm to human health. For this example we have chosen a country that has a strong tradition in science and a long and proud history of combating malaria.

7. Public health insecticides and malaria

The value of PHIs in controlling malaria is best evidenced by historical data on DDT sprayed houses. Brazil, as with other countries with territory within the Amazon Basin, struggles with difficult malaria control issues. The Amazon Basin is the most enduring environment in the Americas for the persistence of endemic malaria. Populated with many rural, poorly housed and mobile inhabitants, the Amazon Basin covers a vast geographical area of warm, humid environments. More importantly, it is populated with the Hemisphere's most dangerous vector of human malaria, *Anopheles darlingi*. In the absence of this species or in regions of the

Americas where it is less common, the chain of malaria transmission is weaker and more easily interrupted. For this reason, malaria often declines to low levels in the face of organized control programs in regions outside the Amazon Basin. In contrast, within the Amazon Basin, malaria exhibited some refractoriness to control measures even during years of the global malaria eradication program. As a consequence, eradication was not achieved. Nevertheless the spraying of DDT on house walls greatly reduced malaria infections and lifted a large part of the burden of malaria from the backs of people in the Amazon Basin.

Successful malaria control by spraying DDT was maintained for many years. Yet, the succession of bio-political events described in the previous section and elsewhere eventually destroyed Brazil's well-orchestrated malaria control program. Malaria cases began to increase when the numbers of houses being sprayed were progressively reduced in the 1980s. The many years of successful control followed by years when the spray program withered away are detailed in Figure 2.

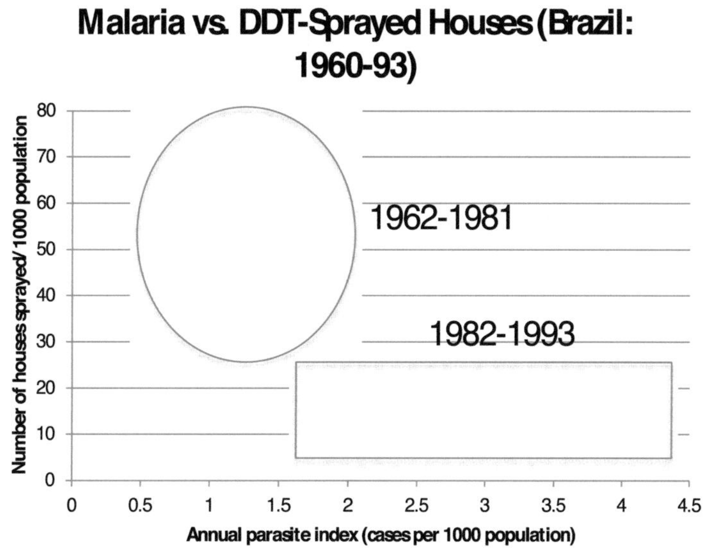

Figure 2. Number of houses sprayed per 1000 population versus the annual parasite index (cases per 1000 population) in Brazil during the years 1962 to 1993. Data for these years were collected under uniform data collection methods (see Roberts et al. 1997. for data sources [34]).

The graph presents annual parasite indices (APIs) and house spray rates (HSRs) from 1962 to 1993. Two clusters of data points are identified. One group represents the years from 1962 to 1981 when house spray rates were high and malaria indices were low. The API is a standard malaria control index, calculated as the annual number of diagnosed malaria cases X 1000/ population size. The HSR represents the number of houses sprayed per 1000 population. As shown in this graph, APIs in years after 1981 increased in response to reductions in numbers of houses being sprayed.

To bring Brazil's story up to date, Figure 3 presents statistics on malaria cases through 2010. As described in the previous section, there has been a global renewal in efforts to control malaria. Thus, in recent years, Brazil expanded its malaria control efforts. But even with increased financial support and availability of new malaria control technologies (e.g., case treatment with the new and effective ACTs, insecticide treated nets and so-called long-lasting nets), the accomplishments of recent years are less than what is needed and certainly far less than what was achieved and sustained during 20 years of spraying houses with DDT. As demonstrated in Figure 3, there was an average of 100,000 cases per year during those 20 years of major reliance on DDT. As DDT use declined in the 1980s, the average number of cases/year increased to 450,000. In the next decade, DDT use was abandoned completely and cases increased to over 500,000 per year. Today, even with an expanded program of control, the average number of cases per year is well over 400,000. The differences in results of the last 30 years over what was achieved with DDT roughly sums to 10.5 million cases that might have been prevented if DDT had not been abandoned. While population growth as an independent variable might account for some growth in numbers of cases, the increased number of cases corresponds, over time, to changes in slide positivity rates. The slide positivity rate is neutral in terms of population size. As a reminder, the estimate of 10.5 million excess malaria cases is for Brazil alone.

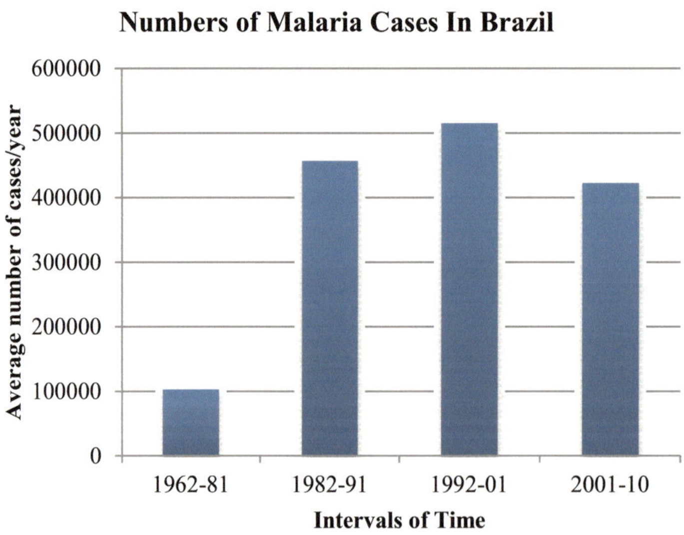

Figure 3. Average number of cases per year in Brazil across defined blocks of years (x-axis). Data for these years were collected under uniform data collection methods (see Roberts et al. 1997 for data sources [34] and PAHO malaria data [57]).

Clearly the great reductions of malaria from 1962 to 1981 compared to later blocks of years reveals the enormous benefit of DDT and other insecticides.

One of the most compelling examples of the usefulness of DDT in malaria control comes from recent experience in South Africa. This country had successfully used DDT in malaria control since the late 1940s and in so doing had dramatically reduced the malarial areas to the regions bordering Mozambique to the east and Zimbabwe to the north. In 1996 South Africa's Malaria Advisory Group (MAG) advised the national malaria control program to begin phasing out DDT. This advice was based on two main factors. First, DDT is best applied to the mud and dung walls of traditional African houses rather than on the plastered and painted walls of western style houses where the DDT can stain the walls. Given the staining, homeowners were often reluctant to allow the spray teams to enter their houses. As the rural areas of South Africa have developed and become wealthier, more and more people have built western style houses, requiring alternative insecticides. Second, the MAG had taken note of the political pressure against the use of DDT and anticipating greater restrictions on the use of DDT, decided to transition over to other chemicals. In the late 1990s therefore the provincial malaria programs began replacing DDT with pyrethroids. The first province to do so was KwaZulu Natal, which borders Mozambique and at the time was the most malarial of the countries three malarial provinces [16].

Almost as soon as the KwaZulu Natal malaria control program changed over to pyrethroids, malaria cases started to rise. By 2000, malaria cases had increased five fold from just over 8,500 cases to almost 42,000 cases. Malaria deaths increased from just 22 in 1996 to 320 in 2000 as malaria patients overwhelmed clinics and hospitals [20].

Research showed that a major driver of the epidemic was resistance to pyrethroid insecticides. In addition, evidence was rising that malaria parasite resistance had grown to SP, or Fansidar. The Department of Health took the decision to reintroduce DDT and change treatment regimen from Fansidar to the newly-available ACT, artemether-lumefantrine, or Coartem. Within a year malaria cases plummeted by around 80 percent [21]. The combination of a proven and effective PHI along with effective treatment reduced malaria transmission so dramatically that within just a few years, malaria elimination was within sight.

Given the benefit and usefulness of DDT and other PHIs in the control of malaria, as described above, how is it possible that PHIs have been so effectively demonized? In the next section we will describe strategies and tactics that have been employed to paralyze malaria control programs in countries around the world. As an aside, it is worth noting that those who ruthlessly campaign against DDT and other PHIs shamelessly deny any responsibility whatsoever for the increasing burdens of disease that inevitably occur when their campaigns succeed.

8. Goals, strategies, and tactics of anti-insecticide campaigns

The goal for environmental campaigns is to reduce or eliminate use of PHIs for the presumed but ambiguous purpose of better environmental health. Another goal, at least for some, appears to be stopping the use of chemicals that protect health and save lives in order to slow growth of human populations.

In the 1960s, the goal of halting or reducing the use of man-made insecticides was laid out in Rachel Carson's unscientific writings in *Silent Spring*. In 1968, the Malthusian rantings of Paul

Ehrlich in *The Population Bomb* focused attention on the contributions of DDT to growth of human populations in malaria-endemic countries. The goal of reducing human populations was never silenced; and it is once again a topic of heated debate, with some claiming billions of people must be eliminated [22].

The goal of today's anti-insecticide activists is still to reduce or eliminate synthetic insecticides. Achieving such a goal requires strategies and tactics. There are three visible strategies for achieving the goal of reducing or eliminating PHIs. The first is to convince people that PHIs are harmful. The second is to claim the chemicals are not needed in order to control diseases. The third strategy is to predict that grave harm will occur if the PHIs continue to be used. In this section we will give background information and three examples of the first strategy. In most cases we will focus on issues of DDT, but the same strategies and tactics are employed against other PHIs.

In a historical context, anti-insecticide advocates used propaganda and emotional arguments to convince people insecticides were dangerous and their use should be stopped. They were helped by science writers of the popular press and their efforts led to public health programs being abandoned around the world – and a resurgence of malaria infections. We have already presented one example of such an outcome (see Figures 2 and 3).

Anti-insecticide activism is an even stronger force today, and anti-insecticide advocates are even more determined to deny developing countries the protections from disease and death that only insecticides can provide. Because of environmental and anti-insecticide advocacy, the WHA adopted a resolution (WHA 50.13) in May 1997 that calls on countries to reduce reliance on use of insecticides for disease control [23]. Then, in 1998, the United Nations Environment Programme (UNEP) began negotiations for a POPs treaty targeting DDT and 11 other chemicals for global elimination [24]. The beginning of those negotiations stimulated malaria scientists and other public health professionals to mount a global campaign to defend the use of DDT in disease control programs. The public health campaign was successful and DDT was listed on Annex B of the Stockholm Convention on Persistent Organic Pollutants, which allowed its continued use. Yet, and despite the public health campaign's success, anti-DDT and anti-insecticide advocacy is unabated in UNEP, the US Environmental Protection Agency, the European Union, and, to lesser extent, in public agencies financing disease control programs. As a result, DDT factories closed their doors. Today, only one in India is still in operation. Also, environmental campaigners have erected formidable international barriers to the purchase and supply of DDT. Countries are under continual pressure from anti-DDT advocacy groups, and they are being enticed by financial mechanisms of Global Environment Facility (GEF) to stop using DDT.

WHA resolution 50.13 and the Stockholm Convention on Persistent Organic Pollutants, described above, are only the most recent in 50 years of efforts to eliminate DDT and other PHIs. Success in anti-PHI campaigns has been achieved by scaring people with false claims. Anti-DDT propaganda typically claims DDT causes all manner of harm to human health. Readily embraced and trumpeted by the popular press, the claims, in reality, never satisfy even the most minimal cause-effect criteria [25]. These internationally accepted criteria are:

http://dx.doi.org/10.5772/55466

- Strength of the association. The stronger an observed association appears over a series of different studies, the less likely this association is spurious because of bias.
- Dose-response effect. The value of the response variable changes in a meaningful way with the dose (or level) of the suspected causal agent.
- Lack of temporal ambiguity. The hypothesized cause precedes the occurrence of the effect.
- Consistency of the findings. Most, or all, studies concerned with a given causal hypothesis produce similar findings.
- Biological or theoretical plausibility. The hypothesized causal relationship is consistent with current biological or theoretical knowledge.
- Coherence of the evidence. The findings do not seriously conflict with accepted facts about the outcome variable being studied.
- Specificity of the association. The observed effect is associated with only the suspected cause (or few other causes that can be ruled out).

In the case of a true cause-effect relationship we can reasonably expect measurable levels of harm as a result of human exposures. Levels of harm will be proportional to harmfulness of the agent and to durations and characteristics of exposures. The more harmful an agent, the more likely it is to produce obvious levels of harm. Harm from weaker agents, on the other hand, will probably not be obvious and be definable only through population-based statistics. Regardless, ending use of a weak, but truly harmful, agent will reduce exposure to the chemical, reduce chemical concentration in the environment, and reduce the levels of harm. This is true even if the chemical is characterized as persistent, as is DDT. Persistence does not mean the chemical does not degrade. It just means that in certain compartments of the environment or living organisms it will degrade or be eliminated more slowly. Levels of DDT in the environment generally decline rapidly after its use is stopped. It is precisely because DDT does degrade that house walls are re-sprayed once or twice a year in order to achieve effective levels of malaria control.

Here, with the example of cigarette smoke and cancer, we illustrate application of cause-effect criteria. The link between smoking and human cancer has been validated through experimentation and vital statistics. In general, the argument that cigarette smoke caused cancer was convincing because patterns of low or high cancer rates consistently correlated with patterns of low or high smoking rates and duration of smoking. Furthermore, as people stopped smoking their risk of cancer actually declined. Consistent and persuasive evidence of cause-effect relationships between cigarette smoking and cancers formed the basis of public health campaigns to reduce or stop cigarette smoking. Unlike those public health campaigns, however, the environmental campaigns against PHIs are not based on persuasive and, certainly not, consistent, scientific evidence. The occasional observational study that suggests use of a public health insecticide harms health is countered by many other studies that suggest otherwise. Nevertheless, and as illustrated below, environmental campaigners readily ignore essential criteria for establishing a cause-effect relationship and greedily grab any new study that suggests some association between PHIs and human disease. The activist community has shown itself to be highly adept at getting such studies widespread national and international media coverage, often with headlines and messages designed to strike fear into people's hearts. These headlines are also very useful in advancing careers and ensuring ongoing research funding. We will describe three examples of how environmental advocates, and in some cases the environmental scientists themselves, ignore the criteria for establishing cause-effect relationships and use preliminary studies to push their anti-PHI agenda, or, more selfishly, their personal research agenda. The three examples are illustrations of the first strategy to convince people that DDT is a public health threat.

Example 1:

Mary Wolff and co-authors (1993) published a paper in which they claimed a statistical association of DDE (a major DDT metabolite) with breast cancer [26]. DDT opponents then used this paper to gain public attention and convince people that DDT caused breast cancer. To be specific, we are talking about anti-insecticide activists, not Dr. Wolff. Years later, with completion of many other studies, and without fanfare or wide publicity, researchers concluded DDE was not a cause of breast cancer. The WHO reassessment of DDT exposures from indoor spray programs states, "Overall, the association between DDT and breast cancer is inconclusive [27]." Regardless, for many years, anti-DDT activists heralded the 1993 paper as final proof of DDT harm and used it to generate funds and recruit new members to campaigns for DDT elimination [28].

Example 2:

Following a different thread of research, Rogan and coauthors reported that DDE was associated with reduced duration of lactation [29,30]. As with the reported association of DDT and breast cancer, this claim was grabbed by the WWF in 1998 and used in the propaganda campaign leading up to the Stockholm Convention on Persistent Organic Pollutants. The stated goal of the WWF campaign was a phase out of DDT by 2007 [28]. In their coverage of this topic, the WWF stated that studies "showed that the duration of lactation was inversely related to the concentration of DDE in milk." Separate from the WWF's use of these claims, the claims were, in part, also the basis for two high-profile publications by Rogan and coauthors in the journals, *Emerging Infectious Diseases* [31] and *The Lancet* [32]. They proposed that the benefits of spraying DDT on house walls to control malaria in Africa would be cancelled out by lowered child survival due to reduced durations of lactation and potential increases in premature births. The claims were used in campaigns against DDT and used to justify more research support.

Once published, the claims became tools for anti-DDT advocacy. For example, the claim is part of a 2005 Physicians for Social Responsibility (PSR) document about DDT and its use in Kenya. The PSR author states, "DDT may have a substantial impact on infant mortality, by increasing the risk of pre-term birth and by decreasing the duration of breast-feeding after birth. In this paper, Chen and Rogan conclude that DDT may cause comparable increase in infant mortality through these mechanisms compared to the decrease in infant mortality it causes by killing mosquitoes and thus reducing malaria cases [33]."

Without doubt the papers had great value for the anti-DDT advocacy community, yet the background studies for those claims did not fulfill the criteria for establishing DDT as the cause of reduced lactation or of pre-term births. In fact, even Chen and Rogan [31] stated the reported associations did not prove DDT caused any of the illnesses they discussed. Regardless, the claims were used as if they proved, beyond any doubt, that DDT was the cause of harm. This was illustrated in an exchange of letters to the Editor of the journal, *Emerging Infectious Diseases*. The exchange was between Roberts [34,35] and the WWF (written by Matteson) [36]. Matteson stated in her letter, "DDT also is associated with reduced lactation, premature births..." Naturally, Matteson used those reported associations to demonize DDT as part of WWF's push for global elimination of DDT by 2007. Misuse of those claims is further illustrated by an article defending Rachel Carson by the Rachel Carson Council. As with the PSR author, this writer used both claims plus the assertions included in the two papers by Rogan and coauthors about the benefits of DDT being canceled out by increased deaths of newborns in Africa. As stated in this very recent online article: "...significant shortening of the lactation cycle-time that human mothers can produce milk for their babies linked to DDT exposure. Based on reports for both premature births and reduced lactation cycles, scientists have predicted that regular DDT exposure could increase the possibility of higher levels of infant mortality for women in Africa who live in treated environments [37]."

There are many other examples of how these claims have been used and continue to be used in anti-insecticide propaganda. As stated in a 2006 article advocating against the use of DDT by the Pesticide Action Network in the UK, "Other studies have linked DDT to reduced breastmilk production, premature delivery and reduced infant birthweights [sic] [38]." Last but not least, Wikipedia includes the following statement:

Human epidemiological studies suggest that exposure is a risk factor for premature birth and low birth weight, and may harm a mother's ability to breast feed. Some 21st-century researchers argue that these effects may increase infant deaths, offsetting any anti-malarial benefits. A 2008 study, however, failed to confirm the association between exposure and difficulty breastfeeding [39].

Mention of the 2008 study is perhaps helpful; but it is not sufficient. Given that DDT produces great benefit in control of malaria, Wikipedia contributors should be careful in comments about DDT lest their written assessments inflict grave harm on poor people in malaria endemic countries. Point of fact, the Wikipedia assessment leaves the reader thinking that DDT causes premature births and reduced duration of lactation, when the weight of scientific evidence shows it does not.

Example 3:

Unfortunately, the false claims against DDT are unabated. One of the more recent and truly tragic examples of a false public image for PHIs occurred in 2009 when researchers in South Africa reported DDT was associated with urogenital birth defects in boys in a region where houses are sprayed with DDT to control malaria [40]. Although the authors, led by Prof. Riana Bornman of the University of Pretoria, suggest that DDT may not have caused the birth defects, the authors still state people should be informed about risks of birth defects if DDT is used.

Their interpretations and claims were aired broadly in the print and electronic media in South Africa. The public's concern over the researcher's claims created difficulties for the malaria control program. DDT, through decades of use in South Africa, had already proven its disease preventing capabilities. Given its proven record of performance, it is hardly reasonable to alarm people unless DDT is proven to be seriously harmful. In this case, the weaknesses of the researcher's claims had been addressed in the journal where the paper was published. Richard Grady addressed this issue in the editorial comment that accompanied the Bornman *et al.* paper [40]. Grady stated that issues of association and causality could not be distinguished in the paper. Grady was right; Bornman and coauthor's claims that DDT caused birth defects did not fulfill criteria for establishing a cause-effect relationship. As point of published fact, there were no statistically significant differences in the proportions of malformed genitalia among boys in sprayed and unsprayed villages. Given this fundamental failing, their pronouncements should not have been published and certainly should not have been used to scare the public away from having their houses sprayed. However, attempts in South Africa to scare people about DDT continue even now.

One of the researchers behind the urogenital birth defects claims recently reported on the levels of DDT in breast milk in sprayed villages in South Africa compared to results of an unsprayed village [41]. During the 70+ years of DDT use, many studies of DDT in breast milk have been performed. Based on those reports, it is expected that residents of DDT sprayed houses will have higher quantities of DDT in breast milk than residents of unsprayed villages. It is expected that intake by some infants will exceed the Provisional Tolerable Daily Intake (PTDI) and, in some cases, the residue levels will exceed the Maximum Residue Limit (MRL). In order to exaggerate the importance of their study, the authors emphasized the outlier measurements beyond confidence limits of mean values, e.g., in the abstract they report their statistics include "the highest ΣDDT level ever reported for breast milk from South Africa." Their control village was not sprayed and had no history of ever being sprayed. Yet the authors fail to mention that mean values of residues were at or above the MRL in the unsprayed village. They fail to mention that outlier data points in the control village, as with sprayed villages, exceeded the PTDI. They fail to mention that confidence limits for measurements from the control village overlap those of some sprayed villages. Authors emphasize gender differences in infants and associated levels of DDT in breast milk even though the differences were not statistically significant. They suggest the results require further research. Additionally, authors [41] report that mean levels of DDT had no impact on duration of lactation.

In press coverage of this paper the headlines read, "Researchers measure highest DDT levels in breast milk from South African nursing mothers [42]." In fact, outlier data points can result from erroneous dilutions, tests, conversions, or other parts of the experimental process, or just uncommon natural variation. For these reasons most researchers give outlier data points little weight. Yet the authors of this study used an outlier data point as a hook for grabbing headlines in the popular media. Media coverage went on to state, "In the region where the measurements were carried out, malformed genitalia among boys was significantly more common in areas treated with DDT compared with untreated areas." The assertion that DDT affects male urogenital development is mentioned in the paper, e.g., referring to the 2009 study they state,

"Research…identified DDT-associated effects on male urogenital parameters…[41]." However, the statement is misleading because, as described above, there were no statistically significant differences in the proportions of malformed genitalia among boys in sprayed and unsprayed villages.

Presented in three examples above is clear and unambiguous demonstration of orchestrated and non-scientific campaigns against PHIs, and DDT in particular. Claims that DDT causes one sort of harm or another are repeated in anti-insecticide propaganda even after published studies show the claims are false, or published rebuttals draw attention to errors in data analyses or research interpretations. A common part of these campaigns is how activists use the term "association" or "associated" as meaning there is a cause-effect relationship between an exposure and disease. In fact, these terms relate only to a statistical association that is often an artifact of study design or a product of systematic bias. Such issues as bias are of particular concern, and are discussed at length in David Savitz's book *Interpreting epidemiologic evidence* [43].

In the history of efforts to preserve use of DDT for public health programs, this chain of events has been repeated over and over, with claims of causation eventually being disproven, but not before they were used to generate funds, recruit new members to anti-insecticide campaigns, and change public health policies. Last but not least, each change in disease control policy has weakened global capacities to control malaria and other diseases. Almost every change is a result of anti-insecticide propaganda that misrepresents the scientific process, as revealed for the three examples described above:

- The breast cancer example reveals a general trend of anti-DDT campaigners railing against DDT while failing to meet minimal evidentiary standards for proof of cause-effect relationships (as defined by the principles of causation [25]). In brief, those who campaign against DDT have failed to show, through replicated and confirmatory studies, that a specific type of public health harm from DDT was a consistent finding across studies, and that it was consistent with current biological or theoretical knowledge of the type of harm and its known risk factors; for example:
    - More common with higher DDT exposure and less common with lower exposure,
    - Less common prior to DDT exposure and appeared or increased in frequency with onset of DDT exposure, and
    - More common with DDT exposure and less common once DDT use was stopped.
- The example of DDT as a reputed cause of reduced duration of lactation illustrates how an unproven claim can be used in scientific literature to assert that an unintended consequence of DDT might cause as much harm as benefit. Also it shows how the claim can continue to appear in anti-insecticide propaganda long after it is disproven.
- The example of malformed male genitalia illustrates how false associations can be used in attempts to scare people away from allowing their houses to be sprayed. Also the example illustrates how tangential studies (a survey of DDT in breast milk) can be used to exaggerate

dangers of DDT and to cast further attention on the results of weak studies. Sadly, the two studies are being used to scare people who live in malarious regions.

9. Dichotomies in patterns/trends of human disease with/without DDT

Decades ago, developed countries used extraordinary quantities of DDT. The richer countries placed DDT in the human food chain through its heavy agricultural use at that time. More explicitly, DDT was used in the environment, around houses, and intensively inside homes. It is now 40 years since being banned for most uses in the US and other developed countries. Yet, recent claims of DDT causing disease or birth defects are not reflected in the historical medical reports and vital statistics for regions and years of broad and heavy DDT usage. The lack of proof that DDT caused harm to human health back in the days of intense exposures goes far in explaining why, to this day, there is no evidence that human health has been improved in any way by stopping public health uses of DDT.

There is a dichotomy in the huge benefit from use of DDT to prevent diseases and deaths versus no definable benefit from stopping its use. For slightly more than three decades (1945-1979) many malaria endemic countries maintained house spray programs. That era was followed by decades, from 1979 through to present time, when most of the same countries phased house spraying out of national programs. The result is a historical record of years when DDT and other insecticides were sprayed in houses followed by almost as many years when spraying was greatly decreased or stopped entirely. An even more drastic stoppage of DDT spraying occurred in agriculture. The dichotomies of outcomes are listed in Table 1.

Benefits versus harms of public health insecticides	1946-79 (period of DDT spraying in houses)	1980-present (period when DDT spraying was reduced or stopped)
Harm from insecticide exposures	Increases in poisonings and deaths from insecticide exposures in houses	Reductions in poisonings and deaths as house spraying is eliminated
Benefits from using insecticides to control malaria and other diseases	Reductions in malaria infections and deaths as a consequence of DDT on house walls	Increases in malaria infections and deaths as house spraying of DDT is eliminated

Table 1. Grid of cause-effect relationships for public health outcomes during periods of use and non-use of DDT in public health programs.

As explained for smoking and human cancers, the relationship of declining risk with reduced exposure attests to a true and meaningful causal relationship. An inverse finding of increasing risk with increasing exposure to a causative agent also attests to a true and meaningful causal relationship. These indicators of causation make it all the more amazing that through decades of anti-insecticide advocacy, insecticide opponents have documented no obvious public health harm as a result of DDT residues on house walls. Likewise, they have documented no meaningful improvements in health or reduced deaths as a direct result of having eliminated

DDT exposure by ending house spray programs. These failings suggest DDT opponents have not been challenged to balance an equation of measurable benefits from preventing the use of DDT and other public health insecticides versus the measurable increases in human deaths and diseases, like malaria, as consequence of stopping use of public health insecticides.

10. Models for modern advocacy against PHIs

Now, on the fiftieth anniversary of *Silent Spring*, the goal of reducing or eliminating DDT and other PHIs is, and has been for decades, entrenched in environmental advocacy literature and in bureaucracies of the UN. In the case of DDT, this goal was clearly enunciated by UNEP in 2000:

WHO and UNEP have joined forces to protect both human health and the environment by promoting strategies to reduce malaria with reduced reliance on DDT. An important first step was taken in March 2000 through a WHO-convened Regional Consultation to Prepare African Countries Towards Reduction of Reliance on DDT for Malaria Control, with UNEP support. [44]

For UNEP bureaucrats, the statement codifies the environmentalist's belief that small quantities of DDT sprayed on house walls harms the environment. Also it codifies the belief that DDT is not needed in malaria control programs. In both cases, the bureaucrats are wrong.

Information presented in Figures 2 and 3 illustrate the enormous danger of forcing countries to abandon DDT and other PHIs. Since the early 1980s over 10.5 million preventable malaria cases were recorded above and beyond what might have occurred if Brazil had not abandoned DDT. There were no DDT resistance issues that caused malaria program managers to abandon DDT, there were no important studies showing DDT repellent properties did not work, there were no malaria trend analyses showing a lack of efficacious control with DDT sprayed walls, and there were no cost-effective insecticides that could be used instead. DDT was abandoned in Brazil and in other countries of South America as a consequence of global environmental policies and anti-insecticide campaigns. DDT was not eliminated from Peru's malaria program until the late 1980s. Peru's malaria problems grew exponentially worse immediately after the country dispensed with DDT spraying. These disastrous outcomes were repeated in many countries.

With the beginning of the 21st Century and infused with renewed support and improved targeting in application of control efforts, malaria control programs are beginning to make some progress. But further progress is needed and malaria continues as a huge public health problem. Meanwhile, as in the 1960s, insecticide opponents are poised to counter the recent progress against malaria. We will now focus on specific tactics that are and will continue to be used in the anti-insecticide campaigns.

As we have described, the first strategy of insecticide opposition is to convince people that DDT or other PHIs are harmful. An important tactic for achieving success is to develop and broadcast widely and repeatedly a list of diverse claims of chemical harm. We have already described examples of how this tactic is implemented. A list of diverse sources of harm is not easy to counter. When an authoritative rebuttal of one claim occurs, the other claims are still in play. Additionally, a broad list of claims allows campaigners to tailor platforms for constituencies, advancing one set of claims with one constituency and a different combination for another. Another tactic is to focus on the most recent study hinting at some health impact of the chemical. It is easier to get the popular media interested in a study that can be presented as a new and sensational finding--a favorite theme of science writers. Regardless, a list of multiple claims of harm is hardly sufficient to achieve a ban of a truly useful PHI. Thus, the second strategy of convincing people the chemical is not needed becomes extraordinarily important. The tactic behind this goal is to argue that alternative chemicals or methods can be used as replacements. We will present two examples of tactics employed in support of this strategy. The third strategy is to predict that grave harm will occur if the chemical continues to be used.

The success of Rachel Carson's *Silent Spring* serves as a model for the three strategies. In *Silent Spring*, Rachel Carson used the strategies on her primary target, DDT. She described a very large list of potential adverse effects of insecticides, including human health and ecological effects. She argued that insecticides were not really needed because their use selected for super bugs that were resistant to the insecticides and that the chemicals only made problems worse. Last but not least, she described scary scenarios of severe harm with continued use of DDT and other insecticides.

Carson focused attention on examples of overuse or misuse of DDT and other insecticides and described the effects of their misuse. Nevertheless, the misuse of chemicals is not a valid reason for banning an insecticide. In the case of DDT, a successful campaign to eliminate it requires that even its proper use will cause a large and systematic adverse effect. However, the proper public health uses of DDT yield no large and systematic adverse effects. Absent such adverse actions, the activists must then rely on claims about insidious effects, particularly insidious effects that scientists will find difficult to prove one way or the other, and that activists can use to predict a future catastrophe.

Rachel Carson relied heavily on possible insidious chemical actions as a means of alarming and scaring the public. Many of those who joined the resulting campaign to ban DDT and other insecticides made extensive use of claims of insidious effects. In particular Carson alluded to insidious effects on reproduction. Her assertions were amplified by the popular press and became part of the public perception about insecticides. Although those perceptions are wrong, they are firmly entrenched in anti-insecticide propaganda.

The three strategies, while largely bogus in terms of their scientific underpinnings, were very effective in anti-insecticide campaigns. The strategies are still used today. Rogan and Chen used these strategies in their two papers against DDT [31,32]. The authors presented strategy number two in the form of a superficial review of the role of DDT in malaria control. They strove to cast doubt on DDT's value in modern malaria control programs. They admitted that

DDT had been very effective in the past, but then argued that malaria control programs no longer needed it and alternative methods of control should be used. Rogan and Chen also employed the first strategy of environmentalism [32]. Their list of potential harms from DDT exposures included toxic effects, neurobehavioral effects, cancers, decrements in various facets of reproductive health, decrements in infant and child development, and immunology and DNA damage. To get the paper past reviewers they presented balanced coverage of their diverse claims of harm, and, as consequence, had to conclude they could not prove that DDT caused any harm at all. Amazingly, they promptly negated this honest conclusion by asserting that if DDT is used for malaria control then great harm might occur. So, while not proving DDT causes harm, the authors still predict severe harm if it is used.

Rogan and Chen end their paper with a call for more research. One could conclude that the intent of the whole paper is merely to lobby for research dollars to better define DDT harm, and what's the harm in that? Surely increasing knowledge is a fine goal. However, having engaged issues of malaria control and what should or should not be done to control the disease, specifying more research funds for research on potential harms of insecticide exposures is unjustified. Large numbers of children and pregnant women die from malaria every year, and the disease sickens hundreds of millions more. Yet, not one death or illness can be attributed to an exposure to the public health use of DDT. Figure 1 illustrates growth in DDT research, with numbers of published papers doubling from one decade to the next. Almost all papers are in environmental literature and many are on potential adverse effects of DDT. Only a small proportion of papers deal with malaria and DDT. It bears repeating that DDT is a spatial repellent, and hardly an insecticide at all, but a search on DDT and repellents will produce even fewer papers. This disparity represents an egregiously disproportionate emphasis on non-sources of harm compared to the enormous harm of malaria.

The US used DDT to eradicate malaria. After malaria disappeared as an endemic disease people in the US became richer. They built better and more enclosed houses. They screened their windows and doors. They air-conditioned their homes. Also, during those early years, the US developed an immense arsenal of mosquito control tools and chemicals. Today, when there is a risk of mosquito borne disease, urban and rural areas can bring this arsenal to bear and quickly eliminate risks. And, as illustrated by aerial spray missions in the aftermath of hurricane Katrina, they can afford to do so. Yet, those modern and very expensive chemicals are not what protect the US from introductions of the old diseases. Use of those chemicals can only respond to a threat; it cannot prevent the old diseases from being reintroduced. What protects US populations is their enclosed, screened, air-conditioned housing, the physical representation of their wealth. Their wealth and living standards stop dengue at the border with Mexico, not the use of insecticides. Stopping mosquitoes from entering and biting people inside their homes is critical in the prevention of malaria and many other insect-borne diseases. This is what DDT does for poor people in poor countries. It stops large proportions of mosquitoes from entering houses. It is, in fact, a form of chemical screening, and until people in disease endemic countries can afford properly enclosed houses and physical screening, or it is provided for them, chemical screening is the only kind they have.

DDT is a protective tool that has been taken away from countries around the world, mostly due to governments acceding to the whims of the anti-pesticide wing of environmentalism, but it is not only the anti-pesticide wing that lobbies against DDT. The activists have a sympathetic lobbying ally in the pesticide industry. DDT opposition was made clear in writings of those within the insecticide industry; a Bayer official stated:

[I speak] Not only as the responsible manager for the vector control business in Bayer, being the market leader in vector control and pointing out by that we know what we are talking about and have decades of experiences in the evolution of this very particular market. [but] Also as one of the private sector representatives in the RBM Partnership Board and being confronted with that discussion about DDT in the various WHO, RBM et al circles. So you can take it as a view from the field, from the operational commercial level - but our companies [sic] point of view. I know that all of my colleagues from other primary manufacturers and internationally operating companies are sharing my view. [45]

The official goes on to say that,

DDT use is for us a commercial threat (which is clear, but it is not that dramatical [sic] because of limited use), it is mainly a public image threat.

However the most damming part of this message was the statement that,

---

...we fully support EU to ban imports of agricultural products coming from countries using DDT...

This email message from Bayer, one of the largest global manufacturers of alternatives to DDT, provides clear evidence of industry applying international and developed country pressures to stop poor countries from using DDT to control malaria. This message also shows the complicity of the insecticide industry in those internationally orchestrated efforts.

The environmental movement lobbied for a WHA resolution that required countries to move away from using insecticides in disease control altogether [23]. The WHA is the premier policy-setting forum for all health issues and is the governing body of the WHO. At that time, 1997, there was no evidence that vector-borne diseases could be controlled without man-made insecticides. The same is true today. The resolution was adopted by the WHA in 1997. Essentially, the lobbying of environmental groups elevated politics and anti-insecticide sentiment above scientific evidence and left hundreds of millions at high risk of death and illness from entirely preventable diseases. As we will show in the next section, UNEP has a particularly odious history of elevating environmental politics over science.

http://dx.doi.org/10.5772/55466

11. UNEP's war against PHIs

The UN Stockholm Convention on POPs, which came into force in 2004, governs the use of DDT. DDT is the only chemical under the POPs Convention that is granted an exemption for use in public health. It is against this background that the Stockholm Convention Secretariat (the Secretariat) and the financial mechanism of the Convention, the GEF, the UNEP, and groups within the Pan American Health Organization (PAHO) and WHO, have engaged in scientific malfeasance to achieve political goals. UNEP's target goal in 2007, now removed from the UNEP website, was DDT elimination by 2020.[1]

The GEF was established in 1991 and is a partnership of 10 agencies, including the World Bank, which houses the GEF. The GEF has allocated over $9bn in funds for projects with the aim of improving the environment and has raised over $40bn from other partners for its projects. At stake is not only increased power over the use of chemicals for the control of diseases but also the reputational benefits of achieving a goal deemed desirable by environmental groups. In addition, one cannot discount the fact that many millions of dollars are programmed by numerous governments via the UN system to rid the world of POPs and find alternatives to DDT. Control over the use of insecticides for public health also gives agencies control over, and benefit from, these funds.

UNEP's and GEF's misrepresentations of scientific records against the use of DDT and other PHIs were exposed in a peer-reviewed paper in *Research and Reports in Tropical Medicine* [46]. The paper exposed the false claims about an insecticide-free malaria control project managed by UNEP and financed by GEF in Mexico and Central America (Mexico/CA). The project was designed to demonstrate successful control of malaria through use of "environmentally sound" methods without DDT and other insecticides. Almost inevitably, the projects' backers claimed it achieved this objective. A proper analysis of epidemiologic data, however, revealed no such success; reductions in malaria cases and deaths in the region were achieved primarily through pharmacosuppression (therapeutic and prophylactic use of anti-malarial drugs). Claims that UNEP's environmental interventions were effective were invalid.

The project, Regional Program of Action and Demonstration of Sustainable Alternatives to DDT for Malaria Vector Control in Mexico and Central America (Mexico/CA Project), was conducted in eight countries (Belize, Costa Rica, Guatemala, Honduras, Mexico, Nicaragua, Panama and El Salvador). It was executed by PAHO's Sustainable Development and Environmental Health Program and implemented by UNEP. It was co-financed by the GEF with additional support from the Commission for Environmental Cooperation of North America (CEC), PAHO, and participating country governments. The project's aim was to improve coordination and national capacity so that new, integrated disease vector (mosquito) control techniques could be implemented, thereby eliminating the need for DDT reintroduction [47]. The objectives of the project (as stated by UNEP) were to: "Demonstrate feasibility of integrated

1 The Stockholm Convention is a UN Convention that arose from UN Environment Program efforts to control and/or ban the production and use of certain persistent organic pollutants. PAHO is an international public health agency and is the Regional Office for the Americas of the WHO and part of the UN.

and environment-friendly methods for malaria vector control without the use of DDT," and "assess the effects of these methods on malaria occurrence [48]."

According to UNEP, the key interventions in the project were as follows: 1) Reduction of contact between mosquitoes and people via treated bed nets; meshes on doors and windows; the planting of repellent trees like neem and oak; and the liming of households. 2) Control of breeding sites by clearing vegetation; draining stagnant water, ditches and channels; and the use of biological controls such as fish and bacteria in some countries. 3) Elimination of places near houses that attract and shelter mosquitoes through, for example, the cleaning and tidying up of areas in and around homes, alongside the promotion of personal hygiene [49].

The project's final evaluation, published in November 2009, mentions various pharmaceutical methods of prophylaxis and treatment within human populations [50]. However, those methods were ongoing components of malaria control in each country prior to the Mexico/CA Project, operating nationally in each country before and during the project. The available evidence suggests national malaria control programs (NMCPs) functioned regardless of the presence or absence of UNEP's project personnel. Thus, anti-malarial treatment (the major component of the NMCPs) in demonstration areas was not part of the epidemiological evaluation of the Mexico/CA Project [51]. Likewise, use of ITNs had no obvious definable role in the Mexico/CA Project. Project successes are therefore advertised as having been achieved without mention of the accompanying use of insecticides.

The project included demonstration areas, where the GEF environmental interventions would be implemented, as well as control areas within epidemiologically similar areas, where the interventions would be excluded, for proper comparisons [51]. As stated by Cesar Chelala, medical consultant affiliated with the Mexico/CA Project, demonstration areas were selected "based on the high incidence of transmission and the persistence of malaria in those places [52]."

An epidemiological evaluation identified 202 demonstration areas and 51 control areas [51]. The former included a total population of 159,018 and the latter 50,834.

The public statements regarding the Mexico/CA Project proclaimed dramatic and very impressive reductions in malaria cases for its environmentally benign interventions. The final report of the Mexico/CA Project, published by the environmental sector of PAHO in December 2008, claims "a 63% reduction in the number of people with the disease without using DDT or any other type of pesticide [53]."

These statistics and claims of success were repeated in an official press release issued by UNEP, WHO and GEF in May 2009 [54]. UNEP Executive Director, Achim Steiner, also repeated these claims and characterized the project as "calculated and tested science [49]." Similar claims have been made in the popular media [52] and used by anti-insecticide activist groups as evidence that malaria control is possible without insecticides [55].

Regrettably, the claims of malaria control through application of GEF interventions were incorrect and fundamentally misleading.

Countries in Latin America were forced away from using DDT in compliance with the North American Free Trade Agreement (NAFTA), wherein the CEC pressured Mexico in the mid-1990s to stop production and use of DDT [56]. Without DDT, countries used more expensive insecticides, which had to be sprayed more frequently, creating problems for malaria control [57]. Over time, the countries in Central America moved to greater use of pharmacosuppression. Malaria cases have fallen as a result of this widespread use of malaria treatments, but not through the environmental controls touted by the UN. Officials of GEF, UNEP and the Secretariat, however, ignored the use of pharmacosuppression in their discussion of successful malaria control in Mexico/CA. Furthermore, these officials falsely attribute changes in malaria burdens to GEF's environmental interventions. A separate epidemiological evaluation which was designed to measure any changes in disease rates, found no statistical differences in malaria rates in demonstration areas versus rates in control areas, and this was consistent across all eight countries [51]. Malaria rates in most countries were falling, but with no difference between the demonstration areas and controls, the decline cannot be attributed to the environmental interventions. But UNEP, GEF, the Secretariat and other officials ignored those findings. Furthermore, despite the fact that the control areas were a crucially important part of the project, they were not even mentioned in the 2008 final report [53]. Ultimately, the successful reduction of malaria was most likely entirely due to pharmacosuppression.

One might wonder why a control program would require insecticides and vector control if pharmacosuppression is such a powerful method of malaria control. This is a complex issue, but it is important to note that even though reductions in malaria cases have been achieved in Mexico and Central America, their model of widespread distribution of the anti-malarial drugs chloroquine and primaquine is not transferable elsewhere and may not be sustainable over the long-term. As a model for malaria control, it is not transferable for several reasons. First, widespread drug resistance to chloroquine in Africa and Southeast Asia would mean the intervention would be largely useless. Second, primaquine is a radical treatment for vivax malaria, whereas in Africa over 90 percent of malaria cases are caused by falciparum malaria, the more deadly form of the disease.[2] Third, pharmacosuppression is expensive and requires more sophisticated health systems than exist in most of Africa, where the greatest burden of malaria lies. So even if UNEP, GEF and their partners were straightforward about the real reasons for the declines in malaria in the project areas, there would be no reasonable argument to claim that pharmacosuppression has any application in most other endemic areas.

Global malaria control policy gives scant notice to pharmacosuppression. In fact, it appears that global leaders are intent on ignoring how countries of the Americas are making use of pharmacosuppression. Yet, and as commonly observed in reports from South America, the only cost-effective insecticides (pyrethroids) they have must be sprayed so frequently as to be of limited value. Thus, countries of the Americas really have no viable cost-effective options for use of PHIs. In absence of an insecticidal solution then, pharmacosuppression becomes the best option for effectively reducing malaria caseloads.

2 In addition, there are concerns about the side effects of using primaquine among people with G6PD deficiency. See Baird K. Eliminating malaria – all of them.Lancet 2010;376(9756): 1883-5. http://www.thelancet.com/journals/lancet/article/PIIS0140-6736%2810%2961494-8/fulltext (accessed 19 September 2012).

If we assume there is a decision to keep quiet on how malaria is being controlled in absence of insecticides, then it is easier to understand why there is less transparency in malaria data for the Americas. Historically PAHO openly reported statistics on the numbers and types of curative treatments dispensed per year in each country. However, transparency of malaria control statistics is down from just two or three years ago. A visit to PAHO's website on interactive malaria control data for the Americas will reveal no data on numbers of treatments with chloroquine or primaquine. Indeed, the only data that is readily available is on use of ACTs for treating cases of falciparum malaria.

12. Conclusion

We have described the systematic and often coordinated campaigns by activists, scientists and UN agencies against essential tools for disease control. We will conclude here with statements that bring our analyses full circle. Rachel Carson started broad scale unscientific attacks on DDT in 1962, with publication of her book, *Silent Spring*. The claims of harm by exposures to DDT, as we describe in this chapter, were not and are not true. In other words, the attributed harms are not caused by DDT exposures. Yet, presented in a 2012 article titled "Critisism [sic] of Carson over DDT unfounded" is a denial of any responsibility whatsoever for the reductions and eliminations of DDT in disease control programs as legacy of her book. In their article the Rachel Carson Council makes the following claims: "DDT has been associated with serious adverse effects in humans, including reduced sperm production in men, shorter lactation times and increasing numbers of pre-term births in women,... breast cancer...[58]."

We ask the reader to compare their claims with those we describe as not meeting even minimal criteria for cause-effect relationships. So the Rachel Carson Council denies responsibility for harm inflicted by Carson's anti-DDT rhetoric, while, at the same time, it continues to implement her strategies for DDT elimination and employs her tactics of falsifying the scientific record to scare the public. Amazingly, when the false statements and fear tactics employed by anti-DDT campaigners succeed in stopping use of DDT to protect health and save lives, the anti-PHI advocacy community, as revealed in the Rachel Carson Council's denial of responsibilities, expects the public to think they had no role in such inhumanely disastrous changes in public health policies. As we have shown, they are, in fact, the very cause of those changes in policy.

We have shown that vast sums of money, mostly from taxpayers, have been spent over many decades undermining and often directly attacking the use of DDT in life-saving disease control programs. These vast expenditures have not delivered alternative strategies or tools to replace DDT. The few alternatives that disease control programs do have for some malaria-endemic regions pale in comparison to the powerful life-saving properties of DDT. It almost goes without saying that if the disease control tool in question were not DDT but were a vaccine or a medicine, there would be a sense of outrage in the general public along with well-funded advocacy to preserve and protect a tool that has the power to save lives. Yet such is the power of the environmental movement, that aside from a few outspoken scientists and individuals,

http://dx.doi.org/10.5772/55466

there has been almost no response from the malaria community or the wider public health community. The strategies employed by anti-DDT activists are anti-science and rely on distortions, half-truths and sometimes outright lies. Ordinarily such behavior would be roundly criticized, yet because DDT is being attacked, such actions are given a free pass.

We are greatly concerned that the majority of private insecticide companies far from opposing the unscientific agenda of the anti-DDT campaigns, support them. These companies may be merely motivated to sell more of their own product, but this is surely one of the most short-sighted strategies imaginable. We already see a growing number of studies finding associations between alternatives to DDT and possible human health harm. As with DDT, the anti-insecticide activists are starting to hype and spread fear about these associations. As the Stockholm Convention adds more and more chemicals to its list of banned or controlled substances, and as the UNEP flexes its regulatory muscles, we fully expect it will become more and more difficult to produce, trade, transport and use all PHIs. It is precisely because of such restrictions that countries of the Americas have had to adopt programs of mass drug distributions (pharmacosuppression) to control vivax malaria. Basically those countries have no cost-effective options for use of PHIs. Continuation of these anti-PHI practices, as we have learned from history, will inflict great harm on disease control efforts and eventually exact a heavy cost in lives from some of the poorest and most vulnerable communities on earth.

We hope this chapter has shed some light on the strategies and tactics of environmental groups, activists, scientists and UN agencies. Well-established patterns of behavior have been set with these groups and individuals and we hope that the malaria community and the wider public health community begin to recognize these patterns and begin to more effectively investigate and respond to claims against PHIs long before the claims become the basis for further restrictions on the efficacy of disease control programs.

List of the acronyms used in the text

ACT-- artemisinin-based combination therapies

API—annual parasite index

CEC—Commission for Environmental Cooperation (The full title is North Americas Commission for Environmental Cooperation. Created as a side agreement of the North American Free Trade Agreement.)

DDT/DDE—Diethyl dichloro trichloroethelene. DDE is a metabolic product of DDT.

EDC-- endocrine disrupting chemicals

GEF—Global Environment Facility

HSR—house spray rate

IRS—indoor residual spray

ITN—insecticide treated net

MRL—maximum residue limit

NAFTA—North American Free Trade Agreement

NGO—Nongovernmental organization

NMCP—National Malaria Control Program

OC—organochlorine compound

PAHO—Pan American Health Organization

PHI—public health insecticide

PMI—President's Malaria Initiative

POP—persistent organic pollutant

PTDI—provisional tolerable daily intake

RBM—Roll Back Malaria

SP-- sulphadoxine-pyrimethamine

UN—United Nations

UNDP—United Nations Development Programme

UNEP—United Nations Environment Programme

UNICEF—United Nations Children's Fund

USAID—United States Agency for International Development

WHA—World Health Assembly

WHO—World Health Organization

WWF—World Wildlife Fund

Author details

Donald R. Roberts[1,2*], Richard Tren[3] and Kimberly Hess[3]

*Address all correspondence to: drdonaldroberts42@gmail.com

1 Uniformed Services University of the Health Sciences, Bethesda, MD, USA

2 Retired, Professor Emeritus, Clifton Forge, VA, USA

3 Africa Fighting Malaria, Washington, DC, USA

References

[1] Roll Back Malaria Partnership: RBM Vision. http://www.rbm.who.int/rbmvision.html (accessed 4 December 2012).

[2] The President's Malaria Initiative: PMI Results. http://www.fightingmalaria.gov/about/results.html (accessed 4 December 2012).

[3] World Health Organization: What is Roll Back Malaria? https://apps.who.int/inf-fs/en/InformationSheet02.pdf (accessed 19 September 2012).

[4] Yamey G. Roll Back Malaria: a failing global health campaign. BMJ 2004;328: 1086. http://www.bmj.com/content/328/7448/1086 (accessed 19 September 2012).

[5] World Health Organization: WHO gives indoor use of DDT a clean bill of health for controlling malaria. http://www.who.int/mediacentre/news/releases/2006/pr50/en/ (accessed 19 September 2012).

[6] The President's Malaria Initiative: Sixth Annual Report to Congress: April 2012. http://www.fightingmalaria.gov/resources/reports/pmi_annual_report12.pdf (accessed 19 September 2012).

[7] The Global Fund to Fight AIDS, TB and Malaria: The Global Fund Annual Report 2011. http://www.theglobalfund.org/en/library/publications/annualreports/ (accessed 19 September 2012).

[8] World Health Organization: World Malaria Report 2011. http://www.who.int/malaria/world_malaria_report_2011/en/index.html (accessed 19 September 2012).

[9] Woodwell GM. Effects of pollution on the structure and physiology of ecosystems. Science 1970;168(3930) 429-433.

[10] World Health Organization: Malaria Fact sheet No. 94: April 2012. http://www.who.int/mediacentre/factsheets/fs094/en/ (accessed 19 September 2012).

[11] World Health Organization: Yellow fever Fact sheet No. 100: January 2011. http://www.who.int/mediacentre/factsheets/fs100/en/ (accessed 19 September 2012).

[12] World Health Organization: World Malaria Report 2009. http://www.who.int/malaria/world_malaria_report_2009/en/index.html (accessed 19 September 2012).

[13] Malaria Site: Malaria in India. http://www.malariasite.com/malaria/MalariaInIndia.htm (accessed 19 September 2012).

[14] Smith D. Worldwide trends in DDT levels in human breast milk. Int J Epidemiol 1999;28(2) 179-88.

[15] Safe S. Clinical correlates of environmental endocrine disruptors. Trends Endocrinol Metab 2005;16(4) 139-44.

[16] Roberts D, Tren R, Bate R, Zambone J. The Excellent Powder, DDT's Political and Scientific History. Indianapolis, IN: Dog Ear Publishing; 2010.

[17] Carson R. Silent Spring. New York: Houghton Mifflin Company; 1962.

[18] World Health Organization. Executive Board, 47th Session, Part II, Appendix 14. "The place of DDT in operations against malaria and other vector borne diseases." Geneva, 1971, p. 176.

[19] World Health Organization. Official Records, 1972, no. 198. Executive Board, 49th Session, Part II. Chapter II, page 23. Under section titled "Report on the Proposed Programme and Budget Estimates for 1973."

[20] South African Department of Health. "Malaria Updates, May 2000." Pretoria.

[21] Barnes KI, Durrheim DN, Little F, et al. Effect of artemether-lumefantrine policy and improved vector control on malaria burden in KwaZulu-Natal, South Africa. PLoS Med 2005;2(11) e330.

[22] Navarro M. Breaking a long silence on population control. The New York Times 2011. http://www.nytimes.com/2011/11/01/science/earth/bringing-up-the-issue-of-population-growth.html?pagewanted=all (accessed 19 September 2012).

[23] World Health Organization: World Health Assembly Resolution 50.13: Promotion of chemical safety, with special attention to persistent organic pollutants: May 1997. http://www.who.int/ipcs/publications/wha/whares_53_13/en/index.html (accessed 19 September 2012).

[24] United Nations Environment Programme: Proceedings of the Governing Council at its Nineteenth Session: Nairobi, 27 January - 7 February 1997. http://www.unep.org/resources/gov/prev_docs/97_GC19_proceedings.pdf (accessed 19 September 2012).

[25] Hill AB. Principles of medical statistics. 9th edition. New York: Oxford University Press; 1971.

[26] Wolff MS, Toniolo PG, Lee EW, Rivera M, Dubin N. Blood levels of organochlorine residues and risk of breast cancer. J Natl Cancer Inst 1993;85(8) 648-52.

[27] World Health Organization: International Programme on Chemical Safety: Environmental Health Criteria 241: DDT in Indoor Residual Spraying: Human Health Aspects. http://whqlibdoc.who.int/publications/2011/9789241572415_eng.pdf (accessed 19 September 2012).

[28] World Wildlife Fund: Resolving the DDT Dilemma: Protecting Biodiversity and Human Health. http://awsassets.panda.org/downloads/resolvingddt.pdf (accessed 19 September 2012).

[29] Rogan WJ, Gladen BC, McKinney JD, et al. Polychlorinated biphenyls (PCBs) and dichlorodiphenyl dichloroethene (DDE) in human milk: effects on growth, morbidity, and duration of lactation. Am J Public Health 1987;77(10) 1294-7.

[30] Gladen BC, Rogan WJ. DDE and shortened duration of lactation in a northern Mexican town. Am J Public Health 1995;85(4) 504-08.

[31] Chen A, Rogan WJ. Nonmalarial infant deaths and DDT use for malaria control. Emerg Infect Dis 2003;9(8): 960-4. http://wwwnc.cdc.gov/eid/article/9/8/03-0082_article.htm (accessed 19 September 2012).

[32] Rogan WJ, Chen A. Health risks and benefits of bis(4-chlorophenyl)-1,1,1-trichloroethane (DDT). Lancet 2005;366(9487): 763-73. http://www.thelancet.com/journals/lancet/article/PIIS0140-6736%2805%2967182-6/fulltext (accessed 19 September 2012).

[33] Physicians for Social Responsibility (PSR) - Kenya: Kenya POPs situation report: DDT, pesticides and polychlorinated biphenyls. http://www.ipen.org/ipepweb1/library/ipep_pdf_reports/1ken%20kenya%20country%20situation%20report.pdf (accessed 19 September 2012).

[34] Roberts DR, Laughlin LL, Hsheih P, Legters LJ. DDT, Global Strategies, and a Malaria Control Crisis in South America. Emerg Infect Dis 1997;3(3): 295–302. http://wwwnc.cdc.gov/eid/article/3/3/97-0305_article.htm (accessed 19 September 2012).

[35] Roberts DR, Laughlin LL. Malaria control in South America-response to P.C. Matteson. Emerg Infect Dis 1999;5(2): 310–311. http://wwwnc.cdc.gov/eid/article/5/2/99-0230_article.htm (accessed 19 September 2012).

[36] Matteson PC. Malaria control in South America. Emerg Infect Dis 1999;5(2): 309–311. http://wwwnc.cdc.gov/eid/article/5/2/99-0229_article.htm (accessed 19 September 2012).

[37] Post D (Rachel Carson Council): DDT, Political Pesticide. http://www.rachelcarsoncouncil.org/uploads/brochures/DDT%20Political%20Pesticide.PDF (accessed 19 September 2012).

[38] Schafer K (Pesticide Action Network North America): What's behind the 'DDT comeback'? http://www.pan-uk.org/pestnews/Issue/pn74/pn74p4.pdf (accessed 19 September 2012).

[39] Wikipedia: DDT. http://en.wikipedia.org/wiki/DDT#Chronic_toxicity (accessed 19 September 2012).

[40] Bornman R, de Jager C, Worku Z, Farias P, Reif S. DDT and urogenital malformations in newborn boys in a malarial area. BJU Int 2010;106(3): 405-11. http://onlinelibrary.wiley.com/doi/10.1111/j.1464-410X.2009.09003.x/full (accessed 19 September 2012).

[41] Bouwman H, Kylin H, Sereda B, Bornman R. High levels of DDT in breast milk: Intake, risk, lactation duration, and involvement of gender. Environ Pollut 2012;170 63-70.

[42] Linköping Universitet. Researchers measure highest DDT levels in breast milk from South African nursing mothers. News-Medical.Net 2012. http://www.news-medi-

cal.net/news/20120903/Researchers-measure-highest-DDT-levels-in-breast-milk-from-South-African-nursing-mothers.aspx (accessed 19 September 2012).

[43] Savitz DA. Interpreting epidemiologic evidence. Strategies for study design and analysis. New York, NY: Oxford University Press; 2003.

[44] United Nations Environment Programme: Contribution of the United Nations Environment Programme to the Implementation of Agenda 21 and the Programme for the Further implementation of Agenda 21: 16 June 2000. http://www.unep.org/malmo/Agenda21.pdf (accessed 19 September 2012).

[45] Email correspondence on file with authors and available upon request.

[46] Roberts DR, Tren R. International advocacy against DDT and other public health insecticides for malaria control. Research and Reports in Tropical Medicine 2011;2011(2): 23-30. http://www.dovepress.com/international-advocacy-against-ddt-and-other-public-health-insecticide-peer-reviewed-article-RRTM (accessed 19 September 2012).

[47] Global Environment Facility: Detail of GEF Project #1591: Regional Program of Action and Demonstration of Sustainable Alternatives to DDT for Malaria Vector Control in Mexico and Central America. http://www.gefonline.org/projectDetailsSQL.cfm?projID=1591 (accessed 19 September 2012).

[48] Betlem J (UNEP), Neira M (WHO), Whyllie P (SSC). Demonstrating and Scaling-up of Sustainable Alternatives to DDT in Vector Management (DSSA - Global Programme). A program implemented by United Nations Environment Program- UNEP and executed by World Health Organization – WHO (Regional Offices) and the governments of participating countries. Approved by GEF Council on 23 April 2008. Presentation on file with authors.

[49] United Nations Environment Programme: Speech by Achim Steiner, UN Environment Programme (UNEP) Executive Director at the Helsinki Chemicals Forum 2009. http://www.unep.org/Documents.Multilingual/Default.asp?DocumentID=588&ArticleID=6191&l=en (accessed 19 September 2012).

[50] Narváez Olalla A: United Nations Environment Programme: Final Evaluation of the UNEP GEF project "Regional Program of Action and Demonstration of Sustainable Alternatives to DDT for Malaria Vector Control in Mexico and Central America". http://www.iwlearn.net/iw-projects/Fsp_112799467892/evaluations/DDT%20Final%20Evaluation%20Report.pdf (accessed 19 September 2012).

[51] Arbeláez Montoya MP. Control de la malaria sin DDT en Mesoamérica: control focalizado y manejo de criaderos como estrategias básicas Aspectos Epidemiológicos. Programa Regional de Acción y Demostración de Alternativas de Control de Vectores de la Malaria sin el Uso de DDT (Proyecto DDT/PNUMA/GEF/OPS). Presentation on file with authors.

[52] Chelala C. Taking a bite out of malaria. Americas 2008; 38-45.

[53] PAHO/WHO, UNEP, GEF: Regional program of action and demonstration of sustainable alternative to DDT for malaria vector control in Mexico and Central America (Project DDT/UNEP/GEF/PAHO): Final Report from September 2003 to December 2008. http://www.paho.org/english/ad/sde/DDT_GEF_Final_Report%282008%29.pdf (accessed 19 September 2012).

[54] UNEP/WHO/GEF: Countries move toward more sustainable ways to roll back malaria. http://www.who.int/mediacentre/news/releases/2009/malaria_ddt_20090506/en/index.html (accessed 19 September 2012).

[55] Pesticide Action Network: Global network calls for safe malaria solutions. http://panna.org/media-center/press-release/global-network-calls-safe-malaria-solutions (accessed 19 September 2012).

[56] North American Commission on Environmental Cooperation: North American Regional Action Plan on DDT: June 1997: Appendix-Presentation by the Mexican Ministry of Health. http://www.cec.org/Page.asp?PageID=924&ContentID=1262#mexhealth (accessed 19 September 2012).

[57] Pan American Health Organization: Report on the situation of malaria in the Americas, 2008: Regional section. http://new.paho.org/hq/index.php?option=com_content&task=view&id=2459&Itemid=2000 (accessed 19 September 2012).

[58] Rachel Carson Council: Critisism of Carson over DDT Unfounded. http://www.rachelcarsoncouncil.org/index.php?page=critisism-of-carson-over-ddt-unfounded (19 September 2012).

Chapter 21

Residual Transmission of Malaria: An Old Issue for New Approaches

Lies Durnez and Marc Coosemans

Additional information is available at the end of the chapter

http://dx.doi.org/10.5772/55925

1. Introduction

Malaria is one of the most serious vector-borne diseases, affecting millions of people mainly in the tropics. Recently, a substantial decline in malaria incidence has been observed all over the world. Vector control is one of the key elements in achieving this world-wide malaria decline, with scaling up of Insecticide Treated Nets (ITNs) and the expansion of Indoor Residual Spraying (IRS) programmes contributing significantly. Besides the personal protection, ITNs confer a community protection when wide coverage is assured, meaning that unprotected persons benefit from the large scale intervention [1]. IRS is only meaningful when applied at a large coverage. In the 2011 World Malaria Report [2], the percentage of households owning at least one ITN in sub-Saharan Africa is estimated to have risen from 3% in 2000 to 50% in 2011 while the percentage protected by indoor residual spraying (IRS) rose from less than 5% in 2005 to 11% in 2010. Household surveys indicate that 96% of persons with access to an ITN within the household actually use it [2]. Although these numbers might overestimate the real ITN use, they show that in recent years, several vector control measures were scaled up substantially. Despite these large increases in coverage, a widely held view is that with the currently available tools, namely vector control tools, intermittent preventive treatment, and early diagnosis and treatment, much greater gains could be achieved, including elimination from a number of countries and regions [3].

When considering vector control tools, even when hypothesizing a full coverage of ITNs and IRS, malaria transmission may still continue. Indeed, IRS only affects endophilic[1] mosquitoes and ITNs only target night biting mosquitoes. Moreover both intervention methods will mainly affect anthropophilic[2] mosquitoes that are endophagic[3]. This leaves ample opportunity

1 Endophily is the tendency for mosquitoes to prefer resting indoors

for more exophilic[4], zoophilic[5] and/or exophagic[6] vectors to escape from contact with insecticide treated surfaces and to maintain a certain level of transmission. Independently of the ITN and/or IRS coverage, outdoor and early malaria transmission occurs in many malaria endemic regions. In the west of Eritrea for example over a two year sampling period 36.4% of infective bites were acquired outdoors [4], in southern Tanzania this was 10% for non ITN users [5]. A study in northeastern Tanzania showed that 12% of the malaria transmission occurred before sleeping time [6]. In Uganda, in 6 sentinel sites throughout the country, up to 36% of indoor transmission and 49 % of outdoor transmission occurred before sleeping time, with the highest proportion of early in- and outdoor transmission in the suburban area of Jinja where *An. gambiae*[7] was the main vector [7]. In central Vietnam, where ITNs are used at large scale, 69% of the infective bites in forest plots were acquired before sleeping time [8]. In a study conducted in the east and west of Cambodia before widespread ITN use, 29% of the bites occurred before sleeping time in villages and forest plots [9]. In North-East India, 21% of the indoor infective bites occurred before 21h [10]. Also in Nicaragua, in an area with mainly Vivax malaria, 50% of the infective bites were acquired before sleeping time [11]. This part of the malaria transmission has the possibility to continue despite high coverage of ITNs and IRS, and is defined for the purpose of this review as 'residual transmission'.

Controlling residual transmission requires a different approach as compared to the currently used vector control measures. This is not new and was already perceived as a major obstacle in the previous malaria eradication era [12]. In 2007 malaria eradication was put as the ultimate goal [3] and renewed attention was given to residual transmission, with vector control models also incorporating outdoor and zoophilic malaria vectors. Recently, an established mathematical model adjusted for human in- and outdoor movements was used to illustrate that even with 50% outdoor biting vectors, transmission suppression can be achieved by a large ITN coverage [13]. However the authors assumed a uniform exposure so that the ITN induced mortality affects equally in- and outdoor biting vectors. When assuming a uniform exposure all individuals of the vector population (belonging to the same or to different species), will exhibit at each gonotrophic cycle a random behaviour (e.g. exo- or endophily, exo-or endophagy, anthropo- or zoophily, early- or late-biting), so that all individual mosquitoes are equally affected by indoor-based vector control measures. In case of non-uniform exposure, two or more subpopulations of vectors (belonging to the same or to different species) are assumed, each exhibiting a specific behaviour. Therefore, each of these subpopulations is affected differently by indoor-based vector control measures [14]. As a result, a fraction of vectors will persist in the presence of these control measures and can be responsible for residual transmission. It was shown that pre-intervention variables reflecting behavior, such as the degree

2 Anthropophily is the tendency for mosquitoes to prefer feeding on human hosts

3 Endophagy is the tendency for mosquitoes to prefer biting indoors

4 Exophily is the tendency for mosquitoes to prefer resting outdoors

5 Zoophily is the tendency for mosquitoes to prefer feeding on animal hosts

6 Exophagy is the tendency for mosquitoes to prefer biting outdoors

7 In this paper, s.l. (sensu lato) is added to the species name when referred to the species complex *(An. gambiae s.l., An. minimus s.l., An. dirus s.l.).* In the absence of s.l., the species is concerned *(e.g. An. gambiae, An. minimus, An. dirus).*

of exophily, may predict the efficacy of a specific intervention [15,16]. Assuming non-uniform exposure, the exophagic fractions of vectors will be less exposed to ITNs, the probability of survival and the vectorial capacity of this subpopulation will be weakly affected, and malaria transmission cannot be reduced further. The model developed in [17] takes into account the non-uniform exposure of the different anopheline species, i.e., the anthropo-endophilic vector species *An. gambiae* and *An. funestus*, and the more zoo-exophilic vector *An. arabiensis*. As would be intuitively expected, this model predicts that even the combination of very effective ITN distribution, twice yearly mass screening and treatment campaigns, and IRS will not succeed in getting the parasite prevalence rate below the 1% threshold if the zoo-exophilic *An. arabiensis* is present. When only *An. gambiae* or *An. funestus* are present, the same combination of interventions are successful in this model [17]. Moreover even within a well-defined species different subpopulations may occur exhibiting different behavioural patterns, resulting in non-uniform exposure within a species.

Therefore, when designing and applying vector control strategies it would be essential to have a good knowledge of the vector behavioural traits particularly those relevant to the chosen control method. However, entomological findings for one region or one anopheline species do not necessarily hold true for the same or different anopheline species encountered in the same or different malaria-endemic regions. In this chapter we will show that even before widespread use of vector control measures, a heterogeneity in behaviour between and within species was present. Because of the heterogeneity in behaviour, mosquitoes have different opportunities to escape from the killing or excito-repellent actions of insecticides used in ITNs or IRS. We will give examples of species shifts, shifts to outdoor- or early biting, shifts to zoophily or to exophily from different malaria endemic regions linked to the use of ITNs and IRS. Although the causes and mechanisms behind these shifts are not yet well understood, we will argue that ITNs and IRS may select for vector populations that predominantly feed early or outdoors, rest outdoors, or that are able to change their behaviour in response to the presence of these insecticides. Therefore, residual transmission will be dominated by vectors that bite outdoors, early or on animals, and that rest outdoors. These vectors require different control strategies, which might also be based on reducing host-vector contact, or target other key environmental resources.

The concept of uniform versus non-uniform exposure is illustrated in Figure 1.

2. Heterogeneity in anopheline behaviour

Heterogeneity in behaviour of anopheline mosquitoes between and within species is present in all malaria endemic regions. In Africa, the two most efficient malaria vector species, *An. gambiae* and *An. funestus,* are very anthropophilic, endophilic, endophagic, and late-night biting [18]. In contrast, *An. arabiensis,* a species belonging to the same complex as *An. gambiae,* is more plastic in its behaviour, exhibiting more often zoophily, exophily, exophagy, and early-night biting as compared to *An. gambiae* and *An. funestus*. However, different factors can influence the behaviour of the anophelines. Host availability for example plays an important

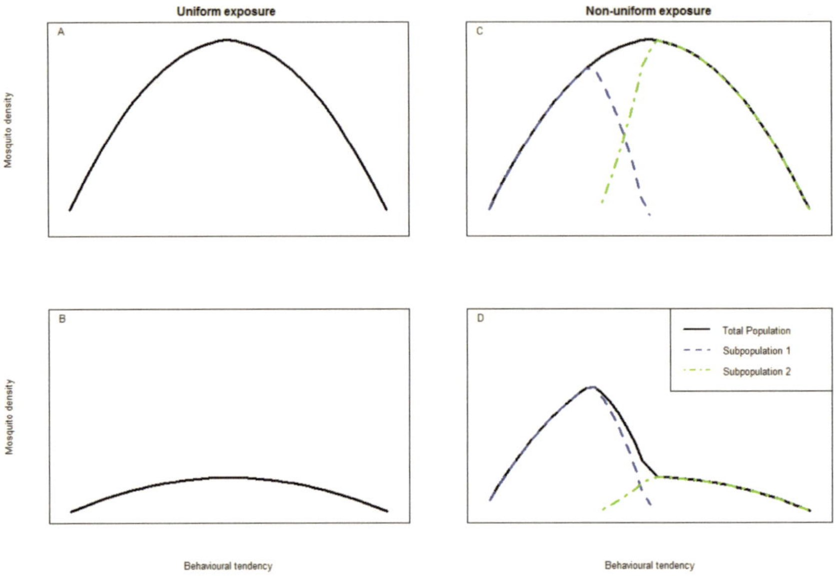

Figure 1. Effect of control measures on mosquito populations in the assumption of uniform exposure and non-uniform exposure. The density of a uniform population (belonging to the same or to different species) A. before applying the control measure. B. after applying the control measure. The control measure reduces the density of the whole population by 80%. The density of a non-uniform population C. before applying the control measure. D. after applying the control measure. The population consists of two subpopulations (Subpopulations 1 and 2, belonging to the same or to different species) each with a different behavioural tendency. Limited contact with the insecticide due to its behavioural tendency makes that Subpopulation 1 is reduced by 20% only, while Subpopulation 2 is reduced by 80% of its initial density. As a result, a fraction of vectors will persist in the presence of these control measures and can be responsible for malaria transmission.

factor in the final host choice of the vector. This has been shown for *An. gambiae* in several study sites. In Burkina Faso for example, a double choice experiment shows that 88% of the *An. gambiae* choose for a human odour baited trap and only 12 % for a cattle odour trap. In contrast, the human blood index of indoor-resting *An. gambiae* collected in the same locality was only 40% [19], showing that this population of *An. gambiae* will adapt its host choice in case of a lower availability of human hosts. *An. gambiae* in São Tomé feeds more on dogs and was observed to be extremely exophagic most probably due to a combination of preference and the ease to reach the dogs sleeping outside under pillar houses [20]. On the Bioko Island (Equatorial Guinea), *An. gambiae* was also observed to be partly exophagic and early-biting [21]. This means that when humans are not available inside, e.g. because of a high bed net use, some populations of *An. gambiae* are observed to feed outside or on animal hosts. In those cases, the frequency of human-vector contact will be lowered although humans will still be bitten in the evening. As a consequence, the longevity of these exophagic or zoophilic vectors will slightly, or not, be affected by ITNs, meaning that the vectorial capacity is not affected and malaria transmission continues.

Also in South-East Asia, heterogeneity of behaviour is observed for the primary and secondary vector species [22]: *An. dirus* is for example very anthropophilic, whereas *An. minimus*, depending on the geographical region, has both anthropophilic and zoophilic tendencies. *An. maculatus* has a high tendency for early biting as compared to *An. dirus* or *An. minimus*, but there are large differences between localities. Different populations of *An. minimus* observed in various localities also differ in their endophilic and endophagic tendencies [22]. Whereas *An. dirus* is generally observed to be very exophagic and exophilic, populations in Lao PDR have shown highly endophilic and endophagic trends [23]. Moreover, as reviewed in [24], *An. dirus* s.l. can even take blood-meals during daylight in the jungle.

In Latin-America, one of the most efficient vectors, *An. darlingi* is mainly anthropophilic, whereas the other dominant vectors, such as *An. albimanus*, *An. nuneztovari*, and *An. aquasalis* also have zoophilic tendencies or are more opportunistic. Most of the vectors in Latin America are mainly exophilic, but within each species, the degree of exophily can vary between geographical regions. *An. albimanus* for example is predominantly exophagic and exophilic, as observed in the Dominican Republic, Colombia, and Haiti. However, in Mexico and Central America, 80% of the *An. albimanus* was observed to have an endophilic resting behaviour [25]. Also the time and place of biting differs between sites for most of the species. In some localities for example, *An. darlingi* bites mostly during sleeping hours, or early in the morning [26], whereas in other localities, the main biting peak is early in the evening [27]. In French Guiana, *An. darlingi* was endo-exophagous with a clear predilection for biting outdoors [28].

3. How can the indoor use of insecticides select for exophilic, exophagic, zoophilic and/or early biting mosquito populations?

Insecticides can elicit different actions with different results on mosquitoes [29–31]. These various modes of action are important when talking about selection of 'insecticide avoiding' mosquitoes. Toxic or cidal actions result in knockdown or death after contact with the insecticide. Excito-repellent actions, including contact irritancy and non-contact repellency, result in above-normal levels of undirected movements coupled with loss of responsiveness to host cues. The insecticidal actions and their results depend among others on the insecticidal product used and on the mosquito species present. Large differences in actions of insecticides used in IRS have been observed: dieldrin for example only elicits a cidal action, while alpha-cypermethrin has both contact-irritant and killing actions, and DDT elicits mainly a repellent effect and secondarily a toxic action. [30]. Pyrethroids, the only family of insecticides used on ITNs, have well-documented excito-repellent actions [21] which are dose-dependent, but with for example higher toxic actions of alphacypermethrin as compared to deltamethrin and permethrin [31].

The general concepts of stress-induced variation in evolution [32] can be applied to the effect of insecticides on mosquito populations. Indoor use of insecticides will pose a stress on the female anopheline population, but only when the insecticides present a barrier for indoor feeding or indoor resting. At least three processes can be at the origin of perceived shifts in mosquito behaviour by insecticides:

1. A first protective mechanism can be behavioural plasticity in response to the presence of the insecticide. The ability to actively remove from the insecticide by either relocation or avoidance requires an ability to detect (either by contact or non-contact) or anticipate the presence of the insecticide and the ability to exhibit insecticide avoidance strategies or adjustments [32]. The insecticide, or the unavailability of the host, can then trigger the expression of gene variants that have been accumulated, but were phenotypically neutral under a normal range of environments [32]. Many mosquitoes indeed naturally possess a high degree of irritability or repellency which is evident at the very first exposure of the population to residual insecticides [29]. Where this irritation is such that mosquitoes settling on the insecticide deposit are activated before they have absorbed a lethal dose of insecticide, and are able to avoid further contact and to escape unharmed, the term "protective avoidance" has been suggested. In the presence of a high coverage of IRS or ITNs, mosquitoes exhibiting this protective avoidance should then be able to redirect their behaviour to low-risk behaviour which also can lower their survival. For example, for a species that is normally endophilic changing its behaviour to resting outdoors, the external environment may be unfavourable to the survival of the species [12].

2. A second protective mechanism for the mosquito is a consistent "protective behaviour" [29] such as exophily, exophagy, zoophily or early-biting resulting in a minimal contact with the insecticides used indoors. As mentioned above, some mosquito populations naturally exhibit this kind of protective behaviour, which is probably genetically determined (see further). Also differences in responses to the insecticides can result in diverse exposure rates of different species or subpopulations to the insecticide. *An. minimus* for example, shows very strong repellency responses to several insecticides and would have a higher survival chance in the presence of insecticides as compared to *An. harrisoni* which shows a much lower repellency response [33]. In this case, insecticides will favour the (sub) populations of mosquitoes that have this innate preference for protective behaviour or for avoidant strategies by which they will escape the exposure to the insecticide. This is probably the mechanism that is occurring for many of the perceived species shifts that are illustrated below.

3. Where these phenomena of protective avoidance or protective behaviour are not evident at the very first exposure of the population to the insecticides, but develop only gradually, perhaps over several years under continued insecticide pressure, the term "behaviouristic resistance" is employed [29]. The presence of the insecticide will in that case result in the selection of mutations and recombination that favour the survival of the mosquito in the presence of the insecticide, eventually leading to a directional selection. This can be compared to the development of insecticide resistance, although selections of many mutations will probably be required before an appropriate behavioural change may occur. Classification as "behaviouristic resistance" is only valid on the basis of accurate comparisons made before and subsequent to the widespread use of residual insecticides in any particular area. As shown below, very few behaviour shifts observed so far, would fit this definition of behaviouristic resistance.

4. Shifts observed in the presence of indoor insecticidal pressure

In the following paragraphs we will review the shifts that were observed in the presence of IRS and ITNs. For the purpose of this review, a 'shift' means an observed change, including relative changes, with a reasonable link to the indoor use of insecticides (ITNs or IRS). A distinction is made between different kinds of shifts: species shifts describe changes in the species composition which can also be within species complexes, whereas shifts to early biting, exophagy, zoophily or exophily describe changes in biting time, biting place, host, or resting place within a species, or within a species complex if no species information was available. Because a large part of the shifts in literature are described in the Afrotropical region, this region will be handled separately.

5. Afrotropical region

5.1. Species shifts

An IRS campaign resulted in the elimination of *An. funestus* from the South Pare District (at the Tanzania-Kenya border), at the same time reducing the numbers of indoor-resting *An. gambiae* s.l. [34]. In the years immediately following this IRS campaign, populations of endophilic *An. gambiae* s.l. slowly regained their former levels, whereas gradual resurgence of *An. funestus* was not observed until almost 10 years after the campaign was abandoned. IRS campaigns in two Kenyan villages resulted in a large decrease (up to total disappearance) of *An. funestus*, with an increase in the more exophagic *An. rivulorum* [35] or *An. parensis* [36], both not considered as malaria vectors in the study sites. In Niger, nation-wide Long-lasting insecticidal net (LLIN) distribution caused a marked decrease of *An. funestus*, without effect on *An. gambiae* s.l. abundance [37]. Following an IRS campaign, *An. gambiae* was completely eliminated from Pemba Island (Tanzania), leaving the salt-water breeding *An. merus*, an exophilic mosquito with a preference for cattle [38]. In Kenya and Tanzania, large scale ITN use significantly decreased the proportion of indoor-resting *An. funestus* [39] and *An. gambiae* [39–42] while the proportion of *An. arabiensis* increased. The shift from *An. gambiae* to *An. arabiensis* was also observed in the larval collections [40,41]. As larvae of *An. gambiae* and *An. arabiensis* show no habitat segregation, larval sampling reflects true proportions of the two species. The change from sub-populations dominated by *An. gambiae* to those dominated by *An. arabiensis* took about a decade, as would be expected if caused by a constant ITN selection pressure [43].

In contrast, in Kenya and on the Bioko Island (Equatorial Guinea), the same species compositions were observed regardless of the use of ITNs or IRS [21,44]. Moreover, in the north-east of Tanzania, a species shift has been observed in the absence of insecticide selective pressure, in a region without organized vector control activities reported [45]: *An. gambiae*, the most dominant in the past, was replaced by *An. arabiensis* without any known reason.

5.2. Shifts to early-evening or early-morning biting

Studies have shown that widespread ITN use increases the proportion of early bites by *An. gambiae* [46] and *An. funestus* [42,46] in Tanzania. Such shift was not observed for *Culex quinquefasciatus* which is highly resistant against pyrethroids [46]. According to the authors [46], this suggests that for anophelines, where there is considerable killing by contact with ITNs, several years of selection has begun to produce an upward shift in the proportions of insects biting at a time when people are accessible. Also in southern Benin, a significant change in host seeking behaviour of *An. funestus* was observed after achieving a universal coverage of ITNs. The shift in biting time was here not to the early evening but to the early morning. Moreover in one locality about 26% of the *An. funestus* bites were observed after sunrise [47].

The use of ITNs resulted in a shift towards earlier biting of *An. gambiae* s.l. in Kenya [48] and Tanzania [42,49], possibly [48,49] or certainly [42] related to a species shift from *An. gambiae* to *An. arabiensis*.

In other studies however, no evidence for a shift in biting time after the introduction of ITNs or IRS was obtained for *An. gambiae* s.l. in Tanzania, Kenya, The Gambia and Nigeria [44,50–52], for *An. gambiae* the Bioko Island (Equatorial Guinea) [21], or for *An. funestus* in Kenya [44]. Widespread use of mostly untreated bed nets did not result in more early biting of *An. gambiae* [5].

Country	Vector control measure [a]	Insecticide [b]	Collection methods [c]	Species shift [d]	Shift to early-biting [d]	Shift to exophagy [d]	Shift to zoophily [d]	Reference
Benin	ITN	Deltamethrin	Indoor/ outdoor HLC	ND	Yes	Yes	ND	[47]
Burkina Faso	ITC	Permethrin	Indoor/ outdoor CDC LT	ND	ND	Not observed	Not observed	[53]
Burkina Faso	ITN	Unspecified	IRC, Odour-baited traps	ND	ND	ND	Yes	[19]
Equatorial Guinea	IRS ITN	Deltamethrin, alpha cypermethrin, bendiocarb. Unspecified LLIN	Indoor/ outdoor HLC	Not observed	Not observed	Yes	ND	[21]
Kenya	IRS	Dieldrin	ORC, IRC, LD, HLC	Yes	ND	ND	ND	[35]
Kenya	IRS	DDT	Indoor/ outdoor HLC	Yes	ND	ND	ND	[36]
Kenya	IRS	Dieldrin	IRC, ORC	Yes	ND	ND	Not observed,	[34]
Kenya	ITN	Permethrin	IRC, indoor and outdoor HLC	ND	Yes	Yes	Yes, but not significant	[48]
Kenya	ITN	Permethrin	IRC, ORC	ND	ND	ND	Yes	[54]
Kenya	ITN	Permethrin	WET, IRC, outdoor bed net traps	Not observed	Not observed	ND	ND	[44]
Kenya	ITN	Permethrin,	IRC	Yes	ND	ND	ND	[39]
Kenya	ITN	Permethrin, alpha cypermethrin, Unspecified LLINs	IRC, LD	Yes	ND	ND	Not observed	[41]

Country	Vector control measure [a]	Insecticide [b]	Collection methods [c]	Species shift [d]	Shift to early-biting [d]	Shift to exophagy [d]	Shift to zoophily [d]	Reference
Kenya	ITN, ITC	Permethrin, alpha cypermethrin, deltamethrin	Bed net traps, IRC, LD	Yes	ND	ND	ND	[43]
Kenya	ITN	Unspecified	IRC, ORC, LD	Yes	ND	ND	Yes, but not significant	[40]
Niger	ITN	Unspecified LLINs	IRC, indoor/ outdoor HLC, indoor/ outdoor CDC LT	ND	ND	Yes	ND	[37]
Nigeria	IRS	Propoxur	Indoor/ outdoor HLC, IRC	ND	ND	Yes	ND	[14]
Nigeria	IRS	Propoxur	Indoor/ outdoor HLC, IRC, ORC, WET	Not observed	Not observed	Yes	Not observed	[52]
Tanzania (Pemba)	IRS	Dieldrin	IRC, ORC, indoor & outdoor HLC	Yes	ND	Not clear	Not clear	[38]
Tanzania	ITN+IRS	Permethrin or lambda cyhalothrin, DDT	Indoor CDC LT, outdoor HLC, IRC, ORC	ND	Inconclusive	Not observed	Inconclusive	[50]
Tanzania	ITN	Lambda cyhalothrin, deltamethrin	IRC, WET, indoor HLC	ND	Yes	ND	ND	[49]
Tanzania	ITN	Majority untreated nets	Indoor/ outdoor HLC	ND	Not observed	Not observed	ND	[5]
Tanzania	ITN	Unspecified	Indoor CDC LTs, Mbita traps	ND	Yes	ND	ND	[46]
Tanzania	ITN	Unspecified	Indoor/ Outdoor HLC	Yes	Yes	Yes	ND	[42]
The Gambia	ITN	Permethrin	Outdoor HLC, IRC, indoor CDC LT, bed net searches	ND	ND	Yes	Not observed	[55]
The Gambia	ITN	Permethrin	Indoor/ outdoor HLC, IRC, WET	ND	Not observed	Not observed	Yes, but not significant	[51]

[a] ITN: Insecticide treated nets; IRC: Indoor residual spraying; ITC: Insecticide treated curtains

[b] LLINs: Long lasting insecticidal nets

[c] IRS: Indoor resting collection; ORC: Outdoor resting collection; CDC LT: Center for Disease Control light trap; HLC: Human landing collection; WET: Window exit trap; LD: Larval dipping; CMR: Capture-Mark-Recapture

[d] ND: Not done

Table 1. Review of the effect of insecticide based indoor vector control measures on malaria vectors in the Afrotropical region

5.3. Shifts to exophagy

In Nigeria, IRS resulted in a threefold increase of the proportion of *An. gambiae* s.l. biting outdoors [14,52]. Several years of vector control by IRS and later ITNs in the Bioko Island, increased the trend for outdoor biting of *An. gambiae* [21] as compared to historical data in the same region of preferred behaviour for indoor biting. Also in Tanzania, high ITN-use resulted in an increased outdoor biting for *An. funestus* [42]. In the latter study the proportion of indoor contact with *An. funestus* bites had dropped to only half of the indoor contact before widespread ITN-use. In southern Benin as well, after achieving universal ITN coverage, a higher proportion of outdoor biting was observed for *An. funestus* [47], although this was only observed in one out of two localities that were studied.

Some studies have shown that distribution of ITNs in Niger, Kenya, and The Gambia decreased the endophagic rate of *An. gambiae* s.l. [37,48,55], and to a lesser extend of *An. funestus* [37]. However, as the species of the *An. gambiae* complex were not determined in these studies, a possible reason for this decrease would be a species shift from *An. gambiae* to *An. arabiensis*.

In other studies however, no evidence for a shift to outdoor biting of *An. gambiae* s.l. due to widespread IRS or ITNs use was found in Tanzania [42,50], Burkina Faso [53] and The Gambia [51]. Also widespread use of mostly untreated bed nets did not result in a higher outdoor biting rate of *An. gambiae* [5].

5.4. Shifts to zoophily

In Kenya, ITN-use caused a shift in host selection of *An. gambiae* s.l. and *An. funestus* [54] from humans towards cattle or other animals. Similar observations were made in Burkina Faso with *An. gambiae* [19]. In other studies in Kenya and The Gambia, the use of ITNs caused only small and insignificant decreases in human blood index (HBI) for *An. gambiae* s.l. [40,48,51] and *An. funestus* [40].

The use of ITNs, IRS, or insecticide treated curtains caused no shift in host selection (or decrease in HBI) for *An. arabiensis* in Zambia [56], for *An. gambiae* s.l. in Nigeria, Burkina Faso, The Gambia, Tanzania and Kenya [34,50,52,53,55], and for *An. funestus* in Tanzania and Kenya [34,50].

5.5. Shifts to exophily

As summarized in [57], different populations of *An. arabiensis*, e.g. in the Pare-Taveta malaria scheme, Mauritius, Madagascar, Zanzibar, Nigeria and other West African localities, became either completely exophilic or, at most, remained only partially endophilic after IRS campaigns. ITN distribution reduced the indoor resting fraction of *An. gambiae* s.l. in Niger and Kenya [37,48], and of *An. funestus* in Kenya [48]. No evidence for a resting place shift after introduction of ITNs or after IRS was observed in Tanzania [50].

6. Australasian, Oriental, and Neotropical Regions

6.1. Species shifts

In the Solomon Islands, IRS in the 1960s has nearly eliminated the major malaria vectors *An. koliensis* and *An. punctulatus*, which are mainly endophagic and late-biters. The density of *An. farauti*, a more exophagic and early-biting malaria vector, remained quite high, particularly in outdoor man-biting situations [58]. The latter species is now the primary vector in the Solomon Islands, with the former major malaria vectors being totally absent. *An. hinesorum*, which is not considered a vector, has now occupied the breeding sites commonly used by *An. koliensis* [59].

In the forested hilly areas of Thailand, IRS resulted in a higher proportional decrease of *An. dirus* s.l. as compared to *An. minimus* s.l. [60]. Widespread use of IRS resulted in a different behaviour of the *An. minimus* s.l. present [61], which probably reflects a species shift from *An. minimus* to *An. harrisoni*, as also observed in Vietnam as a result of widespread use of ITNs [62]. Residual spraying did effectively control indoor resting species in Nepal such as *An. annularis, An. culicifacies, An. splendidus* and *An. vagus*. The abundance of the partially outdoor resting species, *An. fluviatilis* s.l. and *An. maculatus* s.l. also decreased markedly after the spray application, but then rebounded rapidly within 1 or 2 months after treatment [63]. ITN use in China caused a higher decrease of the endophilic and anthropophilic *An. lesteri* (syn. *An. anthropophagus*) [64] and *An. minimus* s.l. [65] than of the exophagic and zoophilic *An. sinensis*.

In British Guiana, the primary malaria vector *An. darlingi* (both larvae and adults) was rapidly eliminated by IRS, whereas larvae and adults of a zoophilic species, *Anopheles aquasalis*, a possible malaria vector, were completely unaffected [66]. In Guatemala, *An. vestitipennis* decreased in abundance in communities with a wide distribution of ITNs, while *An. albimanus* did not change. Whether this change was an effect of the ITNs could not be concluded as the study was not designed for answering that question [67].

6.2. Shifts to early biting

In Papua New Guinea, ITN distribution immediately changed the biting cycles of both *An. farauti* and *An. koliensis* from a post-midnight peak towards a pre-midnight peak [68]. Also on the Solomon Islands, intervention and longitudinal studies have shown that IRS, ITNs, or a combination of both, changed the biting cycle of *An. farauti* to an earlier biting peak [58,69,70].

IRS changed the indoor biting peak of *An. dirus* s.l. in the forested hilly areas of Thailand to one hour earlier. Outdoors, the peak remained the same, but a higher proportion bite earlier. Also for *An. minimus* s.l., a shift to earlier biting was observed [60]. In the foothills on the other hand, where *An. minimus* s.l. was the main vector, no effect of DDT was seen on the already early biting *An. minimus* s.l. population [71]. Also recent studies in Vietnam have shown that in the prolonged presence of impregnated bed nets, 45% of the *Anopheles* bites are acquired before sleeping time in the forest, and 64% before sleeping time in the village [8]. In Cambodia, in a period when ITN coverage was still low, already 29% of the *Anopheles* bites were acquired before sleeping time [9].

Although we have not encountered studies in Latin-America with evidence for shifts to earlier biting, some studies indicated that also in this region, early biting vectors can maintain residual transmission. In an area in Brazil covered by IRS for example, blood-feeding of *An. darlingi* started at sunset, remained high during the first half of the night, and decreased gradually until early morning [72]. Also in the Bolivian Amazon, in an area with high ITN use, peak outdoor biting of *An. darlingi* occurred between 19:00 and 21:00 hours, when 48% of the total night's biting took place, and 83% of the night's biting had occurred by 22:00 hours when most local people go to bed [73].

6.3. Shifts to exophagy

On different islands of the Solomon, proportional shifts to outdoor biting (from 47% to 67%) were observed for *An. farauti* after IRS [58]. Moreover, compared to *An. koliensis* and *An. punctulatus*, the exophagic *An. farauti* population recovered completely within nine months after the spraying campaign. However, in other intervention and longitudinal studies on the Solomon Islands, the shift to outdoor biting of *An. farauti* due to ITNs and/or IRS was not so obvious [59,69].

IRS increased the outdoor biting rate of *An. dirus* s.l. [60,74], and of *An. minimus* s.l. in forested and foothill regions in Thailand [60,61]. In contrast, in another foothill region of Thailand, an initial effect of DDT was seen on the malaria transmission, but this was not sustained for this already outdoor biting *An. minimus* s.l. population [71]. Also wide scale use of ITNs caused a higher decrease in the indoor biting populations as compared to the outdoor biting populations of *An. sinensis*, *An. lesteri* (syn. *An. anthropophagus*) and *An. minimus* s.l. in China [64,65]. In Vietnam, after prolonged ITNs distribution, outdoor biting densities of the main vectors, *An. dirus*, *An. maculatus* s.l. and *An. minimus* s.l. were significantly higher than indoor biting density [8]. In Laos, in contrast, the use of ITNs did not stop *An. dirus* from entering the houses [75].

In an IRS area in Brazil, *An. darlingi* fed more frequently outdoors, whereas in earlier years before IRS this species mainly fed indoors [72]. In contrast, in Colombia, IRS did not stop malaria vectors to bite both indoors and outdoors [76]. The combined use of ITNs and IRS has preceded the collapse of a mainly exophagic *An. darlingi* population in Suriname. However, this collapse can also be attributed to an unusual, extensive flooding which coincided with the onset of the control interventions [77].

6.4. Shifts to zoophily

A significant decrease in HBI of *An. farauti* was observed immediately after the distribution of ITNs in Papua New Guinea, although this shift could be due to a slightly changed sampling method [68].

In Thailand, in the prolonged presence of DDT use in IRS, *An. minimus* s.l. exhibited a marked zoophily, whereas in villages with lower DDT pressure, no preference was observed [61], although this apparent 'change in behaviour' could have been due to a species shift within the *An. minimus* complex as observed in Vietnam [62]. In an intervention study in India, the HBI of *An. culicifacies* was lower in areas with ITNs as compared to areas with untreated bed nets or no nets [78].

In Mexico, a much lower HBI was observed in areas where IRS was implemented as compared to historical data [79]. Also in areas covered by IRS in Brazil, *An. darlingi* was mostly zoophilic [80].

6.5. Shifts to exophily

A very low endophily rate was observed for *An. farauti* after several DDT spraying campaigns in the Solomon Islands [58].

IRS also significantly reduced the indoor resting abundance of all anopheline species except for *An. fluviatilis* s.l. in Nepal [63], and of *An. dirus* s.l. in Thailand [74]. In India, *An. culicifacies* s.l. has been observed to be highly exophilic in areas where residual spraying with DDT was widely used [81]. Also in areas with wide scale use of ITNs in India fewer *An. culicifacies* s.l. were collected indoors (resting collections) as compared to control areas. However, in this area more *An. culicifacies* s.l. were found indoor-resting in individual houses with untreated bed nets as compared to houses with ITNs, both located in the ITN-area [78]. This suggests that this mosquito population did not shift entirely to exophily, but that this behaviour mainly reflects the excito-repellent effect of the permethrin.

IRS has brought the disappearance of *An. darlingi* from the interior of houses in Brazil and French Guiana [28,80]. However, outdoor-resting still persists, either in the vicinity of the houses [80] or outside the peridomestic environment [28]. ITNs as well caused less indoor-resting in an intervention trial in Guatemala [67]. In contrast, in Mexico, after prolonged use of DDT no deterrence was observed anymore for *An. pseudopunctipennis*, with as many mosquitoes seeking shelter in sprayed huts as in unsprayed huts [82].

Country	Vector control measure [a]	Insecticide [b]	Collection methods [c]	Species shift [d]	Shift to early-biting [d]	Shift to exophagy [d]	Shift to zoophily [d]	Reference
Australasian Region								
Papua New Guinea	ITN	Permethrin	Outdoor HLC	Not observed	Yes	ND	Yes?	[68]
Solomon Islands	IRS	DDT	HLC	Yes	Yes	Yes	ND	[58]
Solomon Islands	IRS, ITN	DDT, permethrin	Outdoor HLC, indoor CDC LT, outdoor pig baited traps	ND	Yes	Not clear	ND	[69]
Solomon Islands	IRS, ITN	DDT, lambda cyhalothrin Permethrin, unspecified LLIN	Indoor/ outdoor HLC, LD, animal baited trap	Yes	ND	ND	ND	[59]
Solomon Islands	ITN, IRS	Deltamethrin, lambda cyhalothrin	Indoor/ outdoor HLC, IRC, WET, LD	ND	yes	Yes, small	ND	[59]
Oriental region								

Country	Vector control measure [a]	Insecticide [b]	Collection methods [c]	Species shift [d]	Shift to early-biting [d]	Shift to exophagy [d]	Shift to zoophily [d]	Reference
China	ITN	Deltamethrin	Indoor/ outdoor man-baited nets	Yes	ND	Yes	ND	[64]
China	ITN	Deltamethrin	?	Yes	ND	Yes	ND	In [65]
India	ITN	Lambdacyhalothrin	IRC, Indoor HLC, Outdoor Cattle collection	ND	ND	ND	Yes	[78]
Nepal	IRS	DDT, bendiocarb, malathion	Indoor/ outdoor HLC, IRC, ORC, cattle collections, LD	Yes	ND	?	ND	[63]
Thailand	IRS	DDT	Indoor/ outdoor HLC	Yes	Yes	Yes	ND	[60]
Thailand	IRS	DDT	Indoor/ outdoor HLC	Not observed	Not observed	Not observed	ND	[71]
Thailand	IRS	DDT	Indoor/ outdoor HLC, bovid-baited trap, IRC, ORC	Probably	ND	Yes	Yes	[61]
Thailand	IRS	DDT, fenitrothion	Indoor/ outdoor HLC, IRC	ND	ND	Yes	ND	[74]
Vietnam	ITN	Permethrin	Indoor/ outdoor HLC, IRC, CDC LT	Yes	ND	ND	ND	[62]
Neotropical Region								
Brazil	IRS	DDT	IRC, ORC, animal baited trap,	ND	ND	ND	Yes?	In [80]
Brazil	IRS	DDT	Indoor/ outdoor HLC, outdoor animal baited trap	ND	ND	Yes	ND	[72]
British Guiana	IRS	DDT	IRC, LD	Yes	ND	ND	ND	[66]
Guatemala	ITN	Permethrin	Indoor/ outdoor HLC, IRC, inspection of bed net surfaces, CMR	Yes?	ND	Not observed	ND	[67]
Mexico	IRS	DDT, bendiocarb	IRC, ORC	ND	ND	ND	Yes	[79]
Mexico	IRS	DDT (dieldrin before)	Entry traps, WET	ND	ND	ND	ND	[82]

[a] ITN: Insecticide treated nets; IRS: Indoor residual spraying; ITC: Insecticide treated curtains

[b] LLINs: Long lasting insecticidal nets

[c] IRC: Indoor resting collection; ORC: Outdoor resting collection; CDC LT: Center for Disease Control light trap; HLC: Human landing collection; WET: Window exit trap; LD: Larval dipping; CMR: Capture-Mark-Recapture

[d] ND: Not done

Table 2. Review of the effect of insecticide based indoor vector control measures on malaria vectors in the Australasian, Oriental and Neotropical regions

7. Discussion

7.1. The importance of residual transmission by outdoor and early biting malaria vectors

In this chapter we have shown that outdoor and early biting malaria vectors are widespread among malaria endemic countries and, as relative shifts to outdoor, early or animal-biting and outdoor resting vectors occur due to the use of IRS and ITNs, these vectors will increasingly contribute to malaria transmission in regions with a high coverage of ITNs and IRS. However the reported shifts are not always well documented: species identification of complexes are often missing, and confounding factors such as changes of the environment, habitat, human behaviour and occupation are not considered.

In Africa, most of the species shifts observed resulted in a large decrease of the important endophagic, endophilic and anthropophilic malaria vectors, *An. funestus* and *An. gambiae*, while the more exophagic, exophilic, and/or zoophilic species *An. arabiensis* persists. Reports on such species shift are recently increasing, with most of these shifts described in East-Africa. But also in the other geographical regions, shifts in species abundances have been observed. It is however important to note that the majority of shifts described are shifts in relative abundances, where the more endophagic, endophilic and/or anthropophilic species declines more (or is being eliminated) while the more exophagic, exophilic and/or zoophilic species maintains at the same density or declines less. Only in some cases, the density of the latter species actually increases (e.g. the non-vector species *An. rivulorum* [35] or *An. parensis* [36]), probably because they take over the breeding sites of the declining species. Moreover, as also mentioned in [83], the vectorial capacity of the species predominating after the intervention does not necessarily increase, but persisting species that are malaria vectors, such as *An. arabiensis*, will be responsible for the residual malaria transmission, while the role of e.g. *An. gambiae* or *An. funestus* decreases.

Therefore, one of the most plausible reasons for species shifts to occur in the presence of ITNs or IRS is the non-uniform exposure of the different species to the insecticides, as described above. This hypothesis is supported by a study in Kenya in which the persisting *An. arabiensis* in an area with high ITN coverage had little to no pyrethroid resistance compared to the declining *An. gambiae*, with moderate to high levels of pyrethroid resistance [41,43]. Moreover, in experimental hut trials on northeast Tanzania, the mortality of *An. arabiensis* measured in experimental huts was consistently lower than that of *An. gambiae* and *An. funestus* [83], which probably is a major contributing factor to the species shifts observed in East Africa following scale up of ITNs. The authors state that, as cone tests on the nets prior to the trials produced rather similar levels of mortality among *An. gambiae* and *An. arabiensis*, the most likely explanation for lower *An. arabiensis* mortality was behavioural avoidance of treated net surfaces. As feeding inhibition in this experiment was similar for *An. arabiensis* and *An. gambiae*, outdoor blood-feeding would be the major mechanism to which *An. arabiensis* avoids contact with the ITN, as opposed to abandoning host-searching when confronted with ITNs.

Besides the species shifts, shifts to earlier-, outdoor-, and animal-biting have been observed for primary vectors such as *An. gambiae*, *An. funestus*, *An. farauti*, *An. koliensis*, *An. dirus* s.l., *An.*

minimus s.l., *An. culicifacies*, and *An. darlingi*. These shifts might also be linked to the non-random exposure of subpopulations of vectors to insecticide treated surfaces (ITNs or IRS). Several studies have indeed shown that the feeding and resting behaviour of anophelines is consistent in certain subpopulations and/or linked to certain genetic markers. Most of the studies on genetic determination of biting and resting behaviour are based on chromosomal inversions. Alleles captured within chromosome rearrangements are protected from recombination and can as such favour local adaptation by capturing sets of locally adapted genes which might lead to reproductive isolated entities or subpopulations [84]. In the Garki District in Nigeria, chromosomal arrangements in *An. arabiensis* and *An. gambiae* have been associated with exophagy and exophily [85,86] and with zoophily [87]. Exophagy and exophily were associated with the standard chromosomal arrangements $2R+^a$ for *An. arabiensis* and $2R+^b$ for *An. gambiae*, and the inverted arrangement 2Rbc for *An. arabiensis*. Moreover, the chromosome arrangements associated with indoor biting or resting are the ones adapted to drier environments, while arrangements more frequent in outdoor collected specimens are those associated with more humid environments [85]. In the Zambesi valley, 2Rc *An. arabiensis* heterozygotes were associated with exophily and zoophily [57]. In Ethiopia *An. arabiensis* heterozygotes of the 2La and/or 2Rb chromosomal arrangements tended to bite later at night than the double homozygotes [88]. Also in laboratory experiments an association between chromosomal arrangements and circadian flight activity has been found [89]: female *An. stephensi* homozygotes for the 2Rb inversion showed more activity following light-on (corresponding to early morning) as compared to homozygous females for the standard $2R+^b$ arrangement. Other field-based evidence on the existence of subpopulations showing consistent behaviour was obtained by studying behaviour of *An. balabacensis* in a capture-mark-recapture experiment in Borneo (Malaysia) [90]. This study revealed significant trends of *An. balabacensis* to be recaptured on the same host or resting site of the original capture. In contrast, a similar capture-mark-recapture study on resting behaviour of *An. gambiae* s.l. in Tanzania showed no faithful tendencies of endo- or exophily [91]: the same individuals within the *An. gambiae* s.l. population mixed indoor and outdoor resting. More recent genetic studies are based on the frequencies of enzyme polymorphisms. In the Malaysian study [90], faithfully indoor and outdoor-resting populations showed significant differences in isozyme frequencies (loci *Est-3* and *Idh-3*). Also in Burundi, isozyme frequencies were significantly different between in- and out-door biting *An. arabiensis* (locus *Mdh-2*) and in- and out-door resting *An. gambiae* (*Mpi* and *Got-2* loci) [92]. Such differences were not observed for *An. gambiae* in Burkina Faso [93]. Moreover, mosquitoes carrying a specific genotype [93] or chromosome karyotypes [87] were found to be significantly more infected with sporozoites, suggesting the occurrence of subpopulations having different vector behaviours. These independent genetic studies, either based on karyotyping or on genotyping, provide evidence that active choice for the best place, time or host to bite, or the best place to rest can be associated with specific genotypes. This suggests the existence of subpopulations characterized by specific behavioural patterns which implies a non-uniform exposure to IRS or ITNs. Selection of specific behavioural patterns can then not be excluded.

However, other mechanisms can also explain these kinds of shifts. More early biting could occur as females that fail to obtain a blood meal during the previous night, might be more likely to commence host seeking in the early evening [44]. By disrupting the feeding behaviour,

http://dx.doi.org/10.5772/55925

the ITNs would increase the length of the oviposition cycle of the overall population [68]. This mechanism could explain the immediate change in biting cycles of both *An. farauti* and *An. koliensis* after ITN distribution in Papua New Guinea. Both species shifted from a post-midnight biting peak towards a pre-midnight peak [68], with an extended oviposition cycle. Also in the Solomon Islands, the oviposition cycle was extended from 3 to 4 days due to ITN use, possibly explaining the higher tendency for early biting observed in the village with ITN use [69]. Shifts to outdoor biting by *An. farauti* also occurred immediately after DDT spraying [58]. This first effect would be caused by the deterrent effect of DDT, while only in second instance the endophilic fraction of *An. farauti* is being killed. Moreover, compared to *An. koliensis* and *An. punctulatus*, the *An. farauti* population recovered completely within nine months after the spraying campaign, indicating that this change of behaviour is due to a plastic response to the deterrent effect of DDT. Moreover, it has been shown that the occurrence of a shift in host selection does not necessarily reflect a selection of a more zoophilic vector subpopulation, but can also indicate plasticity in host selection. The *An. gambiae* population in Burkina Faso that showed a high proportion of cattle feeding (HBI of only 40%), had an innate preference for humans (88%) in a choice experiment using an odour-baited trap [19]. The weak accessibility of humans due to the use of ITNs, forces the mosquitoes to feed on cattle. According to the authors of the study, this suggests that in this area a plastic foraging strategy could provide greater benefits than a specialist strategy for this species.

Regardless of the mechanism that causes these behavioural shifts, the case studies show that in several areas the proportion of outdoor-, early- and/or animal biting primary vectors are relatively increasing, which will then be responsible for residual transmission. Moreover, in a similar way, transmission by 'secondary' vectors that have outdoor or early biting behaviour might become more important than transmission by primary vectors in contexts of high coverage of ITNs and IRS. In a malaria endemic region of Thailand, one specimen of the Barbirostris Subgroup (*An. barbirostris/campestris*) was found to contain *Plasmodium* oocysts, in the prolonged absence of the main malaria vectors, showing that *An. barbirostris* s.l., an outdoor biting mosquito [94], might be responsible for maintaining malaria transmission in the absence of the main vectors [95]. As secondary vectors are often less anthropophilic, and might be more exophagic and early biting, planning of vector control should also take into account their behaviour. Moreover, as pointed out in [8], secondary vectors might be better vectors of *P. vivax* as compared to *P. falciparum*, as the extrinsic incubation period of *P. vivax* is shorter. In British Guiana, for example, *An. aquasalis*, a mostly zoophilic and exophilic mosquito species breeding in brackish water, was vector of several Vivax malaria outbreaks after *An. darlingi* was eliminated by DDT spraying [96]. Also more recently in Vietnam, *An. sawadwongporni*, a very early biting secondary vector, was found positive for *P. vivax* [8].

7.2. ITNs and IRS are very effective, but additional measures are needed for reaching malaria elimination

ITNs and IRS have been shown to have a large impact on malaria infection and disease [97,98]. Moreover, several entomological studies have also shown that where the vectors are mostly endophagic, endophilic and anthropophilic, ITNs and IRS are very effective in reducing their population density. This was for example shown for *An. minimus* in India [99] and for *An. dirus* in Laos [100], both of them being anthropophilic, indoor- and late-biting in the respective study sites. A recent study in Zambia also showed that even at a high coverage of ITNs and IRS, the highest probability for malaria transmission based on human and vector behaviour, still occurs indoors [101], making ITNs and IRS valuable tools.

ITNs can also have an effect on malaria transmitted by more zoophilic and exophagic mosquitoes. In Sao Tomé for example, where *An. gambiae* is zoophilic and very exophagic, increased bed net use decreased the malaria prevalence in both bed net users and non-users [102]. The differences in prevalence between users and non-users were greatest in children under 5 years old, who are more likely to use the bed nets in the evening, showing that indeed the bed nets were the cause of the decrease. However, in older age groups, that are more likely to remain outside in the evening, no such difference was observed. Moreover, even at an almost 80% ITN coverage, still a 30% malaria prevalence was observed among bed net users. This means that, as expected, a part of transmission by these zoophilic and exophagic mosquitoes could not be prevented by ITNs [102]. Also in other parts of the world it has been shown that ITNs are less performing in areas with outdoor biting or resting vectors, for example in Peru and Nicaragua [11]. In the Garki District (Nigeria), the impact of the IRS campaign with propoxur was related to the prespraying ratio between the man-biting density and the indoor-resting density and to intraspecific cytogenetic variation [52]. Moreover, as reviewed in [103], even low levels of exophagy, exophily or zoophily may attenuate the impact of ITNs and IRS because this allows mosquitoes to obtain blood while avoiding fatal contact with insecticides.

As we have shown that outdoor-, animal- and early biting behaviour, as well as outdoor resting behaviour is widespread among malaria vectors all over the world and might be increasing as a result of widespread IRS or ITN use, there is an urgent need for additional control measures tackling malaria transmission by these vector populations [103–106]. In other words, there is a 'gap' in protection, not only before sleeping time, but also for people that remain outdoors during the night (Figure 2) and this gap needs to be tackled by additional vector control measures. There are many ways of additionally reducing host-vector contact, including the use of topical repellents, spatial repellents, insecticide treated clothing, long lasting insecticidal hammocks, etc. Recently much research is carried out on the effectiveness of these kind of tools. For example, in the Bolivian Amazon, where the primary vectors *An. darlingi* has a peak biting activity before sleeping time, a household based cluster randomized trial has shown that the combined use of a topical repellent (para-menthane-3,8-diol, PMD) and ITNs can reduce the incidence of malaria by 80%, which was only significant for *P. vivax* and not for *P. falciparum*, as compared to the use of ITNs alone [107]. DEET-based repellents also had an additional protective efficacy against malaria disease in a small scale community based trial in India [108], and DEET-based repellent soap against *P. falciparum* malaria in a household randomized trial in a refugee camp in Pakistan [109]. In an ongoing study in Cambodia, Picaridin based repellents are shown to provide a protection of more than 90% against the bites of the main malaria vectors *An. dirus* and *An. minimus* (MalaResT project led by ITM-Antwerp, preliminary results). Whether the mass use of this repellent will result in a decrease of malaria infection is currently under investigation using a cluster-randomized controlled trial in

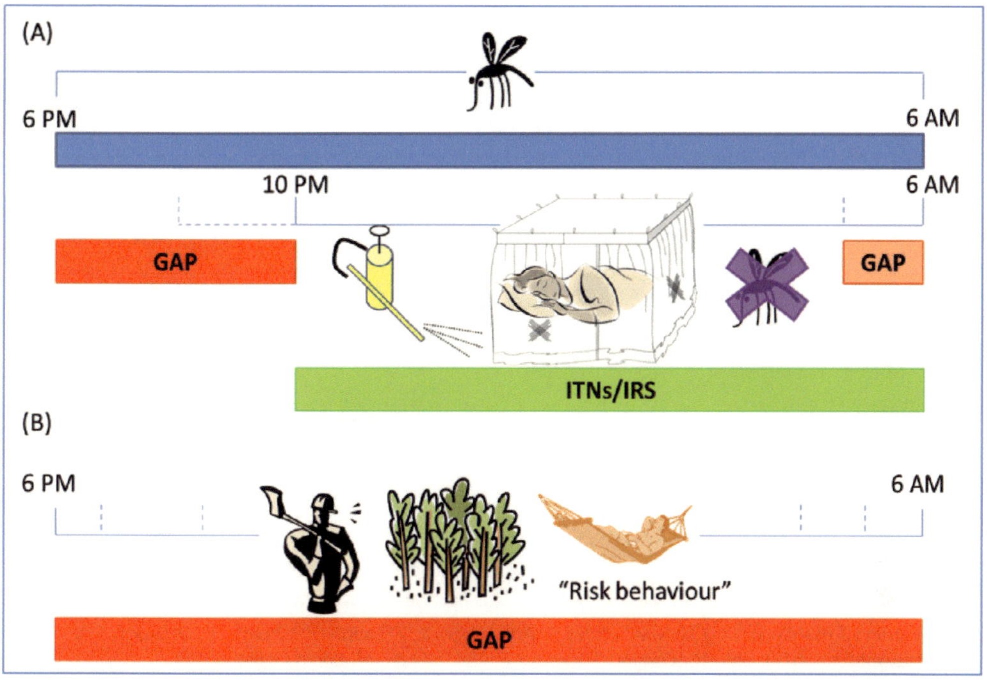

Figure 2. Protection 'gap' when only indoor insecticide-based vector control measures are applied. Anophelines generally bite between 6pm and 6am. ITNs will only protect from infective bites that are acquired indoors, and during sleeping time. IRS only target mosquitoes that rest indoors. Therefore, there is a gap in protection both indoors and outdoors before and after people go to bed (A), but also for people conducting outdoor activities during the night (i.e. 'risk behaviour') (B).

Ratanakkiri province in Cambodia. In a refugee camp in Kenya, permethrin treated clothing and blankets reduced malaria infection significantly [110]. In Southeast Asia, long lasting insecticidal hammocks have been shown to be effective against malaria disease [111] and against *An. minimus* bites, but not *An. dirus* bites [112]. For zoophilic mosquitoes, intervening in the host-vector contact could be more efficient by focusing on its preferred hosts, e.g. by insecticide treatment of cattle. However, killing partly zoophilic mosquitoes in sufficient numbers to suppress malaria transmission would require high protective coverage of both human and animal blood sources [104]. Moreover, it has been observed in Ethiopia that more than 90% of the blood meals taken by zoophilic vectors were taken from the legs of cattle [113], which are more difficult to treat.

Alternative personal protection measures are also of interest for people that work or reside in the forest, a risk area of malaria transmission in Southeast Asia [114]. For temporary shelters in the forest, insecticide treated plastic sheeting could be useful as this has proven to be effective in protecting against malaria disease in emergency camps [115]. Their effectiveness will rely both on their repelling effect and their killing effect, and whether mosquitoes will rest on this sheeting. Alternatively, other more accepted insecticide treated bed net-designs (V-shaped

Tool	Mosquito behaviour that is targeted				Personal (P) or community (C)[b] protection
	Time of biting (E/N)[a]	Host preference (A/Z)[a]	Place of biting (I/O)[a]	Place of resting (I/O)[a]	
Tools relying on host-vector contact					
ITNs	N	A	I	I	P & C
Long lasting insecticidal hammocks & other net designs adapted to outdoor conditions	(E &) N	A	O	O	P & C
Insecticide treated plastic sheeting for shelters in the forest	E & N	A & Z	I & O	O	P
Personal protection including Topical & spatial repellents, Insecticide treated clothing	E & N	A	I & O	I & O	P & C*
Insecticide treatment of cattle	E & N	Z	I & O	I & O	C*
Tools not relying on vector-host contact					
IRS	E & N	A & Z	I & O	I	C
Larval source management	E & N	A & Z	I & O	I & O	C*
Toxic sugar baits	E & N	A & Z	I & O	I & O	C*
Treatment of outdoor resting places, e.g. with fungal biopesticides	E & N	A & Z	I & O	O	C*

[a] E: Early evening & morning biting; N: Night biting; A: Antropophilic; Z: Zoophilic; I: Indoor; O: Outdoor
[b] Community protection can only be achieved if the coverage of the intervention is large enough.
* Community protection is assumed or shown in a limited number of studies, but more evidence is required for confirmation of community protection.

Table 3. Vector control tools and their targets.

nets, long lasting insecticidal hammocks, etc.), could provide protection for people staying in the forest during the night.

The more zoophilic, exophagic, or early biting a mosquito species or population, the more personal protection will act simply by blocking host-vector contact (through lethal or repellent effects). As shown by a mathematical model, malaria transmission involving zoophilic vectors (with 10% feeding on humans) can only be significantly decreased if the personal protection measures confer high levels of individual protection to users (80%) and be used by the majority of human population (80%) [116]. Therefore, the success of any intervention in this context will depend on its entomological efficacy, but also on the human behaviour, including acceptance and adherence to the preventive measures within the community. In São Tomé for example, many people watch communal television outdoors, posing them at risk for early-evening malaria transmission [117]. In Thailand, people do not take their ITN from the village to their farm plot [118]. Also in Vietnam, people often combine living in the village with a second home at their fields located in the forest [119], creating other malaria control needs, such as, for example, long lasting insecticidal hammocks. Taking into account human behaviour when adapting vector control strategies will then be crucial. In Bioko Island (Equatorial Guinea) for example, an increased trend of outdoor biting was observed for the main malaria vector *An. gambiae* [21]. However, the main malaria risk group, namely children under 15 years old, rarely stay outdoors when it is dark, and there is no evidence that children who report to stay outdoors during the night are at higher risk for malaria infection as compared to those who do not [120]. Implementing control measures that target outdoor biting mosquitoes in this age group would then provide no additional benefit and would be a waste of resources, as personal protection tools might be very expensive to implement.

Also other tools not relying on the host-vector contact can supplement ITNs and IRS as they are not specific for indoor biting and indoor resting mosquito populations [105,106]. Vector control tools could for example target key environmental resources such as the aquatic larval habitat, sugar sources, and resting behaviour. Very little is known about how to manipulate these environmental resources so that malaria transmission is interrupted [105]. Knowledge on vector ecology and behaviour therefore remains crucial. However, despite large knowledge gaps, several examples exist of malaria control by targeting non-blood meal related steps of the mosquito cycle. Larval source management has indeed shown to be effective where vectors breed in large water bodies [121]. However, when larval habitats are more dispersed and not permanent, this approach is considered less feasible. Renewed attention has been given to larval source management as complementary tool to ITNs as recent studies in Africa have shown that it provides substantial additional protection with a high cost-effectiveness in specific settings [122]. Moreover, other innovative ideas combined with knowledge on the vector behaviour can lead to successful vector control. Toxic sugar baits for example were successfully used in a targeted way for the control of the cistern dwelling malaria vector *An. claviger* in the desert oases of Israel [123]. Fungal biopesticides also have the potential to significantly reduce densities of malaria vectors [124] as well as associated malaria transmission [125]. These fungi could be delivered through outdoor odour-baited stations, and in this way slowly eliminate a high proportion of outdoor-resting vectors [126].

8. Conclusion

For malaria eradication to succeed, all elements in the transmission cycle must be sufficiently targeted. With the current vector control tools, only indoor- and late-biting, and indoor-resting vectors are tackled. In this paper, we have shown that there is a 'gap' in protection, not only before sleeping time, but also for people that remain outdoors during the night. Moreover, by describing different shifts in vector species, and vector behaviour within species or species complexes, we have shown that the importance of this gap can increase as a result of widespread ITN or IRS use. Therefore, to eliminate residual malaria transmission, additional vector control tools will be needed. These new vector control tools should be designed to target outdoor and early feeding mosquitoes. Moreover, they should be accessible and acceptable for the populations at risk. A specific mosquito behaviour assuring its vectorial status is only relevant in relation to a specific human behaviour and the relation people have with their surrounding environment. Interrupting malaria transmission may than require different combinations of mosquito control methods addressing each mosquito behaviour at risk for transmission, but also taking into account possible changes in soil occupation, housing conditions, sleeping habits, and outdoor occupation. In conclusion, there is no 'silver bullet' in vector control and malaria prevention. New paradigms for controlling and/or interrupting malaria transmission should then be explored for their protective efficacy and adapted to the local context for a good efficiency. Although implementation of such new approaches might be very expensive, they will be crucial if malaria elimination is the final aim.

Acknowledgements

This review was initiated under the impulse of the Roll Back Malaria - Vector Control Working Group – Work Stream Outdoor Malaria Transmission (http://www.rbm.who.int/mechanisms/vcwgWorkstream2.html), the MalaResT research Project (B&M Gates Foundation OPP1032354) and the Third ITM-DGCD Framework Agreement Programme. We would like to thank Vincent Sluydts and Sylvie Manguin for their critical review of this paper.

Author details

Lies Durnez[1] and Marc Coosemans[1,2*]

*Address all correspondence to: mcoosemans@itg.be; ldurnez@itg.be

1 Department of Biomedical Sciences, Institute of Tropical Medicine, Antwerp, Belgium

2 Department of Biomedical Sciences, Faculty of Pharmaceutical, Veterinary and Biomedical Sciences, University of Antwerp, Antwerpen (Wilrijk), Belgium

References

[1] Killeen, G F, Smith, T A, Ferguson, H M, Mshinda, H, Abdulla, S, Lengeler, C, & Kachur, S P. Preventing childhood malaria in Africa by protecting adults from mosquitoes with insecticide-treated nets. PLoS Medicine (2007). 4, e229.

[2] WHO. World Malaria Report 2011. World Health Organisation (2012).

[3] Alonso, P L, Brown, G, Arevalo-herrera, M, Binka, F, Chitnis, C, Collins, F, Doumbo, O K, Greenwood, B, Hall, B F, Levine, M M, Mendis, K, Newman, R D, Plowe, C V, Rodríguez, M H, Sinden, R, Slutsker, L, & Tanner, M. A research agenda to underpin malaria eradication. PLoS Medicine (2011). 8, e1000406.

[4] Shililu, J, Ghebremeskel, T, Seulu, F, Mengistu, S, Fekadu, H, Zerom, M, Asmelash,G, Sintasath, D, Mbogo, C, Githure, J, Brantly, E, Beier, J, & Novak, R. Seasonal abundance, vector behaviour, and malaria parasite transmission in Eritrea. Journal of the American Mosquito Control Association (2004). 20, 155-64.

[5] Killeen, G F, Kihonda, J, Lyimo, E, Oketch, F R, Kotas, M E, Mathenge, E, Schellenberg, J A, Lengeler, C, Smith, T A, & Drakeley, C J. Quantifying behavioural interactions between humans and mosquitoes: evaluating the protective efficacy of insecticidal nets against malaria transmission in rural Tanzania. BMC Infectious Diseases (2006). 6, 161.

[6] Maxwell, C A, Wakibara, J, Tho, S, & Curtis, C F. Malaria-infective biting at different hours of the night. Medical and Veterinary Entomology (1998). 12, 325-7.

[7] Okello, P E, Van Bortel, W, Byaruhanga, A M, Correwyn, A, Roelants, P, Talisuna, A, D'Alessandro, U, & Coosemans, M. Variation in malaria transmission intensity in seven sites throughout Uganda. The American Journal of Tropical Medicine and Hygiene (2006). 75, 219-25.

[8] Van Bortel, W, Trung, H D, Hoi, L X, Van Ham, N, Van Chut, N, Luu, N D, Roelants, P, Denis, L, Speybroeck, N, D'Alessandro, U, & Coosemans, M. Malaria transmission and vector behaviour in a forested malaria focus in central Vietnam and the implications for vector control. Malaria Journal (2010).9, 373.

[9] Durnez, L, Mao, S, Van Bortel, W, Denis, L, Roelants, P, Sochantha, T, & Coosemans, M. Outdoor malaria transmission in forested villages of Cambodia. Manuscript in preparation.

[10] Prakash, A, Bhattacharyya, D, Mohapatra, P, & Mahanta, J. Malaria transmission risk by the mosquito *Anopheles baimaii* (formerly known as *An. dirus* species D) at different hours of the night in North-east India. Medical and Veterinary Entomology (2005). 19, 423-7.

[11] Kroeger, A, González, M, & Ordóñez-González, J. Insecticide-treated materials for malaria control in Latin America: to use or not to use? Transactions of the Royal Society of Tropical Medicine and Hygiene (1999). 93, 565-70.

[12] Mouchet, J, & Hamon, J. Difficulties in malaria eradication campaigns due to the behavior of the vectors. Geneva: World Health Organisation (1963). WHO/Mal/394; WHO/Vector Control/35.

[13] Govella, N J, Okumu, F O, & Killeen, G F. Insecticide-treated nets can reduce malaria transmission by mosquitoes which feed outdoors. The American Journal of Tropical Medicine and Hygiene (2010). 82, 415-9.

[14] Molineaux, L, Shidrawi, G R, Clarke, J L, Boulzaguet, J R, & Ashkar, T S. Assessment of insecticidal impact on the malaria mosquito's vectorial capacity, from data on the man-biting rate and age-composition. Bulletin of the World Health Organization (1979). 57, 265-74.

[15] Molineaux, L, Shidrawi, G R, Clarke, J L, Boulzaguet, R, Ashkar, T, & Dietz, K. The impact of propoxur on *Anopheles gambiae* s.l. and some other anopheline populations,

and its relationship with some pre-spraying variables. Bulletin of the World Health Organization (1976). 54, 379-89.

[16] Smits, A, Coosemans, M, Van Bortel, W, Barutwanayo, M, & Delacollette, C. Readjustment of the malaria vector control strategy in the Rusizi Valley, Burundi. Bulletin of Entomological Research (1995). 85, 541-8.

[17] Griffin, J T, Hollingsworth, T D, Okell, L C, Churcher, T S, White, M, Hinsley, W, Bousema, T, Drakeley, C J, Ferguson, N M, Basáñez, M-G, & Ghani, A C. Reducing *Plasmodium falciparum* malaria transmission in Africa: a model-based evaluation of intervention strategies. PLoS Medicine (2010). 7, e1000324.

[18] Sinka, M E, Bangs, M J, Manguin, S, Coetzee, M, Mbogo, C M, Hemingway, J, Patil, A P, Temperley, W H, Gething, P W, Kabaria, C W, Okara, R M, Van Boeckel, T, Godfray, H C J, Harbach, R E, & Hay, S I. The dominant *Anopheles* vectors of human malaria in Africa, Europe and the Middle East: occurrence data, distribution maps and bionomic précis. Parasites & Vectors (2010). 3, 117.

[19] Lefèvre, T, Gouagna, L-C, Dabiré, K R, Elguero, E, Fontenille, D, Renaud, F, Costantini, C, & Thomas, F. Beyond nature and nurture: phenotypic plasticity in blood-feeding behaviour of *Anopheles gambiae* s.s. when humans are not readily accessible. The American Journal of Tropical Medicine and Hygiene (2009). 81, 1023-9.

[20] Sousa, C A, Pinto, J, Almeida, A P, Ferreira, C, Do Rosário, V E, & Charlwood, JD. Dogs as a favored host choice of *Anopheles gambiae* sensu stricto (Diptera: Culicidae) of São Tomé West Africa. Journal of Medical Entomology (2001). 38, 122-5.

[21] Reddy, M R, Overgaard, H J, Abaga, S, Reddy, V P, Caccone, A, Kiszewski, A E, & Slotman, M A. Outdoor host seeking behaviour of *Anopheles gambiae* mosquitoes following initiation of malaria vector control on Bioko Island, Equatorial Guinea. Malaria Journal (2011). 10, 184.

[22] Trung, H D, Van Bortel, W, Sochantha, T, Keokenchanh, K, Briët, O J T, & Coosemans, M. Behavioural heterogeneity of *Anopheles* species in ecologically different localities in Southeast Asia: a challenge for vector control. Tropical Medicine & International Health (2005). 10, 251-62.

[23] Vythilingam, I, Sidavong, B, Chan, S T, Phonemixay, T, Vanisaveth, V, Sisoulad, P, Phetsouvanh, R, Hakim, S L, & Phompida, S. Epidemiology of malaria in Attapeu-Province, Lao PDR in relation to entomological parameters. Transactions of the Royal Society of Tropical Medicine and Hygiene (2005). 99, 833-9.

[24] Obsomer, V, Defourny, P, & Coosemans, M. The *Anopheles dirus* complex: spatial distribution and environmental drivers. Malaria Journal (2007). 6, 26.

[25] Sinka, M E, Rubio-Palis, Y, Manguin, S, Patil, A P, Temperley, W H, Gething, P W, Van Boeckel, T, Kabaria, C W, Harbach, R E, & Hay, S I. The dominant *Anopheles*

vectors of human malaria in the Americas: occurrence data, distribution maps and bionomic précis. Parasites & Vectors (2010). 3, 72.

[26] Hiwat, H, Issaly, J, Gaborit, P, Somai, A, Samjhawan, A, Sardjoe, P, Soekhoe, T, & Girod, R. Behavioural heterogeneity of *Anopheles darlingi* (Diptera: Culicidae) and malaria transmission dynamics along the Maroni River, Suriname, French Guiana. Transactions of the Royal Society of Tropical Medicine and Hygiene (2010). 104, 207-13.

[27] Moutinho, P R, Gil, LHS, Cruz, R B, & Ribolla, P E M. Population dynamics, structure and behaviour of *Anopheles darlingi* in a rural settlement in the Amazon rainforest of Acre, Brazil. Malaria Journal (2011). 10, 174.

[28] Girod, R, Gaborit, P, Carinci, R, Issaly, J, & Fouque, F. *Anopheles darlingi* bionomics and transmission of *Plasmodium falciparum, Plasmodium vivax* and *Plasmodium malariae* in Amerindian villages of the Upper-Maroni Amazonian forest, French Guiana. Memórias Do Instituto Oswaldo Cruz (2008). 103, 702-10.

[29] Muirhead-Thomson, R C. The significance of irritability, behaviouristic avoidance and allied phenomena in malaria eradication. Bulletin of the World Health Organization (1960). 22, 721-34.

[30] Grieco, J P, Achee, N L, Chareonviriyaphap, T, Suwonkerd, W, Chauhan, K, Sardelis, M R, & Roberts, D R. A new classification system for the actions of IRS chemicals traditionally used for malaria control. PloS One (2007). 2, e716.

[31] Siegert, P Y, Walker, E, & Miller, J R. Differential behavioural responses of *Anopheles gambiae* (Diptera: Culicidae) modulate mortality caused by pyrethroid-treated bednets. Journal of Economic Entomology (2009). 102, 2061-71.

[32] Badyaev, A V. Stress-induced variation in evolution: from behavioural plasticity to genetic assimilation. Proceedings. Biological Sciences / The Royal Society (2005). 272, 877-86.

[33] Pothikasikorn, J, Chareonviriyaphap, T, Bangs, M J, & Prabaripai, A. Behavioural responses to DDT and pyrethroids between *Anopheles minimus* species A and C, malaria vectors in Thailand. The American Journal of Tropical Medicine and Hygiene (2005). 73, 343-9.

[34] White, G. Blood feeding habits of malaria vector mosquitos in the South Pare district of Tanzania 10 years after cessation of a dieldrin residual spraying campaign. Geneva: World Health Organisation (1969). WHO/MAL/69.684 – WHO/VBC/69.144.

[35] Gillies, M, & Smith, A. The effect of a residual house-spraying campaign in East Africa on species balance in the *Anopheles funestus* group. The replacement of *A. funestus* Giles by *A. rivulorum* Leeson. Bulletin of Entomological Research (1960). 51, 243-52.

[36] Gillies, M, & Furlong, M. An investigation into the behaviour of *Anopheles parensis* Gillies at Malindi on the Kenya coast. Bulletin of Entomological Research (1963). 55,1-16.

[37] Labbo, R, Czeher, C, Djibrila, A, Arzika, I, Jeanne, I, & Duchemin, J-B. Longitudinal follow-up of malaria transmission dynamics in two villages in a Sahelian area of Niger during a nationwide insecticide-treated bednet distribution programme. Medical and Veterinary Entomology (2012). 26, 386-95.

[38] Iyengar, R. The bionomics of salt-water *Anopheles gambiae* in East Africa. Bulletin of the World Health Organization (1962). 27, 223-9.

[39] Lindblade, K, Gimnig, J, Kamau, L, Hawley, W, Odhiambo, F, Olang, G, TerKuile, F O, Vulule, J, & Slutsker L. Impact of sustained use of insecticide-treated bednets on malaria vector species distribution and culicine mosquitoes. Journal of Medical Entomology (2006). 43, 428-32.

[40] Mutuku, F M, King, C H, Mungai, P, Mbogo, C, Mwangangi, J, Muchiri, E M, Walker, E D, & Kitron, U. Impact of insecticide-treated bed nets on malaria transmission indices on the south coast of Kenya. Malaria Journal (2011). 10, 356.

[41] Bayoh, M N, Mathias, D K, Odiere, M R, Mutuku, F M, Kamau, L, Gimnig, J E,Vulule, J M, Hawley, W A, Hamel, M J, & Walker, E D. *Anopheles gambiae*: historical population decline associated with regional distribution of insecticide-treated bednets in western Nyanza Province, Kenya. Malaria Journal (2010). 9, 62.

[42] Russell, T L, Govella, N J, Azizi, S, Drakeley, C J, Kachur, S P, & Killeen, G F. Increased proportions of outdoor feeding among residual malaria vector populations following increased use of insecticide-treated nets in rural Tanzania. Malaria Journal (2011). 10, 80.

[43] Mathias, D K, Ochomo, E, Atieli, F, Ombok, M, Bayoh, M N, Olang, G, Muhia, D,Kamau, L, Vulule, J M, Hamel, M J, Hawley, W A, Walker, E D, & Gimnig, J E. Spatial and temporal variation in the kdr allele L*1014*S in *Anopheles gambiae* s.s. and phenotypic variability in susceptibility to insecticides in Western Kenya. Malaria Journal (2011). 10, 10.

[44] Mathenge, E M, Gimnig, J E, Kolczak, M, Ombok, M, Irungu, L W, & Hawley, W A. Effect of permethrin-impregnated nets on exiting behaviour, blood feeding success, and time of feeding of malaria mosquitoes (Diptera: Culicidae) in western Kenya. Journal of Medical Entomology (2001). 38, 531-6.

[45] Derua, Y A, Alifrangis, M, Hosea, K M, Meyrowitsch, D W, Magesa, S M, Pedersen, E M, & Simonsen, P E. Change in composition of the *Anopheles gambiae* complex and its possible implications for the transmission of malaria and lymphatic filariasis in northeastern Tanzania. Malaria Journal (2012). 11, 188.

[46] Braimah, N, Drakeley, C, Kweka, E, Mosha, F, Helinski, M, Pates, H, Maxwell, C, Massawe, T, Kenward, M G, & Curtis, C. Tests of bednet traps (Mbita traps) for mon-

itoring mosquito populations and time of biting in Tanzania and possible impact of prolonged insecticide treated net use. International Journal of Tropical Insect Science (2005). 25, 208-13.

[47] Moiroux, N, Gomez, M B, Pennetier, C, Elanga, E, Djènontin, A, Chandre, F, Djègbé, I, Guis, H, & Corbel, V. Changes in *Anopheles funestus* biting behaviour following universal coverage of Long-Lasting Insecticidal Nets in Benin. The Journal of Infectious Diseases (2012). 206, 1622-9.

[48] Mbogo, C N, Baya, N M, Ofulla, A V, Githure, J I, & Snow, R W. The impact of permethrin-impregnated bednets on malaria vectors of the Kenyan coast. Medical and Veterinary Entomology (1996). 10, 251-9.

[49] Njau, R, Mosha, F, & Nguma, J. Field trials of pyrethroid impregnated bednets in northern Tanzania 1. Effect on malaria transmission. International Journal of Tropical Insect Science (1993). 14, 575-84.

[50] Magesa, S M, Wilkes, T J, Mnzava, A E, Njunwa, K J, Myamba, J, Kivuyo, M D, Hill, N, Lines, J D, & Curtis, C F. Trial of pyrethroid impregnated bednets in an area of Tanzania holoendemic for malaria. Part 2. Effects on the malaria vector population. Acta Tropica (1991). 49, 97-108.

[51] Quiñones, M L, Lines, J D, Thomson, M C, Jawara, M, Morris, J, & Greenwood, B M. *Anopheles gambiae* gonotrophic cycle duration, biting and exiting behaviour unaffected by permethrin-impregnated bednets in The Gambia. Medical and Veterinary Entomology (1997). 11, 71-8.

[52] Molineaux, L, & Gramiccia, G. The Garki Project: Research on the Epidemiology and Control of Malaria in the Sudan Savanna of West Africa. World Health Organisation (1980), 331pp.

[53] Ilboudo-Sanogo, E, Cuzin-Ouattara, N, Diallo, D A, Cousens, S N, Esposito, F, Habluetzel, A, Sanon, S, & Ouédraogo, A P. Insecticide-treated materials, mosquito adaptation and mass effect: entomological observations after five years of vector control in Burkina Faso. Transactions of the Royal Society of Tropical Medicine and Hygiene (2001). 95, 353-60.

[54] Bøgh, C, Pedersen, E M, Mukoko, D A, & Ouma, J H. Permethrin-impregnated bednet effects on resting and feeding behaviour of lymphatic filariasis vector mosquitoes in Kenya. Medical and Veterinary Entomology (1998). 12, 52-9.

[55] Lindsay, S W, Alonso, P L, Armstrong Schellenberg, JR, Hemingway, J, Adiamah, J H, Shenton, FC, Jawara, M, & Greenwood, B M. A malaria control trial using insecticide treated bed nets and targeted chemoprophylaxis in a rural area of The Gambia, west-Africa. 7. Impact of permethrin-impregnated bed nets on malaria vectors. Transactions of the Royal Society of Tropical Medicine and Hygiene (1993). Suppl , 2, 45-51.

[56] Fornadel, C M, Norris, L C, Glass, G E, & Norris, D E. Analysis of *Anopheles arabiensis* blood feeding behaviour in southern Zambia during the two years after introduction of insecticide-treated bed nets. The American Journal of Tropical Medicine and Hygiene (2010). 83, 848-53.

[57] White, G. *Anopheles gambiae* complex and disease transmission in Africa. Transactions of the Royal Society of Tropical Medicine and Hygiene (1974). 68, 278-301.

[58] Taylor, B. Changes in the feeding behaviour of a malaria vector, *Anopheles farauti* Lav., following use of DDT as a residual spray in houses in the British Solomon Islands Protectorate. Transactions of the Royal Entomological Society of London (1975). 127, 277-92.

[59] Bugoro, H, Iro'ofa C, Mackenzie, D O, Apairamo, A, Hevalao, W, Corcoran, S, Bobogare, A, Beebe, N W, Russell, T L, Chen, C-C, & Cooper, R D. Changes in vector species composition and current vector biology and behaviour will favour malaria elimination in Santa Isabel Province, Solomon Islands. Malaria Journal (2011). 10, 287.

[60] Ismail, I A, Notananda, V, & Schepens, J. Studies on malaria and responses of *Anopheles balabacensis balabacensis* and *Anopheles minimus* to DDT residual spraying in Thailand. Acta Tropica (1975). 32, 206-31.

[61] Nustsathapana, S, Sawasdiwongphorn, P, Chitprarop, U, & Cullen, J R. The behavior of *Anopheles minimus* Theobald (Diptera: Culicidae) subjected to differing levels of DDT selection pressure in northern Thailand. Bulletin of Entomological Research (1986). 76, 303-12.

[62] Garros, C, Marchand, R P, Quang, N T, Hai, N S, & Manguin, S. First record of *Anopheles minimus* C and significant decrease of *An. minimus* A in central Vietnam. Journal of the American Mosquito Control Association (2005). 21, 139-43.

[63] Reisen, W K, Pradhan, S P, Shrestha, J P, Shrestha, S L, Vaidya, R G, & Shrestha, J D. Anopheline mosquito (Diptera: Culicidae) ecology in relation to malaria transmission in the inner and outer terai of Nepal, 1987-1989. Journal of Medical Entomology (1993). 30, 664-82.

[64] Li, Z Z, Zhang, M C, Wus, Y G, Zhong, B L, Lin, G Y, & Huang, H. Trial of deltamethrin impregnated bed nets for the control of malaria transmitted by *Anopheles sinensis* and *Anopheles anthropophagus*. The American Journal of Tropical Medicine and Hygiene (1989). 40, 356-9.

[65] Zhang, Z, & Yang, C. Application of deltamethrin-impregnated bednets for mosquito and malaria control in Yunnan, China. The Southeast Asian Journal of Tropical Medicine and Public Health (1996). 27, 367-71.

[66] Giglioli, G. Nation-wide malaria eradication projects in the Americas III. Eradication of *Anopheles darlingi* from the inhabited areas of British Guiana by DDT residual spraying. Journal of the National Malaria Society (1951). 10, 142-61.

[67] Richards, F, Flores, R Z, Sexton, J D, Beach, R F, Mount, D L, Cordon-Rosales, C, Gatica, M, & Klein, R E. Effects of permethrin-impregnated bed nets on malaria vectors of Northern Guatemala. Bulletin of PAHO (1994). 28, 112-21.

[68] Charlwood, J D, & Graves, P M. The effect of permethrin-impregnated bednets on a population of *Anopheles farauti* in coastal Papua New Guinea. Medical and Veterinary Entomology (1987). 1, 319-27.

[69] Hii, J L, Birley, M H, Kanai, L, Foligeli, A, & Wagner, J. Comparative effects of permethrin-impregnated bednets and DDT house spraying on survival rates and oviposition interval of *Anopheles farauti* (Diptera: Culicidae) in Solomon Islands. Annals of Tropical Medicine and Parasitology (1995). 89(1), 521-9.

[70] Bugoro, H, Cooper, R D, Butafa, C,Iro'ofa, C, Mackenzie, DO, Chen, C-C, & Russell, T L. Bionomics of the malaria vector *Anopheles farauti* in Temotu Province, Solomon Islands: issues for malaria elimination. Malaria Journal (2011). 10, 133.

[71] Ismail, I A, Phinichpongse, S, & Boonrasri, P. Responses of *Anopheles minimus* to DDT residual spraying in a cleared forested foothill area in central Thailand. Acta Tropica (1978). 35, 69-82.

[72] Lourenço-de-Oliveira, R, Guimarães, A E, Arlé, M, Da Silva, T F, Castro, M G, Motta, M A, & Deane, L M. Anopheline species, some of their habits and relation to malaria in endemic areas of Rondônia State, Amazon region of Brazil. Memórias Do Instituto Oswaldo Cruz (1989). 84, 501-14.

[73] Harris, A F, Matias-Arnéz, A, & Hill, N. Biting time of *Anopheles darlingi* in the Bolivian Amazon and implications for control of malaria. Transactions of the Royal Society of Tropical Medicine and Hygiene (2006). 100, 45-7.

[74] Suwonkerd, W, Amg-Ung, B, Rimwangtrakul, K, Wongkattiyakul, S, Kattiyamongkool, B, Chitprarop, U, & Takagi, M. A Field Study on the Response of *Anopheles dirus* to DDT and Fenitrothion Sprayed to Huts in Phetchabun Province, Thailand. Tropical Medicine (Nagasaki) (1990). 32, 1-5.

[75] Pongvongsa, T, Ha, H, Thanh, L, Marchand, R P, Nonaka, D, Tojo, B, Phongmany, P, Moji, K, & Kobayashi, J. Joint malaria surveys lead towards improved cross-border cooperation between Savannakhet province, Laos and Quang Tri province, Vietnam. Malaria Journal (2012). 11, 262.

[76] Elliott, R. Studies on man vector contact in some malarious areas in Colombia. Bulletin of the World Health Organization (1968). 38, 239-53.

[77] Hiwat, H, Mitro, S, Samjhawan, A, Sardjoe, P, Soekhoe, T, & Takken, W. Collapse of *Anopheles darlingi* populations in Suriname after introduction of insecticide-treated

nets (ITNs); malaria down to near elimination level. The American Journal of Tropical Medicine and Hygiene (2012). 86, 649-55.

[78] Sampath, T R, Yadav, R S, Sharma, V P, & Adak, T. Evaluation of lambdacyhalothrin impregnated bednets in a malaria endemic area of India. Part 2. Impact on malaria vectors. Journal of the American Mosquito Control Association (1998). 14, 437-43.

[79] Loyola, E G, Rodríguez, M H, González, L, Arredondo-Jimenez, J I, Bown, D N, & Vaca, M A. Effect of indoor residual spraying of DDT and bendiocarb on the feeding patterns of *Anopheles pseudopunctipennis* in Mexico. Journal of the American Mosquito Control Association (1990). 6, 635-40.

[80] Giglioli, G. Biological variations in *Anopheles darlingi* and *Anopheles gambiae*; their effect on practical malaria control in the neotropical region. Bulletin of the World-Health Organization (1956). 15, 461-71.

[81] Barai, D, Hyma, B, & Ramesh, A. The scope and limitations of insecticide spraying in rural vector control programmes in the states of Karnataka and Tamil Nadu in India. Ecology of Disease (1982). 1, 243-55.

[82] Martinez-Palacios, A, & De Zulueta, J. Ethological changes in *Anopheles pseudopunctipennis* in Mexico after prolonged use of DDT. Nature (1964). 203, 940-1.

[83] Kitau, J, Oxborough, R M, Tungu, P K, Matowo, J, Malima, R C, Magesa, S M, Bruce, J, Mosha, F W, & Rowland, M W. Species shifts in the *Anopheles gambiae* complex: do LLINs successfully control *Anopheles arabiensis*? PloS One (2012). 7, e31481.

[84] Ayala, D, Fontaine, M C, Cohuet, A, Fontenille, D, Vitalis, R, & Simard, F. Chromosomal inversions, natural selection and adaptation in the malaria vector *Anopheles funestus*. Molecular Biology and Evolution (2011). 28, 745-58.

[85] Coluzzi, M, Sabatini, A, Petrarca, V, & Di Deco, M A. Behavioural divergences between mosquitoes with different inversion karyotypes in polymorphic populations of the *Anopheles gambiae* complex. Nature (1977). 266, 832-3.

[86] Coluzzi, M, Sabatini, A, Petrarca, V, & Di Deco MA. Chromosomal differentiation and adaptation to human environments in the *Anopheles gambiae* complex. Transactions of the Royal Society of Tropical Medicine and Hygiene (1979). 73, 483-97.

[87] Coluzzi, M. Malaria vector analysis and control. Parasitology Today (1992). 8, 113-8.

[88] White, G B. Biological effects of intraspecific chromosomal polymorphism in malaria vector populations. Bulletin of the World Health Organization (1974). 50, 299-306.

[89] Jones, M. Inversion polymorphism and circadian flight activity in the mosquito *Anopheles stephensi* List. (Diptera, Culicidae). Bulletin of Entomological Research (1974). 64, 305-11.

[90] Hii, J L, Chew, M, Sang, V Y, Munstermann, L E, Tan, S G, Panyim, S, & Yasothornsrikul, S. Population genetic analysis of host seeking and resting behaviours in the

malaria vector, *Anopheles balabacensis* (Diptera: Culicidae). Journal of Medical Entomology (1991). 28, 675-84.

[91] Lines, J D, Lyimo, E O, & Curtis, C F. Mixing of indoor- and outdoor-resting adults of *Anopheles gambiae* Giles s.l. and *A. funestus* Giles (Diptera: Culicidae) in coastal Tanzania. Bulletin of Entomological Research (2009). 76, 171.

[92] Smits, A, Roelants, P, Van Bortel, W, & Coosemans, M. Enzyme polymorphisms in the *Anopheles gambiae* (Diptera: Culicidae) complex related to feeding and resting behaviour in the Imbo Valley, Burundi. Journal of Medical Entomology (1996). 33,545-53.

[93] Coosemans, M, Smits, A, & Roelants, P. Intraspecific isozyme polymorphism of *Anopheles gambiae* in relation to environment, behaviour, and malaria transmission in southwestern Burkina Faso. The American Journal of Tropical Medicine and Hygiene (1998). 58, 70-4.

[94] Sinka, M E, Bangs, M J, Manguin, S, Chareonviriyaphap, T, Patil, A P, Temperley, W H, Gething, P W, Elyazar, I R F, Kabaria, C W, Harbach, R E, & Hay, S I. The dominant *Anopheles* vectors of human malaria in the Asia-Pacific region: occurrence data, distribution maps and bionomic précis. Parasites & Vectors (2011). 4, 89.

[95] Limrat, D, Rojruthai, B, Apiwathnasorn, C, Samung, Y, & Prommongkol, S. *Anopheles barbirostris /campestris* as a probable vector of malaria in Aranyaprathet, Sa Kaeo Province. The Southeast Asian Journal of Tropical Medicine and Public Health (2001). 32,739-44.

[96] Giglioli, G. Ecological change as a factor in renewed malaria transmission in an eradicated area. A localized outbreak of *A. aquasalis*-transmitted malaria on the Demerara river estuary, British Guiana, in the fifteenth year of *A. darlingi* and malaria eradication. Bulletin of the World Health Organization (1963). 29, 131-45.

[97] Lengeler, C. Insecticide-treated bed nets and curtains for preventing malaria. Cochrane Database of Systematic Reviews (2004). 2, CD0003632009.

[98] Pluess, B, Tanscer, F C, Lengeler, C, & Sharp, B L. Indoor residual spraying for preventing malaria. Cochrane Database of Systematic Reviews (2010). 4, CD006657.

[99] Jana-Kara, B R, Jihullah, W A, Shahi, B, Dev, V, Curtis, C F, & Sharma, V P. Deltamethrin impregnated bednets against *Anopheles minimus* transmitted malaria in Assam, India. The Journal of Tropical Medicine and Hygiene (1995). 98, 73-83.

[100] Kobayashi, J, Phompida, S, Toma, T, Looareensuwan, S, Toma, H, & Miyagi, I. The effectiveness of impregnated bed net in malaria control in Laos. Acta Tropica (2004). 89, 299-308.

[101] Seyoum, A, Sikaala, C H, Chanda, J, Chinula, D, Ntamatungiro, A J, Hawela, M, Miller, J M, Russell, T L, Briët, O J, & Killeen, G F. Human exposure to anopheline mos-

quitoes occurs primarily indoors, even for users of insecticide-treated nets in Luangwa Valley, South-east Zambia. Parasites & Vectors (2012). 5, 101.

[102] Charlwood, J D, Alcântara, J, Pinto, J, Sousa, C A, Rompão, H, Gil, V, & Rosário, V E. Do bednets reduce malaria transmission by exophagic mosquitoes? Transactions of the Royal Society of Tropical Medicine and Hygiene (2005). 99, 901-4.

[103] Govella, N J, & Ferguson, H. Why use of interventions targeting outdoor biting mosquitoes will be necessary to achieve malaria elimination? Frontiers in Physiology (2012).3, 199.

[104] Kiware, S S, Chitnis, N, Devine, G J, Moore, S J, Majambere, S, & Killeen, G F. Biologically meaningful coverage indicators for eliminating malaria transmission. Biology Letters (2012). 8, 874-877.

[105] Ferguson, H M, Dornhaus, A, Beeche, A, Borgemeister, C, Gottlieb, M, Mulla, M S, Gimnig, J E, Fish, D, & Killeen, G F. Ecology: a prerequisite for malaria elimination and eradication. PLoS Medicine (2010). 7, e1000303.

[106] The malERA Consultative Group on Vector Control. A research agenda for malaria eradication: vector control. PLoS Medicine (2011). 8, e1000401.

[107] Hill, N, Lenglet, A, Arnéz, A M, & Carneiro, I. Plant based insect repellent and insecticide treated bed nets to protect against malaria in areas of early evening biting vectors: double blind randomised placebo controlled clinical trial in the Bolivian Amazon. BMJ (Clinical Research Ed.) (2007).335, 1023.

[108] Dutta, P, Khan, A M, Khan, S A, Borah, J, Sharma, C K, & Mahanta, J. Malaria control in a forest fringe area of Assam, India: a pilot study. Transactions of the Royal Society of Tropical Medicine and Hygiene (2011). 105, 327-32.

[109] Rowland, M, Downey, G, Rab, A, Freeman, T, Mohammad, N, Rehman, H, Durrani, N, Reyburn, H, Curtis, C, Lines, J, & Fayaz, M. DEET mosquito repellent provides personal protection against malaria: a household randomized trial in an Afghan refugee camp in Pakistan. Tropical Medicine & International Health (2004). 9, 335-42.

[110] Kimani, E W, Vulule, J M, Kuria, I W, & Mugisha, F. Use of insecticide-treated clothes for personal protection against malaria: a community trial. Malaria Journal (2006). 5, 63.

[111] Thang, N D, Erhart, A, Speybroeck, N, Xa, N X, Thanh, N N, Van Ky, P, Hung, L X, Thuan, L K, Coosemans, M, & D' Alessandro, U. Long-lasting Insecticidal Hammocks for controlling forest malaria: a community-based trial in a rural area of central Vietnam. PloS One (2009). 4, e7369.

[112] Sochantha, T, Van Bortel, W, Savonnaroth, S, Marcotty, T, Speybroeck, N, & Coosemans, M. Personal protection by long-lasting insecticidal hammocks against the bites of forest malaria vectors. Tropical Medicine & International Health (2010). 15,336-41.

[113] Habtewold, T, Prior, A, Torr, S J, & Gibson, G. Could insecticide-treated cattle reduce Afrotropical malaria transmission? Effects of deltamethrin-treated Zebu on *Anopheles arabiensis* behaviour and survival in Ethiopia. Medical and Veterinary Entomology (2004). 18, 408-17.

[114] Coosemans, M, & Van Bortel, W. Malaria Vectors in the Mekong Countries: a Complex Interaction between Vectors, Environment and Human Behaviour. In: International Conference Hubs, Harbours and Deltas in Southeast Asia. Royal Academy of Overseas Sciences (2006). 551-569.

[115] Burns, M, Rowland, M, Guessan, R, Carneiro, I, Beeche, A, Ruiz, S S, Kamara, S, Takken, W, Carnevale, P, & Allan, R. Insecticide-treated plastic sheeting for emergency malaria prevention and shelter among displaced populations: an observational cohort study in a refugee setting in Sierra Leone. The American Journal of Tropical Medicine and Hygiene (2012). 87, 242-50.

[116] Kiware, S S, Chitnis, N, Moore, S J, Devine, G J, Majambere, S, Merrill, S, & Killeen, G F. Simplified models of vector control impact upon malaria transmission by zoophagic mosquitoes. PloS One (2012). 7, e37661.

[117] Charlwood, J D, Pinto, J, Ferrara, P R, Sousa, C A, Ferreira, C, Gil, V, & Do Rosário V E. Raised houses reduce mosquito bites. Malaria Journal (2003). 2, 45.

[118] Somboon, P, Lines, J, Aramrattana, A, Chitprarop, U, & Prajakwong, S. Entomological impregnated evaluation of community-wide use of lambdacyhalothrin-bed nets against malaria in a border area of north-west Thailand. Transactions of the Royal Society of Tropical Medicine and Hygiene (1995). 89, 248-54.

[119] Grietens, K P, Xuan, X N, Ribera, J M,Duc, T N, Van Bortel, W, Ba, N T, Van, K P, Xuan, H L, D'Alessandro, U, & Erhart, A. Social Determinants of Long Lasting Insecticidal Hammock-Use Among the Ra-Glai Ethnic Minority in Vietnam: Implications for Forest Malaria Control. PLoS One (2012). 7, e29991.

[120] Bradley, J, Matias, A, Schwabe, C, Vargas, D, Monti, F, Nseng, G, & Kleinschmidt, I. Increased risks of malaria due to limited residual life of insecticide and outdoor biting versus protection by combined use of nets and indoor residual spraying on Bioko Island, Equatorial Guinea. Malaria Journal (2012). 11, 242.

[121] Fillinger, U, & Lindsay, S W. Larval source management for malaria control in Africa: myths and reality. Malaria Journal (2011). 10, 353.

[122] Worrall, E, & Fillinger, U. Large-scale use of mosquito larval source management for malaria control in Africa: a cost analysis. Malaria Journal (2011). 10, 338.

[123] Müller, G C, & Schlein, Y. Efficacy of toxic sugar baits against adult cistern-dwelling *Anopheles claviger*. Transactions of the Royal Society of Tropical Medicine and Hygiene (2008). 102, 480-4.

[124] Scholte, E-J, Ng'habi, K, Kihonda, J, Takken, W, Paaijmans, K, Abdulla, S, Killeen, GF, & Knols, BGJ. An entomopathogenic fungus for control of adult African malaria mosquitoes. Science (2005). 308, 1641-2.

[125] Blanford, S, Chan, BHK, Jenkins, N, Sim, D, Turner, RJ, Read, AF, &Thomas, MB. Fungal pathogen reduces potential for malaria transmission. Science (2005). 308, 1638-41.

[126] Lwetoijera, D W, Sumaye, R D, Madumla, E P, Kavishe, D R, Mnyone, L L, Russell, T L, & Okumu, F O. An extra-domiciliary method of delivering entomopathogenic fungus, *Methariziuman isopliae* IP 46 for controlling adult populations of the malaria vector, *Anopheles arabiensis*. Parasites & Vectors (2010). 3, 18.

Chapter 22

Vector Control: Some New Paradigms and Approaches

Claire Duchet, Richard Allan and Pierre Carnevale

Additional information is available at the end of the chapter

http://dx.doi.org/10.5772/56258

1. Introduction

1.1. Context

The World Malaria Report 2012 [1] summarizes data received from 104 malaria-endemic countries and territories for 2011. Ninety-nine of these countries had on-going malaria transmission. According to the latest World Health Organization (WHO) estimates, there were about 219 million cases of malaria in 2010 and an estimated 660,000 deaths. Africa is the most affected continent: about 90% of all malaria deaths occur there.

Malaria surveillance systems detect now only around 10% of the estimated global number of cases. In 41 countries around the world, it is not possible to make a reliable assessment of malaria trends due to incompleteness or inconsistency of reporting over time.

Actually another estimation of mortality [2] gave the following figures of 1,238,000 (929,000-1,685,000) deaths in 2010. This "one to two" ratio for the same year is matter of concern when considering that the main target of RBM is to reduce by 50% the burden of malaria.

The Lives Saved Tool (LiST) was developed to provide national and regional estimates of cause-specific mortality based on the extent of intervention coverage scale-up in sub-Saharan Africa and it appeared that it "performed reasonably well at estimating the effect of vector control scale-up on child mortality when compared against measured data from studies across a range of malaria transmission settings and is a useful tool in estimating the potential mortality reduction achieved from scaling-up malaria control interventions" [3].

Three major issues deserve special attention: tools for vector control, resistance of mosquito to insecticides, of *Plasmodium* to drugs, of human population to change their behavior, and costs. To tackle these issues new paradigms must be developed with the objectives of efficacy, acceptability and cost-efficiency.

Vector control remains the most generally effective measure to prevent malaria parasite transmission and therefore was one of the four basic technical elements of the Global Malaria Control Strategy [4]. Through the 1980s', vector control was mainly based upon Indoor Residual Spraying (IRS) and, in some circumstances, larval control, but an important break-through occurred with Insecticide Treated Nets (ITNs) then Long Lasting Insecticide treated Nets (LNs) (Figure 1) were introduced. The large scale implementation of ITN has, in several epidemiological settings, produced striking reductions in malaria transmission (-90%), incidence rate of malaria morbidity (-50%) and overall infant mortality (-17%) [5].

For WHO to achieve universal access to long-lasting insecticidal nets (LLINs), 780 million people at risk would need to have access to LLINs in sub-Saharan Africa, and approximately 150 million bed nets would need to be delivered each year. The number of LLINs delivered to endemic countries in sub-Saharan Africa dropped from a peak of 145 million in 2010 to an estimated 66 million in 2012 [1]. This will not be enough to fully replace the LLINs delivered 3 years earlier, indicating that total bed net coverage will decrease unless there is a massive scale-up in 2013. A decrease in LLIN coverage is likely to lead to major resurgences in the disease. In 2011, 153 million people were protected by indoor residual spraying (IRS) around the world, or 5% of the total global population at risk. In the WHO African Region, 77 million people, or 11% of the population at risk were protected through IRS in 2011.

Recent field observations have shown that LLINs may not be as durable as previously estimated and the majority of the most commonly distributed LLINs may have a shorter effective material life, which induce a higher than scheduled cost of global malaria control when LLIN have to be changed more frequently than expected. The problem of cost is a burning issue. International disbursements for malaria control rose steeply during the past eight years and were estimated to be US$ 1.66 billion in 2011 and US$ 1.84 billion in 2012. National government funding for malaria programmes has also been increasing in recent years, and stood at an estimated US$ 625 million in 2011. However, the currently available funding for malaria prevention and control is far below the resources required to reach global malaria targets. An estimated US$ 5.1 billion is needed every year between 2011 and 2020 to achieve universal access to malaria interventions. In 2011, only US$ 2.3 billion was available, less than half of what is needed ([1] fact sheet).

In its 23rd meeting in Senegal, the RBM Partnership Board concluded with an urgent call to governments of malaria endemic countries and development partners to secure the US$2.4 billion needed over the next two years to maintain high levels of coverage with life-saving malaria prevention and treatment interventions in eight African countries. This call follows a decade of success where *malaria deaths have fallen by over one-third in sub-Saharan Africa.*

Overall, out of a total of US$6.8 billion required, US$3.2 billion has been mobilized leaving a US$3.6 billion gap to make sure all affected countries in Africa have enough insecticide treated nets, effective treatments and rapid diagnostic tests for all populations at risk of malaria to achieve the target of near-zero deaths by 2015.

In term of vector control several issues deserve special attention. The change in vector behavior from indoor to outdoor feeding under insecticide pressure may limit the impact of classical

http://dx.doi.org/10.5772/56258

control interventions such as LNs and IRS which target indoor feeding and resting mosquitoes and new tools are obviously needed. On the other hand, species that naturally bite and spend most of their time outdoors such as *Anopheles dirus* in S.E. Asia are poorly controlled by these classical tools and new approaches are urgently needed.

Vector control is also threatened by *the development of insecticide resistance* [4-9]. The frequency of resistance, has risen sharply over the last decade and the relationship between current indicators of resistance and the impact of vector control interventions is still unclear according to the different mechanisms of resistance, though most scientists believe that at some point in the near future resistance will begin to compromise control efforts, and new active ingredients to replace the current ones are urgently needed. Mosquito resistance to at least one insecticide used for malaria control has been identified in 64 countries around the world. In May 2012, WHO and the Roll Back Malaria Partnership released the Global Plan for Insecticide Resistance Management in malaria vectors, a five-pillar strategy for managing the threat of insecticide resistance.

Overcoming insecticide resistance will require novel chemical modes of action or combined interventions, with multiple active agreements, used as part of an integrated vector management strategy or completely new tools to delay the emergence of resistance by reducing selection pressure (e.g. rotations), or kill resistant vectors by exposing them to multiple insecticides (e.g. mixtures, when they become available).

Thus, new paradigms and approaches to vector control will expand the range of species that can be controlled and the chemical modes of action that can be employed, as well as potentially reducing the costs and complications of delivering them.

1.2. Definitions (from Innovative Vector Control Consortium IVCC)

A paradigm can be defined as a mean to deliver an active ingredient to the vector by targeting certain behaviors or ecologies. Paradigms can be associated with general chemical modes of action. Tools that target mosquito resting employ contact toxins. Those based on sugar feeding employ the so-called stomach poisons, etc. New paradigms open the door for exploitation of new chemical modes of action. An intervention paradigm (current examples: Insecticidal Nets or Indoor Residual Spray) is characterized by a primary mode of action (e.g. kills insect that land on the walls) and key characteristics such as the way it applied, its distribution process, economics, user, acceptability etc.

A paradigm may be served by several categories of products, each of which is described by a Target Product Profile (TPP) (e.g. ITNs *vs.* LLINs). The TPP will describe the primary functionality and characteristics that are required of a product to achieve a particular epidemiological outcome. Individual products within the category are defined by specifications.

Figure 1 illustrates the relationship among behaviors, paradigms and chemical mode of action. Where new paradigms do not exist in public health an example from agriculture or home and garden products is listed instead.

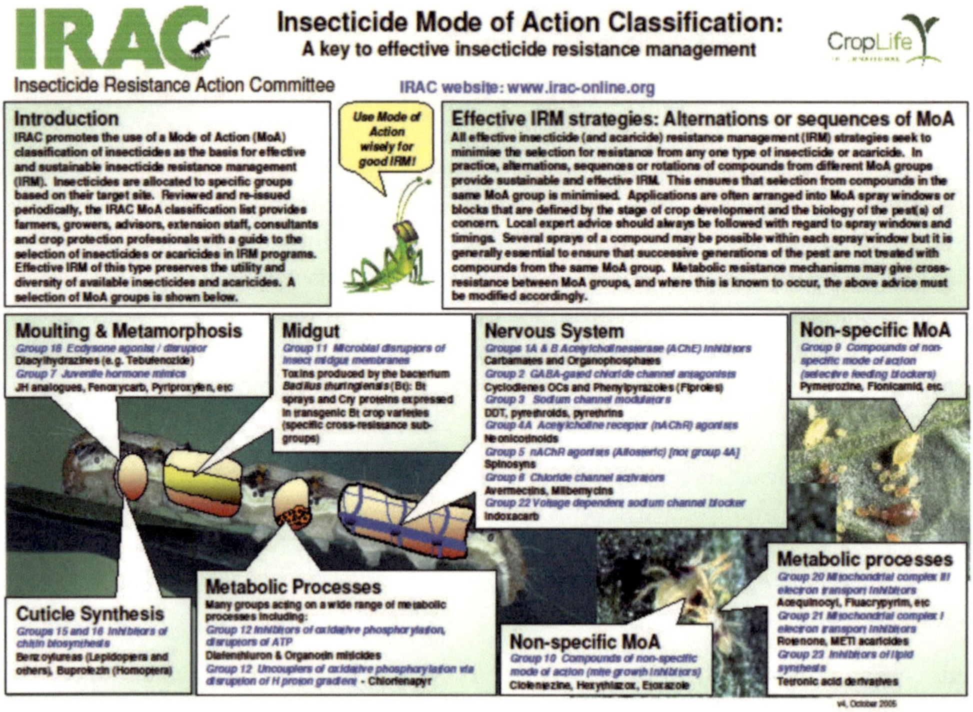

Figure 1. Relationship among behaviors, paradigms and chemical mode of action of insecticides.

2. New approaches to existing paradigms

2.1. New long lasting insecticide formulation for IRS

A microencapsulated formulation (CS) of the organophosphate chlorpyrifos methyl has recently been developed as long lasting i.e., alternative to DDT. In experimental huts in South Benin, against pyrethroid resistant (*kdr* + metabolic resistance) *An. gambiae* M form (and *Cx. quinquefasciatus*), chlorpyrifos methyl (Figure 2) was used to treat mosquito nets, and for IRS, and was compared to other commonly used insecticides: DDT and lambdacyhalothrin [10].

On nets, for N'Guessan et al [10] "the percentage of mortality among *An. gambiae* was 45.2% with the chlorpyrifos methyl-treated net and only 29.8% with the lambacyhalothrin-treated net. Mortality rates among *Cx. quinquefasciatus* were lower than among *An. gambiae* and did not exceed 15% with either type of treated net". While "Mortality of pyrethroid resistant *An. gambiae* was 95.5% with chlorpyrifos methyl-IRS compared to 50.4% in the hut sprayed with DDT and 30.8% in the hut sprayed with lambdacyhalothrin. The mortality of *Cx. quinquefas-*

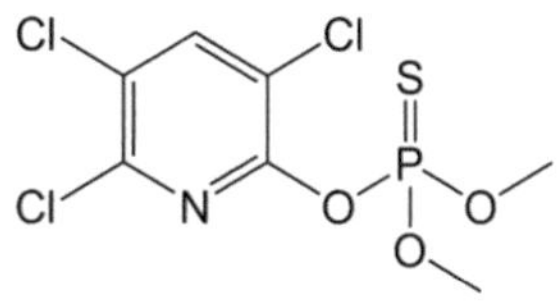

Figure 2. Chemical formula of chlorpyrifos methyl

ciatus in the chlorpyrifos methyl-IRS huts was 66.1% whereas in the DDT and lambdacyhalothrin-IRS huts it was only 14%". Therefore "chlorpyrifos methyl-IRS showed greater potential than DDT of lambdacyhalothrin-IRS for control of pyrethroid resistant *An. gambiae* M form and *Cx. quinquefasciatus* in areas of high *kdr* frequency" [11].

In terms of mortality the short residual activity of chlorpyrifos methyl on ITN is of great concern with a mortality rate decreasing from 100% to 9.7% within just one month while as IRS on cement it was observed "no loss of activity during the nine months of follow-up" compared to the fast decay of DDT and lambdacyhalothrin observed within the first month of spraying. A 9-month efficacy could be very valuable in many West and East African endemic countries with malaria transmission seasons lasting less than 8 months, and where IRS application of chlorpyrifos methyl each year could be adequate. In areas with developing pyrethroid resistance one might envisaged continued use of pyrethroid LLIN in combination with IRS, rotating the use of chlorfenapyr and CS long lasting chlorpyrifos methyl formulation.

2.2. New insecticides paints combining several insecticides and an insect growing regulator for IRS

Insecticide paints are new interesting paradigm for vector control with several advantages regarding classical IRS. It may provide future possibilities to combine several active ingredients in one product and therefore be used to help manage insecticide resistance. Paints can be produced in different colors to fit with people's choice. They may also be potentially implementable by households without the need for a specialized team to deliver the intervention, as is the case with IRS. This could improve community and household acceptance and uptake. Paints may also have the potential of being longer lasting than IRS. Insect growth regulator (IGR), a product usually used as larvicides, is also now being evaluated in Inesfly® 5A IGR™, a paint designed to target adult mosquitoes. Inesfly® 5A IGR™ is composed of two organophosphates (OPs), chlorpyriphos (1.5%), and diazinon (1.5%) and pyriproxyfen (0.063%) an IGR which was successfully used against *Triatoma infestans* [12]. The product is white vinyl paint with an aqueous base. Active ingredients reside within Ca CO3 + resin microcapsules. The formulation allows a gradual release of active ingredients, increasing its persistence.

In Benin the Inesfly® insecticide paint has been tested in laboratory [13] and in field [14] studies. In the laboratory study, the paint was tested against laboratory strains of the urban pest *Cx. quinquefasciatus* the susceptible (S-Lab) strain and the SR homozygote for the ace-1R resistant gene involved in the resistance to OPs and carbamates, with classical bioassay cones (tests on 30 min). Efficacy was measured not only in terms of induced mortality but also in terms of fecundity (number of eggs laid), fertility (% hatching) and larval development (%

pupation and % emergence). Insecticidal paints were tested at different time points: T0, 6 (= 6 months), 9 (= 9 months) and 12 months after application on four different surfaces: softwood, hard plastic (non-porous materials), ready-mixed cement and ready-mixed stucco (porous materials) at two doses, 1kg/6 m^2 (manufacturer's recommended dose to obtain surfaces completely white) and 1 kg/12 m^2. Female mosquitoes were given a blood meal 36 hours after standardized exposure to the painted surfaces. The study showed that the highest rates of mortality were obtained by both doses on susceptible as well as resistant strains even 12 months after treatment, on non-porous surfaces (softwood, plastic), whereas, on porous surfaces (cement, stucco) efficacy was much lower on resistant than on susceptible strain and it dropped to almost 0 at 6 and 12 months in both strains.

Thus long-term efficacy was an issue of porosity of materials rather than the pH of materials or the dose applied. It should be noted that 100% mortality was achieved on non-porous surface even against the OP resistant strain.

In terms of fecundity, fertility, and larval development, "a significant reduction in the number of eggs laid was shown at 0 and 9 months after treatment at either dose. A reduction in egg hatching was observed at T0, but not at T9. An increased mortality from the nymph to the adult stage was shown 9 months after treatment at the higher dose. No differences were found on the duration of the larval development. No IGR effect was observed 12 months after treatment". The percentage of emergence (i.e. adult emerging from pupa) dropped from 80% in control to #53% in samples from exposed females. Hence an adulticide could have impact not only on longevity of females exposed but also on their offspring which is a great advantage for mosquito population control.

Field trials were conducted in area where the local population of *An. gambiae* is composed of the M molecular form with resistance to pyrethroids and DDT, *kdr* is present at a high frequency, but is susceptible to OPs and carbamates, the ace-1R mutation was absent. *Cx. quinquefasciatus* shows high resistance to DDT, pyrethroids and carbosulfan with high *kdr* frequency and elevated levels of esterases and GST activity but the ace-1R mutation was absent [9]. In these trials, experimental huts were treated with either 1 or 2 layers of insecticide paint at one dose (6 kg/m^2). Treatments were applied to either just walls, or to walls plus the ceiling. Unfed females of the lab-reared *An. gambiae* Kisumu strain (sensitive to all insecticides), were tested against local resistant wild strain *An. gambiae* and *Cx. quinquefasciatus*. The *An. gambiae* Kisumu strain mosquitoes were placed inside the huts at a distance of 1 m from two perpendicular walls, and left from 19:00 to 7:00 h [14]. The wild strains were tested using the standard WHO bioassay method.

Mortality of wild resistant *An. gambiae* was high with 83% even 9 months after treatment (2 paint layers on walls). Mortality of wild resistant *Cx. quinquefasciatus* was >50% even 9 months after treatment (2 paint layers on walls). No deterrent or excito-repellent effect was observed against *An. gambiae* nor *Cx. quinquefasciatus*. Mortality rates of exposed *An. gambiae* Kisumu strain in distance experiments in huts (1 m from two perpendicular walls; see above) with 2 layers were most striking, because even one year after treatment 100% of these sensitive mosquitoes were killed (Figure 3C).

Classical cone bioassay showed that in huts with 2 layers "twelve months after treatment mortality rates were of 70-80% against *An. gambiae* and *Cx. quinquefasciatus*". Release of insecticide susceptible unfed *An. gambiae* specimens in huts treated but without net (untreated) showed that 2-13% of females took their blood meal while 72% were well blood fed in control huts. Mortality rates observed in distance experiments were most striking, (Figures 3A & 3B) and even one year after treatment 100% of exposed *An. gambiae* Kisumu strain specimens were killed in huts with 2 layers (Figure 3C).

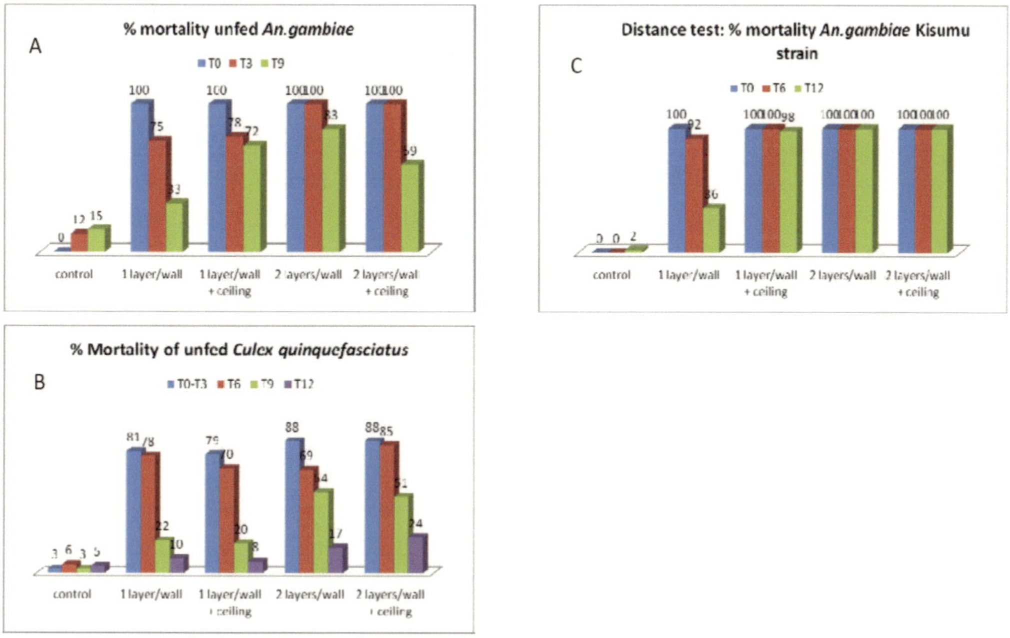

Figure 3. Mortality rates observed in distance experiments of exposed unfed *Anopheles gambiae* (A), unfed *Culex quinquefasciatus* (B), and *Anopheles gambiae* Kisumu strain (C) observed after 3 or 6 or 9 or 12 months after treatment (T3, T6, T9, T12 respectively).

These observations of "volume effect", "layer effect", "substrate effect", residual efficacy duration, and its efficacy against susceptible and resistant strains of the malaria vector *An. gambiae* and the nuisance insect *Culex quinquefasciatus*, are very encouraging. The paints ability to reduce mosquito fecundity and egg hatching opens up interesting new perspectives on malaria and mosquito control for urban settings where walls are commonly constructed with brick, concrete and plaster and provide suitable surfaces for paints, unlike classical mud made wall houses that characterize most rural communities. The paints ability to also reduce *Culex* mosquitoes is likely to increase community acceptance and maintenance of paint.

2.3. New mode of action families for IRS usage: Neonicotinoids

Neonicotinoid insecticides act on the central nervous system of insects by binding of agonist on postsynaptic nicotinic receptors [15]. Discovered in 1998, dinotefuran is a novel neonicotinoid insecticide which belongs to the third-generation neonicotinoids (sub-class: furanicotinyl compounds) [16]. It is a neonicotinoid agonist of the nicotinoid acetylcholine receptor with no cross-resistance to other insecticides such as organochlorine (OC), organophosphate (OP), carbamates or pyrethroids. Its efficiency is not greatly diminished by the presence of resistance mechanisms such as *kdr* or ace-1^R in mosquitoes.

In studies comparing the impact of dinotefuran, permethrin and propoxur on resistant strains of *Cx. quinquefasciatus*, dinotefuran was about 10 times more effective than permethrin on the BKPER strain, and 1000 times more effective than propoxur on resistant R-LAB strain [17]. If this product can be incorporated into material (e.g. LNs) or IRS applications then it should be useful in areas where resistance to pyrethroids and carbamates has developed.

The option of associating insecticides with different modes of action is one of the possible strategies for resistance management (as developed in another Chapter by Corbel & N'Guessan). An interesting approach that has recently been studied, combined Piperonyl butoxide (PBO), organic compound used as pesticide synergist, and dinotefuran in an attempt to restore the efficacy of deltamethrin treated mosquito net against resistant *An. gambiae* [18]. Darriet and Chandre [18] have also conducted classical laboratory cone tests of nets treated with deltamethrin, PBO (the classical synergist, inhibitor of oxidases) and dinotefuran alone or in combination against susceptible ("KIS") and resistant '("VKPR") strains of laboratory reared *An. gambiae*. Results of these tests are summarized in Table 1.

Product/ strain		**KIS**			**VKPR**	
	mortality	KDt50	KDt95	mortality	KDT50	KDT95
Deltamethrin	100%	8'	18'	7.5%	31'	194'
Dinotefuran				39%	No	No
PBO				4%	No	No
Deltamethrin +PBO				58%	13'	36'
Dinotefuran + PBO				28%	No	No
Deltamethrin+ Dinotefuran + PBO				99%	10'	23'

Table 1. Effects of mosquito nets treated with deltamethrin, PBO and dinotefuran on susceptible ("KIS"), and resistant '("VKPR") strains of *Anopheles gambiae*.

WHO's minimum mortality level for insecticides is 80% and this provides a reasonable operational guideline for effectiveness. In this study PBO combined with deltamethrin increased significantly its efficacy (synergistic effect), but not to a level adequate for control against pyrethroid-resistant mosquitoes, "suggesting that the acetylcholine concentration within the synaptic gap probably also increased". Interestingly, PBO had an antagonistic effect when combined with dinotefuran, decreasing this insecticide's efficacy. However, when PBO and Dinotefuran were combined with deltamethrin, the combination resulted in 99% mortality against the pyrethroid resistant mosquito strain, comparable with deltamethrin treated nets (in terms of mortality and KD effect) on the fully susceptible mosquito strain. For Darriet and Chandre [18] "the concomitant action of enhanced acetylcholine concentration in the synaptic gap and inactivation of nicotinic receptors by dinotefuran probably explains the strong synergy observed after exposure to the three-compound mixture, which caused nearly 100% mortality in a pyrethroid-resistant strain of *An. gambiae*".

2.4. New Insecticide Treated Plastic Sheeting (ITPS) and Durable Wall Linings (DL or WL)

Insecticide Treated Plastic Sheeting (ITPS) was developed in 2001 to provide a dual purpose tool capable of providing effective shelter and malaria control to displaced families in humanitarian crises. Durable wall linings (DL), developed in 2005, follow similar principles to ITPS, but are designed to be applied to the surface of existing rural house walls. In both cases these tools were developed to overcome the operational complexities and short comings of IRS, increase user acceptance (as the materials are available in different colors), and to increase residual insecticide activity (from classical 3-6 months with IRS to multiple years with ITPS or DL), and to increase community participation with a tool that households can implement themselves, and finally to provide new tools and new insecticide delivery mechanisms within the framework of insecticide resistance management. To date all factories produced ITPS based on solid format of polyethylene treated with pyrethroid insecticide, either permethrin or deltamethrin. The first generation of DL is also a polyethylene, but in 50% shading material format (woven polyethylene threads, with equal sized spaces between the threads).

One study group [19] has used "plastic sheeting impregnated with carbamates combined with long-lasting insecticidal mosquito nets for the control of pyrethroid-resistant malaria vectors" but this version of ITPS is unlikely to be tested at Phase III level or commercialized due to significant toxicity and fire risk problems associated with carbamates in this format. Different commercial products have been developed with different deltamethrin surface concentrations such as "ZeroVector (DL)" (170 mg a.i./m^2) or "Zero Fly" (360 mg a.i./m^2). Zerofly ITPS have been studied (Phase II) in refugee's camps in Afghanistan [20], in Sierra Leone (Phase III) [21], as well as in India (in endemic area with *An. culicifacies* and *An. fluviatilis* vectors or laborer settlements with *An. culicifacies* and *An. stephensi* as vectors) [22-23].

In Angola, a Phase III field trial was implemented in rural area, 8 villages around Balombo which were paired and received LLIN PermaNet 2.0 (55 mg a.i./m^2; Figures 3) or DL/WL ZeroVector or LLIN + ITPS "Zero Fly" or IRS with lambdacyhalothrin (25 mg a.i./m^2) with comprehensive evaluation: entomology, parasitology and immunology; focus group and KAP surveys were also implemented to follow the household acceptability of the vector control methods introduced.

The main vector in these villages was *An. funestus*. Entomological and parasitological first studies results showed that deltamethrin treated DL ZeroVector alone gave same results as IRS (lambdacyhalothrin) or LLIN (PermaNet®) alone or both PermaNet + ITPS Zero Fly in reducing by 55% the *P. falciparum* prevalence and parasitic load in children 2-9 years old (Figure 5) [24].

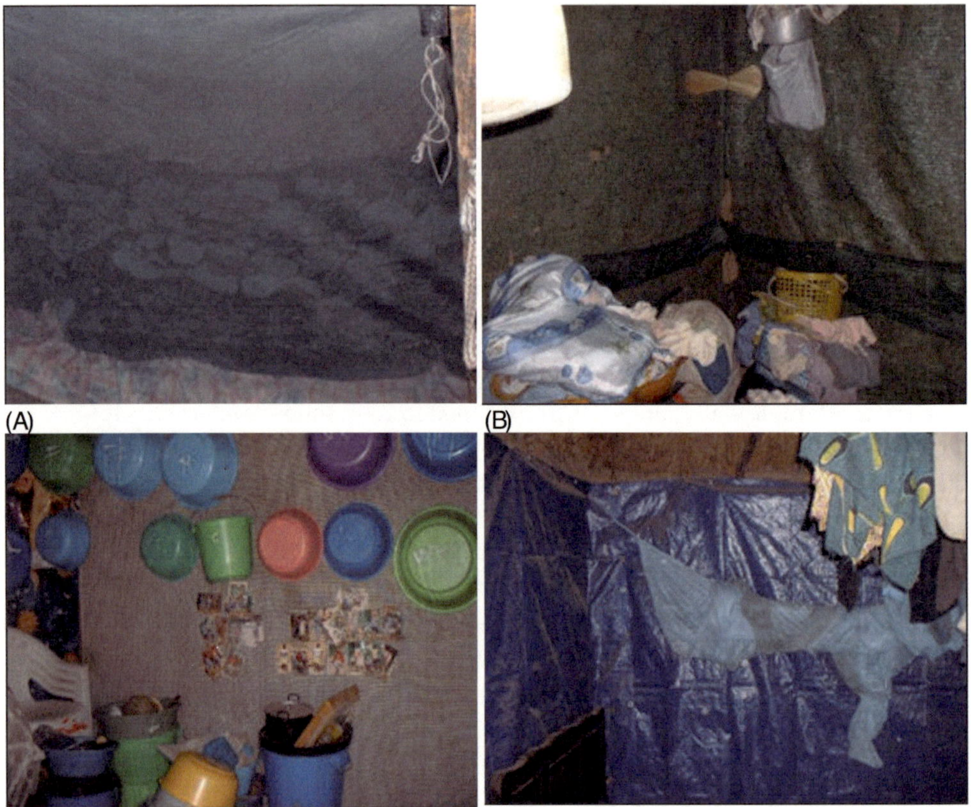

(A) (B) (C) (D)

Figure 4. LLIN PermaNet 2.0 inside a house in Caala village (A); Green DL/WL ZeroVector inside a house in Chisséquélé village (B); Silver DL/WL ZeroVector inside a house in Barragem village (C); LLIN PermaNet 2.0 + ITPS Zero Fly in a house of Capango village (D) (Photos by P. Carnevale).

Entomological data obtained by classical CDC light traps inside houses before/after implementation of vector control measures were in line with the clinical results i.e. similar level of reduction of number of *Anopheles* in each village (Figure 6) such as 79.1% reduction all villages combined [24].

Immunological analysis of antibodies directed against saliva proteins of *Anopheles* [23] (Figure 7) confirmed the actual reduction of man/*Anopheles* contact with ITPS as well as IRS while association LLIN + ZF gave the best result.

A series of smaller Phase II DL/WL feasibility and acceptability studies, with entomological monitoring have also been conducted in Angola and Nigeria [25], Equatorial Guinea, Ghana, Mali, South Africa and Vietnam [26], and Papua New Guinea [27]. In each of these Phase II village studies, DL/WL acceptability data were collected using a standardized household survey used by each of the different study groups, with the conclusive result that DL/WL had an extremely high acceptance level amongst all cultures and communities in which it was

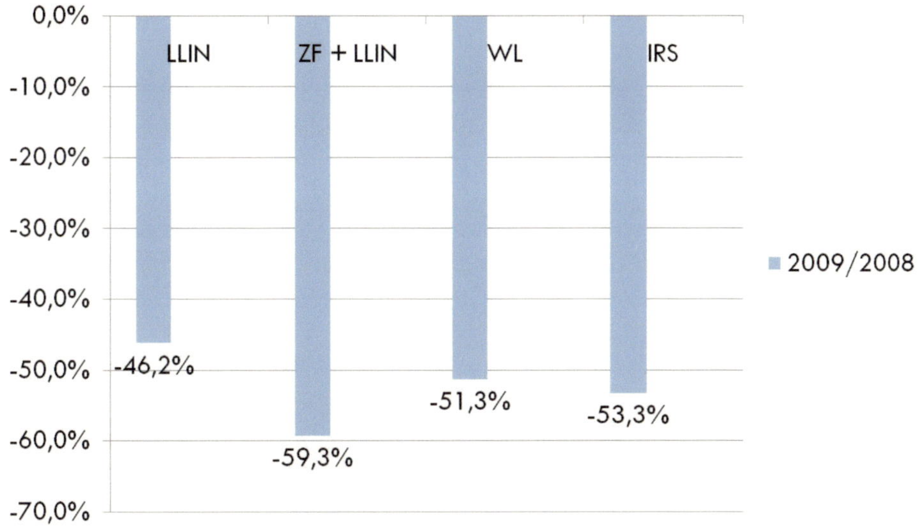

Figure 5. Regressive evolution of endemicity indice (plasmodic indices of 2 – 9 years old children) before/after implementation of each one of the four vector control methods.

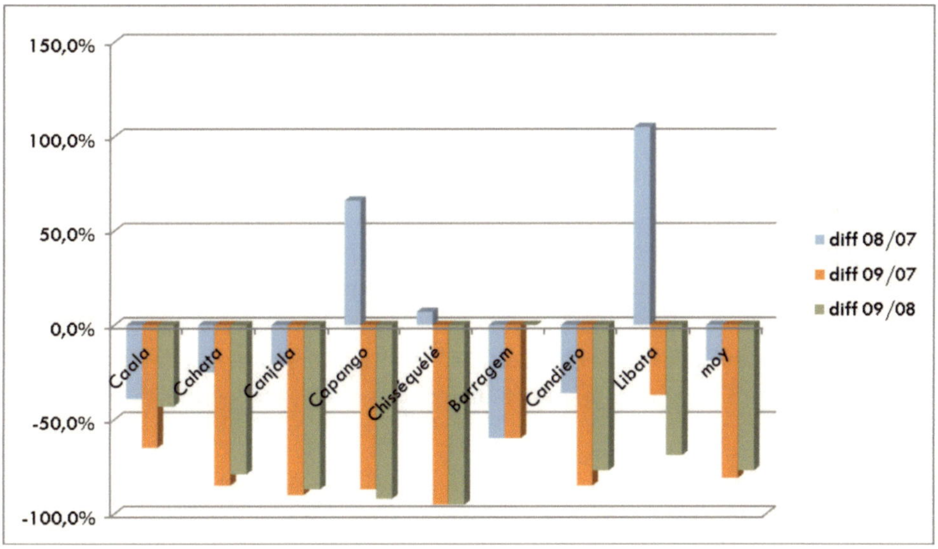

Figure 6. Reduction of number of *Anopheles* in CDC light trap sampling inside houses in villages before (2007-2008) and after (2009) vector control implementation [Caala and Cahata = LLIN alone; Canjala and Capango = LLIN + ZF; Barragem and Chisséquélé = WL alone; Candiero and Libata = IRS.

tested, and that when compared to IRS it was the preferred malaria prevention tool in every study. DL/WL proved feasible in every country study and in all house construction types tested, including brick, mud, wooden, and concrete walled rural houses. In each of these

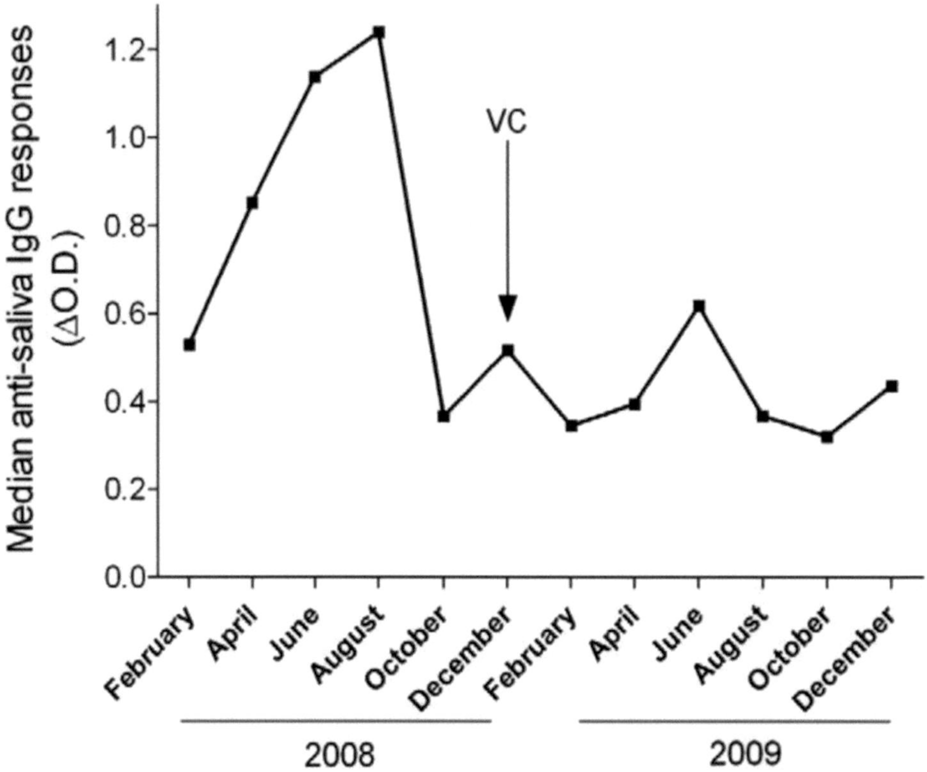

Figure 7. Evolution of the median values of the IgG antibody response to *Anopheles* saliva for all 6 villages combined according to the survey period in 2008 and 2009 (VC: vector control methods implemented in December 2008) [24].

studies, samples of DL/WL were collected at 4 monthly time intervals and were examined for deltamethrin residual content and bioassay impact on vector mosquitoes. The different studies produced very similar results regardless of house construction type, and in all cases DL/WL retained full activity and achieved >90% mortality of vector mosquitoes for the full monitoring periods of each study. The minimum study monitoring period was 6 months and the maximum was 4 years.

In Sierra Leone, Burns et al [21] conducted a Phase III study of ITPS. They constructed two refugee camps, Largo and Tobanda, using ITPS in 50% of each camp for shelter construction. The remaining 50% of each camp had shelter constructed out of untreated plastic sheeting (UPS). In Largo Camp, ITPS/UPS was applied onto walls and the ceiling of each shelter. In Tobanda Camp, ITPS/UPS was used only on ceilings. In Largo, the *Plasmodium falciparum* incidence rate in children up to 3 years of age who were cleared of parasites and then monitored for 8 months, was 163/100 person-years under UPS and 63 under ITPS. In Tobanda, incidence rate was 157/100 person-years under UPS and 134 under ITPS. Protective efficacy was 61% under fully lined ITPS shelters, and 15% under roof lined ITPS alone. Anemia rates improved under ITPS in both camps. Burns et al [21] concluded that "this novel tool proved to be a convenient, safe, and long-lasting method of malaria control when used as a full shelter lining in an emergency setting". Of note Burns et al [21] observed great difference of ITPS on walls + ceiling *versus* ceiling only at *P. falciparum* incidence rate level. Diabate et al [28] found similarly significant entomological difference in experimental huts of Burkina Faso lined with permethrin treated plastic sheeting on walls only or walls + ceiling reporting that "ITPS had a major effect on the mortality of mosquitoes, the proportion killed being dependent upon the surface area covered" and "deterred entry of mosquitoes and inhibition of blood feeding were also correlated with surface area covered."

2.5. New tools for LNs

2.5.1. Combined LN with PBO or two different class of insecticide

Pyrethroid treated LNs are the principle tool upon which malaria control has relied for the last decade, however, the rapid ongoing spread of pyrethroid resistance in Africa, is likely to increasingly compromise their protective efficacy. This concern has highlighted the urgent need to develop alternative active ingredients for LNs. While a study on bitreated (OP or C + pyr) [29] nets showed positive results they have not been commercially developed or operationalised due to safety concerns. To tackle the issue of pyrethroid resistance a new model of LLIN call "Permanet 3" (P3) was recently developed by Vestergaard Frandsen SA, Aarhus, Denmark [30] with *a top panel* made of monofilament polyethylene fabric incorporating deltamethrin (121mg/m^2) and PBO (759mg/m^2) plus side panels made of multifilament polyester fabric coated with a wash-resistant formulation of deltamethrin (85mg/m^2) (while the usual concentration was 55 mg a.i./m^2 in classical Permanet 2 and 25 mg a.i./m^2 in former hand treated nets "ITN"). PBO is the synergist of pyrethrins and pyrethroids without intrinsic insecticidal activity. The action of the synergist PBO is due to inhibition of oxidative enzymes in the insect which can detoxify the insecticide (metabolic resistance). The inhibition or blocking of the detoxification enzyme significantly increases mortality of resistant insects. PBO is used in a ratio ranging generally from 3 to 8 with the active ingredient used, depending on the type of formulation and target insects. LLIN "Permanet 3" (P3) was recently tested in several countries of West, Central [31] and East Africa such as Tanzania [32] and Ethiopia [33].

In southern Benin, N'Guessan et al [11] tested LLIN Permanet 3 against *An. gambiae* M molecular form (highly resistant owing to knockdown resistance (*kdr*) site insensitivity and elevated oxidase and esterase metabolic mechanisms) and *Cx. quinquesfasciatus*, and showed that in experimental huts "the level of personal protection against *An. gambiae* biting from PermaNet 3.0 (50%) was similar to that from PermaNet 2.0 (47%)" and "protection fell significantly after 20 washes to 30% for PermaNet 3.0 and 33% for PermaNet 2.0".

In Côte d'Ivoire, in experimental huts of Yaokoffikro where *An. gambiae* population is mainly composed of S form (90%) *versus* M form (10%) and is strongly resistant with high *kdr* frequency (94%) and Cyt P 450 metabolic resistance, Permanet 3 (unwashed and washed 20x) were compared against the standard Permanet 2 (unwashed and washed 20x), and hand treated ITNs ("CTN") with K Otab® (washed 5x), with untreated nets as control [34]. It appeared that both unwashed and washed P3 reduced entry rate (- 60%) and increased exit rate as well as other treated nets. On the other hand "a significantly higher mortality rate of *An. gambiae* s.s was recorded for unwashed PermaNet® 3.0 (55%) than for unwashed PermaNet® 2.0. However, for washed nets, there was no statistical difference between the mortality rates of *An. gambiae* s.s for washed PermaNet® 2.0, washed PermaNet® 3.0 and the CTN. Classical cone bioassays were conducted with the same nets (testing side panels and roofs) using either susceptible Kisumu strain of *An. gambiae* or local wild resistant population. Against Kisumu strain, all treatments including the washed CTN showed a mean KD rate over the threshold of 95% and a mean mortality rate >80%, (the official cut off).

Against pyrethroid-resistant wild caught *An. gambiae* s.s cone bioassays showed a mean KD rate < 95% and a mean mortality rate < 80% for all treatment arms, except with a mean KD of 94.3% and 98.6% and a mean mortality rate of 93.5% and 99.5%, respectively on side and roof showing a great efficacy even against polyresistant populations. The unwashed PermaNet® 3.0 gave the best results (KD 95.8% and mortality 97.0%)

In Tanzania, laboratory and experimental huts trial compared PermaNet 3.0 (P3), PermaNet 2.0 (P2) and a conventional deltamethrin treated net [32] against pyrethroid susceptible *An. gambiae* and pyrethroid resistant *Cx. quinquefasciatus*, (elevated oxidase and *kdr* mechanisms), Bioassays tests showed that against the susceptible *An. gambiae* P3 and P2 were still efficient after 20 washes while conventionally treated nets lost its efficacy. Against the pyrethroid resistant strain of *Cx. quinquefasciatus* Masimbani strain, it clearly appeared that the treated roof (with PBO) was much more efficient than sides (without PBO) of the LLIN. In experimental huts, general results of P3 and P2 (washed and unwashed) were comparable against pyrethroid susceptible *An. gambiae* and pyrethroid resistant *Cx. quinquefasciatus* and gave high similar personal protection. Mortality induced by unwashed P3 on resistant *Cx. quinquefasciatus* was higher than P2 (both washed and unwashed) and 20x washed P3, showing the increased efficacy achieved by PBO against pyrethroid resistant mosquitoes but this efficacy disappeared after 20 washes. Chemical concentration of the P3 roof decreased from 136 mg a.i./m^2 to 132 mg a.i./m^2 after 20 washes; whereas deltamethrin concentration of the P3 sides decreased from 103-109 mg a.i./m^2 before washing to 53 mg a.i./m^2 after 20 washes. The concentration of PBO decreased from 1142 mg/m^2 before wash to 684 mg/m^2 after 20 washes. Finally, chemical concentration of deltamethrin in P2 decreased from 61- 77 mg a.i./m^2 to 25 77 mg a.i./m^2 after the classical 20 washes.

Tungu et al [32] observed that "the tunnel tests demonstrated a synergistic interaction of PBO and deltamethrin on roof netting against susceptible *An. gambiae* and both susceptible and resistant *Cx. quinquefasciatus* relative to netting from side panels treated with deltamethrin alone. This synergy was manifested in higher mortality, reduced passage through the holes and reduced feeding rates with netting treated with PBO-deltamethrin. The synergy in tunnels against pyrethroid resistant *Cx. quinquefasciatus* was progressively lost over 10 washes and fully lost after 20 washes. Cone bioassays on resistant *Cx. quinquefasciatus* confirmed the loss of synergy over 20 wash".

Sumitomo have also recently released a new LLIN (Olyset Plus®) treated with a combination of permethrin and PBO, and they claim similar increased efficacy against resistant strains of mosquitoes. However, questions do remain about the efficacy of adding PBO and its impact on the development of resistance amongst mosquitoes [35].

2.5.2. New kit: New formulation and binder for long lasting treating net

The efficacy of the long-lasting treatment kits ICON® Maxx (Syngenta) (slow release 10% capsule suspension formulation of lambdacyhalothrin + a polymer binding agent) was evaluated under laboratory conditions and in an experimental hut trial in various situations [36].

Laboratory and field trials were recently implemented in central Côte d'Ivoire, where *Anopheles gambiae* s.s. are resistant to pyrethroid insecticides [37]. In laboratory studies, classical bioassays were conducted on Kisumu SS susceptible *An. gambiae* strain, with polyester and polyethylene nets with up to 20 classical washes. Unwashed the treated polyester net resulted in 89% KD and 52% mortality while the polyethylene treated net achieved 98% KD and 46% mortality. Washing these nets had a serious negative impact on efficacy, in terms of both KD at 1 hour and mortality at 24 hours. After 20 washes, KD rates dropped to 59% with polyethylene and 55% for polyester net i.e. below the mean KD defined for LLINs by WHO Pesticide Evaluation Scheme (WHOPES) guideline (i.e. 95% after 20 washings). After 20 washes the mean mortality also decreased for both netting materials to around 20%, falling well below the WHOPES criteria for long-lasting nets (KD ≥ 95% and/ or mortality ≥ 80% for at least 20 standards WHO washes under laboratory conditions using an *An. gambiae* Kisumu-susceptible strain). Field evaluation of 2 ICON Maxx polyester treated nets and 2 untreated ones (= control) was carried out over one year in the experimental huts of M'bé. The wild *An. gambiae* population (mainly S form, 92%) used in these studies showed a high frequency of *kdr* (# 97% pyrethroid resistant heterozygotes) with 2 ICON Maxx polyester treated nets and 2 untreated one (= control). Blood feeding rate was reduced and mortality was significantly increased (70% for 8 months) in huts with treated nets even against the resistant wild *An. gambiae* population. It is worth noting this impact on insecticide resistant *An. gambiae* population and further epidemiological studies should be carried out.

2.6. New non chemical approaches of larviciding

2.6.1. New formulations of entomopathogen fungus

Laboratory and field bioassays have been implemented "to develop formulations that facilitate the application of *Metarhizium anisopliae* and *Beauveria bassiana* spores (to improve spreading) for the control of anopheline larvae [*An. gambiae* and *An. stephensi*], and also to improve their persistence under field conditions" [36]. These studies showed that the pathogenicity of dry *M. anisopliae* and *B. bassiana* spores against *An. stephensi* larvae is however too short (# 5 days) to have any application in control settings; with ShellSol T fungal spores only somewhat more persistent. In field bioassays (Western Kenya), the percentage of pupation observed in *An. gambiae* larvae treated with ShellSol T formulated spores was much lower than with unformulated treatment: 43 to 49% with *M. anisopliae* and 39 to 50% with *B. bassiana* (at 10 mg and

20 mg respectively). Bukhari et al [38] suggest that "these formulated fungi can be utilized in the field, providing additional tools for biological control of malaria vectors".

2.6.2. *Another new class of product: Spinosad*

Spinosad has been considered as "a new larvicide against insecticide-resistant mosquito larvae" [39] representing a new class of insect control products [40] and it has been tested in several trials [41].

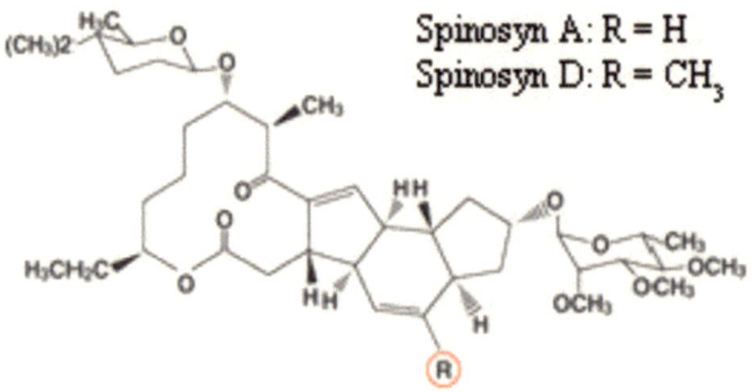

Figure 8. Two toxins of spinosad (Spinosyn A and Spinosyn D).

Spinosad is a fermented product derived from the mixture of two toxins (A and D spinosyns; Figure 8) secreted by soil based bacteria, *Saccharopolyspora spinosa*. It is traditionally used for crop protection [36] against pest insects. In the European Union, the active substance is included in Annex I to Directive 91/414/EEC by Directive 2007/6/EC and the rate of the pesticide residues in food is regulated in Europe. In France, the active substance is authorized for use in approved market products.

Spinosad acts on the nervous system of insects, by external contact or ingestion. It induces involuntary muscle contractions, prostration with tremors and paralysis. An insect stops feeding and paralysis may occur within minutes after ingestion of the product, death ensuing within one to three days. Spinosad has low toxicity to mammals, birds, fish and crustaceans but it is highly toxic to bees and aquatic invertebrates [42]. Spinosad (Group 5 insecticide) when used as a larvicide could be considered in rotation with another insecticide from a different class of pesticides.

Laboratory larval bioassays of spinosad on *Aedes aegypti*, *Cx. quinquefasciatus*, and *An. gambiae* (specimens that were either susceptible or resistant to pyrethroids, carbamates, and organophosphates) have shown that this product has a lethal action (mortality after 24 h of exposure) regardless of the original status, susceptible or resistant, of the mosquito larvae and was significantly more effective against *An. gambiae* than against the two other species and more effective against *Cx. quinquefasciatus* than *Ae. aegypti* [39] (Table2).

http://dx.doi.org/10.5772/56258

species	status	LC_{50}	LC_{100}
An. gambiae	SS	0.01	0.032
	RR (*Kdr*)	0.011	0.073
Cx. quinquefasciatus	SS	0.093	0.49
	RR (Ace-1^R)	0.12	0.59
Ae. aegypti	SS	0.35	0.92
	RR (*Kdr*)	0.32	0.72

Table 2. LC50 and LC100 of spinosad for *An. gambiae*, *Cx. quinquefasciatus*, and *Ae. aegypti* (SS, homozygote susceptible, RR: homozygote resistant).

Several other studies showed the potential of this bioinsecticide against different genera and species of mosquitoes [41, 43-44]. Different concentrations of spinosad were tested against larval instar and pupa of *An. stephensi* [45]. It was observed that "the reduction percentage of *Anopheles* larvae was 82.7%, 91.4% and 96.0% after 24, 48, 72 hours, respectively, while more than 80% reduction was observed after 3 weeks". A CS Spinosad formulation was tested in classical laboratory bioassays and successfully used for the control of *Ae. aegypti* and *An. albimanus* larvae in Mexico [46]. A spinosad shows an absence of cross resistance with insecticides commonly used in Public Health and it may be an interesting product to integrate into vector borne diseases control strategies where vectors are resistant to current insecticides.

3. Other new paradigms

3.1. Slow Acting Product (SAP) — Entomopathogens fungus

A completely new paradigm in vector control would be *slow acting* products called «Late Life Acting products » [47]. As malaria parasite sporogonic development last at least 10 days, any product which kills mosquito vectors within that time frame will automatically reduce the number of infected vectors and therefore almost certainly also reduce *Plasmodium* inoculation rates.

Formulated as biopesticides, fungal entomopathogens may have a great potential for application in indoor residual spraying of house wall surfaces or other resting places in human or animal dwellings. Once infected the fungus physically proliferates within the insect and results in the production of various secondary metabolites that have negative impacts on insect physiology [48-49] and performance and eventual death [50]. Histopathological studies of tissues infected by fungus suggest that the insect dies due to the combination of nutrient depletion, mechanical damage, and toxicosis. These biopesticides, if they can be successfully applied, could be useful for malaria control [51-52] especially if they prove effective against insecticide-resistant mosquitoes [53-55].

3.1.1. *Entomopathogen fungus on clay*

In recent trials [56] adult females of *An. stephensi* mosquitoes were exposed with cone tests to clay tiles sprayed with an oil formulation of spores of the entomopathogenic fungus *Beauveria bassiana* using different concentrations or time of exposure. A mortality rate of 100% was observed in less than one week, even when no KD effect was observed.

In addition to reducing longevity, it was noticed that fungal infection also reduces feeding propensity and fecundity [56-57] which added to the reduction of longevity could have a significant impact on vectorial capacity and therefore also on malaria transmission. Blanford et al [56] showed that "fungal exposed mosquitoes showed a declining response to the feeding stimulus over time, with 77, 60 and 50% of mosquitoes initiating feeding behaviors on days 1, 2 and 3, respectively and no mosquitoes responding on day 4. Combining the proportion of mosquitoes alive with the proportion attempting to feed gives a measure of overall transmission blocking (biting risk) on any given day. For treated mosquitoes, this combination of pre-lethal and lethal effects revealed reductions in biting risk of 36, 52, 72 and 100% on days 1–4, respectively. This represents complete transmission blocking within a feeding cycle".

Fungal infection was also observed to have a negative impact on flight performance which may be an important consideration for malaria control at focal level. Another very important character of entomopathogen fungus is its ability to control insecticide resistant mosquito strains. Exposure to the fungal biopesticide on clay tiles using the standard dose and a 30 minute-exposure period before classical bioassay (WHO cone test) of colonies of 3 species, *An. gambiae s.s.*, *An. arabiensis* and *An. funestus*, (ranging from fully susceptible to resistant to DDT, and/or Bendiocarb, and/or Malathion, and/or Deltamethrin) showed 100% mortality by day 6 irrespective of mosquito species or the level of resistance to insecticides. Blanford et al. [56] who reported that "the *An. gambiae* colony "TONGS", which was fully resistant to all chemical classes, had an Median Lethal Time (MLT) of 4 (3.93–4.07) days and all individuals were dead by day 5 (± 0.0) which was not dissimilar to the fully susceptible *An. gambiae* colony "SUA" which had an MLT of 4 (3.82–4.18) days and were all dead by day 6 "(±0.25)". It clearly appeared that "insecticide resistance confers no cross resistance to fungal pathogens in the key African malaria vectors" and this point must be taken into account in the management of insecticide resistance. For Blanford et al [56] "what is striking here is that when the effects of blood feeding are added in, risk of malaria transmission is essentially reduced to zero within a day of fungal exposure and never recovers".

3.1.2. *Entomopathogen fungus on nets*

Howard et al [58] implemented several classical tube bioassays to compare the fungal-susceptibility of an insecticide-resistant (VKPER) and insecticide-susceptible strain (SKK) of *An. gambiae* and test the activity (and longevity) of *M. anisopliae* and *B. bassiana* conidia on white polyester netting (Table 3). It appeared that *M. anisopliae* and *B. bassiana* significantly increased mortality of both resistant and susceptible strains of *An. gambiae* exposed to 2 or 7 days after treatment of nets (Table 3). *B. bassiana* was significantly more pathogenic than *M. anisopliae* both for SKK and VKPER (Table 3). The insecticide-resistant mosquito strain VKPER was significantly more susceptible to fungal infection than the SKK strain after exposure to 2 or 7 days after treatment of nets (table) while other studies did not find any difference in efficacy of dry conidia of *B. bassiana* on resistant or susceptible strain. It is possible that the discrepancies in data could be due to the mode of formulation of conidia (dry or ShellSol T suspensions in this study). The mosquito pathogenicity was maintained seven days after net application, but the viability of the two fungal species after seven days at 27°C was low, 62% and 2% respectively, for *B. bassiana* and *M. anisopliae,* hampering their practical application in LLINs.

		Days after treatment	
Fungus	*An. gambiae* strain	2	7
M. anisopliae	SKK	3.2	2.6
	VKPER	17.1	29.9
B. bassiana	SKK	11.0	7.4
	VKPER	32.2	43.5

Table 3. Comparison of mortality rates of fungal-susceptibility (*M. anisopliae* and *B. bassiana*) between an insecticide-resistant (VKPER) and insecticide-susceptible strain (SKK) of *Anopheles gambiae*.

Trials of entomopathogen fungus on mosquitoes have generated various results according to the protocol followed: formulation of fungus (dry/suspension); substrata (mud wall, cloth etc); field/lab trials; doses, exposure times; species of fungus; species/strain of mosquitoes, etc. Of note, Howard et al [58] successfully demonstrated the efficacy of nets treated with *B. bassiana* and tested against a resistant strain of *An. gambiae*. Even though the residual efficacy duration was short, the authors logically concluded that "Field trials over a longer trial period need to be carried out to see if wild insecticide-resistant mosquitoes are as susceptible as the colony strain used in this trial". Further studies, against resistant *An. gambiae* VKPER strain showed that "*B. bassiana* infection caused significantly increased mortality with the daily risk of dying being increased by 2.5 × for fungus-exposed mosquitoes compared to control mosquitoes. However, the virulence of the *B. bassiana* conidia decreased with increasing time spent exposed to the tropical field conditions, the older the treatment on the net, the lower the fungus-induced mortality rate. This is likely to be due to the tropical climate because laboratory trials found no such decline within the same trial time period. Conidial viability also decreased with increasing exposure to the net and natural abiotic environmental conditions. After 20 days field exposure the conidial viability was 30%, but the viability of control conidia not exposed to the net or field conditions was 79%" [59].

3.1.3. Influence of temperature

Kikankie et al [55] did several trials "to assess the susceptibility of insecticide-susceptible ("MBN") and resistant ("SENN") laboratory strains and wild-collected *An. arabiensis* to infection with the fungus *B. bassiana* under two different laboratory temperature regimes (21 ± 1°C or 25 ± 2°C)".

It appeared that exposure to dry *B. bassiana* spores resulted in significant reductions in longevity of the wild *An. arabiensis* mosquitoes and virulence was significantly higher at 25°C than 21°C, and exposure to *B. bassiana* spores resulted in significant reductions in longevity in all mosquito colonies regardless of their insecticide susceptibility levels and temperature regimes. Fungal susceptibility was not affected by resistance to insecticides.

It was also noted that "fungus-induced mortality rates were relatively rapid at 25°C, with 100% mortality taking 10-12 days post-fungus exposure in the baseline colonies (MBN and SENN) and field-collected mosquitoes" i.e. a lapse of time shorter than the duration of the sporogonic cycle of *P. falciparum* at this temperature, an important element for actual reduction of malaria transmission through vector control.

3.1.4. Influence of physiological stage and age

Mnyone et al [60] conducted bioassays using fed and unfed adult females of *An. gambiae* maintained in colony for several years with two fungal isolates: *M. anisopliae* and *B. bassiana* I93-825. Mosquitoes were exposed to conidia for 6 hours, with a follow up of 28 days. To study the effect of age, "three different age groups of female mosquitoes were exposed to both fungal isolates (2–4 days, 5–8 days, and 9–12 days post emergence), whereas to study the effect of physiological stage, five groups with differing blood-feeding status were exposed to both fungal isolates (non-fed, 3, 12, 36, or 72 h post-blood feeding). Results showed that, with both fungus, "older mosquitoes died relatively earlier than younger ones" and "blood-fed mosquitoes had a lower risk of dying relative to unfed ones". Increased risk of death in older than younger individuals has also been reported elsewhere [61-62]. Mnyone et al [60] considered that "the fact that blood-fed mosquitoes are less susceptible to fungal infection could be beneficial in terms of evolution proofing against resistance development. Although fungal infection reduces the fecundity of female mosquitoes [57], they are still able to pass their genes to the subsequent generation reducing selection pressure on resistance against fungi [55]. Furthermore, fungal infections suppress the successful development of *Plasmodium* parasites in the vectors [51], and hence both effects (i.e., fungus-induced mortality and parasite resistance) lead to a significantly reduced parasite transmission risk".

3.2. Attractive Toxic Sugar Bait (ATSB) methods

Recent studies on sugar feeding behavior of *Anopheles* [63-73] have been conducted in order "to optimize strategies for malaria vector control in Africa using attractive toxic sugar bait methods" [74] and to develop a new approach for mosquito control [75-78]. Stone et al [79] developed "an effective indoor mesocosm for studying populations of *An. gambiae* in temperate climates" and used the mesocosm concept to "determine whether the sugar-or-blood meal choice of *An. gambiae* females one day after emergence is influenced by blood-host presence and accessibility, nectariferous plant abundance, and female size" [80].

Stone et al. [80] noted that with a sleeping human present in the mesocosm, the majority of one day-old females obtained a blood meal. This was the case even with treated mosquito net use. But when a blood host was not present, or access was restricted through the use of a net, sugar meals became more frequent. The feeding choices of female *An. gambiae* were determined to a great degree by the presence and accessibility of the blood host, and not by the abundance of potential nectar sources in the mesocosm. Concerning the use of sugar baits as a malaria vector control, the strong tendency to feed on blood, even at one day post-emergence, suggests that in areas where larval development sites are close to human habitations, the method may be useful mainly as a complement to mosquito nets. If larval development sites are located at considerable distance from humans, the dominance of blood feeding is a smaller issue. Though females are willing to feed on humans as early as 24 h after emergence, in nature they may not come into contact with humans that early, and attraction to sugar sources would be paramount. Males and small females are particularly likely to seek a sugar meal when access to blood hosts is restricted by mosquito nets, suggesting that a plant-based method may be an effective control tool for such endgame scenarios. The combination of sugar baits (for instance, placed indoors or near a house) and treated mosquito nets, is one of these options. Its feasibility will require bait substantially more attractive than the plant species used in this experiment, such as the one used in Mali [78].

Based on highly successful demonstrations in Israel [75-77, 81] that attractive toxic sugar bait (ATSB) methods can decimate local populations of mosquitoes, Muller et al [78] implemented a study "to determine the effectiveness of ATSB methods for malaria vector control in the semi-arid Bandiagara District of Mali, West Africa". The *Anopheles* vector population was mainly composed of *An. gambiae* s.l. (mainly *An. gambiae* s.s. 86% and *An. arabiensis* 14%) and *An. funestus* [82]. The *Attractive Sugar Bait* (ASB) was composed, among other, by Guava (30%) (*Psidium guajava*) and honey melons (30%) (*Cucumis melo*) highly present in the area of the trial and known to be attractive for *An. gambiae s.l.* [83] while "ATSB was made by adding the boric acid [84-85] 1% (W/V) to ASB liquid". The ASB (in "control areas") and ATSB (in "treated areas") solutions were sprayed on the vegetation around the ponds and rice paddies and mosquitoes collected by CDC Light Traps at fixed positions between the ponds, during the 38 days of the trial, implemented at the end of the peak of malaria transmission period. It was observed that "ATSB treatment reduced densities of female and male *An. gambiae* s.l. by about 90%. After spraying ATSB in the treatment site, population densities of female and male *An. gambiae* s.l. declined rapidly over a week and then stabilized at low levels"; this impact on males is worth underlining as it could have an impact on decreased fertilized females and therefore on progeny. Furthermore, "ATSB treatment correspondingly affected the longevity of female *An. gambiae* s.l."

According to their data, Müller et al [78] considered that "ATSB methods differ from, and potentially complement, LLIN and IRS methods. In terms of malaria vector control in Africa, the ATSB methods when used operationally will likely reduce both total numbers of recently emerged female anophelines before they enter houses to feed on humans, and the proportion of females exiting houses to oviposit and then returning to houses to re-feed on humans. It is likely that ATSB approaches could soon be added as a major component of Integrated Vector Management (IVM) based malaria vector control programs" [86-88].

Along with their studies in Mali on the attractiveness of various local plants, fruits, flowers to mosquitoes *versus* human scents, Müller et al [83] noticed a very interesting "different rhythm of attractivity as plants showed peaks of *An. gambiae* s.l. attraction between 19:30-22:00 and 04:00-05:00, which differed considerably from the response to human odors, which peaked at around midnight". The well-known local *Acacia macrostachya* and *Acacia albida* (Fabaceae) appeared very attractive, and *Hyptis suaveolens* (Lamiaceae) appeared highly repellent.

It is clear that a great lot of questions still remain to be solved about ATSB such as, among others: What is the side effect of spraying vegetation on non-target fauna? What is the actual epidemiological efficacy in various epidemiological settings? Which attractant is the best in different ecological and entomological conditions? Which "toxin" is the most effective in various entomological conditions? And should it be used inside as well as outside and following which method and what about the acceptability and actual community participation, etc?

Nevertheless ATSB is another interesting approach worth further study for potential use, in complement to other classical methods such as IRS and LLIN, to reduce the number and the longevity of vectors i.e. malaria transmission and hence incidence of parasite infection and malaria morbidity.

3.3. New mathematical modeling of impacts of vector control

Since Roos and Macdonald, many mathematical models have been developed [89-90] for example (Figure 9):

- to evaluate the influence of environmental variables (climate, rain, relative humidity etc) [91];
- to facilitate the mathematicians to further develop suitable models and help the biologists and public health personnel to adopt better understanding of the modeling strategies to control the disease [92];
- to evaluate the potential mortality impact achievable by different long lasting, insecticide-treated net delivery strategies [93];
- to develop "a novel, convenient and versatile method to model *Plasmodium falciparum* infection that accounts for the essential in-host processes: parasite replication and its regulation by innate and adaptive immunity" [94];
- to improve malaria elimination strategies in areas where data are still scarce or not fully reliable [95];
- to develop a flexible and user-friendly *website* with an online mathematical model of malaria elimination that is being developed interactively with end users [96]; the website can be accessed at http://www.tropmedres. ac/elimination (see Malaria Elimination Model. http://elimination.tropmedres.ac and Internet Model of Malaria Elimination User Guide http://www.tropmedres.ac/images/modelling/userguide.pdf;
- to inform resistance management practices [97] determining the impact of different mosquito control intervention strategies including the protection conferred by mosquito nets [98];

- to develop new approaches such as the idea of evolution-proof insecticide [99-100].

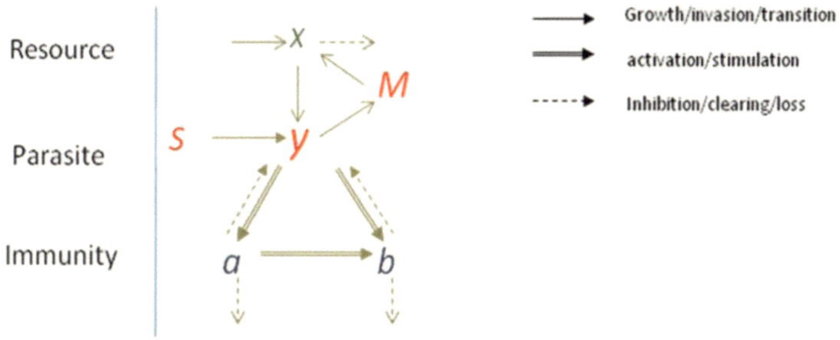

Figure 9. Schematic representation of model. The population of uninfected red blood cells (x) provides the source for the infected population (y). Level I immune effector (a) is stimulated by y. Level II immune effector (b) is stimulated by y interacting with a+b. M represents the number of merozoites, S represents an external source of inoculation

Mathematical models are useful in exposing what may otherwise be non-intuitive results, for example indoor residual spray (IRS) of insecticides in conjunction with mosquito nets can show antagonism, arising via interference of their modes of action while it is generally assumed that the two tools have synergistic benefits in reducing malaria transmission [101]. However, few have considered the spread of resistance in a variable selection pressure context [102]. A mathematical model [35] was recently developed to explore the effects on mosquito populations of spatial heterogeneous deployment of insecticides, to predict changes in mosquito fitness and resistance allele frequency, to identify important parameters in the evolution of insecticide resistance, to examine the contribution of new generation long-lasting insecticidal mosquito nets, that incorporate a chemical synergist on the roof panel, in delaying insecticide resistance.

Four niches were considered:

- Insecticide free (n): it can be an area either inside or outside a household;
- Non public-health related insecticide deployment: typically insecticide use in agriculture and households. These are deployed outwith of public health mosquito control campaigns, and generally out of the control of public health officials; mosquito coils, would also be included in this class;
- Insecticide-treated mosquito nets (ITN);
- Insecticide-treated mosquito nets with synergist on the top of the net (ITN + Synergist).

It appeared that resistance spreads slower in the presence of a synergist. The effect of synergist in males and females was not strictly comparable but was overall similar. The delay in the spread of resistance caused by the synergist was not very large; however, in approximately 10% of cases the rate of allele spread was higher when the synergist was fully effective. The predicted frequency of the resistance allele under different values of k at generation 70, the predicted frequency when the synergist is inefficient ($k = 1$), is 0.11 and when is fully effective ($k = 0$) is 0.26. The synergist has only a small impact in controlling the population, but even small values of *k* will help to recover the effect of the insecticide, and this is may be the main contribution of the synergist. Nevertheless adding synergists to mosquito nets does decrease the rate at which resistance spreads in about 90% of scenarios. If a fully effective synergist ($k = 0$) is present, the fitness of all genotypes inside the house will be zero (*k* affects the 3 genotypes equally, so all mosquitoes die irrespective of their genotype) and the next generation will be mostly composed by progeny of survivors from the niche outside the household where selection for resistance was high. One hypothesis is that in this particular case the synergist removes the refugia of weak selection in the house thereby magnifying the effects of selection for resistance outside the house.

According to Barbosa and Hastings [35], "The finding that a situation can arise in which having a fully effective synergist in place contributes to intensify the spread of resistance is the most interesting result of this work, a very important fact often overlooked in modeling resistance: that it is highly dangerous to consider selection in only a single niche, isolated from other selection pressures, and to then extrapolate the results from the single niche to the whole population. In this case it seems reasonable to conclude that adding effective synergists will reduce selection for resistance in the household niche because all three genotypes are killed. The level of impact that a fully effective synergist could have on disease transmission is a question that cannot be directly answered by the results presented here, because it is not clear how the genetic concept of fitness translates into the demographic factors, such as mosquito population size and longevity that determine the intensity of disease transmission. On the other hand, as noted above, if synergist throws most of the selection pressure onto another niche then overall the rate of selection for resistance may increase. Consequently the impact of the use of insecticide within the home (predominantly as wall sprays and/or mosquito nets) on mosquitoes cannot easily be isolated from other insecticide applications that mosquitoes may encounter during their lifetime. This suggests that the malaria community is correct in being alarmed at the often uncontrolled use of insecticides in applications such as agriculture".

Ghani et al [103] developed a very interesting model to consider the possibility that a large reduction in malaria transmission may result in a loss of immunity, and how useful integrated malaria control measures could be to counterbalance such an eventuality. They prepared "a mathematical model for malaria transmission which incorporates the acquisition and loss of both clinical and parasite immunity", to "explore the impact of the trade-off between reduction in exposure and decreased development of immunity on the dynamics of disease following a transmission-reducing intervention such as insecticide treated nets". It is worth noticing how their model "predicts that initially rapid reductions in clinical disease incidence will be observed as transmission is reduced in a highly immune population. However, these benefits in the first 5–10 years after the intervention may be offset by a greater burden of disease decades later as immunity at the population level is gradually lost. The negative impact of having fewer immune individuals in the population can be counterbalanced either by the implementation of highly-effective transmission-reducing interventions (such as the combined use of insecticide-treated nets and insecticide residual sprays) for an indefinite period, or the concurrent use of a pre-erythrocytic stage vaccine or prophylactic therapy in children to protect those at risk from disease as immunity is lost in the population".

One of the key issues is the still current lack of sound knowledge about "malaria immunity" called "premunition" which involves immunity against the parasite, and therefore against the disease. For Ghani et al [103] "Clinical immunity develops over time dependent on the force of infection in the population and reduces the probability that an individual will develop clinical disease. Parasite immunity develops as individuals' age, and reduces the amount of time spent in the asymptomatic patent infection state (mimicking a reduction in parasite density and hence onward infectiousness)". Their previous model "suggests that the loss of both clinical and parasite immunity occurs over a period of years rather than weeks or months" [104] and according to a study in Madagascar, it seems that "immunity" could be of long duration [105]. In their model, Ghani et al [103] "assume that clinical immunity is developed at a rate proportional to the EIR in each setting and has a half-life of approximately 7 years and that parasite-clearance immunity has a half-life of approximately 14 years". They consider that 3 phrases are crucial: sustain intervention/integrated measures/sustain financial support and "Sustaining both control interventions and effective case management for many years, possibly decades, should remain the primary goal of all intervention programmes and it is essential that these long-term goals are matched with financial commitments".

3.4. New ecological care

Special attention is now devoted to the environment, especially environmental modifications that may result because of the impact of insecticides on the environment and its biodiversity.

3.4.1. Environmental Risk Assessment (ERA) and Insect Pest Management IPM

No pesticide is completely safe. Only through their careful use are we able to gain an understanding of the risks and control them. The environmental impact of biocides is generally studied in the context of scientific investigations conducted beyond the regulatory requirements for approval. This helps to generate better understanding of the biocides and provides opportunity to assess their potential impact and overall effectiveness when used in various control strategies. Although vector control methods are generally confined to urban and suburban areas, these areas may have a significant vegetation cover that provides both refuge and food for wildlife (insects, reptiles, birds, bats etc)...). This shows the need of environmental risk assessments prior to large scale vector control interventions. It also highlights the need for further studies to determine direct, indirect short and long-term potential effects. Risk assessment of control methods must be addressed in an integrated strategy taking into account the relationships between species in regards of the local biodiversity. In fact, environmental risk assessment of these treatments cannot be limited only to consider information on hazards, such as acute toxicity of the biocides used. Every effort needs to be made to minimize the use of chemical pesticides. A great deal of improvement can be made in vector control programs if the existing, methods and materials are more effectively used. The idea of integrated vector control which effectively combines a package of appropriate control methods i.e. insecticidal, environmental, biological and physical, in an orderly and coordinated manner can impact upon insect vectors and diseases with positive results of economic, ecological and sociological consequences [106].

Programs based on Insect Pest Management (IPM) must be designed to reduce vector bites and disease transmission, but also mitigate any potentially negative effects, i.e., such as environmental damage, harm of non-target organisms exposed to insecticides, or increase of insecticide resistant in target organisms [107]. Such programs do already exist notably in the USA (for example in Santa Barbara County) and in Australia [108]. In these programs, process are very well defined step by step: 1) vector surveillance and identification of target vector species to develop species-specific pest management strategies based on developmental and behavioral considerations for each species; 2) threshold measures to determine when action is necessary; 3) public education, control, prevention; 4) monitoring of efficacy and environmental impacts to identify the occurrence of unexpected/unwanted effects of treatments.

3.4.2. Impact of insecticides used for vector control

The impact of insecticides on the environment depends not only on the active substance, but also the formulation and the method of applying: indoor residual spraying, space spraying or treated nets will have different impacts.

3.4.2.1. Indoor Residual Spraying (IRS)

Domestic livestock (particularly chickens) and organisms in the environment may be harmed if operations, cleanup, and disposal are not conducted according to best practices.

Table 4 describes the potential ecological effects of each recommended IRS chemical. There is a lack of data concerning toxicity of IRS insecticides on non-target fauna. However, most insecticides are highly toxic for aquatic and terrestrial arthropods like bees (in particular pyrethroid), and some of them can also be toxic for mammals (some pyrethroids and organophosphates).

3.4.2.2. Space spraying and larviciding

Space spraying has only occasionally been used in malaria epidemic control program and as a complementary measure against exophilic vectors. Nevertheless, pyrethroids, which have a short remanence, have been the predominant insecticides [123], and then care must be taken to avoid applications near fish-bearing water bodies. It is also recommended that such applications should not be carried out directly over water bodies and that a no-treated barrier of 100 m should be maintained to prevent fish mortality. Home owners should be advised to cover domestic fish tanks and bird cages during the applications [123].

Blom [124] examined the effects of aerial, barrier, and ground based ultra-low volume (ULV) sprays with sumithrin and deltamethrin, in Massachusetts on non-target insects. Malaise traps, targeting the flying insect population, were collected in regular intervals before and after sprays, then the captured insects were sorted by order and counted. The results have shown little effect on non-target insects from the ground based sprays, and a temporary knockdown from the aerial spray. However, Coleoptera were affected in the short term by the ULV sprays and, suffered long term effects from aerial spraying.

IRS insecticides	Mammal	Bird	Fish	Aquatic invertebrate	Bee	References
α-cypermethrin	0	0	++	++	++	[109]
Bendiocarb	0	0	+	+	++	[110]
Bifenthrin	+	+	++	++	++	[111], [112]
Cyfluthrin	+	0	++	++	++	[113]
DDT	+	+	++	++	+	[114]
Deltamethrin	+	0	++	++	++	[115]
Etofenprox	0	0	+	+	++	[116], [112]
Fenitrothion	0	+	0	++	++	[117]
λ-cyhalothrin	+	0	++	++	++	[118]
Malathion	+	+	0	++	++	[119], [120], [112]
Pirimiphos-methyl	++	0	++	++	++	[121], [112]
Propoxur	++	++	++	++	++	[122]

Key: 0: non-toxic; +: potentially toxic; ++: highly toxic

Table 4. Toxicity of chemicals used for IRS on non-target organisms

Davis and Peterson [125] assessed long-term impacts of permethrin on non-target terrestrial arthropods after repeat ULV applications in the context of West Nile Virus Management in the USA. The authors concluded that although small flying insects that were active at the same time as mosquitoes were slightly impacted, effects on non-target arthropods exposed to adulticides applied via ULV sprayer would be small in the ecosystem studied.

Several classes of recommended larvicides are used in vector control management such as: the bio-insecticides (*Bacillus thuringiensis* var. *israelensis (Bti)*, *Bacillus sphaericus* (*Bs*) and spinosad), the organophosphates (chlorpyrifos, fenthion, pirimiphos-methyl, and temephos), and the insect growth regulators (diflubenzuron, methoprene, pyriproxyfen). The results of some studies concerning the environmental risk assessment of these larvicides are summarized in the Table 5.

3.4.2.3. Treated net

Long-Lasting Insecticide-Treated Nets (LLINs) have many important advantages as there is no need for re-treatment, the insecticide consumption is reduced, and release of insecticide in natural water bodies during washing is also reduced [142]. However, there is considerable misuse of mosquito nets for drying fish and fishing, in particular along Lake Victoria [143]. In their study, Minakawa et al. [143] surveyed 7 fishing villages along the lake and estimated that 239 LLIN were used for fishing and drying fish from the 1040 LLINs distributed by NGO in these villages. This could have an impact on aquatic organisms while the net are immersed into the lake water. On the other hand, LLIN can also moderately impact non-target household

Larvicides	Mammal	Bird	Fish	Aquatic invertebrate	Bee	References
Bti and *Bs*	0	0	0	0[a]	0	[126]
Spinosad	0	0	0	++	++	[127-129]
Chlorpyrifos	+	++	++	++	++	[130]
Fenthion	++	++	++	++	++	[131-132]
Pirimiphos-methyl	++	0	++	++	++	[133-134]
Temephos	+	0	+	+	++	[135-136]
Diflubenzuron	0	0	+	+	+	[137-139]
Methoprene	0	0	0	++	+	[134]
Pyriproxyfen	+	0	+	++	+	[140-141]

Key: 0: non-toxic; +: potentially toxic; ++: highly toxic

[a] In some cases non-target Nematocera such as Chironomidae can be impacted by *Bti*, depending on the dose and the formulations applied (Boisvert and Lacoursière, 2004)[126].

Table 5. Toxicity of larvicides chemicals on non-target organisms

pests such as house fly, American cockroach, head louse, and mosquito bug after 30-min exposure [144].

3.4.3. *Environmental management*

Mosquitoes breed in shallow-water habitats, so it is not surprising that most environmental management interventions for malaria control are associated with the manipulation of wetland environments. If applied correctly, these strategies can have very good results by modifying vector-breeding habitats [145]. But these habitats can include freshwater wetlands (swamps, flood plains, riverine forest, and swamp forest), mangroves, and coastal wetlands (lagoons, estuaries, and tidal mudflats) [146]. In some geographical regions, there are also semi-arid grasslands, which maintain areas of temporary flooding. Wetlands provide a wide range of ecological services including soil erosion and flood control, water purification and pollutant and nutrient retention, groundwater discharge and recharge, and provision of habitat and breeding grounds for wildlife. Disturbing wetlands through environmental management may alter the quantity and quality of the services that wetlands provide. Increasing water runoff (or, alternatively, a change in the composition or clearing of wetland vegetation by drainage or clearing vegetation) may also decrease the ability of the wetland to take up pollutants, potentially diminishing the quality of water resources. It may also cause higher peak water flows in streams and rivers during rain events, resulting in flood damage. Vegetation clearance may also decrease spawning ground for aquatic species and decrease breeding habitats for migratory birds and animals [147].

Larvivorous fish (such as *Gambusia*) are often introduced for biological control. However, the introduction of exotic fish species into the natural environment (e.g., wetlands and marshes) could disrupt existing predator–prey relationships and alter ecosystem composition. In some cases, the introduction of *Gambusia* has led to the destruction of native fish [145].

3.4.4. Methodological approach for ERA in the context of vector control

Measurements of toxicity based on the impact of a chemical on a species of interest, such as the LC_{50} (concentration that kills 50% of a population), and the no observable effect concentration for reproduction, are used extensively in determining ecological risk. But these methods are too simplistic to establish relationship between the results obtained and the response observed [148] and are not always representative of real life settings. As a consequence, new assessment methodologies to predict and anticipate the risks associated with new chemicals, and improve knowledge about existing chemicals are needed. The last decade has seen some development in this area, but there have been very few studies on the effects of large scale vector control published [149]. Recently, indirect effects of *Bti* treatments on birds such as house martins *Delichon urbicum* have been shown via measuring impact on their insect food sources [150]. In this study, the authors have measured foraging rates and chick diet and have shown that clutch size and fledgling survival were significantly lower at treated sites relative to control. Their hypothesis is that intake of Nematocera (Diptera) and their predators (spiders and dragonflies) decreased significantly in the sites treated with *Bti*, hindering the breeding success of the house martins. Another study on *Bti* monitored Chironomidae populations [151] in three wetlands treated with *Bti*-treatment to control mosquitoes, and three untreated wetlands. Results showed no reduced production of chironomids in *Bti*-treated as compared to untreated wetlands. However, the same authors [152] identified possible indirect effects of *Bti*-treatments in a further study that showed a higher specific richness of chironomids in treated wetlands, compared to control wetlands. They hypothesized that this was the result of reduced competition from mosquito larvae.

These studies demonstrate the need for more suitable methodologies and protocols to be developed for long-term monitoring of ecosystems. Several studies in Europe have monitored long term mosquito control effects, including programmes efforts in western France [153-154], and another in Ramsar area of southern France [155] where the Life-Environment European Program has been studying methods for the sustainable management of mosquito control. The French Ministry for Ecology, Sustainable Development and Spatial Planning via the National Programme for Ecotoxicology (PNETOX; APR2003) are studying the harmonisation of mosquito control methods in terms of their impact on non-target invertebrates in Mediterranean and Atlantic coastal wetlands [156].

A Life-Environment project, sustained by the European Commission, called "Control of noxious or vector mosquitoes: implementation of integrated management consistent with sustainable development (IMCM/n° n°LIFE08 ENV/F/000488)" is also under way in France. Its objective is to validate integrated methodologies and techniques allowing (1) a precise and up to date knowledge of target species' presence, biology, colonized habitats, using GIS/GPS tools, (2) the development of control methods fully appropriate to the health and environmental risks faced, (3) an evaluation of nuisance thresholds based on knowledge of social demands through sociological surveys, in order to optimise the communication strategies, (4) traceability of operations by means of retrospective and prospective analyses, and (5) the adoption of valid procedures and methodologies for the monitoring of the non-intentional effects on Man and the environment that can result from these control methods. This project will implement these decision-making tools with five public bodies that are involved in mosquito control efforts in Metropolitan France (Entente InterDepartementale pour la Démoustication du Littoral méditerranéen, EID Méditerranée, Entente InterDépartementale Rhône-Alpes pour la démoustication, EID Rhône-Alpes, General Council of Southern Corsica) and overseas (General Councils of Martinique and Guyana). The project prioritises environmental care and uses complementary methods for environmental risk assessment (in aquatic and terrestrial compartments) for mosquito control methods in temperate or tropical zones. All these projects have focused on consideration of the indirect possible effects of mosquito control on the invertebrates' communities in order to preserve the local biodiversity and endangered species. These projects have highlighted the importance of using methodologies adapted to the habitats and specific organisms, with relevant bio-indicators, implemented infield settings that represent the context in which the vector control management is to be undertaken. The studies also underlined the necessity of post-approval monitoring of the insecticides used in vector control management.

4. Conclusion — Discussion

The history of vector control for malaria control can roughly be divided in 3 main periods: before DDT: from general control to "eradication"; the DDT era and the "Malaria Eradication Programme" (MEP); after DDT: insecticide treated nets (ITN-LLIN), Integrated Vector Management (IVM) and new paradigms.

4.1. Before DDT

Since his discovery of the role of mosquito as vector of malaria parasite, Ross advocated the vector control for malaria control and in 1899, in Sierra-Leone; he "carried out the first project based on his discovery. His principal weapon was "illuminating oil" (kerosene)". It "was a transient success" not sustained due to lack of funds [157]. "In 1907 Ross was invited to Mauritius to organize antimalaria operations there. His recommendations were sound and the results were good if the government had given them more support" (Bruce-Chwatt, loc.cit.). It is interesting to underline some of the main issues observed at that time: the lack of financial and political support and the financial support is still matter of concerns when referring to the recent RBM statement. The greatest and most successful programme was malaria control in the Panama Canal zone by Gorgas [158] who, helped by Joseph Le Prince, successfully planned and implemented "*sanitation measures*" based on the principle to deal with the situation by all available means based on the role of mosquitoes. He could be therefore considered as the actual precursor of IVM.

Still underlined by Bruce-Chwatt (loc. Cit) "among the early projects one carried out by Malcolm Watson in Malaya deserves special mention, because of the ingenious combination of open and subsoil-drainage with naturalistic methods of control of *Anopheles* [159]. These measures were adapted to the behavioral characteristics of malaria in a given area and formed the basis for the concept of *"species sanitation"* [160].

After the success of Watson, several other "naturalistic methods" were developed such as altering the salinity of breeding site of *An. ludlowae* control in Indonesia, introduction of natural enemies of mosquitoes, use of *Gambusia* in California, Florida, then in Cyprus, Spain, Italy, Russia, Chile, etc [161].

Some of the best example of environmental modifications based upon drainage for successful malaria control were observed in Italy with reclamation of marshy areas (with resettlement of population in new land) for *"bonifica integrale"* of Pontine Marshes of the Roman Campagna [162-164] or Algeria in the marshy area of Mitidja Plaine [165-166].

Such programs could also be considered as precursor in the field of biological control which currently received great attention with the ecological issues of insecticide and insecticide resistance of main vectors.

In term of chemical control, 2 schools of thought were opposed: larva control, based upon Paris Green dust successfully used in Sardinia and Calabria and in several other places such as Brazil to get rid of invaders *An. gambiae* which caused severe epidemics of malaria in 1930s'; and adult control, with the use of the well known oriental daisy *Chrysanthemum cinerariaefolium*, (used for long time as fumigants in China against biting insects) the powder made of it contains powerful insecticide compounds such as pyrethrins and cinerins and as soon as 1932 Park-Ross and De Meillon instituted systematic house to house weekly sprayings of pyrethrum solution in kerosene for the control of adults *Anopheles* in Natal and Zululand and this program is somehow still ongoing with the regular inside resting spraying (with DDT) operations added to case management to control malaria in KwaZulu Natal [167]. Instead of pyrethrins, National Malaria control programme uses now pyrethroid but they are chemically developed from natural pyrethrins used formerly. Somehow history of approaches for malaria control repeats itself.

It is interesting to notice the variety of approaches and techniques involved (species sanitation, sanitation measures, bonifica integrale (reclamation of marshy area and resettlement of populations on the new land), pursued by Italian governments for many years, larval control through different measures from source reduction to Paris Greendust spraying, adult control with spray of pyrethrin, …) based on some knowledge of entomological, ecological and socio-economical situation for improvement of Public Health, control of outbreak or achievement of large constructions (dams, Panama Canal, etc). In a way these measures paved the way for new approaches developed after the failure of the Global Malaria Eradication Programme and the development of IVM with new paradigms for vector control.

4.2. The DDT era 1957 — 1969: Global malaria eradication programme

"In 1874 a Viennese student of chemistry, Othmar Zeidler, published in the Berichtungen (Proceedings) of the German Chemical Society a paper under the title "Verdindungen von

Chlral mit Brom und Chlorbenzol"; the compound described in it was DDT (Bruce-Chwatt, loc cit) but its insecticidal properties remained unknown until 1939 [168].

The first Expert Malaria Committee (Ciuca, Gabaldon, Hamilton, Fairley, Pampana, Russell) met in Geneva in 1947 to deal with "the enormous social and economic damage that malaria was causing to the developing tropical countries", Russell [169] estimating that throughout the world there were some 300 million cases of malaria every year with at least a million deaths, it is interesting to underline that such evaluation of the burden of malaria was regularly reported during the following decades. And as Bruce-Chwatt [157] rightly underlined: "this was also the time when the new concept of malaria control by imagocidal measures was stimulated by the reports of the extraordinary properties of an obscure compound synthesized 65 years before the outbreak of the Second World War. They were observed by a Swiss chemist, Müller who was looking for a substance active against clothes moths, and with the biologist Wiesmann they realized in 1939 the insecticidal properties of this product, named Gesarol or Neocid and first used in agriculture [170] then sent to USA and Britain (where it received the acronym DDT). This product presented 3 important operational properties: long persistence of residues on sprayed surfaces; high toxicity for insects and low for man; killing insects by simple contact. The advent of DDT revolutionized malaria control as the residual indoor spraying as this product appeared simple, and could be successfully and economically used even in rural areas where malaria was the worse. Actually a lot of successful campaigns were done in Sardinia (Italy) (for eradication of *An. labranchiae*), Cyprus, Greece, Venezuela, British Guiana, Bombay State, etc [171]. In 1955, Pampana and Russell [172] underlined the needs of "plans to eradicate malaria from a territory within a few years, so that eventually the recurring item of malaria control could be struck from the annual budget". And the Eighth World Health Assembly in 1955 decided "that the World Health Organization should take the initiative, provide technical advice, and encourage research and co-ordination of resources in the implementation of a programme having as its ultimate objective the world-wide eradication of malaria".

DDT appeared as a "magic bullet" but the great mistake was that the original policy relied only on the use of residual insecticide, DDT then other organochlorines (BHC, dieldrin,...) along with drug use for reducing human reservoir, with the same strategy to be implemented everywhere without taking care of biodiversity, epidemiological diversity, social, economical, entomological diversity. The basic concept was one malaria and therefore one strategy to be implemented faster than insecticide resistance spreading, already noticed in the main vectors such as *An. gambiae*. In 1956, the Ninth World Health Assembly recommended the policy of eradication and stimulation of inter-countries cooperation. The strategy was defined as "operation aimed at cessation of transmission of malaria and elimination of the reservoir of infected cases in a campaign limited in time and carried to such a degree of perfection that, when it comes to an end, there is no resumption of transmission". It was based upon 3 successive steps: "attack phase" with total coverage with inside residual spraying, then "consolidation phase" to eradicate any remaining foci after the IRS rounds, then the "maintenance phase" where the malaria eradication programme doesn't exist as such and comes under the responsibility of general health services involves in "vigilance" to check any imported cases.

http://dx.doi.org/10.5772/56258

During the following decades malaria was actually eradicated from Europe, part of Russia, Middle East, North America, Australia, Japan, Singapore, Korea, Taiwan, almost all West Indies Islands and about 53% of the population of the originally malarious areas became free of malaria. But "the magnitude of the malaria problem in Tropical Africa has been daunting" (Bruce-Chwatt, loc cit). A re-examination of the global strategy of malaria eradication was carried in the 60' and the results presented at the 22nd World Health Assembly in 1969. One of the conclusion was that "in countries where eradication does not appear to be feasible because of the inadequacy of financial resources, manpower requirements or shortcomings of basic health services, malaria control operations should move to a transitional control programme stage, with the aim of launching of an eradication programme in the future". This is political wording that recognizes the failure of the rigid Global Eradication Programme and the reality that this may translate to "malaria control" involving the use of every available effective method to tackle first malaria mortality and morbidity, rather than malaria transmission specifically, as it was targeted by the MEP.

After the illusion of the Malaria eradication came the time of pragmatism, and the recognition of the biodiversity concept with IVM which takes into account all biological but also economical, socio-cultural components of the vector-borne parasitic disease and tools available (or to be developed) to tailor vector control measures to each epidemiological settings, to reach its full efficacy in the aim of sharply reduce, then eliminating malaria steps by steps. In this concept of biodiversity, a flexible and multifaceted approach is requested and paradigms were developed accordingly. For example, it is generally considered that tools for vector control must have a quick action to kill vectors before they transmit the parasites to any other human being, but slow acting products are now envisaged considering that if life is shortening to become less than the duration of the sporogonic cycle there couldn't be any transmission of the pathogenic agent even if this takes slightly more time than the "killing" product. Another approach is to mix different products for LLIN or IRS to deal with insecticide resistance and even to join IGR usually used against larvae in product targeting adults such as insecticide paints and even LLIN. The main impact should therefore be observed in term of reducing fecundity and fertility which would impact new generations of adults and more generally *Anopheles* populations.

Nevertheless for the time being the only new tools operational for vector control at large is insecticide treated nets (ITN) currently industrialized treated to become Long Lasting nets and which clearly showed their efficacy if well used and maintained. But the field is largely open for new tools mainly dealing with insecticide, and sometimes social resistance.

A great attention is now devoted to the cultural and social aspects of vector control methods implemented from outside, the "non usage" or "mis-usage" of mosquito nets are good example of the misfit between International agencies which gave large number of LLIN free of charge and the local social acceptability or local financial constraints.

A great care is also given to ecological impact and Malaria control programme must take lessons from the large multicountries Onchocerciasis Control Programme for managing insecticide resistance and care of non targeted fauna.

We must keep in mind the sentences of late Prof Bruce-Chwatt [173]: "the present approach to the control of this disease envisages a progressive incorporation of all general and specific antimalarial activities into the primary health care structures. This opens up many possibilities for research on the use of different technical resources together with the involvement of indigenous communities. But this is a different story!".

List of abbreviations

ATSB - Attractive toxic sugar bait

ASB - Attractive Sugar Bait

C - Carbamate

CS - Microencapsulated formulation

CTN - hand treated ITN

DL - Durable wall linings

EID - Entente InterDepartementale pour la Démoustication

ERA - Environmental Risk Assessment

IGR - Insect Growth Regulator

IPM - Insect Pest Management

IRS - Indoor Residual Spraying

ITN - Insecticide Treated Nets

ITPS - Insecticide-Treated Plastic Sheeting

IVCC - Innovative Vector Control Consortium

IVM - Integrated Vector Management

KD - KnockDown

KDR - KnockDown Resistance

LC50 - median Lethal Concentration of a substance

LC100 - absolute Lethal Concentration

LiST - Lives Saved Tool

LLIN - Long-Lasting Insecticidal Net

LN - Long lasting insecticide treated Net

MEP - Malaria Eradication Programme

http://dx.doi.org/10.5772/56258

MLT - Median Lethal Time

OC - Organochlorine

OP - Organophosphate

P3 - Permanet 3

PBO - Piperonyl Butoxide

Pyr - Pyrethroid

RBM - Roll Back Malaria

SAP - Slow Acting Product

TPP - Target Product Profile

ULV - Ultra-Low Volume

UPS - Untreated Plastic Sheeting

WHO - World Health Organization

WHOPES - WHO Pesticide Evaluation Scheme

WL - Durable Wall Linings

Acknowledgements

We are grateful to Dr Kate Aultman for her helful suggestions and comments all along the writing of this document.

Author details

Claire Duchet[1,2], Richard Allan[3] and Pierre Carnevale[4]

*Address all correspondence to: pjcarnevale2001@yahoo.fr; cduchet.eid@gmail.com

1 Entente InterDépartementale de Démoustication du Littoral Méditerranéen, Montpellier, France

2 Community Ecology Laboratory, Institute of Evolution and Department of Evolutionary & Environmental Biology, University of Haifa, Israel

3 The MENTOR Initiative, Crawley, UK

4 Portiragnes, France

References

[1] WHO. Global Malaria Report –World Malaria Report. World Health Organization: Geneva; 2012.

[2] Murray CJ, Rosenfeld LC, Lim SS, Andrews KG, Foreman KJ, Haring D, Fullman N, Naghavi M, Lozano R, Lopez AD. Global malaria mortality between 1980 and 2010: a systematic analysis. Lancet Infect Dis 2012; 379: 413–31.

[3] Larsen D, Friberg I, Eisele T. Comparison of Lives Saved Tool model child mortality estimates against measured data from vector control studies in sub-Saharan Africa. BMC Public Health 2011; 11 (3): S34.

[4] WHO. Global malaria control and elimination: report of a technical review. World Health Organization: Geneva; 2009.

[5] Lengeler C, Cattani J, De Savigny D. Net gain - A new method for preventing malaria deaths. IDRC Books; 1996. 189pp.

[6] Ranson H, N'Guessan R. Lines J, Moiroux N, Nkuni Z, Corbel V. Pyrethroid resistance in African anopheline mosquitoes: what are the implications for malaria control? Trends in Parasitology 2011; 27: 91–98.

[7] Nauen R. Insecticide resistance in disease vectors of public health importance. Pest Management Science 2007; 63: 628–633.

[8] Labbé P, Alout H, Djogbénou L, Pasteur N, Weill M. Evolution of Resistance to Insecticide in Disease Vectors. Massachusetts, USA: Elsevier; 2011.

[9] Corbel V, N'Guessan R, Brengues C, Chandre F, Djogbénou L, Martin T, Akogbéto M, Hougard J, Rowland M. Multiple insecticide resistance mechanisms in *Anopheles gambiae* and *Culex quinquefasciatus* from Benin, West Africa. Acta Tropica 2007; 101: 207-16.

[10] N'Guessan R, Boko P, Odjo A, Chabi J, Akogbeto M, Rowland M. Control of pyrethroid and DDT-resistant *Anopheles gambiae* by application of indoor residual spraying or mosquito nets treated with a long-lasting organophosphate insecticide, chlorpyrifos-methyl. Malaria Journal 2010; 9: 44.

[11] N'Guessan R, Asidi A, Boko P, Odjo A, Akogbeto M, Pigeon O, Rowland M. An experimental hut evaluation of PermaNet® 3.0, a deltamethrin–piperonyl butoxide combination net, against pyrethroid-resistant *Anopheles gambiae* and *Culex quinquefasciatus* mosquitoes in southern Benin. Transactions of the Royal Society of Tropical Medicine and Hygiene 2010; 104: 758–765.

[12] Amelotti I, Catalá S, Gorla D. Experimental evaluation of insecticidal paints against *Triatoma infestans* (Hemiptera: Reduviidae), under natural climatic conditions. Parasites & Vectors 2009; 2: 30-6.

[13] Mosqueira B, Duchon S, Chandre F, Hougard J, Carnevale P, Mas-Coma S. Efficacy of an insecticide paint against insecticide-susceptible and resistant mosquitoes - part 1: laboratory evaluation. Malaria Journal 2010; 9: 340.

[14] Mosqueira B, Chabi J, Chandre F, Akogbeto M, Hougard J, Carnevale P, Mas-Coma S. Efficacy of an insecticide paint against malaria vectors and nuisance in West Africa - part 2: field evaluation. Malaria Journal 2010; 9: 341.

[15] Jones A, Sattelle D. Diversity of insect nicotinic acetylcholine receptor subunits. Advances in Experimental Medicine and Biology 2010; 683: 25-43.

[16] Wakita T, Kinoshita K, Yamada E, Yasui N, Kawahara N, Naoi A, Nakaya M, Ebihara K, Matsuno H, Kodaka K. The discovery of dinotefuran: a novel neonicotinoid. Pest Management Science 2003; 59: 1016-22.

[17] Corbel V, Duchon S, Zaim M, Hougard J. Dinotefuran: a potential neonicotinoid insecticide against resistant mosquitoes. Journal of Medical Entomology 2004; 41: 12-7.

[18] Darriet F, Chandre F. Combining piperonyl butoxide and dinotefuran restores the efficacy of deltamethrin mosquito nets against resistant *Anopheles gambiae* (Diptera: Culicidae). Journal of Medical Entomology 2011; 48: 952-5.

[19] Djènontin A, Chandre F, Dabiré K, Chabi J, N'Guessan R, Baldet T, Akogbéto M, Corbel V. Indoor use of plastic sheeting impregnated with carbamate combined with long-lasting insecticidal mosquito nets for the control of pyrethroid-resistant malaria vectors. The American Journal of Tropical Medicine and Hygiene 2010; 83: 266-70.

[20] Graham K, Mohammad N, Rehman H, Nazari A, Ahmad M, Kamal M, Skovmand O, Guillet P, Allan R, Zaim M, Yates A, Lines J, Rowland M. Insecticide-treated plastic tarpaulins for control of malaria vectors in refugee camps. Medical and Veterinary Entomology 2002; 16: 404-8.

[21] Burns M, Rowland M, N'Guessan R, Carneiro I, Beeche A, Ruiz S, Kamara S, Takken W, Carnevale P, Allan R. Insecticide-Treated Plastic Sheeting for Emergency Malaria Prevention and Shelter among Displaced Populations: An Observational Cohort Study in a Refugee Setting in Sierra Leone. The American Journal of Tropical Medicine and Hygiene 2012; 87: 242-50.

[22] Sharma S, Upadhyay A, Haque M, Tyagi P, Mohanty S, Mittal P, Dash A. Field evaluation of ZeroFly--an insecticide incorporated plastic sheeting against malaria vectors & its impact on malaria transmission in tribal area of northern Orissa. Indian Journal of Medical Research 2009; 130: 458-66.

[23] Mittal P, Sreehari U, Razdan R, Dash A. Evaluation of the impact of ZeroFly®, an insecticide incorporated plastic sheeting on malaria incidence in two temporary labour shelters in India. Journal of Vector Borne Disease 2011; 48: 138-43.

[24] Brosseau L, Drame PM, Besnard P, Toto JC, Foumane V, Le Mire J, Mouchet F, Remoue F, Allan R, Fortes F, Carnevale P, Manguin S. Human antibody response to

Anopheles saliva for comparing the efficacy of three malaria vector control methods in Balombo, Angola. PLoS One 2012; 7(9):e44189.

[25] Messenger LA, Miller NP, Adeogun AO, Awolola TS, Rowland M. The development of insecticide-treated durable wall lining for malaria control: insights from rural and urban populations in Angola and Nigeria. Malaria Journal 2012; 11:332.

[26] Messenger LA, Matias A, Manana AN, Stiles-Ocran JB, Knowles S, Boakye DA, Coulibaly MB, Larsen ML, Traoré AS, Diallo B, Konaté M, Guindo A, Traoré SF, Mulder CE, Le H, Kleinschmidt I, Rowland M. Multicentre studies of insecticide-treated durable wall lining in Africa and South-East Asia: entomological efficacy and household acceptability during one year of field use. Malaria Journal 2012; 11(1):358.

[27] Pulford J, Tandrapah A, Atkinson JA, Kaupa B, Russell T, Hetzel MW. Feasibility and acceptability of insecticide-treated plastic sheeting (ITPS) for vector control in Papua New Guinea. Malaria Journal 2012; 11:342 doi:10.1186/1475-2875-11-342.

[28] Diabate A, Chandre F, Rowland M, N'Guessan R, Duchon S, Dabire K, Hougard J. The indoor use of plastic sheeting pre-impregnated with insecticide for control of malaria vectors. Tropical Medicine & International Health 2006; 11: 597-603.

[29] Chandre F, Dabire R, Hougard J, Djogbenou L, Irish S, Rowland M, N'Guessan R. Field efficacy of pyrethroid treated plastic sheeting (durable lining) in combination with long lasting insecticidal nets against malaria vectors. Parasites & Vectors 2010; 3: 65.

[30] WHOPES. Report of the Twelfth WHOPES Working Group Meeting, Review of: Bioflash® GR, Permanet® 2.0, Permanet® 3.0, Permanet® 2.5, Lambda-cyhalothrin® LN. WHO/HTM/NTD/WHOPES/2009.

[31] Corbel V, Chabi J, Dabiré Roch K, Etang J, Nwane P, Pigeon O, Akogbeto M, Hougard J. Field efficacy of a new mosaic long-lasting mosquito net (PermaNet® 3.0) against pyrethroid resistant malaria vectors: a multi centre study in Western and Central Africa. Malaria Journal 2010; 9: 113.

[32] Tungu P, Magesa S, Maxwell C, Malima R, Masue D, Sudi W, Myamba J, Pigeon O, Rowland M. Evaluation of PermaNet 3.0 a deltamethrin-PBO combination net against *Anopheles gambiae* and pyrethroid resistant *Culex quinquefasciatus* mosquitoes: an experimental hut trial in Tanzania. Malaria Journal 2010; 9: 21.

[33] Yewhalaw D, Asale A, Tushune K, Getachew Y, Duchateau L, Speybroeck N. Bio-efficacy of selected long-lasting insecticidal nets against pyrethroid resistant *Anopheles arabiensis* from south-western Ethiopia. Parasites & Vectors 2012; 5: 159.

[34] Koudou B, Koffi A, Malone D, Hemingway J. Efficacy of PermaNet® 2.0 and PermaNet® 3.0 against insecticide-resistant *Anopheles gambiae* in experimental huts in Côte d'Ivoire. Malaria Journal 2011; 10: 172.

[35] Barbosa S, Hastings I. The importance of modeling the spread of insecticide resistance in a heterogeneous environment: the example of adding synergists to bed nets. Malaria Journal 2012; 11: 258.

[36] WHO: Report of the 11th WHOPES Working Group Meeting. Review of Spinosad 7.48% DT, Netprotect®, Duranet®, Dawaplus®, Icon® maxx. World Health Organization, Geneva, WHO/HTM/NTD/WHOPES/2008.1. 2007.

[37] Winkler M, Tchicaya E, Koudou B, Donzé J, Nsanzabana C, Müller P, Adja A, Utzinger J. Efficacy of ICON® Maxx in the laboratory and against insecticide-resistant *Anopheles gambiae* in central Côte d'Ivoire. Malaria Journal 2012; 11: 167.

[38] Bukhari T, Takken W, Koenraadt C. Development of *Metarhizium anisopliae* and *Beauveria bassiana* formulations for control of malaria mosquito larvae. Parasites & Vectors 2011; 4: 23.

[39] Darriet F, Duchon S, Hougard JM. Spinosad: a new larvicide against insecticide-resistant mosquito larvae. Journal of the American Mosquito Control Association 2005; 21: 495-496.

[40] Thompson G, Michel K, Yao R, Myderse J, Mosburg C, Worden T, Chio E, Sparks T, Hutchins S. The discovery of *Saccharopolyspora spinosa* and a new class of insect control products. Down Earth 1997; 52: 1-5.

[41] Bret B, Larson L, Shoonoever J, Sparks T, Thompson G. Biological properties of spinosad. Down Earth 1997; 2: 6-13.

[42] Duchet C, Caquet T, Franquet E, Lagneau C, Lagadic L. Influence of environmental factors on the response of a natural population of *Daphnia magna* (Crustacea: Cladocera) to spinosad and *Bacillus thuringiensis israelensis* in Mediterranean coastal wetlands. Environmental Pollution 2010; 158: 1825-1833.

[43] Romi R, Proietti S, Di Luca M, Cristofaro M. Laboratory evaluation of the bioinsecticide Spinosad for mosquito control. Journal of the American Mosquito Control Association 2006; 22: 93-6.

[44] Kumar A, Murugan K, Madhiyazhagan P, Prabhu K. Spinosad and neem seed kernel extract as bio-controlling agents for malarial vector, *Anopheles stephensi* and non-biting midge, *Chironomus circumdatus*. Asian Pacific Journal of Tropical Medicine 2011; 4: 614-8.

[45] Prabhu K, Murugan K, Nareshkumar A, Bragadeeswaran S. Larvicidal and pupicidal activity of spinosad against the malarial vector *Anopheles stephensi*. Asian Pacific Journal of Tropical Medicine 2011; 4: 610-3.

[46] Bond J, Marina C, Williams T. The naturally derived insecticide spinosad is highly toxic to *Aedes* and *Anopheles* mosquito larvae. Medical and Veterinary Entomology 2004; 18: 50-56.

[47] Read A, Lynch P, Thomas M. How to make evolution-proof insecticides for malaria control. PLoS Biol 2009; 7: e1000058.

[48] Kershaw M, Moorehouse E, Bateman R, Reynolds S, Charnley AK. The role of destruxins in the pathogenicity of *Metarhizium anisopliae* for three species of insect. Journal of Invertebrate Pathology 1999;74: 213–223.

[49] Hajek A, St Leger R. Interactions between fungal pathogens and insect hosts. Annual Review of Entomology 1994; 39: 293–322.

[50] Bell A, Blanford S, Jenkins N, Thomas M, Read A. Real-time quantitative PCR analysis of candidate fungal biopesticides against malaria: Technique validation and first applications. Journal of Invertebrate Pathology 2009; 100: 160–168.

[51] Blanford S, Chan B, Jenkins N, Sim D, Turner R. Fungal pathogen reduces potential for malaria transmission. Science 2005; 308: 1638–1641.

[52] Thomas M, Read A. Can fungal biopesticides control malaria? Nature Reviews Microbiology 2007; 5: 377–383.

[53] Farenhorst M, Mouatcho J, Kikankie C, Brooke B, Hunt R. Fungal infection counters insecticide resistance in African malaria mosquitoes. Proceedings of the National Academy of Sciences 2009; 106: 17443–17447.

[54] Farenhorst M, Knols B, Thomas M, Howard A, Takken W. Synergy of fungal entomopathogens and permethrin against West African insecticide-resistant *Anopheles gambiae* mosquitoes. PLoS One 2010; e12801.

[55] Kikankie C, Brooke B, Knols B, Koekemoer L, Farenhorst M. The infectivity of the entomopathogenic fungus *Beauveria bassiana* to insecticide-resistant and susceptible *Anopheles arabiensis* at two different temperatures. Malaria Journal 2010; 9: 71.

[56] Blanford S, Shi W, Christian R, Marden J, Koekemoer L. Lethal and Pre-Lethal Effects of a Fungal Biopesticide Contribute to Substantial and Rapid Control of Malaria Vectors. PLoS ONE 2011; 6.

[57] Scholte E, Knols B, Takken W. Infection of the malaria mosquito *Anopheles gambiae* with the entomopathogenic fungus *Metarhizium anisopliae* reduces blood feeding and fecundity. Journal of Invertebrate Pathology 2006; 91: 43–49.

[58] Howard A, Koenraadt C, Farenhorst M, Knols B, Takken W. Pyrethroid resistance in *Anopheles gambiae* leads to increased susceptibility to the entomopathogenic fungi *Metarhizium anisopliae* and *Beauveria bassiana*. Malaria Journal 2010; 9: 168.

[59] Howard A, N'Guessan R, Koenraadt C, Asidi A, Farenhorst M, Akogbéto M, Knols B, Takken W. First report of the infection of insecticide-resistant malaria vector mosquitoes with an entomopathogenic fungus under field conditions. Malaria Journal 2011; 10: 24.

[60] Mnyone L, Kirby M, Mpingwa M, Lwetoijera D, Knols B, Takken W, Koenraadt C, Russell T. Infection of *Anopheles gambiae* mosquitoes with entomopathogenic fungi:

effect of host age and blood-feeding status. Parasitological Research 2011; 108: 317–322.

[61] Harrington L, Buonaccorsi J, Edman J, Costero A, Kittayapong P, Clark G, Scott T. Analysis of survival of young and old *Aedes aegypti* (Diptera: Culicidae) from Puerto Rico and Thailand. Journal of Medical Entomology 2001; 38: 537–547.

[62] Styer L, Carey J, Wang J, Scott T. Mosquitoes do senesce: departure from the paradigm of constant mortality. The American Journal of Tropical Medicine and Hygiene 2007; 76: 111–117.

[63] Yuval B: The other habit: sugar feeding by mosquitoes. Bull. Soc. Vector Ecol 1992; 17:150-156.

[64] Foster WA. Mosquito sugar feeding and reproductive energetics. Annual Review of Entomology 1995; 40:443-474.

[65] Beier JC. Frequent blood-feeding and restrictive sugar-feeding behavior enhance the malaria vector potential of *Anopheles gambiae* s.i. and *An. funestus* (Diptera: Culicidae) in western Kenya. Journal of Medical Entomology 1996; 33:613-618.

[66] Gary RE, Foster WA. Effects of available sugar on the reproductive fitness and vectorial capacity of the malaria vector *Anopheles gambiae* (Diptera: Culicidae). Journal of Medical Entomology 2001; 38:22-28.

[67] Gary RE, Foster WA. *Anopheles gambiae* feeding and survival on honeydew and extrafloral nectar of peridomestic plants. Medical and Veterinary Entomology 2004; 18:102-107.

[68] Gary RE, Foster WA. Diel timing and frequency of sugar feeding in the mosquito *Anopheles gambiae*, depending on sex, gonotrophic state and resource availability. Medical and Veterinary Entomology 2006; 20:308-316.

[69] Foster WA, Takken W. Nectar-related vs. human-related volatiles: behavioral response and choice by female and male *Anopheles gambiae* (Diptera: Culicidae) between emergence and first feeding. Bulletin of Entomological Research 2004; 94:145-157.

[70] Müller GC, Schlein Y. Plant tissues: the frugal diet of mosquitoes in adverse conditions. Journal of Veterinary and Medical Entomology 2005; 19:413-422.

[71] Manda H, Gouagna LC, Foster WA, Jackson RR, Beier JC, Githure JI, Hassanali A. Effect of discriminative plant-sugar feeding on the survival and fecundity of *Anopheles gambiae*. Malaria Journal 2007; 6:113.

[72] Manda H, Gouagna LC, Nyandat E, Kabiru W, Jackson RR, Foster WA, Githure JI, Beier JC, Hassanali A Discriminative feeding behavior of *Anopheles gambiae* s.s. on endemic plants in Western Kenya. Medical and Veterinary Entomology 2007; 21:103-111.

[73] Gu W, Müller G, Schlein Y, Novak RJ, Beier JC. Natural plant sugar sources of *Anopheles* mosquitoes strongly impact malaria transmission potential. PLoS One 2011; 6:e15996.

[74] Müller GC, Junnila A, Schlein Y. Effective control of adult *Culex pipiens* by spraying an attractive toxic sugar bait solution in the vegetation near larval habitats. Journal of Medical Entomology 2010; 47:63-66.

[75] Schlein Y, Müller G.C. An approach to mosquito control: Using the dominant attraction of flowering *Tamarix jordanis* trees against *Culex pipiens*. Journal of Medical Entomology 2008; 45:384-390.

[76] Müller G, Schlein Y. Sugar questing mosquitoes in arid areas gather on scarce blossoms that can be used for control. International Journal for Parasitology 2006; 36:1077-1080.

[77] Müller GC, Schlein Y. Efficacy of toxic sugar baits against adult cistern dwelling *Anopheles claviger*. Transactions of Royal Society of Tropical Medicine and Hygiene 2008; 102:480-484.

[78] Müller GC, Beier JC, Traore SF, Toure MB, Traore MM, Bah S, Doumbia S, Schlein Y. Successful field trial of attractive toxic sugar bait (ATSB) plant spraying methods against malaria vectors in the *Anopheles gambiae* complex in Mali, West Africa. Malaria Journal 2010; 9: 210.

[79] Stone CM, Taylor RM, Foster WA. An effective indoor mesocosm for studying populations of *Anopheles gambiae* in temperate climates. Journal of the American Mosquito Control Association 2009; 25:514-516.

[80] Stone CM, Jackson BT, Foster WA. Effects of bed net use, female size, and plant abundance on the first meal choice (blood vs. sugar) of the malaria mosquito *Anopheles gambiae*. Malaria Journal 2012; 11:3.

[81] Müller GC, Kravchenko VD, Schlein Y. Decline of *Anopheles sergentii* and *Aedes caspius* populations following presentation of attractive, toxic (Spinosad), sugar bait stations in an oasis. Journal of the American Mosquito Control Association 2008; 24:147-149.

[82] Sogoba N, Vounatsou P, Bagayoko MM, Doumbia S, Dolo G, Gosoniu L, Traore SF, Toure YT, Smith T. The spatial distribution of *Anopheles gambiae sensu stricto* and *An. arabiensis* (Diptera: Culicidae) in Mali. Geospat. Health 2007; 1:213-22.

[83] Müller GC, Beier JC, Traore SF, Toure MB, Traore MM, Bah S, Doumbia S, Schlein Y. Field experiments of *Anopheles gambiae* attraction to local fruit/seedpods and flowering plants in Mali to optimize strategies for malaria vector control in Africa using attractive toxic sugar bait methods. Malaria Journal 2010; 9:262.

[84] Xue RD, Barnard DR. Boric acid bait kills adult mosquitoes (Diptera:Culicidae). Journal of Economical Entomology 2003; 96:1559-1562.

[85] Xue RD, Kline D, Ali L, Barnard DR. Application of boric acid baits to plant foliage for adult mosquito control. Journal of the American Mosquito Control Association 2006; 22:497-500.

[86] WHO. Global strategic framework for integrated vector management. WHO/CDS/CPE/PVC/2004. World Health Organization, Geneva. 10:1-12. 2004.

[87] WHO. WHO position statement on integrated vector management. Wkly. Epidemiol. Rec. 83:177-181. 2008.

[88] Beier JC, Keating J, Githure JI, Macdonald MB, Impoinvil DE, Novak RJ. Integrated vector management for malaria control. Malaria Journal 2008; 7:54.

[89] Koella J. On the use of mathematical models of malaria transmission. Acta Tropica 1991; 49: 1-25.

[90] Smith D, Battle K, Hay S, Barker C, Scott T, McKenzie F. Ross, Macdonald, and a theory for the dynamics and control of mosquito-transmitted pathogens. PLoS Pathog 2012; 8: e1002588.

[91] Parham P, Pople D, Christiansen-Jucht C, Lindsay S, Hinsley W, Michael E. Modeling the role of environmental variables on the population dynamics of the malaria vector *Anopheles gambiae* sensu stricto. Malaria Journal 2012; 11: 271.

[92] Mandal S, Sarkar R, Sinha S. Mathematical models of malaria--a review. Malaria Journal 2011; 10: 202.

[93] Okell LC, Smith Paintain L, Webster J, Hanson K, Lines J. From intervention to impact: modeling the potential mortality impact achievable by different long lasting, insecticide-treated net delivery strategies. Malaria Journal 2012; 11(1):327.

[94] Gurarie D, Karl S, Zimmerman P, King C, St Pierre T, Davis T. Mathematical modeling of malaria infection with innate and adaptive immunity in individuals and agent-based communities. PLoS One 2012; 7: e34040.

[95] White L, Maude R, Pongtavornpinyo W, Saralamba S, Aguas R, Van Effelterre T, Day N, White N. The role of simple mathematical models in malaria elimination strategy design. Malaria Journal 2009; 8: 212.

[96] Maude R, Saralamba S, Lewis A, Sherwood D, White N, Day N, Dondorp A, White L. Modeling malaria elimination on the internet. Malaria Journal 2011; 10: 191.

[97] Committee on Strategies for the Management of Pesticide Resistant Pest Populations. Pesticide Resistance: Strategies and Tactics for Management. Washington: The National Academies Press. 1986.

[98] Chitnis N, Smith T, Steketee R. A mathematical model for the dynamics of malaria in mosquitoes feeding on a heterogeneous host population. Journal of Biological Dynamics 2008; 2: 259-285.

[99] Koella, J, Lynch P, Thomas M, Read A. Towards evolution-proof malaria control with insecticides. Evolutionary Applications 2009; 2: 469–480.

[100] Gourley S, Liu R, Wu J. Slowing the evolution of insecticide resistance in mosquitoes: a mathematical model. Proceedings of the Royal Society A 2011; 467: 2127–2148.

[101] Yakob L, Dunning R, Yan G. Indoor residual spray and insecticide-treated mosquitonets for malaria control: theoretical synergisms and antagonisms. Journal of the Royal Society Interface 2010; 8: 799–806.

[102] Hermsen R, Hwa T. Sources and Sinks: A Stochastic Model of Evolution in Heterogeneous Environments. Physical Review Letters 2010; 105: 248104.

[103] Ghani AC, Sutherland CJ, Riley EM, Drakeley CJ, Griffin JT, Gosling RD, Filipe JA. Loss of population levels of immunity to malaria as a result of exposure-reducing interventions: consequences for interpretation of disease trends. PLoS One 2009; 4: e4383.

[104] Filipe J, Riley E, Drakeley C, Sutherland C, Ghani AC. Determination of the mechanisms driving the acquisition of immunity to malaria using a mathematical transmission model. PLoS Computational Biology 2007; 3: e255.

[105] Deloron P, Chougnet P. Is immunity to malaria really short-lived? Parasitology Today 1992; 8: 375–378.

[106] Smith R, Reynolds H. Principles, definitions and scope of integrated pest control. Proceeding of the FAO Symposium on Integrated Pest Control 1965; 1: 11-17.

[107] Rajotte E, Kazmierczak RJ, Norton G, Lambur M, Allen W. The National Evaluation of Extension's Integrated Pest Management Programs. Virginia Cooperative Extension Publication 491-010, Blacksburg, VA. 1987.

[108] Government of South Australia. South Australian Integrated Mosquito Management Strategy. Prepared the Environmental Health Service. Department of Health, Adelaide, Australia: 61p. 2007.

[109] WHO, 2006. Alpha-Cypermethrin. World Health Organization, Geneva, 50p.

[110] WHO, 2008. Bendiocarb. World Health Organization, Geneva, 33p.

[111] WHO, 2012. Bifenthrin. World Health Organzitaion, Geneva, 45p.

[112] USAID, 2007. Integrated Vector Management Programs for Malaria Control - Programmatic Environmental Assessment. Prepared for Bureau for Global Health by RTI International, Research Triangle Park, NC. January, 527p.

[113] WHO, 2004. Cyfluthrin. World Health Organization, Geneva, 29p.

[114] WHO, 1989. Environmental Health Criteria 83, DDT and its derivatives – Environmental aspects.

[115] WHO, 1990. Environmental Health Criteria 97, Deltamethrin.

[116] Yaméogo L., Traoré K., Back C., Hougard J.-M., Calamari D., 2001. Risk assessment of etofenprox (vectron®) on non-target aquatic fauna compared with other pesticides used as *Simulium* larvicide in a tropical environment. Chemosphere 42: 965-974.

[117] WHO, 1992. Environmental Health Criteria 133, Fenitrothion.

[118] WHO, 1990. Environmental Health Criteria 99, Cyhalothrin.

[119] WHO, 1986. Environmental Health Criteria 63, Organophosphorus insecticides: a general introduction.

[120] Milam C.D., Farris J. L., Wilhide J. D, 2000. Evaluating mosquito control pesticides for effect on target and non-target organisms. Archives of Environmental Contamination and Toxicology, 39: 324-328.

[121] WHO, 1983. Data sheets on pesticides n°49. Pirimiphos-methyl.

[122] WHO, 1976. Data sheets on pesticides n°25. Propoxur.

[123] Najera J, Zaim M. Malaria vector control decision making criteria and procedures for judicious use of insecticides. World Health Organization, Communicable Disease Control, Prevention and Eradication, WHO Pesticide Evaluation Scheme (WHOPES). WHO/CDS/WHOPES/2002.5. Geneva: 116p. 2003.

[124] Blom A. The effect of mosquito spraying on non-target terrestrial insects. Bachelor degree report. Faculty of the Worcester Polytechnic Institute, 33p. 2011.

[125] Davis R, Peterson R. Effects of single and multiple applications of mosquito insecticides on nontarget arthropods. Journal of the American Mosquito Control Association 2008; 24: 270-280.

[126] Boisvert, J., Lacoursière J.O., 2004. *Bacillus thuringiensis* et le contrôle des insectes piqueurs au Québec. Ministère de l'Environnement Québécois, Québec.

[127] Nasreen, A., Ashfaq, M., Mustafa, G., 2000. Intrinsic toxicity of some insecticides to egg parasitoid *Trichogramma chilonis* (Hym. Trichogrammatidae). Bulletin of the Institute of Tropical Agriculture, Kyushu University 23. 41–44.

[128] WHO, 2007. Spinosad. World Health Organization, Geneva, pp. 32.

[129] Duchet, C., Caquet, Th., Franquet, E., Lagneau, C., Lagadic, L., 2010. Influence of environmental factors on the response of a natural population of *Daphnia magna* (Crustacea: Cladocera) to spinosad and *Bacillus thuringiensis israelensis* in Mediterranean coastal wetlands. Environmental Pollution 158: 1825–1833.

[130] WHO, 1975. Data sheets on pesticides n°18. Chlorpyriphos.

[131] WHO, 1976. Data sheets on pesticides n°23. Fenthion.

[132] Thompson C. Q., Tucker J. W. Jr. 1989. Toxicity of the organophosphate insecticide fenthion, alone and with thermal fog carriers, to an estuarine copepod and young fish. Bulletin of Environmental Contamination and Toxicology 43 (5): 789-796.

[133] WHO, 1983. Data sheets on pesticides n°49. Pirimiphos-methyl.

[134] USAID, 2007. Integrated Vector Management Programs for Malaria Control - Programmatic Environmental Assessment. Prepared for Bureau for Global Health by RTI International, Research Triangle Park, NC. January, 527p.

[135] Gaines T. B., Kimbrough R., Laws ER. Jr. 1967. Toxicology of Abate in laboratory animals. Archives of Environmental Health 14: 283-288.

[136] Sinègre G., Babinot M., Vigo G., Tourenq J. N., 1990. Sensibilité de trois espèces de *Chironomus* (Diptera) à huit insecticides utilisés en démoustication. Annales de Limnologie 26: 65-71.

[137] Tomlin C.D.S. (éd.), 1997. The Pesticide Manual, 11th edition. British Crop Protection Council, Farnham, UK.

[138] Lahr J., Diallo A.O. Gadji B., Diouf P.S., Mosquitoaux J.J.M., Badji A., Ndour K.B., Andreasen J.E., van Straalen, N.M. 2000. Ecological effects of experimental insecticide applications on invertebrates in Sahelian temporary ponds. Environmental Toxicology and Chemistry 19: 1278-1289.

[139] WHO, 1996. Diflubenzuron, WHO, Geneva, 164pp.

[140] Agence de la Santé publique du Canada, 2005. Déclaration relative aux mesures de protection individuelle pour prévenir les piqûres ou morsures d'arthropodes. Relevé des maladies transmissibles au Canada, vol. XXXI, DCC-13.

[141] De Wael L., De Greef M., Van Laere O., 1995. Toxicity of pyriproxyfen and fenoxycarb to bumble bee brood using a new method for testing insect growth regulators. Journal of Agricultural Research 34: 3-8].

[142] Guillet P, Alnwick D, Cham M, Neira M, Zaim M, Heymann D, Mukelabai K. Long-lasting treated mosquito nets: a breakthrough in malaria prevention. Bulletin of the World Health Organization 2001; 79: 998.

[143] Minakawa N, Dida G, Sonye G, Futami K, Kaneko S. Unforeseen misuses of bed nets in fishing villages along Lake Victoria. Malaria Journal 2008; 7: 165-171.

[144] Sharma S, Upadhyay A, Haque M, Padhan K, Tyagi P, Ansari M, Dash A. Wash resistance and bioefficacy of Olyset net – a Long-Lasting Insecticide-Treated mosquito Net against malaria vectors and non-target household pests. Journal of Medical Entomology 2006; 43: 884-888.

[145] Dobrokotov B. Alternatives to chemical methods for vector control. Annales de la Société Belge de Médecine Tropicale 1991; 71: 27-33.

[146] Shumway C. Forgotten Waters: Freshwater and Marine Ecosystems in Africa—Strategies for Biodiversity Conservation and Sustainable Development. Biodiversity Support Program. Washington, D.C.: 167p. 1999.

[147] USAID. Integrated Vector Management Programs for Malaria Control - Programmatic Environmental Assessment. Prepared for Bureau for Global Health by RTI International, Research Triangle Park, NC. January: 527p. 2007.

[148] Calow P, Sibly R, Forbes V. Risk assessment on the basis of simplified life-history scenarios. Environmental Toxicology and Chemistry 1997; 16: 1983-1989.

[149] Caquet T, Roucaute M, LeGoff P, Lagadic L. Effects of repeated field applications of two formulations of *Bacillus thuringiensis* var. *israelensis* on non-target saltmarsh invertebrates in Atlantic coastal wetlands. Ecotoxicolog and Environmental Safety 2011; 74: 1122-1130.

[150] Poulin B, Lefebvre G, Paz L. Red flag for green spray: adverse trophic effects of Bt. on breeding birds. Journal of Applied Ecology 2010; 47: 884-889.

[151] Lundström J, Schäfer M, Petersson E, Persson Vinnersten T, Landin J, Brodinet Y. Production of wetland Chironomidae (Diptera) and the effects of using *Bacillus thuringiensis israelensis* for mosquito control. Bulletin of Entomological Research 2009; 100: 117-125.

[152] Lundström J, Brodin Y, Schäfer M, Persson Vinnersten T, Östman Ö. High species richness of Chironomidae (Diptera) in temporary flooded wetlands associated with high species turn-over rates. Bulletin of Entomological Research 2009; 100: 433-444.

[153] Lagadic L, Caquet T, Fourcy D, Heydorff M. Evaluation à long terme des effets de la démoustication dans le Morbihan: suivi de l'impact écotoxicologique des traitements sur les invertébrés aquatiques entre 1998 et 2001. Rapport Scientifique de fin de programme (Avril 2002) ; Convention de Recherche Conseil Général du Morbihan: 215p. 2002.

[154] Le Goff P, Roucaute M, Lagadic L, Caquet T. Évaluation à long terme des effets de la démoustication dans le Morbihan: suivi de l'impact écotoxicologique d'une nouvelle formulation de larvicide sur les invertébrés aquatiques : étude comparative entre Vectobac® WG et Vectobac® 12AS. Rapport de fin d'étude, Conseil Général du Morbihan, Mars 2009: 26p. 2009.

[155] EID Méditerranée. Contrôle des moustiques nuisant dans les espaces naturels méditerranéens. Proposition méthodologique pour la gestion d'un site "Ramsar" en Languedoc-Roussillon. Programme Life-Environnement n°LIFE99 ENV/F/000489. Actes du Colloque de Restitution du programme Life Environnement, Montpellier, 27 mars 2003. Rapport consultable sur le site: http://www.eid-med.org: 75 p. 2003.

[156] Lagadic L. Évaluation du risque environnemental des traitements de démoustication : harmonisation des méthodes applicables aux invertébrés non-cibles dans les

zones humides littorales méditerranéennes et atlantiques. Rapport Final, Programme PNETOX, Ministère de l'Écologie et du Développement Durable: 41 pp. 2007.

[157] Bruce-Chwatt LJ. History of malaria from prehistory to eradication. In Wernsdorfer W.H. & McGregor I., Malaria. Principles and Practice of Malariology. Churchill Livingstone, Edinburgh London Melbourne & New York. 1988.

[158] Gorgas MD, Hendrick BJ. William Crawford Gorgas: his life and work. Lea & Febiger, Philadelphia. 1924.

[159] Watson M. The Prevention of Malaria in the Federated Malay States. Murray, London. 1921.

[160] Hackett LW, Russell PF, Scharff JW, Senior White R. The present use of naturalistic measures in the control of malaria. Quaterly Bulletin of the Health Organisation of the League of Nations1938; 7: 1016-1064.

[161] Rockfeller Foundation (International Health Board). The use of fish for mosquito control. The Rockfeller Foundation New York 1924.

[162] Celli A. Storia della malaria nell'agro romano. Academia dei Lincei, Roma. 1925.

[163] Ilvento A. The reclamation of the Pontine marshes. Quaterly Bulletin of the League of Nations Health Organization. 1934; 3: 157-201.

[164] Hackett LW. Malaria in Europe. Oxford University Press, London. 1937.

[165] Sergent Ed, Vingt cinq années d'étude et de prophylaxie du paludisme en Algérie. Archives de l'Institut Pasteur d'Algérie 1928; 6: 117-434.

[166] Dedet JP. The Sergent brothers and antimalaria campaigns in Algeria (1902-1948). Parassitologia, 50 (3-4): 221-225.

[167] Blumberg L, Frean J..- Malaria Control in South Africa- challenges and successes. South African Medical Journal 2007; 91: 1193-1197.

[168] Holmstedt B, Liljestrand G. Readings in pharmacology. Pergamon Press, Oxford. 1963.

[169] Russell PF. Malaria and its influence on world health. Bulletin of the New York Academy of Medicine 1943; 1: 559-630.

[170] Müller P. Uber Zusallenhänge zwischen Konstitution und insecticide Wirkung. Helvetia Chemica Acta 1946; 29: 1560-1580.

[171] Pampana EJ. A textbook of malaria eradication. Oxford University Press, London. 1963.

[172] Pampana EJ, Russell PF. Malaria-a world problem. World Health Organization Chronicle 1955; 9: 31-96.

http://dx.doi.org/10.5772/56258

[173] Bruce-Chwatt LJ. Malaria and its control: present situation and future prospects. Annual Review of Public Health 1987; 8: 75-110.

Chapter 23

New Salivary Biomarkers of Human Exposure to Malaria Vector Bites

Papa M. Drame, Anne Poinsignon, Alexandra Marie, Herbert Noukpo, Souleymane Doucoure, Sylvie Cornelie and Franck Remoue

Additional information is available at the end of the chapter

http://dx.doi.org/10.5772/55613

1. Introduction

Mosquitoes are the most menacing worldwide arthropod disease vectors. They transmit a broad range of viral, protozoan and metazoan pathogens responsible of the most devastating human and animal diseases [1]. Among the main frequent mosquito-borne diseases, malaria represents the most widespread and serious infection in terms of heavy burden on health and economic development throughout the world. Despite substantial efforts and increasing international funding to eliminate it, malaria is still a major public health problem with nearly a million of deaths per year, especially in children younger than 5 years old (86%) [2]. Approximately two thirds of the world's population live in areas at risk for malaria [3, 4]. Understanding mechanisms that govern its transmission remains therefore a major scientific challenge, but also an essential step in the design and the evaluation of effective control programs [5, 6].

Entomological, parasitological and clinical assessments are routinely used to evaluate the exposure of human populations to *Anopheles* vector bites and the risk of malaria transmission. However, these methods are labor intensive and difficult to sustain on large scales, especially when transmission and exposure levels are low (dry season, high altitude, urban settings or after vector control) [7, 8]. In particular, the entomological inoculation rate (EIR), the gold standard measure for mosquito–human transmission intensity of *Plasmodium*, is highly dependent on the density of human-biting *Anopheles* [9]. This latter is estimated by using trapping methods such as human-landing catches (HLC) of adult mosquitoes, the commonly used for sampling host-seeking mosquitoes and then for assessing the human exposure level.

HLC may be limited because of ethical and logistical constraints to relevantly apply it to children [10]. Transmission estimates based on the prevalence or density of human infection are susceptible to micro-heterogeneity caused by climatic factors and the socioeconomic determinants of the host-seeking behavior [8]. Incidence of disease may be the closest logical correlate of the burden of disease on health systems. However, it can be subject to variability between sites and may not be appropriate for the evaluation of early phase studies of vector control or reliable for epidemic prediction [10]. More recently, serological correlates of transmission intensity have been described, yet they represent long-term rather than short-term exposure data [8]. They are not then suitable in evaluating the short-term impact of vector control programs. Therefore, it is currently emphasized the need to develop new tools assessing reliably human malaria risk and control interventions, and monitoring changes over time at both population and individual levels [5, 6].

Malaria is a parasitic disease caused by protozoan agents of the genus *Plasmodium* (*Aplicomplexa; Haemosporida*). Five *Plasmodium* species are pathogen for humans: *P. falciparum, P. vivax, P. ovale, P. malariae* and *P. knowlesi*. During their complex life cycle in the female *Anopheles* mosquito (*Insecta; Diptera*), *Plasmodium* parasites go through several developmental transitions, traverse the midgut and reach the salivary gland (SG) epithelium. They acquire their maturity within SGs of the vector and can be then transmitted by the bite of the female mosquito. This latter needs, during the first days after emergence, to feed on sugar to meet the energy demands of basic metabolism and flight, but also to feed on vertebrate blood for its eggs' development and maturation [11], and therefore to keep perennial its life cycle and indirectly malaria transmission cycle.

Anopheles mouthparts comprise six pieces that form a long stylus allowing to perforate human tissues and to suck the internal liquid. However, it is clear that *Anopheles* mosquito acts not only as syringe injecting parasites during the bite. When taking a blood meal, it also injects into human skin avascular tissue [12] a cocktail of bioactive molecules including enzymes that are injected in human skin by saliva [13, 14]. Some of these salivary compounds are essential to the *Plasmodium* life cycle [15]. They have substantial anti-hemostatic, anti-inflammatory, and immunomodulatory activities that assist the mosquito in the blood-feeding process by inhibiting several defense mechanisms of the human host [16]. Furthermore, many of them are immunogenic and elicit strong immune responses, evidenced by the swelling and itching that accompany a mosquito bite [17]. Specific acquired cellular [18, 19] or/and humoral responses are developed by human individuals when exposed to bites of *Anopheles* mosquitoes [20-23]. These immune responses may play several roles in the pathogen transmission ability and the disease outcomes [24]. In addition, recent studies have demonstrated that the intensity of the antibody response specific to salivary proteins could be a biomarker of the exposure level of human to *Anopheles* bites [22, 25]. Therefore, studying *Anopheles*-human immunological relationships can provide new promising tools for monitoring the real human-*Anopheles* contact and identifying individuals at risk of malaria transmission. It can also allow the development of novel methods for monitoring control and mosquito-release programmes' effectiveness.

http://dx.doi.org/10.5772/55613

However, whole saliva could be inadequate as a biomarker tool, because it is a cocktail of various molecular components with different nature and biological functions. Some of these elements are ubiquitous and may potentially cause cross-reactivities with common salivary epitopes of other haematophagous arthropods [26]. In addition, a lack of reproducibility between collected whole *Anopheles* saliva batches has been observed and difficulties to obtain sufficient quantities needed for large-scale studies were highlighted [26]. Therefore, specific and antigenic proteins have been identified in the secretome of *Anopheles* mosquitoes and a specific biomarker of *Anopheles* bites was developed by coupling bioinformatic and immuno-epidemiological approaches. This promising candidate, namely, the gSG6-P1 (*An. gambiae* Salivary Gland Protein-6 peptide 1), has been described to be highly antigenic [26]. It has been then validated as a pertinent biomarker assessing specifically and reliably the exposure level to *Anopheles* bites [27-29] and/or the effectiveness of malaria vector control [30] in all age-classes of human populations (newborns, infants, children and adults) from several malaria epidemiological settings (rural, semi-urban and urban areas…) throughout sub-Saharan Africa countries (Senegal, Angola and Benin).

The present chapter contributes therefore to a better understanding of the human-mosquito immunological relationship. It resumes most of the studies highlighting the roles of mosquito saliva on the human physiology and immunology, approaches, techniques, and methods used to develop and validate specific candidate-biomarkers of exposure to *Anopheles* bites and their applications on malaria control in several different epidemiological settings. Effects of various explanatory variables (age, sex, seasonality, differential use of vector control…) on human antibody responses to *Anopheles* salivary antigens are also discussed in the aim to optimize their use in epidemiological and vector-borne disease (VBD) control studies. Finally, different ways of application of such salivary biomarker of exposure of *Anopheles* vector bites in the field of operational research by National Malaria Control Programmes (NMCP) are highlighted.

2. Human host-mosquito relationship: Roles of mosquito saliva

Arthropods represent the vast majority of described metazoan life forms throughout the world, with species' richness estimated between 5 to 10 million [31]. The blood feeding habit has arisen and evolved independently in more than 14,000 species from 400 genera in the arthropod taxonomy [32]. In mosquitoes, only the adult female is hematophagous, whereas both male and female take sugar meals [33]. During the probing and the feeding stages, like all blood-sucking arthropods, female *Anopheles* must circumvent the highly sophisticated barriers represented by human defense systems (Fig. 1): haemostatic and inflammatory reactions, innate and adaptive immune system defenses. Therefore, they express in their saliva potent pharmacological and immunogenic components.

2.1. Pharmacological properties of mosquito saliva

The first-line of the human host non-specific defense to the insect bite is the haemostatic reaction. It provides an immediate response to the vascular injury caused by the intrusion of

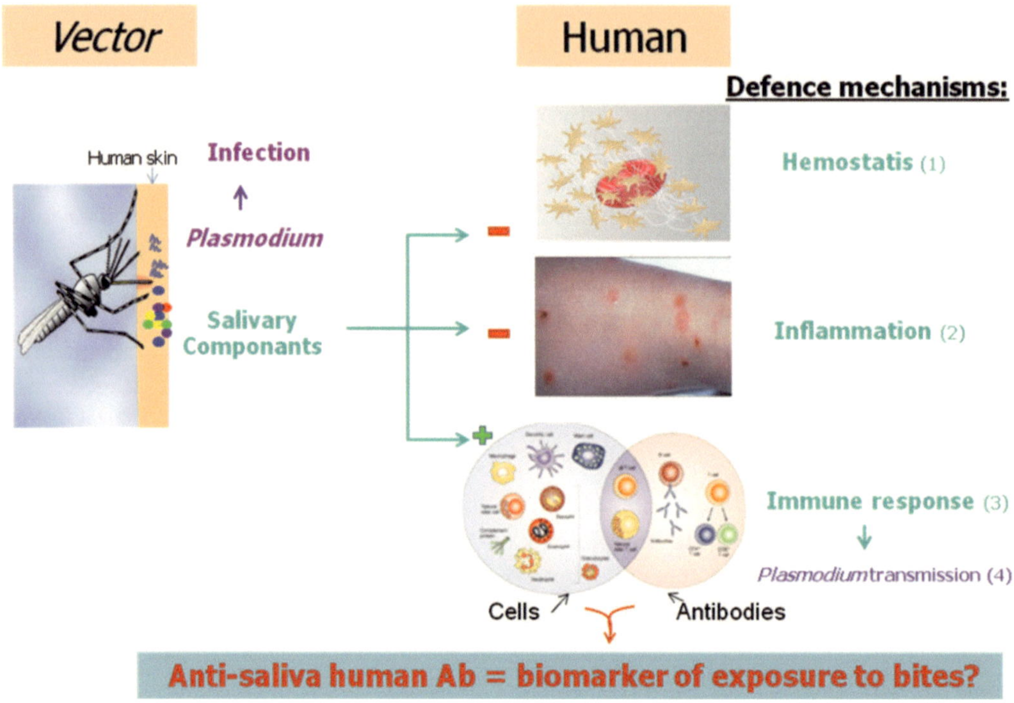

Figure 1. Effects of *Anopheles* saliva on hemostatic, inflammatory and immune reactions of the human to the vector bites.

the mosquito mouthparts in host vessels, thus preventing the extensive loss of host blood [32, 34]. The haemostatic reaction consists of three not physiologically distinct mechanisms: i) the blood coagulation that leads to the production of fibrin clots, ii) the thrombus formation and wound healing mediated by platelet aggregation, and iii) the vasoconstriction that leads to restricted influx of blood to the injured site. Each mechanism is activated by several pathways, in response to different exogenous and endogenous stimuli. Platelet aggregation is the first step in the haemostatic cascade and follows the interaction between blood platelets and the exposed extracellular matrix. This latter contains a large number of adhesive macromolecules such as collagen which is abundant underneath endothelial cells (not found in blood). This interaction results to the activation of platelets by mainly collagen and adenosine diphosphate (ADP, released by damaged cells and by activated platelets), the primary agonists of platelet aggregation. Platelets can be also activated by other agonists such as thrombin (produced by the coagulation cascade) and thromboxane A2 (TXA_2, produced by activated platelets) [35]. Activated platelets release endogeneous secretions such as serotonin and TXA_2, two potent vasoconstrictors. In parallel, the blood coagulation mechanism is getting underway. The main task of the coagulation cascade is to produce fibrin that supports aggregated platelets in a thrombus formation. The coagulation process consists of an enzymatic cascade with two ways of activation, the exogenous and the endogenous, where several amplification points and regulatory mechanisms are known.

However, mosquitoes can successfully engorge on their hosts within a half-minute because antihemostatic components of their saliva facilitate location of blood vessels and the blood sampling [36]. These salivary secretions, named sialogenins (from the Greek *sialo*, saliva; *gen*, origin, source; and *ins* for proteins), are mainly an array of potent anticoagulants, anti-platelets, vasodilators and anti-inflammatory substances [16, 32, 37, 38].

2.1.1. *Inhibition of platelet aggregation*

Compared to other blood-sucking arthropods like ticks and sand flies, only a limited number of *Anopheles* mosquito sialogenins involved in the inhibition of platelet aggregation have been characterized. *Apyrase* (Adenosine triphosphate (ATP)-diphosphohydrolase EC 3.6.1.5) is ubiquitous for hematophagous arthropods (mosquitoes, bugs, sand flies, fleas, triatomines, and ticks) and hydrolyses ATP and ADP into adenosine monophosphate (AMP) and inorganic phosphate (P_i), thus inhibiting platelet aggregation [16]. Three classes of apyrase have been characterized at the molecular level in different blood-sucking arthropods (reviewed by [39]). One named 5′-nucleotidase family is highly expressed in the salivary gland of *Anopheles gambiae* [40]. The *D7 protein family* is one of the most abundantly expressed sialogenins of mosquitoes. Two classes have been described in the saliva of mosquitoes: long (28–30 kDa) and short (15–20 kDa) forms [41-43]. The D7-related proteins may inhibit activation of host plasma. It has been described in *Anopheles* mosquitoes in a short form and may block the platelet activation by scavenging serotonin (agonist-positive feedback loop to increase platelet aggregation), while it principal function is reported to modulate tonus of vessels (vasoconstriction) [44]. *Anophelin* from *An. stephensi* saliva is a 30-kDa protein that directly binds to immobilized collagen and specifically inhibits collagen-induced platelet aggregation and the intracellular Ca^{2+} increase [45]. It can also act by inhibiting the activity of thrombin which plays a role in concentration of platelet aggregation [46].

2.1.2. *Inhibition of blood coagulation cascade*

Arthropod anticoagulants mostly target factor X-active (fXa), which plays a central role at the nexus of the intrinsic and extrinsic pathways, as well as an ultimate role of thrombin in driving production of fibrin from fibrinogen. However, *Anopheles* mosquitoes produce an anti-thrombin [38]. In *An. albimanus* for example, *Anophelin* protein has been shown to be a potent anticoagulant that acts as a specific and tight-binding thrombin inhibitor [46], blocking or delaying then the clot formation process until blood meal completion [34]. In addition, a D7-related protein of *An. stephensi* saliva has been characterized as an inhibitor of fXII [47].

2.1.3. *Vasodilator effect on host blood vessels*

In human, various types of endogenous vasoconstrictors (serotonin, TXA_2, noradrenalin…) are released few seconds after tissue injury in order to stop the blood flow locally at the bite site. Diverse types of vasodilators have been characterized in the saliva of hematophagous arthropods. *Aedes* mosquitoes use sialokinins that mimic the endogenous tachykinin substance P which stimulate the production of nitric oxide (NO), a potent dilator of blood vessels [48, 49]. In contrast, the saliva of the adult female *Anopheles* mosquito has been shown to contain a myeloperoxidase with a vasodilator activity associated with a catechol oxidase/peroxidase activity [50]. This latter drives the H_2O_2-dependent destruction of noradrenalin and serotonin, two important endogenous vasoconstrictors [50]. In addition, some D7 proteins of *Anopheles* have been described to bind to biogenic amines such as serotonin, histamine, and norepinephrine [44]. These strategies remove the human host's ability to maintain vascular tone at the bite site, resulting to a weak but persistent local vasodilatation [14].

2.2. Immunological effects of mosquito saliva

The tissue injury causes an immediate onset of acute inflammation and innate immunity, which promote tissue repair, prevent colonization of the damaged tissues by opportunistic pathogens and initiates adaptive immunity, which is more specific [51]. These responses mobilize multiple elements such as phagocytes and antigen-presenting cells, cytokine-producing cells, T and B lymphocytes (TL and BL) and complement (classical and alternative pathways). It may result to the development of strong cell and humoral immune reactions, thereby altering physiologically the environment at the bite site and leading to the rejection of the blood-sucker [52]. The saliva of *Anopheles* mosquitoes (like blood-feeding arthropods in general) has selected, during evolution, compounds that can counter these host responses by modulating immune cells and cytokines' production [52, 53]. This certainly allows mosquitoes to complete successfully a blood meal in only few seconds. Immunomodulatory effects of *Anopheles* mosquito saliva can therefore affect the transmission of pathogens and the development of associated pathologies [54]. Understanding the mechanisms which govern this immunomodulation could then allow the development of new prevention tools or strategies against malaria transmission [54-56].

2.2.1. *Inhibition of host inflammatory reaction*

The host inflammatory reaction following tissue injury consists of the triple response of Lewis: redness, heat and pain, triggering the awareness of the host to the blood sucker action [16]. If redness and heat are ones of the direct consequences of the dilatation of blood vessels, pain is induced by an increased vascular permeability under the effect of ADP, serotonin and histamine released by platelets and mast cells, following activation of the fXII by tissue-exposed collagen [16]. The fXIIa converts prekallikrein to kallikrein, which hydrolyzes blood kininogen to produce the vasodilator peptide, bradykinin. This latter induces TNF-α (Tumor Necrosis Factor alpha) release by neutrophils [57], which in turn stimulates the release of IL (interleukin)-1β and IL-6 from various cell types. These cytokines contribute to the phenomenon of hyperalgesia (increased sensitivity to pain) that accompanies inflammation. Host inflammatory reaction to bites has been described as mast cells-dependent in individuals bitten by *Anopheles* mosquitoes [58]. In contrast to ticks which need to be attached to their host for several hours (tick *Argasidæ*) or weeks (tick *Ixodidæ*), mosquitoes take just few seconds for a successful blood meal. This certainly explains the poverty of anti-inflammatory components in their saliva in contrast to the ticks' one. Nevertheless, some salivary components of *Anopheles* mosquitoes can inhibit the human inflammatory reaction. In particular, a 16kDa D7 family proteins of *An. stephensi* (Hamadarin) inhibits the contact system by preventing the mutual activation between the fXIIa and the kallikrein in the presence of Zn^{2+} [47].

2.2.2. *Modulation of host immune response*

A role for arthropod saliva in modifying the outcome of transmission and infection is not a novel idea introduced in the context of mosquitoes and malaria parasites. The increased pathogen infectivity in association with ticks, sand flies, and mosquitoes saliva has been described previously [54]. If ticks that take a long time to engorge must additionally necessitate in their saliva anti-inflammatory and immunosuppressive factors, rapidly feeding dipterans, in particular mosquitoes and sand flies, clearly have evolved salivary factors that directly modulate host immune defenses [52]. One possible explanation is that these molecules have evolved because they have long-term beneficial effects for the populations rather than to the individual at the time of feeding [24]. Although the molecular mechanisms by which mosquito saliva induces alteration of the host immune response are unclear [59, 60], data evidently demonstrate that effects depend on the global regulation of the Th1/Th2 cytokines' balance, as it has been described in sand flies/*Leishmania* model, the most studied striking host-parasite vector system [61]. The Th1 response has been described to lead to a protective immunity and the resistance of the host to intracellular pathogens, while the Th2 response might favor the survivor of pathogens (parasites, virus…) and then the disease transmission and evolution [24]. For mosquitoes, studies have globally shown an enhancement of transmission and disease when pathogens are introduced in the presence of vector saliva. Mosquito saliva is commonly associated with a downregulation of the expression of Th1 and an upregulation of the Th2-type cytokines. In mouse models, mosquito saliva can potentiate the infection of arboviruses [24, 62, 63]. The co-inoculation of Sindbis virus with *Aedes aegypti* salivary gland extract resulted on a reduced interferon- gamma (IFN-γ) expression, when compared to injection of virus alone [64]. It has been also shown that *Ae. aegypti* saliva contains multiple factors that can affect various components of the host immune response [65]. For example, factor Xa inhibitor may inhibit complement activation and leukocyte migration to the bite site [24] and other factors inhibit TNF-α release from activated mast cells [66]. Chickens subcutaneously infected with *P. gallinaceum* sporozoites in the presence of *Aedes fluviatillis* salivary gland homogenates showed a higher level of parasitaemia when compared to those that received only sporozoites [67]. For *Anopheles*, mice exposed to mosquito feeding in tandem with the inoculation of sporozoites had higher parasitemia and an elevated progression to cerebral malaria. This was associated with, in particular, elevated levels of IL-4 and IL-10, suppression of overall transcription in response to infection, and decreased mobility of dendritic cells and monocytes [19]. It was also described that *Anopheles stephensi* saliva downregulates specific antibody (Ab) immune responses by a mechanism that is mast cell and IL-10 -dependent [60]. IL-10, by inhibiting pro-inflammatory and Th1 cytokines, stimulates certain T, mast and B cells and has pleiotropic effects in immunoregulation and inflammation, while IL-4 is the prototypical Th2 cytokine (it differentiates $CD4^+$ T-cells and up-regulates MHC class II production). The enhancement of IL-10 expression could account for reduction in secretion of other cytokines because it inhibits antigen presentation, IFN–γ expression, and macrophage activation [68]. However, some data have suggested a paradoxical protective role of mosquito saliva against pathogen transmission and disease infection. *Ae. aegypti* saliva can inhibit infection of dendritic cells by dengue virus, and the pre-sensitization of dendritic cells with saliva prior to infection enhanced this inhibition. Moreover, the proportion of dead cells was also reduced in virus-infected dendritic cell cultures exposed to mosquito saliva, and an enhanced production of IL-12 and TNF-α was detected in these cultures [69]. In addition to these effects on cellular immunity, *Anopheles* saliva can also acts on humoral host immune response. Indeed, specific antibodies (immunoglobulins [Ig] G, M and E) to salivary antigens have been described in several studies [20, 22, 23, 25, 56, 70]. However, the implication of these Ab responses in disease pathogenesis or protection is not yet elucidated.

Therefore, future studies are needed for an overall understanding of mosquito saliva effect, especially *Anopheles* mosquito saliva, in pathogen transmission, disease development and pathogenesis.

2.2.3. *Human host-*Anopheles *vector immune relationship and applications*

The study of immunological properties of salivary proteins of *Anopheles* mosquitoes represents a new research thematic which can significantly improve the understanding of *Plasmodium* transmission mechanisms and therefore help for the effective prevention and control of malaria. It can notably lead to major applications in three areas: i) development of vaccines, diagnosis, treatment, ii) prevention of allergies, and iii) development of biomarkers of exposure to bites and malaria disease risk.

The development of parasite transmission-blocking vaccines, by stimulating the immune response against the vector is an attractive alternative way for malaria control. Several studies targeted the effect of Abs specific to the mosquito midgut antigens have shown promising results [71-73]. The study of the immune response induced by vector saliva at the biting site and its potential effect on the transmission and the development of pathogens suggests the possibility to control parasite transmission by vaccinating the host with immunogenic salivary compounds [54, 74]. In a mouse model, it has been shown that two salivary proteins (29 and 100 kDa) of the female *An. gambiae* can induce production of Ab which can block about 75% of the invasion of *An. stephensi* salivary glands by *P. yoelii* sporozoites [75]. In addition, the prior exposition to non infective *An. stephensi* bites induces a Th1 immune response with increased production of IL-12 and IFN-γ. Its effect can subsequently limit future *P. yoelii* infection (reduced rate of liver and blood parasites) and the development of cerebral malaria in mouse [18]. In this context, saliva can be thought as a non-specific "adjuvant" which could be effective at inducing a Th1-biased environment that is known to be protective against malaria infection. However, the development of such vaccines is complex. For example, Ab produced by immunization (with salivary proteins) must be ingested by the mosquito during a bite, cross it midgut and digestive enzymes, migrate to the salivary glands, before they can block the invasion by sporozoites. Nevertheless, the possibility to develop a pan-arthropod vaccine has been recently demonstrated by another mechanism. Indeed, an immune response directed to salivary proteins that adsorb to pathogens can turn the microorganism into an innocent bystander of anti-salivary immunity as it has been recently reported in a salivary protein (Salp15) from the hard tick *Ixodes scapularis* [76] and vaccine candidate for the control of Lyme disease [77]. Unfortunately, any hematophagous arthropod saliva-based vaccine has not yet been tested on humans.

In the field of allergic reactions to salivary proteins of mosquitoes, the first studies were mainly conducted in Canada and Finland. They concerned *Aedes* and *Culex* mosquitoes which express a panel of allergens in their saliva during the blood feeding time [17, 56, 78]. These proteins can thus be used in recombinant form, as diagnostic tool of the level of human exposure to allergens or in immunotherapy injections for desensitization of human [56, 70, 79]. It exists yet no study highlighting the presence and effect of allergens in the *Anopheles* mosquitoes' saliva.

The study of immunological relationship between human-vector by quantifying specific Ab responses to salivary proteins may also allow the identification and characterization of biological markers for epidemiological assessment of the exposure of individuals and populations to the *Anopheles* bites and thus to the risk of malaria transmission [22]. The development of such biomarkers or indicators (see next chapter) can be a complementary alternative to current referent entomological and parasitological methods which present several limitations especially in low exposure/transmission contexts.

3. Development of biomarkers of human exposure to *Anopheles* bites and indicators of malaria vector control effectiveness

3.1. Validation of concept with whole *Anopheles* saliva

To improve the fight against malaria and regarding numerous limitations described with current entomological and parasitological tools, the World Health Organization (WHO) has emphasized the need of new indicators and methods to evaluate, at individual and population levels, the exposure level to *Anopheles* vectors and the effectiveness of vector control strategies. One promising concept is based on the fact that mosquito saliva injected to the human host during the vector bite is antigenic and can induce an adaptive humoral host response (see Figure 1). Therefore, a logical positive correlation between the human exposure level to *Anopheles* bites and human anti-mosquito saliva Ab level can be expected. In this way, anti-mosquito saliva Ab response can be a pertinent epidemiological biomarker of human exposure to vector bites.

The epidemiological importance of human exposure to the saliva of vectors has been firstly described in Lyme disease [80, 81], leishmaniasis [82] and Chagas disease [83]. During the last decade, studies have provided data on human exposure to anopheline saliva and its interaction with malaria transmission. In particular, Remoue *et al.* [22] have shown that children living in a seasonal malaria transmission region of Senegal developed IgG responses to *An. gambiae* whole saliva (WS). Interestingly, these specific IgG levels were positively associated with an increased rainfall and the *Anopheles* mosquito density, measured by referent entomological methods. Indeed, an increase in the level of IgG was observed according to the *Anopheles* aggressiveness and density in September (Figure 2), the peak of malaria transmission.

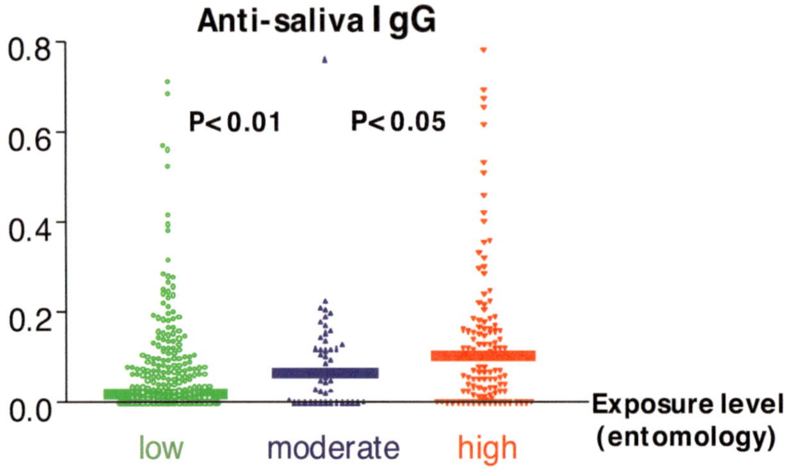

Figure 2. Anti-saliva IgG according to the intensity of exposure [22]. Individual absorbance (OD) values in September are shown for the three groups with different levels of exposure. Bars indicate the median value for each group. Statistical significances between each group by non-parametric Mann–Whitney *U*-test are indicated.

Importantly, IgG response to *An. gambiae* WS can predict clinical malaria cases. Indeed, children who developed a malaria attack in December had higher levels of anti-WS IgG in September of the same year, i.e. three months before they develop the disease (Figure 3) [22].

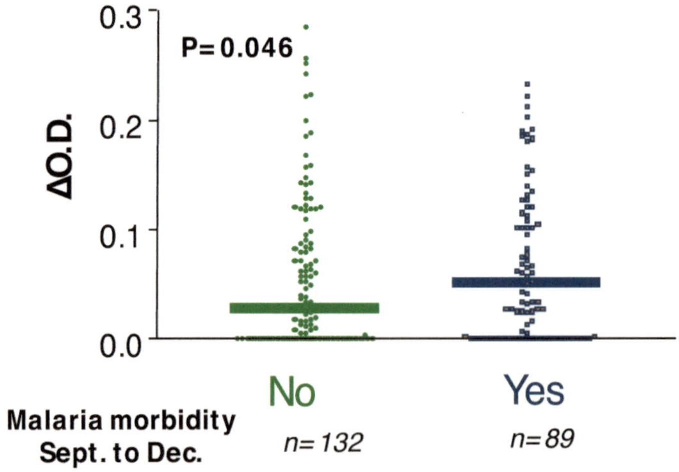

Figure 3. Anti-salivary IgG according to malaria morbidity. The results of individual absorbance (OD) values in September are shown according to subsequent detection of clinical malaria for the age ≥1 year. Bars indicate the median value for each group. Statistical significance between groups is indicated by a non-parametric Mann–Whitney *U*-test).

Anti-mosquito saliva Ab appeared transitional. Soldier travelers transiently exposed to *An. gambiae* bites in endemic areas of Africa (especially Ivory Coast and Gabon) developed specific

IgG responses to anti-*An. gambiae* WS which strongly decreased several weeks after the end of their trip [21]. In addition, anti-*An. gambiae* saliva IgG levels waned rapidly after 6 weeks of Insecticide-Treated Nets (ITNs) well-use in a semi-urban population in Angola, before a new significant increase two months later following the stop of ITN use [84]. Data on human exposure to anopheline saliva and its interaction with malaria were also provided by studies from other none African areas. In South-eastern Asia, it has been described that anti-*An. dirus* salivary protein Ab occur predominantly in patients with acute *P. falciparum* or *P. vivax* malaria; people from non-endemic areas do not carry such Abs [23]. In the Americas, the presence of anti-*Anopheles* saliva Ab has been also described. In adult volunteers from Brazil, anti-*An. darlingi* WS Ab levels increased with *P. vivax* infections [20]. The presence of anti-*An. albimanus* WS Ab with exposure to mosquito bite has been recently described in Haiti [25]. Specific IgG response to *An. gambiae* WS has also been described as an immunological indicator evaluating the efficacy of malaria vector control strategies. Indeed, Drame *et al.* have recently shown in a semi-urban area (Lobito, Provence Benguela) in Angola that specific IgG levels drastically decreased after the introduction of ITNs and this was associated with a drop in parasite load (Figure 4) [84].

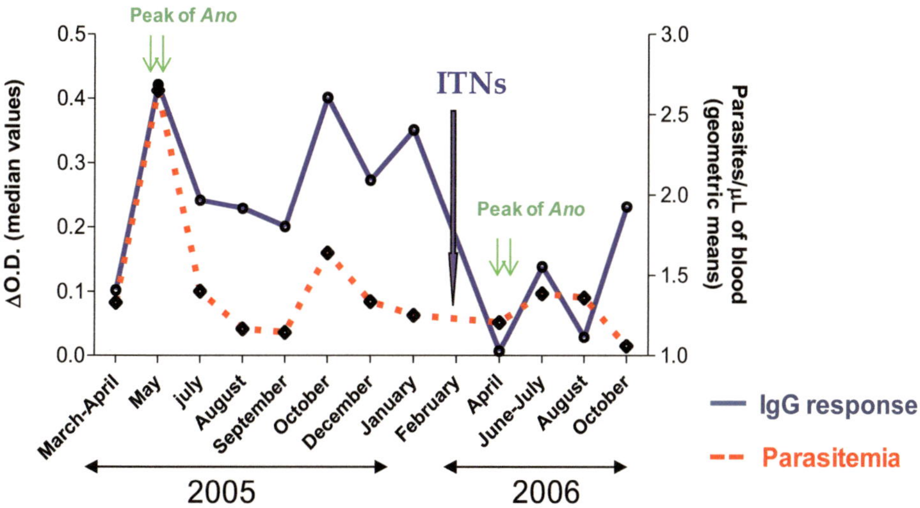

Figure 4. Evolution of anti-*Anopheles* gambiae saliva IgG and *Plasmodium falciparum* infections before and after ITN implementation, (Ano=*Anopheles*).

Anti-*Anopheles* saliva IgG response has also been recently used to evaluate and compare the effectiveness of three malaria vector control strategies in another area (Balombo) of Angola [85]. Indeed, Brosseau *et al.* [85] have investigated over a period of two years (2008-2009) Ab response to *An. gambiae* WS in children between 2 to 9 years old, before and after the introduction of three different malaria vector control methods: deltamethrin treated long lasting impregnated nets (LLIN) and insecticide treated plastic sheeting (ITPS) - Zero Fly®) (ITPS-ZF), deltamethrin impregnated Durable (Wall) Lining (ITPS-DL - Zerovector®) alone, and indoor residual spraying

(IRS) with lambdacyhalothrin alone. They observed considerable decreases in entomological (82.4%), parasitological (54.8%) and immunological criteria analyzed. In particular, the immunological data based on the level of anti-saliva IgG Ab in children of all villages significantly dropped from 2008 to 2009, especially with LLIN+ZF and with IRS (Figure 5).

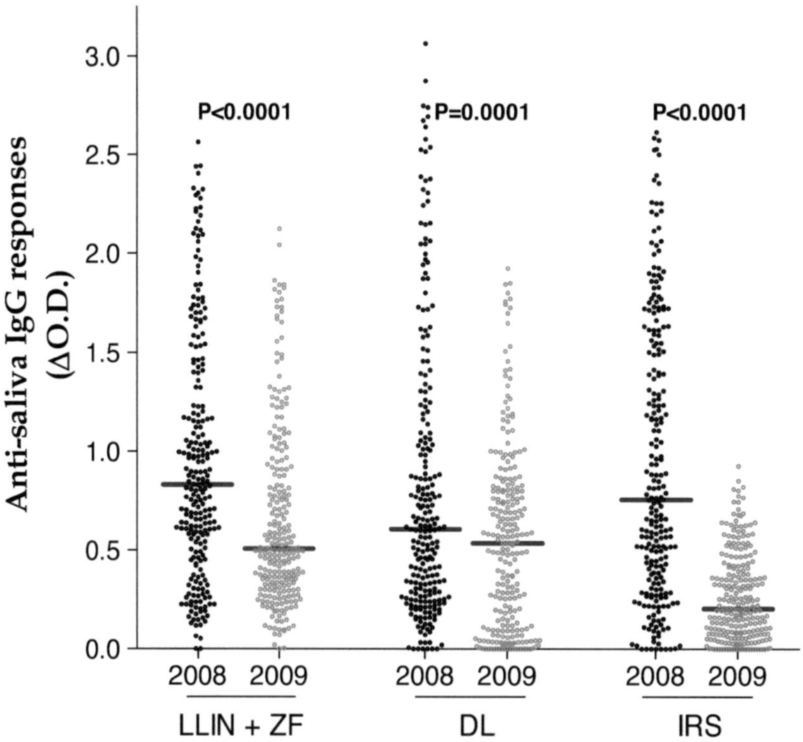

Figure 5. Comparison of median values of the IgG antibody response to *Anopheles* saliva obtained before and after implementation of each vector control method [85].

Taken together, these studies indicated that the estimation of human IgG Ab responses specific to *Anopheles* WS could provide a reliable biomarker for evaluating the *Anopheles* exposure level, the risk of malaria transmission, the disease outcomes and the effectiveness of vector control strategies. However, the pertinence and the practical large-scale application of serological tests for epidemiological purposes have been hampered by several limitations. First, WS is a cocktail of various molecular components with different nature and biological functions. Some components are *Anopheles*-specific and other widely distributed within genus, families, orders or classes of bloodsucking *Diptera* or Arthropods [16]. Therefore, the evaluation of *Anopheles* exposure or vector control effectiveness based on the immunogenicity of WS could be skewed and over or underestimated by possible cross-reactivities between common epitopes between mosquito species or other organisms [26]. Second, the collection of saliva or salivary gland extracts is tedious and time-consuming; therefore it will be difficult or impossible to have an adequate production of mosquito saliva needed for large-scale epidemiological studies [26].

Third, saliva composition can be affected by several ecological parameters such as age, feeding status or infectivity of *Anopheles* [86],which in turn may influence the anti-saliva immune response measured and may cause a lack of reproducibility between saliva batches. An alternative for optimizing the specificity of this immunological test would thus be to identify *Anopheles* genus-specific proteins [87].

3.2. Methods for the identification of specific *Anopheles* salivary proteins

The isolation of salivary components has been a challenge for many years. Many functional active salivary proteins have been isolated following classical biochemical and molecular biology approaches [88]. Protocols mainly consisted of the isolation of salivary components from hundreds of salivary gland pairs, obtaining amino-terminal or internal peptide sequence of the purified component, screening of a salivary gland library with the information obtained, and isolation of the cDNA or gene of interest (Fig. 6).

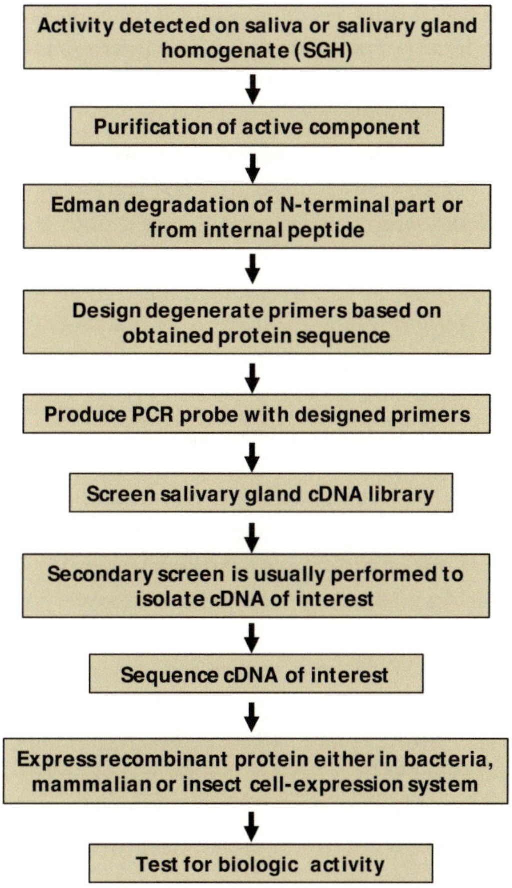

Figure 6. Classical biochemical and molecular biology protocol used for isolation and characterisation of salivary proteins and cDNA from vectors of disease [90].

During the last decade, technical advances in molecular biology have allowed the sequencing of the genome, including transcripts of salivary glands [89], of most disease vectors, comprising *Anopheles* mosquitoes [90]. However, protocols do not allow to obtain entire sequences [89]. Nowadays, researchers have switched from testing one salivary molecule at a time to studying the whole complex of genes and secreted proteins in blood-feeding arthropods using transcriptomic and/or proteomic approaches. The transcriptomic is the complete set of transcripts in an organism for a specific developmental stage or physiological condition. Transcriptomic techniques help to interpret the functional elements of the genome, and to understand the transmission and development of diseases [91]. They aim to catalogue transcript of major *Anopheles* species, including mRNAs, non-coding RNAs and small RNAs; to determine the transcriptional structure of genes and to quantify the changing expression levels of each transcript during development and under different conditions [91]. Proteomic is a large-scale study of the gene expression at the protein level, which ultimately provides direct measurement of protein expression levels [92]. The proteomic revolution is hitting the vector biology field as well as many other fields. The isolation and sequencing of all the proteins from SGs of disease vectors and, more specifically, secreted salivary proteins, is clarifying the complexity of proteins present in the saliva of various blood-feeding arthropods [93]. During the last years, a comprehensive high-throughput approach has been developed (Figure 7) [88]. It combines massive sequencing protocol of high quality full-length salivary gland cDNA libraries, a proteomic approach to isolate a large set of salivary proteins, and high-throughput computational biology and functional assays to analyze and test the biologic activities of these novel molecules. It is a powerful tool which can help easily and rapidly to identify and characterize genes or transcripts encoding for various proteins of SGs (the sialome) of blood-sucking arthropods. This high-throughput approach has then allowed an unprecedented insight into the complexity of salivary gland compounds of mosquito vectors of disease agents, indicating that the diversity of their targets is still larger than previously thought [16].

3.3. Salivary proteins (sialome) of *Anopheles* mosquitoes

The increasing power of large-scale genomic, transcriptomic and proteomic analyses allowed the accumulation of a considerable amount of information on the salivary secretions of blood-sucking arthropods [86]. As far as mosquitoes are concerned, the analysis of salivary transcriptomes of a number of *Anopheles* have allowed the discovery of a variety of genes that matched the sequence of various protein families, providing some clues on the evolution of blood feeding [15, 41-43, 92, 94-100]. Many of the salivary protein sequences are coded by genes related to intrinsic functions of the cell (housekeeping genes). However, the large number of salivary proteins is secreted during plant or blood feeding. Finally, a little number has no similarities to sequences deposited in databases, representing unknown and novel sequences [41, 94, 101]. This emphasizes how much still need to be learned concerning the biological functions of salivary proteins in blood feeding, pathogen transmission and manipulation of host responses.

The analysis of the adult *Anopheles* sialome has shown that secreted proteins and/or peptides (secretome) can be ubiquitous or specific to arthropod classes, orders, families, genus or species

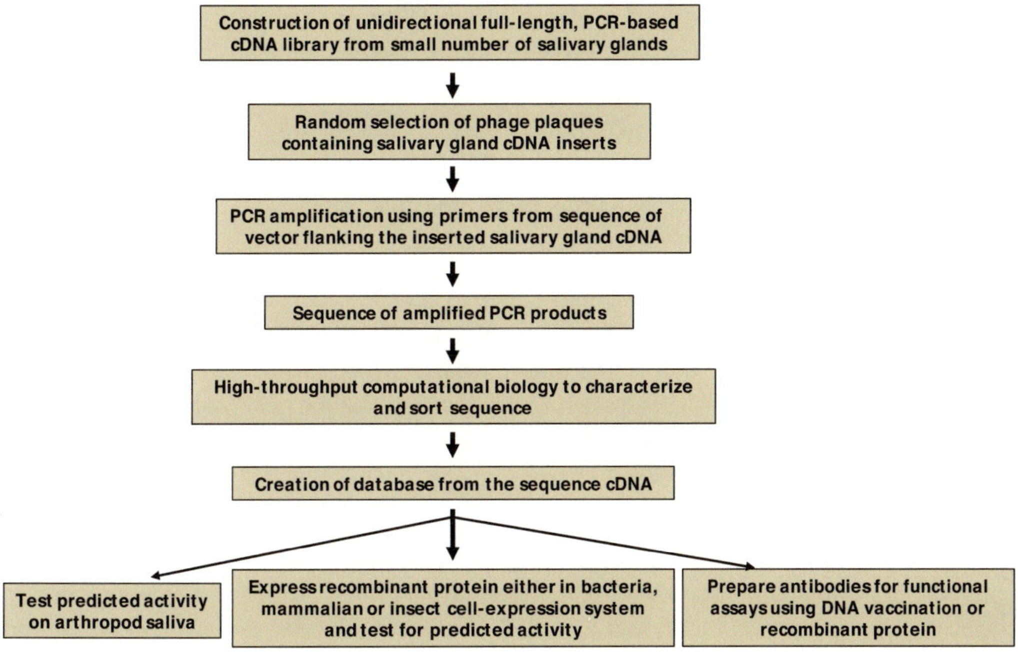

Figure 7. Current high-throughput strategies used for the isolation and characterisation of salivary cDNA and proteins from disease vectors [90].

[44, 101, 102]. In *An. gambiae* salivary gland females over 70 putative secreted salivary proteins have been identified [94].

3.3.1. *Ubiquitous salivary proteins*

AG5 family proteins are found in the salivary glands of many blood-sucking insects and ticks [102, 103]. In *An. gambiae,* four proteins belonging to this family were identified, but only one (putative gVAG protein precursor) was coding for transcripts enriched in the adult female SGs [94]. A precursor of gVAG protein was also described in *An. funestus* (84% sequence identity) and *An. stephensi* (85% sequence identity) sialome [95, 100]. The function of any AG5 protein in the saliva of any blood-sucking arthropod is still unknown.

Enzymes such as maltase, apyrase, 5′ nucleotidase, and adenosine deaminase, are also secreted during the bite of many blood-sucking arthropods, including *Anopheles* mosquitoes [95]. They generally assist in sugar feeding (maltase) or in degradation of purinergic mediators of platelet aggregation (apyrase, 5′ nucleotidases) and inflammation (adenosine deaminase).

3.3.2. *Salivary proteins found exclusively in Diptera*

D7 family proteins are specific to SGs of blood-sucking Nematocera, including mosquitoes and sand flies [104, 105]. They are highly represented in the sialome of *Anopheles* mosquitoes in short and long forms [95, 96, 101, 104, 105]. *An. funestus* D7 proteins vary between 64% and

75% identity with their *An. gambiae* closest match [105]. D7 proteins could act as anti-hemostatic factors by trapping agonists of hemostasis [44, 47]. However, further investigations are needed to clearly describe their function.

Other Diptera-specific protein families or peptides have also been described in the sialome of blood-feeding mosquitoes [95]. However their function is still unknown, even if some were known to play a role in antimicrobial property of mosquito saliva.

3.3.3. Protein families found exclusively in mosquitoes

The 30-kDa antigen family found exclusively in the SGs of adult female mosquitoes has been found in both culicine and anopheline mosquitoes [95, 100, 101, 106-108]. Only one gene enriched in SGs of adult females is known in *An. gambiae*. The *An. funestus* homologue is also abundantly expressed and shares 63% identity with the *An. gambiae* orthologue. The function of this protein family is still unknown [95].

The *gSG (An. gambiae Salivary Gland)-5 family* was first discovered in the SGs of *An. gambiae* and shown to be exclusively expressed in the adult female [94, 109]. This protein shows a high similarity to *Aedes* and *Culex* proteins [101]. Transcripts coding for this family were found in the sialotranscriptome of *An. darlingi* with 46% identical to the *An. gambiae* orthologue and only 26% and 23% identical to the culicine proteins [101]. The function of this mosquito-specific protein remains unknown, but its tissue- and sex-specific expression profile suggests it is possibly related to blood feeding.

The *gSG8 family* is highly divergent with members only found in *An. gambiae* and *Ae. aegypti*. In *An. gambiae*, this protein is specifically expressed in female SGs [109], suggesting a likely role in blood feeding.

Various types of *mucins* have been described in the saliva of adult mosquitoes and may function/act as a lubricant of their mouthparts [15, 41, 94, 102]. Three mucins encoding transcripts have been identified in the *An. gambiae* larval SG [110], suggesting the importance of mucins at multiple developmental stages. Mucins may also play a crucial role in *Anopheles* salivary gland invasion by *P. berghei* sporozoites [111]. Several protein families are also represented in this group, including gSG-3, gSG-10, and 13.5-kDa families [101]. These families were also found abundantly expressed in the sialotranscriptome of *An. gambiae* adult male [112], indicating their function is not related specifically to blood feeding.

3.3.4. Protein families found exclusively in Anophelines

Anophelin was described as a short acidic peptide with strong thrombin inhibitory activity in *An. albimanus* [46]. *An. funestus* anophelin is 59% identical to the *An. gambiae* orthologue [95], and *An. darlingi* anophelin is 86% identical to *An. albimanus* [101].

The 8.2-kDa family is represented in several *Anopheles* species. In *An. funestus* the peptide have 42% identity with the 8.2-kDa salivary peptide of *An. stephensi* and similar proteins from *An. gambiae* and *An. darlingi* [95]. In *An. gambiae*, this peptide was found enriched in adult female SGs, suggesting a role in blood feeding.

The 6.2-kDa family was first described in a sialotranscriptome of *An. gambiae* [94], where it was found enriched in adult female SGs compared to other tissues. The *An. funestus* member of this family is 61% identical to the *An. gambiae* [95], and 53% to an *An. darlingi* [101] homologues.

The SG-1 family proteins appear to be exclusively expressed in the female SGs of *Anopheles* mosquitoes and not observed in other tissues [94, 101]. However, their function remains to be determined.

The SG-2 family proteins were identified from *An. gambiae* saliva and shown to be expressed in female SGs and adult males but not in other tissues [113]. Related, but very divergent, sequences were obtained from salivary transcriptomes of other anopheline species [95, 101]. Because this protein family is expressed in both male and female *An. gambiae*, and due to its relatively small size, it may display antimicrobial function [101].

The *hyp 8.2* and *hyp 6.2 proteins* are similarly enriched in *An. gambiae* adult female SGs [94]. *An. stephensi* and *An. funestus* also have members of these protein families.

The *SG-7/Anophensin family* is also unique to anophelines. In *An. gambiae*, it is highly enriched in female SGs [94]. More recently, the *An. stephensi* homologue was determined to inhibit kallikrein and production of bradykinin, a pain-producing substance [114]. Four putative alleles representing the homologue(s) of gSG7 in *An. darlingi* were identified. These *An. darlingi* transcripts have no more than 45% identity to the *An. gambiae* gSG7 and *An. stephensi* anophensin [101].

The *SG6 protein* is a small protein first described in *An. gambiae* [109] and a unique sequence codes for a mature peptide/protein of ~10 kDa (116 amino-acids) with ten cysteine residues making probably five disulphide bonds. A homologue was later found in the sialotranscriptome of *An. stephensi* [100] and *An. funestus* [95]. *An. funestus* SG6/fSG6 (f for funestus) has 81% and 76% identities with *An. stephensi* and *An. gambiae* polypeptides, respectively. It is not found in the transcriptomes of the Culicinae subfamily members analyzed so far, i.e. *C. pipiens quinquefasciatus*, *Ae. aegypti* and *Ae. albopictus* [108, 115, 116]. In *An. gambiae*, the transcript coding for gSG6 (g for *gambiae*) was found to be 16 times more expressed in SGs of adult females than in males [94]. The gSG6 protein plays some essential blood feeding role and was recruited in the anopheline subfamily most probably after the separation of the lineage which gave origin to *Cellia* and *Anopheles* subgenera [99]. The gSG6 protein, because immunogenic, can be therefore a reliable indicator of human exposure specific to *Anopheles* mosquito bites [99], vectors of malaria.

3.4. Specific salivary biomarker of exposure to *Anopheles* bites: The gSG6-P1 peptide candidate

The SG6 salivary protein has been reported to be immunogenic in travelers exposed for short periods to *Anopheles* bites [21], and in Senegalese children living in a malaria endemic area by an immuno-proteomic, coupling 2D immunoblot and mass spectrometry [117], and by an ELISA [26] approaches. Recently, its immunogenicity has been confirmed in individuals from a malaria hyperendemic area of Burkina Faso [118, 119], by using a recombinant form expressed as purified N-terminal His-tagged recombinant protein in the *E. coli* vector pET28b(+) (Novagen) [99, 119].

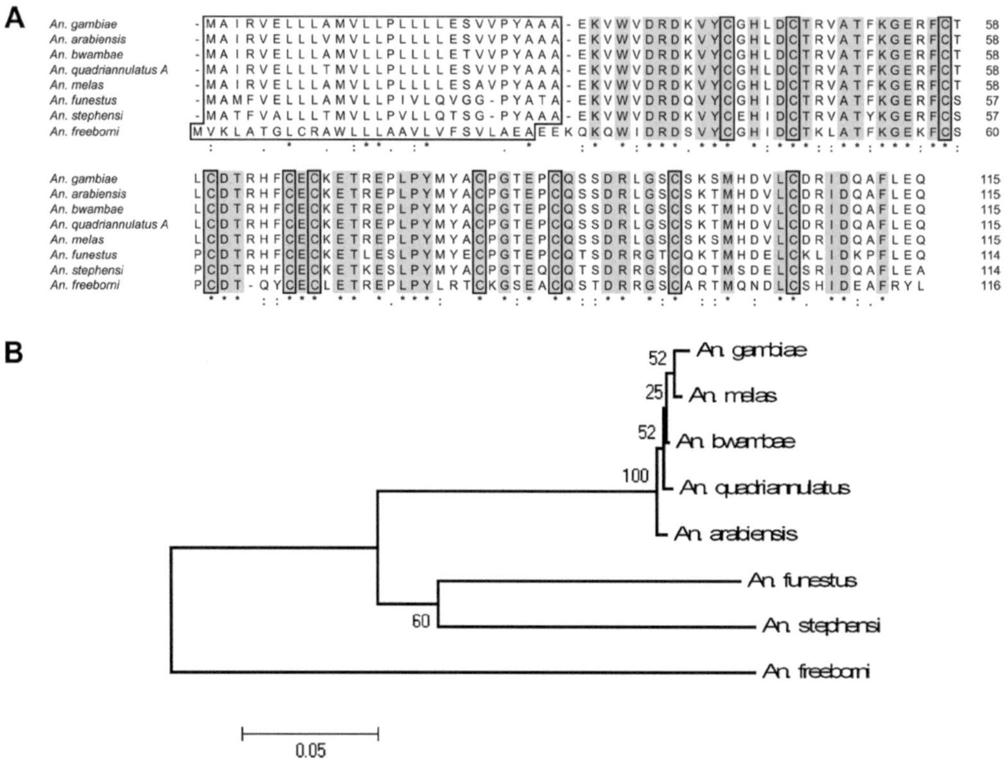

Figure 8. Sequences of the anopheline gSG6 proteins [99]. (A) Clustal alignment of anopheline gSG6 proteins. Signal peptides and conserved Cysteines are boxed. Conserved sites are shaded. (B) Phylogenetic tree (NJ algorithm, bootstrapped 10,000 times) constructed from the alignment of the nucleotide sequence encoding the mature gSG6 polypeptides.

In particular, increased anti-gSG6 IgG levels were observed in exposed individuals during the malaria transmission/rainy season [119]. In addition, anti-gSG6 IgG response appeared to be a reliable serological indicator of exposure to bites of the main African malaria vectors (*An. gambiae, An. arabiensis* and *An. funestus*) in the same area [119]. However, gSG6 recombinant protein has been described to relatively generate a high background in control sera from individuals not exposed to *Anopheles* bites, and considerable variations in specific Ab response between children supposed to be similarly exposed to *Anopheles* bites [26]. Therefore, with the objective of optimizing *Anopheles* specificity and reproducibility of the immunological assay, a peptide design approach was undertaken using bioinformatic tools [26].

3.4.1. Identification and sequence of gSG6-P1 peptide

Several algorithms were employed for prediction of potential immunogenic sites of *the* gSG6 protein by using bioinformatics. The prediction of immunogenicity was based on the determination of physico-chemical properties of the amino-acid (AA) sequences with BcePred and FIMM databases and on the identification of MHC class 2 binding regions using the ProPred-2 online service. This led to define five gSG6 peptides (gSG6-P1 to gSG6-P5) of 20 to 27 AA residues in length (Fig. 9), overlapping by at least 3 residues and spanning the entire sequence of the mature gSG6 protein. Both predictive methods for putative linear B-cell epitopes (FIMM and BcePred) assigned the highest immunogenicity to gSG6-P1, gSG6-P2, gSG6-P3, and then gSG6-P4.

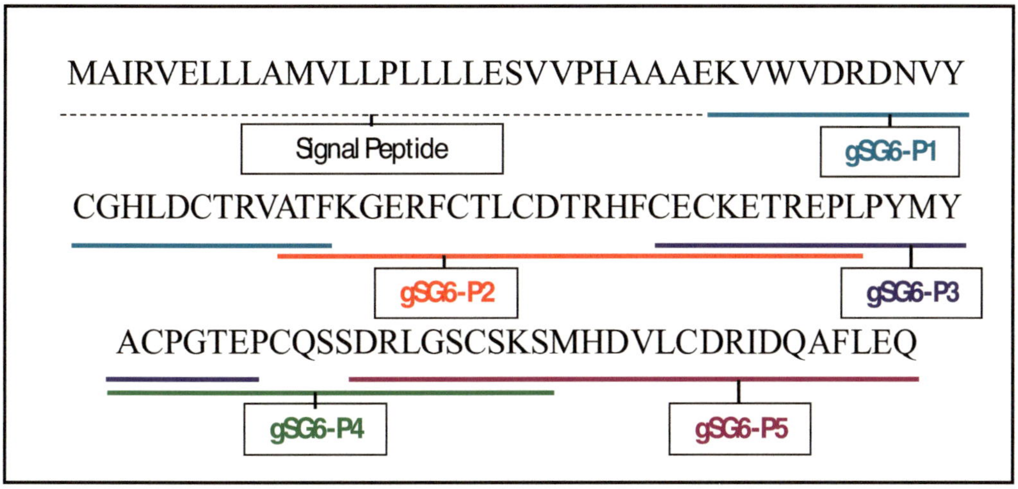

Figure 9. Amino-acid sequence of gSG6 Peptides. Amino-acid sequence of the SG6 protein of *Anopheles gambiae* (gi: 13537666) is presented and sequences of the selected peptides, gSG6-P1 to gSG6-P5, are underlined. Signal peptide (SP) sequence is indicating by dotted underline [26].

Similarities were also searched using the Blast family programs, including both the genome/EST libraries of other vector arthropods available in Vectorbase and of pathogens/ organisms in non-redundant GenBank CDS databases. No relevant identity was found with proteins of other blood-sucking arthropods. Indeed, the longest perfect match was 6 AAs between a putative protein from *Pediculus humanus* and gSG6-P2 and gSG6-P3 peptides. In the case of gSG6-P1, the best match was 4 AAs in length with *Culex pipiens quinquefasciatus* salivary adenosine deaminase. Moreover, no relevant similarity was found with sequences from pathogens or other organisms. The highest hits of gSG6-P1 were with the cyanobacterium *Microcystis aeruginosa* (3 AAs) and with *Ostreococcus* OsV5 virus (4 AAs). Altogether, this analysis confirmed the *bona fide* high specificity of the five selected gSG6 peptides for the *Anopheles* species. Peptides were then synthesized.

3.4.2. Antigenicity of gSG6 peptides

IgG Ab responses to the five gSG6 peptides were evaluated by ELISA in a randomly selected subsample of children (n<30) living in a rural area of Senegal. All peptides were immunogenic, but the intensity of the IgG level was clearly peptide-dependent; weak immunogenicity was observed for gSG6-P3, gSG6-P4 and gSG6-P5, whereas gSG6-P1 and gSG6-P2 appeared highly immunogenic (Fig. 10).

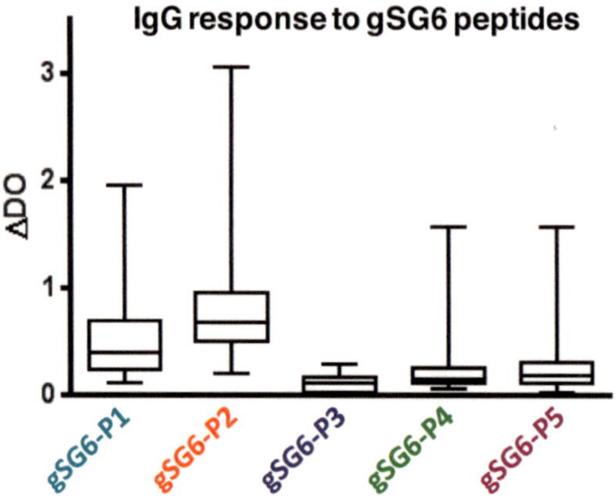

Figure 10. IgG antibody response according to gSG6 peptides [26]. For each peptide, the IgG Ab level was evaluated in a subsample of exposed children. Results at the peak of the season of *Anopheles* exposure are reported according to gSG6 peptides. Results are presented by box plot graph where lines of the boxes represent the 75th percentile, median and 25th percentile of individual average ΔOD values; whiskers represent the lower and upper adjacent values.

3.4.3. Validation as a biomarker of exposure in several epidemiological settings

The specific IgG level to the two most antigenic gSG6 peptides (gSG6-P1 et gSG6-P2) was then evaluated according to the level of exposure (estimated by entomological data) in a larger sample (n=241) of children living in a malaria seasonal area [26]. A positive trend was found for both peptides, but only significant for gSG6-P1 (Figure 11). Altogether, these results indicated that only the IgG response to gSG6-P1 is suitable to be a pertinent biomarker of exposure to *Anopheles* bites and thus to risk of malaria.

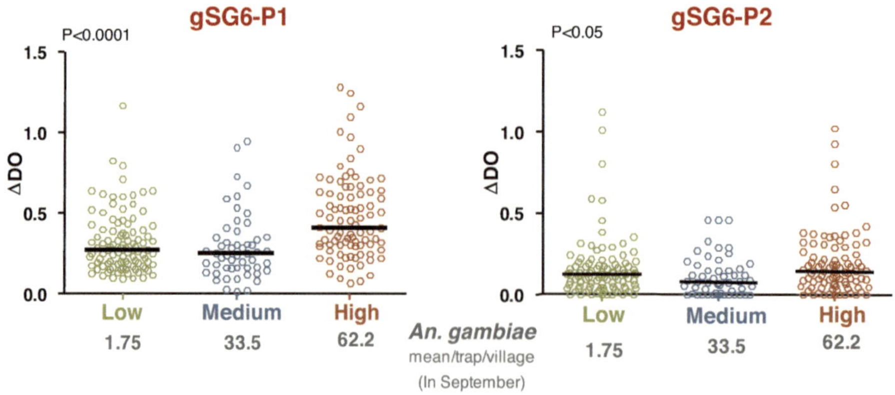

Figure 11. IgG response to gSG6-P1 and gSG6-P2 according to intensity of exposure to *Anopheles* gambiae bites [26]. Individual ΔOD (Optical Density) values in September (peak of the season of *Anopheles* exposure) are shown for the three different exposure groups. Results are presented for the same children (n=241) for gSG6-P1 (A) and gSG6-P2 (B). Exposure groups were defined by entomological data. Bars indicate median value for each exposure group. Statistical significance between the 3 groups is indicated (non-parametric Mann-Whitney U-test).

Therefore, the gSG6-P1 was selected as the most pertinent candidate as marker of exposure. Indeed, this peptide appeared to satisfy several requirements that an exposure biomarker should fulfill. First, it thus far appears to be specific to *Anopheles* genus and therefore, no relevant cross-reactivity phenomena with epitopes from other proteins of arthropods or pathogens would be expected. Second, because it is of a synthetic nature, it guarantees high reproducibility of the immunological assay. Third, it elicits a specific Ab response which correlates well with the level of exposure to *An. gambiae* bites.

3.4.3.1. Biomarker of Anopheles *vector bites*

As previously suggested, anti-gSG6-P1 IgG response was described as a biomarker of *An. gambiae* bites in children living in Senegalese villages where malaria transmission seasonally and moderately occurred [26]. In the same area, a specific IgG response to the peptide has been detected in 36% of children living in villages where very few *An. gambiae*, or none, were collected by classical entomological methods [28]. This deals with a high sensitivity and specificity of the gSG6-P1 epitope(s) after a low immunological boost induced by weak bites exposure. This result points to the potential use of such serological tool as an epidemiological biomarker of *An. gambiae* bites in very low exposure areas, where the sensitivity of current entomological methods of malaria risk assessment is weak.

One study aimed to evaluate the risk of malaria transmission in children and adults living in urban area of Senegal (Dakar region) by using the gSG6-P1 peptide biomarker. Results showed considerable individual variations in anti-gSG6-P1 IgG levels between and within districts, in spite of a context of a global low *Anopheles* exposure level and malaria transmission [27]. Despite this individual heterogeneity, the median level of specific IgG and the percentage of immune responders differed significantly between districts. In addition, a positive association was observed between the exposure levels to *An. gambiae* bites, estimated by classical entomological methods, and the median IgG levels or the percentage of immune responders reflecting the real contact between human populations and *Anopheles* mosquitoes [27]. Differences in exposure levels to *An. gambiae* bites could then partly explain district and/or group-variations in anti-gSG6-P1 IgG Ab response as previously described in a low-exposure rural area of Senegal [28]. Interestingly, in urban Dakar area, immunological parameters seemed to better discriminate the *Anopheles* exposure level between different groups compared to referent entomological data. Moreover, in this study, some discrepancies were observed in the correlation between immunological parameters and the exposure level to *An. gambiae* bites assessed by entomological data in districts. This suggests the main role of the human behavior influencing the contact with vectors. A differential use of Vector Control Measures (ITNs, sprays, curtains) can for example drastically reduce human-vector contact. Many household characteristics (height, type, use of air conditioning, well-closed windows), which can differ between districts, could also be crucial factors. Importantly, the effect of these factors may be not taken into account by assessing the mosquito exposure level and malaria risk with classical entomological tools. This strengthens the usefulness of such biomarker as an alternative tool in the evaluation of exposure levels to *Anopheles* bites, especially in low/very low exposure, where current entomological methods can give inaccurate estimations of the human-mosquito contact [27].

In a population from a malaria hyperendemic area of Burkina Faso, the use of gSG6 recombinant protein as reliable indicator of exposure to the 3 main African malaria vectors (*An. gambiae s.s.*, *An. arabiensis* and *An. funestus*) has been suggested [119]. This probably could be relied to a wide cross-reactivity between SG6 sequences of principal *Anopheles* vectors, which highly share identical epitopes between species. Moreover, the gSG6-P1 peptide has been used to accurately evaluate the exposure level to *An. funestus* bites in a rural area in Senegal [29]. Indeed, two-thirds of 2-9 years old children from this area developed an IgG response to gSG6-P1, in an area where *An. funestus* only was reported. In addition, IgG response increased during the *An. funestus* exposure season, and a positive association was observed with the level of exposure to *An. funestus* bites [29]. This result deals with the cross-reactivity between *An. gambiae* gSG6-P1 and *An. funestus* fSG6-P1 sequences which share a high level of identity. Indeed, these sequences differ only by the substitution of two AAs: asparagine by glutamine (position 9) and leucine by isoleucine (position 15) (Fig. 12).

```
          1       5         10        15        20
fSG6-P1   E K V W V D R D Q V Y C G H I D C T R V A T F
gSG6-P1   E K V W V D R D N V Y C G H L D C T R V A T F
          * * * * * * * * : * * * * * : * * * * * * * *
```

Figure 12. Sequences of the SG6-P1 salivary peptide [29]. Sequences are shown for *An. funestus* (fSG6-P1), for *An. gambiae* (gSG6-P1). Identities are marked with '*' and strong AA conservations with ':'.

AAs from fSG6-P1 are close in terms of polarity and charge to those from *An. gambiae* gSG6-P1. The main consequence is that individuals exposed to *An. funestus* bites can sufficiently develop a specific Ab response against gSG6-P1 *An. gambiae* antigen. This observation, in conjunction with present results, suggests that these substitutions do not alter the synthesis and the recognition of specific Ab because epitope appears to be conserved.

All mentioned studies were conducted on subjects older than 1 year. However, to be more relevant in epidemiological surveys and studies on malaria, such biomarker tool must pertinently be applicable to all human age-classes, including newborns and young infants (<1 year old) who can be also bitten by *Anopheles* and at high risk of malaria transmission [120]. In this way, a recent study has indicated that human Ab responses to gSG6-P1 biomarker help to assess *Anopheles* exposure level and the risk of malaria in younger than 1 year old infants living in moderate to high transmission area of Benin (Drame *et al.*, submitted).

Indeed, the presence of anti-gSG6-P1 IgG and IgM in the blood of respectively 93.28 and 41.79% of 3-months old infants (the majority of infants) and their gradual increasing levels until 12 months (Fig. 13), whatever the *Anopheles* exposure level or the season. These observations are consistent with the development and maturation patterns of the newborn immune system during the first months of life. Indeed, the immature human immune system completes its maturation during infancy following exposition to antigens. Therefore, newborns are naive and increasingly susceptible to infectious agents; their immune system is not or insufficiently

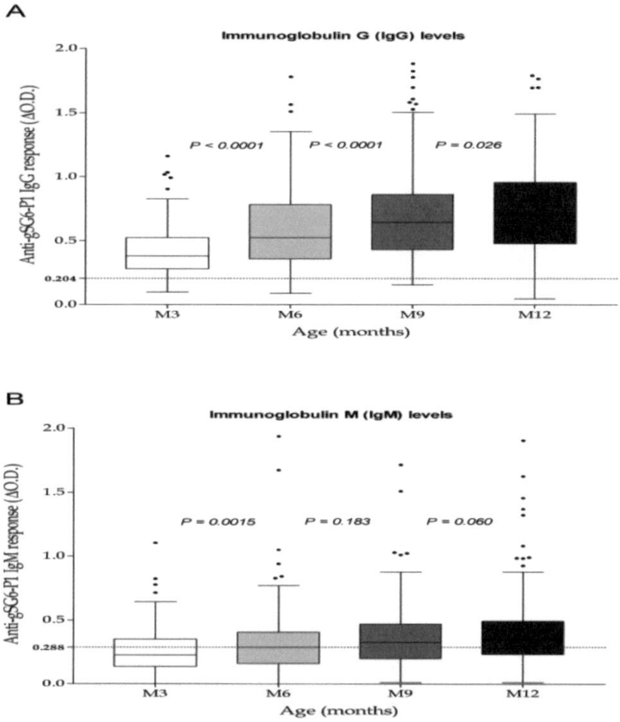

Figure 13. IgG and IgM responses to *Anopheles* gSG6-P1 salivary peptide in the first year-life. Individual IgG (A) and IgM (B) responses to the *Anopheles* gSG6-P1 are represented for infants in months 3 (white), 6 (light-gray), 9 (dark-gray) and 12 (black box) after their birth. Horizontal lines in the boxes indicate medians of the individual data. Horizontal black dotted lines represent the cut-off of IgG (0.204) and IgM (0.288) responder. Statistical significant differences between all age groups (multivariate linear mixed model analysis) are indicated.

stimulated by antigens. In endemic malaria transmission area, they are progressively exposed to salivary antigens of *Anopheles* [121], probably explaining the progressive increase of anti-gSG6-P1 IgG and IgM from 3 to 12 months-old. Individual or population factors and behaviors enhancing the level of the human-*Anopheles* contact with age can play a crucial role on accelerating this gradual acquisition [122, 123].

3.4.3.2. Factors of variation of antibody response to gSG6-P1 and their consequences

Specific gSG6-P1 Ab responses can be influenced by several determinant factors in their variations between individuals, districts, villages, regions... Therefore, identifying effects of human intrinsic (gender, age…) and extrinsic (period of sampling, use of vector control measure…) factors will be useful to the application of the gSG6-P1 biomarker in epidemiological studies or monitoring, evaluation and surveillance of risk of malaria programmes.

Effect of age

Studies have globally reported an increasing anti-gSG6-P1 Ab level according to individual age. In a moderate transmission semi-urban area in Angola, the lowest and highest specific

IgG levels have been described in young children (0-7 years old) and in teenagers/ adults (>14 years old) respectively [30]. In a low malaria transmission urban area (Dakar region) in Senegal, specific IgG levels were significantly higher in adults (>18 years old) compared to 6-10 years old children and in this latter group compared to those aged from 2 to 5 years [27] [124]. In Tori Bossito, moderate-high rural transmission area of Benin, both anti-gSG6-P1 IgG and IgM levels were low at 3 months of age and gradually increased until 12 months after birth (Drame *et al., submitted*). The increase of specific IgG response with age is consistent with the gradual acquired immunity against *Anopheles* mosquito saliva [30] following the development of individual factors and behaviors enhancing the probability of human-vector contact [122, 123]. However, few data have reported a decrease of IgG levels to gSG6-P1 peptide [28] or to SG6 protein [118] with age. In particular, in Senegalese children (0 to 60 months old), the highest specific IgG levels were reported in the youngest children in spite of a probable very weak exposure to *An. gambiae* [30]. It can be explained by a passive IgG transfer from mother to child during pregnancy or breastfeeding as recently reported in young infants from Benin (Drame *et al., submitted*). This represents a way of overestimation of the assessment of human-*Anopheles* contact level and the risk of malaria in young infants by using anti-gSG6-P1 IgG Ab. Therefore, the evaluation of specific IgM Ab levels could be a relevant solution to bias in IgG measurements. Indeed, IgM Ab, in a form of polymers (usually pentamers) in the human organism, could not cross the maternal-foetal barrier [125] and are the first Ab to appear in response to initial or primary exposure to antigen [126]. Interestingly, in Tori Bossito, specific IgM levels seemed to be a serological marker only during the first 6-months of exposure. In infants older to 6 months, the assessment of gSG6-P1-specific IgG showed a more pertinent evaluation of exposure level.

Effect of sex

Some studies have reported higher levels of anti-gSG6-P1 in female individuals (children and women) compared to males (children and men) [27, 30] ([124]; Drame *et al., submitted*). However, this difference was not significant, suggesting that it might be only physiological.

The season of *Anopheles* exposure

The season of individual sampling may be also a factor of confusion in the use gSG6-P1 biomarker in epidemiological studies on malaria risk assessment or control. Indeed, significant seasonally variations in anti-gSG6-P1 IgG or/and IgM levels have been reported in studies conducted in newborns, children or/and adults from endemic malaria areas in Senegal [27-29, 124], Angola [30] and Benin (Drame *et al.*, submitted). In Senegal, in particular, specific gSG6-P1 in urban children and adults steadily waned from the beginning (October) to the end (December) of the study, due to an important drop in human exposure level to *An. gambiae s. l.* bites from the end of rainfalls (October) to the beginning of the dry season (December) [127, 128].

One direct application of a salivary biomarker of exposure could serve in the elaboration of maps representing the risk of exposure to *Anopheles* bites. Such immuno-epidemiological marker might represent a quantitative tool applied to field conditions and a complementary tool to those currently available, such as entomological, ecological and environmental data [59, 129]. It could represent a geographic indicator of the risks of malaria transmission and thus a useful tool for predicting malaria morbidity risk as previously described [22]. Furthermore, it may represent a powerful tool for evaluation of vector control strategies (impregnated bed-net, intradomiciliary aspersion, etc.) and could here constitute a direct criterion for effectiveness and appropriate use (malaria control program) [84].

3.4.3.3. Indicator of malaria vector control effectiveness

Long and short-term evaluation of ITN efficacy

A longitudinal study associating parasitological, entomological and immunological assessments of the efficacy of ITN-based strategies using the gSG6-P1 biomarker has been conducted in a malaria-endemic area in Angola. Human IgG responses to gSG6-P1 peptide were evaluated in 105 individuals (adults and children) before and after the introduction of ITNs and compared to entomo-parasitological data. A significant decrease of anti-gSG6-P1 IgG response was observed just after the effective use of ITNs (Fig. 14). The drop in gSG6-P1 IgG levels was associated with a considerable decrease of *P. falciparum* parasitaemia, the current WHO criterion for vector control efficacy [130]. It was particularly marked in April-August 2006, corresponding to the season peak of *An. gambiae* exposure. Interestingly, the entomological data indicated that this season-dependent peak was of similar intensity before (2005) and after (2006) ITN use, suggesting ITN installation had no impact on *An. gambiae* density, probably because of the low percentage of the overall human population covered in the studied area [131]. This study indicated also that the drop of anti-gSG6-P1 IgG response was associated with correct ITN use and not due to low *Anopheles* density. In addition, this was observed in all age groups studied (<7 years, 7–14 years, and >14 years), suggesting that this biomarker is relevant for ITN evaluation in all age groups. This rapid decrease after correct ITN usage appears to be a special property of anti-gSG6-P1 IgG which is short-lived (4-6 weeks) in the absence of ongoing antigenic stimulation, at/for all age classes.

The response does not seem to build up but wanes rapidly, when exposure failed. This property represents a major strength when using such salivary biomarker of exposure for evaluating the efficacy of vector control. In addition, using a response threshold (ΔOD=0.204) combined with ΔOD_{ITNs} - the difference between April (after ITNs) and January 2006 (before) - makes possible the use of this operational biomarker at individual level (Fig. 15). The threshold response (TR) represents the non-specific background IgG response (the cut-off of immune response) and was calculated in non-*Anopheles* exposed individuals (n= 14- neg; North of France) by using this formula: TR= mean (ΔDO_{neg}) + 3SD = 0.204. An exposed individual was then classified as an immune responder if its ΔOD> 0.204. If the ΔOD_{ITNs} value is comprised between -0.204 and +0.204, no clear difference in exposure level to *Anopheles* bites can be defined.

In contrast, if the individual ΔOD_{ITNs} value <–0.204, it could be concluded with a high level of confidence that this individual is benefiting from ITN installation. The ΔOD_{ITNs} parameter could therefore provide a measure of ITN efficacy at the individual level. An individual biomarker would also be relevant at the large-scale operational studies or surveillance in the field, e.g. in National Malaria Control Programs (NMCP). In addition, the high sensitivity and specificity of the gSG6-P1 Ab response make it ideal for the evaluation of low-level ex-

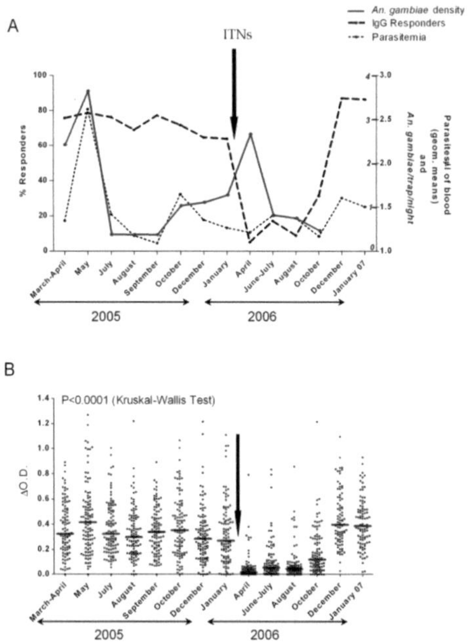

Figure 14. IgG Ab responses to gSG6-P1 before and after ITN use [30]. The percentage (%) of anti-gSG6-P1 IgG immune responders (thick-dotted line) in the "immunological" sub-population (n=105), before (2005) and after (2006 and January 2007) the installation of ITNs (A). These results are presented together with the intensity of *P. falciparum* infection (mean parasitaemia – fine-dotted line) measured in the same population and the mean of number of *An. gambiae* (solid line) in the studied area (A). Entomological data were not available in December 2006 and January 2007 (the last two months of the study). Arrows indicate the installation of Insecticide Treated Nets (ITNs) in February 2006. Individual anti-gSG6-P1 IgG levels (ΔOD) are presented before (2005) and after (2006) the installation of ITNs (B). Bars indicate the median value for each studied month. Statistically significant differences between months are indicated.

posure to *Anopheles bites* [27, 28], even when exposure or transmission is curtailed by NMCP efforts. Taken together, the estimation of human IgG responses to *Anopheles* gSG6-P1 could provide a reliable indicator for evaluating the efficacy of ITN-based strategies against malaria vectors, at individual and population levels, even after vector control generating particular low exposure/transmission contexts. This salivary biomarker is a relevant tool for the evaluation of short-term efficacy as well as longer-term monitoring of malaria VCMs.

Evaluation of effectiveness of diverse vector control measures

A recent cross-sectional study conducted from October to December 2008 on 2,774 residents (children and adults) of 45 districts of urban Dakar (Senegal) has validated IgG responses to gSG6-P1 as an epidemiological indicator evaluating the effectiveness of a range of VCMs. Indeed, in this area, IgG levels to gSG6-P1 as well as the use of diverse malaria VCMs (ITNs, mosquito coils, spray bombs, ventilation and/or incense) highly varied between districts [124]. This difference of use suggests some socio-economical and cultural discrepancies between householders as described in large cities of Ivory Coast [132] and Tanzania [123]. At the district level, specific IgG levels significantly decreased with VCM use in children as well as in adults.

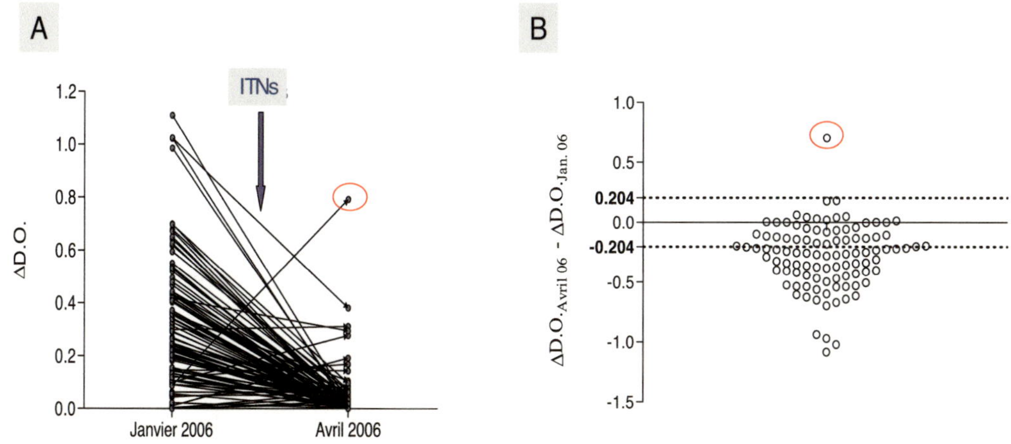

Figure 15. IgG response to gSG6-P1 as biomarker for short-term ITN efficacy. Changes in individual IgG levels (ΔOD) are presented between "just before" (January 2006) and "just after" (April 2006) ITN introduction (n=105; children and adults) (A). The arrow indicates the installation of Insecticide Treated Nets (ITNs) in February 2006. Individual IgG level changes from January (before) to April are presented (B) by individual $\Delta OD_{ITNs,}$ value ($\Delta OD_{ITNs=}\Delta OD_{April06}$, - $\Delta OD_{January06}$). The threshold of specific IgG responders (TR=0.204) is indicated (dotted line). Significant positive (ΔOD>0.204) or negative (ΔOD<–0.204) changes are therefore individually presented.

Among used VCM, ITNs, the 1st chosen preventive method (43.35% rate of use), by reducing drastically the human-*Anopheles* contact level and specific IgG levels in children as well as in adults, were by far the most efficient whatever age, period of sampling or the exposure level to mosquito bites. Spray bombs were secondarily associated to a decrease of specific IgG level, due certainly to their power and fast knock-down action. But, their effects can be limited by the non-persistence of used products and some socio-economic considerations [133]. In addition, they only have been recently adopted and are more expensive in the majority of sub-Saharan Africa cities [133], explaining their less frequent use (9.57% rate of use) in the Dakar area. The non-effect of mosquito coil use is surprising, regardless to their well-adoption by residents (36.68% of rate of use), but it can be explained by their power deterrent effect which tends to push *Anopheles* vectors outside where they can remain active [133]. However, the protection ensured by ITN use seemed to be insufficient because anti-gSG6-P1 IgG levels in ITN users were specifically high in some periods of fairly high exposure to *Anopheles* bites. Changes in *An. arabiensis* behaviour, the major malaria vector in the area, can also explain this lack of protection. It can bite outside the rooms/ habitations with a maximal activity around 10.00 pm, when people are not in bed and ITNs not hanged [123]. Therefore, ITNs must be associated to a complementary VCM for an effective protection against *Anopheles* bites.

Taken together, these results suggest that the assessment of human IgG responses to *Anopheles* gSG6-P1 salivary peptide can provide a reliable evaluation of the effectiveness of malaria vector control in urban settings of Dakar whatever the age, sex, level of exposure to bites or period of malaria transmission. Therefore, this salivary biomarker can be used to compare the effectiveness of different anti-malaria vector strategies in order to identify the most suitable for a given area.

Comparing effectiveness of combined or not vector control measures

In parallel to an entomological and parasitological evaluation, IgG responses to gSG6-P1 were also used to assess, in a randomized controlled trial in 28 villages in southern Benin, four malaria vector control interventions: Long-Lasting Insecticide-treated Net (LLIN) targeted coverage to pregnant women and children younger than 6 years (TLLIN, reference group), LLIN universal coverage of all sleeping units (ULLIN), TLLIN plus full coverage of carbamate-indoor residual spraying (IRS) applied every 8 months (TLLIN+IRS), and ULLIN plus full coverage of carbamate-treated plastic sheeting (CTPS) lined up to the upper part of the household walls (ULLIN+CTPS). Results from this study have shown that specific IgG levels were similar in the 4 groups before intervention and only significantly lower in the ULLIN group compared to the others after intervention. In contrast to immunological data, clinical incidence density of malaria, the prevalence and parasite density of asymptomatic infections, and the density and aggressiveness of *Anopheles* mosquitoes, were not significantly different between the four groups before as well as after interventions [134]. These findings mean that LLIN used along by all the population of a given area may be more suitable in reducing the contact between human populations and the *Anopheles* vectors, even if any effect on malaria morbidity, infection, and transmission was not observed. Therefore, combining anti-vector tools do not undeniably reduce individual exposure to malaria vectors, even if significant effect on reducing more rapidly malaria transmission and burden has been reported [135]. These findings confirm that anti-vector saliva Ab response as a biomarker of exposure is also important for NMCPs and should help the design of more cost-effective strategies for malaria control and elimination.

3.4.4. Importance to develop a specific biomarker of infecting Anopheles *bites*

Recent data have shown that the use of the gSG6-P1 biomarker for the assessment of the differential risk of the disease transmission may have some limitations in high exposure areas (Drame *et al.*, submitted). Indeed, the gSG6-P1 assesses the exposure level to both infective and not infective *Anopheles* bites. In malaria hyperendemic areas, resident people are highly exposed to mainly not infective bites and present almost all Ab specific to gSG6-P1 levels relatively high. Therefore it should be relevant to develop a biomarker of exposure specific to infective bites in order to assess the human risk of malaria transmission in such contexts. Such epidemiological parameter would be important to define in the context of malaria control. The transmission depends on the density of competent *Anopheles*, of their *Plasmodium* infective rate and of the intensity of human-vector contact. In addition, current methods to measure the intensity of malaria transmission show several limitations, especially in low transmission areas. The EIR (entomological inoculation rate) is a commonly used metric rate that estimates the number of bites by infectious mosquitoes per person per unit time. It is the product of the "human biting rate" – the number of bites per person per day by vector mosquitoes – and the fraction of vector mosquitoes that are infectious (the "sporozoite rate"). The classical method to estimate the density of sporozoites in mosquitoes is the dissection of salivary glands and the sporozoites counting under microscope. But in area of low exposure and because few mosquitoes are infected, many mosquitoes must be caught and dissected. The salivary glands dissection is a tedious technique which required well trained and studious personnel. Moreover this technique cannot differentiate *Plasmodium* species. Another technique named CSP-ELISA detects the CSP (Circumsporozoite protein) parasite surface protein and is generally done on head/thorax of mosquitoes. However the CSP protein is expressed at the oocyst stage, consequently the CSP can be detected in the mosquito before the sporozoites have reached the salivary glands (until 2-3 days) [136, 137]. Therefore, this method induced a bias with an overestimation of sporozoites index [138, 139]. Other traditional epidemiological estimates mainly based on parasitological tests are very sensitive and specific allowing the determination of parasite species, but the examination of finger prick and thick blood smear is also labour intensive and time-consuming requiring well trained staff for a reliable examination [140]. To improve the measure of transmission, antibody responses against parasite proteins (CSP, AMA1, MSP1, MSP3, etc…) could be used but several studies have highlighted limits of this approach. Actually, people exposed to malaria can be seropositive during several months [141, 142], even after transmission has stopped [141] or in the context of low transmission [143]. So by using this method we are not able to distinguish old and new infection which is particularly important in the context of evaluation of the effectiveness of vector control program. Considering these limits, these serological parameters seem inappropriate to assess the malaria exposure at the individual level. Some proteomic and transcriptomic studies highlighted that the composition of *Anopheles* salivary glands could be modified with the presence of *Plasmodium* parasite [15, 144, 145]. Therefore, the development of a biomarker specific of infective bites based on the analysis of antibody response against salivary proteins should represent an alternative method to assess the parasite transmission to the human.

The principle of biomarker of infective bites is based on the use of immunogenic salivary protein like marker of transmission. The expression of some salivary proteins could be induced or regulated when the salivary glands are infected. Therefore, if one of such protein presents also immunogenic properties, we can probably use the specific immune response to this protein like a marker of transmission in human. Such a biomarker will be also particularly relevant in the context of re-emergence after malaria transmission reduction or in area of low exposure. This tool will allow focusing the intervention (vector control strategies and drugs distribution) on the most exposed and the most susceptible population.

4. Conclusions

In the present chapter, we have described the development of a biomarker (the *An. gambiae* gSG6-P1 peptide) of *Anopheles* mosquito bites by using an original approach coupling bioinformatic tools and immuno-epidemiological assays. Then, measurements of IgG level specific to gSG6-P1 at individual as well as population level, represent a tool/biomarker for accurately evaluate the level of human exposure to *Anopheles* bites and the risk of malaria in all age-classes of populations (newborns, infants, children, adults) living in various settings (very-low, low, moderate, and high malaria transmission areas) of rural, semi-urban and urban regions of Senegal, Angola and Benin. In the majority of these areas, this biomarker appeared to be promising and complementary to classical entomological methods, because it can give a reliable evaluation of the individual contact with anthropophilic *Anopheles* even if exposure to bites is low/very low (urban area). Therefore, such biomarker would be particularly relevant in places where malaria transmission is low, e.g. in foci of urban, high-altitude or seasonal malaria, and in travelers in endemic areas. This chapter has also shown that the availability of such a biomarker could allow the evaluation of the exposure to the main *P. falciparum* vectors (*An. gambiae s.s., An. arabiensis, An. funestus, An. melas*) in Africa where different species of malaria vector co-inhabit. One direct application of such a gSG6 peptide marker of exposure could be in the elaboration of maps representing the risk of exposure to *Anopheles* bites. It could represent a geographic indicator of the risks of malaria transmission and thus a useful tool for predicting malaria morbidity risk as previously described. Furthermore, it represents a powerful and reliable tool for the evaluation of the effectiveness of vector control strategies. Such an indicator could also represent an alternative to classical entomological-parasitological monitoring methods for measuring and following the effectiveness of vector control strategies used by the National Malaria Control Programmes in various settings across Africa. Finally, this biomarker approach could be similarly applied to vector-control strategies for other mosquito-borne diseases such as emergent or re-emergent arbovirus diseases and trypanosomiasis.

Author details

Papa M. Drame[1*], Anne Poinsignon[1], Alexandra Marie[1], Herbert Noukpo[2], Souleymane Doucoure[1], Sylvie Cornelie[1,2] and Franck Remoue[1,2]

*Address all correspondence to: drpapamak@gmail.com

1 Universités Montpellier 1 et 2, Institut de Recherche pour le Développement (IRD), Montpellier, France

2 Universités Montpellier 1 et 2, Centre de Recherche Entomologique de Cotonou (CREC), Cotonou, Bénin

References

[1] Gubler DJ. Resurgent vector-borne diseases as a global health problem. Emerg Infect Dis 1998;4:442-50.

[2] WHO. 2011. In: Organization WH, ed. Geneva: World Health Organization, World Malaria Report 2011.

[3] Guerra CA, Gikandi PW, Tatem AJ, et al. The limits and intensity of *Plasmodium falciparum* transmission: implications for malaria control and elimination worldwide. PLoS Med 2008;5:e38.

[4] Hay SI, Guerra CA, Gething PW, et al. A world malaria map: *Plasmodium falciparum* endemicity in 2007. PLoS Med 2009;6:e1000048.

[5] WHO. Global Malaria Action Plan World Health Organization. Geneva, Switzerland: World Health Organization, 2009.

[6] The MalERA Consultative group on Monitoring EaS. A research agenda for malaria eradication: monitoring, evaluation, and surveillance. PLoS Med. 2011;8:e1000400.

[7] Beier JC, Killeen GF and Githure JI. Short report: entomologic inoculation rates and *Plasmodium falciparum* malaria prevalence in Africa. Am J Trop Med Hyg 1999;61:109-13.

[8] Drakeley CJ, Corran PH, Coleman PG, et al. Estimating medium- and long-term trends in malaria transmission by using serological markers of malaria exposure. Proc Natl Acad Sci U S A 2005;102:5108-13.

[9] Hay SI, Rogers DJ, Toomer JF and Snow RW. Annual *Plasmodium falciparum* entomological inoculation rates (EIR) across Africa: literature survey, Internet access and review. Trans R Soc Trop Med Hyg 2000;94:113-27.

[10] Smith DL, Dushoff J, Snow RW and Hay SI. The entomological inoculation rate and *Plasmodium falciparum* infection in African children. Nature 2005;438:492-5.

[11] Clements AP, Ferry JG. Cloning, nucleotide sequence, and transcriptional analyses of the gene encoding a ferredoxin from *Methanosarcina thermophila*. J Bacteriol 1992;174:5244-50.

[12] Vanderberg JP, Frevert U. Intravital microscopy demonstrating antibody-mediated immobilisation of *Plasmodium berghei* sporozoites injected into skin by mosquitoes. Int J Parasitol 2004;34:991-6.

[13] Champagne DE. Antihemostatic strategies of blood-feeding arthropods. Curr Drug Targets Cardiovasc Haematol Disord 2004;4:375-96.

[14] Champagne DE. Antihemostatic molecules from saliva of blood-feeding arthropods. Pathophysiol Haemost Thromb 2005;34:221-7.

[15] Choumet V, Carmi-Leroy A, Laurent C, et al. The salivary glands and saliva of *Anopheles gambiae* as an essential step in the *Plasmodium* life cycle: a global proteomic study. Proteomics 2007;7:3384-94.

[16] Ribeiro JM, Francischetti IM. Role of arthropod saliva in blood feeding: sialome and post-sialome perspectives. Annu Rev Entomol 2003;48:73-88.

[17] Peng Z, Simons FE. Mosquito allergy: immune mechanisms and recombinant salivary allergens. Int Arch Allergy Immunol 2004;133:198-209.

[18] Donovan MJ, Messmore AS, Scrafford DA, Sacks DL, Kamhawi S and McDowell MA. Uninfected mosquito bites confer protection against infection with malaria parasites. Infect Immun 2007;75:2523-30.

[19] Schneider BS, Mathieu C, Peronet R and Mecheri S. *Anopheles stephensi* saliva enhances progression of cerebral malaria in a murine model. Vector Borne Zoonotic Dis 2011;11:423-32

[20] Andrade BB, Rocha BC, Reis-Filho A, et al. Anti-*Anopheles darlingi* saliva antibodies as marker of *Plasmodium vivax* infection and clinical immunity in the Brazilian Amazon. Malar J 2009;8:121.

[21] Orlandi-Pradines E, Almeras L, Denis de Senneville L, et al. Antibody response against saliva antigens of *Anopheles gambiae* and *Aedes aegypti* in travellers in tropical Africa. Microbes Infect 2007;9:1454-62.

[22] Remoue F, Cisse B, Ba F, et al. Evaluation of the antibody response to *Anopheles* salivary antigens as a potential marker of risk of malaria. Trans R Soc Trop Med Hyg 2006;100:363-70

[23] Waitayakul A, Somsri S, Sattabongkot J, Looareesuwan S, Cui L and Udomsangpetch R. Natural human humoral response to salivary gland proteins of *Anopheles* mosquitoes in Thailand. Acta Trop 2006;98:66-73.

[24] Schneider BS, Higgs S. The enhancement of arbovirus transmission and disease by mosquito saliva is associated with modulation of the host immune response. Trans R Soc Trop Med Hyg 2008;102:400-8.

[25] Londono-Renteria BL, Eisele TP, Keating J, James MA and Wesson DM. Antibody response against *Anopheles albimanus* (Diptera: Culicidae) salivary protein as a measure of mosquito bite exposure in Haiti. J Med Entomol 2010;47:1156-63.

[26] Poinsignon A, Cornelie S, Mestres-Simon M, et al. Novel peptide marker corresponding to salivary protein gSG6 potentially identifies exposure to *Anopheles* bites. PLoS One 2008;3:e2472

[27] Drame PM, Machault V, Diallo A, et al. IgG responses to the gSG6-P1 salivary peptide for evaluating human exposure to *Anopheles* bites in urban areas of Dakar region, Senegal. Malar J 2012;11:72.

[28] Poinsignon A, Cornelie S, Ba F, et al. Human IgG response to a salivary peptide, gSG6-P1, as a new immuno-epidemiological tool for evaluating low-level exposure to *Anopheles* bites. Malar J 2009;8:198.

[29] Poinsignon A, Samb B, Doucoure S, et al. First attempt to validate the gSG6-P1 salivary peptide as an immuno-epidemiological tool for evaluating human exposure to *Anopheles funestus* bites. Trop Med Int Health 2010;15:1198-203.

[30] Drame PM, Poinsignon A, Besnard P, et al. Human antibody responses to the *Anopheles* salivary gSG6-P1 peptide: a novel tool for evaluating the efficacy of ITNs in malaria vector control. PLoS One 2010;5:e15596.

[31] Odegaard F. How many species of arthropods? Erwin's estimate revised. Biological Journal of the Linnean Society 2000;71:583-597.

[32] Ribeiro JM. Blood-feeding arthropods: live syringes or invertebrate pharmacologists? Infect Agents Dis 1995;4:143-52.

[33] Foster WA. Mosquito sugar feeding and reproductive energetics. Annu Rev Entomol 1995;40:443-74.

[34] Ribeiro JM. Role of saliva in blood-feeding by arthropods. Annu Rev Entomol 1987;32:463-78.

[35] Francischetti IM, Sa-Nunes A, Mans BJ, Santos IM and Ribeiro JM. The role of saliva in tick feeding. Front Biosci 2009;14:2051-88.

[36] Ribeiro JM, Rossignol PA and Spielman A. Role of mosquito saliva in blood vessel location. J Exp Biol 1984;108:1-7.

[37] Champagne DE. The role of salivary vasodilators in bloodfeeding and parasite transmission. Parasitol Today 1994;10:430-3.

[38] Stark KR, James AA. Salivary gland anticoagulants in culicine and anopheline mosquitoes (Diptera:Culicidae). J Med Entomol 1996;33:645-50.

[39] Francischetti IM. Platelet aggregation inhibitors from hematophagous animals. Toxicon 2010;56:1130-44.

[40] Lombardo F, Di Cristina M, Spanos L, Louis C, Coluzzi M and Arca B. Promoter sequences of the putative *Anopheles gambiae* apyrase confer salivary gland expression in *Drosophila melanogaster*. J Biol Chem 2000;275:23861-8.

[41] Arca B, Lombardo F, Capurro M, et al. Salivary gland-specific gene expression in the malaria vector *Anopheles gambiae*. Parassitologia 1999;41:483-7.

[42] Arca B, Lombardo F, de Lara Capurro M, et al. Trapping cDNAs encoding secreted proteins from the salivary glands of the malaria vector *Anopheles gambiae*. Proc Natl Acad Sci U S A 1999;96:1516-21.

[43] Calvo E, Andersen J, Francischetti IM, et al. The transcriptome of adult female *Anopheles darlingi* salivary glands. Insect Mol Biol 2004;13:73-88.

[44] Calvo E, Mans BJ, Andersen JF and Ribeiro JM. Function and evolution of a mosquito salivary protein family. J Biol Chem 2006;281:1935-42.

[45] Yoshida S, Sudo T, Niimi M, et al. Inhibition of collagen-induced platelet aggregation by anopheline antiplatelet protein, a saliva protein from a malaria vector mosquito. Blood 2008;111:2007-14.

[46] Francischetti IM, Valenzuela JG and Ribeiro JM. Anophelin: kinetics and mechanism of thrombin inhibition. Biochemistry 1999;38:16678-85.

[47] Isawa H, Yuda M, Orito Y and Chinzei Y. A mosquito salivary protein inhibits activation of the plasma contact system by binding to factor XII and high molecular weight kininogen. J Biol Chem 2002;277:27651-8.

[48] Champagne DE, Ribeiro JM. Sialokinin I and II: vasodilatory tachykinins from the yellow fever mosquito *Aedes aegypti*. Proc Natl Acad Sci U S A 1994;91:138-42.

[49] Ribeiro JM. Characterization of a vasodilator from the salivary glands of the yellow fever mosquito *Aedes aegypti*. J Exp Biol 1992;165:61-71.

[50] Ribeiro JM, Valenzuela JG. Purification and cloning of the salivary peroxidase/catechol oxidase of the mosquito *Anopheles albimanus*. J Exp Biol 1999;202:809-16.

[51] Fontaine A, Pascual A, Diouf I, et al. Mosquito salivary gland protein preservation in the field for immunological and biochemical analysis. Parasit Vectors 2011;4:33.

[52] Wikel SK. Immune responses to arthropods and their products. Annu Rev Entomol 1982;27:21-48.

[53] Konik P, Slavikova V, Salat J, Reznickova J, Dvoroznakova E and Kopecky J. Anti-tumour necrosis factor-alpha activity in *Ixodes ricinus* saliva. Parasite Immunol 2006;28:649-56.

[54] Titus RG, Bishop JV and Mejia JS. The immunomodulatory factors of arthropod saliva and the potential for these factors to serve as vaccine targets to prevent pathogen transmission. Parasite Immunol 2006;28:131-41.

[55] Andrade BB, Barral-Netto M. Biomarkers for susceptibility to infection and disease severity in human malaria. Mem Inst Oswaldo Cruz 2011;106 Suppl 1:70-8.

[56] Peng Z, Estelle F and Simons R. Mosquito allergy and mosquito salivary allergens. Protein Pept Lett 2007;14:975-81.

[57] Poole S, Lorenzetti BB, Cunha JM, Cunha FQ and Ferreira SH. Bradykinin B1 and B2 receptors, tumour necrosis factor alpha and inflammatory hyperalgesia. Br J Pharmacol 1999;126:649-56.

[58] Demeure CE, Brahimi K, Hacini F, et al. *Anopheles* mosquito bites activate cutaneous mast cells leading to a local inflammatory response and lymph node hyperplasia. J Immunol 2005;174:3932-40

[59] Billingsley PF, Baird J, Mitchell JA and Drakeley C. Immune interactions between mosquitoes and their hosts. Parasite Immunol 2006;28:143-53.

[60] Depinay N, Hacini F, Beghdadi W, Peronet R and Mecheri S. Mast cell-dependent down-regulation of antigen-specific immune responses by mosquito bites. J Immunol 2006;176:4141-6.

[61] Gillespie RD, Mbow ML and Titus RG. The immunomodulatory factors of blood-feeding arthropod saliva. Parasite Immunol 2000;22:319-31.

[62] Edwards JF, Higgs S and Beaty BJ. Mosquito feeding-induced enhancement of Cache Valley Virus (Bunyaviridae) infection in mice. J Med Entomol 1998;35:261-5.

[63] Schneider BS, Soong L, Girard YA, Campbell G, Mason P and Higgs S. Potentiation of West Nile encephalitis by mosquito feeding. Viral Immunol 2006;19:74-82.

[64] Schneider BS, Soong L, Zeidner NS and Higgs S. *Aedes aegypti* salivary gland extracts modulate anti-viral and TH1/TH2 cytokine responses to sindbis virus infection. Viral Immunol 2004;17:565-73.

[65] Esmon CT. Interactions between the innate immune and blood coagulation systems. Trends Immunol 2004;25:536-42.

[66] Bissonnette EY, Rossignol PA and Befus AD. Extracts of mosquito salivary gland inhibit tumour necrosis factor alpha release from mast cells. Parasite Immunol 1993;15:27-33.

[67] Rocha AC, Braga EM, Araujo MS, Franklin BS and Pimenta PF. Effect of the *Aedes fluviatilis* saliva on the development of *Plasmodium gallinaceum* infection in *Gallus* (*gallus*) *domesticus*. Mem Inst Oswaldo Cruz 2004;99:709-15.

[68] Thomson SA, Sherritt MA, Medveczky J, et al. Delivery of multiple CD8 cytotoxic T cell epitopes by DNA vaccination. J Immunol 1998;160:1717-23.

[69] Ader DB, Celluzzi C, Bisbing J, et al. Modulation of dengue virus infection of dendritic cells by *Aedes aegypti* saliva. Viral Immunol 2004;17:252-65.

[70] Remoue F, Alix E, Cornelie S, et al. IgE and IgG4 antibody responses to *Aedes* saliva in African children. Acta Trop 2007;104:108-15.

[71] Ramasamy MS, Srikrishnaraj KA, Wijekoone S, Jesuthasan LS and Ramasamy R. Host immunity to mosquitoes: effect of antimosquito antibodies on *Anopheles tessellatus* and *Culex quinquefasciatus* (Diptera: Culicidae). J Med Entomol 1992;29:934-8.

[72] Siden-Kiamos I, Louis C. Interactions between malaria parasites and their mosquito hosts in the midgut. Insect Biochem Mol Biol 2004;34:679-85.

[73] Suneja A, Gulia M and Gakhar SK. Blocking of malaria parasite development in mosquito and fecundity reduction by midgut antibodies in *Anopheles stephensi* (Diptera: Culicidae). Arch Insect Biochem Physiol 2003;52:63-70.

[74] Gomes R, Teixeira C, Teixeira MJ, et al. Immunity to a salivary protein of a sand fly vector protects against the fatal outcome of visceral leishmaniasis in a hamster model. Proc Natl Acad Sci U S A 2008;105:7845-50.

[75] Brennan JD, Kent M, Dhar R, Fujioka H and Kumar N. *Anopheles gambiae* salivary gland proteins as putative targets for blocking transmission of malaria parasites. Proc Natl Acad Sci U S A 2000;97:13859-64.

[76] Ramamoorthi N, Narasimhan S, Pal U, et al. The Lyme disease agent exploits a tick protein to infect the mammalian host. Nature 2005;436:573-7.

[77] Dai J, Wang P, Adusumilli S, et al. Antibodies against a tick protein, Salp15, protect mice from the Lyme disease agent. Cell Host Microbe 2009;6:482-92.

[78] Peng Z, Beckett AN, Engler RJ, Hoffman DR, Ott NL and Simons FE. Immune responses to mosquito saliva in 14 individuals with acute systemic allergic reactions to mosquito bites. J Allergy Clin Immunol 2004;114:1189-94.

[79] Peng Z, Ho MK, Li C and Simons FE. Evidence for natural desensitization to mosquito salivary allergens: mosquito saliva specific IgE and IgG levels in children. Ann Allergy Asthma Immunol 2004;93:553-6.

[80] Schwartz BS, Ford DP, Childs JE, Rothman N and Thomas RJ. Anti-tick saliva antibody: a biologic marker of tick exposure that is a risk factor for Lyme disease seropositivity. Am J Epidemiol 1991;134:86-95.

[81] Schwartz BS, Ribeiro JM and Goldstein MD. Anti-tick antibodies: an epidemiologic tool in Lyme disease research. Am J Epidemiol 1990;132:58-66.

[82] Barral A, Honda E, Caldas A, et al. Human immune response to sand fly salivary gland antigens: a useful epidemiological marker? Am J Trop Med Hyg 2000;62:740-5.

[83] Nascimento RJ, Santana JM, Lozzi SP, Araujo CN and Teixeira AR. Human IgG1 and IgG4: the main antibodies against *Triatoma infestans* (Hemiptera: Reduviidae) salivary gland proteins. Am J Trop Med Hyg 2001;65:219-26.

[84] Drame PM, Poinsignon A, Besnard P, et al. Human antibody response to *Anopheles gambiae* saliva: an immuno-epidemiological biomarker to evaluate the efficacy of insecticide-treated nets in malaria vector control. Am J Trop Med Hyg 2010;83:115-21.

[85] Brosseau L, Drame PM, Besnard P, et al. Human antibody response to *Anopheles* saliva for comparing the efficacy of three malaria vector control methods in Balombo, Angola. PLoS One 2012;7:e44189.

[86] Ribeiro JM. A catalogue of *Anopheles gambiae* transcripts significantly more or less expressed following a blood meal. Insect Biochem Mol Biol 2003;33:865-82.

[87] Lombardo F, Lanfrancotti A, Mestres-Simon M, Rizzo C, Coluzzi M and Arca B. At the interface between parasite and host: the salivary glands of the African malaria vector *Anopheles gambiae*. Parassitologia 2006;48:573-80.

[88] Valenzuela JG. High-throughput approaches to study salivary proteins and genes from vectors of disease. Insect Biochem Mol Biol 2002;32:1199-209

[89] Charlab R, Valenzuela JG, Rowton ED and Ribeiro JM. Toward an understanding of the biochemical and pharmacological complexity of the saliva of a hematophagous sand fly *Lutzomyia longipalpis*. Proc Natl Acad Sci U S A 1999;96:15155-60

[90] Holt RA, Subramanian GM, Halpern A, et al. The genome sequence of the malaria mosquito *Anopheles gambiae*. Science 2002;298:129-49

[91] Wang Z, Gerstein M and Snyder M. RNA-Seq: a revolutionary tool for transcriptomics. Nat Rev Genet 2009;10:57-63

[92] Jariyapan N, Roytrakul S, Paemanee A, et al. Proteomic analysis of salivary glands of female *Anopheles barbirostris* species A2 (Diptera: Culicidae) by two-dimensional gel electrophoresis and mass spectrometry. Parasitol Res 2012. 111(3), 1239-49.

[93] Valenzuela JG, Belkaid Y, Garfield MK, et al. Toward a defined anti-*Leishmania* vaccine targeting vector antigens: characterization of a protective salivary protein. J Exp Med 2001;194:331-42

[94] Arca B, Lombardo F, Valenzuela JG, et al. An updated catalogue of salivary gland transcripts in the adult female mosquito, *Anopheles gambiae*. J Exp Biol 2005;208:3971-86

[95] Calvo E, Dao A, Pham VM and Ribeiro JM. An insight into the sialome of *Anopheles funestus* reveals an emerging pattern in anopheline salivary protein families. Insect Biochem Mol Biol 2007;37:164-75

[96] Das S, Radtke A, Choi YJ, Mendes AM, Valenzuela JG and Dimopoulos G. Transcriptomic and functional analysis of the *Anopheles gambiae* salivary gland in relation to blood feeding. BMC Genomics 2010;11:566.

[97] Jariyapan N, Baimai V, Poovorawan Y, et al. Analysis of female salivary gland proteins of the *Anopheles barbirostris* complex (Diptera: Culicidae) in Thailand. Parasitol Res 2010;107:509-16.

[98] Jariyapan N, Choochote W, Jitpakdi A, et al. Salivary gland proteins of the human malaria vector, *Anopheles dirus* B (Diptera: Culicidae). Rev Inst Med Trop Sao Paulo 2007;49:5-10.

[99] Lombardo F, Ronca R, Rizzo C, et al. The *Anopheles gambiae* salivary protein gSG6: an anopheline-specific protein with a blood-feeding role. Insect Biochem Mol Biol 2009;39:457-66.

[100] Valenzuela JG, Francischetti IM, Pham VM, Garfield MK and Ribeiro JM. Exploring the salivary gland transcriptome and proteome of the *Anopheles stephensi* mosquito. Insect Biochem Mol Biol 2003;33:717-32.

[101] Calvo E, Pham VM, Marinotti O, Andersen JF and Ribeiro JM. The salivary gland transcriptome of the neotropical malaria vector *Anopheles darlingi* reveals accelerated evolution of genes relevant to hematophagy. BMC Genomics 2009;10:57.

[102] Francischetti IM, Valenzuela JG, Pham VM, Garfield MK and Ribeiro JM. Toward a catalog for the transcripts and proteins (sialome) from the salivary gland of the malaria vector *Anopheles gambiae*. J Exp Biol 2002;205:2429-51.

[103] Li S, Kwon J and Aksoy S. Characterization of genes expressed in the salivary glands of the tsetse fly, *Glossina morsitans morsitans*. Insect Mol Biol 2001;10:69-76.

[104] Arca B, Lombardo F, Lanfrancotti A, et al. A cluster of four D7-related genes is expressed in the salivary glands of the African malaria vector *Anopheles gambiae*. Insect Mol Biol 2002;11:47-55.

[105] Valenzuela JG, Charlab R, Gonzalez EC, et al. The D7 family of salivary proteins in blood sucking Diptera. Insect Mol Biol 2002;11:149-55.

[106] Simons FE, Peng Z. Mosquito allergy: recombinant mosquito salivary antigens for new diagnostic tests. Int Arch Allergy Immunol 2001;124:403-5.

[107] Jariyapan N, Choochote W, Jitpakdi A, et al. A glycine- and glutamate-rich protein is female salivary gland-specific and abundant in the malaria vector *Anopheles dirus* B (*Diptera: Culicidae*). J Med Entomol 2006;43:867-74.

[108] Ribeiro JM, Arca B, Lombardo F, et al. An annotated catalogue of salivary gland transcripts in the adult female mosquito, *Aedes aegypti*. BMC Genomics 2007;8:6.

[109] Lanfrancotti A, Lombardo F, Santolamazza F, et al. Novel cDNAs encoding salivary proteins from the malaria vector *Anopheles gambiae*. FEBS Lett 2002;517:67-71.

[110] Neira Oviedo M, Ribeiro JM, Heyland A, VanEkeris L, Moroz T and Linser PJ. The salivary transcriptome of *Anopheles gambiae* (Diptera: Culicidae) larvae: A microarray-based analysis. Insect Biochem Mol Biol 2009;39:382-94.

[111] Okulate MA, Kalume DE, Reddy R, et al. Identification and molecular characterization of a novel protein Saglin as a target of monoclonal antibodies affecting salivary gland infectivity of *Plasmodium* sporozoites. Insect Mol Biol 2007;16:711-22.

[112] Shen Z, Jacobs-Lorena M. A type I peritrophic matrix protein from the malaria vector *Anopheles gambiae* binds to chitin. Cloning, expression, and characterization. J Biol Chem 1998;273:17665-70.

[113] Calvo E, Pham VM, Lombardo F, Arca B and Ribeiro JM. The sialotranscriptome of adult male *Anopheles gambiae* mosquitoes. Insect Biochem Mol Biol 2006;36:570-5.

[114] Isawa H, Orito Y, Iwanaga S, et al. Identification and characterization of a new kallikrein-kinin system inhibitor from the salivary glands of the malaria vector mosquito *Anopheles stephensi*. Insect Biochem Mol Biol 2007;37:466-77.

[115] Arca B, Lombardo F, Francischetti IM, et al. An insight into the sialome of the adult female mosquito *Aedes albopictus*. Insect Biochem Mol Biol 2007;37:107-27.

[116] Ribeiro JM, Charlab R, Pham VM, Garfield M and Valenzuela JG. An insight into the salivary transcriptome and proteome of the adult female mosquito *Culex pipiens quinquefasciatus*. Insect Biochem Mol Biol 2004;34:543-63.

[117] Cornelie S, Remoue F, Doucoure S, et al. An insight into immunogenic salivary proteins of *Anopheles gambiae* in African children. Malar J 2007;6:75.

[118] Rizzo C, Ronca R, Fiorentino G, et al. Humoral response to the *Anopheles gambiae* salivary protein gSG6: a serological indicator of exposure to Afrotropical malaria vectors. PLoS One 2011;6:e17980.

[119] Rizzo C, Ronca R, Fiorentino G, et al. Wide cross-reactivity between *Anopheles gambiae* and *Anopheles funestus* SG6 salivary proteins supports exploitation of gSG6 as a marker of human exposure to major malaria vectors in tropical Africa. Malar J 2011;10:206.

[120] Larru B, Molyneux E, Ter Kuile FO, Taylor T, Molyneux M and Terlouw DJ. Malaria in infants below six months of age: retrospective surveillance of hospital admission records in Blantyre, Malawi. Malar J 2009;8:310.

[121] Rogier C. [Childhood malaria in endemic areas: epidemiology, acquired immunity and control strategies]. Med Trop (Mars) 2003;63:449-64.

[122] Carnevale P, Frezil JL, Bosseno MF, Le Pont F and Lancien J. [The aggressiveness of *Anopheles gambiae* A in relation to the age and sex of the human subjects]. Bull World Health Organ 1978;56:147-54.

[123] Geissbuhler Y, Chaki P, Emidi B, et al. Interdependence of domestic malaria prevention measures and mosquito-human interactions in urban Dar es Salaam, Tanzania. Malar J 2007;6:126.

[124] Drame PM, Diallo A, Poinsignon A, et al. Evaluation of the effectiveness of malaria vector control measures in urban settings of Dakar by a specific *Anopheles* salivary biomarker. PLoS One (2013). In press.

[125] Palmeira P, Quinello C, Silveira-Lessa AL, Zago CA and Carneiro-Sampaio M. IgG placental transfer in healthy and pathological pregnancies. Clin Dev Immunol 2012;2012:985646.

[126] Kinyanjui SM, Bull P, Newbold CI and Marsh K. Kinetics of antibody responses to *Plasmodium falciparum*-infected erythrocyte variant surface antigens. J Infect Dis 2003;187:667-74.

[127] Gadiaga L, Machault V, Pages F, et al. Conditions of malaria transmission in Dakar from 2007 to 2010. Malar J 2011;10:312.

[128] Machault V, Gadiaga L, Vignolles C, et al. Highly focused anopheline breeding sites and malaria transmission in Dakar. Malar J 2009;8:138.

[129] Kalluri S, Gilruth P, Rogers D and Szczur M. Surveillance of arthropod vector-borne infectious diseases using remote sensing techniques: a review. PLoS Pathog 2007;3:1361-71.

[130] Smith T, Killeen G, Lengeler C and Tanner M. Relationships between the outcome of *Plasmodium falciparum* infection and the intensity of transmission in Africa. Am J Trop Med Hyg 2004;71:80-6.

[131] Corran P, Coleman P, Riley E and Drakeley C. Serology: a robust indicator of malaria transmission intensity? Trends Parasitol 2007;23:575-82

[132] Doannio JM, Doudou DT, Konan LY, et al. [Influence of social perceptions and practices on the use of bednets in the malaria control programme in Ivory Coast (West Africa)]. Med Trop (Mars) 2006;66:45-52.

[133] Pages F, Orlandi-Pradines E and Corbel V. [Vectors of malaria: biology, diversity, prevention, and individual protection]. Med Mal Infect 2007;37:153-61.

[134] Corbel V, Akogbeto M, Damien GB, et al. Combination of malaria vector control interventions in pyrethroid resistance area in Benin: a cluster randomised controlled trial. Lancet Infect Dis 2012;12:617-26.

[135] Okumu FO, Moore SJ. Combining indoor residual spraying and insecticide-treated nets for malaria control in Africa: a review of possible outcomes and an outline of suggestions for the future. Malar J 2011;10:208.

[136] Beier JC. Malaria parasite development in mosquitoes. Annu Rev Entomol 1998;43:519-43.

[137] Lombardi S, Esposito F, Zavala F, et al. Detection and anatomical localization of *Plasmodium falciparum* circumsporozoite protein and sporozoites in the Afrotropical malaria vector *Anopheles gambiae* s.l. Am J Trop Med Hyg 1987;37:491-4.

[138] Burkot TR, Williams JL and Schneider I. Identification of *Plasmodium falciparum*-infected mosquitoes by a double antibody enzyme-linked immunosorbent assay. Am J Trop Med Hyg 1984;33:783-8.

[139] Fontenille D, Meunier JY, Nkondjio CA and Tchuinkam T. Use of circumsporozoite protein enzyme-linked immunosorbent assay compared with microscopic examination of salivary glands for calculation of malaria infectivity rates in mosquitoes (Diptera: Culicidae) from Cameroon. J Med Entomol 2001;38:451-4.

[140] Siala E, Ben Abdallah R, Bouratbine A, Aoun K. Current biological diagnosis of malaria. Revue Tunisienne d'Infectiologie 2010;4:5-9.

[141] Druilhe P, Pradier O, Marc JP, Miltgen F, Mazier D and Parent G. Levels of antibodies to *Plasmodium falciparum* sporozoite surface antigens reflect malaria transmission rates and are persistent in the absence of reinfection. Infect Immun 1986;53:393-7.

[142] Greenhouse B, Ho B, Hubbard A, et al. Antibodies to *Plasmodium falciparum* antigens predict a higher risk of malaria but protection from symptoms once parasitemic. J Infect Dis 2011;204:19-26.

[143] Clark EH, Silva CJ, Weiss GE, et al. *Plasmodium falciparum* malaria in the Peruvian Amazon, a region of low transmission, is associated with immunologic memory. Infect Immun 2012;80:1583-92.

[144] Dixit R, Sharma A, Mourya DT, Kamaraju R, Patole MS and Shouche YS. Salivary gland transcriptome analysis during *Plasmodium* infection in malaria vector *Anopheles stephensi*. Int J Infect Dis 2009;13:636-46.

[145] Rosinski-Chupin I, Briolay J, Brouilly P, et al. SAGE analysis of mosquito salivary gland transcriptomes during *Plasmodium* invasion. Cell Microbiol 2007;9:708-24.

Chapter 24

Transgenic Mosquitoes for Malaria Control: From the Bench to the Public Opinion Survey

Christophe Boëte and Uli Beisel

Additional information is available at the end of the chapter

http://dx.doi.org/10.5772/56193

1. Introduction

The recent field releases of genetically modified mosquitoes in inter alia The Cayman Islands, Malaysia and Brazil have been the source of intense debate in the specialized press [1, 2] as well as in the non-specialized mass media. For the first time in history (to our knowledge), transgenic *Aedes aegypti* were released in the Cayman Islands in 2010 by a private company, Oxitec, in collaboration with the local Mosquito Research and Control Unit (MRCU) [3]. The releases were followed by other releases in Malaysia in 2010/11 and then in Brazil in 2011 [4]. While the releases in Malaysia and Brazil were publicised beforehand, the releases in The Cayman Islands were only announced publicly one year after the fact [1, 5]. This lack of transparency, not to say the secrecy, in the way the first trial was conducted is without much doubt the major reason for the controversy that emerged. Brushing aside years of discussion in the scientific world and a shared recognition of the importance to consider ethical, legal and social issues this first trial could be read as a fait-accompli: the cage of transgenic mosquitoes has now been opened [6]. Oxitec faced harsh criticism for these releases, both within the scientific community, as well as from non-governmental organisations, such as GeneWatch that accused the company of acting like "a last bastion of colonialism". A vector-borne diseases method for control has rarely been the subject of such discussion not even concerning its potential efficacy at reducing the burden associated with a vector-borne disease.

Focusing on malaria control, this chapter reviews the major technological milestones associated with this technique from its roots to its most recent development. Key-points in the understanding of mosquito ecology are going to be presented, as well as their use in models whose major aim is to determine the validity of the transgenic approach and to help designing successful strategies for disease control.

Furthermore, the ethical and social points related to both field trials and wide-scale releases aiming at modifying mosquito populations (and thus controlling vector-borne diseases) are going to be discussed as well as the question of public engagement and the role scientists might play in fostering debate and public deliberation. While large part of the laboratory research is done in the Global North, most of the vector-borne diseases are endemic in the Global South. We suggest that the geopolitics related to the genetically modified (GM) mosquitoes as well as the specificity of Southern contexts needs to be considered when discussing the application of this technology.

2. Why acting on the vector population: How efficient are transgenic methods for malaria control?

When discussing the epidemiology of malaria the gold standard is the description of the R_0 [7-9]. Focusing on the vector compartment suggests that the spread of malaria can be curved either by reducing the mosquito population or by decreasing their vectorial capacity. In other words, one either aims to decrease the number of mosquitoes or to make them less efficient in transmitting the parasites. These two strategies can both be addressed by vector control including through a transgenic approach: population reduction or population replacement. However, when looking closely at R_0 one can notice that the parameters that are affected by those strategies are not the most likely ones to curve transmission efficiently. The mortality of mosquitoes (μ) and their biting rate (a) are indeed affecting R_0 in an exponential and in a quadratic manner respectively. In this respect, they are the parameters whose modifications affect R_0 and consequently the human prevalence mostly (see Box 1). This means that modifying a linear parameter is less likely to lead to a drastic change in malaria epidemiology. For example halving the vector population density (m) is going to reduce R_0 by two but because of the non-linear relationship between R_0 and the human prevalence (y) the decrease of the latter one is not going to be affected in such a manner especially in a context of high transmission.

3. Technology: What has lead to GM mosquitoes for malaria control?

The roots of the technology can be traced back to the early 80's/90's when the knowledge gained in genetics in *Drosophila* research sparked the development of new tools in the fight of vector-borne diseases. The plan was straightforward with three milestones to be achieved in a decade: i) the stable transformation of *Anopheles* mosquitoes by 2000 ii) the engineering of a mosquito unable to carry malaria parasites by 2005 and iii) the development of controlled experiments to understand how to drive this genotype of interest into wild populations by 2010 [10].

Regarding malaria most recent research has concentrated on the development of an *Anopheles* strain that has the ability to interrupt transmission through the synthesis and production of molecules able to block the development of the parasite. A few years ago, the SM1 peptide was shown to reduce malaria oocysts number by about 80% [11]. More recently, it was

http://dx.doi.org/10.5772/56193

$$R_0 = \frac{ma^2 b_1 b_2 e^{-\mu T}}{r\mu} \quad \text{(equation 1)}$$

m : Number of mosquitoes per host.
a : Biting rate of mosquitoes on their host.
μ : Mortality of adult mosquitoes
T : Incubation time of the the parasite in the mosquito vector
r : Recovery rate of humans
b1 : Infectiousness of hosts to mosquitoes.
b2 : Susceptibility of humans

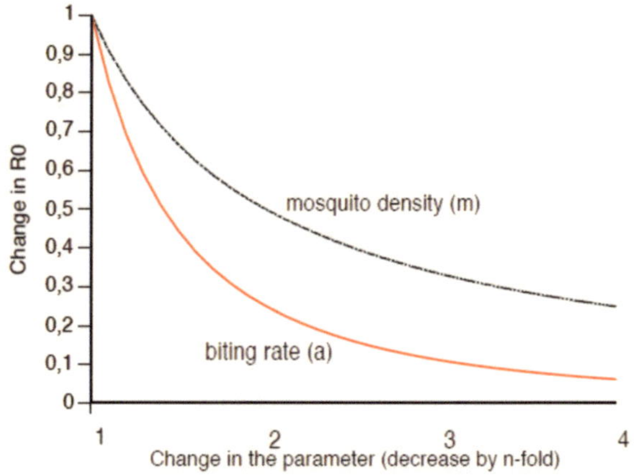

Evaluating the impact of several parameters on R0 permits to determine that a decrease in the biting rate is affecting R0 in a greater manner than a change of the same magnitude in mosquito density. The biting rate (a) appears indeed quadratically whereas the mosquito density (m) is a linear factor in equation 1.

$$y = \frac{R_0 - 1}{R_0 + \frac{a}{\mu}} \quad \text{(equation 2)}$$

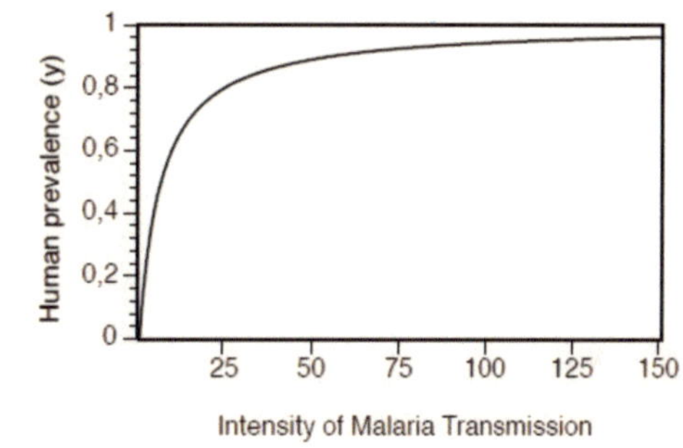

Box 1. The Ross-MacDonald model permits to describe R0 which is the number of secondary case arising from a single one in an otherwise uninfected population (Macdonald 1957; Koella, 1991). It permits to determine the relative importance of the different parameters implicated in the transmission of malaria (equation 1). From the R0 value, a simple expression permits to determine the prevalence in the human population (equation 2). As seen on the graph above, only a large decrease in the intensity of transmission (estimated by R0) can affect significantly the human prevalence (y).

synthesised from a transgenic entomopathogenic fungi [12], this later one is by-itself (in its natural version) already considered as a potentially interesting method to develop [13-15]. Other potential solutions currently developed rely on single-chain antibodies [16-18]. Using the φC31 integration system for the first time in *An. stephensi* it is now possible to insert the transgene of interest in a permanent manner at chromosomal 'docking' site using site-specific recombination and to have a tissue- and sex-specific expression. The authors have then shown that the prevalence and number of oocysts decreased when the transgenic mosquitoes were challenged with *Plasmodium falciparum* [17]. If technology has been able to determine how the insertion of a transgene can be made to change a vector to a quasi non-vector, the next question to answer concerns the spread of this construction in natural populations of mosquitoes.

4. Mosquito ecology: First hurdle at the door of the Lab

When the ecological and evolutionary issues related to the potential use and impact of *Plasmodium*-resistant transgenic mosquitoes started to be discussed about a decade ago [19, 20], most studies aimed at providing information on the fitness of genetically-modified mosquitoes were based on the use of natural mosquito immune responses as a model system. This was mainly driven by the fact that using the natural immune system of mosquitoes in a transgenic approach was considered of some potential interest [21], and also because the only fully effective system against malaria parasite was the melanization response (also known as melanotic encapsulation) in selected lines of mosquitoes [22]. The mechanism leading to the death of the parasite because of melanization remains unclear. It seems that death can occur because of starvation (by isolation from the hemolymph) as well as because of the cytotoxic function of melanin [21, 23]. The melanization response was then considered as a model of what could happen with an artificial peptide mimicking an immune response and thus aiming at reducing the number of parasites in the mosquito.

Before considering the cost associated with resistance that could impair the spread of resistance in mosquito populations, it is important to notice that the sole insertion of an exogenous gene (not even conferring any anti-parasitic advantage) leads to a drastic decrease in *Anopheles stephensi* fitness [24]. However, recent work with site-specific insertion seems to bring a less negative outcome in term of fitness [18]. This even seems to be the case when all different groups including the control group (called wild) derive from a lab colony and the fitness reduction due to the colonisation process is probably significant. Concerning the cost of resistance, mosquitoes are no exception and reduced fitness associated with the absence of parasite can be observed. Thus, several studies have measured the associated cost in *Anopheles stephensi* carrying a transgene conferring resistance again the rodent malaria parasite *P. gallinaceum*. Regardless if resistance was provided by the expression of SM1 (termed for salivary gland- and midgut binding peptide 1) [25] or the phospholipase A2 gene (PLA2) [26], a fitness cost was associated with it. Even in conditions where harbouring an allele conferred an advantage i.e. when mosquitoes were fed on *Plasmodium*-infected blood, the SM1 transgene could not reach fixation revealing that the benefit of resistance was counterbalanced by the cost of resistance in the transgenic homozygotes [27]. In any case the construction needs to follow a couple of requirements for the promoter and the gene of interest for the method to have some chances of success [28]. The gene of interest needs to express in a temporal manner i.e. after a blood-meal is taken, but also only in the tissues where it could efficiently impact the parasite life cycle, such as the midgut epithelium and the salivary glands.

Recent work on GM mosquitoes have also been done with *Aedes* that are not resistant towards a pathogen but that are carrying a gene that makes nearly all their offspring non-viable in a natural environment [29-31]. To date such a strategy has not been developed for the *Anopheles* genus.

For the strategy considering the replacement of malaria vector by their modified non-vector version, this question of a cost associated with resistance leads necessarily to the idea of the need to use a driving system in order to favour the spread of resistance in natural populations of mosquitoes.

5. Driving an allele of interest in natural populations of mosquitoes

The idea of using a gene drive to affect the epidemiology of vector-borne diseases is not a recent idea as the use of chromosomal translocation to reduce mosquito populations was already proposed in 1940 by Serebrovskii [32]. It was revived later with the idea to use those translocations to drive alleles conferring refractoriness in mosquito populations [33].

Thus the spread of refractoriness in mosquito populations could be facilitated if the allele, conferring resistance but also associated with a cost, was linked with an element whose spread is not Mendelian. One of the techniques for which various models provide information is the use of transposable elements. A tandem made of a transposon and an allele of interest can spread easily and fixation can be reached [34, 35], even if the cost of resistance is particularly high [36].

Using intracellular bacteria associated with cytoplasmic incompatibility, such as *Wolbachia,* is also an idea that has been explored. Modifying them so that they could harbour the allele of interest would permit, at least in theory, to favour the spread of the allele of interest [37, 38]. There is no natural infection of *Anopheles* by *Wolbachia* but work is in progress trialling infections of *Anopheles gambiae* cells by *Wolbachia pipientis* (strains wRi and wAlbB) in the lab [39]. However, up to now no such sustainable transformation has been done [40].

Other constructions that would favour the spread of resistance have also been considered [41, 42]. Among them the use of HEG (Homing Endonuclease Genes) has been the centre of a lot of attention in the last years [43-45]. Apart from those systems another approach relies on the use of pairs of unlinked lethal genes. In this case, each gene is associated with the repressor of the lethality of the other one and this system is called engineered underdominance [46]. With respect to those methods a number of recent papers have been focusing on theoretical work aiming at spreading an allele conferring resistance as well as containing it. If the aim of a GM approach is to favour the spread of an allele conferring resistance it is also important to consider that self-limitation could be a real advantage to avoid the establishment of the transgene in non-target populations. Such an approach has been studied in theoretical analysis with the *Inverse Medea* gene drive system [47] and with the *Semele* one [48].

If the speed at which the construction of interest can spread in mosquito populations is a major issue, authors have also shown that in the case of the use of transposable elements one of the problems is the stability of the system with the probability of disruption [49].

However, if the spread of an allele conferring resistance is a target that can be reached, the real aim should be a strong decrease in the prevalence of the disease or even its elimination. Two models merging population genetics and epidemiology have pointed out the major importance of the efficacy of resistance [36, 50]. They have shown that a significant reduction in malaria prevalence can only be obtained if the efficacy is close to 1 especially when a release of resistant mosquitoes is done in high transmission areas.

If recent work claims that the engineered-mosquito do not suffer too much from carrying a resistant allele [17], this remain only valid under lab conditions where environmental conditions remain fairly stable and usually favourable. It is interesting to note that the survival of the mosquitoes in Isaacs et al. study reaches about 35 to 40 days which is probably far more that what happens under natural conditions.

As shown with natural immune responses, environmental conditions experienced at the larval or at the adult stage can greatly affect the host-parasite interactions and thus the outcome of an infection [51]. A reduction of 75% on food availability at the larval stage in lines selected for refractoriness [22] leads to a decrease in the proportion of the mosquitoes able to melanize half of the surface of a foreign body (a Sephadex bead) of more than 50% of it [52]. Even more worryingly, a recent paper [53] revealed the complex effects of temperature on both the cellular and humoral immune responses on the malaria vector *Anopheles stephensi*. What is highly interesting in this study is that not only temperature can affect immune responses but also that different immune responses are affected in different manners by temperature. The authors have studied the melanization response, the phagocytosis (a cellular immune response that lead to the destruction of small organisms or apoptotic cells) and the defensin (an antimicrobial peptide) expression. The three of them are higher at 18°C while the expression of Nitric Oxide Synthase (active against a large number of pathogens [54]) peaks at 30°C and the one of cecropin (an antimicrobial peptide) seems to be temperature-independent. Concerning melanization it is important to note that if the melanization rate is higher at 18°C, the percentage of melanised beads -introduced inside the mosquito to measure its immunocompetence- (at least partly) was higher when the temperature increased (fig. 1).

This result highlights the difficulties to define what is an optimal temperature for the melanization response especially as it is also involved in developmental processes. The complexity of the immune function appears also with cecropin expression that despite being independent from temperature was affected by the administration of an injury or the injection of heat-killed *E. coli*. Other works have also revealed that the immune function is affected in a complex manner by a variety of environmental parameters such as the density of conspecifics or the quality of food resources [55]. Apart from showing the need to better understand the impact of the complex interactions between temperature and other variables on the vector competence, this work also highlights the crucial importance to take them into account when determining the potential outcome of the interactions between the natural immune function, the allele conferring resistance in a GM mosquito and finally the resulting vectorial competence under a large variety of ecological conditions.

What appears to be clear is that the expression of genes involved in the anti-parasitic response are not only influenced by the sole host-parasite interactions but that the environment is a

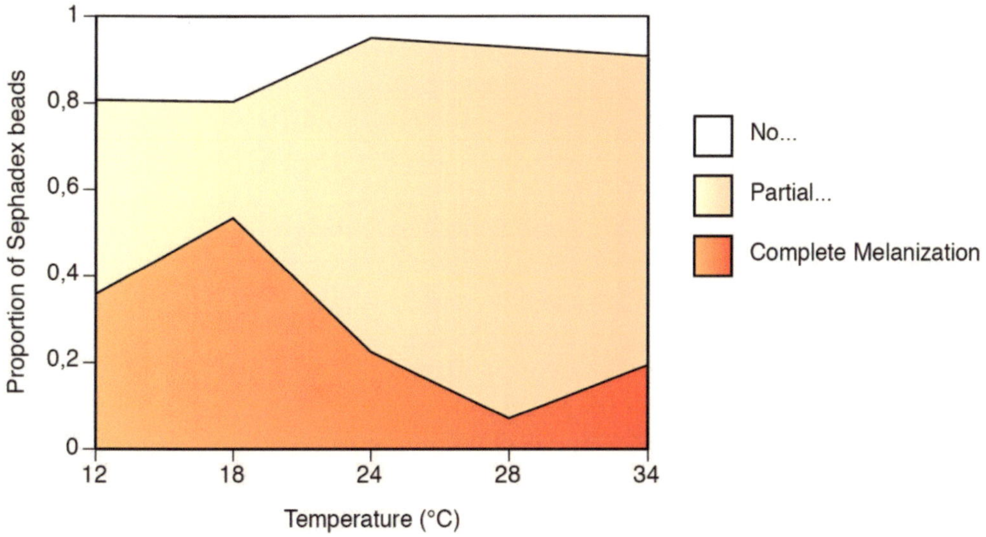

Figure 1. Influence of the temperature on the melanization response of Sephadex beads in the malaria vector Anopheles stephensi. The melanization of beads was measured 24h after the injection. The proportion of completely melanized beads was the highest at 18°C whereas the higher proportion of beads being at least partially melanized occurs at higher temperatures (modified after Murdock et al. 2012)[53].

crucial factor be it the abiotic conditions, such as temperature and its daily variations, or biotic factors, such as parasites encountered at the larval or adult stage [56, 57].

On the side of the parasite it would be naïve not to consider an evolutionary response in the face of selective pressure represented by any (natural or artificial) resistance. The quick selection of resistance against artemisinin in South-East Asia in the last years [58] and the evidence of its genetic basis [59] suggests that it is reasonable to envision the selection of parasite strains able to overcome any engineered resistance mechanism. Using transgenic *Plasmodium*-resistant mosquitoes can be considered equivalent to artificially increasing the investment of the mosquito in an immune response. Referring to some theoretical work [60] this is assumed to be followed by an increase in the parasite investment to avoid resistance. In the long term this would lead to a decrease in the effectiveness of the programme aiming at decreasing malaria prevalence or the need to 'play evolution' by monitoring the parasite population and releasing transgenic mosquitoes for which resistance could be modified as in an arm race with parasite evasion.

What is then important is to determine the longer-term of such a strategy regarding parasite virulence. Some answers have already been provided by theoretical work concerning the impact on parasite virulence to humans and mosquitoes in the case of dengue [61]. The authors examined four distinct situations: blocking transmission, decreasing mosquito biting rate, increasing mosquito background mortality or increasing the mortality due to infection; if all of them are associated with a benefit in terms of disease incidence, only the ones affecting mosquito mortality seem to pose the smallest risk in term of virulence to humans. It is important to note the scarcity of studies aiming at providing empirical data on this topic even if experimental evolution with mosquitoes and parasite can provide interesting results in a reasonable number of generations [62]. This lack of data not only concerns dengue but also malaria as has already been discussed in a paper on possible outcomes of the use of transgenic *Plasmodium*-resistant mosquitoes [63].

6. Vector control: To be or not to be transgenic-based

As mentioned earlier one of the major points to consider with transgenic mosquitoes used for malaria control are the ethical and societal issues and public acceptance of this high-tech method. Even though the importance of societal acceptance of GM mosquitoes has been recognised for a decade [64], studies on acceptability remain scarce. One first study conducted in Mali mapped out several crucial aspects of potential acceptance or rejection of GM mosquitoes [65]. While Marshall reports that his interviewees were generally "pragmatic" about the technology, acceptance was dependent on several conditions.

If people were supportive of a release of transgenic mosquitoes for malaria control, they first wanted to see evidence of safety for human health and the environment prior to releases. In addition, proof of efficacy of the technology in reducing malaria prevalence was requested. Lastly people declared that they would prefer the trial to be done outside of their village and when comparing GM crops and GM mosquitoes, people were more sceptical of the latter. Even if this not a rejection of the idea of using a GM technology for health purpose, it is important to note that a population, even if at risk of contracting malaria, remains cautious about the idea of using such a technology. This should remind us how, in the 70's, a decade-long programme conducted by the WHO in India utilising the sterile insect technique (SIT) ended in a chaotic way after the publication of inaccurate information in the Indian press [66].

Secondly, the question of regulation has recently been highlighted as crucial [5, 67]. Because the social and environmental implications of GM mosquitoes are significant and potentially irreversible, and as the regulatory attention that GMOs have received in Europe suggests broad-based trials and releases require robust legislation and international agreements. These regulations are still under development, and it is important to note that at the time of the first releases in The Cayman Islands international guidance on open field releases of GM mosquitoes was still in preparation [67, 68]. While the existing Cartagena Protocol on Biosafety is considered to be applicable to GM crops, it is in need of specific amendments in order to work for GM mosquitoes [69].

Furthermore, in terms of regulation one has to distinguish between two different types of GM mosquitoes. While regulation and tracking might be possible for genetically sterilised mosquitoes as they are self-limiting in their spread, tracking and containment of GM mosquitoes with self-spreading genetics, i.e. fertile mosquitoes that block disease transmission, is considered almost impossible, or at the very least extremely difficult [70, 71]. This distinguishes GM mosquitoes from earlier GM technologies, such as for the modification of crops. GM and non-GM crops can be separated from each other and marked by labels on GM products, it can thus be seen as a technology of choice. However, the accuracy of this argument is only limited. As

http://dx.doi.org/10.5772/56193

for instance Lezaun has shown, bees have proven to be effective agents of cross-pollination between GM and non-GM crops, thus subverting regulations that aim to keep GM and non-GM crops separate [72]. GM insects, however, are markedly different. The elusiveness of mosquitoes will likely be a major impediment to tracking, containment and comprehensive regulation, as for instance the spread of *Aedes albopictus* and herewith the increased risk of arboviral transmission in new locations across the world has shown, mosquitoes are hard to contain. This renders GM mosquitoes as a no-choice technology – once released, GM mosquitoes will stay in our environments.

A second major issue in terms of the social and ethical implications of GM mosquitoes is the question by whom and how they are produced and implemented. GM modification of insects is an expensive high-tech intervention and research so far has mainly been located in resource rich laboratories in the Global North, rather than in disease-endemic developing countries [73]. This enrols the technology thoroughly into discussions about technology transfer and development initiatives from North to South, and sits uncomfortably with the West's history in colonial exploitation and tropical medicine. Aside from this imbalance in bio-capital and agenda setting, GM mosquitoes are as much a product of the biotech industry as they are tools for public or global health. Are GM mosquitoes currently seen as a public good or a commercial product? While most of the research and development of GM mosquitoes has so far been funded by public institutions –both national research foundations -such as the US National Science Foundation- and philanthropic organisations -such as the Bill and Melinda Gates Foundation and the Wellcome Trust, the mosquitoes that have been released were part of a commercial project. The emerging GM mosquito industry has caught the interest of private biotech firms. The first company to produce and market GM mosquitoes is Oxford Insect Technologies (Oxitec), founded by a group of entomologists as a spin-off company of Oxford University. The company is a for-profit-enterprise, so far has mainly been funded by public entities and venture capitalists, and is one of the main drivers of high-end developments in the field. As discussed in the introduction, Oxitec was the first to release sterile GM mosquitoes into the wild in the field trials in The Cayman Islands. A fundamental issue that is raised through the dominance of Oxitec in the field is the tension between GM mosquitoes as a public health tool and a commercial product [74-76]. While GM mosquitoes in malaria control would be used as a tool of disease control and to foster public health, companies like Oxitec follow different aims – they have to become profitable and eventually make profits with their GM entities. This tension brings another social issue of GM mosquitoes to the forefront, namely the question of how one conducts field trials with GM mosquitoes in an ethical way?

As we alluded to in the introduction, the first releases in The Cayman Islands were conducted in a rather secretive fashion. Oxitec only published the news about the release with a one-year delay [1], leading to accusations that the releases were deliberately done in secret [75, 76]. Oxitec stated the trials were prepared and conducted in close cooperation with local Mosquito Control and Research Unit, had conformed to the British Overseas Territory's biosafety rules, and that information had been sent to local newspapers preceding the trials. However, many locals claimed they were not informed and no risk assessment documents were made available to the public on the internet. The only risk assessment document that can be found was published by the UK parliament in 2011, over one year after the releases started [5]. The Cayman Island releases have triggered fears for entomologists working on GM mosquitoes that such secretive trials might lead to a public backlash and undermine their own extensive efforts at public engagement, some scientists for instance claimed they have spent years preparing a study site through "extensive dialogues with citizen groups, regulators, academics and farmers"[1].

GeneWatch argued that Oxitec purposefully bypassed existing international GM regulations (developed mainly for GM crops), because Cayman Islands does not have biosafety laws and is not a signatory to the Cartagena Protocol on Biosafety or the Aarhus Convention (even though since the UK is a signatory to the protocol, Oxitec had a duty to report the export of GM eggs to UK government). As a result GeneWatch reads Oxitec's actions as colonialist tactics: "the British scientific establishment is acting like the last bastion of colonialism, using an Overseas Territory as a private lab" [76].

All in all, this raises the question what ethically and socially responsible research on GM mosquitoes means? Here, the ability of researchers and stakeholders to communicate with each other is key for meaningful public engagement. In this respect, a recent survey has focused on the willingness of scientists to have interactions with a non-scientific audience [77]. One of the main findings of the survey indicates that more than 90% of scientists working on GM mosquitoes are agreeable to interactions with the public on their research. However, communication might not be enough and real discussion might not be easy between researchers and a non-scientific audience. This has been underlined by the reluctance of a fraction of the research community to have their research project evaluated by a non-scientific public [77]. Thus, while a significant proportion of researchers are ready to interact with a non-scientific audience, they seem to be less likely to accept an evaluation and a prior-agreement of a research proposal by the general public, interestingly especially researchers from the Global North are hesitant. On the other hand, many scientists in malarious countries do welcome exchanges with publics and are more willing to negotiate their research project with members of the disease-endemic communities.

In summary, the GM mosquito technology in malaria control raises a set of challenging questions. Challenges from a biological and ecological perspective are interlinked with questions about democratic decision-making, local acceptance and international regulation of these emerging entities. Such a potentially controversial technology cannot afford to skip these debates and time is ripe to focus on the ethical and sociological aspects governing the potential use of GM mosquitoes. Furthermore, it is crucial that the development of transgenic methods does not lead to a decrease in funding of classical, accepted and efficient vector control methods – indeed, they should be favoured and enhanced to continue curbing the malaria burden today.

Acknowledgements

Thanks to Sylvie Manguin for the kind invitation to write this chapter. Thanks to Courtney C Murdock for providing necessary data and to Silke Fuchs for a preprint. We are also grateful to Luisa Reis de Castro and Guy Reeves for helpful comments on a previous version of this paper. Both authors wish also to thank the Institut des Sciences de la Communication, CNRS (France) for financial support.

Author details

Christophe Boëte[1*] and Uli Beisel[2]

*Address all correspondence to: cboete@gmail.com

1 UMR 190 "Emergence des Pathologies Virales", Aix Marseille Université IRD (Institut de Recherche pour le Développement) EHESP (Ecole des Hautes Etudes en Santé Publique), France

2 Lancaster Environment Centre, Lancaster University, Lancaster LA1 4YQ, UK

References

[1] Enserink M. Science and society. GM mosquito trial alarms opponents, strains ties in Gates-funded project. Science 2010;330:1030-1031.

[2] Subbaraman N. Science snipes at Oxitec transgenic-mosquito trial. Nature Biotechnology 2011;29:9-11.

[3] Harris AF, Nimmo D, McKemey AR, Kelly N, Scaife S, Donnelly CA, et al. Field performance of engineered male mosquitoes. Nature Biotechnology 2011;29:1034-1037.

[4] Harris AF, McKemey AR, Nimmo D, Curtis Z, Black I, Morgan SA, et al. Successful suppression of a field mosquito population by sustained release of engineered male mosquitoes. Nature Biotechnology 2012;30:828-830.

[5] Reeves RG, Denton JA, Santucci F, Bryk J, Reed FA. Scientific standards and the regulation of genetically modified insects. PLoS Neglected Tropical Diseases 2012;6:e1502. doi: 10.1371/journal.pntd.0001502

[6] Boëte C. Moustiques Transgéniques: La cage est ouverte. Les blogs du Diplo (http://blog.mondediplo.net/2011-02-10-Moustiques-transgeniques-la-cage-est-ouverte) (accessed 20 February 2013).

[7] Koella JC. On the use of mathematical models of malaria transmission. Acta Tropica 1991;49:1-25.

[8] Smith DL, Battle KE, Hay SI, Barker CM, Scott TW, McKenzie FE. Ross, Macdonald, and a theory for the dynamics and control of mosquito-transmitted pathogens. PLoS Pathogens 2012;8:e1002588. doi: 10.1371/journal.ppat.1002588.

[9] Smith DL, McKenzie FE, Snow RW, Hay SI. Revisiting the basic reproductive number for malaria and its implications for malaria control. PLoS Biology2007;5:e42. doi: 10.1371/journal.pbio.0050042.

[10] World Health Organization. Prospects for malaria control by genetic manipulation of its vectors TDR/BCV/ MAL-ENT/91.3. Geneva; 1991.

[11] Ito J, Ghosh A, Moreira LA, Wimmer EA, Jacobs-Lorena M. Transgenic anopheline mosquitoes impaired in transmission of a malaria parasite. Nature 2002;417:452-455.

[12] Fang W, Vega-Rodriguez J, Ghosh AK, Jacobs-Lorena M, Kang A, St Leger RJ. Development of transgenic fungi that kill human malaria parasites in mosquitoes. Science 2011;331:1074-1077.

[13] Scholte EJ, Knols BG, Takken W. Infection of the malaria mosquito *Anopheles gambiae* with the entomopathogenic fungus *Metarhizium anisopliae* reduces blood feeding and fecundity. Journal of Invertebrate Pathology 2006;91:43-49.

[14] Scholte EJ, Ng'habi K, Kihonda J, Takken W, Paaijmans K, Abdulla S, et al. An entomopathogenic fungus for control of adult African malaria mosquitoes. Science 2005;308:1641-1642.

[15] Scholte EJ, Njiru BN, Smallegange RC, Takken W, Knols BG. Infection of malaria (*Anopheles gambiae* s.s.) and filariasis (*Culex quinquefasciatus*) vectors with the entomopathogenic fungus *Metarhizium anisopliae*. Malaria Journal 2003;2:29. doi: 10.1186/1475-2875-2-29

[16] de Lara Capurro M, Coleman J, Beerntsen BT, Myles KM, Olson KE, Rocha E, et al. Virus-expressed, recombinant single-chain antibody blocks sporozoite infection of salivary glands in *Plasmodium gallinaceum*-infected *Aedes aegypti*. American Journal of Tropical Medicine and Hygiene 2000;62:427-433.

[17] Isaacs AT, Jasinskiene N, Tretiakov M, Thiery I, Zettor A, Bourgouin C, et al. Transgenic *Anopheles stephensi* coexpressing single-chain antibodies resist *Plasmodium falciparum* development. Proceedings of the National Academy of Sciences U S A 2012;109:E1922-1930.

[18] Isaacs AT, Li F, Jasinskiene N, Chen X, Nirmala X, Marinotti O, et al. Engineered resistance to *Plasmodium falciparum* development in transgenic *Anopheles stephensi*. PLoS Pathogens 2011;7:e1002017. doi:10.1371/journal.ppat.1002017

[19] Boëte C, Koella JC. Evolutionary ideas about genetically manipulated mosquitoes and malaria control. Trends in Parasitology 2003;19:32-38.

[20] Scott TW, Takken W, Knols BG, Boëte C. The ecology of genetically modified mosquitoes. Science 2002;298:117-119.

[21] Christensen BM, Li J, Chen CC, Nappi AJ. Melanization immune responses in mosquito vectors. Trends in Parasitology 2005;21:192-199.

[22] Collins FH, Sakai RK, Vernick KD, Paskewitz S, Seeley DC, Miller LH, et al. Genetic selection of a *Plasmodium*-refractory strain of the malaria vector *Anopheles gambiae*. Science 1986;234:607-610.

[23] Nappi AJ, Christensen BM. Melanogenesis and associated cytotoxic reactions: applications to insect innate immunity. Insect Biochemistry and Molecular Biology 2005;35:443-459.

[24] Catteruccia F, Godfray HC, Crisanti A. Impact of genetic manipulation on the fitness of *Anopheles stephensi* mosquitoes. Science 2003;299:1225-1227.

[25] Marrelli MT, Li CY, Rasgon JL, Jacobs-Lorena M. Transgenic malaria-resistant mosquitoes have a fitness advantage when feeding on *Plasmodium*-infected blood. Proceedings of the National Academy of Sciences U S A 2007;104:5580-5583.

[26] Moreira LA, Wang J, Collins FH, Jacobs-Lorena M. Fitness of anopheline mosquitoes expressing transgenes that inhibit *Plasmodium* development. Genetics 2004;166:1337-1341.

[27] Lambrechts L, Koella JC, Boëte C. Can transgenic mosquitoes afford the fitness cost? Trends in Parasitology 2008;24:4-7.

[28] Fuchs S, Nolan T, Crisanti A. Mosquito transgenic technologies to reduce *Plasmodium* transmission. Methods in Molecular Biology 2013;923:601-622.

[29] Bargielowski I, Nimmo D, Alphey L, Koella JC. Comparison of life history characteristics of the genetically modified OX513A line and a wild type strain of *Aedes aegypti*. PLoS One 2011 6(6): e20699. doi:10.1371/journal.pone.0020699

[30] Bargielowski I, Kaufmann C, Alphey L, Reiter P, Koella J. Flight Performance and Teneral Energy Reserves of Two Genetically-Modified and One Wild-Type Strain of the Yellow Fever Mosquito *Aedes aegypti*. Vector Borne Zoonotic Diseases 2012.

[31] Bargielowski I, Alphey L, Koella JC. Cost of mating and insemination capacity of a genetically modified mosquito *Aedes aegypti* OX513A compared to its wild type counterpart. PLoS One 2011 6(10) :e26086. doi:10.1371/journal.pone.0026086

[32] Serebrovskii AS. On the possibility of a new method for the control of insect pests. (In Russian). Zoologichesky Zhurnal 1940;19:618-630.

[33] Curtis CF. Possible use of translocations to fix desirable genes in insect pest populations. Nature 1968;218:368-369.

[34] Kiszewski AE, Spielman A. Spatially explicit model of transposon-based genetic drive mechanisms for displacing fluctuating populations of anopheline vector mosquitoes. Journal of Medical Entomology 1998;35:584-590.

[35] Ribeiro JM, Kidwell MG. Transposable elements as population drive mechanisms: specification of critical parameter values. Journal of Medical Entomology 1994;31:10-16.

[36] Boëte C, Koella JC. A theoretical approach to predicting the success of genetic manipulation of malaria mosquitoes in malaria control. Malaria Journal 2002;1:3. doi: 10.1186/1475-2875-1-3

[37] Curtis CF, Sinkins SP. *Wolbachia* as a possible means of driving genes into populations. Parasitology 1998;116 Suppl:S111-115.

[38] Rasgon JL, Scott TW. Impact of population age structure on *Wolbachia* transgene driver efficacy: ecologically complex factors and release of genetically modified mosquitoes. Insect Biochemistry and Molecular Biology 2004;34:707-713.

[39] Rasgon JL, Ren X, Petridis M. Can *Anopheles gambiae* be infected with *Wolbachia pipientis*? Insights from an in vitro system. Applied and Environmental Microbiology 2006;72:7718-7722.

[40] Hughes GL, Koga R, Xue P, Fukatsu T, Rasgon JL. *Wolbachia* infections are virulent and inhibit the human malaria parasite *Plasmodium falciparum* in *Anopheles gambiae*. PLoS Pathogens 2011 7(5): e1002043. doi:10.1371/journal.ppat.1002043

[41] Sinkins SP, Gould F. Gene drive systems for insect disease vectors. Nature Reviews Genetics 2006;7:427-435.

[42] Hay BA, Chen CH, Ward CM, Huang H, Su JT, Guo M. Engineering the genomes of wild insect populations: challenges, and opportunities provided by synthetic *Medea* selfish genetic elements. Journal of Insect Physiology 2010;56:1402-1413.

[43] Burt A. Site-specific selfish genes as tools for the control and genetic engineering of natural populations. Proceedings of the Royal Society B: Biological Sciences 2003;270:921-928.

[44] Deredec A, Godfray HC, Burt A. Requirements for effective malaria control with homing endonuclease genes. Proceedings of the National Academy of Sciences U S A 2011;108:E874-880.

[45] Windbichler N, Menichelli M, Papathanos PA, Thyme SB, Li H, Ulge UY, et al. A synthetic homing endonuclease-based gene drive system in the human malaria mosquito. Nature 2011;473:212-215.

[46] Davis S, Bax N, Grewe P. Engineered underdominance allows efficient and economical introgression of traits into pest populations. Journal of Theoretical Biology 2001;212:83-98.

[47] Marshall JM, Hay BA. Inverse *Medea* as a novel gene drive system for local population replacement: a theoretical analysis. Journal of Heredity 2011;102:336-341.

[48] Marshall JM, Pittman GW, Buchman AB, Hay BA. *Semele*: a killer-male, rescue-female system for suppression and replacement of insect disease vector populations. Genetics 2011;187:535-551.

[49] Curtis CF, Coleman P, Kelly DW, Campbell-Lendrum DH. Advantages and Limitations of Transgenic Vector Control: Sterile Males versus Gene Drivers. In: Boëte C. (ed.). Genetically Modified Mosquitoes for Malaria Control. Georgetown, TX, USA: Landes Biosciences - Eurekah 2006. p60-78.

[50] Koella JC, Zaghloul L. Using evolutionary costs to enhance the efficacy of malaria control via genetically manipulated mosquitoes. Parasitology 2008;135:1489-1496.

[51] Lambrechts L, Chavatte JM, Snounou G, Koella JC. Environmental influence on the genetic basis of mosquito resistance to malaria parasites. Proceedings of the Royal Society B: Biological Sciences 2006;273:1501-1506.

[52] Suwanchaichinda C, Paskewitz SM. Effects of larval nutrition, adult body size, and adult temperature on the ability of *Anopheles gambiae* (Diptera: Culicidae) to melanize Sephadex beads. Journal of Medical Entomology 1998;35:157-161.

[53] Murdock CC, Paaijmans KP, Bell AS, King JG, Hillyer JF, Read AF, et al. Complex effects of temperature on mosquito immune function. Proceedings of the Royal Society B: Biological Sciences 2012;279:3357-3366.

[54] Rivero A. Nitric oxide: an antiparasitic molecule of invertebrates. Trends in Parasitology 2006;22:219-225.

[55] Triggs A, Knell RJ. Interactions between environmental variables determine immunity in the Indian meal moth *Plodia interpunctella*. Journal of Animal Ecology 2012;81:386-394.

[56] Boëte C. *Anopheles* mosquitoes: not just flying malaria vectors... especially in the field. Trends in Parasitology 2009;25:53-55.

[57] Aliota MT, Chen CC, Dagoro H, Fuchs JF, Christensen BM. Filarial worms reduce *Plasmodium* infectivity in mosquitoes. PLoS Neglected Tropical Diseases 2011;5:e963.

[58] Dondorp AM, Nosten F, Yi P, Das D, Phyo AP, Tarning J, et al. Artemisinin resistance in *Plasmodium falciparum* malaria. New England Journal of Medicine 2009;361:455-467.

[59] Anderson TJ, Nair S, Nkhoma S, Williams JT, Imwong M, Yi P, et al. High heritability of malaria parasite clearance rate indicates a genetic basis for artemisinin resistance in western Cambodia. Journal of Infectious Diseases 2010;201:1326-1330.

[60] Koella JC, Boëte C. A model for the coevolution of immunity and immune evasion in vector-borne diseases with implications for the epidemiology of malaria. The American Naturalist 2003;161:698-707.

[61] Medlock J, Luz PM, Struchiner CJ, Galvani AP. The impact of transgenic mosquitoes on dengue virulence to humans and mosquitoes. The American Naturalist 2009;174:565-577.

[62] Legros M, Koella JC. Experimental evolution of specialization by a microsporidian parasite. BMC Evolutionary Biology 2010;10:159.

[63] Ferguson HM, Gandon S, Mackinnon MJ, Read AF. Malaria parasite virulence in mosquitoes and its implications for the introduction of Efficacy of GMM malaria Control Programs. In: Boëte C. (ed.). Genetically Modified Mosquitoes for Malaria Control. Georgetown, TX, USA: Landes Biosciences - Eurekah 2006. p103-116.

[64] Touré YT, Oduola AMJ, Sommerfeld J, Morel CM. Biosafety and risk assessment in the use of genetically modified mosquiotes for disease control. In: Takken W, Scott TW, editors. Ecological Aspects for Application of Genetically Modified Mosquitoes. Wageningen: Kluwer Academic Publishers; 2003.

[65] Marshall JM, Toure MB, Traore MM, Famenini S, Taylor CE. Perspectives of people in Mali toward genetically-modified mosquitoes for malaria control. Malaria Journal 2010;9:128. doi:10.1186/1475-2875-9-128.

[66] Anonymous Oh New Delhi, Oh Geneva. Nature 1975;256:355-357.

[67] Mumford JD. Science, regulation, and precedent for genetically modified insects. PLoS Neglected Tropical Diseases 2012 6(1): e1504. doi:10.1371/journal.pntd.0001504

[68] World Health Organization. Progress and prospects for the use of genetically modified mosquitoes to inhibit disease transmission. Geneva; 2009.

[69] Marshall JM. The Cartagena Protocol and genetically modified mosquitoes. Nature Biotechnology 2010;28:896-897.

[70] Angulo E, Gilna B. International law should govern release of GM mosquitoes. Nature 2008;454:158.

[71] Angulo E, Gilna B. When biotech crosses borders. Nature Biotechnology 2008;26:277-282.

[72] Lezaun J. Bees, beekeepers, and bureaucrats: parasitism and the politics of transgenic lifeEnvironment and Planning D: Society and Space 2011;29(4):738-756.

[73] Mshinda H, Killeen GF, Mukabana WR, Mathenge EM, Mboera LE, Knols BG. Development of genetically modified mosquitoes in Africa. The Lancet Infectious diseases 2004;4:264-265.

[74] Beisel U, Boëte C. The Flying Public Health Tool: Genetically Modified mosquitoes in malaria control. Science as Culture 2013 22(1).

[75] Genewatch UK Oxitec's genetically-modified mosquitoes: in the public interest? http://tinyurl.com/by8vsvd (accessed 20 February 2013)

[76] Genewatch UK British Overseas Territory used as private lab for GM mosquito company. 2010. http://www.genewatch.org/uploads/f03c6d66a9b354535738483c1c3d49e4/Oxitecbrief_fin.pdf (accessed 20 February 2013)

[77] Boëte C. Scientists and public involvement: a consultation on the relation between malaria, vector control and transgenic mosquitoes. Transactions of the Royal Society of Tropical Medicine and Hygiene 2011;105:704-710.